Orthobiologics

Scientific and Clinical Solutions for Orthopaedic Surgeons

Orthobiologics

Scientific and Clinical Solutions for Orthopaedic Surgeons

Editors

Scott P. Bruder, MD, PhD, FORS
Founder and CEO
Bruder Consulting & Venture Group, LLC
Franklin Lakes, New Jersey

Roy K. Aaron, MD, FAAOS, FORS
Professor, Orthopedic Surgery
Director, Orthopedic Program in Clinical/Translational Research
Research Director, Miriam Hospital Joint Replacement Center
Warren Alpert Medical School of Brown University
Providence, Rhode Island

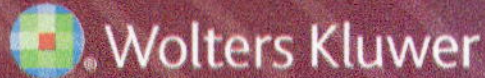

Philadelphia • Baltimore • New York • London
Buenos Aires • Hong Kong • Sydney • Tokyo

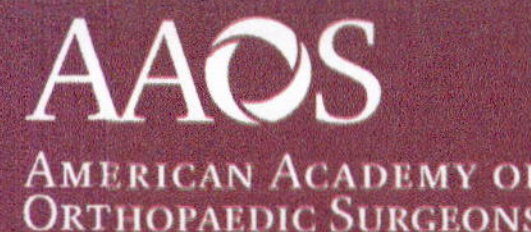

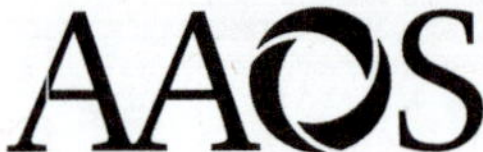

AMERICAN ACADEMY OF ORTHOPAEDIC SURGEONS

Staff

American Academy of Orthopaedic Surgeons
Anna Salt Troise, MBA, *Chief Commercial Officer*
Hans Koelsch, PhD, *Director, Publishing*
Lisa Claxton Moore, *Senior Manager, Editorial*
Steven Kellert, *Senior Editor*

Wolters Kluwer Health
Brian Brown, *Director, Medical Practice*
Tulie McKay, *Senior Content Editor, Acquisitions*
Stacey Sebring, *Senior Development Editor*
Chester Anthony Gonzalez, *Editorial Coordinator*
Erin Cantino, *Product Marketing Manager*
Alicia Jackson, *Senior Production Project Manager*
Stephen Druding, *Design Coordinator*
Beth Welsh, *Senior Manufacturing Coordinator*
TNQ Technologies, *Prepress Vendor*

Orthobiologics: Scientific and Clinical Solutions for Orthopaedic Surgeons

ISBN: 978-1-9751-7545-0

Library of Congress Control Number: Cataloging in Publication data available on request from publisher.

Printed in the United States of America

Published 2024 by the American Academy of Orthopaedic Surgeons
9400 West Higgins Road
Rosemont, Illinois 60018

1 2 3 4 5 6 7

Editorial Board

Editorial Board
Orthobiologics: Scientific and Clinical Solutions for Orthopaedic Surgeons

Contributors

Ishan Agarwal, BS
Department of Orthopaedic Surgery
Division of Spine Surgery
Rush University Medical Center
Chicago, Illinois

Raquel Ajalik, MSc
Center for Musculoskeletal Research
Department of Biomedical Engineering
University of Rochester
Rochester, New York

Koji Akeda, MD, PhD
Department of Orthopaedic Surgery
Mie University Graduate School of Medicine
Tsu, Japan

Rahul Alenchery, MSc
Center for Musculoskeletal Research
Department of Biomedical Engineering
University of Rochester
Rochester, New York

Hani Awad, PhD
Professor, Department of Orthopaedics
University of Rochester Medical Center
Rochester, New York

Stephen F. Badylak, DVM, PhD, MD
McGowan Institute for Regenerative Medicine
Department of Surgery
University of Pittsburgh
Pittsburgh, Pennsylvania

Hyun W. Bae, MD
Professor of Surgery
Department of Orthopaedic Surgery
Cedars-Sinai Medical Center
Los Angeles, California

Spencer B. Bailey, MBA, CPC
Director of Reimbursement and Health Economics
Bruder Consulting & Venture Group, LLC
New York, New York

Kevin C. Baker, PhD
Associate Scientist, Bone & Joint Center
Department of Orthopaedic Surgery
Henry Ford Health
Detroit, Michigan

Elizabeth Rosado Balmayor, PhD
Professor and Head of Experimental Orthopaedic and Trauma Surgery
Clinic for Orthopaedic, Trauma, and Reconstructive Surgery
University Hospital Aachen
Aachen, Germany

Frank Barry, PhD
Professor of Cellular Therapy
Regenerative Medicine Institute
National University of Ireland Galway
Galway, Ireland

Bryce A. Basques, MD
Department of Orthopaedics
Division of Spine Surgery
Warren Alpert Medical School of Brown University
Providence, Rhode Island

Hannah Bradsell, BS
Department of Orthopaedic Surgery
University of Colorado School of Medicine
Aurora, Colorado

Robert H. Brophy, MD, FAAOS
Professor, Department of Orthopaedic Surgery
Washington University School of Medicine
St. Louis, Missouri

Alissa J. Burge, MD
Radiology, Hospital for Special Surgery
New York, New York

Camila B. Carballo, PhD, PT
Postdoctoral Research Fellow
Hospital for Special Surgery
New York, New York

Jorge Chahla, MD, PhD
Division of Sports Medicine
Midwest Orthopaedics at Rush
Rush University Medical Center
Chicago, Illinois

Julie L. Chan, MD, PhD
Neurosurgery Resident, Department of Neurosurgery
Cedars-Sinai Medical Center
Los Angeles, California

George J. Christ, PhD
Departments of Biomedical Engineering and Orthopaedic Surgery
University of Virginia
Charlottesville, Virginia

Justin D. Cohen, MD
Neurosurgery Resident
Department of Neurosurgery
Cedars-Sinai Medical Center
Los Angeles, California

James L. Cook, DVM, PhD
William & Kathryn Allen Distinguished Chair in Orthopaedic Surgery
Vice Chair, Orthopaedic Research
Director, Thompson Laboratory for Regenerative Orthopaedics & Mizzou BioJoint Center
University of Missouri
Missouri Orthopaedic Institute
Columbia, Missouri

Kevin Credille, BSE, MS
Orthopedic Research Fellow
Rush University and Medical Center
Chicago, Illinois

Suhas P. Dasari, MD
Division of Sports Medicine
Midwest Orthopaedics at Rush
Rush University Medical Center
Chicago, Illinois

Kathleen A. Derwin, PhD
Department of Biomedical Engineering
Lerner Research Institute
Cleveland Clinic
Cleveland, Ohio

Sarah E. Dyer, BS
Department of Biomedical Engineering
University of Virginia
Charlottesville, Virginia

Claire D. Eliasberg, MD
Orthopaedic Surgery Resident
Hospital for Special Surgery
New York, New York

Michael Eng, MD
Orthopaedic Surgery Resident
Department of Orthopaedic Surgery
Cedars-Sinai Medical Center
Los Angeles, California

Vahid Entezari, MD, MSc
Department of Orthopaedic Surgery
Orthopedic and Rheumatologic Institute
Cleveland Clinic
Cleveland, Ohio

Christopher H. Evans, PhD
Consultant, Department of Physical Medicine & Rehabilitation
Professor of Physical Medicine and Rehabilitation
Professor of Orthopedics
Mayo Clinic
Rochester, Minnesota

Niloofar Farhang, PhD
Medical Writer/Editor II
Arup Laboratories
Salt Lake City, Utah

Rachel M. Frank, MD, FAAOS
Department of Orthopaedic Surgery
University of Colorado School of Medicine
Aurora, Colorado

Christopher Frey, MD
Resident Physician, Orthopaedic Surgery
Redwood City, California

Erica G. Gacasan, MS
University of California San Diego
San Diego, California

Joel J. Gagnier, ND, MSc, PhD
Associate Professor, Orthopaedic Surgery
Associate Professor, Epidemiology
School of Public Health
University of Michigan
Ann Arbor, Michigan

Steven C. Ghivizzani, PhD
University of Florida College of Medicine
Gainesville, Florida

Juliane Glaeser, PhD
Program Manager, Research Instructor
Regenerative Orthobiologics Center
Orthopedic Stem Cell Research Lab
Board of Governors Regenerative Medicine Institute
Department of Orthopaedics
Cedars-Sinai Medical Center
Los Angeles, California

S. Raymond Golish, MD, PhD, MBA, FAAOS
Chief Medical Officer
HCA Healthcare JFK Medical Center
Palm Beach, Florida

Laurie Goodrich, DVM, MS, PhD
Professor of Orthopedics in the Department of Clinical Sciences
Colorado State University
College of Veterinary Medicine and Biomedical Sciences
Fort Collins, Colorado

Daniel A. Grande, PhD
Professor, Institute of Bioelectronic Medicine
Feinstein Institutes for Medical Research
Northwell Health
Manhasset, New York

Kevin Grassie, BS
Department of Biomedical Engineering
Connecticut Convergence Institute for Translation in Regenerative Engineering
University of Connecticut Health Center
Farmington, Connecticut

Robert E. Guldberg, PhD
Professor and Executive Director
Knight Campus for Accelerating Scientific Impact
University of Oregon
Eugene, Oregon

Safa Gursoy, MD, PhD
Division of Sports Medicine
Midwest Orthopaedics at Rush
Rush University Medical Center
Chicago, Illinois

Matthew J. Hadad, MD
Orthopaedic Surgery Resident
Department of Orthopaedic Surgery
Cleveland Clinic Foundation
Cleveland, Ohio

Joseph Harrington, BS
Graduate Research Assistant
Department of Biomechanics
University of Nebraska Omaha
Omaha, Nebraska

Janice Havasy, BS, MD
Hospital for Special Surgery
New York, New York

Michael W. Heffner, MD
Stanford University
Stanford, California

Emily Dianne Henderson, BS
McGowan Institute for Regenerative Medicine
University of Pittsburgh
Pittsburgh, Pennsylvania

Mario Hevesi, MD, PhD
Physician
Orthopedic Surgery
Midwest Orthopaedics at Rush
Chicago, Illinois

Angelica Adrian Highsmith, MS
Senior Bioprocess Scientist
Discgenics
Salt Lake City, Utah

Jason C. Ho, MD
Department of Orthopaedic Surgery
Orthopedic and Rheumatologic Institute
Cleveland Clinic
Cleveland, Ohio

Wellington K. Hsu, MD, FAAOS
Clifford C. Raisbeck Distinguished Professor of Orthopaedic Surgery
Director of Research
Professor, Department of Orthopaedic Surgery
Professor, Department of Neurological Surgery
Northwestern University Feinberg School of Medicine
Chicago, Illinois

Clark T. Hung, PhD
Professor of Biomedical Engineering and Orthopedic Science (in Orthopedic Surgery)
Columbia University
Department of Biomedical Engineering
New York, New York

Shepard Hurwitz, MD, FAAOS
Department of Orthopaedic Surgery
University of Virginia
Charlottesville, Virginia

Joseph P. Iannotti, MD, PhD, FAAOS
Department of Orthopaedic Surgery
Orthopedic and Rheumatologic Institute
Cleveland Clinic Florida
Weston, Florida

Jie Jiang, PhD
Department of Orthopaedics
University of Maryland School of Medicine
Baltimore, Maryland

Aric Kaiser, MS
Expert Biomedical Engineer
US Food and Drug Administration
Silver Spring, Maryland

Linda E. A. Kanim, MA
Clinical and Translational Research Specialist
Spine Center
Orthopaedic Stem Cell Research Lab
Cedars-Sinai Medical Center
Los Angeles, California

Kenji Kato, MD, PhD
Department of Orthopedic Surgery
Nagoya City University Graduate School of Medical Sciences
Nagoya, Japan

Regis J. O'Keefe, MD, PhD, FAAOS
Fred C. Reynolds Professor and Chair
Department of Orthopaedic Surgery
Washington University School of Medicine
St. Louis, Missouri

Yusuf Khan, PhD
Department of Biomedical Engineering
University of Connecticut
Storrs, Connecticut
Connecticut Convergence Institute for Translation in Regenerative Engineering
Department of Orthopaedic Surgery
University of Connecticut Health Center
Farmington, Connecticut

Evangeline Fumina Kobayashi, MD
Orthopaedic Surgery Resident
Michigan Medicine
University of Michigan
Ann Arbor, Michigan

Robert F. LaPrade, MD, PhD, FAAOS
Complex Knee Surgeon
Twin Cities Orthopedics
Edina, Minnesota

Cato T. Laurencin, MD, PhD, FAAOS
Department of Materials Science and Engineering
Department of Biomedical Engineering
University of Connecticut
Connecticut Convergence Institute for Translation in Regenerative Engineering
Department of Orthopaedic Surgery
University of Connecticut Health Center
Farmington, Connecticut

Natalie L. Leong, MD, FAAOS
Baltimore VA Medical Center
University of Maryland School of Medicine
Baltimore, Maryland

Jay R. Lieberman, MD, FAAOS
Professor and Chair of Orthopaedic Surgery
Keck School of Medicine of the University of Southern California
Los Angeles, California

Robert G. Marx, MD, FAAOS
Sports Medicine
Hospital for Special Surgery
New York, New York

Koichi Masuda, MD
Department of Orthopaedic Surgery
School of Medicine
University of California San Diego
San Diego, California

Allan Mishra, MD, FAAOS
Adjunct Clinical Associate
Professor, Orthopedic Surgery
Menlo Medical Clinic
Stanford Healthcare
Stanford, California

Amy M. Moore, MD
Professor and Chair
Robert L. Ruberg, MD Alumni Endowed Chair
The Ohio State University Wexner Medical Center
Columbus, Ohio

Mary Murphy, PhD, DSc
Regenerative Medicine Institute
School of Medicine
National University of Ireland Galway
Galway, Ireland

Minh Hoang Nguyen, MD
Department of Plastic and Reconstructive Surgery
The Ohio State University Wexner Medical Center
Columbus, Ohio

Clayton W. Nuelle, MD, FAAOS
University of Missouri
Columbia, Missouri

Kenneth S. Ogueri, PhD
Department of Materials Science and Engineering
University of Connecticut
Connecticut Convergence Institute for Translation in Regenerative Engineering
University of Connecticut Health Center
Farmington, Connecticut

Joseph T. Patterson, MD
Assistant Clinical Professor of Orthopaedic Surgery
Keck School of Medicine of the University of Southern California
Los Angeles, California

Frank M. Phillips, MD
Ronald DeWald Endowed Professor of Spinal Deformity
Director, Spine Surgery
Department of Orthopaedic Surgery
Rush University Medical Center
Chicago, Illinois

Nicolas S. Piuzzi, MD
Director of Research, Adult Joint Reconstruction
Department of Orthopaedic Surgery
Cleveland Clinic
Cleveland, Ohio

Jennifer Racine-Avila, MBA
Program Manager, Clinical/Translational Research
Department of Orthopaedic Surgery
Warren Alpert Medical School of Brown University
Program Manager, Clinical/Translational Research
Department of Orthopaedic Surgery
Warren Alpert Medical School of Brown University
Providence, Rhode Island

Anthony Ratcliffe, PhD
President and CEO
Synthasome Inc.
San Diego, California

Eric T. Ricchetti, MD, FAAOS
Department of Orthopaedic Surgery
Orthopedic and Rheumatologic Institute
Cleveland Clinic
Cleveland, Ohio

Scott A. Rodeo, MD, FAAOS
Director, Center for Regenerative Medicine
Hospital for Special Surgery
New York, New York

Daniel Rodriguez-Granrose, PhD
Senior Manager of Bioprocess Development
DiscGenics
Salt Lake City, Utah

Vicki Rosen, PhD
Professor and Chair
Department of Development Biology
Harvard School of Dental Medicine
Boston, Massachusetts

Robert L. Sah, MD, ScD
Professor, University of California San Diego
Department of Bioengineering
San Diego, California

Daisuke Sakai, MD, PhD
Department of Orthopaedic Surgery
Tokai University School of Medicine
Isehara, Japan

Michael J. Sayegh, MD
Department of Orthopaedic Surgery
Zucker School of Medicine at Hofstra/Northwell
Long Island Jewish Medical Center
New Hyde Park, New York

Ryan W. Schmucker, MD
Assistant Professor
Department of Plastic Surgery
The Ohio State University Wexner Medical Center
Columbus, Ohio

Jordy Schol, MSc
Department of Orthopaedic Surgery
Tokai University School of Medicine
Isehara, Japan

Edward M. Schwarz, PhD
Professor, Department of Orthopaedics
Director, Center for Musculoskeletal Research
University of Rochester Medical Center
Rochester, New York

Nicholas A. Sgaglione, MD, FAAOS
Northwell Health Orthopaedic Institute
Donald and Barbara Zucker School of Medicine at Hofstra/Northwell
New York, New York

Lara Ionescu Silverman, PhD
Principal Consultant
LIS BioConsulting
Salt Lake City, Utah

Caroline Taber, AB
Research Assistant
Hospital for Special Surgery
New York, New York

David P. Trofa, MD
Assistant Professor of Orthopaedic Surgery
Division of Sports Medicine
Columbia University Medical Center
Brownsville, New York

Mirtijn van Griensven, MD, PhD
Professor of Regenerative Medicine
Chair Department Cell Biology-Inspired Tissue Engineering
Vice-Director, MERLN Institute for Technology-Inspired Regenerative Medicine
Associate at Department of General Surgery, Division of Trauma Surgery
Maastricht University, The Netherlands

J. Tracy Watson, MD, FAAOS
Professor, Orthopaedic Surgery
Chief, Orthopaedic Trauma Service
Department of Orthopaedic Surgery
Saint Louis University School of Medicine
St. Louis, Missouri

Brian C. Werner, MD, FAAOS
Associate Professor of Orthopaedic Surgery
Department of Orthopaedic Surgery
University of Virginia
Charlottesville, Virginia

Adam Yanke, MD, PhD, FAAOS
Orthopedic Surgeon
Midwest Orthopedics at Rush Oak Park Hospital
Oak Park, Illinois

Kenneth R. Zaslav, MD, FAAOS
Attending Orthopedic Surgeon
Northwell Orthopedic Institute
Professor Orthopedic Surgery
Zucker School of Medicine Hofstra University
Director, Center for Regenerative Orthopedic Medicine
Lenox Hill Hospital New York
New York, New York

Athan G. Zavras, BA, MD
Department of Orthopaedic Surgery
Rush University Medical Center
Chicago, Illinois

Victor Z. Zhang, BSc
Department of Biomedical Engineering
The Center for Musculoskeletal Research
University of Rochester
Rochester, New York

Foreword

I feel deeply honored to have the opportunity to compose the foreword to this book. This is a landmark text with a unique group of expert and thoughtful contributors and an exhibition of subject material that is relevant to the current practice of orthopaedics. Both Dr. Aaron and I have been in orthopaedics for over 50 years each and we were initiated into our professional careers in the era of the physician-scientist, where in medical school we had to engage in laboratory research as part of the curriculum. Young Dr. Bruder had the unique pleasure, beginning in 1982, of being sequentially Dr. Aaron's student (Honors ScB at Brown University) and then my student (MD, PhD at Case Western Reserve University). Dr. Bruder has spent almost his entire career associated with orthobiologics, but from a very different, product development perspective. We all have witnessed the evolution of orthopaedics from a hardware/implant-based surgery to the biologic approaches of the 21st century, the age of orthobiologics, and with the recent start of robotic-assisted surgery.

From the days of Aristotle until 1999 when William Haseltine coined the term regenerative medicine, orthopaedic surgery involved the use of a variety of surgical techniques for musculoskeletal reconstruction. Regenerative medicine implies the premise that biologic techniques will be used to stimulate injured tissue to slowly regenerate the afflicted segments themselves, such as in a long bone fracture in humans. Orthobiologics, in this context, provides exogenously added natural and manmade materials to assist in more complex, multiple fractures of long bones.

The previous eras in orthopaedics have involved the use of hard materials such as ivory and metal with an emphasis on mechanics. In the case of hip replacement surgery, this dates back to 1891 when Gluck used ivory, Smith-Petersen cup arthroplasty in the 1920s, and Wiles total hip replacement with stainless steel parts in 1938. The modern arthroplasty era was pioneered by Charnley in 1962 when he replaced a total hip joint with implants made of metal and plastic and used polymethyl methacrylate cement for anchorage. For knee replacement, Gluck used ivory in the 1860s, and Walldius introduced the hinged joint in 1951 that was redesigned and constructed of cobalt-chromium in 1958. The modular metal-polyethylene knees came into their own in the 1970s and 1980s with cobalt-chromium and titanium elements.

Orthobiologics are coming to maturity in the 21st century for orthopaedics. Our fascination with the biologic concepts and mechanisms of regenerative medicine represents long-term interests, which date back to anthropologists who studied regenerating limbs of amphibian fossils called *Micromelerpeton* from 300 million years ago. For me, orthobiologics started with the experiments reported by Marshall Urist, MD in 1965 where this talented young orthopaedic surgeon (physician-scientist) placed demineralized bone chips into the muscle pouch of an adult mouse. Six weeks later, he observed newly formed bone in this muscle site. Dr. Urist hypothesized that the demineralized bone placed in situ released bioactive molecules that stimulated the formation of newly fabricated bone in the heterotopic muscle site. Dr. Urist coined the term bone morphogenetic proteins, or BMPs, as the responsible bioactive elements and started on a 25-year quest to purify and characterize these molecules. Many of us were drawn into the challenge of identifying, characterizing, and using demineralized bone and, thus, BMPs to restore and regenerate skeletal tissue in orthotopic sites.

The modern era of molecular regenerative medicine and orthobiologics started in the late 1980s when John Wozney and his team at the Genetics Institute (a biotech company in Cambridge, Massachusetts) cloned and patented the BMP-transforming growth factor beta family of proteins and in doing so, proved that all of the studies previously done by Dr. Urist were correct. I am an author of a patent (not maintained by my university) from the 1980s that used a collagen sponge to deliver BMP-like molecules to surgical sites. This combination-orthobiologic product (BMP-2 and a collagen sponge) eventually became the FDA-approved product for bringing recombinant BMP to a bony site (spinal fusion).

For centuries, orthopaedic surgeons have been transplanting bone, tendon, and muscle to regenerate function in injured tissues. Thus, the field of orthobiologics has always been intrinsic to orthopaedic surgery. Because no body part stands alone, a single tissue, a femur for example, is a composite variety of tissues including ligaments, tendons, vasculature, marrow, and neural elements, etc. The orthopaedic physician, either currently or in the time of Aristotle, had to choose from available materials to use in reconstructions. In today's context, taking a piece of tissue in an operating room from one part of the body and bring it into use in another part of the body (using the principles of minimal manipulation) is considered standard practice. The orthopaedic physician must be creative in every single surgery in reconnecting and reforming the damaged tissue. Such approaches are invented with every single surgery because every single patient is different. If you have a 100-lb slender female and a 250-lb football player who shatter their femurs, the surgical approach will require creativity and patient-specific reconstructions.

Technology development involves understanding how and why a tissue fails or becomes injured and deducing a healing sequence and integrating orthobiologic materials or reagents. Such additive material can come from the patient themselves (autologous), from a donor whether the donor is alive or newly deceased (allogenic), or from a xenogeneic donor that appropriately integrates into and functions in the host. The subsequent steps of using an appropriate experimental animal model to test the surgical procedure or injected material, designing clinical trials to optimize the procedure and document its efficacy in cooperation and collaboration with the FDA are currently required.

The commercialization of any product must involve the detailed development and testing of the product in the context of its health care use. Of course, such products must first fill an unmet health care need. That unmet need will already have a standard of care that will have a cost associated with it. The new product must not only be more efficacious than the current standard of care, but it also must be competitive on a cost basis. A number of products have been approved by the FDA for use, but the cost structure of those products may prove disadvantageous to the company and the number of products with sales directly related to the perceived enhanced therapeutic capabilities of the new product.

Upper extremity surgery including rotator cuff, tendon management, complex fracture repair, and muscle regeneration are quite different in their anatomic complexity compared with lower extremities. Lower extremities involve large pieces of bone, tissues that do not regenerate normally as does meniscus or cartilage, and very complex outcome parameters that influence the surgical and medical approaches used by the orthopaedic physician. The spine adds additional complexity because it is a multifaceted, multicomponent anatomic structure and because it houses neural elements. Interrupting the spinal cord (ie, affecting spinal ganglia that send axonal projections into or out of the spinal cord) must be avoided. Moreover, the unique union between the cartilaginous end plates and each bony facet with its central spinal cord is unmatched by any other orthopaedic component in its complexity and sensitivity to disruption. A small angular displacement of one vertebra can not only affect the nerve roots and ganglia coming in and out of the spinal cord but affect the spinal cord itself and, thus, coordinate function. Thus, minor injuries to the spine can have profound neurologic and organismal effects. The entry into the vertebral column including the injection of bioactive molecules has to be done with high degrees of precision. An entire section of the book concerns itself with placement of these orthobiologic reagents into and onto the spine.

This is an ambitious and noteworthy volume that is uniquely constructed by knowledgeable section editors with important summaries, perspectives, and commentaries at the end of each section. Because of the choice of contributors to each of the sections and the interaction with the section editors, Drs. Aaron and Bruder have done a masterful job of bringing together a large body of useful evidence and medical considerations in this new era of orthobiologics. Successfully integrating the scientific and clinical considerations by both young and seasoned investigators is, itself, an admirable and thoughtful undertaking. This volume will be the gold standard for many years to come.

Arnold I. Caplan, PhD
Skeletal Research Center
Biology Department
Case Western Reserve University
Cleveland, Ohio

Acknowledgments

To Roy Aaron, my undergraduate thesis advisor, thank you for introducing me to the thrill of scientific discovery and opportunities to influence the biology of musculoskeletal tissue repair 40 years ago. Your early guidance and lifelong interest in my development as a physician-scientist has been fundamental to my personal journey, and editing this textbook together is an extraordinarily meaningful bookend to our professional alliance and friendship. To Arnold Caplan, my graduate thesis advisor, collaborator, and friend, thank you for always encouraging me to undertake "the heroic experiment" and make bold career choices. Your partnership in the development of MSC therapies and more has been the bedrock of my clinical and scientific career. And to Lisa Bruder, my wife and partner, thank you for your unwavering support through an odyssey of unconventional academic, industrial, and geographic transitions. You and our daughters, Hannah and Emma, are at the core of what inspires me and I have boundless gratitude for what the three of you have taught me about balance and being "present."

Scott P. Bruder, MD, PhD, FORS

I have been fortunate to have had inspiring mentors and teachers at several stages in my professional life. In residency, Henry Mankin was a charismatic educator whose words echo to this day, almost 50 years later, as he seems to practice along with me. Both in residency and later as my department chairman, Michael Ehrlich brought me to the intersection of medicine and humanity. I gratefully acknowledge how much I've learned from my students and my patients. The generous, gifted clinicians and scientists of many disciplines who were my teachers led and inspired by example. To them I owe the ability of working at the interface of science and clinical medicine. They provided me with insights into what would be my medical life—about discovery, about working on the edge of what is known and what is yet unknown, and perhaps creating some new truth that may lead those who will succeed me in new directions. My wonderful wife, Judy, has been steadfast in her support throughout the tender journey that is academic medicine, and our gifts to the future are our two extraordinary sons, David and Daniel, who I know will carry on.

Roy K. Aaron, MD, FAAOS, FORS

Introduction

For nearly 40 years the American Academy of Orthopaedic Surgeons (AAOS) has been at the forefront of educating the clinical and scientific communities on the potential of biologic intervention in the management of musculoskeletal pathology. Our field has moved from the practice of removing, and then replacing, diseased or injured tissue to a mindset embodied by the pursuit of repairing or regenerating the affected tissue in situ. The evolution of this perspective is a direct result of the emergence of powerful tools in cell and molecular biology during the late 20th and 21st century. The Editorial Board and Contributors to this volume represent some of the most influential pioneers in the discovery and implementation strategies that improve human health using cutting-edge biological tools in orthopaedics. The intersection of these disciplines is what clinical and scientific innovators have termed orthobiologics, and the AAOS has increased their sponsorship of symposia, workshops, monographs, and committee efforts over the last two decades to address the safe and effective use of these technologies to treat musculoskeletal disorders in patients. This treatise is the first comprehensive text sponsored by the AAOS, and stems from a recommendation by the Education Council.

Our approach for the construction of this text underwent several iterations, landing on a final blueprint aimed at first describing the fundamental technologies and tools available for the creation of orthobiologic products in Part 1. By first setting the framework for an appreciation of the cellular, molecular, and biomaterial underpinnings, we provided an overview of the major strategies for both hard and soft tissue repair and regeneration in Section 1. Next, we turned our focus to an exposition of the process and challenges associated with advancing basic science technology through the product development, clinical evaluation, regulatory approval, and reimbursement processes in Section 2. Understanding what is required to bring an idea from the bench to the bedside, and eventually into broad clinical use, is something not generally taught in medical education but is at the heart of translational medicine. Successful navigation of this product development pathway can be elusive, and understanding the implications of clinical study design and its limits on broad applicability outside of the controlled environment of FDA registered studies will help physicians critically analyze data and make wise choices in their management of patients.

In Part 2 of the book we asked leading clinical specialists familiar with commercially available, and other promising, technologies to provide updates and guidance on the use of orthobiologics across the spectrum of pathologies treated. We organized these recommendations by simple anatomic distinction of upper extremity, lower extremity, and spine conditions, recognizing still that some approaches would be applicable across many surgical sites. For example, management of challenging bone repair and nonunions is addressed in the Upper Extremity section, but the astute reader will appreciate that the solutions presented also have applicability in the lower extremity and spine. Likewise, though articular cartilage repair is addressed in Section 4: Solutions for Lower Extremity Pathology, we know that the shoulder represents another joint amenable to such an intervention. The same is true for management of tendon and ligament defects and osteoarthritis. On the contrary, current approaches for intervertebral disk repair and regeneration are limited to that complex tissue and anatomic location.

In each of the Clinical Applications sections, we have included a chapter on some of the unique considerations for designing and interpreting clinical studies. Clearly, every target tissue should have a set of patient-reported and objective outcome parameters that are embraced by specialists in that pathology, such as the WOMAC Pain and Function scales validated for use in osteoarthritis studies. However, not all clinical measurement tools or instruments are applicable for every type of pathology within the same joint. The WOMAC instrument, for example, is not useful for studies of articular cartilage repair in the knee, so an appreciation for the subtle issues related to clinical study design and interpretation become paramount. When members of the clinical community, or Value Assessment Committees in hospitals, need to evaluate the strength of outcome data to guide the delivery of orthobiologic products overall, it is essential for them to understand the limitations of study design and potential biases introduced by the investigator or sponsor.

The final, common design element of all sections is a Summary and Perspectives chapter written by the Section Editors. The intent of such a review is to highlight those areas where clinical and scientific consensus may have been established and illuminate those areas where uncertainty remains and more work is required. The very nature of assembling a textbook during a period of intense scientific, clinical, and product development efforts subjects itself to criticism and controversy of opinions expressed. Clearly there will be more than one possible solution for many conditions treatable with orthobiologic products, but performing comparative studies between approved products is a very difficult undertaking without support from industry sponsors who themselves may not want to underwrite such a study. New data sets are emerging every month in the literature, at conferences and in personal clinics around the world. Practitioners using similar technologies on different patient populations may see variations in outcomes relative to the latest publication, which may add confusion to the clinical justification for adopting any particular product or technology. Just during the assembly of this book, we have seen dozens of products in development fail in FDA-registered studies while others have successfully navigated the approval or clearance process. Further still, there is a segment of orthobiologic offerings based on human cellular and tissue products (HCT/Ps) that are legally available without compelling clinical evidence to support their broad use, raising a number of ethical issues.

In conclusion, we have sought to provide a contemporary review of the burgeoning field of orthobiologics with a focus on scientific and clinical solutions for the orthopaedic community. We recognize that technologies will evolve, data will emerge that support or refute the use of products described in this volume, and commercial success will depend on the ability to demonstrate meaningful outcomes that can be justified by health economic analyses of broad populations and covered lives. Our health care systems cannot absorb more expensive interventions that fail to deliver meaningful improvements to morbidity and quality-of-life measures. We believe that this compendium of chapters will help arm the current generation of scientists and practitioners with the knowledge and tools necessary to make informed decisions on patient care. Our hope is that the next generation of investigators will see far beyond where we are today, just as the Editors and Contributors to this exposition did over the course of their careers with tremendous joy, enthusiasm, wonder, and amazement at the power of biology.

Scott P. Bruder, MD, PhD, FORS
Roy K. Aaron, MD, FAAOS, FORS

Contents

Section 5: Solutions for Spinal Pathology

Section Editors: Wellington K. Hsu, MD, FAAOS; Kevin C. Baker, PhD

PART

1

Foundational Principles

SECTION

1

Biologic Options for Tissue Repair and Regeneration

Section Editors
Robert E. Guldberg, PhD
Edward M. Schwarz, PhD
Christopher H. Evans, PhD

CHAPTER 1

Cell Biology and Cell Sources

Frank Barry, PhD • Mary Murphy, PhD, DSc

INTRODUCTION

Cell therapy is a clinical protocol involving the transplantation of living cells for the treatment of tissue injury or disease. It involves a number of different cell types, mainly derived from postnatal tissues, which may be either isolated and expanded in a defined culture format or presented as an unexpanded cell concentrate derived from a tissue biopsy. In many broader applications, cells are delivered to the circulation by infusion. This includes the use of transplanted bone marrow or expanded hematopoietic stem cells (HSCs) for the treatment of blood disorders and malignancies, or T cells and natural killer cells genetically modified to express a chimeric antigen receptor to target specific tumor cells. The use of cell therapy in orthopaedic applications most commonly involves local delivery to the site of tissue damage, for example, to treat focal cartilage defects, degenerative disk disease, osteoarthritis, or spine fusion or for fracture repair. In devising a cellular therapy for use in these clinical targets, it is apparent that a clear understanding of the biologic phenotype and therapeutic mechanism of action is essential for successful translation.

LIVING CELLS AS MEDICINAL PRODUCTS

Cell therapy can be used in the treatment of musculoskeletal conditions. The selection of the expanded cell type generally depends on the specific application and includes chondrocytes for cartilage repair, nucleus pulposus cells for disk repair, and mesenchymal stromal cells (MSCs) as a potential (but not yet fully proven) cell type for wider application in a number of different targets. In many cases, the protocols involve autologous (patient-derived) cells but allogeneic use, where the cells are derived from a mismatched donor or pool of donors, is also common. It is obvious that the allogenic use involves deployment of cells that are nonimmunogenic and tolerated by an immunocompetent recipient without the need for any pretreatment regimen involving immunosuppression.

The use of expanded cell therapy in orthopaedics presents significant logistical and regulatory hurdles that are not easily overcome. These include access to aseptic tissue culture suites and technical expertise in the isolation, culture, characterization, formulation, storage, and transport of the expanded cell dose. In addition, because culture-expanded cells do not meet regulatory criteria relating to minimally manipulated transplant materials, their use requires adoption of stringent standards of manufacturing compliance and clinical proof. Because of this, recent attention has focused on the use of minimally manipulated, autologous, unexpanded cell preparations, generally prepared as concentrates taken from blood, bone marrow, or adipose tissue, which are more easily prepared in an intraoperative setting. The historical development of cellular repair strategies in human medicine is described, as well as the evolution of biologic understanding underpinning clinical practice. In addition, the major cell types used in orthopaedic cell-based treatment strategies, with consideration of both expanded and nonexpanded methods, are reviewed. The essential biologic attributes of each cell type are described as a rationale for their specific use. The tissue source of the cells is also discussed, as well as the relative advantages of autologous versus allogeneic use.

EVOLUTION OF CELL THERAPY

In discussing the applications of cell therapy in modern orthopaedics, it is useful to consider how current principles and practices evolved. In this context, a great deal can be learned from the fields of bone marrow transplant (BMT) and tissue engineering because these are now recognized as pioneering efforts that established many of the biologic principles that surgeons currently rely on.

Cell therapy has its origins in the search for treatment options for radiation-induced disease, an issue of great urgency in the nuclear age and at a time when the threat of exposure to ionizing radiation was significant. It was understood that bone marrow was especially vulnerable to the effects of radiation, and, in the 1950s, BMT was pioneered by Thomas et al[1] for the restoration of hematopoiesis following radiation-induced ablation of the bone marrow. At this time, there was limited understanding of transplant antigens and the host immune response to these. However, with the development of treatment strategies to encourage graft acceptance, BMT became more and more successful with the survival of patients who

Neither of the following authors nor any immediate family member has received anything of value from or has stock or stock options held in a commercial company or institution related directly or indirectly to the subject of this chapter: Dr. Barry and Dr. Murphy.

would otherwise have died from hematologic malignancies.[2] This was essentially a two-stage process, involving destruction of the patient's blood system using lethal whole-body irradiation to eradicate leukemic cells, followed by the regeneration of the patient's blood system by the transplantation of healthy and histocompatible donor marrow. To date, approximately one million BMTs have been successfully carried out, and this has extended to umbilical cord blood transplants for pediatric patients.[3] This was the first clinically proven application of cell transplantation as an effective therapy, and many of the principles currently applicable in the field of cell transplantation had their origins in those first applications.

The successful use of BMT as a therapeutic strategy for patients with leukemia, and subsequently for immune deficiency disorders, demonstrated that healthy, viable cells could be used for the functional restoration of diseased tissue. In addition to these clinical innovations, there was a substantial focus on understanding the cell biology and genesis of the hematopoietic system. Key among these was the early realization that the entire repertoire of cells that constitute the blood and immune systems were derived from a single precursor HSC. The work of Civin et al[4] identified a molecular label—the CD34 surface marker—that was specific for a population of stem cells resident in human bone marrow and was of particular significance. This provided a means of enrichment for HSCs from among the millions of other blood cells found in the bone marrow, which up to that moment had been a major challenge. The effect of these discoveries has been profound and far reaching, providing the initial understanding of the role of stem cells in tissue homeostasis, laying the foundation for future efforts in stem cell therapy, and demonstrating that tissue regeneration is possible when cell preparations are selected, expanded in culture, and transplanted to the patient. **Figure 1** provides a historical timeline relating to the evolution of concepts in cellular therapies.

The field of tissue engineering had its genesis in the 1980s and at that time represented a new paradigm, based firmly on the principle of combining living cells with biologically friendly materials to create new implants for repair of damaged organs.[5] Among the early innovations in this arena were the application of keratinocytes and

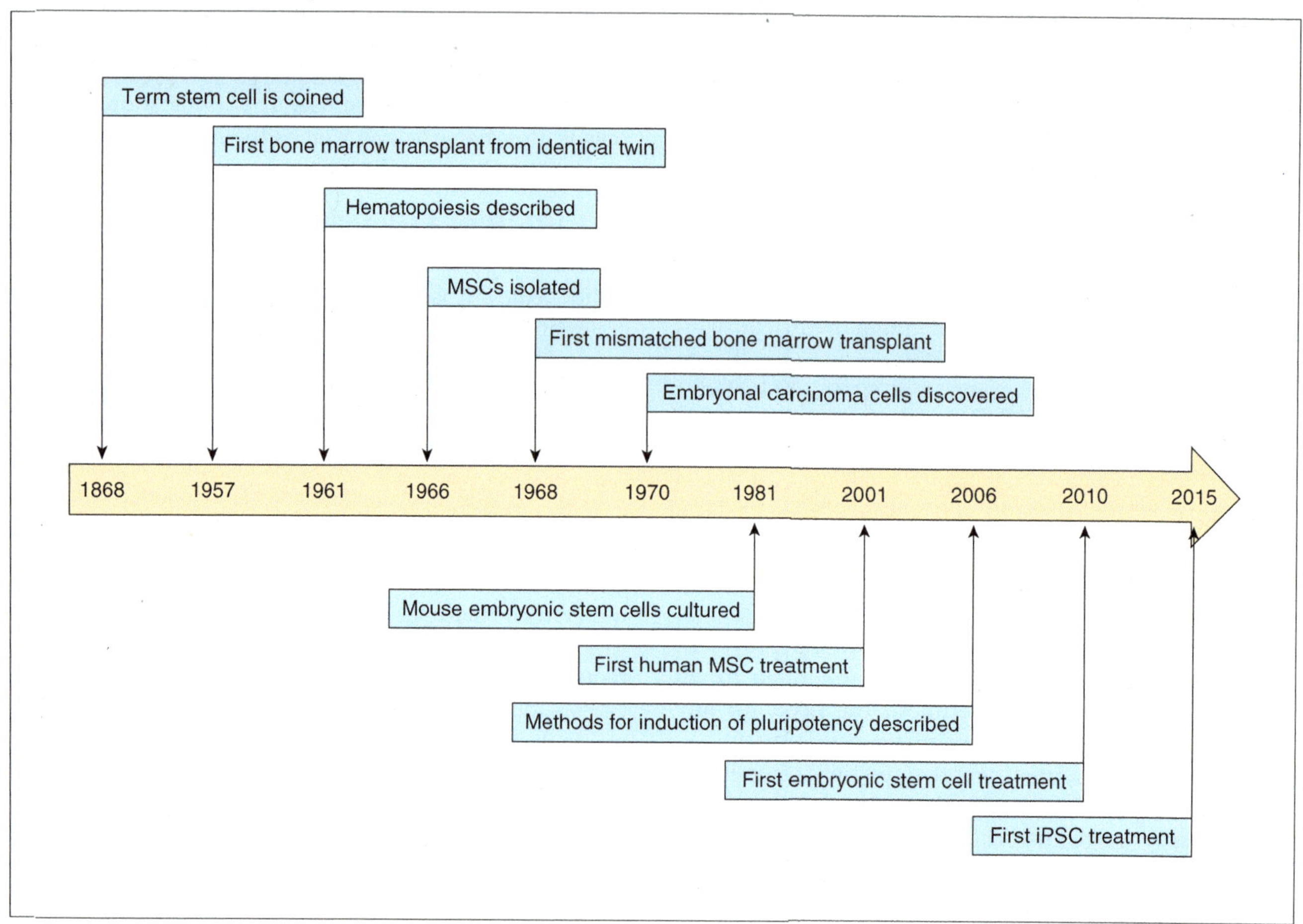

FIGURE 1 Timeline of key developments in cell therapy. iPSC = induced pluripotent stem cell, MSC = mesenchymal stromal cell

fibroblasts seeded on collagen gels for the treatment of burns[6] and the use of polymers containing chondrocytes as a transplantable modality for cartilage repair.[7] Many other applications were suggested, and it was proposed at the time that tissue engineering would provide a solution to the chronic shortage of organs needed for transplantation—at that time, and currently, a major issue in the management of organ failure. Examples included liver[8] and pancreas[9] regeneration, nerve replacement,[10] and reconstruction of urologic tissues including the bladder.[11] It is probably fair to state that many of these ideas have not been effectively translated into wide clinical uptake and the construction of engineered organs for transplantation is still challenging, although there are some striking examples of innovation in this arena.

As a general consideration, it can be stated that the tremendous success of cell-based treatment strategies for bone marrow reconstitution probably relates to the plastic nature of that tissue with its very high cell turnover as well as the clear biologic understanding of the roles of HSCs. In contrast, the relative lack of progress in cell-based reconstitution of solid organs can be attributed to their complex architecture, terminally differentiated state with low cells, and the poorer understanding of the nature and role of progenitor cells. Many of these considerations still find strong relevance in orthopaedic cell therapy.

USE OF CULTURE-EXPANDED CELLS IN ORTHOPAEDIC TISSUE REPAIR

A number of different cell types have been widely used in expanded cell therapy applications in orthopaedics, including chondrocytes, nucleus pulposus cells, notochord cells, and stromal cells derived from adipose tissue, bone marrow, or umbilical cord. The phenotypic attributes, tissue source, and possible mechanistic elements are summarized in **Figure 2**. In the following section, each of these is addressed in detail.

Chondrocytes

Chondrocytes have occupied a dominant position in orthopaedic tissue engineering and cell transplantation protocols for the past few decades.[12,13] These are the sole cellular component of the articular cartilage and produce the abundant extracellular matrix (ECM), including the collagens and proteoglycans that confer on the tissue its unique biomechanical properties. Within the healthy cartilage matrix, chondrocytes are of low abundance (occupying less than 10% of the tissue volume), quiescent, and maintain the matrix components at a low rate of turnover.[14] In terms of developmental origin, cell-type specification and differentiation are mediated by groups of transcription factors, with SRY-related HMG-box 9 (SOX9) playing an essential role.[15] SOX9, in association with SOX5/SOX6, actively drives the expression of many

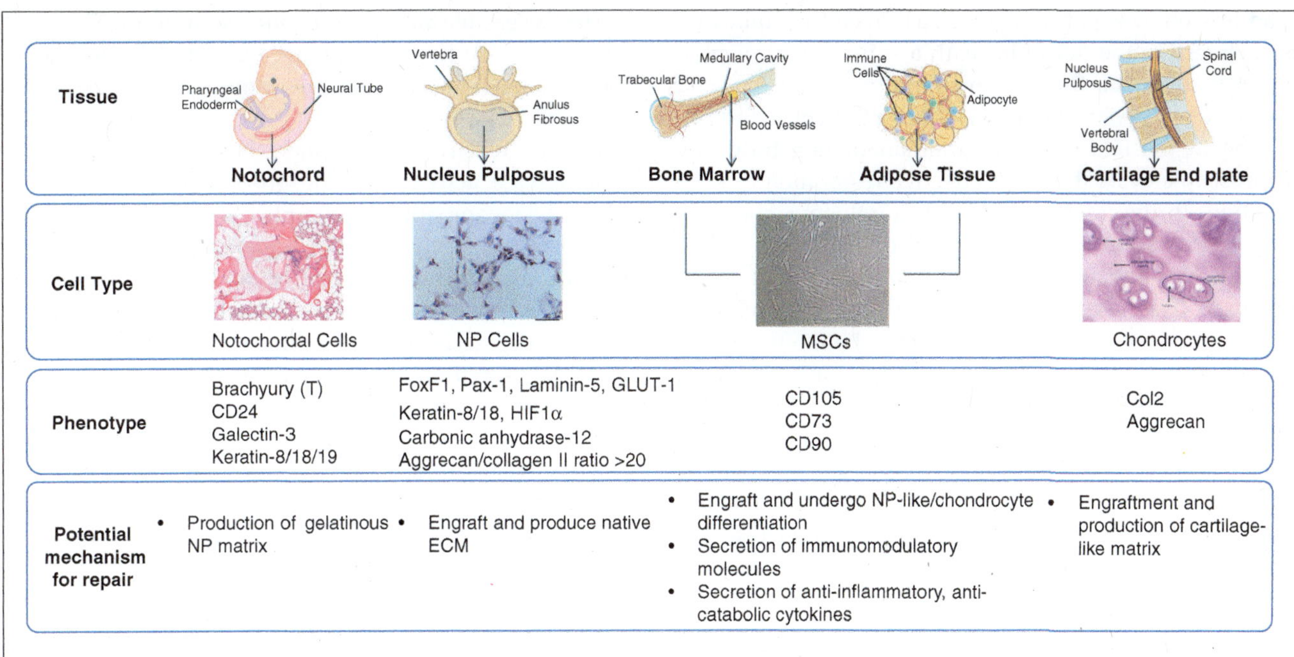

FIGURE 2 Schematic illustration shows tissue sources and cell types used in expanded cell therapies, with reference to cell-specific phenotypic markers and potential therapeutic mechanism. COL2 = collagen type II, DDD = degenerative disk disease, ECM = extracellular matrix, GLUT1 = glucose transporter 1, HIF1α = hypoxia-inducible factor 1 alpha, MSCs = mesenchymal stromal cells, NP = nucleus pulposus.

cartilage-specific genes and maintains cartilage homeostasis. This SOX trio inhibits entry to a hypertrophic state, preserving the articular phenotype. On development of a prehypertrophic state within the epiphyseal plate, the SOX RNAs disappear, whereas SOX9 protein remains and is required for the expression of prehypertrophic genes.[15] These gene expression pathways and their control by the transcription factor networks are of profound importance in chondrocyte-based therapeutic applications because they are key elements in retention of the articular phenotype.

Chondrocytes can be extracted from the cartilage with relative ease by enzymatic digestion and expanded under standard expansion conditions either in monolayer or in three-dimensional constructs composed of alginate or other materials.[14] The quiescent and terminally differentiated nature of chondrocytes and the avascular and aneural characteristics of cartilage allow for very limited capacity for self-repair. The clinical need for effective treatment strategies that regenerate or replace chondrocytes following acute cartilage injury is therefore compelling because of the effect that these injuries have and the frequent progression to osteoarthritis. Chondrocytes have been widely used to treat articular cartilage defects since the original studies of Brittberg et al were published in 1994,[16] and this represented a progressive step in the development of cellular therapies. In this method, chondrocytes are extracted from a cartilage biopsy harvested from a non–weight-bearing region of knee cartilage. The low density of chondrocytes in native articular cartilage is addressed by expansion of the cells in culture, followed by delivery to the defect beneath a sutured flap of periosteal tissue taken from the medial tibia. Early reported results were positive with evidence of cartilage regeneration at the site of transplantation demonstrated by arthroscopic evaluation and effective restoration of knee function. In the intervening years, autologous chondrocyte implantation has been carried out in thousands of patients and has become a common treatment in sports medicine. The success of this approach has been qualified by a number of compounding factors. Foremost among these is questionable efficacy[17] relating to assessment of clinical outcomes compared with standard treatments. In this regard, the failure of the technique to reproduce collagen structure and, therefore, mechanical characteristics of the cartilage is of prime importance.[18] Other factors include the complex surgical intervention required to harvest the cartilage biopsy and a second procedure for preparation of the periosteal flap and delivery of the cells. Both procedures are separated by a period of 14 to 21 days, the time needed for cell expansion.

The technique has been refined by the use of various biomembrane scaffolds to replace the periosteal tissue.[19] A second, and more serious, obstacle is provided by the phenotypic instability of cultured chondrocytes, which have a well-described tendency to dedifferentiate, thereby losing their capacity to build an ECM.[20,21] Because healthy cartilage is composed mostly of ECM, which is responsible for the critical biomechanical properties of the tissue, this is a distinct disadvantage. Furthermore, chondrocytes from aged donors have more limited capacity to proliferate compared with those from younger donors.[22] A solution to this problem has been available in the application of chondrocytes from neonatal tissue, which have greater proliferative capacity and phenotypic stability and overcome immunogenic obstacles.[23] Recent approaches involving the use of chondrocytes obtained from patients with polydactyly in cross-linked hyaluronan gels represent one such approach.[24] An analogous allograft approach involves the use of particulated cartilage obtained from neonates up to 13 weeks old and delivered with a fibrin adhesive. This product, DeNovo NT Graft from Zimmer Biomet, is a fresh allograft viable for 40 days after harvest and has the effect of delivering chondrocytes to the defect without a requirement for cell expansion.[25]

The question of allogenicity in chondrocyte transplantation is of major significance. Although there has been a strong focus on the use of autologous cells—based on the premise that nonautologous cell transplantation induces an immune response—the complexity of the surgical approach and logistics associated with cell expansion provide a strong rationale for considering allogeneic cell transplants. There is now an abundance of information that suggests that allogeneic delivery of chondrocytes is perfectly feasible and does not elicit an immune response. In contrast, studies with rat and human allogeneic chondrocytes indicate that they are immunomodulatory, with a potent ability to suppress T-cell proliferation, evade cytotoxic reactivity, and modulate pro-inflammatory macrophage activity.[26,27] The absence of expression of major histocompatibility complex class II molecules on chondrocytes further supports their utility in an allogeneic context.[28] Thus, the use of allogeneic chondrocyte cell banks as an off-the-shelf treatment for acute cartilage injury may well be a feasible clinical strategy with distinct advantages in terms of reduced cost and complexity.

A further and potentially more robust approach involves the use of chondrocytes derived from neural crest cells rather than those derived from the mesoderm. Cartilage tissue in the cranial skeleton is derived from neural crest cells of the mesoectoderm, whereas articular cartilage in joints has a distinct, mesodermal origin.[29] Nasal chondrocytes, isolated from the mature nasal septum, are neural crest-derived cells with a high proliferative capacity. Although they tend to dedifferentiate in monolayer culture, similar to articular chondrocytes, they have a clear capacity to redifferentiate in three-dimensional culture after expansion.[30] Thus, nasal chondrocytes provide advantages compared with articular chondrocytes as a self-renewing cell population capable of forming cartilage tissue. These cells have been assessed in patient studies and, although limited in scale, nonetheless provide positive outcomes.[31]

Mesenchymal Stromal Cells

MSCs have been tested in cell therapy applications across a wide range of disease conditions. They were first identified in rat bone marrow as fibroblastic, colony-forming cells with a capacity to form bone and support hematopoiesis.[32] Although MSCs were first defined as a cellular entity some 50 years ago[33] and first proposed as a therapeutic entity 30 years ago,[34] clinical translation has been remarkably slow. Many clinical trials have been registered and reported, and a vast literature has emerged describing the biologic attributes of these cells, their differentiation propensity, and immunomodulatory capacity. In addition, thousands of preclinical reports have described the results of testing in animal models of human disease. In most cases, and in a wide spectrum of models—including cardiac repair, nerve regeneration, vascular repair, and kidney repair as well as musculoskeletal indications—positive results were reported. Despite this, only a handful of market authorizations has been granted. This highlights a number of issues surrounding the translational process and the use of small animal models as indicators of therapeutic efficacy, lacking more comprehensive preclinical approaches and robust investigation.

The earliest reports of MSCs as a therapeutic agent described their use in the management of bone[35] and cartilage[36] defects. In these preclinical studies, the cells were generally applied with a scaffold for the repair of superficial and full-thickness cartilage defects and critical-sized bone defects. MSCs have a well-defined trilineage differentiation capacity and can readily form the bone, fat, and cartilage tissue.[37] This was seen as the essential characteristic of the cells underpinning their repair potential, essentially as a cell replacement strategy, whereby the delivered undifferentiated cells would respond to local cues and differentiate to the appropriate cell type. These efforts were underpinned by the idea that MSCs are multipotent stem cells with a capacity for self-renewal and differentiation. Subsequently, the concept of MSCs as stem cells was corrected, and it is now clear that they do not have the self-renewing capacity of true stem cells and readily undergo senescence when expanded in culture through many generations. At this time, the accepted nomenclature changed from mesenchymal stem cells to MSCs, a term that is widely used and still the subject of some disagreement. It also quickly became clear that MSC-derived chondrocytes develop an ECM more closely resembling hypertrophic rather than articular cartilage, a distinct disadvantage if the intention is to repopulate the articular surface.[38]

The most successful clinical uses of MSCs to date have been in the treatment of graft-versus-host disease[39] and Crohn disease.[40] These applications—in immune-related disorders—reveal the true therapeutic value of MSCs as cells capable of interacting with host immune cells and providing anti-inflammatory and immunomodulatory signals. Subsequently, the wider use of MSCs would be in conditions where there was an element of inflammation. It further became clear that MSCs have allogeneic tolerance, whereby donor-derived cells can be delivered to a fully mismatched and immunocompetent host without rejection or any evidence of an immune response. These observations were transformative and opened the field of MSC therapy to a staggering array of clinical applications, some logical and based on rational biologic principles and many lacking a clear biologic premise. In a few cases, such as those cited previously, market authorizations have been granted. In orthopaedic use, MSCs remain an attractive treatment option for osteoarthritis, and this is an approved use in several countries. In this treatment, the cells are delivered by intra-articular injection into the joint[41] space and the therapeutic mechanism most likely involves an immune-mediated response rather than differentiation of the delivered cells.

It is useful to explore further the relative lack of progress in the translation of MSC therapies toward widespread clinical use compared with, for example, HSC treatment. It seems clear that a major element relates to the lack of definitive understanding of potency and mechanism of action. The absence of a cell-specific, robust, and biologically relevant potency assay is an obstacle that hinders clinical development. In the absence of a useful and quantitate potency test, it is not possible to calibrate dose, optimize treatment strategies, or indeed provide a meaningful release test in manufacturing. In the case of HSCs, a realistic and targeted potency test is available, namely marrow reconstitution in lethally irradiated mice. Although this is a cumbersome bioassay, it nonetheless represents a validated and specific test. The absence of an MSC-specific molecular label, analogous to the CD34 marker, is another deficiency that has so far remained unfulfilled. These deficiencies represent severe obstacles to translation and, thus far, the field is deprived of a biologically meaningful premise that underpins therapeutic application, and it seems likely that progress will be hindered until these issues are robustly addressed.

Nucleus Pulposus Cells

Diseases of the intravertebral disk (IVD) are common and contribute greatly to lower back pain, a condition of high prevalence and severe socioeconomic burden. IVDs are located between the vertebrae of the spinal column and are composed of distinct anatomic regions: the gelatinous nucleus pulposus located within and constrained by thick layers of radially aligned collagen fibers forming the anulus fibrosus. A thin layer of hyaline cartilage, the cartilaginous end plate, lies between the vertebrae and the disk. The region-specific ECM structures—a proteoglycan-rich nucleus pulposus surrounded by a collagen-rich anulus fibrosus, each maintained by distinct cell populations (nucleus pulposus cells, anulus fibrosus cells, and notochordal cells)—contribute to the exceptional biomechanical resilience of the tissue. During degeneration, IVDs become subject to biochemical and inflammatory changes that subsequently lead to painful outcomes. In terms of cell-based strategies for repair of the diseased IVD, the three cell types are legitimate candidates. Because nucleus pulposus cells are rapidly lost during degeneration, most efforts to date have focused on MSCs, nucleus pulposus cells, and notochordal cells. Nucleus pulposus cells are the resident cells of the disk (**Figure 2**), are phenotypically similar to chondrocytes, and are adapted to these environments and programmed to produce tissue-specific matrices, making them a sensible option for transplantation. Both nucleus pulposus cells and chondrocytes, expanded ex vivo, have been tested in clinical studies. However, limitations around their availability affect their feasibility as a therapeutic option for cell delivery.[42] Newly identified nucleus pulposus progenitors might be the basis for a valuable additional strategy.[43] These are notochordal cells, the embryonic precursors of nucleus pulposus cells, which persist in the nucleus pulposus during postnatal development. Isolated and expanded notochordal cells may represent an effective strategy, somewhat analogous to neonatal chondrocytes.

Induced Pluripotent Stem Cells

The discovery of induced pluripotent stem cells (iPSCs) has been a key breakthrough in stem cell biology and regenerative medicine. The properties of pluripotent differentiation and long-term self-renewal in vitro exhibited by these cells are of great significance and potential value in developing new therapeutic strategies without encountering ethical obstacles associated with embryonic stem cells. iPSCs have the same genetic background as the somatic cells from which they were derived, giving rise to the prospect of generating constantly renewable immunoprivileged cell populations for autologous cell therapy. Another opportunity of value is provided by the prospect

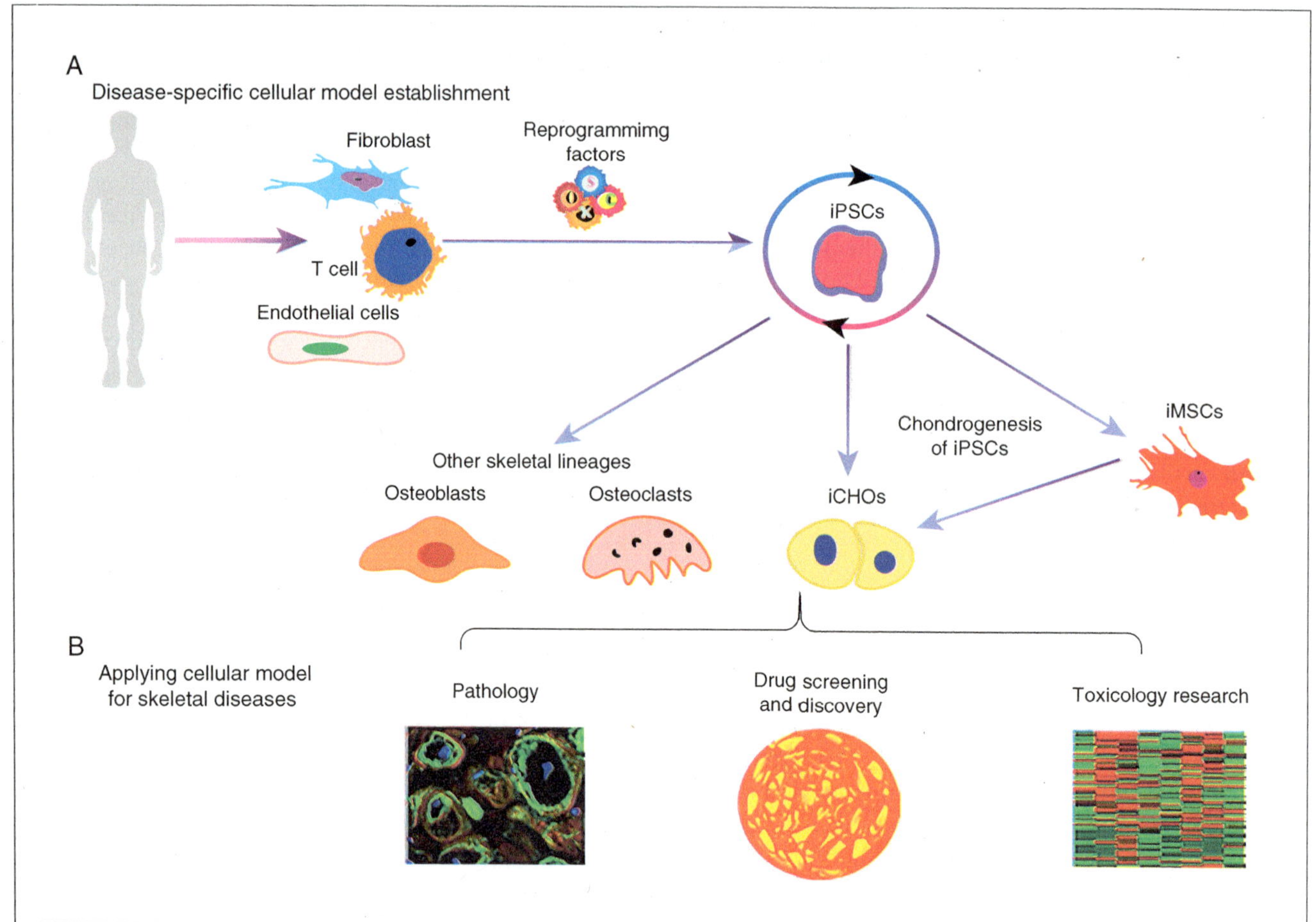

FIGURE 3 Schematic illustrations show the generation of induced pluripotent stem cells (**A**) and of differentiated progeny for use in orthopaedic applications (**B**). iCHOs = iPSC-derived chondrocytes, iMSCs = iPSC-derived mesenchymal stromal cells, iPSCs = induced pluripotent stem cells. (Reprinted from Xu M, O'Brien A, Barry F: Chondrocytes derived from pluripotent stem cells: applications in cartilage repair, in Birbrair A, ed: *Current Progress in iPSC-Derived Cell Types*. Copyright (2021), with permission from Elsevier.)

of using iPSCs to uncover the origin and pathogenesis of human diseases (**Figure 3**).

It is likely that the use of iPSC-derived cells will become the dominant strategy in expanded cell therapies in the future. Protocols now exist for the generation of all the cell types listed previously. For example, mesengenic differentiation strategies give rise to MSC-like cells, termed iPSC-derived MSCs, with morphologic features, growth characteristics, immunophenotype, and trilineage differentiation capacity similar to those of primary tissue-derived MSCs.[44] Commonly used protocols include (1) transferring iPSCs to a suspension culture to form embryoid bodies followed by culturing on gelatin-coated plates; (2) directly seeding dissociated iPSC colonies in precoated culture surfaces such as gelatin, collagen type I, or synthetic polymers; or (3) simply replacing iPSC culture medium with MSC medium. In addition, inhibitors of kappa-B kinase epsilon, transforming growth factor beta receptor type 1, activin A, and bone morphogenetic protein 4 have been used to enhance early mesodermal induction in culture. The successful direct differentiation of iPSCs to chondrocytes has also been reported,[45] as well as generation of cells with a nucleus pulposus cell phenotype,[46] and generally requires complex multistep differentiation conditions, which at this time will provide obstacles in terms of scalability and good manufacturing practice–compliant manufacturing.

Several concerns exist relating to the safe use of iPSCs as transplanted cells in human medicine. These include a risk of tumor formation, migration, and ectopic tissue formation.[47] Elaborate strategies now exist to eliminate these harmful effects, for example, by using genome engineering to create a cell death response by linking the cell division gene cyclin-dependent kinase 1 to the suicide gene herpes simplex virus thymidine kinase.[48]

Tissue Sources for Expanded Cell Therapy

The selection of cell source is an important biologic variable that has not received enough attention. In the past, the tissue source of the cells was probably driven by convenience and ease of access rather than by a full understanding of their biologic attributes. As insight into the phenotype, plasticity, genomic, and epigenomic characteristics of these cells improves, it is becoming increasingly clear that there are critical variables that are likely to affect clinical outcomes. In the case of chondrocytes, much attention has been focused on the use of expanded autologous cells isolated from the tibial plateau. More recently, alternative tissue sources have been identified, namely nasal and auricular tissue as well as juvenile tissues such as neonatal cartilage and polydactyly cartilage as mentioned previously. In the case of nucleus pulposus and notochordal cells, the only source is the disk itself. Recent exciting discoveries of nucleus pulposus progenitor cells have provided a broader range of opportunities.

For MSCs, the choice of tissue source is critical. MSCs have generally been isolated from bone marrow, adipose tissue, umbilical cord, dental pulp, and other tissues. Most therapeutic uses have involved cells from the bone marrow, adipose tissue,[49] and umbilical cord. To a large extent, the interest in MSCs has been driven by their ease of isolation and expansion and the use of a panel of tests, proposed as international standards, which represent an exceptionally low threshold in terms of quality compliance. Essentially, the biologic attributes of cells selected for therapeutic use must be assessed in the context of the target disease. This requires an understanding of the therapeutic mechanism, and this is now becoming clearer. For example, the concept of licensing is now widely accepted, relating to the fact that the cell phenotype in the transplant environment will differ greatly from the culture phenotype. Therefore, assessment of gene expression, release of paracrine factors, and interaction with other cells must be understood in the context of the target disease. A great deal of progress has been made in this area including, for example, the use of in vitro models of therapeutic licensing that involve exposure of cells to inflammatory mediators such as interleukin (IL)-1, tumor necrosis factor alpha, and interferon gamma. Conditioning experiments such as this reveal important biologic properties of cells that are not discernible using standard cell surface and differentiation assays. A 2019 study, carried out using bone marrow–derived MSCs and adipose-derived stem cells (ASCs) for the same donors, suggested that ASCs, rather than bone marrow–derived MSCs, provided an optimal repair response.[50] The objective was to define an in vitro milieu that would resemble or replicate the degenerate disk environment (**Figure 4**), containing elevated levels of inflammatory cytokines, blood vessel ingrowth, and loss of ECM. Conditioning of the cells with common inflammatory cytokines IL-1α and tumor necrosis factor alpha elicited a response involving marked upregulation of anti-inflammatory molecules IL-1RA, IL-4, and IL-10. The quantitative response was higher in the ASCs, and although such studies need to be carefully replicated in vivo, the results suggest that ASCs may be a preferred choice for treatment of degenerative disk disease. These data illustrate the importance of probing the phenotypic response of therapeutic cells under the conditions that mimic the transplanted environment.

CELL ISOLATES AND CONCENTRATES

Stromal Vascular Fraction

An alternative and more accessible strategy has been the use of tissue preparations and cell concentrates instead of expanded cells. The distinct advantage of these preparations is that they are instantly obtainable, can be processed easily in an intraoperative setting, and are of low cost. In addition, because these are classified into minimally manipulated therapeutic agents, they are subject to

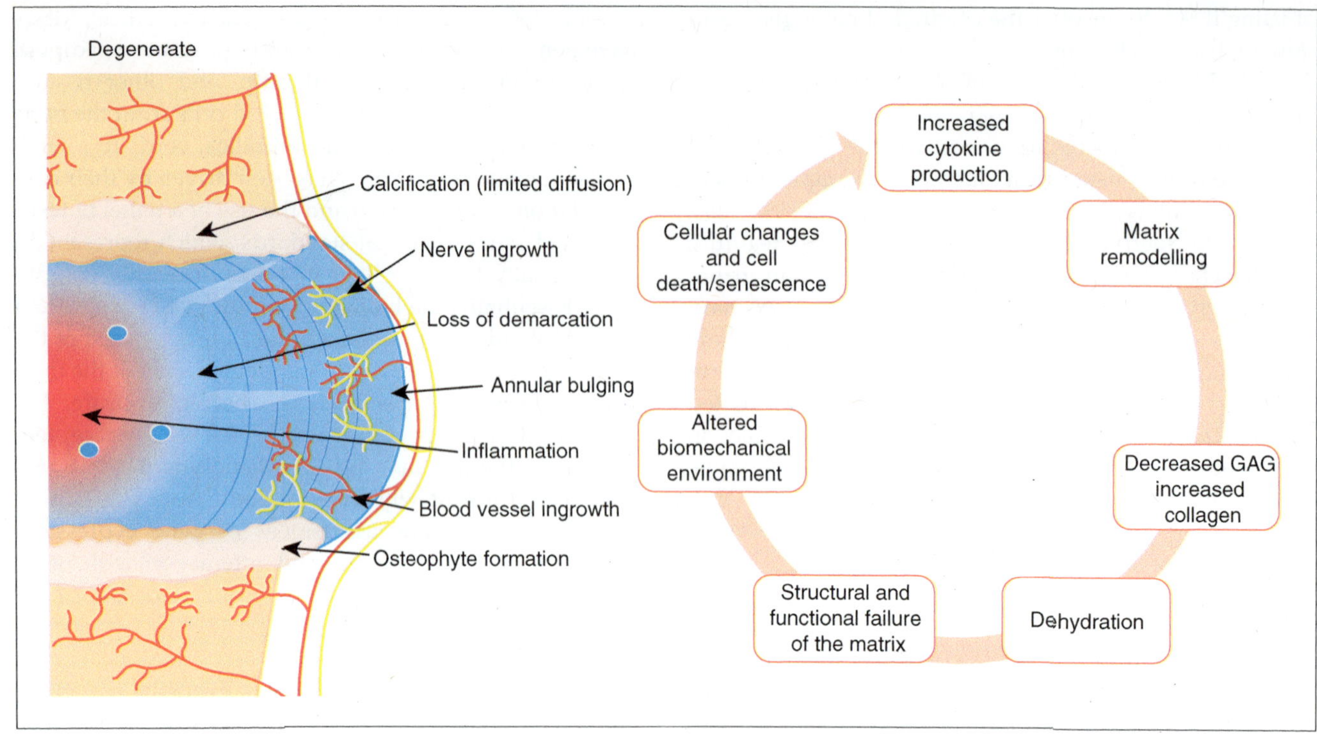

FIGURE 4 Schematic illustration shows definition of the inflammatory niche in the degenerate nucleus pulposus as a guide to develop in vitro models to predict the response of transplanted cells. GAG = glycosaminoglycan

less-stringent regulatory criteria. For example, stromal vascular fraction (SVF) is a cellular isolate from lipoaspirate tissue produced by enzymatic digestion and centrifugation. The cell fraction contains a multiplicity of cell types, including ASCs, mesenchymal and endothelial progenitor cells, leukocyte subtypes, lymphatic cells, pericytes, and vascular smooth muscle cells, and has been used for many years in plastic surgery.[51] The heterogenous nature of the concentrated cell population may in fact be responsible for superior clinical outcomes. There is a multiplicity of examples of autologous SVF use, and in recent years, there has been an interest in allogeneic application and the establishment of human adipose tissue biobanks. SVF was initially used in cosmetic breast augmentation[52] and in the management of radiation injury following radiation therapy for breast cancer.[53]

SVF has been used in the management of knee osteoarthritis, and several studies have reported clinical improvement. In 2013, Pak et al[54] reported a retrospective cohort study involving 91 patients with osteoarthritis treated with autologous SVF and platelet-rich plasma (PRP). In a 3-month follow-up, there were no serious adverse effects and pain, measured using the visual analog scale score, was significantly improved. In a clinical study of 18 patients aged between 18 and 75 years, Mehranfar et al[55] found that a high-dose (1.0×10^8 cells) SVF injection resulted in a mean reduction of Western Ontario and McMaster Universities Osteoarthritis Index function scores of 39% after 6 months. MRI showed cartilage regeneration. Pak et al have provided a summary of current results from several clinical trials.[54] In all cases, there was a positive outcome, but in general, the studies were of insufficient scale to allow a definitive conclusion.

As is the case with PRP, the lack of standardization of prepared SVF is an obstacle that affects its consistent application and accurate comparison of different clinical studies. Therefore, the International Federation for Adipose Therapeutics and Science and the International Society for Cell & Gene Therapy have issued a joint statement proposing a set of standards that define the crucial quality attributes of SVF. This standard proposes that SVF is identified using the markers $CD45^-$, $CD235a^-$, $CD31^-$, and $CD34^+$. Additional testing may identify the cells within the SVF using the common SVF markers CD90, CD73, CD105, and CD44.

Bone Marrow Concentrates

Similar to SVF, bone marrow concentrates are obtained by enriching the cellular fraction of a bone marrow biopsy, usually taken from the superior iliac crest. The cells are concentrated by centrifugation, often with the use of a density gradient fractionation or thixotropic gel. Bone marrow concentrate has been regarded as a minimally manipulated material and has been widely used in the treatment of fractures, meniscal injury, tendinopathy, and osteoarthritis.

Platelet-Rich Plasma

PRP is an autologous product derived from whole blood.[56] It consists of a concentration of platelets, several times larger than is present in whole blood, obtained by centrifugation and suspended in a small volume of plasma. It contains high concentrations of growth factors that are active components involved in tissue repair, angiogenesis, mitogenesis, and chemotaxis. Platelets are anuclear cell fragments derived from megakaryocytes present in the bone marrow, and their normal function is to react to bleeding by initiating a blood clot. The alpha granules of platelets contain concentrated mixtures of growth factors and cytokines, and the therapeutic benefit of the product is apparently associated with the release of these.[57] The range of growth factors that are present in PRP includes those involved in a number of physiologic responses associated with wound repair, such as revascularization of damaged tissue, connective tissue formation, proliferation, and differentiation of mesenchymal precursor cells into tissue-specific cell types.[58] PRP has been used for about the past decade in a wide range of applications in cardiac repair, dermatology, wound repair, and orthopaedics.[59] Although PRP is very attractive because of its low cost and simplicity, it is not without controversy and there is still considerable debate regarding its effectiveness. Nonetheless, there are many reports in the literature that describe a positive outcome when PRP is delivered to the osteoarthritic knee by intra-articular injection. It has also been tested in a variety of other musculoskeletal applications, including rotator cuff injury,[60] anterior cruciate ligament reconstruction,[61] Achilles tendinopathy,[62] and fracture healing.[63] However, in many cases, these studies are of insufficient scale or lack suitable control patients to allow for definitive assessment. It is worth noting that a recent meta-analysis, looking at data comparing PRP with hyaluronan injections, suggested that PRP was superior in terms of the treatment of symptomatic knee pain, but failed to improve clinical outcomes indicating that, as with other biologic treatment strategies, it is a symptom-modifying rather than a disease-modifying intervention.[64]

Another concern has been the lack of standardization in protocols for the preparation of PRP, meaning that different batches of material may have different composition of growth factors, further complicating the interpretation of clinical results. Many published clinical trials, carried out for the evaluation of the effectiveness of PRP, fail to include detailed protocols on the preparation of the material or detailed analysis of its composition. This compounds the inherent variability associated with an autologous blood product when individual donor characteristics are taken into account.

It is appropriate to provide a general comment regarding selection of outcome measures in clinical studies involving either expanded or concentrated cell isolates. This is very important because of a potentially serious disconnect between outcome measures in preclinical versus clinical studies. In preclinical assessment, histology and morphologic assessment are commonplace, whereas in clinical studies, these are naturally more difficult to obtain and there may be a tendency to rely on outcomes that refer to pain rather than structural improvement. It is indeed critical that clinical studies of cell therapies in orthopaedics involve outcome measures that distinguish between symptom-modifying and disease-modifying effects. This is essential to determine that the therapeutic application is regenerative rather than merely analgesic.

Within the past several decades, new and previously unimagined therapeutic modalities have become available to orthopaedic surgeons based on live cell products. There now exist opportunities for tissue regeneration and repair and treatment of degenerative and inflammatory conditions, which have the capacity to change clinical outcomes. There is still a long way to go. The complex and variable nature of cell-based products is an obstacle still to be overcome. The precise nature of the therapeutic mechanism needs clearer understanding. Finally, production standards and compliant manufacturing models need to be put in place to ensure greater reliability and better prediction of outcomes. The new era of cell-based therapeutics in orthopaedics has arrived and will provide newer and more effective tools.

SUMMARY

Cell therapy is a clinical protocol involving the transplantation of living cells for the treatment of tissue injury or disease. It includes a number of different cell types, derived from postnatal tissues, which may be either isolated and expanded in culture or presented as an unexpanded cell concentrate derived from a tissue biopsy. In many nonorthopaedic applications, cells are delivered to the circulation by infusion and MSCs, chondrocytes, and nucleus pulposus cells have all been used in this context. In recent years, MSCs have been at the forefront of investigation, but successful clinical translation has been difficult to achieve in all but a handful of disease targets. This may be due to a number of factors, including the limited scale and design of clinical testing protocols. The absence of a validated and biologically meaningful potency test may represent a significant obstacle to successful transplantation. Some of the current impediments may well be overcome by the use of cells derived from iPSCs rather than primary cells isolated from tissue biopsies.

ACKNOWLEDGMENT

The assistance of Tarlan Eslami Arshaghi, Joan Fitzgerald, and Abbie Binch in the preparation of figures is gratefully acknowledged.

REFERENCES

1. Thomas ED, Lochte HL, Lu WC, Ferrebee JW: Intravenous infusion of bone marrow in patients receiving radiation and chemotherapy. *N Engl J Med* 1957;257:491-496.
2. Simpson E, Dazzi F: Bone marrow transplantation 1957-2019. *Front Immunol* 2019;10:1246.

3. Ballen KK, Gluckman E, Broxmeyer HE: Umbilical cord blood transplantation: the first 25 years and beyond. *Blood* 2013;122(4):491-498.
4. Civin CI, Trischmann T, Kadan NS, et al: Highly purified CD34-positive cells reconstitute hematopoiesis. *J Clin Oncol* 1996;14(8):2224-2233.
5. Langer R, Vacanti JP: Tissue engineering. *Science* 1993;260(5110):920-926.
6. Przekora A: A concise review on tissue engineered artificial skin grafts for chronic wound treatment: Can we reconstruct functional skin tissue in vitro? *Cells* 2020;9(7):1622.
7. Green WT Jr. Articular cartilage repair. Behavior of rabbit chondrocytes during tissue culture and subsequent allografting. *Clin Orthop Relat Res* 1977;124:237-250.
8. Fiegel HC, Kaufmann PM, Bruns H, et al: Hepatic tissue engineering: from transplantation to customized cell-based liver directed therapies from the laboratory. *J Cell Mol Med* 2008;12(1):56-66.
9. Chaikof EL: Engineering and material considerations in islet cell transplantation. *Annu Rev Biomed Eng* 1999;1:103-127.
10. Bourzac K: Neuroscience: New nerves for old. *Nature* 2016;540:S52-S54.
11. Atala A: Tissue engineering of human bladder. *Br Med Bull* 2011;97:81-104.
12. Grande DA, Singh IJ, Pugh J: Healing of experimentally produced lesions in articular cartilage following chondrocyte transplantation. *Anat Rec* 1987;218(2):142-148.
13. Lindahl A: From gristle to chondrocyte transplantation: Treatment of cartilage injuries. *Philos Trans R Soc Lond B Biol Sci* 2015;370(1680):20140369.
14. Goldring MB: Human chondrocyte cultures as models of cartilage-specific gene regulation. *Methods Mol Med* 2005;107:69-95.
15. Lefebvre V, Angelozzi M, Haseeb A: SOX9 in cartilage development and disease. *Curr Opin Cell Biol* 2019;61:39-47.
16. Brittberg M, Lindahl A, Nilsson A, Ohlsson C, Isaksson O, Peterson L: Treatment of deep cartilage defects in the knee with autologous chondrocyte transplantation. *N Engl J Med* 1994;331(14):889-895.
17. Institute for Quality and Efficiency in Health Care (IQWiG): Autologous chondrocyte implantation in the knee joint: IQWiG Reports – Commission No. N19-02 [Internet]. Cologne (Germany): *Institute for Quality and Efficiency in Health Care (IQWiG)* 2021.
18. Långsjö TK, Vasara AI, Hyttinen MM, et al: Quantitative analysis of collagen network structure and fibril dimensions in cartilage repair with autologous chondrocyte transplantation. *Cells Tissues Organs* 2010;192(6):351-360.
19. Zeifang F, Oberle D, Nierhoff C, Richter W, Moradi B, Schmitt H: Autologous chondrocyte implantation using the original periosteum-cover technique versus matrix-associated autologous chondrocyte implantation: A randomized clinical trial. *Am J Sports Med* 2010;38(5):924-933.
20. von der Mark K, Gauss V, von der Mark H, Müller P: Relationship between cell shape and type of collagen synthesised as chondrocytes lose their cartilage phenotype in culture. *Nature* 1977;267:531.
21. Benya PD, Padilla SR, Nimni ME: Independent regulation of collagen types by chondrocytes during the loss of differentiated function in culture. *Cell* 1978;15:1313-1321.
22. Bobacz K, Erlacher L, Smolen J, Soleiman A, Graninger WB: Chondrocyte number and proteoglycan synthesis in the aging and osteoarthritic human articular cartilage. *Ann Rheum Dis* 2004;63(12):1618-1622.
23. Saha S, Kirkham J, Wood D, Curran S, Yang X: Comparative study of the chondrogenic potential of human bone marrow stromal cells, neonatal chondrocytes and adult chondrocytes. *Biochem Biophys Res Commun* 2010;401(3):333-338.
24. Cavalli E, Levinson C, Hertl M, et al: Characterization of polydactyly chondrocytes and their use in cartilage engineering. *Sci Rep* 2019;9:4275.
25. Yanke AB, Tilton AK, Wetters NG, Merkow DB, Cole BJ: DeNovo NT particulated juvenile cartilage implant. *Sports Med Arthrosc Rev* 2015;23(3):125-129.
26. Lohan P, Treacy O, Lynch K, et al: Culture expanded primary chondrocytes have potent immunomodulatory properties and do not induce an allogeneic immune response. *Osteoarthritis Cartilage* 2016;24(3):521-533.
27. Fahy N, Farrell E, Ritter T, Ryan AE, Murphy JM: Immune modulation to improve tissue engineering outcomes for cartilage repair in the osteoarthritic joint. *Tissue Eng Part B Rev* 2015;21(1):55-66.
28. Abe S, Nochi H, Ito H: Alloreactivity and immunosuppressive properties of articular chondrocytes from osteoarthritic cartilage. *J Orthop Surg* 2016;24(2):232-239.
29. Li T, Chen S, Pei M: Contribution of neural crest-derived stem cells and nasal chondrocytes to articular cartilage regeneration. *Cell Mol Life Sci* 2020;77(23):4847-4859.
30. Pelttari K, Mumme M, Barbero A, Martin I: Nasal chondrocytes as a neural crest-derived cell source for regenerative medicine. *Curr Opin Biotechnol* 2017;47:1-6.
31. Mumme M, Barbero A, Miot S, et al: Nasal chondrocyte-based engineered autologous cartilage tissue for repair of articular cartilage defects: an observational first-in-human trial. *Lancet* 2016;388(10055):1985-1994.
32. Friedenstein AJ, Petrakova KV, Kurolesova AI, Frolova GP: Heterotopic of bone marrow. Analysis of precursor cells for osteogenic and hematopoietic tissues. *Transplantation* 1968;6(2):230-247.
33. Friedenstein AJ, Piatetzky-Shapiro, Petrakova KV: Osteogenesis in transplants of bone marrow cells. *J Embryol Exp Morphol* 1966;16(3):381-390.
34. Caplan AI: Mesenchymal stem cells. *J Orthop Res* 1991;9(5):641-650.
35. Bruder SP, Kurth AA, Shea M, Hayes WC, Jaiswal N, Kadiyala S: Bone regeneration by implantation of purified, culture-expanded human mesenchymal stem cells. *J Orthop Res* 1998;16(2):155-162.

36. Wakitani S, Goto T, Pineda SJ, et al: Mesenchymal cell-based repair of large, full-thickness defects of articular cartilage. *J Bone Joint Surg Am* 1994;76(4):579-592.

37. Barry FP, Murphy JM: Mesenchymal stem cells: Clinical applications and biological characterization. *Int J Biochem Cell Biol* 2004;36(4):568-584.

38. Kavalkovich KW, Boynton RE, Murphy JM, Barry F: Chondrogenic differentiation of human mesenchymal stem cells within an alginate layer culture system. *In Vitro Cell Dev Biol Anim* 2002;38(8):457-466.

39. Markov A, Thangavelu L, Aravindhan S, et al: Mesenchymal stem/stromal cells as a valuable source for the treatment of immune-mediated disorders. *Stem Cell Res Ther* 2021;12(1):192.

40. Panés J, García-Olmo D, Van Assche G, et al: Expanded allogeneic adipose-derived mesenchymal stem cells (Cx601) for complex perianal fistulas in Crohn's disease: A phase 3 randomised, double-blind controlled trial. *Lancet* 2016;388(10051):1281-1290.

41. Pers YM, Rackwitz L, Ferreira R, et al: Adipose mesenchymal stromal cell-based therapy for severe osteoarthritis of the knee: A phase i dose-escalation trial. *Stem Cells Transl Med* 2016;5(7):847-856.

42. Sakai D, Nakamura Y, Nakai T, et al: Exhaustion of nucleus pulposus progenitor cells with ageing and degeneration of the intervertebral disc. *Nat Commun* 2012;3:1264.

43. Potier E, de Vries S, van Doeselaar M, Ito K: Potential application of notochordal cells for intervertebral disc regeneration: an in vitro assessment. *Eur Cell Mater* 2014;28:68-80.

44. Xu M, Shaw G, Murphy M, Barry F: Induced pluripotent stem cell-derived mesenchymal stromal cells are functionally and genetically different from bone marrow-derived mesenchymal stromal cells. *Stem Cell* 2019;37(6):754-765.

45. Dicks A, Wu CL, Steward N, Adkar SS, Gersbach CA, Guilak F: Prospective isolation of chondroprogenitors from human iPSCs based on cell surface markers identified using a CRISPR-Cas9-generated reporter. *Stem Cell Res Ther* 2020;11(1):66.

46. Chen J, Lee EJ, Jing L, Christoforou N, Leong KW, Setton LA: Differentiation of mouse induced pluripotent stem cells (iPSCs) into nucleus pulposus-like cells in vitro. *PLoS One* 2013;8(9):e75548.

47. Lee AS, Tang C, Rao MS, Weissman IL, Wu JC: Tumorigenicity as a clinical hurdle for pluripotent stem cell therapies. *Nat Med* 2013;19(8):998-1004.

48. Liang Q, Monetti C, Shutova MV, et al: Linking a cell-division gene and a suicide gene to define and improve cell therapy safety. *Nature* 2018;563(7733):701-704.

49. Zuk PA, Zhu M, Mizuno H, et al: Multilineage cells from human adipose tissue: implications for cell-based therapies. *Tissue Eng* 2001;7(2):211-228.

50. Binch ALA, Richardson SM, Hoyland JA, Barry FP: Combinatorial conditioning of adipose derived-mesenchymal stem cells enhances their neurovascular potential: Implications for intervertebral disc degeneration. *JOR Spine* 2019;2(4):e1072.

51. Bora P, Majumdar AS: Adipose tissue-derived stromal vascular fraction in regenerative medicine: A brief review on biology and translation. *Stem Cell Res Ther* 2017;8(1):145.

52. Yoshimura K, Sato K, Aoi N, et al: Cell-assisted lipotransfer for cosmetic breast augmentation: Supportive use of adipose-derived stem/stromal cells. *Aesthetic Plast Surg* 2008;32:48-55.

53. Rigotti G, Marchi A, Galie M, et al: Clinical treatment of radiotherapy tissue damage by lipoaspirate transplant: A healing process mediated by adipose-derived adult stem cells. *Plast Reconstr Surg* 2007;119:1409-1422.

54. Pak J, Lee JH, Pak N, et al: Cartilage regeneration in humans with adipose tissue-derived stem cells and adipose stromal vascular fraction cells: Updated status. *Int J Mol Sci* 2018;19(7):2146.

55. Mehranfar S, Abdi Rad I, Mostafavi E, Akbarzadeh A: The use of Stromal Vascular Fraction (SVF), Platelet-Rich Plasma (PRP) and stem cells in the treatment of osteoarthritis: An overview of clinical trials, *Artif Cell Nanomed Biotechnol* 2019;47(1):882-890.

56. Everts P, Onishi K, Jayaram P, Lana JF, Mautner K: Platelet-rich plasma: New performance understandings and therapeutic considerations in 2020. *Int J Mol Sci* 2020;21(20):7794.

57. Etulain J: Platelets in wound healing and regenerative medicine. *Platelets* 2018;29(6):556-568.

58. Krüger JP, Hondke S, Endres M, Pruss A, Siclari A, Kaps C: Human platelet-rich plasma stimulates migration and chondrogenic differentiation of human subchondral progenitor cells. *J Orthop Res* 2012;30(6):845-852.

59. Chahla J, Cole BJ: Editorial commentary: Platelet-rich plasma for knee osteoarthritis – A "Novel" and effective symptomatic approach. *Arthroscopy* 2019;35(1):118-120.

60. Barber FA: PRP as an adjunct to rotator cuff tendon repair. *Sports Med Arthrosc Rev* 2018;26(2):42-47.

61. Bailey L, Weldon M, Kleihege J, et al: Platelet-rich plasma augmentation of meniscal repair in the setting of anterior cruciate ligament reconstruction. *Am J Sports Med* 2021;49(12):3287-3292.

62. Dragoo JL, Wasterlain AS, Braun HJ, Nead KT: Platelet-rich plasma as a treatment for patellar tendinopathy: A double-blind, randomized controlled trial. *Am J Sports Med* 2014;42(3):610-618.

63. Calori GM, Tagliabue L, Gala L, d'Imporzano M, Peretti G, Albisetti W: Application of rhBMP-7 and platelet-rich plasma in the treatment of long bone non-unions: A prospective randomised clinical study on 120 patients. *Injury* 2008;39(12):1391-1402.

64. Filardo G, Previtali D, Napoli F, Candrian C, Zaffagnini S, Grassi A: PRP Injections for the treatment of knee osteoarthritis: A meta-analysis of randomized controlled trials. *Cartilage* 2020;13(1 suppl):364S-375S.

CHAPTER 2

Materials Science and Biodegradable Scaffolds

Kenneth S. Ogueri, BS, MSc, PhD • Kevin Grassie, BS • Yusuf Khan, PhD • Cato T. Laurencin, MD, PhD, FAAOS

INTRODUCTION

Recent advances in materials science and engineering have spurred the design and development of sophisticated biomaterials with various properties and diverse functionalities. The advancements present leverage that ensures the fulfillment of the continuous demands and the understanding of the intricacies of regenerative engineering. Polymeric materials, including natural, synthetic, and composite, are poised to play a leading role in ensuring the effectiveness and success of matrix-based regenerative engineering. A holistic overview of the use of polymeric scaffolds in matrix-based strategies for tissue regeneration is provided, highlighting the underlying concepts and principles of several aspects of the regenerative process, such as osteoconductivity, osteoinductivity, and osseointegration. Moreover, the different fabrication methods typically used to ensure optimal scaffold geometry for enhanced biomaterial-tissue interactions and integration are discussed. The technology outlook and future direction of biodegradable scaffolds is outlined.

MATRIX-BASED REGENERATIVE ENGINEERING AND ITS COMPONENTS

The approach of regenerative engineering has seen consistent growth and advancements in recent decades. The progress is due to the quest for a new frontier in advancing the treatment of bone loss or failure. Regenerative engineering is an innovative and transdisciplinary approach that amalgamates and maximizes the principles of several areas of study such as advanced materials science and engineering, stem cell science, developmental biology, biophysics, and clinical translation for the regeneration of complex tissues and biologic systems[1-3] (**Figure 1**). Essentially, the approach provides a platform that uses the expertise in these areas to design and develop the next-generation bone grafts. It encompasses bringing together stem cells, biocompatible and biomimetic scaffolds, and appropriate biochemical and mechanoelectrical cues to regenerate bone tissues. Scaffolding materials are used in matrix-based regenerative engineering as a structural template to arouse the body's self-healing mechanism, leading to functional tissue development.[4] The ultimate goal is to have a scaffold with appropriate instructive cues that can induce favorable cellular responses and regulate the formation of tissues. Considerable material science effort has been expended on the design of ideal biomaterials that can be used to fabricate biomimetic scaffolds with optimal topographic, biologic, and mechanical features required for effective tissue regeneration. A suitable scaffold possesses sufficient initial mechanical strength and presents a degradation rate that matches with the regeneration process while degrading into benign and resorbable degradation products. These scaffolding material attributes will be discussed in detail in the next section. Developmental biology provides a solid theoretic and practical basis in the processing of bone healing, unveiling the molecular and morphogenetic events fundamental to the formation and development of bone tissues. The functional insights gained from the field can be leveraged as a conceptual framework for directing and moderating early-stage tissue formation in regenerative engineering.

Developmental biology encompasses osteoinduction by using growth factors and small bioactive molecules to stimulate certain physiologic processes toward tissue formation. Bone morphogenetic proteins (BMPs)

Dr. Ogueri or an immediate family member serves as a paid consultant to or is an employee of Pfizer. Dr. Khan or an immediate family member serves as a board member, owner, officer, or committee member of the Regenerative Engineering Society. Dr. Laurencin or an immediate family member has received royalties from CT Biotech and Globus Medical; is a member of a speakers' bureau or has made paid presentations on behalf of Johnson & Johnson, Society for Science and the Public, Southern University of Science and Technology (SUSTech), Technion Israel Institute of Technology, University of California - San Diego, University of Oklahoma, University of Texas MD Anderson Cancer Cente, Vail Scientific Summit, and Western University of Health Sciences; serves as a paid consultant to or is an employee of Biorez, Bioventus, DePuy, Endo Pharmaceuticals, Johnson & Johnson, and Soft Tissue Regeneration; has stock or stock options held in Alkermes, BioBind, Healing Orthopaedic Technologies, HOT Bone, and Soft Tissue Regeneration, Inc.; has received research or institutional support from BioBind, Endo Pharmaceuticals, Healing Orthopaedic Technologies, and HOT Bone; and serves as a board member, owner, officer, or committee member of the National Academies, the National Academy of Inventors, and the Regenerative Engineering Society. Neither Kevin Grassie nor any immediate family member has received anything of value from or has stock or stock options held in a commercial company or institution related directly or indirectly to the subject of this chapter.

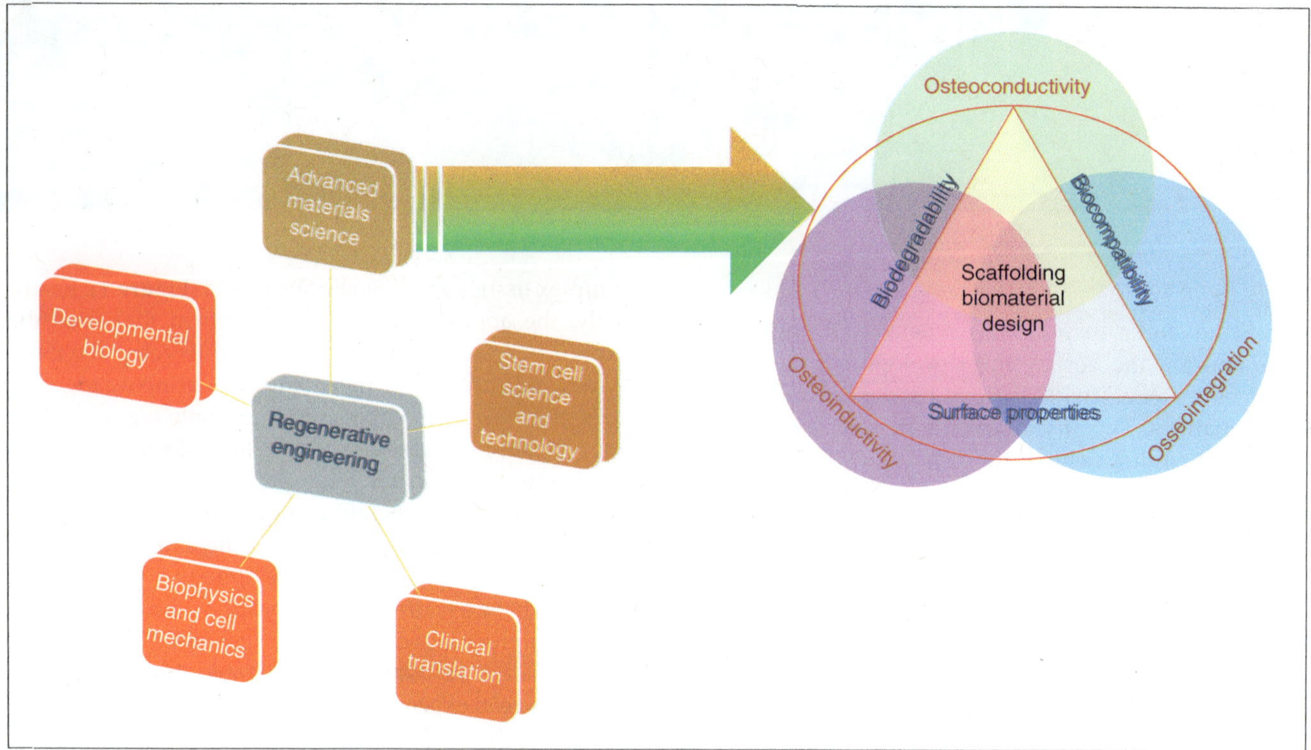

FIGURE 1 Schematic diagram showing the five different components of regenerative engineering. Biomaterial design constitutes a significant aspect of regenerative engineering, and its molecular understanding informs the rational development of scaffolds for tissue regeneration.

are commonly used as potent osteoinductive factors because they facilitate stem cell mitogenesis that ultimately leads to cell division and differentiation toward osteoblasts. Stem cell technology is an essential component of regenerative engineering with remarkable traits of self-renewal and a tendency to differentiate into all types of cells. Stem cells used in regenerative engineering include mesenchymal stem cells (MSCs), embryonic stem cells, and induced pluripotent stem cells.[4,5] Stem cell research and therapy have blossomed in recent years, and more stem cells are expected to be identified and developed, ensuring an unlimited source for a wide range of human cells needed for regenerative purposes. Biophysics has added another dimension to the regenerative toolbox because it aids in providing a good understanding of the cell mechanics and response to external stimuli such as stress within a bioengineered construct. The mechanical behavior of living cells relates to their functions because the cells produce and sustain mechanical stresses within their microenvironment as part of their normal physiology. This biomechanical stimulation plays a critical role in controlling and directing the morphogenetic actions of the cells, leading to the conversion of such forces into chemical signals that influence cellular behaviors. Several recent studies have illustrated that cells have the inherent ability to detect mechanical signals in their immediate environment. For example, the mechanical features of a cultured substrate can influence and manipulate the cellular fate because the cells tend to maneuver their ways to suit the mechanical profile of the substrate. Sometimes, they exhibit durotaxis, a phenomenon by which cells tend to drift toward specific mechanical conditions. As such, the control of the cell mechanics could be a valuable facet of regenerative engineering that can be exploited to optimize cell growth and organization.

As the last component, clinical translation entails the part of the regenerative tool that ensures the actual execution of the regenerative concepts in bone tissue repair and regeneration. It bridges the gap between science and clinical practice because it connects the findings of these different research areas to each other and ultimately to the patients. Clinical translation sets the pragmatic tone for investigating new techniques that can facilitate the effective translation of discovery into real applications. This also includes the navigation of the regulatory obstacles, ensuring safety and success of technology transfer. So, conglomerate expertise and knowledge from these various facets of regenerative engineering are leveraged to present a game-changing platform for positive clinical outcomes during the design process of bioengineered tissue constructs.

BIOMATERIAL DESIGN FOR BONE REGENERATIVE ENGINEERING

Bone regeneration is a complex and well-organized cascade of the physiologic process of bone formation that commonly takes place during routine healthy healing of fractures and bone remodeling. Certain medical conditions and disease states (such as infections, trauma, tumor resection, genetic defects, significant bone defects, and hormonal imbalance) can compromise the normal regenerative process in affected individuals. This necessitates substantial bone regeneration beyond the standard self-healing potential for skeletal reconstruction of significant bone defects. Several strategies such as allografts, autographs, and xenografts exist to augment the weakened regenerative process. Nonetheless, the effectiveness and availability of these treatment options are limited. An autograft is most widely used as a gold standard but has limited availability and potential donor morbidity. However, there are high chances of potential disease transmission for allografts and xenografts, and they could induce unfavorable immunogenic responses from the new host. To overcome the limitations of current treatment strategies, bone scaffolds based on biomaterials have been designed for bone regenerative engineering. Biomaterial-based scaffolds must meet certain critical criteria for them to be appropriate for bone regenerative engineering: (1) the material must be biodegradable, biocompatible, bifunctional, and completely benign; (2) the material must possess preprogrammed and predetermined degradation rates that correspond to the regeneration rates with adequate dimensional integrity; (3) the material should have suitable surface chemistry that could allow optimal cellular attachment and proliferation (osteoconductive); (4) the material should exhibit physicochemical features that mimic native bone tissues; (5) the material should be able to present three-dimensional (3D) porous microstructures with efficient interconnectivity and optimal pore size (150 to 350 μm) for accommodation of cell infiltration, tissue ingrowth, oxygen diffusion, vascularization, nutrient transport, and enhanced surface area for improved cell-material interactions; (6) the material should be able to encapsulate growth factors and small bioactive molecules such as BMPs and anti-inflammatory agents; and (7) the material should be capable of recruiting progenitor cells that promote the induction of bone growth (they are osteoinductive).[1,6] It is important to note that the complexity and variations that exist for biologic tissues make it very difficult for a material to meet and satisfy all the requirements, as mentioned previously. For this reason, it can be categorically postulated that no one-size-fits-all material exists for bone scaffold design. As a result, it becomes valuable to have a design platform that allows the customization and modification of scaffolding materials' attributes. For example, the pore size and distribution can be tailored and personalized to meet specific application requirements because living cells and biologic tissues differ in compositions, chemistries, and physical properties for different patients and body parts.[6]

Generally, tissues are composed of a cluster of cells embedded in extracellular matrix (ECM), and the ECM plays a vital role in the overall well-being of the cells. The main functions of ECM are to support cell growth, promote differentiation, and supply essential nutrients to the cells. Several studies have demonstrated these characteristics where ECM was used as a structural template and an avenue to supply essential nutrients and growth factors for optimal cell growth.[6,7] Thus, effective regeneration cannot be achieved by just supplying cells to the site of injury because both ECM and cells are lost because of injury when it comes to large-size defects.[1] So, it becomes necessary to devise an environment that architecturally looks similar to the ECM environment for the seeded cells. Biomaterials can be used as a substitute for ECM because they can be designed to exhibit physical attributes that mimic ECM proteins. Scaffold fabricated from biomaterial aims to mimic the ECM in a regenerating bone environment. Several biomaterials, including biopolymers, bioceramics, and composites, have shown great promise in regenerative engineering. These regenerative materials have unique properties that make them good candidates and appropriate for cell recruitment purposes. They have to be informative to cells and also provide structural support. Polymers are well known for their excellent tunability and mechanical properties, and ceramics have well-investigated effectiveness as bone scaffolds due to their similarity (in structure and chemical composition) with the main mineral phase of bone.

Mechanical competence is an essential requirement for regenerative materials as the biomaterial scaffolds must present mechanical attributes that correspond with the anatomic site they are meant to be implanted. Sometimes, pure materials may not be capable of providing all the needed mechanical attributes by themselves. However, the mechanical properties can be enhanced by designing composite materials that synergistically combine the desirable properties of two different materials. At least one of the components will provide biocompatibility, and the other will offer mechanical strength, making the composite suitable for tissue regeneration. Despite the versatile design tools and a continuum of materials at the orthopaedic surgeon's disposal, no material developed over recent decades can boast of having an exact footprint of the native bones.

ROLES OF BIOMATERIALS IN BONE REGENERATIVE ENGINEERING

Osteoconduction

For a biomaterial to be suitable for matrix-based regenerative engineering, it must have a certain degree of osteoconductivity that allows the formation of new bones on its surface.[8] Specifically, an osteoconductive surface of a bone implant stimulates and supports cell attachments, migration, proliferation, differentiation, and deposition of ECM of osteoprogenitor cells within the defect area. These are critical early stages of new bone formation. The formation of thin carbonated hydroxyapatite on a material surface causes protein adsorption, and this is instrumental to the attachment of bone-forming cells and subsequent activities related to bone matrix deposition. The integration of the newly formed bone into the bone tissue microenvironment or the stable anchorage of an implant obtained by the direct bone-to-implant contact is instigated by osteoconductivity of material through the apposition of bone mineral. Hence, osteoconductivity is essential to achieving functional bone regeneration. The physicochemical properties of biomaterials have a controlling influence on their osteoconductivity during bone healing, and as such, they can be used to exert control on cellular behavior. The osteoconductivity-controlling features of biomaterials include chemical composition, surface chemistry, morphology, architectural geometry, etc.[8] As mentioned previously, certain biomaterials such as bioceramics (hydroxyapatite and tricalcium phosphate) and bioglass depict enormous osteoconductivity due to their similarity to natural bone minerals. In addition, some natural polymers such as collagen could possess excellent osteoconductivity, attributable to their compositional and structural characteristics that foster mineral deposition and mineralization through binding of non-collagenous matrix proteins.[1,6]

Conversely, biomaterials of low biocompatibility, such as copper and silver, could generally exhibit little to no osteoconduction. Meanwhile, it is a common practice to introduce osteoconductive attributes to materials (such as metals, ceramics, and synthetic polymers) that generally have poor osteoconductivity through several methods such as coating and composite. Several studies have reported the feasibility of improving the osteoconductivity of synthetic polymers by the surface treatment with calcium phosphate (CaP) or the integration of CaP as the second phase in a composite system.[9]

Osteoinduction

Osteoinductivity is the biomaterial property that entails the induction of osteogenesis, which is regularly seen in any bone-healing process.[10] The osteoinduction process practically involves the mesenchymal and osteoprogenitor cell recruitment and their stimulation to more specialized bone-forming osteoblasts in an ectopic bone formation in vivo. Although the exact mechanism behind osteoinduction remains elusive, innovative biomaterials with osteoinductive potential have emerged. In recent years, cell and molecular biology advancements have dramatically improved understanding of the phenomena.[6] Two general prerequisites facilitate the phenomenon: (1) the presence of a matrix/scaffold that constitutes 3D porous structures that could accommodate and foster cell filtration; and (2) the cell recruitment to the defect site for the elevation of osteogenesis.[6,11] Osteogenic bone formation is activated through the local accumulation of growth and differentiation factors such as BMP families, fibroblast growth factors, and bone-associated ions (calcium and phosphate).[9] The influence of osteoinductive biomaterials on bone regeneration occurs at multiple levels. At the tissue level, osteoinductive biomaterials serve as active facilitators for oxygen diffusion, nutrient transport, and waste exchange between the material and tissue. Vascularization of the materials, which enhances tissue growth, is also stimulated. At the cellular level, osteoinductive biomaterials tend to initiate the differentiation of stem cells/osteoprogenitor cells toward osteogenic lineage by forming a carbonated apatite layer. The release of calcium and phosphate ions could signal cell chemotaxis, which involves the migration and direction of multiple cell types at the implantation sites. At the molecular level, osteoinductive materials tend to accrue osteogenic proteins such as BMP-2 and BMP-7 because of their great affinity with the surrounding proteins (osteoinductive) within the tissue microenvironment. A sequence of cellular activities on the biomaterial surface could be coordinated and encouraged by the accumulation and supplementation of local growth factors.[12] Moreover, the enrichment of calcium and phosphate ions could result in supersaturation in the void of implants, accelerating the mineralization in bone formation. To date, CaP-based bioceramics are the most commonly used osteoinductive biomaterials for tissue regeneration.

Another noteworthy and essential feature of osteoinductive biomaterials is their porous macrostructure. Essentially, porosity is necessary for osteoinductivity because bone induction has not been observed on a flat surface. Instead, bone formation has always transpired in the pores within implants, where there is supersaturation of calcium and phosphate ions. This concept was confirmed in a study by Barradas et al,[10] in which they demonstrated a direct correlation between microstructure and osteoinductivity of biomaterials. Based on the study, changes in porosity and roughness of the implants induced different levels of bone formation. For instance, surface-treated titanium implants with microstructural porosity could cause enormous bone induction as opposed to the untreated titanium that showed no sign of bone formation.[13] Thus, the importance of adequate osteoinductivity of a biomaterial for regenerative engineering cannot be overemphasized.

Vascularization

Vascularization is an essential aspect of bone regeneration as the formation of blood vessels is needed for tissues with a size greater than 200 μm (oxygen diffusion limit in vivo). The development of the vascular system allows the integration of newly formed vessels with the host blood supply, presenting a driving force for functional bone formation. The newly formed vessels play a role in ensuring an adequate supply of nutrients such as glucose and oxygen to the surrounding cells and the removal of metabolic by-products, such as carbon dioxide, lactate, and urea. The vascular network also participates in the regeneration process by helping to recruit progenitor cells to the defect sites.[14-17] When bone injury or trauma occurs, a local oxygen deficiency (local hypoxia microenvironment) causes the blood vessels to invade the bone defects.[5,18] However, this spontaneous process occurs much slower than the tissue healing rates, resulting in severe hypoxia and ultimately failure of bone regeneration.[9,19] Given the pressing need to establish a functional vascular network during bone regeneration, various biomaterials demonstrated the ability to improve several aspects of vessel network formation. These materials have been used to fabricate scaffolds for bone regenerative engineering.[1,6] Bone scaffolds could serve as a provisional framework that mediates the progenitor cells and the pericyte migration, offering structural support for nascent capillary sprouts. The architecture of the scaffolds during fabrication can be fine-tuned to optimize their effect on tissue-engineered constructs.[20] A 2013 study by Choi et al[21] reported a significant improvement in vascular network formation using inverse opal scaffolds with tiny pores. Recent advancements in scaffold fabrication techniques have spurred the development of 3D printing, which is being used to design more perfusable engineered tissue constructs. 3D-printed perfusable vascular systems populated with endothelial cells have shown good maintenance of metabolic function of tissue during regeneration of primary hepatocytes. There is a direct interaction between the endothelial cells and the chemical components of the biomaterials, and as such, vascularization can be influenced by the chemical composition of the scaffolding materials. Although most of the biomaterials used as regenerative materials exhibit high biocompatibility with endothelial cells, some have a proangiogenic potential for tissue healing. For example, silicate bioceramic (akermanite) has been shown to induce angiogenesis successfully by releasing an optimal amount of silicon ion that stimulated human aortic endothelial cell proliferation and gene expression. Hydroxyapatite biomaterials are capable of regulating vascularization due to their high affinity to angiogenic cytokines such as vascular endothelial growth factor (VEGF), endothelial growth factor, and basic fibroblast growth factor. Inspired by the interaction between these biomaterials and bioactive molecules, there is the sequestration of endogenous growth factors at the defect sites and the ultimate improvement of bone formation via an enhanced vascular network development. Techniques such as the integration of growth factors (VEGF and basic fibroblast growth factor) with biomaterial scaffolds have been used to increase the vascularization of the tissue-engineered construct.[7,20] The VEGF-encapsulated biomaterials intend to achieve a certain level of vascularization by promoting the proliferation of endothelial cells and the formation of a vascular network. Hence, the need to develop a vascular network may require that the biomaterial possess the ability to regulate and maintain VEGF release.

CELL-BIOMATERIAL INTERACTIONS

At the cellular level, the interaction of biomaterials and surrounding cells has a controlling or modifying influence on bone regenerative engineering because the nature and characteristics of biomaterials determine the regeneration outcome.[11] Cell-biomaterials interactions occur in sequential manners that involve three different stages: adhesion, proliferation, and differentiation. As an integral aspect of the cell-material interactions, cell adhesion plays a central role of mediating and dictating the cellular behaviors on the surface of biomaterials. Integrins, heterodimeric and transmembrane receptors, are responsible for the adhesion between cells and substrate through the activation of a series of intracellular signaling pathways that transmit the character of the matrix to the cells.[9] Integrins are composed of a diverse family of glycoproteins highly organized as heterodimers. These heterodimers can specifically bind onto the surface of a variety of matrix constituents. Integrin-mediated cell adhesion is a critical determinant of subsequent cell activities including cell morphology, motility, proliferation, and differentiation.[20]

In general, most of these interactions occur on the surface of the biomaterials, and hence the surface properties such as chemical composition, hydrophilicity, and topography of biomaterials have an enormous effect on cell fates.[11,19] The chances of attaining optimal cell responses are maximized by directing the adsorption of proteins at the cell-biomaterial interface because the materials are immediately covered with protein layers from the environment once implanted.[7,20] This mechanism has motivated the development of a series of surface modification and functionalization strategies that have been vastly extended to integrin-ECM molecule interactions. Numerous ECM macromolecules such as collagens, laminins, fibronectin, and vitronectin have been coated on various biomaterial surfaces to precisely control cellular performance on these surfaces. For example, bone substitutes based on collagen and its derivatives have been extensively used as implants to facilitate and improve material-cell interactions on implantation. The arginine-glycine-aspartic acid motif derived from fibronectin is the most widely investigated cell-binding peptide and has been used in several studies to enhance cell attachments. Arginine-glycine-aspartic acid motif has been blended with some bioinert systems, such as poly(ethylene glycol) (PEG), to control material property for selective cell behavior studies.[6]

Outside of protein-mediated interactions, other material surface characteristics can also have a remarkable effect on bone-forming capability by mediating cellular behaviors during bone regeneration. The importance of surface chemistry and chemical composition has been demonstrated in various orthopaedic devices and bone scaffolds surface treated with CaP.[6] The surface energy of biomaterials can influence the capacity for new bone formation by affecting the response of the osteoblasts. Olivares-Navarrete et al[19] found that osteoblast differentiation was improved on titanium surface with increasing surface energy. The topography of biomaterials has also been proven to affect bone formation. Lu et al[22] pioneered the work that confirmed this topographic effect, showing enhanced osteoblast alignment on grooved titanium (without a compositional change) as opposed to titanium without groove. More recent studies have channeled efforts in microfabrication and nanofabrication methods that have the potential to create multiscale physical features that favor bone formation. Webster et al[23,24] identified that nanoscale features (<100 nm) of biomaterials could be recognized by osteoblasts, leading to altered cellular responses and activities.

Furthermore, cell-material interactions depend on the mechanical properties of biomaterials because the cells react to mechanical stimuli such as the stiffness gradient of ECM via mechanotransduction.[1] The mechanotransduction process occurs through mechanosensitive ion channels, the forced unfolding of proteins, and remodeling of focal adhesion sites. In particular, changes in the stiffness of the matrix could induce different cellular responses, which could serve as an important driving force for cellular behaviors.[25-27] For example, MSCs seeded on a matrix with the stiffness of the brain differentiated into neural cells, whereas the same MSCs turned to osteogenic cells when they were brought in contact with a matrix whose stiffness is the same as the bone.[11]

Integration With Host Tissue

The integration of newly formed bone tissue with the native microenvironment is one of the requirements for functional bone regeneration.[28] During the course of this process, biomaterials assume an essential role because they serve as a scaffold for cell infiltration and tissue deposition and provide an avenue for the release of inductive signals. These biochemical cues facilitate tissue connection with the surrounding host networks, including the vasculature and the nervous system.[13,19,29] The initial step of tissue integration entails supporting cell adhesion on the surface of scaffolds fabricated by various biomaterials. These biomaterial-based scaffolds are designed to present porous structures that support adequate nutrient transport and oxygen diffusion, allowing cell migration and population within the scaffolds. In the next stage, infiltrated endothelial cells and pericytes reorganize and form capillaries, which are critical to sustaining the viability of newly formed tissues.[11] Ideal biomaterials support the formation and stabilization of vascular networks with an appropriate combination of chemistry and microstructure.[11] Meanwhile, osteoblasts may begin to deposit a large amount of tissue matrix such as collagen and minerals on the structure of the scaffolds. Finally, the remodeling process regulated by osteoblasts connects the newly formed ECM to the natural ECM. The remodeling process must match the degradation rate of the scaffold for optimal integration of the newly formed bone with the host bone tissue. Generally, biomaterials have a bearing influence on bone tissue integration because they serve as mediators and regulators in multiple stages of bone formation.

Various strategies have been devised to facilitate and improve the integration of biomaterials into the host bone tissue during bone regenerative engineering. Interconnected porosity of scaffolds is one of such approaches that have demonstrated the feasibility to improve tissue integration by way of efficiently promoting nutrient and oxygen transport.[30] Optimal pore size increases surface area for improved cell-material interactions, resulting in enhanced tissue integration.[21] Another method to enhance tissue integration is to redesign or modify the intrinsic chemical structure or surface chemistry of materials via techniques such as grafting, coating, and patterning.[6] Improvements in tissue integration have been observed with the incorporation of cell adhesive molecules, and this approach has witnessed exponential growth lately due to the associated positive outcome. Furthermore, the addition of biologic components into scaffolds has been used to enable cell-mediated remolding, which presents an excellent prospect to attain satisfactory bone integration.[9,31] The practicality of this approach was proven by Ehrbar and colleagues[32,33] where the group incorporated a variety of cell-cleavable peptide sequences into hydrogel-based biomaterials, yielding favorable integration and regeneration results.

POLYMERIC BIOMATERIALS FOR BONE TISSUE SCAFFOLDS

Polymers and polymer-based composites have been widely used to design bone grafts because of their chemical structure flexibility, biocompatibility, tailorable degradability, functional diversity, and processability.[6,20] Polymeric biomaterials undergo enzymatic or hydrolytic degradation through the cleavage of their functional linkages, yielding smaller molecules. The hydrophobicity and crystallinity of the polymeric biomaterials can be modulated to precisely control their degradation rates and profiles.[6] Copolymerization and blending, along with the compositional changes of the respective components, could offer a broader possibility for the design of a polymer-based system that fully capitalizes on the benefits of each component while minimizing the demerits of polymers.[2,34] This approach can be used to further customize the rate of degradation of biomaterials to specific needs. Typical polymers used as scaffolding materials can be classified into synthetic and natural polymers. Synthetic polymers exhibit relatively high mechanical strength, whereas natural polymers tend to be chemically and structurally identical to macromolecules present in the ECM, making them more biocompatible than their synthetic counterparts.[1,6]

As stated previously, bone regenerative engineering applications require particular physicochemical, biologic, and degradation properties for effective therapy.[6,11] Hence, the optimal and desirable characteristics could be achieved by blends of two synthetic polymers, natural polymers, or both in an ideal ratio. Since the first introduction of polymers to biomedical fields, a broader range of natural and synthetic polymers have been developed and investigated for tissue regeneration.[6,35] The following sections will discuss the different types of natural and synthetic polymers explored as substrates for bone regenerative engineering.

NATURAL POLYMERS

Various natural biodegradable polymers have been used to fabricate scaffolds with predetermined properties.[6,35] Because of the similarity of natural polymers with macromolecular compounds found in the body, they possess enormous benefits for applications in tissue regeneration. Natural polymers, including collagen, alginate, chitosan, hyaluronic acid, gelatin, and silk, are the most extensively investigated for the design of bone scaffolds.[9,11] Some of the natural polymers are discussed in the next section.

Collagen

Collagen is the most abundant protein in the body of humans, attributable to being the main component of ECM in most musculoskeletal tissues. It is the compound that holds the body together, providing strength and structure.[6,11]

These proteins are rodlike structures 300 nm in length and with a molecular weight of 300,000 Da. Thus far, 29 distinct types of collagen have been identified, and they all display a typical triple-helix structure, which encompasses three polypeptide subunits arranged in elongated fibrils.[6] Collagen types I, II, III, V, and XI tend to form collagen fibers, and type I has been extensively investigated because it constitutes more than 90% of the collagen in the human body. Type I is a trimeric molecule in which the three polypeptides have similar amino compositions and sequences. Each polypeptide contains 1,050 amino acids with approximately 33% glycine, 25% proline, and 25% hydroxyproline with a relative abundance of lysine. The amino acids are organized in repeating triplets of $(\text{glycine-X-Y})_n$, where X and Y are often proline and hydroxyproline. The repeating sequence lends collagen its predictable mechanical strength and helical structure. The presence of glycine makes the collagen flexible, and the flexibility increases with increasing glycine content. The reactive center on the chemical structure of the amino acids can be used for cross-linking and functionalization to enhance the mechanical properties of collagen.[1,6]

Collagen can be obtained from various sources and it presents low immunogenicity, a porous structure, good permeability, biocompatibility, and biodegradability. Because of these excellent properties, collagen scaffolds have been widely used in tissue regeneration. However, their poor mechanical strength and structural stability pose limitations to their applications to some extent. This associated drawback can be addressed by cross-linking collagen scaffolds via chemical or physical methods (amino acid's reactive center), improving their mechanical properties. In addition, the mechanical issues can be overcome by modifying collagen biomaterials with natural and/or synthetic polymers or inorganic materials, resulting in blends or composites with enhanced mechanical competence. Meanwhile, biochemical factors can be incorporated into the scaffold to enhance its biologic activity and cellular outcome.[20,35]

The structure of collagen is relatively stable because of covalent cross-link formation within the collagen fibrils. The nature of its structure, however, dictates biodegradability. Collagen degrades within the body by catabolic processes, involving enzymolysis of collagenase and yielding amino acids as degradation products. Based on previous studies, degradation rates of collagen can be fine-tuned by cross-linking (introduction of cross-links within the fibrils) or through enzymatic pretreatment. This capability offers the possibility of tailoring the degradation profile to a variety of regenerative needs.

Collagen is a primary element of ECM in many tissues, and it plays a critical role in tissue development and the maintenance of typical tissue architecture and function.[36] Because they serve as a natural substrate for cell attachment, proliferation, and differentiation, there is renewed interest in their use as a matrix for tissue regeneration. For instance, Inzana et al[37] demonstrated that 3D-printed scaffolds based on collagen-CaP interaction exhibited optimal cytocompatibility, osteoconductivity, and mechanical strength appropriate for effective bone regeneration.

Another exciting aspect is that the high reactivity of collagen makes it capable of exhibiting dual functions because it could be used to fabricate drug delivery scaffolds for regenerative engineering.[6,26,38] Geiger et al[39] illustrated the feasibility of using cross-linked absorbable collagen sponges as protein delivery scaffolds. In this study, bioactive proteins, such as recombinant human

BMP-2, were encapsulated in the collagen-based matrix. As a result of the affinity of collagen to the protein molecules, the protein release was sustained, leading to improved bone healing. This combination product is in the market with a titanium interbody spinal fusion cage as INFUSE Bone Graft/LT-Cage Lumbar Tapered Fusion Device. This product is used in anterior lumbar spinal fusion and for the treatment of acute tibia fractures in adults.[6] Absorbable collagen sponges exhibit excellent biocompatibility, biodegradability, and porosity, and for these reasons, they have been extensively investigated as a matrix for accelerated tissue regeneration. A collagen-based composite of fibrillar collagen, hydroxyapatite, and tricalcium phosphate is commercially available as a biodegradable bone graft substitute. Several other forms of collagen-based biomaterials have been exploited for the fabrication of optimal bone scaffolds.[1,9,13]

Collagens used in biomedical applications are generally extracted from bovine, porcine, or equine tissue.[6] These animal-based collagens carry a risk of disease-causing contaminants and may cause allergic reactions. Variations in immune responses are attributed to parameters such as processing techniques, production site, and isolation species.[13,35] Given the variations in collagen compositions, the cost of pure collagen tends to be exorbitant, and the biologic properties tend to differ. The introduction of recombinant human collagens provides a promising strategy for the mass production of collagen. This approach has been facilitated by the development of genetic engineering, which enables the design of recombinant human collagens by host cells, such as yeast, bacteria, mammalian/insect cells, transgenic animals, and transgenic plants.[6]

Gelatin

Gelatin is a natural polymeric biomaterial obtained from the denaturation or disintegration of insoluble collagen. Unlike collagen, which comes in several types, gelatin is only derived from alkaline or acidic hydrolysis of type I collagen.[13,35] Typically, it can be extracted from animal collagen, bones, skins, and tendons using pH-dependent hydrolyses. The extraction techniques determine the surface charge of the gelatin: partial acid hydrolysis yields type A gelatin, and alkaline hydrolysis results in type B gelatin. Gelatin type A exhibits an isoelectric point around a pH level of 9, identical to that of collagen, whereas gelatin type B displays an isoelectric point around a pH level of 5.[1,6] The modulation of the isoelectric points of gelatin allows it to bind with either positively or negatively charged therapeutic agents. This comes into play when different types of gelatins are appropriated for various regenerative needs. Type A gelatin, with an isoelectric point of pH 5.0, could be used in vivo as a carrier for proteins, and type B gelatin, with an isoelectric point of pH 9.0, could be applied to physiologic conditions for constant release of acidic materials.[40] The discrepancies in collagen sources and preparation techniques complicate its physicochemical characteristics and heterogeneity. Gelatin is composed of 19 amino acids that are partially organized and possess polyampholyte surface properties. The nature of their surface charges and the polymer architecture control their mechanical properties and cellular responses.[6,40] In addition, gelatin's surface charge changes accordingly because it shows a negatively charged surface at high pH and a positively charged surface at lower pH. The fast degradation rate of gelatin is a limitation for its use and is caused by enzymatic digestion and high physiologic solubility, which can be implicated for its typical low mechanical stability. The mechanical instability usually leads to a significant difference between the new bone formation and the scaffold degeneration.[41] There are many unanswered questions regarding the role of higher-order gelatin structures and the bioactivity of scaffolds. It is essential to consider and evaluate the possibility of the cells becoming reactive to the secondary and higher-order gelatin structures in the scaffolds. At the same time, the presence of active chemical groups (eg, NH_2 and COOH) offers a leeway that can be explored for optimal and augmented degradation periods.[42]

Chitosan

Chitosan-based biomaterials are attractive candidate materials for regenerative engineering applications because their promising properties such as nontoxicity, biodegradability, and biocompatibility distinguished them as suitable biomaterials for most tissue repair studies. Their chemical and structural characteristics exhibit a wide range of properties. These unique chemicals and structural features include reactive hydroxyl and amino groups, high charge density, broad hydrogen-bonding capacities, and a single chemical structure. Because of its charge density, chitosan enables the interaction with several negatively charged molecules and membranes. Chitosan is a linear positively charged polysaccharide that is commercially produced from chitin by alkali deacetylation. It consists of randomly distributed N-acetyl glucosamine and D-glucosamine linked by 1,4-β-glycosidic bonds. As a precursor of chitosan, chitin is obtained from crustaceans and insects, making it abundant in nature. The applicability of chitosan includes implantable and injectable orthopaedic substrates, drug delivery systems, and scaffolds for regenerative engineering because of its diverse biologic activity and unique interactions with ECM components and growth factors. For the regeneration of tissues, chitosan promotes osteoblast growth and matrix mineralization. However, their poor mechanical properties limit them from being used alone. For this reason, they are often used in combination with different materials, such as CaP, hydroxyapatite, and silk, to improve mechanical strength. For instance, Maji and Dasgupta[15] developed a biomaterial scaffold containing chitosan, hydroxyapatite, and gelatin. The composite scaffold exhibited excellent compressive strength of 1.2 MPa, which is within the range of the trabecular bones. Moreover, chitosan-based materials are integrated with other molecules or compounds to enhance biologic functions and increase osteoactivity. An explicative example is the coating of chitosan on other biomaterials to improve hydrophilicity and biocompatibility. These chitosan-coated composites encourage cell adhesion and proliferation. In addition, another set of studies demonstrated the positive effects of chitosan-based hybrid scaffolds loaded with BMP on large-scale bone defects. BMP release from the hybrid scaffolds stimulated new bone formation, osseointegration, and complete bone healing.[18,43,44] The in vivo degradation pathways of chitosan are known to be triggered by lysozymes that depolymerize the polysaccharide molecular chains. The rate at which the breakdown occurs depends on the acetyl content, which varies for different chitosan grades. The ease with which the modification of chitosan can be carried out has yielded a variety of chitosan biomaterials with enhanced properties as required by the complex regeneration process.

Alginate

In contrast to chitosan, alginate is a negatively charged polysaccharide. It is a natural multifunctional polymer that has been well investigated for regenerative engineering because of its excellent biocompatibility and mild gelation conditions. Alginate-based biomaterials comprise (1,4)-linked-D mannuronic acid and (1,4)-linked-L-guluronic acid, whose compositional changes permit the customization of their mechanical and biologic properties, affirming its regenerative potentials. These traits, coupled with cytocompatibility and controlled gelation, make alginate an interesting and promising biomaterial for minimally invasive bone regenerative engineering application and drug/cell delivery.[6]

Hyaluronic Acid

Hyaluronic acid is a linear polysaccharide known for its biocompatibility, degradability, and viscoelasticity. Hyaluronic acid is a glycosaminoglycan commonly found in many areas of the body in the extracellular tissue. It is increasingly becoming a vital biomaterial, and its main application is in hydrogel design, which can be used in various areas such as tissue culture scaffolds and wound dressing.

Hyaluronic acid exhibits sought-after physical and biochemical properties both in solution and hydrogel, and as such, it is highly desirable in different body repair technologies. Generally, hyaluronic acid constitutes a vital part of connective tissue, where it plays an essential role in cell growth, cell differentiation, and lubrication. Thus, it can be used to regulate cell differentiation, cellular fate, and subsequent bone formation. The chemical structure of hyaluronic acid contains carboxylic acid and alcohol groups, which allow further functionalization to yield smart hydrogels with tunable properties. It belongs to a particular category of regenerative biomaterials that not only possess excellent biocompatibility but also show the ability to positively affect its biologic surroundings. In other words, scaffolds based on hyaluronic acid are ideally bioactive and biodegradable with nontoxic degradation products. It is worth noting that hyaluronic displays low nonspecific protein adsorption and can be personalized to enable robust growth and repair of tissues via cell receptors.

Silk

Silk is a natural protein-based polymer composed mainly of fibroin, and it is derived from various Lepidoptera larvae, such as silkworms (cocoon of larvae), and from spiders. Inherently, silk displays variable composition, structural multiplicity, and functional dynamism induced by its source and environment. Silk is a rare emblem of high strength, low weight, excellent durability, and toughness, all combined appropriately.

Apart from possessing extraordinary mechanical behavior, silk exhibits excellent biocompatibility, high thermostability (up to 250°C), customizable degradation rates, and good processibility within a broader temperature range. The manufacturing of silk presents parameters that allow the fabrication of scaffolds with varying configurations. This design flexibility tends to result in a controlled degradation profile and enhanced cell-material interactions. The fibroin diameter, failure strength, and mass degradation could be used to predict the proteolysis of silk fibroin-based scaffolds.

Silk fibroin has been used in several tissue regenerative applications, including the healing and regeneration of critical-size femur defects. Several scientists have explored the feasibility of integrating silk with other materials to attain optimal characteristics modulated by changes in the component compositions and the silk-producing source. This approach has proven suitable for tissue regeneration because silk could be applied as a bulk part or as a coating or reinforcement of scaffolds with low biocompatibility. As a blend or hybrid system component, silk fiber inclusion increases the compression strength (in both in vivo and in vitro tests), thereby shortening the setting time without compromising the injectability and cytocompatibility. This was demonstrated by Gao et al,[29] who showed that tussah silk fibroin–poly(L-lactic-*co*-glycolic acid) composites improved cytocompatibility, osteoblast differentiation, and mechanical properties. Because of its moderate mechanical properties, controllable degradation rate compared with many other natural polymers, and high biologic compatibility, silk fibroin is a promising biomaterial for scaffold-based regenerative engineering.

SYNTHETIC POLYMERS

Synthetic polymeric biomaterials constitute the most considerable portion of the biomaterials market, and a reasonable number of them have been used to fabricate bone scaffolds for various musculoskeletal tissues. Synthetic polymers offer substantial advantages such as tunable, reproducible, and predictable properties and well-established structures over natural polymers. The benefits associated with synthetic biomaterials ensure the effective regeneration of damaged/diseased tissues and restoration of their structure and functions. The flexible polymerization techniques (copolymerization), pliable interlinkage and functionality, and adjustable molecular weights and crystallinity make them easy to synthesize compared with natural polymers. The demerits of synthetic polymeric biomaterials are that they lack adequate cell attachment sites and need modification to improve cell adhesion (and ultimately, the bioactivity). Commercially available and widely used degradable synthetic polymers and copolymers for regenerative engineering include aliphatic polyesters (such as polycaprolactone [PCL], poly(propylene fumarate) [PPF], poly(glycolic acid) [PGA], poly(lactic acid) [PLA], and their copolymer [poly(lactic-*co*-glycolic acid) (PLGA)]), polyanhydrides, polyphosphazenes (PPHOs), polyurethanes, and poly(glycerol sebacate), among others. These polymers possess different levels of biodegradability, biocompatibility, and mechanical properties, but as mentioned previously, no single polymer enjoys all three of these essential properties at ideal level.

Aliphatic Polyesters (PLA, PGA, PLGA, PCL, and PPF)

Poly(α-hydroxyl esters) constitute a vital subgroup of synthetic biodegradable polymers known for their capacity to undergo hydrolysis through the cleavage of the ester linkage in their backbone. However, when the aliphatic chains between the ester linkages are too long, their degradation may be hindered, rendering them unsuitable for tissue regeneration. Conversely, polyesters with reasonably short aliphatic chains have optimal degradation rates and profiles that suit most biomedical applications. For instance, the hydrophilicity of degradable polymers is influenced by $-CH_2-$ groups, which retard hydrolytic degradation. The chemistry and synthetic flexibility of polyesters distinguished them as a top-tier class of synthetic biomaterials for regenerative engineering. In regenerative engineering, PLA, PGA, and their copolymer PLGA are commonly used biomaterials to manage damaged or destroyed tissues. Historically, they have demonstrated their biocompatibility, breakdown into benign products, and reputable record of use in scaffold fabrication and degradable surgical sutures. The processibility of PLA and PGA is relatively easy because their physicochemical properties and degradation rates can be modulated using different molecular weights and compositions of their copolymers over a specific time frame. PLGA copolymers degrade at a rate that depends on the ratio of PLA and PGA. In general, the PLGA with higher PGA content degrades too rapidly, whereas the one with higher content of PLA degrades too slowly. So, the different molecular weights and wide-ranging compositions of the copolymers dictate the physical and mechanical properties and degradation rates of PLGA. PCL is a semicrystalline and aliphatic polymer with excellent toughness and sufficient biocompatibility. Its main limitation is hydrophobicity, which prevents cell adhesion and cell proliferation. The slow degradation rate (3 or 4 years) of PCL is also attributed to the issue of hydrophobicity. In this regard, the approach of copolymerization has been investigated to improve the PCL bioactivity because scaffolds based on PCL copolymers were able to increase biologic activities such as osteogenic differentiation, cell viability, calcium deposition, and cell seeding efficiency in comparison with pure PCL scaffolds.

Another biodegradable copolyester polymer is PPF, a high-strength polymeric biomaterial engineered for orthopaedic applications. PPF is a linear polymer chain with repeating ester units. The double bonds of fumarates in PPF can cross-link at room temperature, resulting in polymer networks. The high mechanical strength that results from this cross-linking makes PPF suitable for orthopaedic applications. The hydrolytically sensitive ester bond makes PPF amenable to degradation, and the degradation rate depends on molecular weight, type of curing agent, and cross-linking density. When in contact with an aqueous medium, PPF hydrolyzes into propylene glycol and fumaric acid, both of which are quickly excreted from the human body by natural metabolic processes. PPF is typically used to enhance the hydrophobicity of PLA, PGA, or PCL. One common issue among all the polyesters discussed is that they exhibit bulk erosion and release acidic degradation products. The accumulation of these acidic products in the tissue microenvironment may cause local inflammatory responses, leading to abrupt failure of the scaffold and foreign body reaction. Thus, regenerative biomaterials must present neutral degradation products on hydrolysis. Several studies have illustrated that the addition of other polymers (PPHO) or substances (alkaline salts) to polyester polymers could go a long way in addressing the issue of acidic degradation products.

Poly(Ethers) (PEG, PEO, PVA, and Polyurethane)

Poly(ethers), including PEG, poly(ethylene oxide) (PEO), polyurethane, and poly(vinyl alcohol) (PVA), are an indispensable class of regenerative biomaterials, and their popularity has grown over the past decades. These are the most known examples, although there are currently others that are currently being developed.[13]

PEG-based polymers are nonionic, are biocompatible, and have optimal physicochemical and biologic properties suitable for biomedical applications. PEG is regarded to have an inadequate immune response after implantation. Various cross-linking techniques are used to produce hydrophilic PEG scaffolds, and the selected technique can influence the scaffold's physicochemical properties, including permeability, molecular diffusion, elasticity, and modulus, or degradation rate. However, PEO is a longer molecular form of PEG, and it possesses a molecular mass above 20,000 g/mol. PEO is a hydrophilic polymer that is chemically inert with negligible antigenicity, immunogenicity, cell adhesion, and protein binding. The absence of hydrogen-rich groups triggers the low protein-binding tendency. PEG, with a low molecular mass below 20,000 g/mol, also inhibits the absorption of proteins, and this attribute is of interest in the medical field. The photopolymerization abilities of both PEO and PEG present a platform for tailoring the mechanical features and controlling the architecture of scaffolds and chemical composition. These capabilities make PEG and PEO attractive scaffolding biomaterials for the fabrication of 3D regenerative templates. PVA is a semicrystalline polyhydroxy polymer, prepared through the hydrolysis of poly(vinyl acetate). Although some of the synthetic polymeric biomaterials mentioned previously undergo enzymatic and/or hydrolytic degradation, several other polymers including PVA, PEO, and PEG are used to instill faster degradation tendency and characteristics in biomaterials. Polyurethane contains a urethane moiety in its repeating units, and the polycondensation of diisocyanate and polyol synthesizes them. Polyurethane polymers are widely used in the production of blood-contacting devices such as artificial veins and arteries or heart valves and the design of tissues such as bones, heart muscles, heart valves, blood vessels, skin, skeletal muscles, and cartilages. The urethane linkage in the long molecular chain in this large family of materials provides a pathway for developing various bonds such as allophane, biuret, acyl urea, or isocyanurate. These bonds could result in further branching and cross-linking, which affect the overall physicochemical properties and biocompatibility of these biomaterials. Biodegradable polyurethane can be synthesized using alternative diisocyanine compounds, usually based on biodegradable diisocyanates, such as lysine diisocyanate or hexamethylene diisocyanate. On degradation, the degradable polyurethane releases nontoxic products, making it suitable for regenerative engineering.[6,13,35]

Polyphosphazene

Since its discovery and utility in biomedicine, PPHO polymers have enjoyed tremendous growth and expansion in regenerative engineering because of their unique chemical behaviors. Polyphosphazenes are one of the few classes of inorganic-organic hybrid polymers that have been thoroughly investigated for tissue regeneration. The nature of the inorganic backbone and the chemical structure of the organic side groups influence and dictate the polymer properties. Polyphosphazenes with hydrolytically sensitive side groups (such as amino acid ester, peptide ester, glucosyl, glyceryl, glycolate, lactate, and imidazole) are susceptible to degradation and are often used for scaffold fabrication for tissue regeneration. The side group chemistry can be used to modulate the degradation rates and profile. Unlike the widely used polyesters, the degradation products of PPHOs are near neutral and can constitute a natural buffer in the local tissue microenvironment, preventing adverse effects. The physiologically benign and neutral pH of these degradation products has motivated researchers to blend PPHOs with other clinically relevant polymers such as polyesters. These studies show that the degradation products of PPHOs were able to neutralize or stabilize the acidic degradation products of polyesters. Another interesting observation of the PPHO-polyester blending was that the blend system exhibited a unique erosion profile, quite distinct from any other biodegradable systems currently available. The degradation occurred in such a way that the coherent blended biomaterial turned to an assemblage of microspheres with interconnected porous structures. The intrinsic pore formation enhances cell infiltration, tissue ingrowth, and nutrient transport, resulting in effective tissue regeneration. The design flexibility, neutral bioactivity, and unique erosion mechanism of PPHOs would be a game changer for biomaterial design in the nearest future.[2,30]

POLYMER-CERAMIC COMPOSITE

Given the multifaceted and copious requirements of the scaffold design for bone regenerative engineering, composite materials have been widely used to synergistically combine the benefits of two or more materials to meet these needs. Inorganic-organic composites are an important biomaterial for bone regenerative engineering that combines the ductility of a polymer phase with the stiffness and strength of inorganic components, generating advanced biomaterials with enhanced mechanical properties and desirable degradation profiles. Moreover, the integration of polymers with composites provides an avenue for controlling and influencing the structure and uniformity of composites. Bioceramics including hydroxyapatite, bioactive glass (eg, bioglass), alumina, TiO_2 (titanium dioxide), and CaP have been extensively investigated for bone regenerative engineering because they have the capability to enhance the mechanical properties and bioactivity of these composite biomaterials. For instance, both the mechanical strength and bioactivity of PLA, PLGA, and PCL could be improved by many folds when hydroxyapatite is added to them. Interestingly, numerous studies have illustrated that nanohydroxyapatite incorporation into porous PLGA matrix significantly encouraged preosteoblast proliferation, differentiation, and mineralization. For bone regenerative engineering applications, CaP-based bioceramics are the most commonly used additives for scaffold fabrication due to their similarity with bone minerals. They tend to stimulate bone bridge formation and induce CaP precipitation and deposition, forming a direct bone between implants and natural bone.[9]

SCAFFOLD FABRICATION METHODOLOGY

Numerous methods have been developed for the fabrication of biomaterial-based scaffolds for musculoskeletal tissue regeneration (**Table 1**). Many of these methods resemble or repurpose industrial material processing technologies but are either modified or miniaturized to produce tissue scaffolds with high architectural and compositional precision. Each of the methods that follow can be used either alone or in combination, to produce scaffolds that are biodegradable and possess complex biomimetic porous microstructures with sufficient mechanical strength to support musculoskeletal tissue regeneration.

Solvent Casting and Particulate Leaching

Solvent casting and particulate leaching are two of the simplest and most commonly used scaffold fabrication methods. Solvent casting involves the dissolution of polymers in organic solvents and depositing the mixture onto or into a mold to produce membranes or 3D scaffolds, respectively, on evaporation of the solvent. Particulate leaching is combined with this process to obtain highly porous scaffolds with more favorable microstructures for tissue regeneration. Salt or sugar crystals, the sugar crystal considered less toxic, are uniformly distributed within the polymer solution as a water-soluble sacrificial porogen phase. After the solvent evaporates, the polymer-porogen composite is submerged in water and the porogen phase leaches out, creating interconnected cavities within the polymer scaffold. The pore size and porosity can be controlled by the particle size and quantity of porogen added. For example, Mao et al[45] synthesized PLA/ethyl cellulose/hydroxyapatite scaffolds for bone regeneration using dichloromethane as a solvent and NaCl as a porogen with final pore sizes and porosities ranging from 150 to 250 μm and 74% to 89%, respectively. Although this method is straightforward and does not require special equipment, sufficient vacuum drying is required to remove residual toxic solvent that can harm cells and denature growth factors or ECM proteins that are incorporated onto the scaffold. Moreover, there is a risk of residual porogen that does not leach out, leaving salt or sugar particles or even noninterconnected pores.

Freeze-Drying or Lyophilization

During the solvent casting process, thorough removal of organic solvents can be achieved by freeze-drying or lyophilization. The polymer solution is cooled below its freezing point and subjected to a low-pressure environment to induce sublimation of ice crystals and solvent, resulting in a solid scaffold with interconnected pores. Increased control over scaffold porosity can be achieved by lyophilizing emulsions of organic polymer solutions and water that undergo phase separation during the sublimation process.[58]

Melt Molding

Melt molding is an alternative to solvent casting for fabricating polymeric tissue scaffolds. Instead of using toxic organic solvents, polymers are heated to a glassy or liquid state, cast into or coated onto a mold, and cooled to form a solid structure. This method can also be used in combination with particulate leaching to obtain adequate scaffold porosity via removal of the porogen phase. Oh et al[47] used this method to construct PLGA/PVA scaffolds with 200 to 300 μm pores and approximately 90% porosity by compression molding layered stacks of thin polymer disks and NaCl porogen particles at 180°C. It is important to note, however, that melt molding is not compatible with the incorporation of any biomolecules into the scaffold because the high temperatures can destroy the bioactivity or chemical structure of these sensitive factors.

Microsphere Emulsions and Sintering

Polymer-ceramic composite microspheres are useful scaffold materials because of their tunable porosity, high mechanical strength, and ability to encapsulate and deliver bioactive molecules that aid in tissue regeneration. The standard emulsion technique for fabricating microspheres involves dripping a biopolymer/ceramic solution into a rapidly rotating immiscible liquid phase containing a surfactant and allowing the solvents to evaporate. The size of the resulting microspheres can be controlled by tuning the stirring rate and the surfactant concentration. The microspheres can then be packed into a mold and sintered at elevated temperatures to partially fuse them to one another. The resulting bulk scaffold has a porous microstructure and high mechanical strength, which are controlled by the sintering temperature and duration.[48] For example, Lv et al[49] created strong and highly porous composite scaffolds from PLGA/nanohydroxyapatite microspheres that improved osteogenic differentiation in human MSCs.

Gas Foaming

This simple and low-cost technique is also used to produce porous 3D polymeric scaffolds while avoiding the use of organic solvents. Rather than using a solid porogen phase, nontoxic inert gases such as CO_2 or N_2 are either injected into the polymer solution at elevated pressures or generated from acidic reactions with foaming agents such as sodium bicarbonate. Saturation of these gases enables bubble nucleation and growth within the

TABLE 1 Summary of Tissue Scaffold Fabrication Methods

Scaffold Fabrication Method	Description of Method	Example Studies
Solvent casting/particulate leaching	Polymer solution cast into a mold with embedded water-soluble particles that leave interconnected pores in the final scaffold	Mao et al 2018[45]
Freeze-drying	Polymer solutions or emulsions cooled under vacuum to remove solvents and create porous structures	Aranaz et al 2104[46]
Melt molding	Polymer is heated to a glassy or liquid state and cast into a mold	Oh et al 2003[47]
Microsphere sintering	Water-oil emulsions produce polymer-based microspheres that partially fuse into porous scaffolds at elevated temperatures	Shi et al 2011[48] Lv et al 2009[49]
Gas foaming	Pressurized injection and subsequent depressurization of inert gas within polymer solutions create highly porous scaffolds	Annabi et al 2011[50]
Thermally induced phase separation	Homogeneous polymer solutions split into multiple phases on cooling to yield scaffolds with complex porous microstructures	Munir and Callanan, 2018[51]
Membrane lamination	Biodegradable membranes are cut, stacked, folded or rolled, and fused to form complex three-dimensional scaffold geometries	Chen et al 2017[52]
Fiber mesh/fiber bonding	Polymer fibers are woven into meshes or heated to fuse them at fiber intersections to produce biomimetic tissue scaffolds	Mikos et al 1993[53]
Electrospinning	High electrostatic forces are used to overcome cohesive forces in polymer solutions and extract a thin jet that produces biomimetic nanofibrous sheets on a collection surface	Choi et al 2008[21] Zhang et al 2008[54]
Rapid prototyping	Complex scaffolds are manufactured layer-by-layer from computer-aided designs via precise material deposition or curing	Yuan et al 2017[55]
3D bioprinting	Living scaffolds are printed from cell-laden and biomaterial-laden bioinks to mimic tissue composition, architecture, and function	Chae et al 2021[56]
Self-assembly	Amphiphilic biomolecules, copolymers, or extracellular matrix components spontaneously organize into ordered structures	Hairfield-Stein et al 2007[57]

solidifying polymer solution, thereby creating pores in the final scaffold. However, inhomogeneity in the scaffold foams can result from buoyant forces that carry the bubbles upward and yield a steep gradient in porosity.[59] In one example, high-pressure CO_2 was injected into molten poly(ε-caprolactone)/NaCl mixtures and then used again to spray bovine ligament–derived elastin to obtain 3D porous scaffolds capable of facilitating chondrocyte adhesion and cartilage repair.[50]

Thermally Induced Phase Separation

In this method, a homogeneous polymer solution is cooled to form a complex arrangement of separate polymer-rich and polymer-poor phases. A microporous polymer scaffold is formed after a coarsening process and removal of the solvent. The pore morphology and composition of the scaffold can be tuned by varying the polymer concentration, solvent type, and cooling path within the phase diagram of the system. This technique was used to produce porous poly(ε-caprolactone) scaffolds with 0.2% w/v collagen type I that supported chondrocyte proliferation and had compressive properties similar to native cartilage tissue.[51]

Membrane Lamination

This scaffold fabrication method is a simple way to construct complex anatomic 3D structures from individual porous biodegradable membranes. The procedure involves digitally converting a 3D shape into a series of two-dimensional slices that are cut out from the membranes, stacked layer by layer, and fused together using solvents such as chloroform or seeded cells.[60] Membranes can also be folded or rolled into cylindrical structures before lamination to form different scaffold architectures.

Fiber Mesh/Bonding

Fiber mesh scaffolds consist of interwoven fibers made from biodegradable polymers such as PGA that create 3D patterns with large surface area to support cell attachment and nutrient/oxygen diffusion. Similarly, fiber bonding involves heating polymer fibers slightly above their melting temperature to fuse them at their intersection points in nonwoven meshes.[53] These mesh scaffolds are sometimes combined with a secondary polymer matrix to improve structural integrity.

Electrospinning

Electrospinning uses strong electric fields to draw out thin turbulent jets of a charged solution of synthetic and/or natural polymers that deposit nanofibers onto a platform or rotating mandrel. These scaffolds are highly porous and biomimetic in structure, and the thickness and orientation of the nanofibers can be controlled by the polymer composition, ambient conditions, electric potential difference, and motion of the collecting platform. In a 2008 study, poly(ε-caprolactone)/collagen nanofibers were produced and aligned via electrospinning and showed potential for guiding myotube formation, muscle cell alignment, and regeneration of functional muscle tissue.[61]

Rapid Prototyping

This category of fabrication methods, also known as solid freeform fabrication, involves the precise construction of complex 3D scaffolds using computer-controlled tools that can be customized for individual patients and defect geometries. Rapid prototyping methods include stereolithography, selective laser sintering, fused deposition modeling, and 3D printing.[37,55]

3D Bioprinting

3D bioprinting is a novel scaffold fabrication method that deposits mixtures of cells, biopolymers, and/or bioactive molecules, collectively termed bioinks, to form complex living scaffolds that imitate native tissue architecture and function. Various cell types can also be printed without scaffold materials to mimic the conditions of embryonic tissue development. A new study by Chae et al[56] printed a graded scaffold from tendon-derived and bone-derived ECM bioinks that accelerated tendon-bone interface repair in a rat rotator cuff tear model.

Self-Assembly

This new approach for synthesizing tissue scaffolds exploits the ability of cells and/or certain biomolecules such as hydrogels to block copolymers and polymeric dendrimers to spontaneously organize into well-ordered nanoscale structures that serve as a framework for tissue regeneration. For instance, porcine bone marrow stromal cells cultured on SYLGARD/laminin-coated dishes between silk suture anchors were able to self-assemble into aligned, ligamentlike tissues that, on maturation, could serve as mechanically suitable ligament replacements.[57]

SUMMARY

The emergence of regenerative engineering has sparked a paradigm shift in the design strategy for ideal biomaterials and scaffolds. Matrix-based regenerative engineering is a vital and revolutionary approach to addressing clinical challenges such as musculoskeletal tissue injury and disease. The success of this innovative approach immensely depends on factors such as material choice, scaffold geometry, cell type, and signals (biologic, chemical, and mechanical). The material choice is based on the currently available biomaterials, comprising natural and synthetic polymers as well as polymer-ceramic composites. Advancements in materials science have enabled and guaranteed the development of ideal biomaterial scaffolds that serve as a basic framework and regulate various aspects of regenerative engineering. With the ever-changing demands of this complex regenerative approach, the need for an optimal graft with precise cues (as well as spatial and temporal control) will indisputably set the ground for polymeric biomaterials for a leading and increasingly prominent role in translational medicine.

The direction for the future in this field is to develop an integrated technology strategy that fosters close and scientific collaboration between orthopaedic surgeons, biologists, materials scientists, regulatory entities, and patients. It will be interesting to consider a patient-centric effort that allows the customization and personalization of biomaterial design for precision and personalized medicine. As regenerative engineering continues to evolve, biomaterial properties can be tailored to accommodate patient-to-patient variations, ensuring the administration of suitable therapies based on individual patient complexity and personal characteristics such as sex, age, race, and ancestry.

REFERENCES

1. Ogueri KS, Laurencin CT: Nanofiber technology for regenerative engineering. *ACS Nano* 2020;14(8):9347-9363.
2. Ogueri KS, Allcock HR, Laurencin CT: Generational biodegradable and regenerative polyphosphazene polymers and their blends with poly(lactic-co-glycolic acid). *Prog Polym Sci* 2019;98:101146.
3. Laurencin CT, Khan Y: *Regenerative Engineering*. American Association for the Advancement of Science, 2012, vol 4.
4. Laurencin CT, Nair LS: Regenerative engineering: Approaches to limb regeneration and other grand challenges. *Regen Eng Transl Med* 2015;1(1):1-3.
5. Quintero AJ, Wright VJ, Fu FH, Huard J: Stem cells for the treatment of skeletal muscle injury. *Clin Sports Med* 2009;28(1):1-11.
6. Ogueri KS, Jafari T, Ivirico JLE, Laurencin CT: Polymeric biomaterials for scaffold-based bone regenerative engineering. *Regen Eng Transl Med* 2019;5(2):128-154.
7. Zhang Y, Di Wu XZ, Pakvasa M, et al: Stem cell-friendly scaffold biomaterials: Applications for bone tissue engineering and regenerative medicine. *Front Bioeng Biotechnol* 2020;8:598607.

8. Khan WS, Rayan F, Dhinsa BS, Marsh D: An osteoconductive, osteoinductive, and osteogenic tissue-engineered product for trauma and orthopaedic surgery: How far are we? *Stem Cell Int* 2012;2012:236231.
9. Yu X, Tang X, Gohil SV, Laurencin CT: Biomaterials for bone regenerative engineering. *Adv Healthc Mater* 2015;4(9):1268-1285.
10. Barradas A, Yuan H, van Blitterswijk CA, Habibovic P: Osteoinductive biomaterials: current knowledge of properties, experimental models and biological mechanisms. *Eur Cell Mater* 2011;21(407):29.
11. Ogueri KS, Laurencin CT: Matrix-based bone regenerative engineering, in Zaidi M, ed: *Encyclopedia of Bone Biology*. Academic Press, Oxford, 2020, pp 135-148.
12. Barradas AM, Fernandes HA, Groen N, et al: A calcium-induced signaling cascade leading to osteogenic differentiation of human bone marrow-derived mesenchymal stromal cells. *Biomaterials* 2012;33(11):3205-3215.
13. Rao SH, Harini B, Shadamarshan RPK, Balagangadharan K, Selvamurugan N: Natural and synthetic polymers/bioceramics/bioactive compounds-mediated cell signalling in bone tissue engineering. *Int J Biol Macromol* 2018;110:88-96.
14. He D, Zhao AS, Su H, et al: An injectable scaffold based on temperature-responsive hydrogel and factor-loaded nanoparticles for application in vascularization in tissue engineering. *J Biomed Mater Res* 2019;107(10):2123-2134.
15. Maji K, Dasgupta S: Hydroxyapatite-chitosan and gelatin based scaffold for bone tissue engineering. *Trans Indian Ceram Soc* 2014;73(2):110-114.
16. Marchini A, Gelain F: Synthetic scaffolds for 3D cell cultures and organoids: Applications in regenerative medicine. *Crit Rev Biotechnol* 2022;42(3):468-486.
17. Ding Y, Zhao A-S, Liu T, et al: An injectable nanocomposite hydrogel for potential application of vascularization and tissue repair. *Ann Biomed Eng* 2020;48(5):1511-1523.
18. Wu H, Lei P, Liu G, et al: Reconstruction of large-scale defects with a novel hybrid scaffold made from poly (L-lactic acid)/nanohydroxyapatite/alendronate-loaded chitosan microsphere: In vitro and in vivo studies. *Sci Rep* 2017;7(1):1-14.
19. Olivares-Navarrete R, Raines AL, Hyzy SL, et al: Osteoblast maturation and new bone formation in response to titanium implant surface features are reduced with age. *J Bone Miner Res* 2012;27(8):1773-1783.
20. Shoichet MS: Polymer scaffolds for biomaterials applications. *Macromolecules* 2010;43(2):581-591.
21. Choi SW, Zhang Y, MacEwan MR, Xia Y: Neovascularization in biodegradable inverse opal scaffolds with uniform and precisely controlled pore sizes. *Adv Healthc Mater* 2013;2(1):145-154.
22. Lu X, Leng Y, Zhang X, Xu J, Qin L, Chan C-W: Comparative study of osteoconduction on micromachined and alkali-treated titanium alloy surfaces in vitro and in vivo. *Biomaterials* 2005;26(14):1793-1801.
23. Webster TJ, Ejiofor JU: Increased osteoblast adhesion on nanophase metals: Ti, Ti6Al4V, and CoCrMo. *Biomaterials* 2004;25(19):4731-4739.
24. Webster TJ, Ergun C, Doremus RH, Siegel RW, Bizios R: Enhanced functions of osteoblasts on nanophase ceramics. *Biomaterials* 2000;21(17):1803-1810.
25. Teasdale I: Stimuli-responsive phosphorus-based polymers. *Eur J Inorg Chem* 2019;2019(11-12):1445-1456.
26. Ulery BD, Nair LS, Laurencin CT: Biomedical applications of biodegradable polymers. *J Polym Sci B Polym Phys* 2011;49(12):832-864.
27. Woodard JR, Hilldore AJ, Lan SK, et al: The mechanical properties and osteoconductivity of hydroxyapatite bone scaffolds with multi-scale porosity. *Biomaterials* 2007;28(1):45-54.
28. Clark PA, Moioli EK, Sumner DR, Mao JJ: Porous implants as drug delivery vehicles to augment host tissue integration. *Faseb J* 2008;22(6):1684-1693.
29. Gao Y, Shao W, Qian W, et al: Biomineralized poly(L-lactic-co-glycolic acid)-tussah silk fibroin nanofiber fabric with hierarchical architecture as a scaffold for bone tissue engineering. *Mater Sci Eng C* 2018;84:195-207.
30. Ogueri KS, Ogueri KS, McClinton A, et al: In vivo evaluation of the regenerative capability of glycylglycine ethyl ester-substituted polyphosphazene and poly(lactic-co-glycolic acid) blends: A rabbit critical-sized bone defect model. *ACS Biomater Sci Eng* 2021;7(4):1564-1572.
31. Yang G, Mahadik B, Choi JY, Fisher JP: Vascularization in tissue engineering: fundamentals and state-of-art. *Prog Biomed Eng* 2020;2(1):012002.
32. Ehrbar M, Rizzi SC, Hlushchuk R, et al: Enzymatic formation of modular cell-instructive fibrin analogs for tissue engineering. *Biomaterials* 2007;28(26):3856-3866.
33. Ehrbar M, Rizzi SC, Schoenmakers RG, et al: Biomolecular hydrogels formed and degraded via site-specific enzymatic reactions. *Biomacromolecules* 2007;8(10):3000-3007.
34. Ogueri KS, Ivirico JLE, Nair LS, Allcock HR, Laurencin CT: Biodegradable polyphosphazene-based blends for regenerative engineering. *Regen Eng Transl Med* 2017;3(1):15-31.
35. Reddy M, Ponnamma D, Choudhary R, Sadasivuni KK: A comparative review of natural and synthetic biopolymer composite scaffolds. *Polymers* 2021;13(7):1105.
36. Cunniffe GM, Dickson GR, Partap S, Stanton KT, O'Brien FJ: Development and characterisation of a collagen nano-hydroxyapatite composite scaffold for bone tissue engineering. *J Mater Sci Mater Med* 2010;21(8):2293-2298.
37. Inzana JA, Olvera D, Fuller SM, et al: 3D printing of composite calcium phosphate and collagen scaffolds for bone regeneration. *Biomaterials* 2014;35(13):4026-4034.
38. Titorencu I, Georgiana Albu M, Nemecz M, V Jinga V: Natural polymer-cell bioconstructs for bone tissue engineering. *Curr Stem Cell Res Ther* 2017;12(2):165-174.
39. Geiger M, Li R, Friess W: Collagen sponges for bone regeneration with rhBMP-2. *Adv Drug Deliv Rev* 2003;55(12):1613-1629.

40. Kuttappan S, Mathew D, Nair MB: Biomimetic composite scaffolds containing bioceramics and collagen/gelatin for bone tissue engineering-A mini review. *Int J Biol Macromol* 2016;93:1390-1401.
41. Bhattarai DP, Aguilar LE, Park CH, Kim CS: A review on properties of natural and synthetic based electrospun fibrous materials for bone tissue engineering. *Membranes* 2018;8(3):62.
42. Ranganathan S, Balagangadharan K, Selvamurugan N: Chitosan and gelatin-based electrospun fibers for bone tissue engineering. *Int J Biol Macromol* 2019;133:354-364.
43. Shi S, Cheng X, Wang J, Zhang W, Peng L, Zhang Y: RhBMP-2 microspheres-loaded chitosan/collagen scaffold enhanced osseointegration: an experiment in dog. *J Biomater Appl* 2009;23(4):331-346.
44. Hou J, Wang J, Cao L, et al: Segmental bone regeneration using rhBMP-2-loaded collagen/chitosan microspheres composite scaffold in a rabbit model. *Biomed Mater* 2012;7(3):035002.
45. Mao D, Li Q, Bai N, Dong H, Li D: Porous stable poly(lactic acid)/ethyl cellulose/hydroxyapatite composite scaffolds prepared by a combined method for bone regeneration. *Carbohydr Polym* 2018;180:104-111.
46. Aranaz I, Gutiérrez MC, Ferrer ML, Del Monte F: Preparation of chitosan nanocompositeswith a macroporous structure by unidirectional freezing and subsequent freeze-drying. *Mar Drugs* 2014;12(11):5619-5642.
47. Oh SH, Kang SG, Kim ES, Cho SH, Lee JH: Fabrication and characterization of hydrophilic poly(lactic-co-glycolic acid)/poly(vinyl alcohol) blend cell scaffolds by melt-molding particulate-leaching method. *Biomaterials* 2003;24(22):4011-4021.
48. Shi X, Su K, Varshney RR, Wang Y, Wang D-A: Sintered microsphere scaffolds for controlled release and tissue engineering. *Pharm Res* 2011;28(5):1224-1228.
49. Lv Q, Nair L, Laurencin CT: Fabrication, characterization, and in vitro evaluation of poly(lactic acid glycolic acid)/nano-hydroxyapatite composite microsphere-based scaffolds for bone tissue engineering in rotating bioreactors. *J Biomed Mater Res A* 2009;91(3):679-691.
50. Annabi N, Fathi A, Mithieux SM, Martens P, Weiss AS, Dehghani F: The effect of elastin on chondrocyte adhesion and proliferation on poly(ε-caprolactone)/elastin composites. *Biomaterials* 2011;32(6):1517-1525.
51. Munir N, Callanan A: Novel phase separated polycaprolactone/collagen scaffolds for cartilage tissue engineering. *Biomed Mater* 2018;13(5):051001.
52. Chen Z, Song Y, Zhang J, et al: Laminated electrospun nHA/PHB-composite scaffolds mimicking bone extracellular matrix for bone tissue engineering. *Mater Sci Eng C* 2017;72:341-351.
53. Mikos AG, Bao Y, Cima LG, Ingber DE, Vacanti JP, Langer R: Preparation of poly(glycolic acid) bonded fiber structures for cell attachment and transplantation. *J Biomed Mater Res* 1993;27(2):183-189.
54. Zhang Y, Venugopal JR, El-Turki A, Ramakrishna S, Su B, Lim CT: Electrospun biomimetic nanocomposite nanofibers of hydroxyapatite/chitosan for bone tissue engineering. *Biomaterials* 2008;29(32):4314-4322.
55. Yuan B, Zhou S-Y, Chen X-S: Rapid prototyping technology and its application in bone tissue engineering. *J Zhejiang Univ Sci B* 2017;18(4):303-315.
56. Chae S, Sun Y, Choi Y-J, Ha D-H, Jeon I, Cho D-W: 3D cell-printing of tendon-bone interface using tissue-derived extracellular matrix bioinks for chronic rotator cuff repair. *Biofabrication* 2021;13(3):035005.
57. Hairfield-Stein M, England C, Paek HJ, et al: Development of self-assembled, tissue-engineered ligament from bone marrow stromal cells. *Tissue Eng* 2007;13(4):703-710.
58. Eltom A, Zhong G, Muhammad A: Scaffold techniques and designs in tissue engineering functions and purposes: A review. *Adv Mater Sci Eng* 2019;2019.
59. Dehghani F, Annabi N: Engineering porous scaffolds using gas-based techniques. *Curr Opin Biotechnol* 2011;22(5):661-666.
60. Tran RT, Thevenot P, Zhang Y, Gyawali D, Tang L, Yang J: Scaffold sheet design strategy for soft tissue engineering. *Materials* 2010;3(2):1375-1389.
61. San Choi J, Lee SJ, Christ GJ, Atala A, Yoo JJ: The influence of electrospun aligned poly(ε-caprolactone)/collagen nanofiber meshes on the formation of self-aligned skeletal muscle myotubes. *Biomaterials* 2008;29(19):2899-2906.

CHAPTER 3

Bioactive Factors and Designer Molecules

Vicki Rosen, PhD

INTRODUCTION

Successful healing and regeneration of orthopaedic tissues after injury requires highly orchestrated interactions between cell types responding to multiple signaling inputs. Bioactive factors will be defined here as signals that have the potential to help injuries heal and tissues regenerate. A bioactive factor may be a naturally occurring protein or may be an engineered moiety created to mimic the action of a naturally occurring molecule. The targets of bioactive factors are cells with the potential to engage in the healing process. These cells may be present at the injury site, recruited to the tissue during the repair process, or added from exogenous sources to enhance healing. Additionally, a bioactive factor might be secreted into the extracellular space by resident cells, or could be tethered to or embedded in native extracellular matrix (ECM), or might be provided exogenously in engineered biocompatible tissue-specific matrices. Figuring out the most effective combinations of bioactive factors, biomaterials, and tissue-specific target cells able to initiate and sustain repair until a tissue returns to homeostasis remains both the biggest challenge and best opportunity for advancing the regeneration of orthopaedic tissues. The molecules chosen for discussion[1-26] (**Table 1**) meet an important set of criteria: each is a known component of a tissue repair cascade or mimetic of a naturally occurring repair component; each has been tested for the ability to enhance repair in relevant preclinical and/or clinical models; each can be produced using good manufacturing practices. What remains to be determined is how to best use each alone or in combination to achieve successful repair and regeneration in a tissue-specific manner.

AUTOLOGOUS PLATELET-RICH PLASMA

Platelet-rich plasma (PRP) is the designation given to preparations of autologous human plasma with increased platelet concentration produced by centrifuging the patient's blood to concentrate contents. As platelets contain many growth factors including transforming growth factor beta, platelet-derived growth factor (PDGF), basic fibroblast growth factor, vascular endothelial growth factor, epidermal growth factor, and insulinlike growth factor-1 (**Figure 1**), using PRP would deliver combinations of these bioactive proteins to the wound site in a greater than normal amount.[27,28] The ability of PRP to provide anabolic stimulus for healing by exerting mitogenic, chemoattractant, and proliferative effects would depend on the presence of growth factors in PRP known to mediate these processes. Plasma processing can be tailored to remove specific blood cell components, which would then change the combination of bioactive factors present in the final PRP.[29]

There is no general consensus in the orthopaedic community as to what constitutes optimal PRP and it is likely that the optimal PRP for individual tissue-specific healing indications would need to be determined based on information about the healing and/or regenerative process in that tissue. For example, knowledge of the strength and duration of the inflammatory environment immediately after tissue injury would be key data when designing PRP. As leukocyte-rich PRP is thought to be proinflammatory by containing elevated catabolic cytokines, Zitsch et al[30] conducted a prospective randomized double-blind clinical trial for leukocyte-reduced PRP for patients undergoing surgery for pilon fractures and found that a single intra-articular injection of leukocyte-reduced PRP significantly reduced proinflammatory and degradative biomarkers while increasing anabolic biomarkers.

Several confounding factors exist for proving the efficacy of PRP for enhancing tissue repair and regeneration. There is inherent variability in blood contents collected from patients based on age, sex, medication status, and general overall individual health. In fact, PRP collected from the same patient has been found to change throughout the day.[31,32] Additionally, commercial concentrating systems differ on platelet capture efficiency, platelet isolation method, centrifugation speed, and collection tubes.[28] These variations led Obana in a 2021 review of the previous 11 years of PRP clinical data to conclude that there is a dearth of high-level evidence and methodologic standardization about PRP despite the trend upward in use of PRP.[33] Future developments to be considered for optimizing PRP use include: creating a test kit that would be available before PRP administration that can determine if the PRP meets specific quality standards; creating

Dr. Rosen or an immediate family member serves as a paid consultant to or is an employee of Keros Therapeutics and has stock or stock options held in Keros Therapeutics.

TABLE 1 FDA Approval Status of Bioactive and Designer Molecules

Bioactive or Designer Agent	Clinical Indications
Preclinical Development	
rhBMP-6	Spine fusion and large segmental defects
rhGDF-5	Articular cartilage defect repair
BV-265/CM	Fibular osteotomy and critically sized ostectomy
rhPTH	Osteoarthritis
Nell-1	Fracture healing
Sck/DKK-1 bispecific antibody	Fracture healing, osteoporosis
Clinical Development	
rPDGF-BB	Rotator cuff repair augmentation
rPDGF-BB	Periodontal repair
rhBMP-6	Distal radial fractures, tibial wedge osteotomy defects
rhPTH	Forteo: osteoporosis
PTH with fibrin matrix	Spine fusion, tibial plateau fractures
Nell-1	Degenerative disk disease
Wnt3A	Autograft enhancement in posterolateral lumbar spinal fusion
DKK-1	Postmenopausal osteoporosis, myeloma-induced bone disease
Scl-Ab	Fracture healing, osteogenesis imperfecta
P-15L	Degenerative disk disease
Commercially Available	
rPDGF-BB	Regranex: topical soft-tissue wound healing
rPDGF-BB	Augment: foot and ankle fusions
rhBMP-2	InFuse: spine fusion, tibial fracture, sinus augmentation, localized alveolar ridge augmentation
rhBMP-7	OP-1: recalcitrant long bone nonunions (via humanitarian device exemption)
PTHrP	Abaloparatide: osteoporosis
P-15	i-Factor: spine fusion
Scl-Ab	Romosozumab: osteoporosis

DKK-1 = Dickkopf-1, PTH = parathyroid hormone, rhBMP-6 = recombinant human bone morphogenetic protein 6, rhGDF-5 = recombinant human growth differentiation factor 5, rhPTH = recombinant human parathyroid hormone, Scl-Ab = sclerostin antibody, PTHrP = parathyroid hormone–related protein.

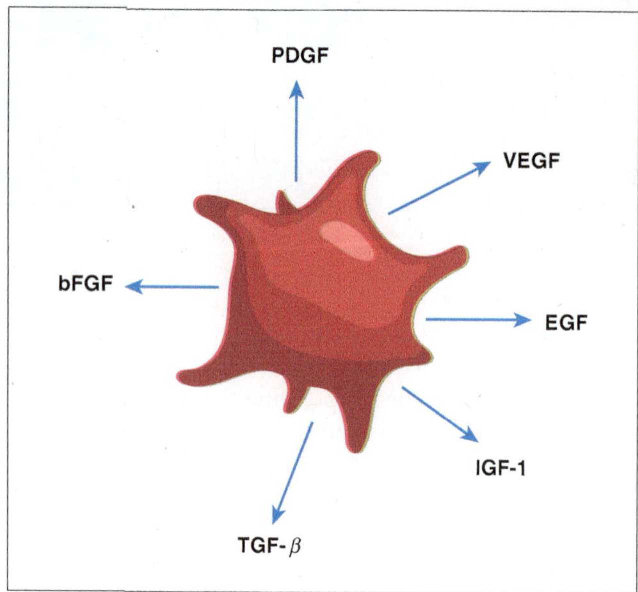

FIGURE 1 Platelet-rich plasma contains a mixture of bioactive factors. In this schematic illustration, each platelet (red) produces bioactive factors that are released when platelets are activated. These include platelet-derived growth factor (PDGF), vascular endothelial growth factor (VEGF), epidermal growth factor (EGF), basic fibroblast growth factor (bFGF), insulinlike growth factor 1 (IGF-1), and transforming growth factor beta (TGF-β). As these molecules individually regulate many different cell behaviors, the combinatorial interactions possible may produce a potent tissue repair stimulus.

a point-of-care blood test that can determine if a donor's PRP will be of high quality; and combining PRP with tissue-compatible carriers specific to the repair site.

PLATELET-DERIVED GROWTH FACTOR-BB

PDGFs are a family of dimeric isoforms: PDGF-AA, PDGF-BB, PDGF-C, and PDGF-D.[34] PDGF-BB is the isoform that binds both PDGF receptors, PDGF receptor alpha and PDGF beta, so it is considered the most universal of PDGF proteins.[35] PDGF was originally identified as a product made and stored in the alpha granules of platelets that is released into serum during blood clotting.[36] Although platelets are a major storage site for PDGF, PDGF is also produced by many other cell types, including macrophages, osteoblasts, and fibroblasts.[37] PDGF has many functions in target cells and has been shown to stimulate proliferation, control chemotaxis (directed cell movement), enhance cell survival, and induce differentiation, all functions that are integral components of the tissue repair process.[36,37] It is not surprising then that PDGF also has many target cells including smooth muscle, pericytes, connective tissue fibroblasts, and mesenchymal stem cells (MSCs).[38] As such, successful use of PDGF as a bioactive factor is highly dependent on controlling where and when it acts during the healing cascade.

The current clinical product, recombinant human (rh) PDGF-BB, is made in yeast in a commercial process that first gained FDA approval for use in topical indications in soft-tissue wound healing (Regranex).[39] PDGF-BB has a short half-life when delivered without a carrier, but biologic activity can be extended by the use of a carrier such as tricalcium phosphate (TCP).[40] PDGF-BB interactions with specific carriers also prevent large amounts of growth factor from entering systemic circulation and initiating off-target effects. PDGF-BB has shown positive effects on healing in numerous animal studies including osteoporotic rat fracture healing, diabetic rat fracture healing, and rodent distraction osteogenesis.[41] These preclinical successes led to multicenter trials to ascertain the safety and efficacy of using rhPDGF-BB in foot and ankle fusion surgery as an alternative to autograft. Based on clear efficacy, FDA approval of rhPDGF-BB applied using TCP as carrier for foot and ankle fusions was achieved in 2012. Currently, AUGMENT, the drug name for rhPDGF-BB, is available in two formulations: as an injectable containing rhPDGF-BB, beta-TCP particles, and collagen or as an implant consisting of PDGF-BB and beta-TCP.[21] rhPDGF-BB has also demonstrated preliminary efficacy in clinical trials for periodontal repair.

There continue to be substantial efforts to expand the potential uses of rhPDGF-BB in tendon reattachment surgeries such as rotator cuff repair. However, successful enhancement of healing appears to be dependent on the specifics of the surgical model used in the study, the mode of rhPDGF-BB delivery, the concentration of PDGF-BB used, and the timing of factor application. For example, Condron et al[8] concluded in 2021 that there was no difference in strength after treatment of animal/human rotator cuff with PDGF-BB. PDGF-BB has also been unsuccessful in driving fusion in the setting of spine surgery, although the reasons for this lack of success remain to be determined. Niemiec et al[42] in a 2021 study noted that the presence of a polymorphism in the patient's PDGF-BB gene was associated with effectiveness of PDGF-BB therapy, suggesting that gene sequencing before treatment may make a difference in the successful use of PDGF-BB for shoulder injuries. An additional concern for using PDGF-BB is the fact that overactivity of PDGF has been linked to certain malignancies and other disorders that involve an excess of cell proliferation, including atherosclerosis, and fibrotic conditions.[43]

Future expansion of the uses of PDGF-BB depends on a greater understanding of the circumstances that allow for strong responses to this factor. Additionally, pairing PDGF-BB with an osteogenic stimulus may optimize the efficacy of both bioactive factors. Subbiah et al[44] suggested the potential use of PDGF in combination with vascular endothelial growth factor and low-dose bone morphogenetic protein (BMP)-2 in a model of vascularized tissue regeneration.

DEMINERALIZED BONE MATRIX

The therapeutic potential of active biologic factors present in bone matrix has long been recognized in orthopaedic settings. This realization led first to the individual use of allografts as substitutes for autografts in challenging orthopaedic surgical procedures and then to the development of demineralized bone matrix (DBM) as a product central to bone repair.[45] DBM is prepared by decalcifying cortical bone. The removal of calcium is thought to make more accessible the bioactive factors that are stored within the collagen matrix of bone. The fact that DBM has both collagen ECM and biologically active factors has led to its classification as both an osteoconductive and osteoinductive material.[46]

Currently, there are more than 50 commercially available DBM products. Forms of DBM include sponges, strips, injectable putty, paste, and paste mixed with chips. Properties of individual DBM formulations vary based on how the starting bone material was processed for demineralization, sterilization, and storage.[46] As the FDA considers DBM products to be minimally manipulated tissue rather than a biologic or device, no agency approval is required, and this fact has allowed for the lack of standardization of DBM products. The comparisons of the biologic factor content of individual DBM preparations that have taken place have found high variability in the bioactive factors present within DBM and in the amounts of factor available when present. Most constant for all DBMs subjected to analysis has been the presence of BMP-2 and BMP-7. Based on the available information, it is unclear why variability exists in the bioactive factor content of DBM. Possible sources of variability include how the bone used to make DBM was originally processed and sterilized; it may also be due to the source of the bone starting material itself as age, health, harvest methods, and site of harvest are known effectors of growth factor DBM content.

From a tissue repair/regeneration perspective, the best way to think about DBM may be to consider it as an autograft extender in spine, trauma, and bone defects where the lack of biomechanical strength of DBM would not allow for use as a bone graft substitute. Considering the fact that using DBM is highly cost effective and very safe, future uses that modulate DBM to best fit therapeutic need are likely to expand the therapeutic indications for this product. Possibilities include decorating DBM with mRNAs or DNAs for the bioactive factors discussed here, or creating designer ECMs from cartilage, tendon, and meniscus that could be used as autograft extenders or delivery systems for repair/regeneration of these tissues.[47] These specialized DBMs would be highly tissue specific, in the manner of the partially demineralized product created by Arthrex that targets restoration of a tendon-bone enthesis.[48]

THE BMP SUPERFAMILY

Urist was first to recognize that an interfibrillar protein complex purified from bone was able to induce de novo bone formation when implanted ectopically in rodents, and named this activity BMP in 1965. One of the most intriguing aspects of this finding was that the process initiated by the implantation of BMP resembled to a great degree the cellular events seen during embryonic endochondral ossification and in adult fracture repair. The first human BMP genes were cloned in 1988. It was at that time that it was realized that the BMP activity first identified by Urist was a combination of multiple individual related gene products that are deposited into bone matrix and individually possess osteoinductive activity.[49]

Many investigators using a variety of models provided substantial preclinical data to support the ability of recombinant human BMPs to induce de novo bone formation in a clinically relevant manner. These efforts led to eventual FDA approval for BMP-2 as an alternative for bone graft during spine fusion (2002), to augment tibial fracture repair (2006) and to aid bone regeneration in the oral cavity (2007).[22] OP-1 (recombinant human BMP-7) was granted a humanitarian device exemption for use as an alternative to bone grafting during management of recalcitrant long bone nonunion around this same time. In these settings, BMPs are used with a carrier that aids in retaining BMP at the site of application and helps to define the shape and volume of new bone produced.

There is now much information about the strengths and weaknesses of using recombinant human BMP-2; for some, the weaknesses of cost, difficulty in delivery, and potential for unwanted side effects outweigh the benefits of enhanced healing. For others, the opposite is true. There has been time to learn a great deal about the specific physiologic roles that BMP family members play in the body and this knowledge will be exceptionally useful in developing better indication-specific BMP products. An example of an indication-specific therapy based on a novel biology is the use of growth differentiation factor (GDF)-5 for cartilage repair/regeneration. Expression of GDF-5 during development suggests it has a fundamental role in synovial joint formation, consistent with the finding that single-nucleotide polymorphisms located in the 5′ untranslated region of the human GDF-5 gene are associated, at the genome-wide level, with osteoarthritis susceptibility.[50,51] Testing of GDF-5 in rodent models of articular cartilage injury and osteoarthritis demonstrated that intra-articular injection of recombinant human GDF-5 attenuated cartilage lesions, whereas implantation of GDF-5 gene-transfected autologous bone marrow stromal cells enhanced repair of full-thickness articular cartilage defects.[2] These findings provide a rationale for continued exploration of using exogenous GDF-5 to maintain cartilage homeostasis during osteoarthritis progression.

Another example of using knowledge of biology to develop better therapies is the recent success of BMP-6 for bone repair. BMP-6 is resistant to antagonism by noggin, a potent BMP antagonist made by skeletal cells. By evading capture by noggin, the amount of BMP-6 required for successful healing would be predicted to be much less than that of BMP-2, a molecule that binds to noggin with high affinity.[52] Recent studies have reported that low doses of recombinant human BMP-6 dispersed within an autologous blood coagulum successfully induced healing in distal radial fractures and tibial wedge osteotomy defects in patients enrolled in phase 1 trials.[10] The combination of BMP-6 and autologous blood coagulum was also shown to be efficacious in animal models of spine fusion and large segmental defects.[1]

Another approach, based on using knowledge of the specific ligand-receptor interactions that occur to promote BMP signaling, is the design of chimeric recombinant proteins, composed of specific regions of individual BMP family members that allow for enhanced receptor specificity. Allendorph et al[53] reported a strategy for creating chimeric BMP variants possessing unique receptor binding and cell signaling properties. They also reported that, like BMP-6, all of the highly potent chimeras possessed insensitivity to noggin. Using these findings as a starting point, Seeherman et al[3] detailed the construction of BMP chimeras with increased receptor binding by substituting BMP-6 and activin A receptor-binding domains into BMP-2 (BV-265/CM). When tested in a nonhuman primate bone repair model with a carrier optimized for chimera retention and tissue ingrowth, BV-265/CM was efficacious at concentrations ranging from $^1/_{10}$ to $^1/_{30}$ of the BMP-2/absorbable collagen sponge concentration approved for clinical use. Future uses of this chimera strategy may be a means to create BMP-like molecules tailored to specific clinical needs in orthopaedics.

An exciting potential future approach for therapies dependent on modulating BMP activity is the development of ligand traps that can be delivered systemically to regulate availability of specific BMP family molecules. Ligand traps are composed of the extracellular ligand-binding domain of a BMP receptor fused to an immunoglobulin fragment crystallizable domain (**Figure 2**). Once injected, ligand traps act as decoy receptors, capturing proteins that exhibit high-affinity binding to the receptor extracellular ligand-binding domain, thus preventing these molecules from activating target cells.[54] Preclinical studies using ligand traps to BMP family proteins collectively demonstrate that modulating signaling of these molecules can be highly beneficial in reducing disease burden in mouse models of chronic illnesses.[55] Many if not most of these chronic illnesses have skeletal manifestations and are confounding issues when treating patients with orthopaedic conditions. Because ligand traps are

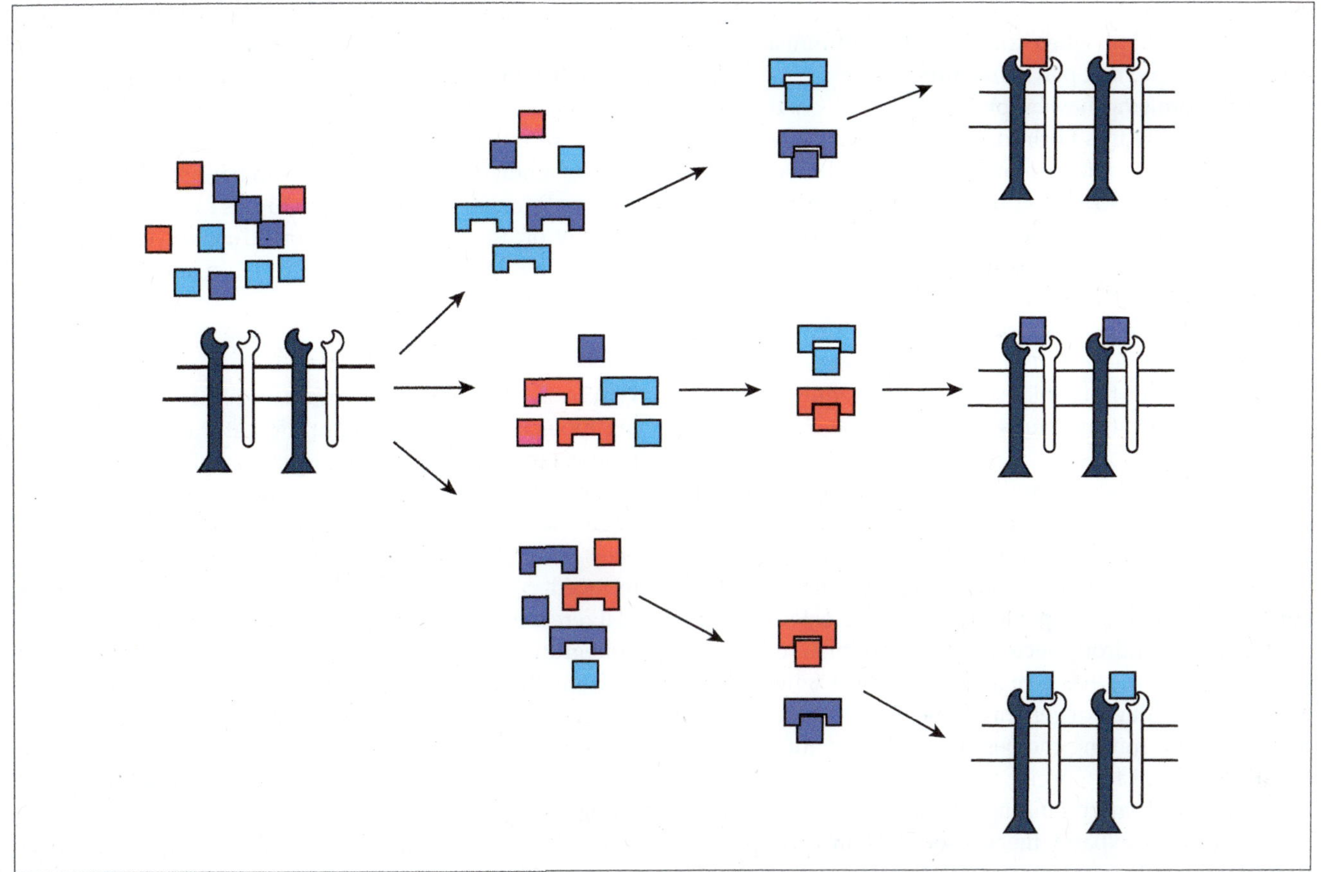

FIGURE 2 Schematic illustration shows ligand traps allow for specificity in receptor: ligand interactions. In the bone morphogenetic protein (BMP) signaling family, ligands compete for shared receptors. To direct specific interactions, ligand traps (shown as bridge-shaped moieties) can be engineered to interact with high specificity to single BMP-like molecules (shown as squares of specific colors). By altering the ligand traps present so that they capture BMPs that are not wanted, BMPs that are needed bind receptor and initiate signaling. As an example, if growth differentiation factor (GDF)-5 was the ligand of choice, ligand traps for BMP-2 and BMP-4 could be used to guarantee that GDF-5 binds receptor.

administered systemically, the need for carrier is obviated, allowing ease of use in combination with more invasive therapies.

PARATHYROID HORMONE AND FIBRIN-PARATHYROID HORMONE

Parathyroid hormone (PTH) is a peptide secreted by the parathyroid glands that regulates serum calcium concentration through effects on the bone, kidney, and intestine. Naturally occurring PTH consists of 84 amino acids; PTH (1-34) is a recombinant form consisting of the first 34 amino acids that retains all of the biologic activities of native PTH. PTH exerts its actions by binding to PTH receptors; PTHR1 is present at high levels on bone and kidney cells, whereas PTHR2 is present on cells of the central nervous system, pancreas, testes, and placenta.[56] The stimulatory effects of PTH on bone formation led to the development of teriparatide (recombinant PTH (1-34)) as a bone anabolic therapy for patients with osteoporosis. Also approved is abaloparatide, a 34-amino-acid synthetic PTH-related protein analog.[57]

PTH (1-34) has been evaluated as a potential therapy in a large number of animal models for skeletal repair including fracture healing, allografting, spinal arthrodesis, inflammatory arthritis, glucocorticoid-induced bone loss, and distraction osteogenesis.[11] In these studies, treatment with PTH enhances and accelerates the skeletal repair process, including improving the fusion rate and fusion mass in the setting of spine fusion. However, human clinical trials have not demonstrated a consistent positive influence of PTH in aiding or enhancing repair. A detailed analysis by Yamashita and McCauley[58] reviewed efficacy of PTH and concluded that although results were not overwhelming with regard to fracture healing, there was a general trend to promotion of repair. These results are consistent with a 2019 report by Jespersen et al,[59] who concluded that 90-day subcutaneous administration of PTH did not increase fusion volume or improve quality of fusion mass in elderly patients after noninstrumented spinal fusion surgery for degenerative spondylolisthesis. Conflicting results have also been reported when intact PTH is administered to patients with hip and pelvic fractures.[58]

One promising new approach is based on the local delivery of PTH in a fibrin matrix.[12] In vivo experiments evaluating bone defect filling in animals showed dose-dependent bone formation using the PTH-fibrin matrix, with evidence of both osteoconductive and osteoinductive bone-healing mechanisms. Based on promising animal data, Fibrin-PTH (KUR-113) has entered a phase 2 clinical trial for efficacy in spine fusion in humans in the United States. Phase 2 trials using fibrin-PTH alone or with a carrier in tibial plateau fractures requiring grafting and tibial shaft fractures have also shown promising results.[13]

PTH has also been examined for its chondroprotective and chondroregenerative activities. Studies in rodents have shown that systemic PTH administration decelerates cartilage matrix degradation and stimulates matrix synthesis in models of posttraumatic knee osteoarthritis where it is chondroprotective when administered at the time of injury and has a regenerative effect when delivered once cartilage degeneration begins.[4] Future studies aimed at determining the best time for systemic administration of PTH for specific orthopaedic indications and those that look at combining PTH with locally applied PTH may also expand the use of PTH in orthopaedic practice.

NELL-1

Nell-1 is a 90K protein, secreted as a trimer. It is made by many cell types and found at low levels in many tissues.[60] In the skeleton, Nell-1 is secreted by bone-forming cells as they begin to lay down ECM.[61] This observation coupled with loss-of-function and gain-of-function studies in transgenic mice led to the evaluation of Nell-1 in a variety of bone regeneration settings. Nell-1 was shown to enhance repair in calvarial defects, spine fusion, and critical size femoral defects when implanted with carriers such as TCP and DBM.[62-64] Unlike BMP-2, the target cell responding to Nell-1 is thought to be a committed osteoprogenitor and not a skeletal stem cell or MSC.[65] It has also been suggested that Nell-1 exerts its effects by binding to beta integrin and enhancing osteoprogenitor cell attachment to ECM, thus promoting osteoblast differentiation and inducing vascularization.[66] Data from these preclinical studies form the basis for the recent Human Research Ethics Committee approval for bone biologics to evaluate Nell-1 in degenerative disk disease in Australia.[14]

Although most preclinical studies use Nell-1 loaded onto a carrier, recent reports have suggested that Nell-1 can be effective when delivered systemically. James et al[65] observed that systemic administration of Nell-1 in mice induces expansion of MSC subset with Sca1 expression, whereas Tanjaya et al reported that a pegylated version of Nell-1, administered systemically, can promote fracture healing.[5,6]

Nell-1 may also have a role in cartilage. It is highly expressed in cartilage tumors,[67] and has been reported to aid repair of rabbit femoral condylar osteochondral defects when delivered on chitosan nanoparticles embedded in alginate gels.[67,68] Future studies focusing more specifically on the Nell-1 signal transduction pathway may provide a rationale for testing Nell-1 in additional orthopaedic indications.

WNT3A

Wnt3A is a member of a large family of secreted signaling molecules.[69] It is a potent regulator of stem cell self-renewal in a variety of organ systems where the addition of Wnt3a enables postnatal progenitors with modest innate regenerative capacity to proliferate.[70] Wnt3a has been used to expand the MSC produced from human-induced pluripotent stem cells in vitro and has been delivered via liposome encapsulation to accelerate osseointegration around implants placed in mouse femur.[71,72] Current clinical trials include the use of a liposomal formulation of recombinant human Wnt3A protein that is applied ex vivo, to harvested autologous bone grafts (autograft) to enhance the osteogenic properties of the autograft before reimplantation in patients undergoing posterolateral lumbar spinal fusion.[15] Because it is the only bioactive factor currently being tested for efficacy in expanding stem cell populations at skeletal sites, future studies using Wnt3A might target elderly patients or those individuals in whom healing responses have failed. Wnt3A might also be used to expand stem cell populations at the site of repair before treatment with agents that induce differentiation to bone-forming cells, or to articular chondrocytes, or to tenocytes.

ANTIBODIES TO THE WNT SIGNALING ANTAGONISTS SCLEROSTIN AND DICKKOPF-1

Several Wnt signaling antagonists regulate bone formation by binding to Wnt ligands or by competing with Wnt ligands for binding to Lrp5 and Lrp6, thus reducing levels of Wnt signaling.[69] This endogenous means of regulating Wnt activity raises the possibility that blocking Wnt antagonists might enhance bone formation. Antibodies that neutralize sclerostin (Scl-Ab, ramucirumab) have been shown to potently increase bone formation and are currently approved by the FDA for use as an osteoporosis therapy.[73,74] However, the drug's label carries a black box warning noting an increased risk of myocardial infarction, stroke, and cardiovascular death, making its use in bone regeneration dependent on patient comorbidities.[75] Dickkopf (DKK)-1 antibody treatment has shown benefits in fracture repair preclinical studies, consistent with the finding that DKK-1 expression is elevated in fracture tissues of patients with nonunion.[76] Paradoxically, sclerostin inhibition leads to a compensatory increase in DDK-1 expression.[7] To address antagonism of Wnt signaling by both sclerostin and DKK-1, a bispecific heterodimeric antibody that inhibits both molecules has been developed and has demonstrated efficacy in preclinical models where it potently increased bone formation and bone strength in intact bones and in bone fracture.[7] Future studies are required to support the therapeutic efficacy of this bispecific antibody for patients requiring augmentation of healing.

P-15 PEPTIDE

P-15 is a synthetic, non–arginine-glycine-aspartate-containing, 15-amino-acid peptide that is inexpensive to produce.[20] It is an analog of the cell-binding domain of type I collagen and mimics that native ability of collagen to direct cell attachment and oriented migration to a specific location.[77] MSCs cultivated on anorganic bone mineral (ABM) matrices coated with P-15 show increased expression of osteogenic genes as well as increased expression of factors that direct osteoblastic differentiation and osteoprogenitor cell differentiation.[78] This led to the development of P-15 combined with ABM for several orthopaedic indications. P-15 showed positive results when tested for efficacy for anterior lumbar interbody fusion in humans; it demonstrated solid fusion faster than autologous bone graft, with a low complication rate, and was deemed equivalent to results with BMP-2.[79-81] Regulated as a device, P-15, under the commercial name i-Factor Flex, was given breakthrough device designation for use in degenerative disk disease by the FDA.[82] Future developments include embedding P-15/ABM in a hydrogel carrier to evaluate as replacement for bone graft and expanding use in the spine setting by modifying the handling characteristics of the ABM carrier.

SUMMARY

Based on years of study of bioactive factors discussed in this chapter and the promising results obtained in specific tissue repair settings, it is likely that multiple strategies can be used to optimize bone repair depending on the desired cost, ease of delivery, and individual patient characteristics. Using bioactive factors in combinations, or in a temporal sequence, or as spatially restricted components of implantable matrices is a logical next step for molecules known to be safe and to have demonstrated efficacy for enhancing skeletal healing. To find the therapeutic agents with the best chance of successfully regenerating musculoskeletal tissues other than bone, the powerful genomic, metabolomic, and proteomic tools available are needed to allow more accurately define repair signaling cascades in the tissue of interest and systems biology used to determine how signaling networks govern repair cell behavior in that tissue. Because many of the bioactive factors discussed here are highly conserved signaling molecules, it would not be surprising to learn that they are part of the repair process in tissues other than bone, but they may need to be combined with yet-to-be identified factors to achieve successful repair. Inherent for success in cartilage, meniscus, tendon, and ligament will be a better understanding of the relationships between tissues attempting to repair and neighboring tissues that need to maintain homeostasis in the face of a changing local environment. Finally, by careful selection of patient populations through gene profiling, physicians may eventually have the ability to design individual instead of universal approaches that enhance healing.

REFERENCES

1. Grgurevic L, Erjavec I, Gupta M, et al: Autologous blood coagulum containing rhBMP6 induces new bone formation to promote anterior lumbar interbody fusion (ALIF) and posterolateral lumbar fusion (PLF) of spine in sheep. *Bone* 2020;138:115448.
2. Kania K, Colella F, Riemen AH, et al: Regulation of Gdf5 expression in joint remodelling, repair and osteoarthritis. *Sci Rep* 2020;10:157.
3. Seeherman HJ, Berasi SP, Brown CT, et al: A BMP/activin A chimera is superior to native BMPs and induces bone repair in nonhuman primates when delivered in a composite matrix. *Sci Transl Med* 2019;11:eaar4953.
4. Sampson ER, Hilton MJ, Tian Y, et al: Teriparatide as a chondroregenerative therapy for injury-induced osteoarthritis. *Sci Transl Med* 2011;3:101ra93.
5. Kwak J, Zara JN, Chiang M, et al: NELL-1 injection maintains long-bone quantity and quality in an ovariectomy-induced osteoporotic senile rat model. *Tissue Eng Part A* 2013;19:426.
6. Tanjaya J, Lord EL, Wang C, et al: The effects of systemic therapy of PEGylated NEL-Like protein 1 (NELL-1) on fracture healing in mice. *Am J Pathol* 2018;188:715.
7. Florio M, Gunasekaran K, Stolina M, et al: A bispecific antibody targeting sclerostin and DKK-1 promotes bone mass accrual and fracture repair. *Nature Commun* 2016:7;11505.
8. Condron NB, Kester BS, Tokish JM, et al: Nonoperative and operative soft-tissue, cartilage, and bony regeneration and orthopaedic biologics of the shoulder: An orthoregeneration network foundation review. *Arthroscopy* 2021;37:3200.
9. Sarment DP, Cooke JW, Miller SE, et al: Effect of rhPDGF-BB on bone turnover during periodontal repair. *J Clin Periodontol* 2006;33(2):135.
10. Chiari C, Grgurevic L, Bordukalo-Niksic T et al: Recombinant human BMP6 applied within autologous blood coagulum accelerates bone healing: Randomized controlled trial in high tibial osteotomy patients. *J Bone Miner Res* 2020;35:1893-1903.
11. Sain A, Bansal H, Pattabiraman K, Sharma V: Present and future scope of recombinant parathyroid hormone therapy in orthopaedics. *J Clin Orthop Trauma* 2021;17:54.
12. Arrighi I, Mark S, Alvisi M, von Rechenberg B, Hubbell JA, Schense JC: Bone healing induced by local delivery an an engineered parathyroid hormone prodrug. *Biomaterials* 2009;30:1763-1771.

13. Kuros Bio. Available at: https://kurosbio.com/fibrin-pth/. Accessed June 26, 2022.
14. Bone Biologics. Available at: https://www.bonebiologics.com/. Accessed June 26, 2022.
15. Clinical trial. Search parameters "Ankasa" and "liposomal formulation of recombinant human Wnt3A protein". Available at: https://clinicaltrials.gov/ct2/show/NCT04378543. Accessed June 26, 2022.
16. Padhi D, Jang G, Stouch B, Fang L, Posvar E: Single-dose, placebo-controlled, randomized study of AMG 785, a sclerostin monoclonal antibody. *J Bone Miner Res* 2011;26:19.
17. Munshi NC, Abonour R, Beck JT, et al: Early evidence of anabolic bone activity of BHQ880, a fully human anti-DKK1 neutralizing antibody: Results of a phase 2 study in previously untreated patients with smoldering multiple myeloma at risk for progression. *Blood* 2012;120:331.
18. Edenfield WJ, Richards DA, Vukelja SJ, et al: A phase 1 study evaluating the safety and efficacy of DKN-01, an investigational monoclonal antibody (Mab) in patients (pts) with advanced non-small cell lung cancer. *J Clin Oncol* 2014;32(suppl 15):8068.
19. Search terms "Romosozumab, bone, United States". Available at: www.clinicatrials.gov. Accessed June 26, 2022.
20. Qian JJ, Bhatnagar RS: Enhanced cell attachment to anorganic bone mineral in the presence of a synthetic peptide related to collagen. *J Biomed Mater Res* 1996;31:545.
21. Solchaga LA, Hee CK, Roach S, Snel LB: Safety of recombinant human platelet-derived growth factor-BB Augment bone graft. *J Tissue Eng* 2012;3(1):2041731412442668.
22. Rosen V, Gamer LW, Lyons KM: Bone morphogenetic proteins and the skeleton, in *Principles of Bone Biology*, ed 3. Academic Press-Elsevier, 2008, vol 2, p 1167.
23. Steed DL: Clinical evaluation of recombinant human platelet-derived growth factor for the treatment of lower extremity diabetic ulcers. *J Vasc Surg* 1995;21(1):71.
24. Vaccaro AR, Chiba K, Heller JG, et al: Bone grafting alternatives in spinal surgery. *Spine J* 2002;2:206.
25. Arnold PM, Sasso RC, Janssen ME, et al: Efficacy of i-Factor bone graft versus autograft in anterior cervical discectomy and fusion: Results of the prospective, randomized, single-blinded food and drug administration investigational device exemption study. *Spine* 2016;41(13):1075.
26. Package insert. Available at: https://www.accessdata.fda.gov/drugsatfda_docs/label/2017/208743lbl.pdf. Accessed June 26, 2022.
27. Foster TE, Puskas BL, Mandelbaum BR, Gerhardt MB, Rodeo SA: Platelet-rich plasma: From basic science to clinical applications. *Am J Sports Med* 2009;37:2259.
28. Le ADK, Enweze L, DeBaun MR, Dragoo JL: Current clinical recommendations for use of Platelet-Rich plasma. *Curr Rev Musculoskelet Med* 2018;11:624.
29. Castillo TN, Pouliot MA, Kim HJ, Dragoo JL: Comparison of growth factor and platelet concentration from commercial platelet-rich plasma separation systems. *Am J Sports Med* 2011;39:266.
30. Zitsch BP, James CR, Crist BD, Stoker AM, Della Rocca GJ, Cook JL: A prospective randomized double-blind clinical trial to assess the effects of leukocyte-reduced platelet-rich plasma on pro-inflammatory, degradative, and anabolic biomarkers after closed pilon fractures. *J Orthop Res* 2022;40(4):925-932.
31. Mazzocca AD, McCarthy MBR, Chowaniec DM, et al: Platelet-rich plasma differs according to preparation method and human variability. *J Bone Joint Surg Am* 2012;94:308.
32. Sundman EA, Cole BJ, Fortier LA: Growth factor and catabolic cytokine concentrations are influenced by the cellular composition of platelet-rich plasma. *Am J Sports Med* 2011;39:2135.
33. Obana KK, Schallmo MS, Hong IS, et al: Current trends on orthobiologics. An 11-year review of the orthopedic literature. *Am J Sports Med* 2021;50(11):3121-3129.
34. Heldin CH: Platelet-derived growth factor (PDGF), in *Encyclopedia of Hormones*. Academic Press, 2003, p 231.
35. Fredriksson L, Hong L, Eriksson U: The PDGF family: Four gene products form five dimeric isoforms. *Cytokine Growth Factor Rev* 2004;4:197.
36. Heldin CH, Westermark B: Mechanism of action and in vivo role of platelet derived growth factor. *Physiol Rev* 1999;79:1283.
37. Alvarez RH, Kantarjian HM, Cortes JE: Biology of platelet derived growth factor and its involvement in disease. *Mayo Clin Proc* 2006;81:1241.
38. Andrae J, Gallini R, Betsholtz C: Role of platelet-derived growth factors in physiology and medicine. *Genes Dev* 2008;22:1276.
39. Borena BM, Martens A, Broeckx SY, et al: Regenerative skin wound healing in mammals: State-of-the-art on growth factor and stem cell based treatments. *Cell Physiol Biochem* 2015;36(1):1-23.
40. DiGiovanni CW, Lin S, Pinzur M: Recombinant human PDGF-BB in foot and ankle fusion. *Expert Rev Med Devices* 2012;9(2)111-122.
41. Hollinger JO, Hart CE, Hirsch SN, Lynch S, Friedlaender GE: Recombinant human platelet-derived growth factor: Biology and clinical applications. *J Bone Joint Surg Am* 2008;90(suppl 1):48.
42. Niemiec P, Szyluk K, Balcerzyk A, et al: Why PRP works only on certain patients with tennis elbow? Is PDGFB gene a key for PRP therapy effectiveness? A prospective cohort study. *BMC Musculoskelet Disord* 2021;22:710.
43. Roskoski R Jr. The role of small molecule platelet-derived growth factor receptor inhibitors in the treatment of neoplastic disorders. *Pharmacol Res* 2018;129:65.
44. Subbiah R, Ruehle MA, Klosterhoff BS, et al: Triple growth factor delivery promotes functional bone regeneration following composite musculoskeletal trauma. *Acta Biomater* 2021;127:180.

45. Zhang H, Yang L, Yang X-G, et al: Demineralized bone matrix carriers and their clinical applications: An overview. *Orthop Surg* 2019;11:725.

46. Gruskin E, Doll BA, Futrell FW, Schmitz JP, Hollinger JO: Demineralized bone matrix in bone repair: History and use. *Adv Drug Deliv Rev* 2012;64:1063.

47. Pigeot S, Klein T, Gullotta F, et al: Manufacturing of human tissues as off-the-shelf grafts programmed to induce regeneration. *Adv Mater* 2021;33(43):e2103737.

48. Sundar S, Pendergrass CJ, Blunn GW: Tendon bone healing can be enhanced by demineralized bone matrix: A functional and histological study. *J Biomed Mater Res B Appl Biomater* 2009;88(1):115.

49. Salazar VS, Gamer LW, Rosen V: BMP signaling in skeletal development, disease and repair. *Nature Rev Endocrinol* 2016;12:203.

50. Muthuirulan P, Zhao D, Young M, et al: Joint disease-specificity at the base-pair level. *Nat Commun* 2021;12:4161.

51. Jia B, Jiang Y, Xu Y, Wang Y, Li T: Correlation between growth differentiation factor 5 (rs143383) gene polymorphism and knee osteoarthritis: An updated systematic review and meta-analysis. *J Orthop Surg Res* 2012;16:146.

52. Song K, Krause C, Shi S, et al: Identification of a key residue mediating bone morphogenetic protein (BMP)-6 resistance to noggin inhibition allows for engineered BMPs with superior agonist activity. *J Biol Chem* 2010;285:12169.

53. Allendorph GP, Read JD, Kawakami Y, Kelber JA, Isaacs MJ, Choe S: Designer TGFß superfamily ligands with diversified functionality. *PLoS One* 2011;6:e26402.

54. Martinez-Hackert E, Sundan A, Holien T: Receptor binding competition: A paradigm for regulating TGF-beta family action. *Cytokine Growth Factor Rev* 2021;57:39-54.

55. Yung LM, Yang P, Joshi S, et al: ACTRIIA-Fc rebalances activin/GDF versus BMP signaling in pulmonary hypertension. *Sci Transl Med* 2020;12(543):eaaz5660.

56. Leder B: Parathyroiid hormone and parathyroid hormone-related protein analogs in osteoporosis therapy. *Curr Osteoporos Rep* 2017;15:110.

57. Forteo approved for osteoporosis treatment. *FDA Consum* 2003;37:4.

58. Yamashita J, McCauley LK: Effects of intermittent administration of parathyroid hormone and parathyroid hormone-related protein on fracture healing: A narrative review of animal and human studies. *JBMR Plus* 2019;3:e10250.

59. Jespersen AB, Andresen ADK, Jacobsen MK, Andersen MØ, Carreon LY: Does systemic administration of parathyroid hormone after noninstrumented spinal fusion surgery improve fusion rates and fusion mass in elderly patients compared to placebo in patients with degenerative lumbar spondylolisthesis? *Spine* 2019;44:157.

60. Kuroda S, Oyasu M, Kawakami M, et al: Biochemical characterization and expression analysis of neural thrombospondin-1 like proteins NELL1 and NELL2. *Biochem Biophys Res Commun* 1999;265:79.

61. Zhang X, Carpenter D, Bokui N, Soo C, Miao S, Truong T: Overexpression of Nell-1 a craniosynostosis-associated gene, induces apoptosis in osteoblasts during craniofacial development. *J Bone Miner Res* 2003;18:2126.

62. Aghaloo T, Cowan CM, Chou YF, et al: Nell-1-induced bone regeneration in calvarial defects. *Am J Pathol* 2006;169:903.

63. Li W, Lee M, Whang J, et al: Delivery of lyophilized Nell-1 in a rat spinal fusion model. *Tissue Eng Part A* 2010;16(9):2861.

64. Lai K, Xi Y, Du X, et al: Activation of Nell-1 in BMSC sheet promotes implant osseointegration through regulating Runx2/Osterix axis. *Front Cell Dev Biol* 2020;8:868.

65. James AW, Shen J, Tsuei R, et al: NELL-1 induces Sca-1+ mesenchymal progenitor cell expansion in models of bone maintenance and repair. *JCI Insight* 2017;2:e92573.

66. Shen J, James AW, Chung J, et al: NELL-1 promotes cell adhesion and differentiation via Integrinβ1. *J Cell Biochem* 2012;113:3620.

67. Shen J, LaChaud G, Shrestha S, et al: NELL-1 expression in tumors of cartilage. *J Orthop* 2015;12:S223.

68. Siu RK, Zara JN, Hou Y, et al: NELL-1 promotes cartilage regeneration in an in vivo rabbit model. *Tissue Eng Part A* 2012;18:252.

69. Baron R, Kneissel M: WNT signaling in bone homeostasis and disease: From human mutations to treatments. *Nat Med* 2013;19:179.

70. He L, Zhou J, Chen M, et al: Parenchymal and stromal tissue regeneration of tooth organ by pivotal signals reinstated in decellularized matrix. *Nat Mater* 2019;18:627.

71. Bruschi M, Sahu N, Singla M, et al: A quick and efficient method for the generation of immunomodulatory MSC from human iPSC. *Tissue Eng Part A* 2022;28(9-10)433.

72. Li Z, Yaun X, Arioka M, et al: Pro-osteogenic effects of WNT in a mouse model of bone formation around femoral implants. *Calcif Tissue Int* 2021;108:240.

73. Ominsky MS, Vlasseros F, Jolette J, et al: Two doses of sclerostin antibody in cynomologous monkeys increases bone formation, bone mineral density, and bone strength. *J Bone Miner Res* 2010;25:948-959.

74. McClung MR, Grauer A, Boonen S, et al: Romosozumab in postmenopausal women with low bone mineral density. *N Engl J Med* 2014;370;412-420.

75. Mullard A: FDA approves first-in-class osteoporosis drug. *Nat Rev Drug Discov* 2019:18;411.

76. Li X, Grisanti M, Fan W, et al: Dickkopf-1 regulates bone formation in young growing rodents and upon traumatic injury. *J Bone Miner Res* 2011:26;2610.

77. Bhatnagar RS, Qian JJ, Wedrychowska A, Sadeghi M, Wu YM, Smith N: Design of biomimetic habitats for tissue engineering with P-15, a synthetic peptide analogue of collagen. *Tissue Eng* 1999;5:53.

78. Hanks T, Atkinson BL: Comparison of cell viability on anorganic bone matrix with or without P-15 cell binding peptide. *Biomaterials* 2004;25:4831.

79. Lindley EM, Guerra FA, Krauser JT, Matos SM, Burger EL, Patel VV: Small peptide (P-15) bone substitute efficacy in a rabbit cancellous bone model. *J Biomed Mater Res B Appl Biomater* 2010;94:463.

80. Mobbs RJ, Maharaj M, Rao PJ: Clinical outcomes and fusion rates following anterior lumbar interbody fusion with bone graft substitute i-FACTOR, an anorganic bone matrix/P-15 composite. *J Neurosurg Spine* 2014;21:867.

81. Hestehave Pedersen R, Rasmussen M, Overgaard S, Ding M: Effects of P-15 peptide coated hydroxyapatite on tibial defect repair in vivo in normal and osteoporotic rats. *Biomed Res Int* 2015;2015:253858.

82. Cerapedics. Available at: https://cerapedics.com/i-factor-and-p-15. Accessed June 26, 2022.

CHAPTER

4 Gene Therapy

Steven C. Ghivizzani, PhD • Christopher H. Evans, PhD

INTRODUCTION

Gene therapy was developed as a means of treating, and potentially curing, so-called mendelian diseases resulting from mutations in single genes (monogenic diseases). However, in the field of orthopaedics, rather than rare monogenic conditions, gene transfer is being developed for targeted, sustained delivery of therapeutic gene products for treatment of common, yet problematic, multigenic diseases and injuries involving the musculoskeletal system.[1] Following injury, endogenous repair or regenerative processes in connective tissues can be slow and often result in repair tissue of inferior quality and strength. Skeletal structures are also susceptible to chronic inflammatory and degenerative conditions that present significant clinical challenges.

The concept of using gene therapy to address such conditions arose in concert with advances in molecular biology and DNA sequencing technologies that identified a wide array of gene products with the potential to augment skeletal repair and inhibit or reverse degenerative disease. However, there was no clinically reasonable way to deliver these products for a period of time that matched the needs of skeletal tissue repair, typically requiring weeks to months, or degenerative conditions, such as osteoarthritis, tendinosis, and degenerative disk disease, which are chronic, lifelong conditions. With the exception of monoclonal antibodies, most gene products have brief half-lives in vivo (minutes to hours).

By delivering the coding sequence for a therapeutic protein (typically in the form of a complementary DNA [cDNA]) under independent control to cells in the pathologic environment, the biosynthetic machinery of the modified cells can be directed to overexpress the therapeutic gene product for an extended duration, in some cases indefinitely.[1] The ability to target gene delivery specifically to sites of need limits unwanted exposure of nonaffected tissues to transgene products. Successful of proof-of-concept studies in rheumatoid arthritis[2] and subsequent progression to clinical trial[3] inspired exploration of similar strategies for a wide range of orthopaedic conditions, including osteoarthritis, skeletal fracture, cartilage repair, intervertebral disk degeneration (IVDD), and ligament and tendon repair, among others.

COMPONENTS OF A SUCCESSFUL GENE THERAPY

The development of an effective gene-based therapy is a highly complex undertaking, requiring the integration of multiple biologic components into a treatment platform that addresses the clinical need while avoiding adverse consequences. At a minimum, there is a need to identify a therapeutic transgene, design and construct an expression cassette, select and manufacture an appropriate vector, confirm in vitro potency, determine a preferred delivery route, and perform preclinical studies in animal models. Each of these components is described. Gene editing and RNA therapeutics are discussed only briefly.

Selection of Transgene Product: Secreted Versus Intracellular

To date, investigations of orthopaedic gene therapy have primarily focused on the delivery of cDNA-encoding bioactive proteins that are secreted from the modified cells. Several distinct advantages favor this approach. First, the cDNA of signaling molecules tend to be small and can be inserted fairly easily in the limited space available in most viral vectors. Second, a relatively small population of genetically modified cells can release transgene products into the extracellular fluids to affect regional cell populations in a paracrine manner. Further, the soluble gene products present in conditioned media, biologic fluids, and tissue homogenates can be quantified by enzyme-linked immunosorbent assay, allowing compilation of dose response and pharmacokinetic profiles of both vector and gene product to define the functional parameters of the procedure.[4]

Alternatively, numerous gene products with therapeutic potential function intracellularly. Because there is no common mechanism by which exogenous proteins can be taken in by a cell and retain function, gene transfer is the only method by which the activities of certain types of molecules, for example, nuclear receptors, transcription factors etc., can be exploited for clinical use. Because

Dr. Ghivizzani or an immediate family member has stock or stock options held in Genascence Inc. Dr. Evans or an immediate family member serves as a paid consultant to or is an employee of Cellastra Inc., L&J Inc., and Orthogen AG and has stock or stock options held in Cellastra Inc., Genascence Inc., Orthogen AG, and TissueGene.

the effects of the gene product are limited specifically to the population of modified cells, the chance of adverse response from unintended diffusion to a nontarget tissue is eliminated. On the downside, overexpression of various transcription factors essential for chondrogenic differentiation and bone formation, such as RUNX2 and SOX9, has been shown to induce adverse skeletal phenotypes[5] and tumorigenic activation.[6] From a technical standpoint, for procedures involving direct in vivo gene delivery, for an intracellular gene product to induce a meaningful response at the tissue level or organ level, a large proportion of the resident cell population must be genetically modified by the vector. Regardless of vector type, functional in vivo gene delivery of this magnitude is an extremely challenging undertaking, even with viral systems in small laboratory animals. Further, because efficacy is a function of the number and locations of the cell populations modified by the vector (rather than total protein expression), exhaustive marker studies are required to assess and optimize dosing relative to the density and distribution of transduced cell populations in the target environment.

Expression Cassette

Transgene

Once a candidate gene product is selected, commercial synthesis of the coding sequence permits codon optimization to enhance translation efficiency and additional sequence modifications to facilitate subcloning into the transfer vector. Following synthesis, the designer transgene is inserted into an expression cassette containing the appropriate cis-acting DNA sequences (promoter, enhancer, etc.) for efficient transcription, RNA processing, and protein translation in the milieu of the target tissue.

Promoter

The greatest hurdle to an effective treatment platform is making enough transgene products for a sufficient length of time to mediate a meaningful response. Because problems with overproduction are somewhat rare, for most applications, a strong constitutively active promoter sequence is used to drive RNA synthesis. Those used most often include the human elongation factor 1 alpha and chicken beta actin promoters, the immediate-early cytomegalovirus promoter/enhancer and the CAG hybrid promoter composed of the cytomegalovirus enhancer, the chicken beta actin promoter and first intron, and the splice acceptor site of the rabbit beta globin gene.[7,8] Each has high basal level of activation and provides near maximal levels of constitutive expression. Though continuously active, expression levels often vary among cell types and fluctuate with metabolic state. Empirical testing in vivo is recommended.

Inducible promoter systems engineered with response elements for specific transcription factors can enable selective activation of transgene expression under specific growth conditions, such as inflammation or hypoxia, or in the presence of an exogenous activator such as tetracycline as in the tetracycline/on system.[8] Alternatively, tissue-specific promoters provide the advantage of limiting transgene expression to a desired cell type or tissue, but low activity and/or large size can limit their use.

Auxiliary Elements

Additional transcribed but noncoding sequence elements can be inserted into the DNA template of the expression cassette, including artificial introns for RNA splicing, polyadenylation sequences, and post-transcriptional response elements that provide signals for enhanced nuclear export, translation, and mRNA stability.[7] Additional regulatory elements (eg, Kozac sequences, micro RNA-binding sequences) can be engineered into the 5′ and 3′ untranslated regions of the transcript to fine-tune mRNA translation.

VECTORS FOR GENE TRANSFER

Because the uptake of exogenous nucleic acids by mammalian cells, both in vivo and in culture, is highly inefficient, a delivery vehicle, or vector, is required to ferry the expression cassette into the target cell, facilitate its trafficking to the nucleus, and then stabilize its expression. Vector development over the past 50 years or so has followed two distinct tracks: (1) vectors derived from viruses[9] and (2) those that are not.[10] For the sake of clarity, viral-mediated gene transfer occurs through the process of transduction, whereas nonviral gene delivery occurs through transfection.

Viral Vectors

A virus is a biologic entity composed of genetic material (RNA or DNA) packaged in a protective shell (capsid). Through evolution, viruses have fine-tuned both their genome and capsid components for peak transduction efficiency making them attractive as vectors. The challenges lie with engineering a recombinant vector that is technically manipulable, maintains efficient transduction, and can be manufactured at high titer while at the same time eliminating its ability to reproduce in the host and cause pathology.[9]

In general, a viral vector is created by removing the coding sequences from its genome while leaving in place the noncoding, cis-acting sequence elements required for efficient replication and packaging into the viral capsid. Because the genome length of the wild type virus approximates the maximum amount of genetic material that can be efficiently inserted into the viral capsid, the removal of viral genes creates room for insertion of an exogenous expression cassette. Transfer and expression of the viral coding sequences required for replication in a complementing cell line allows for selective replication and packaging of the vector DNA containing the cis-acting recognition sequences. The resulting recombinant viral particles can infect and transduce target cells but can only replicate in the complementing cell line. Removal of viral coding sequences from the vector genome precludes their expression in transduced cell populations, which reduces their immunogenicity and prolongs transgene expression (discussed later). As each viral vector is unique, with different genomes, host-cell range (tropism), and molecular mechanisms for transduction, the key to a successful platform involves tailoring the vector and expression cassette to the therapeutic needs of the target disease. The following sections describe the salient features of the most common viral vector systems in clinical gene therapy: adenovirus, adeno-associated virus (AAV), and retrovirus (gamma retrovirus [γ-retrovirus] and lentivirus) (**Table 1**).

Adenovirus

Vectors derived from adenovirus have been widely used in orthopaedic research because of their broad tropism, high-level infectivity, and ease of propagation. Wild-type adenovirus is common in nature and generally associated with self-limiting respiratory tract infections. The viral capsid is a nonenveloped icosahedron approximately 80 to 100 nm in diameter that encases a linear, double-stranded DNA genome approximately 35 kb in length. The genome is flanked on either end by inverted terminal repeat (ITR) sequences, with a short psi sequence positioned immediately downstream from the 5′ (left hand) ITR that marks the DNA for packaging into the adenovirus capsid. The wild type genome encodes approximately 35 proteins, which are sequentially expressed in the early (E) and late phases of viral infection and replication.[9]

Early-generation adenovirus vectors were created by removing the immediate E1A and E1B genes, and later the E3 gene, creating room for insertion of an expression cassette of approximately 7.5 kb. Because expression of the E1A gene is required for transcription of the other viral genes, removal of the E1 locus from the adenovirus genome renders the vector replication deficient in normal cells. The vector is propagated by infection of the widely used 293 cells, derived from a human embryonic kidney cell line. A total of 293 cells were engineered to stably harbor the left hand in 11% of the wild-type adenovirus genome, and constitutively express the E1A and E1B proteins required for activation of the remaining viral genes that reside on the vector genome.[11] Infection of 293 cells with recombinant adenovirus provides the E1 proteins in trans-, complementing the defective vector genome to allow its replication. The ease of propagating recombinant adenovirus vectors in this way is very convenient but requires vigilant quality control because serial propagation selects for virions that have jettisoned their transgene cassette baggage to replicate more efficiently.

Adenovirus vectors offer several advantages for gene transfer applications: (1) highly efficient transduction of dividing and nondividing cells from a wide range of species and tissues, (2) a nonintegrating genome maintained as an extrachromosomal (episomal) element in nondividing cells; (3) high-level transgene expression with rapid onset; (4) a relatively large packaging capacity; and (5) technically straightforward methods of vector propagation. A distinct limitation of adenovirus vectors is the tendency to provoke immune responses against transduced cell populations in vivo. Despite removal of the E1 locus, leaky readthrough transcription allows low-level expression of the residual adenovirus coding sequences in transduced cells leading to neutralizing immune reactions.

To reduce the immunogenicity of vector-modified cells, third-generation vectors were developed in which all viral coding sequences were removed from the vector genome, leaving only the flanking ITRs and the *psi* packaging sequence. These gutted or high-capacity vectors accommodate up to 36 kb of exogenous DNA but require coinfection with a helper adenovirus for replication. Although removal of the viral coding sequences reduces the immunogenicity of the transduced cells and prolongs transgene expression, innate immune responses to the capsid protein and viral infection cause the vector to be inflammatory;[12] elimination of the helper virus from vector preparations presents an additional challenge.[13]

Because of the prevalence of wild-type adenovirus in nature, much of the human population is seropositive for neutralizing antibodies (NAbs) against one or more human variants, which renders common adenoviral vectors ineffective. To address this, vector systems have been developed from nonhuman variants common in other species. Currently, adenoviral vectors account for approximately 50% of the clinical trials worldwide, primarily for vaccination and anticancer protocols. Notably, two different adenoviral vectors, both developed from variants found in chimpanzees, are used to deliver and express the coding sequence for the SARS-CoV-2 spike protein and are in widespread use as vaccines against COVID-19.[14]

Adeno-associated Virus

Recombinant adeno-associated virus (rAAV) is another nonintegrating viral vector with the ability to transduce both dividing and nondividing cells.[15] Compared with other prominent viral vector systems, rAAV is accepted as the least toxic and, relative to adenovirus vectors, induces relatively low innate and adaptive immunity against transduced cells in vivo. Though its genome remains episomal, rAAV is capable of achieving long-term (>10 years) transgene expression in quiescent cell populations in vivo.[16] The first human trial of AAV-mediated gene delivery was reported in 1998 for cystic fibrosis. Because of its favorable safety profile in this and more than 200 subsequent clinical studies, rAAV is currently the

TABLE 1 Properties of the Main Classes of Vectors Used for Gene Therapy

Vector System	Composition	Advantages	Limitations
Viral			
Adenovirus	dsDNA virus	Broad tropism Infects dividing and nondividing cells High efficiency High levels of transgene expression Ease of production Mid-size cDNA capacity Best suited for applications requiring brief expression	Leaky expression of viral antigens Activates innate and adaptive immunity Transient gene expression Capsid-specific NAb from wt infection or previous vector delivery limits readministration
High-capacity Adenovirus	dsDNA virus	High efficiency Reduced immunogenicity of transduced cells Large cDNA capacity	Innate immune response Capsid-specific NAb from wt infection or previous vector delivery limits readministration Difficult to manufacture Transient expression Contaminating helper adenovirus
AAV	ssDNA virus sc dsDNA	Infects dividing and nondividing cell types No viral coding sequences Straightforward vector composition Vector genome can be packaged in alternate capsids Long-term expression in postmitotic cells Excellent safety profile at moderate dose Self-complementary variant provides increased expression with rapid onset	Small packaging capacity Capsid-specific NAb from wild type infection or previous vector delivery may limit readministration
Lentivirus	RNA virus	Integrating virus: Stable expression Highly efficient transduction Infects dividing and nondividing cells Amplification in proliferating cells In vivo and ex vivo applications Immune stealthy In multiple clinical trials Pseudotyping allows broad tropism, increased stability	Integrating potential for insertional oncogenesis Concerns over replication competent virus 4 plasmid cotransfection, variable titer
γ-Retrovirus	RNA virus	Integrating virus: Stable expression Amplification in proliferating cells Immune stealthy In multiple clinical trials Pseudotyping allows broad tropism, increased stability	Requirement for proliferating cells limits applications to ex vivo approaches Potential for insertional oncogenesis
Nonviral			
Plasmid DNA	Circular DNA	Large capacity Stability Inexpensive to produce No adaptive immune response	Inefficient uptake Transient expression Inflammatory—innate immune reactivity

AAV = adeno-associated virus; cDNA = complementary DNA, dsDNA = double-stranded DNA, NAb = neutralizing antibody, sc dsDNA = self-complementary double-stranded DNA, ssDNA = single-stranded DNA, wt = wild type preferred vector system for human protocols involving in vivo gene delivery.

Wild-type AAV is a small (<50 nm diameter), nonenveloped, single-stranded DNA virus that is nonpathogenic in humans. Naturally replication defective, wild-type AAV requires coinfection with a second virus (eg, adenovirus or herpes simplex virus) to provide helper functions necessary for replication.[17] The 4.7 kb genome harbors four open reading frames that contain the *rep* and *cap* genes and coding sequences for two accessory proteins. ITR sequences flank the viral genome and are the only required sequence elements for vector replication and packaging; thus, the vector genome is remarkably simple and comprises an expression cassette with an ITR sequence on either end. The packaging limit of approximately 5 kb precludes the use of large cDNA and promoter sequences and complex multigenic cassettes. The viral vector is propagated by cotransfection of 293 cells with the vector plasmid and plasmid(s) harboring the AAV *rep* and *cap* genes and the adenoviral helper functions.[15]

More than 1,000 naturally occurring wild-type AAV variants have been identified, along with at least 12 natural serotypes, which preferentially bind to various cell surface glycans and secondary receptors.[18] Following entry into the cell, the virus is trafficked through late endosomal and lysosomal compartments before being shuttled into the nucleus where the genome is unencapsidated. The single-stranded DNA genome of both wild-type AAV and the conventional rAAV vector requires second-strand synthesis before it can be recognized by the transcriptional apparatus of the infected cell.[15] The ITR sequences facilitate intermolecular and intramolecular recombination to form concatenated double-stranded DNA circles, which provide stability and enable the vector genomes to be maintained as episomal elements. In mesenchymal tissues, where the resident cell populations are largely quiescent, the requirement for second-strand DNA synthesis can limit transgene expression. However, double-stranded self-complementary AAV genomes have been engineered that are fully functional at the time of infection.[15,19] The transduction efficiency of self-complementary AAV vectors is substantially higher than that of single-stranded AAV vectors in mesenchymal cells and tissues, with rapid onset of expression—often within 24 hours of delivery.[20] However, the self-complementary modification reduces the vector genome by one-half (approximately 2.5 kb),[19] which further restricts the size and composition of the expression cassette.

Wild-type AAV is prevalent in nature and, though nonpathogenic, childhood infections are common and typically induce a potent humoral immune response and life-long production of NAb specific to the capsid of the infecting serotype. Depending on location, anywhere from 30% to 70% of the human population have circulating NAb to one or multiple AAV variants. The ability to cross-package (or pseudotype) the vector genome in different capsids alters its tropism, providing the opportunity to increase the efficiency of gene transfer in specific tissues, as well as the potential to evade recognition by preexisting capsid-specific NAb. Engineering the AAV capsid to obtain designer vectors with enhanced properties for specific applications is currently an area of intense investigation.[15]

Retroviral Vectors

Vectors derived from members of the retrovirus family, γ-retrovirus and lentivirus, are spherical enveloped viruses approximately 100 nm in diameter whose genomes are composed of two copies of single-stranded RNA of the sense (+) strand.[21] Nonenveloped viruses, for example, adenovirus and AAV, reproduce by lytic infection, releasing thousands of viral progeny in a burst that kills the host cell. Retroviruses, in contrast, are enveloped and reproduce by continuous budding from the surface of the infected cell. Though the genome is encased in a protective capsid, the outer envelope comprises lipid bilayer pilfered from the plasma membrane of the host cell as the virus is released from the surface.

Retroviruses can be classified as either simple or complex based on the composition and organization of their genome. γ-retroviruses, which harbor only three genes, are considered to be simple, whereas lentiviruses with nine overlapping coding regions are complex.[9] The genome of the retrovirus family is flanked on each end by complex long terminal repeat (LTR) sequences containing strong promoter/enhancer elements that drive expression of the entire viral genome. Other cis-acting elements positioned downstream of the 5′ LTR include sequences for replication priming and a *psi*-sequence for encapsidation. All retroviral genomes contain three core genes: *gag*, *pol*, and *env*. For both types of retroviral vectors, the endogenous *env* gene, which codes for the surface glycoprotein used for cell-surface receptor binding, is often replaced with the coding sequence for the vesicular stomatitis virus glycoprotein.[22] Pseudotyping the virus in this manner dramatically expands the tropism of the vector, enhances infectivity, and increases the stability of the vector particle during production. The *pol* gene codes for reverse transcriptase and integrase proteins that are carried within the viral envelope.[22] The viral reverse transcriptase converts the RNA genome to double-stranded DNA, which the integrase inserts into the host genome as a provirus, preferentially targeting regions that are transcriptionally active.[23] Vector integration provides the potential for stable expression of the transgene, which can be amplified with subsequent cell divisions in vitro and in vivo. Retroviral vectors are highly infectious, elicit relatively weak immune responses, and, depending on the biology of the target cell, can support long-term expression of therapeutic gene products.

γ-Retrovirus

The vector derived from the genome of Moloney murine leukemia virus was among the first γ-retroviral vector systems developed and the first used successfully in a clinical trial.[24,25] As γ-retroviruses are unable to penetrate the nuclear envelope of an infected cell, they can only gain access to the host genome during mitosis, when the nuclear envelope is disassembled.[24] This limits their host range to cells that are actively dividing and confines their use to ex vivo applications. In early vectors, the *gag*, *pol*, and *env* genes were replaced by the cDNA of interest, and expression of the transgene was driven by the endogenous promoter/enhancer of the 5′ LTR.[25] The viral vector was propagated in complementing cell lines where the *gag*, *pol*, and *env* genes are stably expressed and supplied in trans. In later self-inactivating vector generations, a more conventional expression cassette is used.

γ-retroviral vectors preferentially integrate near the transcription start sites of active genes, with a particular affinity for proto-oncogenes, which raises the potential for insertional mutagenesis and oncogenic activation of the infected cell.[23] In one of the earliest gene therapy clinical trials, a γ-retroviral vector was used to modify hematopoietic stem cells to treat X-linked severe combined immunodeficiency. Though the treatment was successful and stably reversed disease in 9 of 10 male infants, within a few years of treatment, four of the boys went on to develop T-cell acute lymphocytic leukemia. DNA sequence analysis of the leukemic cells revealed insertional mutagenesis of the vector genome leading to aberrant activation of proto-oncogenes LMO2 and BMI1.[26,27] Based on this and similar adverse events in other trials using γ-retroviral vectors, modifications have been made to the genome, including deletion/inactivation of the LTR enhancers to create self-inactivating vectors incapable of generating replication competent retrovirus with reduced risk of vector-induced oncogenesis.[28] As one of the earliest viral vector systems, γ-retroviral vectors have been used in numerous clinical trials, including gene therapy for rheumatoid arthritis,[3] some of which are currently ongoing.

Lentivirus

Distinct from γ-retrovirus, lentiviral vectors are more complex and use active transport mechanisms that enable the viral assembly to traverse the pores of the nuclear envelope to access the host chromosomes. This endows lentiviral vectors with the ability to transduce both dividing and nondividing cells with similarly high efficiency and expands the utility of lentiviral vectors to both ex vivo and in vivo applications.[29] Although lentiviruses also preferentially integrate in genes that are transcriptionally active, they target the gene body rather than the start site, which reduces the likelihood of insertional oncogenesis.[23] Because of their increased versatility and reduced genotoxicity, recombinant lentivirus has emerged as the preferred retroviral system for gene delivery, especially for clinical ex vivo applications.

Nonviral Gene Delivery

Historically, the motivation for pursuing nonviral gene transfer has been based on several theoretical advantages over viral-based systems[30] specifically (1) ease of manipulation, (2) lower production costs, (3) lack of immune response, (4) increased safety, and (5) large payload capacity. With advancements in viral vector technology over the past several years, the extent to which these benefits still exist is highly questionable. Although exogenous nucleic acids do not provoke adaptive immune responses, they are potent inducers of innate immune pathways[31] and are characteristically inflammatory following delivery in vivo. Regarding safety, available data from over 200 clinical trials involving more than 3,000 patients indicate that AAV gene therapy when administered at moderate doses is safe, well-tolerated, and efficacious: a profile compatible with use in common, non–life-threatening disorders.[32] Finally, although it is possible to create plasmid DNA constructs that are large and complex, transfection efficiency is inversely proportional to size of the DNA, such that plasmid uptake and expression drops precipitously with constructs over 3 kb in length and is most efficient with minicircles of 650 bp or less.[33,34] Although nonviral vectors are perhaps easier to manipulate and somewhat less costly to produce than recombinant virus, these advantages are irrelevant considering the functional limitations of nonviral gene transfer in vivo. Central among these is the inefficient delivery and brief duration of transgene expression. Plasmid DNA must be taken into the cell either through endocytosis or pinocytosis then passively find its way to the nucleus and traverse the nuclear envelope before it can be transcribed. Much like γ-retrovirus, transfection efficiency is far higher in mitotic cells, which strongly favors transfection in vitro. Technologies such as electroporation, hydrodynamic injection, and ultrasonography, which perturb or temporarily disrupt the cellular membranes, can enhance uptake and gene expression in vivo. In larger tissues, these technologies are difficult to administer effectively and, in some cases, provoke significant tissue damage. Regardless of the transfection reagent or method of delivery, gene expression in vivo is modest and transient. These limitations effectively restrict nonviral applications to vaccine development and ex vivo procedures.

In 1999, the concept of a gene-activated matrix was introduced, whereby plasmid DNA containing the cDNA for human parathyroid hormone 1 to 34 (teriparatide) was linked to a scaffold and subsequently implanted into critical-size bone defects in a canine model.[35] It was theorized that local progenitor cells would infiltrate the matrix, acquire the plasmid, and express the transgene to stimulate local osteogenesis and enhance repair of critical size defects. Unfortunately, the early reports of efficacy have not been widely reproducible. Attaching or incorporating exogenous genetic material into a scaffold reduces its bioavailability, such that the already inefficient process of DNA uptake becomes even more so. The problem with nonviral gene transfer is not a matter of controlled release but inefficient uptake. Newer iterations of the gene-activated matrix concept include viral vectors.

GENE EDITING

Over the past decade, technologies for targeted editing of eukaryotic genomes have been developed from bacterial defense systems that use clustered regularly interspaced short palindromic repeat (CRISPR) sequences. The CRISPR system used for genomic editing comprises two core components: a small guide RNA approximately 125 nucleotides in length and a CRISPR-associated nuclease (Cas9), which makes a double-strand break in the genomic DNA. This triggers the induction of endogenous DNA repair pathways whose activities are co-opted for specific editing functions.[36]

Discussion of gene editing lies outside the scope of this text, but it offers the opportunity to obviate concerns about insertional mutagenesis that accompany the use of retroviruses. However, many significant technical and biologic hurdles impede the application of gene editing in clinical orthopaedics. These include low efficiency, off-target effects, immune responses to the bacterial Cas9 protein, and long-term safety concerns.[36] However, the greatest obstacle is with delivery and the inability to transduce enough cells in situ. This is especially problematic in orthopaedics, where the target tissues are surrounded by a dense extracellular matrix (ECM) and the predominant monogenic disorders are skeletal dysplasias (eg, achondroplasia and osteogenesis imperfecta) that generate abnormalities throughout the entire skeletal system.

RNA THERAPY

RNA can be used therapeutically to enhance or inhibit the synthesis of specific proteins.[37] To enhance protein synthesis, the mRNA is engineered to encode the desired protein. It is often easier to deliver mRNA than DNA and it does not need to be transported to the nucleus of the cell where the transcriptional machinery resides. Instead, it needs only to enter the cytoplasm where translation occurs. Because mRNA tends to degrade quickly, various modifications to its composition are often used to increase its stability and, depending on the application, reduce its inflammatory properties. This produces chemically modified RNA that can be used for vaccination (Pfizer and Moderna vaccines for COVID-19 are RNA vaccines) or applications where short-term expression is therapeutic, such as initiating tissue regeneration. Impressive preclinical data using chemically modified RNA to promote bone healing in animal models have recently been published.[38]

Various types of noncoding RNA can be used to inhibit the synthesis of proteins that contribute to disease. In this context, several RNA drugs have recently been approved by the FDA for diseases such as hereditary transthyretin (TTR)–mediated amyloidosis. This disease is caused by the accumulation of mutant TTR that accumulates in different organs. The drug Tegsedi is an antisense RNA oligonucleotide that hybridizes to the mutant TTR mRNA and prevents synthesis of the mutant protein. The TTR gene product has also been targeted by small interfering RNA, leading to approval of the drug patisiran for the treatment of patients with polyneuropathy caused by hereditary TTR-mediated amyloidosis. Another small interfering RNA drug, givosiran, received recent FDA approval for the management of acute hepatic porphyria.[37]

To improve the stability and uptake of therapeutic RNA molecules, they are incorporated into delivery systems, of which lipid nanoparticles are used clinically both to deliver vaccine RNA and noncoding RNA.[39]

IMMUNE RESPONSES TO VECTOR AND TRANSGENE

Mammals have developed a multilayered network of immune mechanisms, both innate (rapid, nonspecific) and adaptive (slower, antigen targeted) to defend against infectious agents. However, therapeutic gene delivery has all the characteristics of a microbial invasion, and these overlapping defense systems can be formidable barriers to efficacy.[40] To the extent that the vector or transgene product persists in the target tissues and is recognized as nonself, a corresponding adaptive, antigen-specific immune response (cellular and humoral) will result.

The rapidity and efficacy of the adaptive immune response can vary with the vector, dose, delivery route, animal strain, species, target tissue, and anatomic location. For example, the synovial lining of arthrodial joints tends to be hyperimmune sensitive,[41] whereas the dense ECM in articular cartilage and intervertebral disks largely excludes T cell entry and surveillance, enabling prolonged expression of foreign proteins in the resident cells.[42] As immune reactivity can vary with each tissue and species, the immunogenicity of the vector platform in the target tissue must be evaluated empirically in an appropriate immune-competent animal model. Comparison of expression patterns following vector delivery in immune competent animals with those obtained in animals with various forms of immune deficiency can be used to determine the immunogenicity of the vector, transgene, and genetically modified cells.[41]

Although ex vivo methods (discussed below) avoid concerns related to the administration of free virus into the host, the implantation of modified cells expressing foreign antigens, either in the form of viral proteins or xenogenic gene products, will provoke adaptive cytotoxic T lymphocyte responses against the implanted cells. The same principle applies to the use allogeneic cells. Even if the transgene product is homologous to the host (species matched), allogeneic cells expressing mismatched major histocompatibility complex molecules will appear to the immune system as virally infected and will be eliminated within several days of implantation.

Immune reactions to vector antigens not only limit the duration of transgene expression and prevent repeat dosing, but also cause severe adverse side effects in certain settings. They thus limit the reach of gene therapy and remain the subject of considerable research.

EX VIVO VERSUS IN VIVO DELIVERY

Depending on the application, gene transfer can be achieved by either in vivo or ex vivo methods (**Figure 1**).

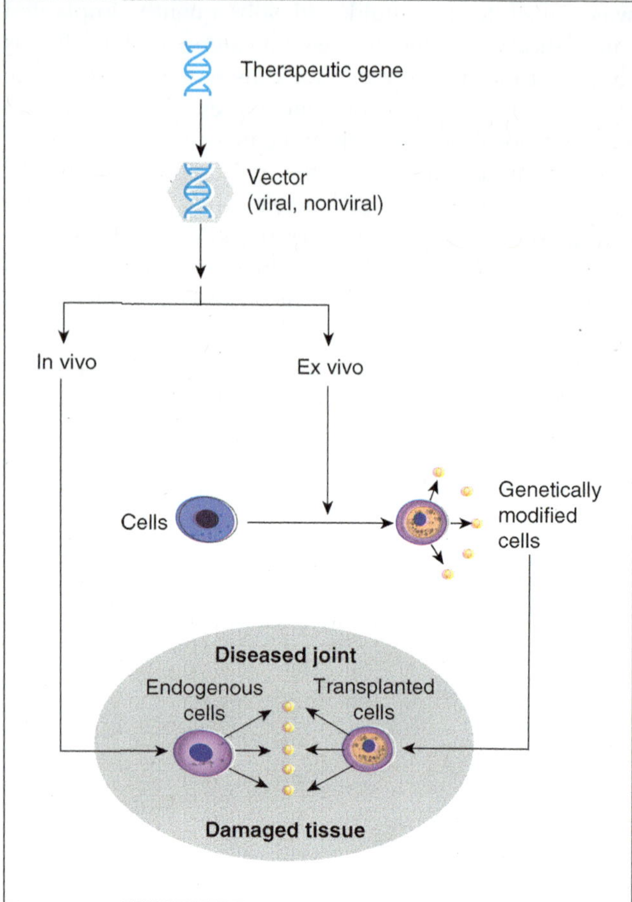

FIGURE 1 Principles of local gene therapy for the treatment of orthopaedic conditions. The therapeutic gene, usually in its complementary DNA form, is incorporated into a viral or nonviral vector and delivered to a site of disease or damage in an in vivo or ex vivo fashion. For in vivo delivery, the vector is administered directly to the relevant site. For ex vivo delivery, the vector transfers genes to cells outside the body, and the genetically modified cells are then administered to the relevant site. (Reproduced with permission from Evans CH, Ghivizzani SC, Robbins PD: Orthopaedic gene therapy: Twenty-five years on. *JBJS Rev* 2021;9[8]. https://journals.lww.com/jbjsreviews.)

In Vivo Gene Delivery

For in vivo gene transfer, a suspension of recombinant vector is injected directly into the recipient host to modify accessible, receptive cell populations in situ. Depending on the clinical application, the vector can be administered using either systemic or local delivery methods. Regarding systemic administration, counter to numerous reports, there is no mechanism by which recombinant vectors (viral or nonviral), nucleic acids, nanoparticles, or genetically modified cells can be delivered into the bloodstream (or peritoneum) to achieve targeted delivery at meaningful levels in damaged or diseased skeletal tissues. With limited exception, the genetic agents will be filtered or trapped by the organs that handle or process the blood (ie, the heart, liver, lungs, spleen, and kidneys). For most orthopaedic applications, gene therapy is used to inhibit disease pathology or augment healing responses at a specific anatomic location (eg, a bone fracture, arthritic knee, cartilage lesion, torn tendon, etc.). For these applications, local vector delivery is the more rational approach, where a defined quantity of recombinant virus is applied/injected directly into the affected tissues at the site of pathology. By targeting the vector and transgene product specifically to the site of need, the vector dose required for efficacy is reduced, as is the chance of adverse side effects in uninvolved healthy tissues from incidental exposure to vector or gene products. With regard to clinical application, in vivo gene delivery strategies provide significant practical benefits including (1) timely, expedient application; (2) straightforward, minimally invasive delivery; and (3) substantially lower costs relative to protracted ex vivo methods or cellular engineering strategies. On the downside, the prospect of injecting free viral particles into human patients raises concerns over safety and the incidence of adverse side effects from ectopic transgene expression in vital organs. Concerns over unwanted trafficking of vector to vital organs can be mitigated to a large degree by precise anatomic positioning of the injection needle via fluoroscopic, or ultrasonographic guidance, use of minimal injection volumes, and delivery at a controlled flow rate to ensure targeted vector placement with minimal dispersion to off-target locations.

Ex Vivo Gene Transfer

For ex vivo gene transfer, cells isolated from the tissues of the intended host are genetically modified in the laboratory and returned to the donor to engraft in the target tissues to express the therapeutic gene product.[29] Depending on therapeutic need, the modified cells can be delivered in suspension or seeded into a biocompatible matrix or scaffold to enhance retention at the site of pathology. Relative to in vivo gene transfer, ex vivo methods offer additional layers of control and safety. Because genetic modification is performed in the laboratory, no free vector is administered into the host. Before delivery, the modified cells can be analyzed for transgenic expression, adventitious agents, or as appropriate, replication-competent virus. In these respects, the practitioner controls the phenotype, dose, and expression levels of the modified cells and (at least in theory) can manage their administration to provide a fairly consistent therapeutic product.

For orthopaedic applications, ex vivo methods have significant technical hurdles and concerns of real-world utility. The number and quality of the cells recovered from individual human donors can vary widely, as can their growth rate, receptiveness to modification, and levels of transgene expression, especially among older patients.[43] In many cases, cells adapted to in vitro culture die soon after implantation because of the stress of the sudden change in growth environment. From a practical standpoint, ex vivo methods involve serial invasive medical procedures, are time consuming, labor intensive, and require dedicated good manufacturing practices facilities with certified technical personnel, all of which amount to a dramatic increase in cost, often to the extent that the procedure becomes impractical.

Although plasmid DNA is largely ineffective for in vivo delivery, it has much greater potential in ex vivo applications, where cells in culture can be transfected with reasonable efficiency. Integrating vectors, such as lentivirus, are especially useful.[29] As the vector genome is stably inserted in the host genome, it will be copied and passed on to both daughter cells with each round of cell division. A few thousand cells can be modified with a nominal amount of recombinant lentivirus and expanded in culture to generate tens of millions of modified cells that express the transgene.[29] For vector DNA that remains episomal (eg, AAV, adenovirus, plasmid DNA), the genetic payload will not be copied, neither will it segregate with the host chromosomes during mitosis and will often be excluded from the nucleus following reassembly of the nuclear envelope.[44] As each round of cell division results in the progressive loss of vector DNA and transgene expression, the entire cell population required for a procedure must be generated first and then transduced/transfected just before delivery. For procedures requiring large volumes of cells, efficient modification can be technically challenging and consume large quantities of vector, increasing costs substantially.

Abbreviated Ex Vivo Delivery

As mentioned previously, for an experimental therapy to transition into the clinical mainstream, in addition to being effective, it must be both practical and cost effective.[45] In this respect, gene delivery approaches that are simple, efficient, and involve the least handling and manipulation of patient tissues and cells have the greatest clinical potential. When pursuing translational research, applicability is key. As will be discussed later, some groups are exploring abbreviated ex vivo methods of gene delivery that can be performed intraoperatively. Cells or tissues are isolated from the anesthetized patient, genetically modified in the operating room, and immediately implanted, bypassing the need for multiple procedures, transport of patient materials, processing, and prolonged culture in good manufacturing practice facilities.[45-47]

Stromal Cells

Mesenchymal stromal cells (MSCs), more commonly referred to as mesenchymal stem cells or adult stem cells, are well suited for ex vivo gene therapy in orthopaedics,[48] particularly in applications that involve tissues that are difficult to access, or exist in limited quantities. MSCs are relatively abundant in most somatic tissues and with appropriate environmental and growth factor signaling can be guided to differentiate along most mesenchymal lineages. Although the use of MSCs in orthopaedic gene therapy holds great potential, investigators are encouraged to view most of the published literature with a considerable dose of skepticism.

MSCs were first identified in the 1960s as plastic-adherent, colony-forming unit fibroblasts. Subsequent rebranding of the colony-forming unit fibroblasts as a mesenchymal stem cell[49] helped to elevate the status of the MSC among the research and lay communities to that of miracle cure-all.[50] Following delivery in immune competent hosts, allogeneic major histocompatibility complex–mismatched MSCs elicit potent humoral and cytotoxic T lymphocyte responses.[51-53] When administered systemically, MSCs do not home to bone marrow or sites of disease or injury at appreciable levels but instead become trapped in the organs that process the blood (the lungs, liver, heart, spleen, and kidney), such that most cells die within 48 hours of injection.[54,55]

In gene-based and cell-based strategies for healing and regeneration of skeletal tissues, MSCs can fulfill two important roles: (1) as cellular factories genetically engineered for prolonged synthesis and release of therapeutic and/or bioactive gene products; and (2) as a readily available cell source capable of adopting chondrocytic, osteoblastic, and related mesenchymal phenotypes and elaborating the characteristic ECM components. Although there is optimism that MSCs can be used effectively in gene-enhanced repair protocols, clinical translation will require methods that support their directed differentiation, retain the modified cells at the site of repair, and maintain the desired end-stage phenotype in vivo. For each intended application, detailed tracking studies are required (with objective, unbiased reporting) to establish the fate of transplanted MSCs, to determine their density, distribution, lifespan, and contributions, if any, to healing or repair.

Induced Pluripotent Stem Cells

Induced pluripotent stem cells (iPSCs) offer an additional source of cells for potential use in ex vivo gene therapy. The transient delivery and expression of the cDNA for a cocktail of transcription factors that control pluripotency and cell division (OCT4, KLF4, NANOG, and c-MYC) induces wholesale epigenomic reprogramming to render terminally differentiated cells into a primordial pluripotent state.[56,57] The advent of iPSC technology obviated the need for the isolation of pluripotent cells from human embryos and defused an area of intense public controversy. Once reprogrammed, iPSCs can be directed to differentiate along any lineage to generate cell populations of any desired phenotype(s). In theory, this would allow generation of a boundless supply of patient autologous cells of a specific phenotype otherwise available only in limited quantities, or correction of a genetic defect in the patient's own cells, which could then be expanded, differentiated, and reimplanted, avoiding issues of immune incompatibility from cells isolated from allogeneic donors.

IPS technology has been used to reprogram and transdifferentiate fibroblasts into cells of varied mesenchymal lineages, including chondrocytes,[58] osteoblasts,[59] tenocytes,[60] and nucleus pulposus cells,[61] whose phenotypes appear to remain stable following implantation into syngeneic animals. Although the use of iPSCs in orthopaedic medicine has considerable downstream potential, much work remains before they can be legitimately considered for routine clinical use.[62] Reprogramming efficiency and cellular phenotype after differentiation are still highly variable. iPSCs routinely form teratomas following implantation into mammalian hosts, which brings the risk of tumor formation from undifferentiated subpopulations. Further, the extensive handling and manipulation required for cellular reprogramming, expansion, and redifferentiation currently render this technology impractical. Although advances in technology may alter the economic landscape, iPSCs likely will remain as experimental tools for the foreseeable future.

EXPERIMENTAL MODELS

Toward the development of a gene-based therapy, conventional in vitro studies are useful for general verification of vector function and transgene expression, but the results obtained are not illustrative of the efficiency of gene delivery in vivo. With limited exception, cells in culture are far more amenable to genetic modification than they are in vivo. Importantly, in vitro systems are simplistic and artificial; they lack the inherent complexity, organization, and architecture of living tissues that have a profound effect on vector distribution, uptake, and transgene expression in vivo. The influence of the surrounding fluids, the ECM and three-dimensional growth environment, the diverse cellularity, vasculature, and importantly, the immune system is impossible to accurately simulate in vitro.

Therapeutic gene transfer is an extraordinarily complex process that can only be evaluated in the context of an immune competent animal in a relevant disease/injury model. When attempting to treat a condition with molecular tools, it is vital that the pathogenesis and pathology of the experimental model reflect the human condition as closely as possible at the organ, tissue, cellular, and molecular levels. Common laboratory animals (eg, mice, rats, rabbits) are useful for entry-level, proof-of-concept studies and development of basic methodology. They are relatively inexpensive and can be housed and manipulated in large numbers. Small animals, though, have a remarkable capacity for self-repair and frequently exaggerate the efficacy of repair/regenerative strategies and the facility with which they can be performed. In these respects, large animal models (eg, sheep, horses, goats, pigs, cows) are essential to the clinical advancement of orthopaedic gene therapies. They have skeletal tissues of a similar scale, thickness and architecture as humans, and thus provide valuable insight into dosing and efficacy of treatment, as well as the local and systemic distribution of vector and gene product and any associated toxicity. In orthopaedics, experimental therapies typically involve surgical application. Large animal studies better depict the logistics, ergonomics, and efficacy of the experimental procedure in a clinical setting on a scale relevant to human application. Further, because most large animals are outbred, they more closely resemble the genetic and phenotypic diversity of the human population, as well as the variability of the pathologic condition and its response to treatment. Large animal studies are pivotal to clinical translation and are required by the FDA for testing advanced therapeutic medicinal products in human subjects.[63]

EXPERIMENTAL PROGRESS

Rheumatoid Arthritis

The use of gene transfer in orthopaedics was first conceived in the early 1990s to tap into the therapeutic potential of the growing list of proteins with promising activities in the management of rheumatoid arthritis.[64] The inherent instability of recombinant proteins in vivo, coupled with the continuous turnover of synovial fluid in diarthrodial joints, provided only transient effects following intra-articular injection, a profile incompatible with management of a chronic erosive disease. Further, as many of the candidate proteins blocked inflammation and cytokine signaling, elevated levels in the circulation brought the potential for systemic immune suppression and increased vulnerability to infection. However, by delivering the respective cDNA to the cells in the joint tissues, the gene products could be continuously synthesized and secreted locally within the diseased joints to inhibit ongoing erosive pathologies.[64]

Limited by the state of vector technology at the time, the initial approach used an ex vivo procedure involving transduction of autologous synovial fibroblasts with a γ-retroviral vector (MFG) containing the cDNA for interleukin-1 receptor antagonist (IL-1Ra).[65] Following transduction and expansion in culture, the modified cells were assayed for IL-1Ra expression, replication-competent retrovirus, and sterility and then injected into the arthritic joints of the respective donors to engraft in the synovial lining and express the IL-1Ra transgene. The success of early preclinical studies,[2,66] followed later by a phase I trial, showed that local gene delivery was feasible, safe, and effective.[43] Unfortunately, the logistics and expense associated with the harvest and manipulation of human cells made the procedure impractical for mainstream use.

Osteoarthritis

With the development of recombinant tumor necrosis factor receptors and antitumor necrosis factor antibodies (eg, etanercept and adalimumab), whose systemic delivery proved effective in treating rheumatoid arthritis in most patients, the focus of arthritis gene therapy shifted toward osteoarthritis, which is likely better suited to a local gene therapy. Unlike rheumatoid arthritis, which is a systemic autoimmune disease, osteoarthritis is a progressive degenerative condition that affects few joints per patient and has no known extra-articular component.[67] Existing medications for osteoarthritis are palliative and have no effect on the ongoing degenerative processes that progressively erode the articular cartilage.[67]

To make gene transfer more clinically applicable and cost effective, methods for local in vivo delivery, involving direct intra-articular injection of candidate vectors, have been extensively explored. To date, patterns of intra-articular transgene expression have been characterized from every well-developed vector system available, both viral and nonviral.[1] The anatomy of the arthrodial joint is well suited for in vivo delivery. Vectors delivered intra-articularly diffuse through the synovial fluid and interact primarily with the synovium, because of its disproportionately large surface area. As there is no basement membrane separating the intimal fibroblasts from the joint fluids, the abundant synovial fibroblasts are immediately available and receptive to modification from most viral vectors.[1] With a secreted gene product, such as IL-1Ra, temporal analysis of synovial fluid IL-1Ra content by using enzyme-linked immunosorbent assay reveals the efficiency of gene delivery and the cumulative levels of transgene expression and persistence over time. With the use of homologous transgenes and vectors such as AAV with a low immunogenic profile, the articular cell populations are capable of supporting transgene expression at high levels for well over 1 year[4,68] (**Figure 2**).

Of the available vector systems, rAAV is currently the most promising for in vivo gene transfer in osteoarthritis. Following injection into the joints of large animal models, rAAV can modify cells resident in the synovium and articular cartilage with high efficiency to provide expression of a homologous IL-1Ra transgene at levels 50- to 100-fold greater than endogenous production. Because of its uniquely small size (<50 nm in diameter), AAV is the only vector system capable of penetrating the cartilage ECM to provide efficient, stable modification of articular chondrocytes in situ[4] (**Figure 3**). This feature is particularly valuable in osteoarthritis, because cartilage degradation is the characteristic pathology, and the resident chondrocytes are directly responsible for cartilage matrix homeostasis.

Although a wide range of cDNA and gene products have been delivered to joints with experimental osteoarthritis and reported to have therapeutic activity, IL-1Ra has been used most frequently, and has consistently shown marked anti-inflammatory and chondroprotective effects.[1] Currently, two clinical trials of osteoarthritis gene therapy are listed as active with clinical trials.gov (https://clinicaltrials.gov/ct2/home). Both involve direct in vivo delivery of IL-1Ra cDNA. The first is via scAAV (NCT02790723), whereas the second uses a high-capacity adenovirus (NCT04119687).

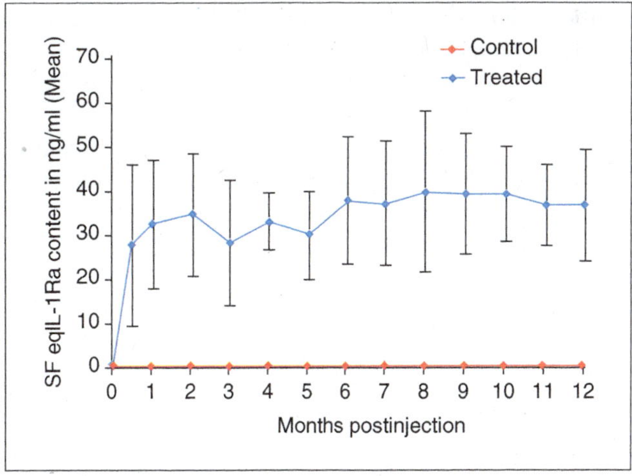

FIGURE 2 Long-term gene expression in equine joints following a single injection of vector. Adeno-associated virus encoding equine interleukin-1 receptor antagonist (eqIL-1Ra) was delivered by intra-articular injection. Synovial fluid was aspirated at monthly intervals and the concentration of eqIL-1Ra measured by enzyme-linked immunosorbent assay.

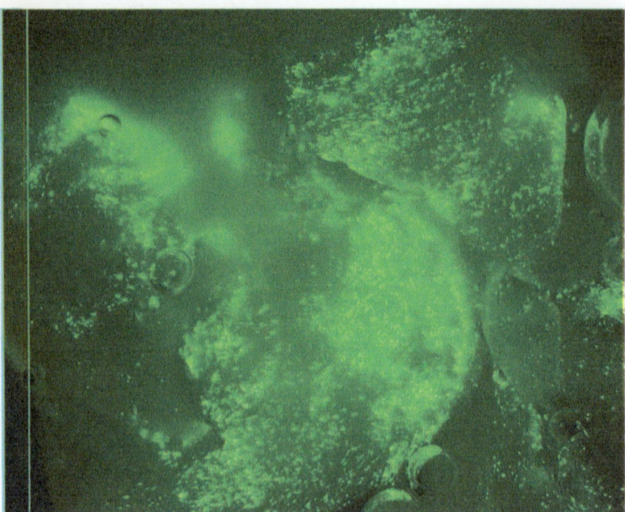

FIGURE 3 Transgene expression in equine articular cartilage following a single injection of vector. Adeno-associated virus encoding green fluorescent protein was delivered by intra-articular injection. Two weeks later, articular cartilage was recovered from the injected joint. Freshly excised cartilage was placed under a fluorescent microscope without processing. The view shown is looking down on the articular surface.

A third trial whose status is listed as unknown on clinicaltrials.gov describes an ex vivo approach promoted as a disease-modifying osteoarthritic drug. The procedure involves intra-articular injection of irradiated allogeneic chondrocytes modified with a γ-retroviral vector to express transforming growth factor beta 1 (TGF-ß1), mixed 1:3 with unmodified irradiated cells (NCT03383471). The conceptual basis for this trial is of particular concern. Several independent tracking studies have shown that cells injected into the joint do not adhere to cartilage surfaces, damaged or otherwise, but primarily engraft in the synovial lining, and to a much lesser extent the surface of the meniscus.[69,70] Overexpression of TGF-ß1 intra-articularly induces severe synovial fibrosis.[71] Moreover, allogeneic cells injected intra-articularly are recognized as foreign and are killed by CD8 + T cells in immune-competent hosts.[51,72] Analysis of the modified cells used in a series of clinical trials in South Korea and the United States revealed that they were not actually chondrocytes, but instead were 293 cells. Although initial approval in South Korea has been revoked; atypically, the once-suspended phase III study in the United States has been allowed by the FDA to resume. The extent to which this protocol will go forward is unclear.

Cartilage Repair

Most gene-based repair strategies look to augment the efficacy of existing surgical techniques to repair cartilage. However, although large volumes of studies have described repair strategies and the delivery of cDNA that influence cartilage healing, the best platform (combination of cell, gene, scaffold, delivery method, etc) for durable repair remains elusive.[73]

Because of the inability of exogenous cells to adhere to and colonize cartilage surfaces[69,70] and the inability of resident chondrocytes to migrate to sites of damage, there is no readily apparent mechanism by which suspensions of modified chondrocytes or MSCs injected into the joint can affect repair of a cartilage lesion of significant scale or regenerate cartilage loss in osteoarthritis. Moreover, anabolic growth factors released from genetically modified cells in the synovium stimulate rapid proliferation of the fibroblast cells in the joint lining and the formation of massive volumes of fibrotic tissue which progressively undergo endochondral ossification.[71] To avoid the formation of chondro-osseous metaplasia in the synovial lining, gene delivery strategies are required that limit growth factor production and signaling activity specifically to the cells within cartilage lesions. Along these lines, several strategies involving in vivo and ex vivo gene delivery localized specifically to cartilage lesions have been investigated.[73] These include the ex vivo implantation of genetically modified chondrocytes or MSCs and the intraoperative administration of vectors via in vivo or expedited ex vivo strategies. Distinct from an acute focal injury, cartilage loss in osteoarthritis is the product of a progressive degenerative process. Successful regeneration under these circumstances will require the diseased environment of the osteoarthritis joint to be addressed.

Bone

Distinct from other connective tissues, bone is endowed with a robust capacity for self-repair. However, compound open fractures or loss of significant bone volume from severe trauma or tumor resection can create large skeletal lesions that exceed the regenerative capacity of even healthy individuals. Spinal fusion and implant fixation present additional scenarios where the capacity to augment local bone synthesis could improve surgical outcome.

In 1998, identification and initial cloning of the osteoinductive factors in demineralized bone matrix,[74] the bone morphogenetic proteins (BMPs), revealed a novel family of osteoinductive ligands closely related to the TGF-ß superfamily. Because of their short half-lives and reduced activity in vivo, recombinant forms of these proteins can be difficult to administer clinically to repair bone, often requiring extremely high doses (with high costs and associated side effects) for prolonged effect. Gene transfer provides a delivery approach that may be more favorable for clinical use—and more economical to patient consumers. By delivering cDNA-encoding osteoinductive growth factors to cells within the repair milieu, prolonged local stimulation can be achieved by ongoing synthesis of the gene product in a more physiologic range. BMP-2 expressed as a transgene product by mammalian cells is processed, glycosylated, and transmitted to neighboring cell populations in a more natural form and context, providing enhanced bioactivity at 100 to 1,000-fold lower concentrations.[75,76]

Following initial demonstrations that local gene delivery methods could be used to induce bone deposition in rodents,[77,78] numerous gene delivery strategies involving both direct and ex vivo approaches have been tested and shown to stimulate osteogenesis in vivo. Direct gene delivery of an adenoviral vector containing the cDNA human BMP-2 into an open fracture model was found to provide robust transgene expression that peaked around 2 weeks after delivery and then declined during weeks 3 through 6. Expression levels were sufficient to heal critical-size bone defects following direct administration into rabbits,[79] and percutaneous injection in rats[80] and later in a fracture model in sheep with experimental osteoporosis.[81] In addition to the BMPs, factors such as vascular endothelial growth factor, Nell-1, insulinlike growth factor (IGF-1), and TGF-ß1 have been shown to stimulate bone synthesis in vivo, as well as cyclooxygenase 2 and ex vivo delivery of osteogenic transcription factors, RUNX-2 and Osterix.[76]

Ex vivo strategies using genetically modified MSCs have the potential to enhance bone repair from two directions.[82] First, the modified MSCs serve as local factories for prolonged synthesis and secretion of osteoinductive gene products. Second, they provide a supplemental source of osteoprogenitor cells receptive to autocrine stimulation, to expand the regenerative, osteogenic capacity of the endogenous repair milieu in defects that suffer substantial loss of bone volume and soft-tissue support. To this end, most well-characterized viral vector systems have been shown to transduce preparations of MSCs with reasonable efficiency.[83]

Lieberman et al[82] are examining the capacity of recombinant lentivirus to induce high-level BMP-2 expression in MSCs across multiple human donors. This allows an abridged procedure for the lentiviral transduction and delivery of autologous bone marrow cells, whereby the standard multiweek ex vivo process of surgical harvest, transduction, expansion, and delivery is condensed to a 1-day[46] or 2-day[84] protocol, applicable to both preplanned surgical procedures and acute trauma.

A second abbreviated method involves the implantation of autologous (syngeneic) grafts from muscle or adipose tissue genetically modified to overexpress BMP-2. Both provide natural three-dimensional support matrices, preloaded with populations of MSCs. Particularly, muscle is a well-established rich source of osteogenic cell and is highly susceptible to heterotopic ossification. Although implantation of Ad.BMP-2-modified grafts from muscle and fat[47,85] was noted to mediate bridging repair of critical-size femoral defects in rats, muscle was found to provide more robust bone formation and consistent repair. This conceptually and technically straightforward approach is highly efficient and simultaneously solves multiple challenges that continue to plague tissue engineering strategies in skeletal tissue repair.[76]

An allograft approach in which genetically modified allogeneic cells are encapsulated in hydrogel microspheres to protect from immune engagement and cytotoxic T lymphocyte activation has also shown promise. Poly(ethylene glycol) diacrylate microspheres[86] were found to be appropriately permeable to allow diffusion of a secreted gene product, for example, BMP-2, but sufficiently dense to shield the modified major histocompatibility complex–mismatched cells from immune recognition. Effective immune suppression or shielding of allogeneic cells would truncate the process of ex vivo gene delivery considerably, to allow its use in cases of acute trauma, providing an off-the-shelf source of modified allogeneic cells whose transgenic expression and osteoinductive activity have been previously quantified and validated.[76]

Intervertebral Disk

The pathophysiology of intervertebral disk degeneration has certain similarities to osteoarthritis and, similar to osteoarthritis, studies of IVD gene therapy follow two directions: halting the degenerative progression by inhibiting inflammatory signaling and/or ECM proteolysis or disk repair/regeneration by inducing mitotic expansion of the resident cell populations and enhanced ECM synthesis to restore IVD cellularity, volume, and mechanical properties.

Prior investigations of IVD biology, degeneration, and repair identify a list of gene products whose activities have therapeutic potential, but diminished bioactivity in recombinant form and brief half-life in vivo limit their clinical potential. Moreover, the simple act of inserting a needle into the IVD can cause or exacerbate disk degeneration. Indeed, experimental models of disk degeneration are routinely induced solely by inserting a needle into the IVD of an experimental animal.[87] Although it is reported that adverse effects can be prevented with the use of needles with proportionally small diameter,[88] biologic agents that require high doses or repeat administration are clearly ill-suited to the IVD. Gene transfer offers an attractive alternative, as it provides the capacity for sustained targeted delivery of therapeutic gene products following a single injection.

Initial investigations of the feasibility of in vivo gene transfer to the IVD involved marker studies with a first-generation adenovirus vector containing the LacZ reporter gene.[42] These studies showed clear evidence of gene delivery and expression in nucleus pulposus cells in situ. However, reporter activity was decidedly focal and limited to cell populations adjacent to the needle track.

Remarkably, despite the use of an immunogenic vector and xenogenic marker gene, reporter activity was sustained in the nucleus pulposus for 12 months confirming that the cells are largely quiescent, that the dense ECM of the healthy disk sequesters the cells from immune surveillance.[42]

Despite the limited vector dissemination observed in these studies, enhanced matrix production and protection in experimental models of disk degeneration has been reported following intradiscal gene delivery of anabolic factors, such as TGF-ß1, TGF-ß3, IGF-1, BMP-2, growth differentiation factor (GDF-5), TIMP-1, and various RNAi molecules, with several viral vectors including AAV, lentivirus, and adenovirus.[89]

Gene delivery methods need to be addressed before a gene-based treatment strategy can be viewed as clinically viable.[90] Intradisk injection is favored, but because of the low permeability of the ECM, the increase in fluid volume from injection can elevate the pressures in the local tissue. On withdrawal of the needle, the increase in pressure can force suspensions of virus or cells backward through the needle track[91] to be expelled from the disk where the materials can engage the regional cells and tissues. Safety studies of off-target growth factor expression and toxicity following vector dispersal from the rabbit disk found that administration of Ad.TGF-ß1 at high dose induced a pronounced fibrotic inflammatory response causing bilateral lower limb paralysis. Similarly, high-dose Ad.BMP-2 was found to cause loss of hind limb sensory perception and foci of chondro-osseous metaplasia.[92] Similar responses at the tissue and histologic levels are seen following gene delivery and overexpression of both TGF-ß1 and BMP-2 intra-articularly.[71] However, their ectopic expression in the central nervous system[93] provides a warning that intradiscal gene delivery of anabolic growth factors should be avoided.

Ex vivo gene delivery is complicated by results from several studies confirming the migration of injected cells from the disk.[94] The limited number of cells that remain in the disk is localized in clusters at the injection site and is unable to traverse the ECM to migrate to distal locations. The implanted cells die within a few weeks of delivery, likely because of the harsh growth conditions (low oxygen, high osmolarity, nutritional deficits, low pH), and do not add to the cellularity nor meaningfully contribute to repair.[95,96] To date, there is no proven method by which exogenous cells, genetically modified or otherwise, can be delivered to the IVD and substantively mediate tissue regeneration.

Tendon and Ligament Tissue

Exploratory work demonstrated the ability of commonly used viral vectors to deliver and support expression of marker genes and reporters to the ligaments and tendons of animal models by both in vivo and ex vivo methods.[97,98] As with other tissues, repair strategies have most often involved the delivery cDNA for growth or transcription factors associated with tendon/ligament development, such as BMP-12/GDF-7, BMP-14/GDF-5, scleraxis, mohawk homeobox, RUNX-2, periostin, and tenomodulin alone and in combination.[99] These protein factors are known to induce differentiation of tenocyte or ligament fibroblast progenitor cells and stimulate synthesis of relevant ECM components. Other cDNA-encoding growth factors and signaling molecules, including BMP-2, BMP-4, Smad-8, TGF-β1, and vascular endothelial growth factor known to increase cellularity, vascularity, and ECM deposition, have also been tested.[99,100] IGF-1 gene transfer has been explored as a way of augmenting tendon structure in tendinitis. The use of gene transfer to aid in the assimilation of transplanted ligament or tendon tissue to bone to augment engraftment following ligament reconstruction surgery has also been explored.[1]

Although articles can be found in the literature regarding tendon and ligament repair, much of the work is difficult to evaluate or compare because of inconsistencies among models, differences in methods of delivery, and lack of dosing studies. Although evidence of gene-induced tendon/ligament synthesis is convincing, there appears to be little progression toward clinical testing.

CLINICAL APPROVAL OF GENE THERAPIES

As reflected in the history of the field, bringing gene therapies into clinical translation has been a long and tortuous process. The theoretical framework was established over 50 years ago, but the first human clinical trial did not occur until 1989 and the first gene therapeutic product was not approved by the FDA until 2015. There are multiple reasons for such slow progress, including technologic hurdles, especially vector development, issues with attaining appropriate levels and duration of in vivo transgene expression, immunologic barriers, cell targeting, and safety. The last of these has been a particular problem, and the well-publicized deaths of patients in gene therapy trials for ornithine transcarbamylase deficiency in 1998[101] and X-linked severe combined immunodeficiency in 2004[27] provided major setbacks at times when data were beginning to show robust evidence of efficacy. Of relevance to the musculoskeletal field, the FDA determined that the 2007 death of a trial patient receiving intra-articular gene therapy for rheumatoid arthritis was not directly related to the vector and the trial was allowed to proceed with certain modifications.[102]

The fortunes of gene therapy improved dramatically in 2017 when the FDA approved the first two chimeric antigen receptor T-cell therapies for cancer and an in vivo, AAV-based gene therapy for a rare, inherited form of retinal dystrophy. These advances triggered renewed academic and, crucially, commercial interest in using gene therapy for cancer and rare mendelian disorders, despite the high cost of such treatments.

At the time of writing, the field is burgeoning. Indeed, gene therapy is now becoming mainstream, and the FDA expects to be approving 10 to 20 new cell and gene therapy products per year within 5 years. This sea change has created space for additional clinical applications of gene transfer to thrive, including the use of adenovirus to express viral antigens for vaccination, as used in the COVID-19 vaccines of Johnson & Johnson and AstraZeneca. Orthopaedic gene therapy should benefit from this assimilation, such that several of the applications described in this review could enter the orthopaedic armamentarium within 1 decade.

SUMMARY

Few orthopaedic conditions are caused by single-gene defects, so they are not obvious targets for gene therapy. Nevertheless, orthopaedics provides many opportunities to harness gene transfer to provide focal, local, and sustained delivery of therapeutic gene products, both RNA and protein, to sites of injury and disease. The main potential applications are in the management of complex, degenerative conditions such as arthritis and intervertebral disk degeneration, and the regeneration of damaged tissues such as bone, cartilage, ligaments, and tendons. A variety of viral and nonviral vectors are available for orthopaedic gene therapy and the scope of the field has been expanded by the recent introduction of gene editing and RNA therapeutics.

Because most orthopaedic conditions are not life threatening, safety is of particular importance and the bar to clinical translation is set very high accordingly. The resulting long time lines, high costs, and regulatory complexity help explain why, despite 30 years of development, there have been very few clinical trials in orthopaedic gene therapy, all of them for arthritis.

Other than arthritis, bone healing has attracted the most attention as a target for gene therapy. Although fractures to long bones normally heal well, nonunions, segmental defects, and cranial defects are problematic; improved ways to grow bone would also be useful in spinal fusion and implant fixation. Unlike many other potential applications of gene therapy in regenerative orthopaedics, bone healing has a clearly identified therapeutic gene: *BMP2*. Recombinant BMP-2 has provided incremental benefit in clinical cases where it is necessary to promote osteogenesis, but the received view suggests that a better clinical result could be achieved if it were possible to deliver more BMP-2 for a longer duration in a targeted fashion that avoided side effects. Gene transfer has the potential to satisfy this need. Progress has been slow, for the reasons mentioned previously, but an eventual successful outcome is likely.

Clinical application of gene therapy in orthopaedics will be accelerated by the recent explosion of interest in gene therapy as a whole. Both venture capital groups and large pharmaceutical companies are now providing increasing resources and expertise to the field, and the regulatory authorities are becoming more accepting of gene therapy. Orthopaedic applications of gene therapy will benefit from these trends, leading to FDA-approved gene medicines in the foreseeable future.

REFERENCES

1. Evans CH, Ghivizzani SC, Robbins PD: Orthopaedic gene therapy: Twenty-five years on. *JBJS Rev* 2021;9(8).
2. Bandara G, Mueller GM, Galea-Lauri J, et al: Intraarticular expression of biologically active interleukin 1-receptor-antagonist protein by ex vivo gene transfer. *Proc Natl Acad Sci USA* 1993;90(22):10764-10768.
3. Evans CH, Robbins PD, Ghivizzani SC, et al: Clinical trial to assess the safety, feasibility, and efficacy of transferring a potentially anti-arthritic cytokine gene to human joints with rheumatoid arthritis. *Hum Gene Ther* 1996;7(10):1261-1280.
4. Watson Levings RS, Broome TA, Smith AD, et al: Gene therapy for osteoarthritis: pharmacokinetics of intra-articular self-complementary adeno-associated virus interleukin-1 receptor antagonist delivery in an equine model. *Hum Gene Ther Clin Dev* 2018;29(2):90-100.
5. Liu W, Toyosawa S, Furuichi T, et al: Overexpression of Cbfa1 in osteoblasts inhibits osteoblast maturation and causes osteopenia with multiple fractures. *J Cell Biol* 2001;155(1):157-166.
6. Panda M, Tripathi SK, Biswal BK: SOX9: An emerging driving factor from cancer progression to drug resistance. *Biochim Biophys Acta Rev Cancer* 2021;1875(2):188517.
7. Powell SK, Rivera-Soto R, Gray SJ: Viral expression cassette elements to enhance transgene target specificity and expression in gene therapy. *Discov Med* 2015;19(102):49-57.
8. Qin JY, Zhang L, Clift KL, et al: Systematic comparison of constitutive promoters and the doxycycline-inducible promoter. *PLoS One* 2010;5(5):e10611.
9. Bulcha JT, Wang Y, Ma H, Tai PWL, Gao G: Viral vector platforms within the gene therapy landscape. *Signal Transduct Target Ther* 2021;6(1):53.
10. Zu H, Gao D: Non-viral vectors in gene therapy: Recent development, challenges, and prospects. *AAPS J* 2021;23(4):78.
11. McGrory WJ, Bautista DS, Graham FL: A simple technique for the rescue of early region I mutations into infectious human adenovirus type 5. *Virology* 1988;163(2):614-617.
12. Carlin CR: New insights to adenovirus-directed innate immunity in respiratory epithelial cells. *Microorganisms* 2019;7(8):216.
13. Alba R, Bosch A, Chillon M: Gutless adenovirus: last-generation adenovirus for gene therapy. *Gene Ther* 2005;12(suppl 1):S18-S27.
14. Barrett JR, Belij-Rammerstorfer S, Dold C, et al: Phase 1/2 trial of SARS-CoV-2 vaccine ChAdOx1 nCoV-19 with a booster dose induces multifunctional antibody responses. *Nat Med* 2021;27(2):279-288.

15. Li C, Samulski RJ: Engineering adeno-associated virus vectors for gene therapy. *Nat Rev Genet* 2020;21(4):255-272.

16. Nathwani AC, Reiss UM, Tuddenham EG, et al: Long-term safety and efficacy of factor IX gene therapy in hemophilia B. *N Engl J Med* 2014;371(21):1994-2004.

17. Linden RM, Berns KI: Molecular biology of adeno-associated viruses. *Contrib Microbiol* 2000;4:68-84.

18. Mietzsch M, Broecker F, Reinhardt A, Seeberger PH, Heilbronn R: Differential adeno-associated virus serotype-specific interaction patterns with synthetic heparins and other glycans. *J Virol* 2014;88(5):2991-3003.

19. McCarty DM, Fu H, Monahan PE, Toulson CE, Naik P, Samulski RJ: Adeno-associated virus terminal repeat (TR) mutant generates self-complementary vectors to overcome the rate-limiting step to transduction in vivo. *Gene Ther* 2003;10(26):2112-2118.

20. Kay JD, Gouze E, Oligino TJ, et al: Intra-articular gene delivery and expression of interleukin-1Ra mediated by self-complementary adeno-associated virus. *J Gene Med* 2009;11(7):605-614.

21. Robbins PD, Tahara H, Mueller G, et al: Retroviral vectors for use in human gene therapy for cancer, Gaucher disease, and arthritis. *Ann N Y Acad Sci* 1994;716:72-88.

22. Hanawa H, Kelly PF, Nathwani AC, et al: Comparison of various envelope proteins for their ability to pseudotype lentiviral vectors and transduce primitive hematopoietic cells from human blood. *Mol Ther* 2002;5(3):242-251.

23. Mitchell RS, Beitzel BF, Schroder AR, et al: Retroviral DNA integration: ASLV, HIV, and MLV show distinct target site preferences. *PLoS Biol* 2004;2(8):E234.

24. Mann R, Mulligan RC, Baltimore D: Construction of a retrovirus packaging mutant and its use to produce helper-free defective retrovirus. *Cell.* 1983;33(1):153-159.

25. Maetzig T, Galla M, Baum C, Schambach A: Gammaretroviral vectors: biology, technology and application. *Viruses* 2011;3(6):677-713.

26. Howe SJ, Mansour MR, Schwarzwaelder K, et al: Insertional mutagenesis combined with acquired somatic mutations causes leukemogenesis following gene therapy of SCID-X1 patients. *J Clin Invest* 2008;118(9):3143-3150.

27. Hacein-Bey-Abina S, Garrigue A, Wang GP, et al: Insertional oncogenesis in 4 patients after retrovirus-mediated gene therapy of SCID-X1. *J Clin Invest* 2008;118(9):3132-3142.

28. Suerth JD, Maetzig T, Galla M, Baum C, Schambach A: Self-inactivating alpharetroviral vectors with a split-packaging design. *J Virol* 2010;84(13):6626-6635.

29. Naldini L: Ex vivo gene transfer and correction for cell-based therapies. *Nat Rev Genet* 2011;12(5):301-315.

30. Hardee CL, Arevalo-Soliz LM, Hornstein BD, Zechiedrich L: Advances in non-viral DNA vectors for gene therapy. *Genes (Basel)* 2017;8(2):65.

31. Turvey SE, Broide DH: Innate immunity. *J Allergy Clin Immunol* 2010;125(2 suppl):S24-S32.

32. Kuzmin DA, Shutova MV, Johnston NR, et al: The clinical landscape for AAV gene therapies. *Nat Rev Drug Discov* 2021;20(3):173-174.

33. Kreiss P, Cameron B, Rangara R, et al: Plasmid DNA size does not affect the physicochemical properties of lipoplexes but modulates gene transfer efficiency. *Nucleic Acids Res* 1999;27(19):3792-3798.

34. Yin W, Xiang P, Li Q: Investigations of the effect of DNA size in transient transfection assay using dual luciferase system. *Anal Biochem* 2005;346(2):289-294.

35. Bonadio J, Smiley E, Patil P, Goldstein S: Localized, direct plasmid gene delivery in vivo: Prolonged therapy results in reproducible tissue regeneration. *Nat Med* 1999;5(7):753-759.

36. Rees HA, Minella AC, Burnett CA, Komor AC, Gaudelli NM: CRISPR-derived genome editing therapies: Progress from bench to bedside. *Mol Ther* 2021;29(11):3125-3139.

37. Damase TR, Sukhovershin R, Boada C, Taraballi F, Pettigrew RI, Cooke JP: The limitless future of RNA therapeutics. *Front Bioeng Biotechnol* 2021;9:628137.

38. De La Vega RE, van Griensven M, Zhang W, et al: Efficient healing of large osseous segmental defects using optimized chemically modified messenger RNA encoding BMP-2. *Sci Adv* 2022;8(7):eabl6242.

39. Hou X, Zaks T, Langer R, Dong Y: Lipid nanoparticles for mRNA delivery. *Nat Rev Mater* 2021;6(12):1078-1094.

40. Shirley JL, de Jong YP, Terhorst C, Herzog RW: Immune responses to viral gene therapy vectors. *Mol Ther* 2020;28(3):709-722.

41. Gouze E, Gouze JN, Palmer GD, Pilapil C, Evans CH, Ghivizzani SC: Transgene persistence and cell turnover in the diarthrodial joint: Implications for gene therapy of chronic joint diseases. *Mol Ther* 2007;15(6):1114-1120.

42. Nishida K, Kang JD, Suh JK, Robbins PD, Evans CH, Gilbertson LG: Adenovirus-mediated gene transfer to nucleus pulposus cells. Implications for the treatment of intervertebral disc degeneration. *Spine (Phila Pa 1976)* 1998;23(22):2437-2442.

43. Evans CH, Robbins PD, Ghivizzani SC, et al: Gene transfer to human joints: Progress toward a gene therapy of arthritis. *Proc Natl Acad Sci U S A* 2005;102(24):8698-8703.

44. Dunbar CE, High KA, Joung JK, Kohn DB, Ozawa K, Sadelain M: Gene therapy comes of age. *Science* 2018;359(6372):eaan4672.

45. Evans CH, Palmer GD, Pascher A, et al: Facilitated endogenous repair: making tissue engineering simple, practical, and economical. *Tissue Eng* 2007;13(8):1987-1993.

46. Virk MS, Sugiyama O, Park SH, et al: "Same day" ex-vivo regional gene therapy: A novel strategy to enhance bone repair. *Mol Ther* 2011;19(5):960-968.

47. Evans CH, Liu FJ, Glatt V, et al: Use of genetically modified muscle and fat grafts to repair defects in bone and cartilage. *Eur Cell Mater* 2009;18:96-111.

48. Bianco P, Robey PG, Simmons PJ: Mesenchymal stem cells: revisiting history, concepts, and assays. *Cell Stem Cell* 2008;2(4):313-319.

49. Caplan AI: Mesenchymal stem cells. *J Orthop Res* 1991;9(5):641-650.

50. Sipp D, Robey PG, Turner L: Clear up this stem-cell mess. *Nature* 2018;561(7724):455-457.

51. Berglund AK, Fortier LA, Antczak DF, Schnabel LV: Immunoprivileged no more: Measuring the immunogenicity of allogeneic adult mesenchymal stem cells. *Stem Cell Res Ther* 2017;8(1):288.
52. Zangi L, Margalit R, Reich-Zeliger S, et al: Direct imaging of immune rejection and memory induction by allogeneic mesenchymal stromal cells. *Stem Cell* 2009;27(11):2865-2874.
53. Nauta AJ, Westerhuis G, Kruisselbrink AB, Lurvink EG, Willemze R, Fibbe WE: Donor-derived mesenchymal stem cells are immunogenic in an allogeneic host and stimulate donor graft rejection in a nonmyeloablative setting. *Blood* 2006;108(6):2114-2120.
54. Prockop DJ: Repair of tissues by adult stem/progenitor cells (MSCs): Controversies, myths, and changing paradigms. *Mol Ther* 2009;17(6):939-946.
55. Makela T, Takalo R, Arvola O, et al: Safety and biodistribution study of bone marrow-derived mesenchymal stromal cells and mononuclear cells and the impact of the administration route in an intact porcine model. *Cytotherapy* 2015;17(4):392-402.
56. Takahashi K, Tanabe K, Ohnuki M, et al: Induction of pluripotent stem cells from adult human fibroblasts by defined factors. *Cell* 2007;131(5):861-872.
57. Wernig M, Meissner A, Foreman R, et al: In vitro reprogramming of fibroblasts into a pluripotent ES-cell-like state. *Nature* 2007;448(7151):318-324.
58. Craft AM, Rockel JS, Nartiss Y, Kandel RA, Alman BA, Keller GM: Generation of articular chondrocytes from human pluripotent stem cells. *Nat Biotechnol* 2015;33(6):638-645.
59. Li F, Bronson S, Niyibizi C: Derivation of murine induced pluripotent stem cells (iPS) and assessment of their differentiation toward osteogenic lineage. *J Cell Biochem* 2010;109(4):643-652.
60. Nakajima T, Nakahata A, Yamada N, et al: Grafting of iPS cell-derived tenocytes promotes motor function recovery after Achilles tendon rupture. *Nat Commun* 2021;12(1):5012.
61. Tang R, Jing L, Willard VP, et al: Differentiation of human induced pluripotent stem cells into nucleus pulposus-like cells. *Stem Cell Res Ther* 2018;9(1):61.
62. Yamanaka S: Pluripotent stem cell-based cell therapy-promise and challenges. *Cell Stem Cell* 2020;27(4):523-531.
63. Ribitsch I, Baptista PM, Lange-Consiglio A, et al: Large animal models in regenerative medicine and tissue engineering: To do or not to do. *Front Bioeng Biotechnol* 2020;8:972.
64. Evans CH, Robbins PD: Progress toward the treatment of arthritis by gene therapy. *Ann Med* 1995;27(5):543-546.
65. Boggs SS, Patrene KD, Mueller GM, Evans CH, Doughty LA, Robbins PD: Prolonged systemic expression of human IL-1 receptor antagonist (hIL-1ra) in mice reconstituted with hematopoietic cells transduced with a retrovirus carrying the hIL-1ra cDNA. *Gene Ther* 1995;2(9):632-638.
66. Evans CH, Robbins PD: Possible orthopaedic applications of gene therapy. *J Bone Joint Surg Am* 1995;77(7):1103-1114.
67. Martel-Pelletier J, Barr AJ, Cicuttini FM, et al: Osteoarthritis. *Nat Rev Dis Primers* 2016;2:16072.
68. Goodrich LR, Grieger JC, Phillips JN, et al: scAAVIL-1ra dosing trial in a large animal model and validation of long-term expression with repeat administration for osteoarthritis therapy. *Gene Ther* 2015;22(7):536-545.
69. Grady ST, Britton L, Hinrichs K, Nixon AJ, Watts AE: Persistence of fluorescent nanoparticle-labelled bone marrow mesenchymal stem cells in vitro and after intra-articular injection. *J Tissue Eng Regen Med* 2019;13(2):191-202.
70. Murphy JM, Fink DJ, Hunziker EB, Barry FP: Stem cell therapy in a caprine model of osteoarthritis. *Arthritis Rheum* 2003;48(12):3464-3474.
71. Watson RS, Gouze E, Levings PP, et al: Gene delivery of TGF-beta1 induces arthrofibrosis and chondrometaplasia of synovium in vivo. *Lab Invest* 2010;90(11):1615-1627.
72. Ankrum JA, Ong JF, Karp JM: Mesenchymal stem cells: immune evasive, not immune privileged. *Nat Biotechnol* 2014;32(3):252-260.
73. Bougioukli S, Evans CH, Alluri RK, Ghivizzani SC, Lieberman JR: Gene therapy to enhance bone and cartilage repair in orthopaedic surgery. *Curr Gene Ther* 2018;18(3):154-170.
74. Urist MR: Bone: Formation by autoinduction. *Science* 1965;150(3698):893-899.
75. Bessho K, Kusumoto K, Fujimura K, et al: Comparison of recombinant and purified human bone morphogenetic protein. *Br J Oral Maxillofac Surg* 1999;37(1):2-5.
76. De la Vega RE, Atasoy-Zeybek A, Panos JA, Griensven MV, Evans CH, Balmayor ER: Gene therapy for bone healing: Lessons learned and new approaches. *Transl Res* 2021;236:1-16.
77. Lieberman JR, Le LQ, Wu L, et al: Regional gene therapy with a BMP-2-producing murine stromal cell line induces heterotopic and orthotopic bone formation in rodents. *J Orthop Res* 1998;16(3):330-339.
78. Boden SD, Titus L, Hair G, et al: Lumbar spine fusion by local gene therapy with a cDNA encoding a novel osteoinductive protein (LMP-1). *Spine (Phila Pa 1976)* 1998;23(23):2486-2492.
79. Baltzer AW, Lattermann C, Whalen JD, et al: Genetic enhancement of fracture repair: Healing of an experimental segmental defect by adenoviral transfer of the BMP-2 gene. *Gene Ther* 2000;7(9):734-739.
80. Betz OB, Betz VM, Nazarian A, et al: Direct percutaneous gene delivery to enhance healing of segmental bone defects. *J Bone Joint Surg Am* 2006;88(2):355-365.
81. Egermann M, Baltzer AW, Adamaszek S, et al: Direct adenoviral transfer of bone morphogenetic protein-2 cDNA enhances fracture healing in osteoporotic sheep. *Hum Gene Ther* 2006;17(5):507-517.
82. Lieberman JR, Daluiski A, Stevenson S, et al: The effect of regional gene therapy with bone morphogenetic protein-2-producing bone-marrow cells on the repair of segmental femoral defects in rats. *J Bone Joint Surg Am* 1999;81(7):905-917.
83. Virk MS, Conduah A, Park SH, et al: Influence of short-term adenoviral vector and prolonged lentiviral vector mediated bone morphogenetic protein-2 expression on the quality of bone repair in a rat femoral defect model. *Bone* 2008;42(5):921-931.

84. Bougioukli S, Alluri R, Pannell W, et al: Ex vivo gene therapy using human bone marrow cells overexpressing BMP-2: "Next-day" gene therapy versus standard "two-step" approach. *Bone* 2019;128:115032.

85. Betz OB, Betz VM, Abdulazim A, et al: The repair of critical-sized bone defects using expedited, autologous BMP-2 gene-activated fat implants. *Tissue Eng Part A* 2010;16(3):1093-1101.

86. Sonnet C, Simpson CL, Olabisi RM, et al: Rapid healing of femoral defects in rats with low dose sustained BMP2 expression from PEGDA hydrogel microspheres. *J Orthop Res* 2013;31(10):1597-1604.

87. Cuellar JM, Stauff MP, Herzog RJ, Carrino JA, Baker GA, Carragee EJ: Does provocative discography cause clinically important injury to the lumbar intervertebral disc? A 10-year matched cohort study. *Spine J* 2016;16(3):273-280.

88. Kang JD: Does a needle puncture into the annulus fibrosus cause disc degeneration? *Spine J* 2010;10(12):1106-1107.

89. Sampara P, Banala RR, Vemuri SK, Av GR, Gpv S: Understanding the molecular biology of intervertebral disc degeneration and potential gene therapy strategies for regeneration: A review. *Gene Ther* 2018;25(2):67-82.

90. Tibiletti M, Kregar Velikonja N, Urban JP, Fairbank JC: Disc cell therapies: critical issues. *Eur Spine J* 2014;23(suppl 3):S375-S384.

91. Varden LJ, Nguyen DT, Michalek AJ: Slow depressurization following intradiscal injection leads to injectate leakage in a large animal model. *JOR Spine* 2019;2(3):e1061.

92. Levicoff EA, Kim JS, Sobajima S, et al: Safety assessment of intradiscal gene therapy II: Effect of dosing and vector choice. *Spine (Phila Pa 1976)* 2008;33(14):1509-1516.

93. Kadow T, Sowa G, Vo N, Kang JD: Molecular basis of intervertebral disc degeneration and herniations: What are the important translational questions? *Clin Orthop Relat Res* 2015;473(6):1903-1912.

94. Maidhof R, Rafiuddin A, Chowdhury F, Jacobsen T, Chahine NO: Timing of mesenchymal stem cell delivery impacts the fate and therapeutic potential in intervertebral disc repair. *J Orthop Res* 2017;35(1):32-40.

95. Loibl M, Wuertz-Kozak K, Vadala G, Lang S, Fairbank J, Urban JP: Controversies in regenerative medicine: Should intervertebral disc degeneration be treated with mesenchymal stem cells? *JOR Spine* 2019;2(1):e1043.

96. Binch ALA, Fitzgerald JC, Growney EA, Barry F: Cell-based strategies for IVD repair: Clinical progress and translational obstacles. *Nat Rev Rheumatol* 2021;17(3):158-175.

97. Hildebrand KA, Deie M, Allen CR, et al: Early expression of marker genes in the rabbit medial collateral and anterior cruciate ligaments: The use of different viral vectors and the effects of injury. *J Orthop Res* 1999;17(1):37-42.

98. Gerich TG, Kang R, Fu FH, Robbins PD, Evans CH: Gene transfer to the patellar tendon. *Knee Surg Sports Traumatol Arthrosc* 1997;5(2):118-123.

99. Abat F, Alfredson H, Cucchiarini M, et al: Current trends in tendinopathy: Consensus of the ESSKA basic science committee. Part II – Treatment options. *J Exp Orthop* 2018;5(1):38.

100. Ilaltdinov AW, Gong Y, Leong DJ, et al: Advances in the development of gene therapy, noncoding RNA, and exosome-based treatments for tendinopathy. *Ann N Y Acad Sci* 2021;1490(1):3-12.

101. Raper SE, Chirmule N, Lee FS, et al: Fatal systemic inflammatory response syndrome in a ornithine transcarbamylase deficient patient following adenoviral gene transfer. *Mol Genet Metab* 2003;80(1-2):148-158.

102. Evans CH, Ghivizzani SC, Robbins PD: Arthritis gene therapy's first death. *Arthritis Res Ther* 2008;10(3):110.

CHAPTER

5

Clinically Applicable and Translatable Animal Models in Orthobiologic Research for Cartilage Repair and Osteoarthritis in Humans

Laurie Goodrich, DVM, MS, PhD

INTRODUCTION

The burgeoning field of biologic therapies for cartilage repair and osteoarthritis has resulted in an explosion of information in this area and reports of success, but also failures, abound. As most orthopaedic surgeons know, there are few patients who do not inquire about stem cells or blood products for their multitude of orthopaedic conditions. Orthopaedic surgeons are frequently challenged by their patients on whether to pursue biologics or surgery or both to improve their musculoskeletal pain and long-term outcomes. Although there is expanding information regarding these therapies, there are many more reports of level II and higher studies (of low scientific rigor) and an unending supply of anecdotal claims of success that delve further into the field and layperson reports that pique the interest of patients, who may be uninformed or worse, misinformed. However, the need for double-blind, randomized controlled clinical trials is immense; interestingly, funding for these types of trials in the field of orthobiologics is low and even lower is the number of meticulously carried-out studies in preclinical models to scientifically track the physiologic and long-term healing of these therapies for cartilage repair and osteoarthritis. The need for relevant animal models is considerable because often research in rodent or lower phylogenetic species is associated with lower costs, shorter time lines, and quicker turnaround times to complete the project, but the resultant data gained from these studies often are not translatable to the human condition and therefore much time, effort, and cost are incurred with very little application or relevant information to how, why, and whether physicians should be using these therapies for the musculoskeletal condition being treated.

The various animal models to consider for testing orthobiologics for cartilage repair and osteoarthritis are reviewed, starting with rodent models and moving up to larger animal species. For reasons that will be described in more detail, larger animal species are closer to humans in clinical relevance, whereas smaller species are great for initial proof-of-concept work. There is increasing evidence that species with fewer phylogenetic comparisons with humans are less relevant.[1,2] Additionally, larger animal models have both the advantage of similar anatomic comparisons and also the benefits of studying orthobiologics in naturally occurring diseases such as cartilage degeneration and osteoarthritis.[3-6] This is leading the field of orthobiologics to embrace more relevant large animal models in preclinical research. The most rigorous level of evidence in medicine will continue to be double-blind, randomized controlled clinical trials; however, properly designed studies in this area are expensive and unfortunately often take years to properly execute. With the quickly developing and broadening options in orthobiologics development, the science commonly lags behind the hype. Clinicians and clinician scientists who want to further study specific orthobiologics should consider the main objectives of their questions, the preclinical animal model they are considering, and the translatability to their patients.

BROAD CONSIDERATIONS OF PRECLINICAL MODELS IN ORTHOPAEDIC RESEARCH

When considering what preclinical models to use in cartilage repair and osteoarthritis, surgeons should first review FDA, American Society for Testing and Materials International, International Cartilage Regeneration & Joint Preservation Society, and Osteoarthritis Research Society International (OARSI) guidelines because each organization offers both regulatory and helpful recommendations for specific approaches of the therapy to be

Dr. Goodrich or an immediate family member is a member of a speakers' bureau or has made paid presentations on behalf of AlloSource; serves as a paid consultant to or is an employee of AlloSource; has stock or stock options held in ART and EqCell; has received research or institutional support from AlloSource; and serves as a board member, owner, officer, or committee member of North American Veterinary Regenerative Medicine and Orthopaedic Research Society.

studied. Each organization, especially the FDA, also has specific divisions that concentrate on whether the orthobiologic is considered a drug, device, biologic, or gene therapeutic type of treatment.[7,8] Importantly, the FDA and its members recognize that no perfect animal model exists. For these reasons, clinician scientists are encouraged to contact these groups before embarking on investigations in a preclinical animal model for ultimate translation to humans.

Another important consideration in orthobiologic research is the intersection of the specific animal model and the orthobiologic to be studied. Some animal models may have components of the orthobiologic being tested that are not suitable (or translatable) to humans. Specifically, some preclinical models have mesenchymal stromal cell populations that are difficult to harvest and expand due to size (mice) or have limited adipogenic sources readily able to harvest. Investigators should ensure that properties such as phenotypic, molecular, and growth characteristics of various species of mesenchymal stromal cell populations in the preclinical population being studied should be appropriate for human translation.[9] Some animal models such as sheep tend to have very different platelet-rich plasma characteristics than humans, which could directly affect translation to humans if properties of the biologic are not acknowledged or taken into consideration.[10,11] Unique characteristics of each preclinical model should be considered before embarking on the model.

When surgeons are recruiting key members of the scientific team for preclinical research, several issues should be considered. Naturally, the surgeon/clinician who is interested in studying the orthobiologic should combine their expertise and clinical experience with that of a veterinary surgeon (many are board certified with the American College of Veterinary Surgeons and also have orthopaedic fellowship training and certification) who also has surgical expertise in the method or approach in the specific preclinical model to be used. A biostatistician should be included to assist in power calculations and the crucial task of determining animal numbers and data analysis. Centers that are carrying out the studies should have a team experienced in anesthesia, postoperative animal care, and husbandry and experts in testing important outcomes such as biomechanical engineers, imaging experts (veterinary radiologists are also board certified with the American College of Veterinary Radiology), and histologic processing experts. Furthermore, some institutions also have regulatory expertise and industrial partners who can also work alongside the team of investigators to assist and guide in the approval pipeline. Finally, for many projects, it may be the first time a biologic is studied in a specific preclinical animal model, and there is considerable value in performing pilot studies. Pilot studies can inform the pivotal study and ensure that all procedures (surgical or medical induction of pathologic changes that induce disease), tests, outcome measures (physical, histologic, imaging, etc), and team dynamics are worked out well in advance of the main pivotal preclinical study. The pivotal study can be carried out in larger and more relevant animal models, but the cost is justified if the results of the studies enhance translation to humans.

THE THREE Rs AND ARRIVE GUIDELINES IN ETHICAL PRECLINICAL RESEARCH

The three Rs principle (replacement, reduction, and refinement) in animal research refers to guidelines put in place in 1959 and has become an important objective of many academic and research institutes across the United States and Europe.[12] These guidelines specify that experiments may not be performed if another scientifically satisfactory method of obtaining the result sought, not entailing the use of an animal, is reasonably and practically available. Furthermore, the choice of species should be carefully considered and experimentation should not only use the minimum number of animals with the lowest degree of neurophysiologic sensitivity and cause the least amount of pain, suffering, distress, and harm but also result in satisfactory results. All experiments shall be designed to avoid distress and unnecessary pain and suffering to the animals. These principles are important to abide by in any preclinical model research and surgeons looking to use the animals should ensure the groups they partner with practice these values. Also contributing to ethical preclinical research are the ARRIVE (Animals in Research: Reporting In Vivo Experiments) guidelines originally developed in 2010 and updated in 2020.[13] The guidelines ensure that reproducibility of research findings by flawed study design, data analysis, and variability in reagents, materials, and results is minimized. Many research journals are strictly adhering to these guidelines by requiring authors to report the details of study design including sample size, inclusion/exclusion criteria, randomization, blinding, outcome measures, statistical methods, experimental animal, and procedures as well as reporting results gathered from listed statistical methods. Research groups that practice these principles most commonly have the most reproducible and clinically important data.

CLINICALLY RELEVANT ANIMAL MODELS FOR CARTILAGE AND OSTEOCHONDRAL REPAIR

Cartilage repair is used as an example of the many preclinical approaches used in other tissues including bone, ligament, and tendon. When considering animal models to study cartilage, subchondral defects, and attendant diseases, there are many important aspects to consider. The principal investigator needs to focus not only on the main tissue of interest but also all articular tissues contributing to joint physiology. When lesions are induced in cartilage, not only is the repair tissue important but also the surrounding cartilage, remote cartilage, apposing cartilage, meniscus, subchondral bone, synovium, joint capsule, muscle, and tissues surrounding the joint and even remote tissues such as lymph nodes and nerves/vessels may be important.[14-16] The joint should be considered as an organ, and inclusion of these tissues is paramount to have a complete and global view of any orthobiologic an individual may be investigating.

Two major challenges that exist in the field of cartilage repair and should be acknowledged are as follows: (1) The goal of treatment of articular cartilage defects is improvement in structure and function and inhibition of the known accelerated degeneration of adjacent (to the lesion) cartilage. Quantitative outcomes at specific and defined time points that might demonstrate superiority over the standard of care (microfracture) do not currently exist. Because of this lack of international consensus, a consensus meeting is needed to define the end points that could lead to validated outcomes on which superiority versus standard of care could be based. (2) Pain, physical function, and patient satisfaction are the outcome measures on which success is based in human clinical trials; patients with microfracture in 3-year patient-reported outcomes (Western Ontario and McMaster Universities Osteoarthritis Index and Patient-Reported Outcomes Measurement Information System) generally have excellent success. Therefore, demonstrating orthobiologic superiority to microfracture in phase 3 clinical trials may be untenable. Furthermore, it is also unclear that the FDA would approve an orthobiologic based on structural outcomes only unless they were significantly correlated with long-term outcomes such as reduction in total joint replacements at 15 years, for example. These hurdles must be considered when orthobiologics are being evaluated for further studies in focal cartilage defects.

There are many variables and peculiarities relating to animal models of cartilage repair. The FDA, International Cartilage Regeneration & Joint Preservation Society, and other agencies recognize that there is no perfect animal model, and only models that may approximate what disease and what orthobiologic is best studied for the specific defect(s) to be analyzed. Through the decades, animal models from rodents and rabbits to larger models such as dogs, sheep, goats, and horses have been frequently used for cartilage repair strategies. Each has its benefits and also limitations. Defects often are surgically created in the stifle (knee joint), which is most similar to the human knee, but in other joints as well. There are many variables to clinical translation with each animal model including anatomic similarities to humans (cartilage and subchondral bone thickness), size of joint, age of musculoskeletal maturity of the animal (physeal closure and endochondral ossification), and gait and movement characteristics, and how those affect the biomechanics of cartilage repair. In the field of orthobiologics, other considerations relating to blood or bone marrow harvest in the smaller animal models may prove difficult due to the small size and/or blood/cell volume.[17]

Critical-size cartilage defects in each animal model, according to American Society for Testing and Materials International, are defined as the smallest size defects that will not heal without intervention.[16] Furthermore, historically American Society for Testing and Materials International has suggested that defect size should not exceed 20% of the articulating surface, 60% of width, and depth of 1 to 10 mm depending on the animal model chosen. These suggestions are based on the need to create a critical-size defect that stays within the depth of the chosen animal model. Control groups and cohorts are also very important when considering study design.[16,18] Postoperative exercise should be considered for all models to most closely approximate the human condition. For instance, horses can commonly be exercised on a treadmill to simulate training that a human athlete may be instructed to follow; very few animal models would allow a non–weight-bearing period postoperatively to simulate a person on crutches or limited weight bearing. Furthermore, therapies such as continuous passive motion devices that are applied to human knees immediately after surgery are also very difficult to mimic in animal models.

Imaging is also an important component to longitudinal monitoring in preclinical model research. Before the time or at the time of sacrifice, imaging such as MRI (including T2 mapping and T1rho, CEST, T2star, and CT)[19] should be performed. Ideally, several time points of imaging could be performed throughout the study to assess defect filling.[18] In addition, longitudinal arthroscopic scoring (recheck/second-look arthroscopy) in appropriate animal models allows gross assessment as well as the potential to biopsy the defect. Furthermore, validated macroscopic scoring systems developed by the International Cartilage Regeneration & Joint Preservation Society can also be used at the time of sacrifice.[20] In addition to macroscopic grading, biomechanical analysis should be accomplished on fresh tissues (**Figure 1**) including aggregate modulus, Poisson ratio, permeability, creep, or indentation.[20-22] Complete analysis of the joint organ should occur, including but not limited to gross and/or arthroscopic scoring, harvest of synovial fluid, synovial tissue, joint capsule, repair tissue and perilesional and remote tissue, osteochondral blocks, and osteophytes. Histologic analysis should include validated scoring systems with which the principal investigators have a high level of comfort. There are many different scoring systems, and, currently, some groups recommend using more than one because there are also no perfect histologic scoring systems.[14] All data should be analyzed with appropriate statistical analysis decided on a priori.[18]

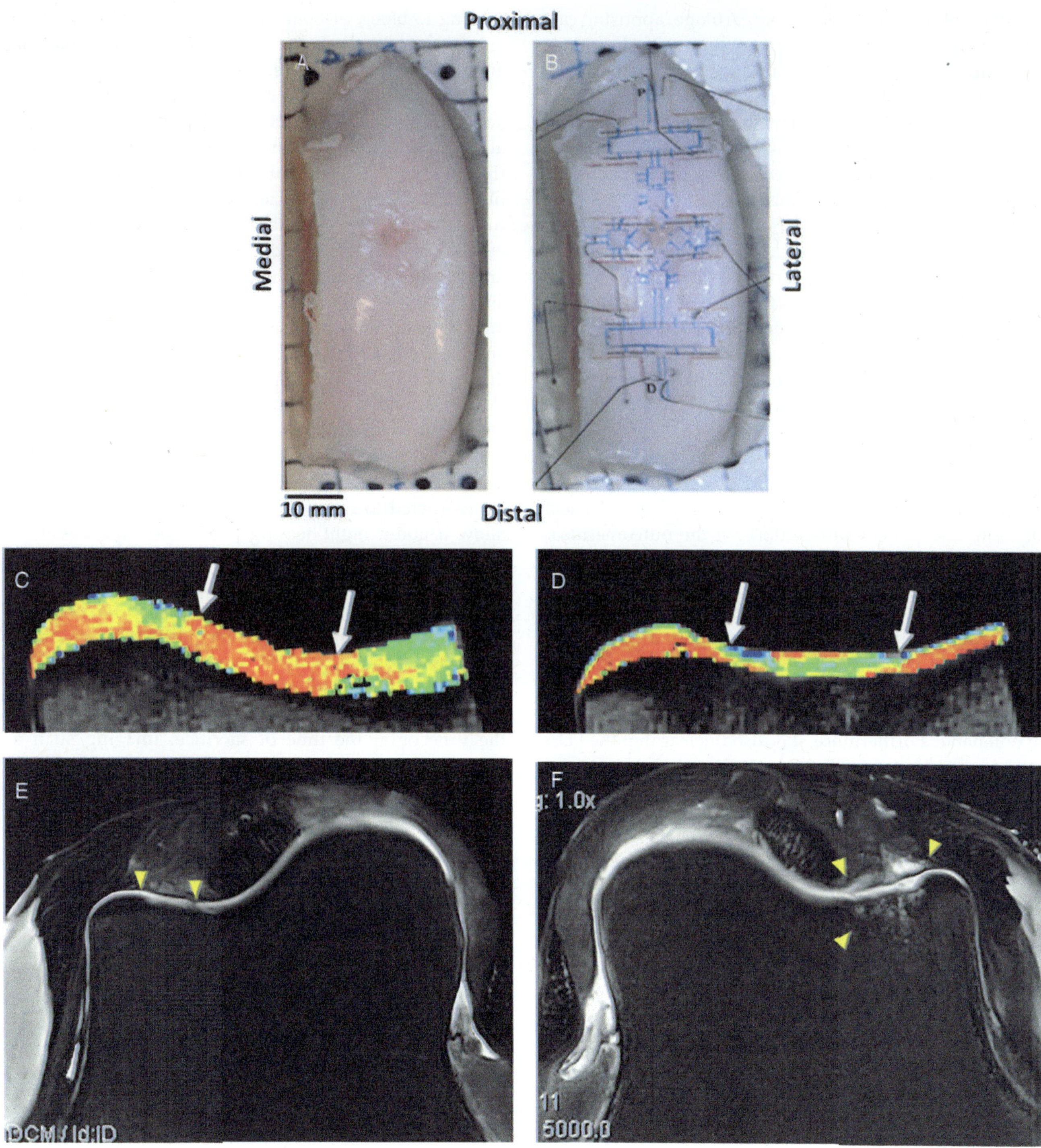

FIGURE 1 Example of an equine femoropatellar joint used in a osteochondral defect study. The following images demonstrate various aspects of assessments: photos (**A** and **B**) showing gross anatomy, mapping on T2 MRI (**C** and **D**), and MRI (**E** and **F**); histologic imaging (**G** through **V**) and biomechanical analysis (**W**) that can be performed on all regions of a relevant large animal model (horse). Arrows mark where the cartilage regeneration/repair (**E**, **G** through **V**) or subchondral bone repair (**F**) is occurring following creation of an osteochondral defect. (Modified with permission from Goodrich LR, Chen AC, Werpy NM, et al: Addition of mesenchymal stem cells to autologous platelet-enhanced fibrin scaffolds in chondral defects: Does it enhance repair? *J Bone Joint Surg Am* 2016;98[1]:23-34.)

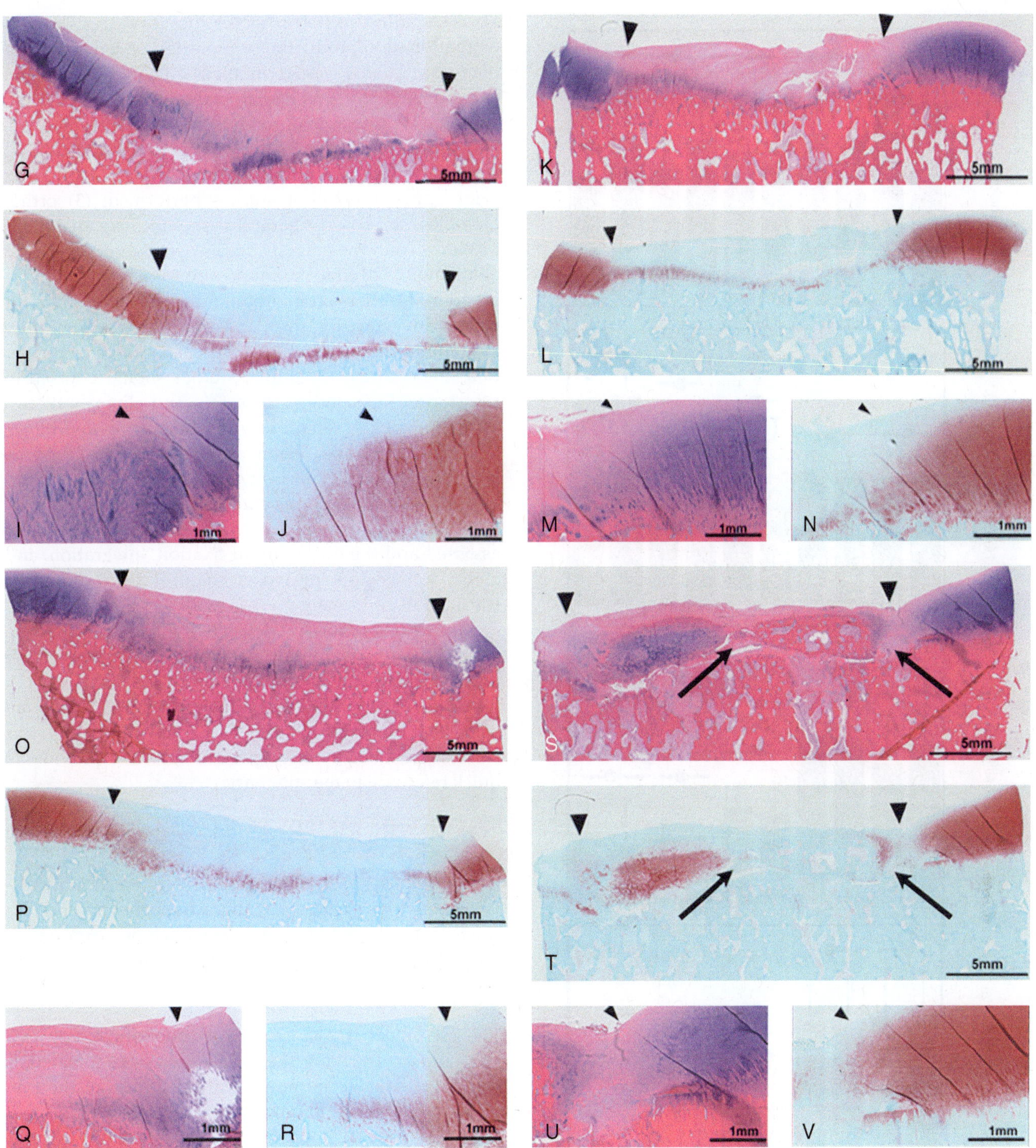

FIGURE 1 *(Continued)*

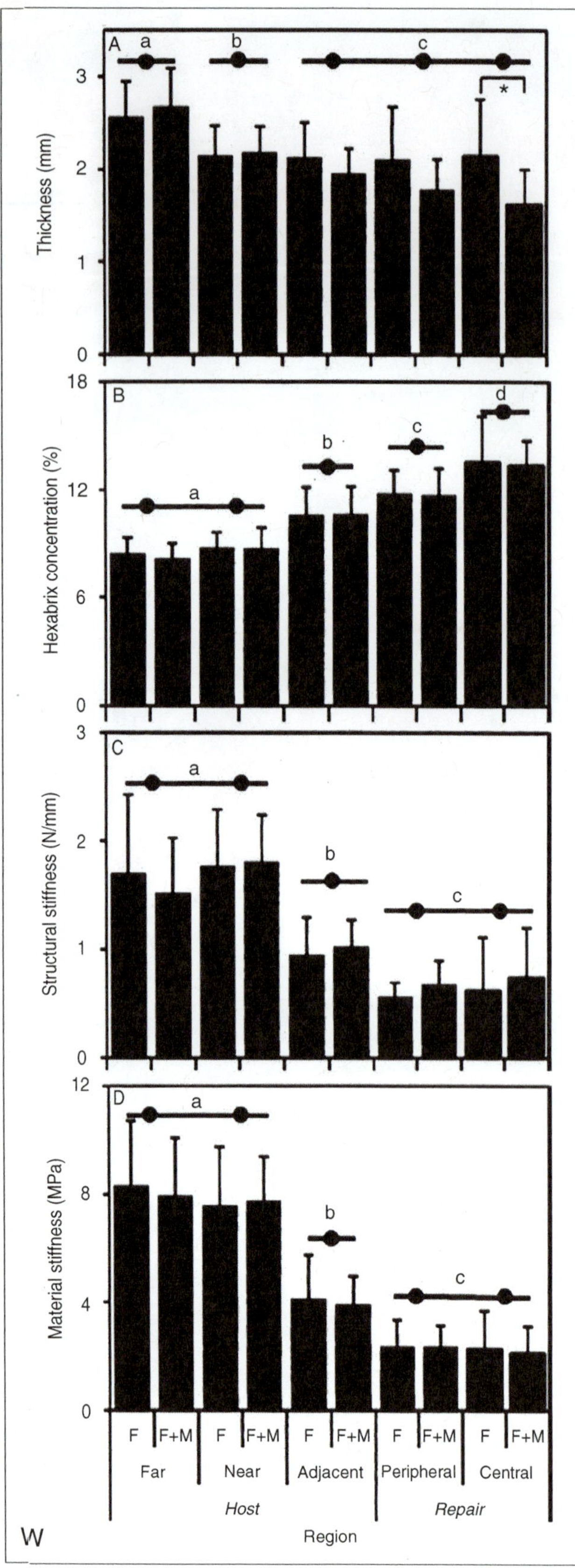

FIGURE 1 *Continued*

FDA pathways for orthobiologics (or drugs, devices, or combination products) for repairing or replacing cartilage are clearly stated in their guidance document. Components of preclinical animal model research include (1) large animal models that are recommended, and further, the model should reflect intended use; (2) studies should be a minimum of 1 year in length with prior appropriate pilot studies performed; (3) orthobiologics/cell-based therapies should use analogous products from the animal species being studied so as to eliminate the need for immunosuppressive drug administration; (4) there should be nonclinical safety data for clinical investigation in the preclinical model, and ideally, animal and mechanical testing should be combined in a single study; (5) animal studies should be used to assess proof of concept for safety and clinical efficacy, durability of the repair, local and systemic toxicology, dose response, and lesion size, and there should be location similarity to people; and (6) end points should approximate the end point in humans, and, at sacrifice, gross examination and mechanical testing should be assessed and the durability of fixation, integration, and ability to sustain expected mechanical loads should be translatable to humans.[16]

The average chondral defect in the human is approximately 550 mm^3 in volume, with 95% of defects involving only cartilage and not subchondral bone.[23,24] Although no model precisely mimics human conditions, there are some that come fairly close. The following paragraphs summarize each model type, and **Table 1** provides a quick reference to the summary.

SPECIFICS OF VARIOUS PRECLINICAL MODELS FOR CARTILAGE REPAIR STUDIES

Examples of the use of various species for preclinical cartilage studies are presented with the hope that the specifics can be extrapolated to preclinical models and experimental considerations for other tissues as well.

Murine

The rat model is often used for proof-of-concept data and studies involving the implantation of biomaterials subcutaneously or intramuscularly. Because of the thin nature of the cartilage (three to five cells thick) and small joint size, rodents do not offer great relevance to cartilage defects in humans, although they have been used in a limited number of studies. Furthermore, their epiphyseal plates do not close through their lifetimes. Rodents require limited space and housing/husbandry logistics, and they are easy to handle. However, time to end points is relatively short (10 weeks); because of the difficulty of producing a surgical defect that is suitable for comparison with humans, they are not highly recommended models in cartilage repair studies.

TABLE 1 Comparison of Common Currently Used Animal Models for Articular Cartilage Repair

Species	Joint(s)	Cartilage Thickness (mm)[a]	Defect Type/Size	Primary Use	Arthroscopy/ Second-Look Arthroscopy	Postoperative Management Capabilities	Outcome Assessments
Rat	Knee	~0.1[b]	Surgically created, 0.75 to 3 mm chondral/osteochondral; critical size = unknown	Mechanisms of action; use of xenogeneic cells or tissues; screening of treatment strategies for pivotal study in large animal model	–	Laboratory rat caging; running wheel; hindlimb suspension	MRI if 7T or greater capabilities or micro-CT; gross; histology; biochemical; biomechanical
Rabbit	Knee, shoulder	0.21-0.56	Surgically created, 2 to 4 mm (3 mm most common) chondral/osteochondral; critical size = 3 mm	Mechanisms of action; screening of treatment strategies for pivotal study in large animal model	–	Laboratory rabbit caging	MRI if 7T or greater capabilities or micro-CT; gross; histology; biochemical; biomechanical
Sheep/goat	Knee	0.4-1.5	Surgically created, 4 to 15 mm chondral/osteochondral; impact injury; critical size = 6 to 7 mm	Pivotal studies using surgically created defects for which postoperative management variables are not critical	+/–	Stall/pasture; Schroeder–Thomas splint	MRI, CT, or radiography; subjective function; gross; India ink staining; histology; biochemical; biomechanical
Pig	Knee	2.0	Surgically created to 6 mm	Surgically created lesions for cartilage repair	+	Pens	Arthroscopic scoring; MRI, CT, or radiography; gross; India ink staining; histology; biochemical; biomechanical
Dog	Knee, shoulder, elbow, hip, ankle	0.95-1.3	Surgically created, 3 to 12 mm chondral/osteochondral; impact injury; osteochondrosis; secondary osteoarthritis; elbow dysplasia; critical size = 4 mm	Pivotal studies using surgically created or spontaneous defects; postoperative assessments and management most closely mimic human	+	Kennel/run/group housed; bandages, casts, splints, orthotics, external skeletal fixators, or non–weight-bearing slings; dedicated exercise; physical therapy	Arthroscopic scoring; MRI, CT, or radiography; VAS for pain, function, effusion, and QoL; ROM; muscle mass; kinetics and kinematics; gross; India ink staining; histology; biochemical; biomechanical
Horse	Knee, carpus, ankle	1.5-2.0	Surgically created, 6 to 20 mm chondral/osteochondral; chip fracture; osteochondrosis; critical size = 9 mm	Pivotal studies using surgically created or spontaneous defects; cartilage thickness and cartilage biomechanics most closely resemble those of human	+	Stall/pasture; treadmill exercise	Arthroscopic scoring; MRI and CT if special capabilities or radiography; subjective function; kinetics and kinematics; gross; India ink staining; histology; biochemical; biomechanical

[a]Human range, 2.2 to 2.5 mm.

[b]Indicates approximation.

ROM = range of movement, VAS = visual analog scale, QoL = quality of life

Modified with permission from Cook JL, Hung CT, Kuroki K, et al: Animal models of cartilage repair. *Bone Joint Res* 2014;3(4):89-94.

Laprine

Rabbits, like rodents, are relatively inexpensive and require simple husbandry, but reach skeletal maturity at 9 months. Defects should not be created before 9 months because remarkable spontaneous regeneration has been seen in younger animal models prior to this time point.[2] Critical-size defects have been considered to be 3 to 5 mm in diameter, and the cartilage thickness in femoral condyles is approximately 0.3 mm. This often results in 90% of the defect volume involving subchondral bone.[2] Defect location in rabbits has involved femoral trochlea and medial and lateral femoral condyles. Rabbits also possess an acute angulation and a relatively light body weight, which further decreases their approximation to large animal models.

Canine

Dogs as preclinical models are subject to intense scrutiny due to the companion animal status and the fact that skeletal maturity occurs between ages 12 and 24 months, at which point most human–animal bonds are very strong. Cartilage thickness in the canine model is an average of 1.15 mm and defect diameters have been reported from 2 to 10 mm, with 4 mm being most common.[25,26] Although the cartilage thickness in dogs allows for only chondral defects (in which the volume would still be considerably less than that for defects in humans), most studies use osteochondral defects.[24,27] Sites of defects commonly induced in the dog are femoral trochlea and medial and lateral femoral condyles.[2,28,29] Cartilage defect volume of 10 mm in diameter and of 10 mm in depth is still considerably smaller than that of humans.[30]

The dog is considered a reasonable preclinical model due to somewhat similar anatomy, ability for cartilage-only lesions, the option to have second-look arthroscopy, and ease of trainability on treadmills. Further testing in the canine model may also be translated to clinical patients with naturally occurring disease (naturally occurring disease models). However, because of ethical reasons and public perceptions of the human–animal bond, it is still not a widely used species.[2]

Ovine

Sheep are used broadly in biomedical research and certainly in musculoskeletal studies including cartilage repair. Anatomic similarity to the human joint is high and second-look arthroscopy capabilities exist. However, a technically proficient arthroscopist is required because of the extensive fat pad and high degree of flexion required to observe the femoral condyles. Sheep also have variable thickness of their cartilage with varying degrees of biochemical content,[2,31] which may lead to variability in defect volume for both cartilage and subchondral bone. Average thickness in sheep is 0.45 mm. It is also well known that sheep have extremely dense and firm subchondral bone, which does not allow reproducible pathology of the subchondral surface.[2,32] Furthermore, without a healthy bleeding subchondral bone surface, orthobiologics that need to be applied to such a surface are difficult to study. The average 7.4-mm-diameter defect that is often created on the medial or lateral condyles or femoral trochlea still results in a dissimilar removal of cartilage volume that is equivalent to volumes of cartilage missing in human osteochondral defects. Skeletal maturity in sheep is between ages 2 and 3 years, although frequently age range in musculoskeletal studies in sheep is not reported, departing from what the ARRIVE guidelines suggest. In summary, sheep are often a readily accessible animal model for cartilage repair studies; however, because of the aforementioned limitations, they are still lacking good translatability to human cartilage repair.

Caprine

The goat is commonly used and relatively close to human joint anatomy, and while there is variability in cartilage thickness throughout, cartilage thickness is on average 0.8 to 2 mm on the medial femoral condyle.[33] Furthermore, full-thickness and partial-thickness defects can be created, and the goat is also a species in which second-look arthroscopy is possible. The subchondral bone is softer in the goat model, lending itself to surgical techniques that create osteochondral defects. Cartilage defects of 12 mm diameter can result in 150 mm^3, which allows some correlation between caprine and human defects. A critical-size defect in the goat, on average, has been reported to be 6 mm in diameter because defects that are 3 mm in diameter have been reported to heal spontaneously.[2,34] Cartilage defects have been made on the medial condyles and trochlear groove, and studies in which defects have been made in goats typically extend to 26 weeks. Skeletal maturity in goats, as in sheep, occurs at approximately age 2 to 3 years.

Porcine

Pigs are a species that have cartilage thickness similar to humans, and although the normal-size porcine makes their handling difficult, minipigs are a great alternative because they are significantly smaller and the cartilage thickness is relatively similar to that in humans. Various reports have listed pigs with cartilage that is 1.5 to 2.0 mm thick on the medial femoral condyle,[2,35,36] which also allows for the study of partial-thickness cartilage defects. Pigs, similar to goats, have also been used to study partial-thickness cartilage defect therapies,[37] and the potential of only studying the cartilage (versus the subchondral bone) also exists. Minipigs reach musculoskeletal maturity at 42 to 52 weeks, and defect size of 6 mm or less can spontaneously heal. Lesions have been reported to be created in the trochlear grove and medial and lateral condyles. The pig is a reasonable model to approximate human cartilage defects; however, researchers must contend with animals that are harder to handle and housing dilemmas that are less problematic than other animals already mentioned.

Equine

The horse has been shown to be the most closely approximated animal model to humans in terms of cartilage thickness, subchondral bone characteristics, overall joint anatomy, and weight bearing.[2,20,35] Cartilage thickness of 1.75 to 2 mm is consistent and allows the study of both full-thickness and partial-thickness defects.[38] Many studies have validated gross, histologic, and biochemical assays using the horse model.[20,39,40]

Horses are also athletes with musculoskeletal injuries similar to humans, and this has initiated many studies in the equine sports medicine world. Furthermore, clinical trials in equine veterinary patients allow the equine model to have applied research in naturally occurring equine conditions. This allows the horse to be an excellent preclinical model and also facilitates parallel studies to be performed in humans and clinical equine patients that have naturally occurring disease. This alone can be extremely valuable because approximating the human condition in clinical cases following intense study in preclinical models often closes the loop in clinical relevance. The large size of the horse also allows for second-look arthroscopy, and further, cartilage defects can be made between 8 and 15 mm in diameter that result in 350 mm^3 with no subchondral bone involvement. These observations suggest close approximation to the human chondral defect; therefore, the horse has been statistically found to be the most similar to humans for cartilage repair studies.[2,35] Defects have been made on the lateral and medial trochlea, the femoral condyles, and also the metacarpophalangeal joint and middle carpal joint. The length of cartilage healing studies is usually 12 months but has taken up to 46 months as well.[2] Last, because of the ease and practicality of being able to simply harvest synovial fluid in a sedated horse, biomarker analysis is also a benefit of using this model. Housing requirements, expense, and specialty requirements of working with this model make it more difficult to use; however, specific groups around the United States and internationally have facilities and programs built around this species to practically execute these studies.

SUMMARY OF CARTILAGE REPAIR MODELS

In summary, preclinical animal models for cartilage repair range in practicality, cost, and translatability to the human cartilage or osteochondral defect. **Figure 2, A** is a helpful reference of the average size of the critical defect in each animal model and in particular species, how much cartilage and subchondral bone are removed. **Figure 2, B** is a reference to the average cartilage volume removed in a critical-size defect compared with average reported studies (assuming both are full-thickness defects) in each animal species. This is important because in cartilage repair studies, the volume of cartilage that is removed is of higher priority than just the cartilage diameter.[2] As stated previously, rodent models are good for screening studies but because of the lack of utility, large animal models offer much greater relevance to human study of orthobiologic therapies.

CLINICALLY RELEVANT PRECLINICAL MODELS OF OSTEOARTHRITIS

Osteoarthritis is of great importance in healthcare. With more than 25 million people affected in the United States alone, the healthcare industry sustains costs upward of more than $180 billion annually.[5,41-43] Osteoarthritis is a difficult disease to study partially because of its poorly understood pathogenesis, the disease is often slow and unpredictable, and effective diagnostic tools are not available for the early stages of the disease process.[44] Furthermore, clinical symptoms often arise later during the course of the disease and may not completely reflect structural abnormalities within the joint.[5] The lack of correlation of symptoms with structural disease is an important challenge in studying disease progression. To overcome some of this lack of understanding, animal models of osteoarthritis have been developed over the past 50 years.[13,45] Researchers have sought understanding into disease pathogenesis, diagnosis, and treatment. Many animal models currently exist to better understand osteoarthritis; however, the greatest challenge lies in selecting the model that most closely approximates the human condition but also realizing that there exists no single gold standard that mimics all aspects of disease in humans.

A widely perceived and documented discrepancy in research into osteoarthritis is that animal models have poor translatability to clinical human disease.[46-49] Many reasons exist for the pervasive feeling regarding animal models, but two of the primary reasons are (1) mistakes made in choosing the correct animal model and (2) bias and a lack of rigor in designing studies and/or reporting the outcomes of those studies.[50] The subject of poor predictive value of animal models for osteoarthritis has been extensively reviewed[51,52] and, in summary, highlights the requirement that animal models must accurately reflect the specific type of osteoarthritis (posttraumatic osteoarthritis, juvenile, end stage, etc), the phenotype, and the stage of disease progression.[14] Very often in animal research, poor outcomes and lack of translatability are due to deficient attention to rigorous experimental design. A helpful and concise review of DEPART (Design and Execution of Protocols for Animal Research and Treatment) guidelines is listed in **Tables 1** through **4**.[13] As was mentioned previously, strict attention and practice of ARRIVE guidelines will enhance the likelihood of success when choosing the correct animal model for the study of

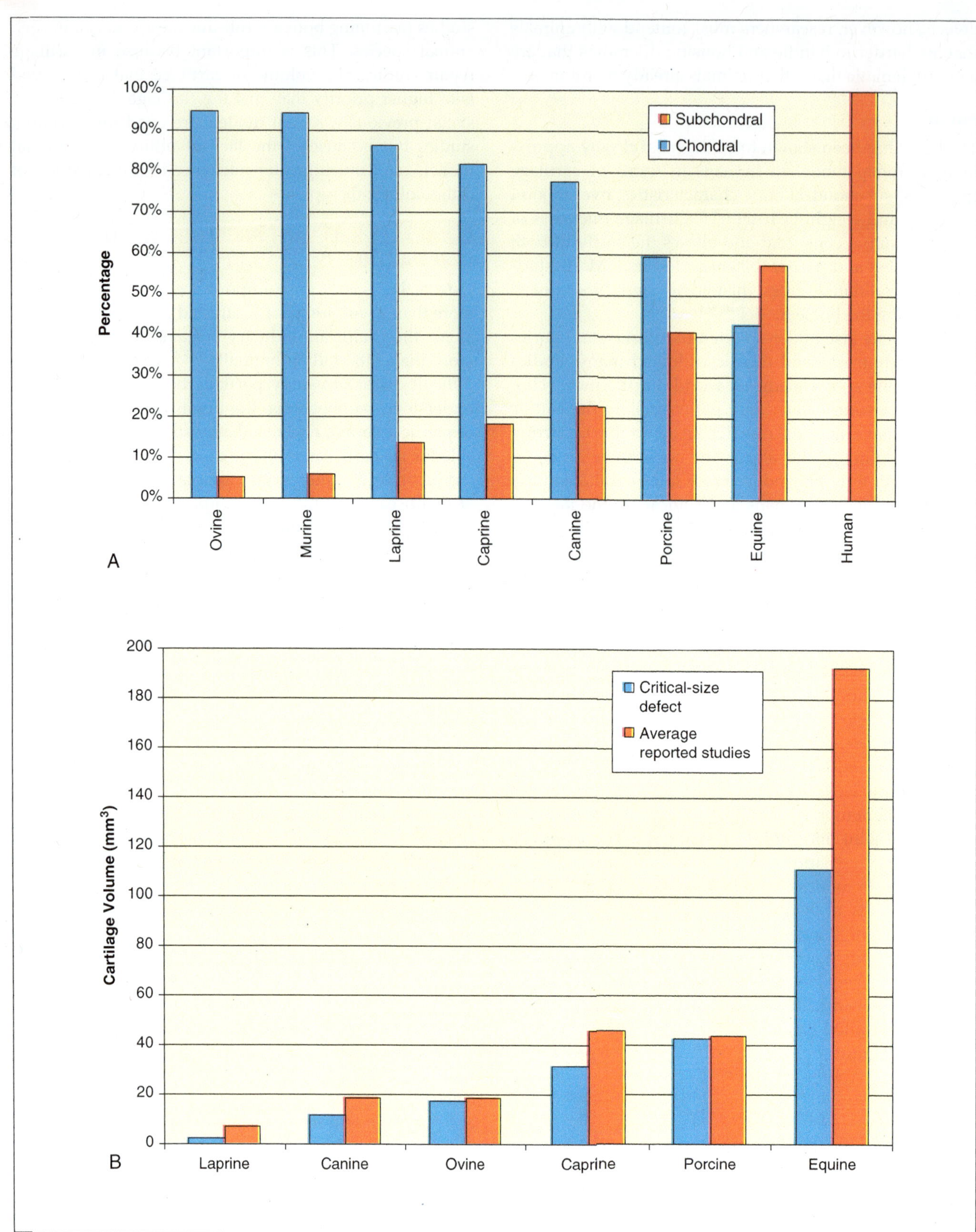

FIGURE 2 Graphs of proportion of chondral versus subchondral bone of preclinical animal model defects as a percentage of total defect compared with that of a human patient (**A**) and a comparison of the cartilage volume of critical-size defect with average reported cartilage defect volume assuming both are full thickness (**B**). (Reproduced with permission from Ahern BJ, Parvizi J, Schaer TP, et al: Preclinical animal models in single site cartilage defect testing: A systematic review. *Osteoarthritis Cartilage* 2009;17[6]:705-713; with permission from Elsevier.)

TABLE 2 DEPART: Design Considerations Before the Animal Experiment Begins

Issue	GRADE Domain[a]	Comments and Questions

Objective of study	1, 2, 4	• Is the objective to investigate disease pathophysiology or test a treatment? The answer may change the model used and study design (eg, genome-wide expression available in mice, intra-articular therapy easier in large animals).
		• Treatment trial design questions:
		  • How and how often is the drug administered (this may alter the choice of species, eg, daily intravenous may be problematic in mice; oral may be an issue in ruminants; systemic versus local may allow bilateral disease to minimize animal use)?
		  • Should a dose response be performed (this is an upgrade for GRADE and may alter the study design, sample numbers, and data analysis method)?
		  • When will the therapy be applied (eg, prophylactic to stop disease onset, therapeutic to stop disease progression)? This may affect the choice of model (eg, slowly progressive to allow intervention after onset but before maximal damage), time points examined, and if longitudinal outcomes are appropriate.
		  • What is the drug target (eg, pain versus structure; in the latter, cartilage degradation versus bone remodeling)? This may affect the choice of model (eg, differential level of bone remodeling alters cartilage response to diphosphonate in mouse versus rat), outcome measures (eg, imaging methods to detect the cartilage versus bone), and animal husbandry (eg, analgesics interfere with pain assessment; all analgesics even opioids can alter inflammation and potentially disease course).
		• Experimental design may be altered if there are one or more treatment strategies (eg, superiority versus equivalence to treatment/control). Longitudinal, cross-sectional, and crossover designs are possible and may determine or be determined by outcome measures (eg, histology versus imaging) and must include consideration of the 3 Rs of animal use.

Choice of outcome measures	1, 2, 3, 4	• Select a primary outcome measure to meet the study objective and then select secondary outcomes. • Outcomes should, where possible, be standardized to improve reliability and reproducibility. • Can all outcomes be performed in an individual or are separate animals needed (eg, biomechanics may not be compatible with subsequent histology or gene expression)? This will affect the sample size and study design. • As there can be regional variations (eg, cartilage gene expression, synovial pathology), sampling sites should be prespecified and standardized. • In cross-sectional design, multiple time points may be necessary (eg, to show progressive disease versus injury and repair of cartilage damage) and may need different time points for different aspects of progression (eg, cartilage proteoglycan loss versus erosion; cartilage damage versus bone sclerosis; structural disease versus pain). • Determine methods for allocation of animals to treatment and outcome groups and blinding of inducers (if preassigned allocation) and assessors. Failure to do this may lead to detection bias. • Predetermine the inclusion/exclusion criteria for outcome assessment and/or termination/removal of animal from study to prevent attrition bias from incomplete outcome data. • Outcome measures should be directly relevant to the human disease/intervention (eg, imaging used in both animal and human studies); histopathology and certain pain outcomes (eg, mechanical allodynia versus gait or weight bearing) may only indirectly relate to structural and clinical assessments in humans. • Consider whether longitudinal assessment of outcomes is possible (eg, imaging versus histology) and if this is more directly translatable to human trials (eg, would translation of the research question to human trials involve longitudinal assessment or cross-sectional comparison?).
Arthritis model	2	• Select the most appropriate model for applicability to human disease/population of interest and to meet study objectives. The osteoarthritis phenotype (eg, posttraumatic versus age-associated versus metabolic; more or less inflammatory) and joint (eg, knee versus hip versus hand) may affect disease pathogenesis and response to therapy.

(Continued)

TABLE 2 DEPART: Design Considerations Before the Animal Experiment Begins (Continued)

Issue	GRADE Domain[a]	Comments and Questions
Animals	2, 3	• Select appropriate animal characteristics to meet the study objective and target human population (eg, age, sex, species suitability for chosen model, and outcome measures [eg, larger species better for cartilage imaging or surgical therapy]). • Ensure a consistent source of animals: different sourcing of groups might affect disease outcomes (eg, wild-type versus genetically modified mice from different homozygous strains; genetic drift may change disease outcome). If animals are sourced from different locations, ensure adequate acclimatization period to avoid different disease outcome (eg, stress of shipping; animals from different sources may have disparate microbiomes). • Predetermine any criteria for inclusion/exclusion of animals entering the study and report this (eg, minimum weight; excitable animals excluded from analysis of pain outcome measures).
Control groups	1, 2	• Select same comparator group as that of interest in the human disease for direct applicability to human trial translation (eg, consider including non–disease-positive/healthy control, nontreated disease-negative/maximal disease control, as well as sham-induced and sham-treated groups). • The contralateral limb may not be appropriate as a control—altered load bearing induces remodeling in normal joint, which may be exacerbated or reduced with therapy. • For treatment studies, what is the appropriate control (eg, immunoglobulin G [IgG] rather than carrier/saline as control for biologic trial because IgG alone could affect disease outcome especially in more inflammatory arthropathy)?
Treatment strategies	2	• Select the same intervention method as of interest in the human disease, including type, timing, and route of administration (eg, intraperitoneal convenient in mouse but not in patients) to increase translational relevance.
Sample size	4	• Calculate the sample size (independent samples versus replicates) from previous studies or pilot studies, based on the variability of the primary outcome measure using an accepted method, and a clinically relevant and translatable effect size (eg, effects on pain in animal studies are known to be greater than human; unclear how cartilage erosion scored by histopathology relates to joint-space narrowing on MRI in patients).

[a]GRADE domain: 1 = risk of bias, 2 = indirectness, 3 = inconsistency, 4 = imprecision, and 5 = publication bias.

DEPART = Design and Execution of Protocols for Animal Research and Treatment

Modified with permission from Smith MM, Clarke EC, Little CB: Considerations for the design and execution of protocols for animal research and treatment to improve reproducibility and standardization: "DEPART well-prepared and ARRIVE safely". *Osteoarthritis Cartilage* 2017;25(3):354-363.

TABLE 3 DEPART: Design Considerations During the Animal Experiment

Issue	GRADE Domain[a]	Comments and Questions
Allocation of animal groups	1	• Animal identification and allocation should be performed by a different person than both those inducing disease and the observers assessing outcomes, to ensure blinding and avoid bias. • Randomization procedure must be specified (eg, coin flip, random number): simple randomization may be problematic with small sample size; block design ensures group equipoise (stratified block if covariates, eg, sex, weight, and age, also need equal distribution in treatment strategies/genotypes). • Ideally identify and allocate animals before starting disease induction (eg, taking animals in order of capture may select most docile/least mobile first) because this may alter the disease severity and pain/behavior outcomes.

TABLE 3 DEPART: Design Considerations During the Animal Experiment (Continued)

Issue	GRADE Domain[a]	Comments and Questions
Animal housing	1, 3	• Consider and report on animal housing density—is this maintained and consistent across study groups? • Consider solitary versus multiple animal/cage because activity may affect disease severity, sequential animal removal from cages stresses the remainders, and cohousing or single housing of groups (eg, genotypes, naïve/sham/osteoarthritis; different treatment strategies) may affect behavioral/pain responses (eg, mice display empathy). • Consider issues of cohousing male and female animals (eg, even housing both sexes in the same room can affect behavior in mice) because this may alter the activity and disease severity and pain/behavior outcomes.
Animal husbandry	1, 3	• All groups/treatment strategies should be performed simultaneously rather than sequentially to avoid changes in temperature and humidity (eg, season can be sensed even within sealed facility), food and water (eg, constituents may change with time or supplier), noise/vibrations (eg, building works at different times), staff (eg, change in sex or different cologne use by animal handlers/observers), facility disease status, schedules (eg, light/dark), suppliers (eg, bedding), etc. All of these issues may affect animal stress, immunity, and pain outcomes. • Ensure equivalent husbandry of all animals (eg, different light, temperature, vibration in different rooms/stalls in animal facility, even with cage locations in a rack in a single room [eg, top or bottom], and environmental enrichment in cages, etc) because this may alter the activity and disease severity, stress, and pain/behavior outcome.

Blinding of inducers, treaters, and observers	1, 3	• Avoid risk of unblinding and unconscious bias in:
		  • Inducers, for example, randomize and blind until intraoperative to avoid less invasive surgery for sham control mice.
		  • Treaters, for example, placebo and drug injection/solution/tablet, should be identical and unidentifiable to the person administering to avoid differences in animal handling or surety of intra-articular injection.
		  • Observers, particularly for subjective outcomes, such as pain, for example, groups cohoused in cages and placed in observation cages by separate person and identical appearance of groups (eg, shaved leg, skin incision in naïve/sham/osteoarthritis) so observer does not have expectation of similar outcome for a given group.

Disease induction and treatment	1, 3, 4	• Reagent differences may change the model severity or outcome measure (eg, induction materials—different sources/types of antigens, anesthetics, antibiotics, suture material; treatment efficacy—drug source may alter its activity; palatability of food/water may change and affect health/weight gain). • Personnel differences (eg, surgical skill levels) may change model severity and time course. • Consider if the model or treatment may have secondary effects (eg, weight loss, sedation, joint fibrosis, muscle atrophy) that may confound activity, disease severity, and pain outcomes.
Outcome measures	1, 3, 4	• Consider euthanasia method that will not influence any outcome measure (eg, stress and serum biomarkers, including sequential animal removal from groups). • Observer differences (eg, subjective pain measures) may change outcome measures. This may be avoided/reduced by randomization of observers and training to ensure standardization. • Multiple measures in one individual may change outcome measures (eg, pain responses affected by repeated handling from multiple pain outcomes or prior interference such as blood sampling; order of testing—ipsilateral versus contralateral limb first for allodynia). • The aforementioned issues may require separate groups to be used for different outcomes. If this is the case, consider how animals are assigned to different outcome measures (eg, randomization, blinding, preallocation). • Timing of observations may alter the outcome measure (eg, weekend versus midweek may change facility noise, number of people, etc, may change pain/behavior measures; morning, midday, or evening may change noise, etc, as aforementioned but also in nocturnal species, this may affect behavioral outcomes or diurnal variation in biomarkers with different day/night cycle than humans).

[a]GRADE domain: 1 = risk of bias, 2 = indirectness, 3 = inconsistency, 4 = imprecision, and 5 = publication bias.

DEPART = Design and Execution of Protocols for Animal Research and Treatment

Reproduced with permission from Smith MM, Clarke EC, Little CB: Considerations for the design and execution of protocols for animal research and treatment to improve reproducibility and standardization: "DEPART well-prepared and ARRIVE safely". *Osteoarthritis Cartilage* 2017;25(3):354-363.

TABLE 4 DEPART: Analysis Considerations After the Animal Work is Performed

Issue	GRADE Domain[a]	Comments
Outcomes as prespecified	1, 2	• Outcomes to be analyzed are all those specified before the experiments began and that were adequately powered to detect differences between treatment groups (any others are speculative and should be designated pilot data for future follow-up): avoid [b]HARKing and [c]p-hacking. • Changing/adding/deleting outcomes after initiation of experiments must not be performed without adequate justification.
Outcome measures: Analysis and Specific Considerations		
Blinding of assessors	1	• Blinding (eg, group, genotype, time, treatment) must continue for analyses conducted after animal termination (eg, histopathology scoring, imaging analysis, biomechanical measures) to reduce bias.
Histopathology	1, 4	• Slides should be assessed in a randomized order (if serial sections from individual animal, these can be grouped) by more than one blinded observer using a validated scoring system for which interobserver and intraobserver variation has already been reported. Any unpredicted interesting features found during analysis can be reported as pilot or preliminary data for follow-up in a subsequent study. • Predetermine what joint regions (eg, medial femorotibial joint versus both medial and lateral), what pathology outcomes (eg, cartilage, subchondral bone, osteophytes, synovitis), and how many sections will be scored.
Imaging	1, 2, 3, 4	• Regardless of whether outcome quantitation is manual or automated by computer program, images should be evaluated in a randomized order by one or more blinded observers according to a prespecified protocol for predetermined pathologies or measurements. Any unpredicted interesting features can be reported as pilot or preliminary data for follow-up in a subsequent study.
Biomechanics	1, 2, 3, 4	• Gait analyses require consistent standardization because different systems vary markedly and individual gait parameters may measure different disease pathologies. • Describe in full the isolated joint/tissue biomechanical measures because there is no standardized terminology (eg, laxity, range of motion), normalization (eg, size, cross section), or testing parameters (eg, defining neutral position, speed, preconditioning). • Consider how well the chosen outcomes match definitions and methods used in human studies to optimize translation.
Gene expression	1, 2, 3, 4	• Consider the most appropriate method for normalization (eg, correct for total RNA versus one or more reference genes) because housekeeping genes may be regulated by biomechanical loading and disease stage.
Data Analysis and Visualization		
Blinding of data analysis	1	• Ideally, the data analyst should be blinded (eg, to group, genotype, time, treatment, etc—these can be designated X and Y, A and B) to reduce bias.
Distribution of outcome data	1, 4	• It may be that data have a different distribution (nonnormal) than were expected/predicted and data transformation and/or nonparametric testing will need to be performed (distinct from p-hacking, this is performed to ensure appropriate analysis).
Statistical analysis for each outcome	1, 3	• Statistical tests should be specified before experimentation (see caveat above redistribution) and detailed fully in the methods. • Tests/models should be appropriate for the type of data and outcome measure (eg, noncontinuous scores may be used for activity, morphology/pathology, histopathology, etc, and these require nonparametric comparison tests or logistic regression models; if data have been collected at a number of time points, investigators should consider using a longitudinal regression model, survival analysis, or mixed-model regression).

TABLE 4 DEPART: Analysis Considerations After the Animal Work is Performed (Continued)

Issue	GRADE Domain[a]	Comments
Adjustments for plausible confounders and multiple comparisons	1	• A direct comparison between groups may not be valid without correction for plausible confounders (ie, those that may influence the primary outcome such as weight, age of the animals, time postinduction). This is particularly important if there are differences between groups at baseline. • Predetermine whether correction for multiple comparisons will be applied and if so which method. Is the experiment exploratory/hypothesis generating (correction will reduce detection of potentially interesting findings) or confirmatory/hypothesis testing (correction ensures detection of robust/reproducible findings)?
Data visualization	1, 4	• Graphs should be carefully chosen to match the type of data (eg, for continuous variables such as cartilage glycosaminoglycan content or biomechanics, raw data points with a mean and standard deviation or confidence intervals; for categorical variables such as histology, scoring tables or box plots showing the median and the 25/75 and 10/90 percentiles may be clearer; for ratios like fold changes in gene expression, use of logarithmic scales to avoid positive change visual bias—note if bar/column graphs are used for these ratios, the origin is one, not zero).

[a]GRADE domain: 1 = risk of bias, 2 = indirectness, 3 = inconsistency, 4 = imprecision, and 5 = publication bias.

[b]HARKing = Hypothesizing after the result is known.

[c]p-Hacking = applying multiple statistical analyses until hitting on a significant finding.

DEPART = Design and Execution of Protocols for Animal Research and Treatment

Modified with permission from Smith MM, Clarke EC, Little CB: Considerations for the design and execution of protocols for animal research and treatment to improve reproducibility and standardization: "DEPART well-prepared and ARRIVE safely". *Osteoarthritis Cartilage* 2017;25(3):354-363.

orthobiologic therapies.[53] Both the DEPART and ARRIVE guidelines should be read and contemplated fully before launching any project with these treatment strategies.

Models of osteoarthritis are generally divided into spontaneous (genetically or naturally occurring) and induced (surgical or intra-articular injection).

Spontaneously occurring osteoarthritis in species such as the dog and horse (in the naturally occurring disease process) closely mimics that in human osteoarthritis. However, they take time to develop and are variable in outcomes; therefore, these types of studies are hard to standardize to have adequate power.[5] Other models of naturally and spontaneously occurring disease exist with many distinct strains of rodent models, but these often oversimplify the disease and therapeutic interventions such as orthobiologics may not be specifically well studied in these models. For example, if osteoarthritis does not develop normally in a knockout mouse with an aggrecanase deletion, this would not necessarily account for the many variables around aggrecanases or other catabolic molecules that may also be at play in developing disease. Osteoarthritic therapies have been developed and have been successful in mice; however, they are rarely successfully translated to clinically relevant therapies in humans.[5,45]

Surgical induction in rodents and large animal models encompasses many different techniques including meniscectomy (partial or total), destabilization of the medial meniscus, meniscal defect, anterior cruciate ligament (ACL) tear or posterior cruciate ligament tear, medial or lateral collateral transection, creation of an articular groove, osteotomy, impact, and osteochondral fragmentation.[1,5,54] All of these procedures rely on either joint instability, altered joint mechanics, or inflammation to induce osteoarthritic lesions.[54] Most of these procedures are performed in the stifle (human equivalent to the knee), with the exception of the horse model, which is performed in the carpal or metacarpophalangeal joint. Osteoarthritis reliably develops in surgical models and may have a shorter timeline versus spontaneous osteoarthritis in genetically modified models, which may be easier for budgeting and project planning as well.[55,56]

Chemically induced models of osteoarthritis (such as monosodium iodoacetate, collagenase, carrageenan, and Freund adjuvant) also exist; however, their validity is often questioned because of widespread cell death and rapid joint destruction.[14]

Few studies, interestingly, evaluate pain in an in-depth manner, which is surprising because pain is the most common reason for which people seek treatment.

Ignoring the measurement and validation of improvement of pain in these studies is a serious oversight in researching this disease process.[1,5,57] There are significant technical and ethical difficulties in pain studies because pain is variable in all species including humans. Each species feels and exhibits pain differently, and the nonverbal nature of any animals raises issues with validation as well as ethical concerns. Each institution has animal care and use committees that oversee and are responsible for scoring the level of pain that is acceptable for each species; however, there certainly exist inconsistencies in teams between institutions and that also introduces variability across studies performed at different centers.

Other techniques that are important in osteoarthritic assessments are imaging, biomarkers, and histopathology. Imaging modalities that can significantly improve quantification of outcomes are MRI and CT. The field of imaging for relevant osteoarthritic models continues to be developed, and it is now clearly recognized that improved measurement of cartilage characteristics through various imaging modalities is of great importance in longitudinal assessments in cartilage treatment.[58] Radiographic assessment is only beneficial for progressive or end-stage disease.[54,59] Mostly, MRI (and to a lesser extent, CT) is looked at for incorporation into studies to assess progression through time of response to therapies.[5,54,60,61]

Biochemical biomarkers are measured either systemically (serum or urine) or locally (in synovial fluid).[54,60] Biomarkers is also a burgeoning field within the study of osteoarthritis. OARSI published a consensus report in 2011, but most of these are measured in the urine or serum and therefore are subject to influence by systemic factors as well.[62] A wide array of biomarkers also exist for synovial fluid and have been published extensively throughout the recent literature; however, there is no consensus yet on best markers to measure. Another important factor in considering biomarkers is that, depending on species, various biomarker assays may not be available for that animal species. Last, because of their size, small animal models of osteoarthritis have limitations or, based on handling, synovial fluid aspiration is often unrewarding except by lavage, which then adds another component of complexity. Likely, the biomarker field will continue to develop, and although an array of biomarkers will be recommended, there will be no single biomarker thought of as the gold standard.[60]

Histopathologic outcomes are integral to almost all preclinical models of osteoarthritis. Histologic grading systems have been widely published with several in the early stages with the Mankin scoring system and many modifications thereof widely used through several decades.[14,63] Because of the concern of the reliability of that scoring system, most notably in early stages of osteoarthritis, OARSI published a better grading system that would exemplify the principles of simplicity, utility, scalability, extendibility, and comparability.[63] While that system was validated in animal and human articular cartilage, a follow-up initiative of OARSI further developed other grading scales that standardized scoring systems for each major species used in osteoarthritic research.[64] In these OARSI guidelines, recommendations were made for processing histologic samples, histomorphometry, terminology for reporting, and statistical analysis recommendations.[63,65-67]

SUMMARY OF SPECIFIC ANIMAL MODELS FOR THE STUDY OF OSTEOARTHRITIS

Small Animal Models

Mouse

As mentioned in the section discussing cartilage repair, mouse models are inexpensive, easy to handle, and have cost-effective housing strategies. These models are good for drug screening and altering genetic properties to screen for molecular targets of pathways; however, for studying orthobiologics, they are less relevant. Many different strains of the mouse exist, and because of variability in genetic backgrounds, they should always be reported.[68] There are more than 135 distinct strains of mice genetically modified for osteoarthritis that have been reviewed.[45] The mouse cartilage surface is only a few cells thick compared with that of the human (**Figure 3**); therefore, surgical manipulations are not correlated with the human condition. Therapeutics have attempted to be developed in mice based on specific genes in the mouse; however, replication and translatability are reported to be poor.[45] Furthermore, biomechanical loading is drastically different, and the aforementioned anatomy is also different, leaving this species to have low translatability for the study of orthobiologics.

Rat

The rat has had surgically and chemically induced disease widely reported in the osteoarthritic arena; however, similar to mice, epiphyseal plates remain open into adulthood. Rat articular cartilage is slightly (0.1 mm) thicker than that of the mouse; however, biomechanics are still vastly different from the human. Furthermore, spontaneous healing has been reported, which further decreases their utility in orthobiologic research.[16] Although advanced imaging techniques such as MRI, micro-CT, and phase-contrast radiographic imaging have been developed for the rat, the model still leaves large gaps in translatability to human osteoarthritis.[16]

Guinea Pig

The Dunkin Hartley guinea pig is a commonly used strain for modeling osteoarthritis because of strong similarities to human primary idiopathic osteoarthritis. Similarly, the size of the joint is much greater than that of the mouse or the rat, and their size allows collection of joint and body fluids

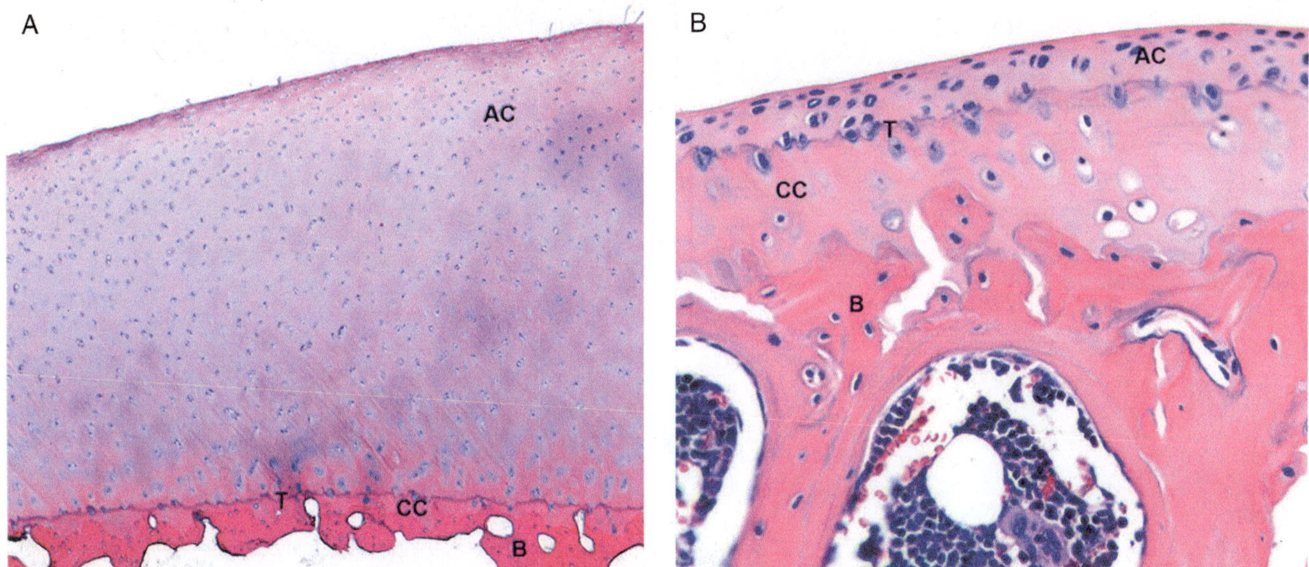

FIGURE 3 Histologic photomicrographs of normal adult human cartilage of the knee (**A**) and mouse (stifle/knee equivalent) (**B**) revealing the large differences of thickness of articular cartilage (AC) between species. B = bone, CC = calcified cartilage. (Reproduced with permission from McCoy AM: Animal models of osteoarthritis: Comparisons and key considerations. *Vet Pathol* 2015;52[5]:803-818.)

to evaluate biomarkers, they are suitable for a number of imaging techniques, they are easy to handle, and their time to skeletal maturity is reasonable versus larger spontaneous models.[5,69,70] Furthermore, osteoarthritis develops in guinea pigs that are not diet restricted, similar to people with obesity, making them an appropriate model to study obesity.[71] Surgical models are also developed with the Dunkin Hartley strain; however, these lesions then more rapidly affect the progression of osteoarthritis.[5] OARSI also has a guinea pig working group, and a complete and validated scoring system is available.[70]

Rabbit

Rabbits have been used for osteoarthritis studies for decades;[5,16,69] however, their biomechanical (much higher flexion angles) and gait differences to humans make their translatability questionable. Additionally, important structural differences exist because the rabbit cartilage is 10 times thinner than the human cartilage but curiously has a higher chondrocyte density.[5,60,72] In addition, the cartilage zones are very different between the two because the transitional and radial zones differ tremendously throughout sites in the joint.[72] In addition, rabbits, like other small animal models, experience spontaneous healing especially in the young,[2,16,69] so importantly, rabbits younger than 8 to 9 months should be used for any osteoarthritic studies. Radiographic verifications to ensure epiphyseal plate closure can be considered. Histologic cartilage grading scales and the rabbit working group within OARSI have been established and have proven the utility of osteoarthritic degeneration.

The Relevance of Large Animal Models in Studying Orthobiologic Therapies for Osteoarthritis

Larger animal models are fairly established to be more relevant animal models for studying osteoarthritis, especially for the study of orthobiologics due to the translational accuracy and the important ability to easily access synovial fluids and assess pain. Furthermore, there is a widespread occurrence of naturally occurring primary idiopathic and secondary posttraumatic osteoarthritis in these species. Diagnostic imaging, arthroscopic intervention, and second-look arthroscopies as well as postoperative management of these models make them much more favorable in studying therapeutic intervention with orthobiologics. Some drawbacks that are associated with large animal models are expense, longer time to maturity, progression of disease, and ethical considerations, especially companion animals. The general consensus for many, however, is that large animal models are worth the greater expense if translation is important to humans. A relevant example is how the extensive study of intra-articular corticosteroids in the equine athlete can translate to the human athlete in a very realistic manner.[73] Decades of published studies in equine preclinical models have lent themselves to relevant observations by many orthopaedic clinicians treating people with osteoarthritis. A quick reference to advantages and disadvantages of the animal models is summarized in **Table 5**.

Canine

The dog model has anatomic similarities and good translational value to humans because there is amenability to

TABLE 5 Advantages and Disadvantages of Osteoarthritic Animal Models

	Advantages	Disadvantages	Models Used
Mouse	Low cost Easy to use Genome sequenced Can view whole knee on slides	Thin cartilage Postoperative management difficult	Genetic Meniscal destabilization Chemical
Rat	Low cost Easy to use Thicker cartilage than mouse Can view whole knee on slides	Small joints Postoperative management difficult	Medial meniscus tear Partial medial meniscectomy Anterior cruciate ligament (ACL) transection ACL transection with partial medial meniscectomy Chemical
Rabbit	Easy to use	Knee biomechanics Cartilage capable of regeneration Different histology from human Postoperative management difficult	ACL transection Meniscectomy Chemical
Guinea pig	Similar histopathology to human Prone to spontaneous osteoarthritis	Sedentary lifestyle Arthroscopy not possible	Spontaneous Meniscectomy Chemical
Dog	Prone to spontaneous osteoarthritis Arthroscopy feasible MRI feasible Gastrointestinal physiology Genome sequenced Validated outcome measures	Cost Public perception	Spontaneous ACL transection Meniscal release Focal cartilage defect
Pig	Large joint Arthroscopy feasible MRI feasible Gastrointestinal physiology Validated outcomes	Cost Handling	ACL transection Focal cartilage defect
Sheep/goat	Large joint Easy to use Arthroscopy feasible MRI feasible	Cost Gastrointestinal physiology	Partial/total meniscectomy
Horse	Spontaneous osteoarthritis Can induce osteoarthritis without instability Arthroscopy feasible MRI feasible	Cost Anatomy	Spontaneous Osteochondral fragment exercise model

Modified with permission from Gregory MH, Capito N, Kuroki K, Stoker AM, Cook JL, Sherman SL: A review of translational animal models for knee osteoarthritis. *Arthritis* 2012;2012:764621.

ACL = anterior cruciate ligament

postoperative strategies such as bandaging, splinting, and various postoperative exercise regimens.[5,69] Commonly, in dog models, the stifle is used; however, naturally occurring diseases occur in this joint in dogs and in the hip and elbow as well. For this reason, therapies studied in canine preclinical model can also be taken into clinical trials naturally occurring in dog populations. Because of widespread clinical disease in dogs, gait and kinematic analysis and MRI (up to 7T magnets) have been developed and clinically applied in dogs.[74]

Histologic outcomes in dogs continue to be the gold standard, and the OARSI dog working group validated a new scoring system in 2021[75] that validates a macroscopic and microscopic scoring of cartilage, synovium, and meniscus. The advantages of this system have been described as versatile and comprehensive.[75] As in other preclinical models, the dog stifle has much more flexion than that of humans, and skeletal maturity can vary widely by breed and sex. Closure of epiphyseal plates should be validated radiographically. As previously mentioned, because of the dog being a companion animal that forms strong human–animal bonds, many research facilities are not willing to use the dog model for osteoarthritic research; therefore, they are not as widely used as other preclinical models.

Sheep/Goat

Sheep and goats are highly used species as models for osteoarthritic study because of their ease of handling and low cost (compared with some of the other larger animal models). They are considered to be the best large animal model for studying ACL repair and subsequent osteoarthritis secondary to ACL rupture. Goats have menisci that are highly similar to humans as well.[76] Their cartilage can be up to 2 mm but is also highly variable throughout the stifle, which is important regarding consistency, and principal investigators should be aware that this inconsistency can play out in data analysis.[31]

The OARSI sheep/goat working group formed a total joint scoring system that combined both medial and lateral femoral condyles and tibial plateaus. Separate from that, osteophytes may be graded as well. An additional grade of 0 to 5 is assigned based on the percentage of area of the tibial plateau or femoral condyle that can be assessed. Furthermore, imaging using MRI has been reported to be well correlated to macroscopic scoring systems that have been developed in sheep and goats and thus longitudinal analysis could be highly informative to progression of therapies over time.[77] Sheep and goats also do not experience spontaneous osteoarthritis, although severe joint degeneration can develop in goats because of caprine arthritis encephalitis virus so should be negative for testing to this virus before osteoarthritic studies.[78] The most frequently used osteoarthritis induction model in both sheep and goats is destabilization or meniscectomy/partial meniscectomy followed by forced exercise.[79-81] Forced exercise has been determined to be a pivotal component of osteoarthritic development, and without exercise only mild osteoarthritic ensues.[78,82,83]

Porcine

Pigs, especially minipigs, have included ACL transection and medial meniscectomy.[84] Anatomically, the stifle of the pig and the human knee are very similar with some variability in meniscus width (that of the pig is wider) and the cruciate ligaments are longer.[76,85] The thickness of cartilage is similar, and importantly, the gastrointestinal physiology of pigs is similar to that of humans, therefore making the pig a good model for oral biologic interventions.[54]

Equine

The horse has been cited as being the closest or one of the closest models to human osteoarthritis due to similar joint anatomy, cartilage thickness and subchondral bone characteristics, biochemical makeup, and biomechanical characteristics.[2,35,86] Interestingly, horses are used as athletes and sustain injuries highly correlative to those of humans, thus making the horse both an excellent translational model and a model by which clinical studies can be carried out for similar conditions in people. Furthermore, the veterinarians who treat musculoskeletal conditions in equine athletes use orthobiologics frequently, making the preclinical study of these drugs very translational to both the equine patient and the human patient.[4,87] Similar to humans, osteoarthritis develops in horses in the stifle and also in the carpus and metacarpophalangeal joint. Intensive studies have been performed on the horse regarding diagnostics (such as imaging and biomarker analysis) and therapeutics, especially in the area of orthobiologics research.

In addition to second-look arthroscopy, ease of harvesting serial synovial fluids, and performing in-depth imaging such as MRI, CT, and radiographic analysis, rehabilitation practices have made the horse model very popular for osteoarthritis studies.[20,40,88] Similar to cartilage repair studies in the horse, the equine osteoarthritis model has been tested and validated through many published studies regarding orthobiologic osteoarthritis therapies, further demonstrating the utility of this species for studying orthobiologics.[89] The most popular and well-studied model is the osteochondral chip fragment model in the middle carpal joint, where a small fragment is created prior to horses exercising on the treadmill to induce low-grade osteoarthritis. Another model has been an osteochondral fragment induced in the metacarpophalangeal joint[90,91] and an impact model.[92] The OARSI histology horse working group published recommendations for histologic evaluation through a modified Mankin score.[93] In addition to this synovial score, an equine synovial membrane score was developed. A slightly different scoring system was verified for the metacarpophalangeal joint by Boyce et al.[91] Together with the in-depth physical, histologic, imaging, and biomarker analysis validation in relation to osteoarthritis, the horse, although more expensive than some of the other large animal models, yields much information that is highly translational and can be quickly applied to naturally occurring disease processes in horses with osteoarthritis.[5,94]

It is important to also acknowledge that the study of orthobiologics in treating osteoarthritis in naturally occurring models in horses (horses that have some form of posttraumatic osteoarthritis) absolutely exists.[4,87,95,96]

Although these studies in naturally occurring animal models, as in humans, lack the ability to control variability, they reduce the translatability issue around induced defects or disease that may not entirely mimic the clinical scenario or disease progression in people.

SUMMARY OF OSTEOARTHRITIS MODELS

There exist various animal models to study osteoarthritis, and no model is perfect. Asking the targeted questions, designing a comprehensive study by first reviewing DEPART and ARRIVE guidelines can be hugely beneficial.[13] The responsibility of using animals in preclinical models falls on the principal investigator and the entire team to make sure animals are ethically treated and the three Rs principle is followed. Large animal models ultimately provide the most relevant information and will be required for verification of findings before moving to human clinical studies.[5] Because large animal models can be expensive, considerations of cost, adequate power, housing availability, and outcome measures need to be weighed against the question being asked. Surgically induced osteoarthritis in large animal models more closely assimilates to the study of posttraumatic osteoarthritis (PTOA). Additionally using orthobiologics in both surgically induced disease and then naturally occurring PTOA can then be an added benefit as a follow-up to those preclinical models in which disease was surgically induced. Parallel studies can be performed using both FDA and Center for Veterinary Medicine guidelines. Some academic institutions will also be good laboratory practice/good manufacturing practice certified, so research institutions and centers that have that capability are often the most expeditious route to get the approval. Ultimately, it is important to work with a group in which communications and partnerships can be formed that can lead fast-tracking therapies such as orthobiologics into the human market to benefit both animals and people.

SUMMARY

Animal models, specifically large animal models of cartilage repair and osteoarthritis, can be quite relevant in the study of orthobiologics because the large size, anatomic similarities of cartilage and subchondral bone, and the ability to sample joint fluid and perform gait analysis studies allow for translatable preclinical studies relevant to the human condition. Naturally occurring cartilage defects and/or osteoarthritis allow additional studies in less controlled conditions but may more naturally mimic disease in humans and can also be performed in parallel to further confirm preclinical findings. Guidelines for researchers and clinician scientists exist for studies in all animal models in the ARRIVE and DEPART descriptions and can be beneficial in elaborating on preclinical models. Furthermore, abiding by the three Rs recommendation of reducing, replacing, and refining animal models based on the specifics of the orthobiologic selected to study is also important. Understanding the animal model and suitability of a particular biologic that may be derived from that model is also of paramount importance to ensure that translatable information results. Regulatory agencies such as the FDA and United States Department of Agriculture should be consulted, and expertise in the chosen animal model should be sought before settling on the final preclinical model to use. Although large animal preclinical models are more expensive to use than rodent models for the study of orthobiologics in joint disease, translatable information and relevant results that can inform efficacy can be tremendously valuable when using orthobiologics for humans and often justify greater costs.

REFERENCES

1. Little CB, Zaki S: What constitutes an "animal model of osteoarthritis" – The need for consensus? *Osteoarthritis Cartilage* 2012;20(4):261-267.
2. Ahern BJ, Parvizi J, Boston R, Schaer TP: Preclinical animal models in single site cartilage defect testing: A systematic review. *Osteoarthritis Cartilage* 2009;17(6):705-713.
3. Ferris D, Frisbie D, Kisiday J, McIlwraith CW: In vivo healing of meniscal lacerations using bone marrow-derived mesenchymal stem cells and fibrin glue. *Stem Cell Int* 2012;2012:691605.
4. Bertone AL, Ishihara A, Zekas LJ, et al: Evaluation of a single intra-articular injection of autologous protein solution for treatment of osteoarthritis in horses. *Am J Vet Res* 2014;75(2):141-151.
5. McCoy AM: Animal models of osteoarthritis: Comparisons and key considerations. *Vet Pathol* 2015;52(5):803-818.
6. Olsen A, Johnson V, Webb T, Santangelo KS, Dow S, Duerr FM: Evaluation of intravenously delivered allogeneic mesenchymal stem cells for treatment of elbow osteoarthritis in dogs: A Pilot Study. *Vet Comp Orthop Traumatol* 2019;32(3):173-181.
7. McGowan KB, Stiegman G: Regulatory challenges for cartilage repair technologies. *Cartilage* 2013;4(1):4-11.
8. ASTM American Society for Testing and Materials: *ASTM F2451-05 Standard Guide for In Vitro Assessment of Implantable Devices Intended to Repair or Regenerate Articular Cartilage.* 2010. https://www.astm.org/f2451-05.html.
9. Casado JG, Gomez-Mauricio G, Alvarez V, et al: Comparative phenotypic and molecular characterization of porcine mesenchymal stem cells from different sources for translational studies in a large animal model. *Vet Immunol Immunopathol* 2012;147(1-2):104-112.
10. Greif G, Mrowietz C, Meyer-Sievers H, Ganter M, Jung F, Hiebl B: Differences in human and sheep platelet adherence, aggregation and activation induced by glass beads in a modified chandler loop-system. *Clin Hemorheol Microcirc* 2021;79(1):129-136.
11. Zhang Y, Xing F, Luo R, Duan X: Platelet-rich plasma for bone fracture treatment: A systematic review of current evidence in preclinical and clinical studies. *Front Med* 2021;8:676033.

12. Gorzalczany SB, Rodriguez Basso AG: Strategies to apply 3Rs in preclinical testing. *Pharmacol Res Perspect* 2021;9(5):e00863.
13. Smith MM, Clarke EC, Little CB: Considerations for the design and execution of protocols for animal research and treatment to improve reproducibility and standardization: "DEPART well-prepared and ARRIVE safely". *Osteoarthritis Cartilage* 2017;25(3):354-363.
14. Zaki S, Blaker CL, Little CB: OA foundations – Experimental models of osteoarthritis. *Osteoarthritis Cartilage* 2021;30(3):357-380.
15. Goodrich LR, Grieger JC, Phillips JN, et al: scAAVIL-1ra dosing trial in a large animal model and validation of long-term expression with repeat administration for osteoarthritis therapy. *Gene Ther* 2015;22(7):536-545.
16. Cook JL, Hung CT, Kuroki K, et al: Animal models of cartilage repair. *Bone Joint Res* 2014;3(4):89-94.
17. Liebig BE, Kisiday JD, Bahney CS, Ehrhart NP, Goodrich LR: The platelet-rich plasma and mesenchymal stem cell milieu: A review of therapeutic effects on bone healing. *J Orthop Res* 2020;38(12):2539-2550.
18. *ASTM F3224-17 Standard Test Method for Evaluating Growth of Engineered Cartilage Tissue Using Magnetic Resonance Imaging*. American Society for Testing and Materials, 2021.
19. Nelson BB, Goodrich LR, Barrett MF, Grinstaff MW, Kawcak CE: Use of contrast media in computed tomography and magnetic resonance imaging in horses: Techniques, adverse events and opportunities. *Equine Vet J* 2017;49(4):410-424.
20. Goodrich LR, Chen AC, Werpy NM, et al: Addition of mesenchymal stem cells to autologous platelet-enhanced fibrin scaffolds in chondral defects: Does it enhance repair? *J Bone Joint Surg Am* 2016;98(1):23-34.
21. Mow VC, Kuei SC, Lai WM, Armstrong CG: Biphasic creep and stress relaxation of articular cartilage in compression? Theory and experiments. *J Biomech Eng* 1980;102(1):73-84.
22. Mow VC, Ateshian GA, Spilker RL: Biomechanics of diarthrodial joints: A review of twenty years of progress. *J Biomech Eng* 1993;115(4B):460-467.
23. Hjelle K, Solheim E, Strand T, Muri R, Brittberg M: Articular cartilage defects in 1,000 knee arthroscopies. *Arthroscopy* 2002;18(7):730-734.
24. Bouwmeester PS, Kuijer R, Homminga GN, Bulstra SK, Geesink RGT: A retrospective analysis of two independent prospective cartilage repair studies: Autogenous perichondrial grafting versus subchondral drilling 10 years post-surgery. *J Orthop Res* 2002;20(2):267-273.
25. Breinan HA, Minas T, Hsu H-P, Nehrer S, Shortkroff S, Spector M: Autologous chondrocyte implantation in a canine model: Change in composition of reparative tissue with time. *J Orthop Res* 2001;19(3):482-492.
26. Lee CR, Grodzinsky AJ, Hsu H-P, Spector M: Effects of a cultured autologous chondrocyte-seeded type II collagen scaffold on the healing of a chondral defect in a canine model. *J Orthop Res* 2003;21(2):272-281.
27. Hunziker EB: Articular cartilage repair: Basic science and clinical progress. A review of the current status and prospects. *Osteoarthritis Cartilage* 2002;10(6):432-463.
28. Breinan HA, Minas T, Hsu H-P, Nehrer S, Sledge CB, Spector M: Effect of cultured autologous chondrocytes on repair of chondral defects in a canine model. *J Bone Joint Surg Am* 1997;79(10):1439-1451.
29. Nehrer S, Breinan HA, Ramappa A, et al: Chondrocyte-seeded collagen matrices implanted in a chondral defect in a canine model. *Biomaterials* 1998;19(24):2313-2328.
30. Hunziker EB: Articular cartilage repair: Are the intrinsic biological constraints undermining this process insuperable? *Osteoarthritis Cartilage* 1999;7(1):15-28.
31. Risch M, Easley JT, McCready EG, et al: Mechanical, biochemical, and morphological topography of ovine knee cartilage. *J Orthop Res* 2021;39(4):780-787.
32. Hurtig MB, Buschmann MD, Fortier LA, et al: Preclinical studies for cartilage repair: Recommendations from the International Cartilage Repair Society. *Cartilage* 2011;2(2):137-152.
33. Brehm W, Aklin B, Yamashita T, et al: Repair of superficial osteochondral defects with an autologous scaffold-free cartilage construct in a caprine model: Implantation method and short-term results. *Osteoarthritis Cartilage* 2006;14(12):1214-1226.
34. Jackson DW, Lalor PA, Aberman HM, Simon TM: Spontaneous repair of full-thickness defects of articular cartilage in a goat model. A preliminary study. *J Bone Joint Surg Am* 2001;83(1):53-64.
35. Frisbie DD, Cross MW, McIlwraith CW: A comparative study of articular cartilage thickness in the stifle of animal species used in human pre-clinical studies compared to articular cartilage thickness in the human knee. *Vet Comp Orthop Traumatol* 2006;19(3):142-146.
36. Hembry RM, Dyce J, Driesang I, et al: Immunolocalization of matrix metalloproteinases in partial-thickness defects in pig articular cartilage. A preliminary report. *J Bone Joint Surg Am* 2001;83(6):826-838.
37. Vasara AI, Hyttinen MM, Pulliainen O, et al: Immature porcine knee cartilage lesions show good healing with or without autologous chondrocyte transplantation. *Osteoarthritis Cartilage* 2006;14(10):1066-1074.
38. Nelson BB, Mäkelä JTA, Lawson TB, et al: Cationic contrast-enhanced computed tomography distinguishes between reparative, degenerative, and healthy equine articular cartilage. *J Orthop Res* 2021;39(8):1647-1657.
39. Fortier LA, Balkman CE, Sandell LJ, Ratcliffe A, Nixon AJ: Insulin-like growth factor-I gene expression patterns during spontaneous repair of acute articular cartilage injury. *J Orthop Res* 2001;19(4):720-728.
40. Fortier LA, Chapman HS, Pownder SL, et al: BioCartilage improves cartilage repair compared with microfracture alone in an equine model of full-thickness cartilage loss. *Am J Sports Med* 2016;44(9):2366-2374.
41. Kotlarz H, Gunnarsson CL, Fang H, Rizzo JA: Insurer and out-of-pocket costs of osteoarthritis in the US: evidence from national survey data. *Arthritis Rheum* 2009;60(12):3546-3553.
42. Lawrence RC, Felson DT, Helmick CG, et al: Estimates of the prevalence of arthritis and other rheumatic conditions in the United States. Part II. *Arthritis Rheum* 2008;58(1):26-35.

43. Neogi T, Zhang Y: Epidemiology of osteoarthritis. *Rheum Dis Clin North Am* 2013;39(1):1-19.
44. Matthews GL: Disease modification: Promising targets and impediments to success. *Rheum Dis Clin North Am* 2013;39(1):177-187.
45. Little CB, Hunter DJ: Post-traumatic osteoarthritis: from mouse models to clinical trials. *Nat Rev Rheumatol* 2013;9(8):485-497.
46. Greek R, Menache A: Systematic reviews of animal models: Methodology versus epistemology. *Int J Med Sci* 2013;10(3):206-221.
47. Pound P, Bracken MB: Is animal research sufficiently evidence based to be a cornerstone of biomedical research? *BMJ* 2014;348:g3387.
48. Whiteside GT, Pomonis JD, Kennedy JD: An industry perspective on the role and utility of animal models of pain in drug discovery. *Neurosci Lett* 2013;557(pt A):65-72.
49. Cook D, Brown D, Alexander R, et al: Lessons learned from the fate of AstraZeneca's drug pipeline: A five-dimensional framework. *Nat Rev Drug Discov* 2014;13(6):419-431.
50. Perel P, Roberts I, Sena E, et al: Comparison of treatment effects between animal experiments and clinical trials: Systematic review. *BMJ* 2007;334(7586):197.
51. Malfait AM, Little CB: On the predictive utility of animal models of osteoarthritis. *Arthritis Res Ther* 2015;17:225.
52. Hunter DJ, Little CB: The great debate: Should osteoarthritis research focus on "Mice" or "Men"? *Osteoarthritis Cartilage* 2016;24(1):4-8.
53. Percie du Sert N, Hurst V, Ahluwalia A, et al: The ARRIVE guidelines 2.0: Updated guidelines for reporting animal research. *BMJ Open Sci* 2020;4(1):e100115.
54. Teeple E, Jay GD, Elsaid KA, Fleming BC: Animal models of osteoarthritis: Challenges of model selection and analysis. *AAPS J* 2013;15(2):438-446.
55. Gibson M, Li H, Coburn J, et al: Intra-articular delivery of glucosamine for treatment of experimental osteoarthritis created by a medial meniscectomy in a rat model. *J Orthop Res* 2014;32(2):302-309.
56. Glasson SS: In vivo osteoarthritis target validation utilizing genetically-modified mice. *Curr Drug Targets* 2007;8(2):367-376.
57. Malfait AM, Little CB, McDougall JJ: A commentary on modelling osteoarthritis pain in small animals. *Osteoarthritis Cartilage* 2013;21(9):1316-1326.
58. Nelson BB, Kawcak CE, Barrett MF, McIlwraith CW, Grinstaff MW, Goodrich LR: Recent advances in articular cartilage evaluation using computed tomography and magnetic resonance imaging. *Equine Vet J* 2018;50(5):564-579.
59. Palmer AJ, Brown CP, McNally EG, et al: Non-invasive imaging of cartilage in early osteoarthritis. *Bone Joint J* 2013;95-B(6):738-746.
60. Poole R, Blake S, Buschmann M, et al: Recommendations for the use of preclinical models in the study and treatment of osteoarthritis. *Osteoarthritis Cartilage* 2010;18(suppl 3):S10-S16.
61. Chan DD, Neu CP: Probing articular cartilage damage and disease by quantitative magnetic resonance imaging. *J R Soc Interface* 2013;10(78):20120608.
62. Kraus VB, Burnett B, Coindreau J, et al: Application of biomarkers in the development of drugs intended for the treatment of osteoarthritis. Osteoarthritis and cartilage/OARS. *Osteoarthritis Cartilage* 2011;19(5):515-542.
63. Pritzker KP, Aigner T: Terminology of osteoarthritis cartilage and bone histopathology – A proposal for a consensus. *Osteoarthritis Cartilage* 2010;18(suppl 3):S7-S9.
64. Aigner T, Cook JL, Gerwin N, et al: Histopathology atlas of animal model systems – Overview of guiding principles. *Osteoarthritis Cartilage* 2010;18(suppl 3):S2-S6.
65. Schmitz N, Laverty S, Kraus VB, Aigner T: Basic methods in histopathology of joint tissues. *Osteoarthritis Cartilage* 2010;18(suppl 3):S113-S116.
66. Pastoureau PC, Hunziker EB, Pelletier JP: Cartilage, bone and synovial histomorphometry in animal models of osteoarthritis. *Osteoarthritis Cartilage* 2010;18(suppl 3):S106-S112.
67. Pearce GL, Frisbie DD: Statistical evaluation of biomedical studies. *Osteoarthritis Cartilage* 2010;18(suppl 3):S117-S122.
68. Vincent TL, Williams RO, Maciewicz R, Silman A, Garside P: Mapping pathogenesis of arthritis through small animal models. *Rheumatology* 2012;51(11):1931-1941.
69. Gregory MH, Capito N, Kuroki K, Stoker AM, Cook JL, Sherman SL: A review of translational animal models for knee osteoarthritis. *Arthritis* 2012;2012:764621.
70. Kraus VB, Huebner JL, DeGroot J, Bendele A: The OARSI histopathology initiative – Recommendations for histological assessments of osteoarthritis in the guinea pig. *Osteoarthritis Cartilage* 2010;18(suppl 3):S35-S52.
71. Bendele AM, Hulman JF: Effects of body weight restriction on the development and progression of spontaneous osteoarthritis in guinea pigs. *Arthritis Rheum* 1991;34(9):1180-1184.
72. Pedersen DR, Goetz J, Kurriger GL, Martin JA: Comparative digital cartilage histology for human and common osteoarthritis models. *Orthop Res Rev* 2013;2013(5):13-20.
73. McIlwraith CW, Lattermann C: Intra-articular corticosteroids for knee pain-what have we learned from the equine athlete and current best practice. *J Knee Surg* 2019;32(1):9-25.
74. Pepin SR, Griffith CJ, Wijdicks CA, et al: A comparative analysis of 7.0-Tesla magnetic resonance imaging and histology measurements of knee articular cartilage in a canine posterolateral knee injury model: A preliminary analysis. *Am J Sports Med* 2009;37(suppl 1):119S-1124S.
75. Cook JL, Kuroki K, Visco D, Pelletier J-P, Schulz L, Lafeber FPJG: The OARSI histopathology initiative – Recommendations for histological assessments of osteoarthritis in the dog. *Osteoarthritis Cartilage* 2010;18(suppl 3):S66-S79.
76. Proffen BL, McElfresh M, Fleming BC, Murray MM: A comparative anatomical study of the human knee and six animal species. *Knee* 2012;19(4):493-499.
77. Goebel L, Orth P, Müller A, et al: Experimental scoring systems for macroscopic articular cartilage repair correlate with the MOCART score assessed by a high-field MRI at 9.4 T--comparative evaluation of five macroscopic scoring systems in a large animal cartilage defect model. *Osteoarthritis Cartilage* 2012;20(9):1046-1055.

78. Little CB, Smith MM, Cake MA, Read RA, Murphy MJ, Barry FP: The OARSI histopathology initiative – Recommendations for histological assessments of osteoarthritis in sheep and goats. *Osteoarthritis Cartilage* 2010;18(suppl 3):S80-S92.
79. Appleyard RC, Burkhardt D, Ghosh P, et al: Topographical analysis of the structural, biochemical and dynamic biomechanical properties of cartilage in an ovine model of osteoarthritis. *Osteoarthritis Cartilage* 2003;11(1):65-77.
80. Armstrong SJ, Read R, Ghosh P, Wilson D: Moderate exercise exacerbates the osteoarthritic lesions produced in cartilage by meniscectomy: A morphological study. *Osteoarthritis Cartilage* 1993;1(2):89-96.
81. Cake MA, Read RA, Corfield G, et al: Comparison of gait and pathology outcomes of three meniscal procedures for induction of knee osteoarthritis in sheep. *Osteoarthritis Cartilage* 2013;21(1):226-236.
82. Maher AD, Coles C, White J, et al: 1H NMR spectroscopy of serum reveals unique metabolic fingerprints associated with subtypes of surgically induced osteoarthritis in sheep. *J Proteome Res* 2012;11(8):4261-4268.
83. Moody HR, Heard BJ, Frank CB, Shrive NG, Oloyede AO: Investigating the potential value of individual parameters of histological grading systems in a sheep model of cartilage damage: the Modified Mankin method. *J Anat* 2012;221(1):47-54.
84. Murray MM, Fleming BC: Use of a bioactive scaffold to stimulate anterior cruciate ligament healing also minimizes posttraumatic osteoarthritis after surgery. *Am J Sports Med* 2013;41(8):1762-1770.
85. Sandmann GH, Adamczyk C, Garcia EG, et al: Biomechanical comparison of menisci from different species and artificial constructs. *BMC Musculoskelet Disord* 2013;14:324.
86. Malda J, Benders KEM, Klein TJ, et al: Comparative study of depth-dependent characteristics of equine and human osteochondral tissue from the medial and lateral femoral condyles. *Osteoarthritis Cartilage* 2012;20(10):1147-1151.
87. Ferris DJ, Frisbie DD, Kisiday JD, et al: Clinical outcome after intra-articular administration of bone marrow derived mesenchymal stem cells in 33 horses with stifle injury. *Vet Surg* 2014;43(3):255-265.
88. Wilke MM, Nydam DV, Nixon AJ: Enhanced early chondrogenesis in articular defects following arthroscopic mesenchymal stem cell implantation in an equine model. *J Orthop Res* 2007;25(7):913-925.
89. McIlwraith CW, Fortier LA, Frisbie DD, Nixon AJ: Equine models of articular cartilage repair. *Cartilage* 2011;2(4):317-326.
90. McCoy AM, Kemper AM, Boyce MK, Brown MP, Trumble TN: Differential gene expression analysis reveals pathways important in early post-traumatic osteoarthritis in an equine model. *BMC Genom* 2020;21(1):843.
91. Boyce MK, Trumble TN, Carlson CS, Groschen DM, Merritt KA, Brown MP: Non-terminal animal model of post-traumatic osteoarthritis induced by acute joint injury. *Osteoarthritis Cartilage* 2013;21(5):746-755.
92. Delco ML, Bonnevie ED, Bonassar LJ, Fortier LA: Mitochondrial dysfunction is an acute response of articular chondrocytes to mechanical injury. *J Orthop Res* 2018;36(2):739-750.
93. McIlwraith CW, Frisbie DD, Kawcak CE, Fuller CJ, Hurtig M, Cruz A: The OARSI histopathology initiative – Recommendations for histological assessments of osteoarthritis in the horse. *Osteoarthritis Cartilage* 2010;18(suppl 3):S93-S105.
94. McIlwraith CW, Frisbie DD, Kawcak CE: The horse as a model of naturally occurring osteoarthritis. *Bone Joint Res* 2012;1(11):297-309.
95. Broeckx S, Zimmerman M, Crocetti S, et al: Regenerative therapies for equine degenerative joint disease: A preliminary study. *PLoS One* 2014;9(1):e85917.
96. Broeckx S, Suls M, Beerts C, et al: Allogenic mesenchymal stem cells as a treatment for equine degenerative joint disease: A pilot study. *Curr Stem Cell Res Ther* 2014;9(6):497-503.

CHAPTER

6 Overview of Orthobiologics for Articular Cartilage Repair

Erica G. Gacasan, MS • Robert L. Sah, MD, ScD

INTRODUCTION

The predilection of articular cartilage to be damaged, along with its biology and extracellular matrix (ECM) structure, renders it a target for orthobiologics. Throughout an adult's life, articular cartilage normally functions as a key component of diarthrodial joints, withstanding years of repetitive loading and facilitating pain-free motion. However, with injury and aging, articular cartilage is often damaged; it then exhibits a limited intrinsic repair response and often deteriorates (**Figure 1**), making it an attractive candidate for orthobiologics.[1] Orthobiologics address tissue repair, protection, healing, and regeneration based on individual or combination products comprising cells, biomaterials, and/or bioactive factors. Orthobiologics can be classified using one or more of the three classic components: cells, scaffolds, and signals. These components can be derived from naturally occurring substances, such as tissues or blood, or consist of synthesized or modified materials or cells, such as engineered proteins, gene therapies, and culture-expanded cells. Effective orthobiologic treatment strategies may induce repairs that range from the ideally regenerated normal adult articular cartilage to tissues that variably restore function.

An overview of orthobiologics for articular cartilage repair is provided. It begins with summaries of the hierarchal structure of articular cartilage, the biology of indwelling chondrocytes and their precursors, and its ECM composition, turnover, and function. It is important to review the three major components of cartilage orthobiologics: scaffolds, cells, and signals. In addition, within this context, established and emerging orthobiologic approaches to cartilage repair are described.

BRIEF BIOLOGY OF CARTILAGE

The biology of articular cartilage is fundamentally coupled through its ECM to its biomechanical and biotransport properties, which vary during growth, homeostasis, and disease. Articular cartilage is a component of joints that functions as an organ, with interactions and cross-talk between tissues, including articular cartilage, synovium, and underlying bone, mediated by synovial fluid (**Figure 2**). Chondrocytes, the indwelling cells of cartilage, elaborate and remodel the cartilage ECM, affecting their microenvironment. Conversely, chondrocytes are regulated by the milieu of insoluble (ECM), soluble (cytokines, growth factors, and extracellular vesicles), and mechanical factors (due to joint loading). Thus, chondrocytes interact reciprocally with their surrounding matrix and fluid to form and maintain the structure and function of cartilage tissue.

The articular surface is bathed in synovial fluid that affects cartilage biology and physiology. Synovial fluid is a dialysate of plasma that contains substances originating from the local joint tissues. Synovial fluid helps lubricate the articulating joint surfaces, due to its high concentration of hyaluronic acid and lubricin/proteoglycan 4 (PRG4) lubricant molecules. Synovial fluid also mediates regulation and degradation of articular cartilage through synovium-secreted cytokines and proteases. In general, synovial fluid acts as a transport medium to provide cartilage with basic nutrients, including carbohydrates such as glucose, lipids, proteins, vitamins, minerals, and water.[2]

Cartilage growth, remodeling, maturation, and morphogenesis typically occur concurrently during joint development. During postnatal growth, the overall size and volume of joints increase (**Figure 3**). In skeletally immature individuals, the covering of bone ends includes a layer of epiphyseal growth cartilage and articular cartilage, which are collectively known as the articular–epiphyseal cartilage complex.[3,4] This complex grows before being either replaced by mineralized tissue via endochondral ossification or retained as articular cartilage. The overall growth of the joint involves expansion of the joint surface with concomitant thinning of the articular cartilage. The normal homeostatic balance between matrix synthesis and loss may become disrupted not only by direct damage or infiltrating enzymes but also by dysregulated chondrocytes, displaying an aberrant or development-like phenotype.[5] Common regulatory pathways of matrix turnover in normal joint development and joint pathology can provide avenues for orthobiologic interventions.

Dr. Sah or an immediate family member has stock or stock options held in GlaxoSmithKline, Johnson & Johnson, and Medtronic. Neither Erica Gacasan nor any immediate family member has received anything of value from or has stock or stock options held in a commercial company or institution related directly or indirectly to the subject of this chapter.

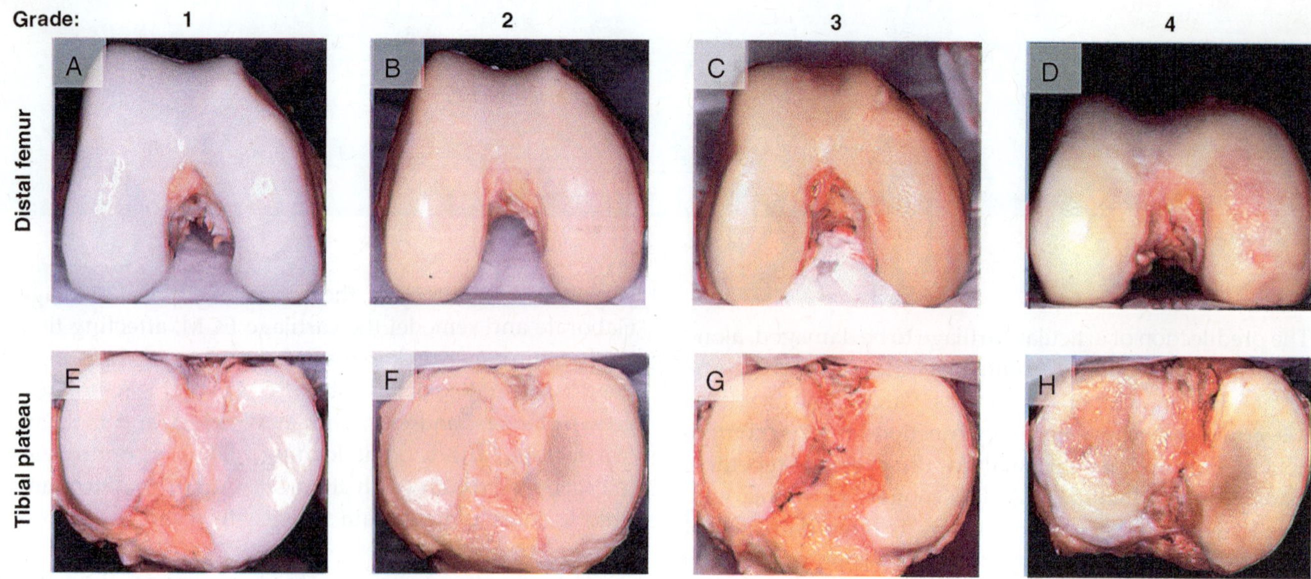

FIGURE 1 Photographs show human knee articular cartilage with signs of aging and osteoarthritis-related deterioration. Human distal femur (**A** through **D**) and tibial plateau (**E** through **H**). Diffuse cartilage degeneration due to chronic wear or osteoarthritis at the International Centre for Consortium Research: (**A** and **E**) grade 1, (**B** and **F**) grade 2, (**C** and **G**) grade 3, and (**D** and **H**) grade 4.

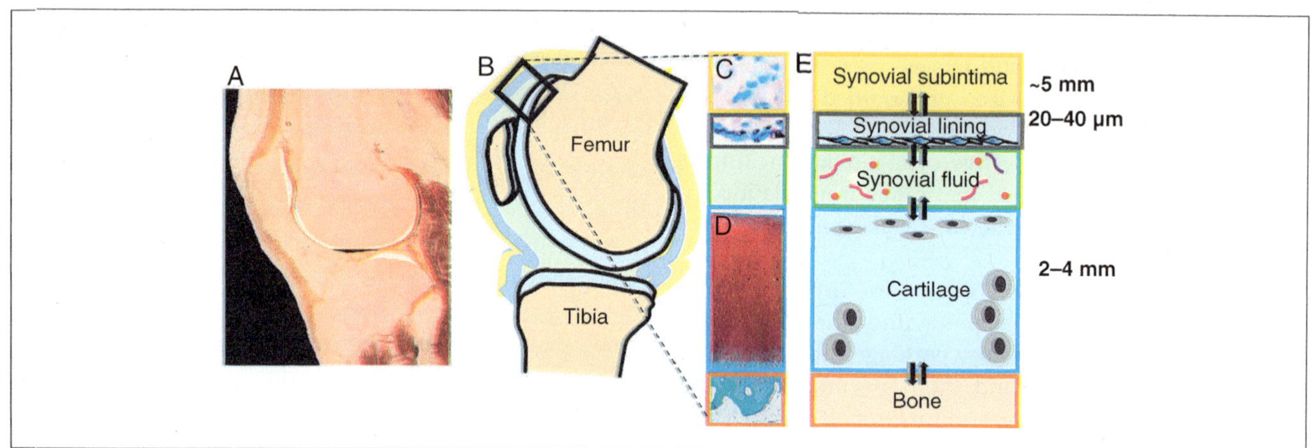

FIGURE 2 Cross-talk between the cartilage and synovium is mediated by synovial fluid. **A**, MRI of the knee in the sagittal view. **B**, Schematic representation of knee joint. Photomicrographs of human synovial lining (**C**) and articular cartilage and bone (**D**). **E**, Compartmental model of cross-talk between joint tissues. (Panel [A] courtesy of Dr. Walter Carpenter, PhD, MD, Panels [B] and [E] adapted with permission from Raleigh AR, McCarty WJ, Chen AC, Meinert C, Klein TJ, Sah RL: 6.7 Synovial joints: Mechanobiology and tissue engineering of articular cartilage and synovial fluid, in Dycheyne P, Grainger DW, Healy KE, Hutmacher DW, Kirkpatrick CJ, eds: *Comprehensive Biomaterials II*, ed 2. Elsevier, 2017, pp 107-34, Panel [C] adapted with permission from Freemont AJ: 5 – Histopathology of the Rheumatoid joint, in Henderson B, Edwards JCW, Pettipher ER, eds: *Mechanisms and Models in Rheumatoid Arthritis*. Academic Press, 1995, pp 83-113.)

Cartilage homeostasis is sensitive to mechanical stimuli, depending on magnitude, duration, and nature, in part through receptors that are responsive to mechanical stimulation. In vivo, articular cartilage is subjected to time-averaged static and time-varying dynamic cyclic compression, articulation-inducing shear stress, and resultant hydrostatic pressure, and compressive, shear, and tensile strain.[6] Mechanosensitive receptors can transmit mechanical information from the ECM to the chondrocyte and may activate or repress a variety of mechanotransduction pathways that alter the balance between catabolic and anabolic activity.[7] Catabolic activation may occur through both reduced loading and overloading as well as chronic pathologic joint loading. Net cartilage degradation and thinning are induced by high levels of peak stress, high strain rates, and long-term

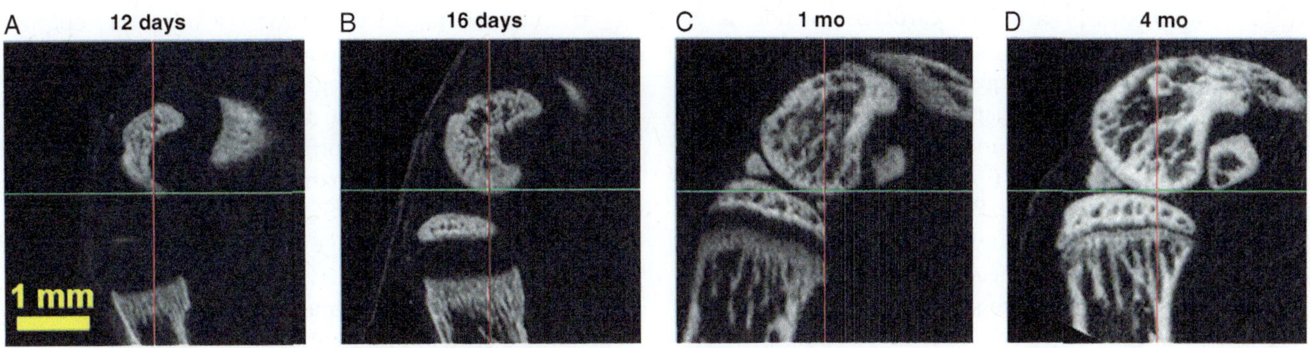

FIGURE 3 Growth and mineralization of the distal femur and proximal tibia. Micro-CT scans of C57BL/6 wild-type mouse knees from 12 days (**A**), 16 days (**B**), 1 month (**C**), and 4 months (**D**) postnatal.

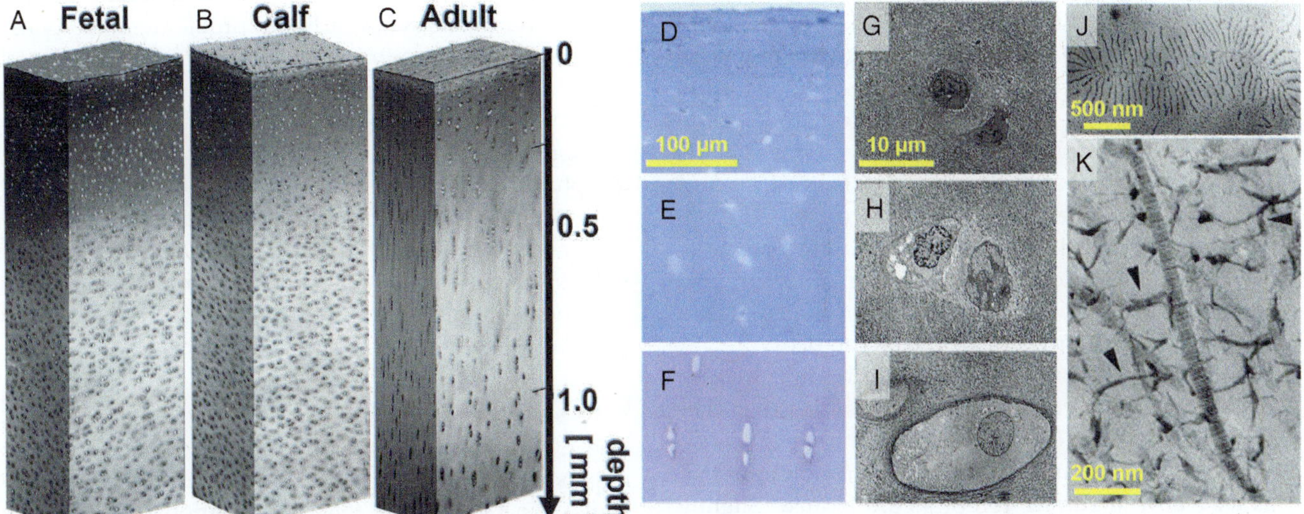

FIGURE 4 Age- and depth-varied cell and matrix organization of articular cartilage. Three-dimensional rendering of bovine fetal (**A**), calf (**B**), and adult (**C**) tissue. Light (**D** through **F**) and transmission electron (**G** through **I**) micrographs of chondrocytes within the superficial (**D** and **G**), transitional middle (**E** and **H**), and deep (**F** and **I**) zones. **J**, Electron micrograph of proteoglycan aggregate isolated from bovine cartilage. **K**, Micrograph of hyaline cartilage with type II collagen fibril lying parallel to the section plane and proteoglycans (arrowheads). Magnification is the same among panels (**D** through **F**) and among panels (**G** through **I**). (Panels [**A** through **C**] adapted with permission from Jadin KD, Bae WC, Schumacher BL, Sah RL: Three-dimensional (3-D) imaging of chondrocytes in articular cartilage: Growth-associated changes in cell organization. *Biomaterials* 2007;28[2]:230-239, Panels [**D** through **I**] adapted with permission from Quinn TM, Häuselmann HJ, Shintani N, Hunziker EB: Cell and matrix morphology in articular cartilage from adult human knee and ankle joints suggests depth-associated adaptations to biomechanical and anatomical roles. *Osteoarthritis Cartilage* 2013;21[12]:1904-1912, Panel [J] adapted with permission Buckwalter JA, Roughley PJ, Rosenberg LC: Age-related changes in cartilage proteoglycans: Quantitative electron microscopic studies. *Microsc Res Tech* 1994;28[5]:398-408, Panel [K] adapted with permission from Keene DR, Tufa SF: Transmission electron microscopy of cartilage and bone. *Methods Cell Biol* 2010;96:443-473.)

pathologic mechanical loading (eg, joint malalignment) as well as prolonged immobilization.[6]

Hierarchy of Cartilage Structure

The primary load-bearing structure of synovial joints is the osteochondral unit, consisting of articular cartilage, calcified cartilage, and underlying subchondral bone. The calcified cartilage is a thin tissue layer between the articular cartilage and subchondral bone and is bounded histologically by the tidemark, between the uncalcified hyaline cartilage and calcified cartilage, and the cement line, between the calcified cartilage and subchondral bone. The calcified cartilage provides load transfer, structural integration, and a barrier to solute transport between the uncalcified cartilage and the subchondral bone.[8]

The cartilage matrix has zonal, regional, and site variation that facilitates tissue function under complex loading and changes with growth (**Figure 4**). The main

ECM components of articular cartilage include large aggregates of the proteoglycan aggrecan and fibrils of predominantly type II collagen, which contribute to the cartilage's unique biomechanical properties. Aggrecan associates with hyaluronan and link protein to form large multimolecular aggregates (~10^9 Da) that are effectively retained within the cartilage. Because of the large number of polyanionic glycosaminoglycan chains on aggrecan, and the restraining and space-filling nature of the dense collagen network, the aggregates provide a high negative fixed charge density and osmotic swelling pressure within the tissue, with a high water content and compressive resistance.[9,10] In contrast to its dense matrix and compared with other tissues, normal adult articular cartilage has a relatively low density of cells and is also avascular, alymphatic, and aneural.

Articular cartilage exhibits depth-wise variation, with (1) superficial, (2) middle, and (3) deep zones, as well as (4) calcified cartilage. Within the superficial zone, chondrocytes are flattened and aligned parallel to the surface, collagen fibrils run parallel to the articular surface, and aggrecan content is relatively low. With depth, cell density decreases, chondrocytes exhibit a larger and more rounded hypertrophic appearance, collagen orientation is increasingly perpendicular to the articular surface, and the matrix becomes progressively aggrecan rich.

The cartilage matrix surrounding chondrocytes also exhibits distinctive arrangements at increasing distances from the cell surface. The pericellular matrix lies immediately around the cell and is the zone where molecules that interact with cell surface receptors are located. Slightly further from the cell is the territorial matrix, and even further is the interterritorial matrix. The types of collagen and the collagen-binding proteins that form the matrices are different in each zone.[11] Furthermore, the compositional, structural, and functional properties of articular cartilage vary across joint surfaces, consistent with modulation by the extent and pattern of joint loading.[12]

Chondrocyte Biology and Lineage

Articular chondrocyte biology varies with depth from the articular surface, in health and disease. For example, superficial zone chondrocytes are a major source of the synovial fluid lubricant, PRG4. Furthermore, gene expression profiles may help to elucidate stages of disease by reflecting the evolving expression of anabolic and catabolic genes during different phases of maturation and disease.[13] In normal adult articular cartilage, the greatest differences in gene expression occurs between the superficial and deep zones, which reflects the differing functional roles of the superficial zone, in maintaining the low-friction articulating surface, and the deep zone, where an enhanced biosynthetic capacity is necessary to form and maintain the dense cartilaginous matrix.[14,15]

The natural transitional growth of immature epiphyseal cartilage to adult articular cartilage provides a paradigm for regenerative strategies of orthobiologics. Mature articular chondrocytes arise from multiple pools of progenitor cells from the superficial zone and perichondral tissues. Synovial joint formation involves descendants of mesenchymal stem cells (MSCs) from the interzone area of embryonic limbs, which give rise to joint tissues. Articular cartilage maturation is driven mainly by increase in cell volume, cellular rearrangement, and matrix deposition, with limited cellular proliferation in the neonatal stages[16,17] (**Figure 5**). In mice, superficial zone PRG4+ cells expressing stem cell markers facilitate appositional and interstitial growth of articular cartilage and entirely reconstitute adult cartilage during growth and maturation.[18] PRG4+ cells found in the synovial lining proliferate in response to injury and may contribute to healing.[17] A population of cells positive for progenitor markers in the perichondral groove of Ranvier have also been identified and contribute appositionally to the articular cartilage from the joint periphery.[19] In mature tissue, MSCs from bone marrow and adipose tissue are capable of differentiating into chondrocytes and may contribute to cartilage repair. Thus, lineage-tracing studies have substantial implications for how orthobiologics may target endogenous and exogenous cell populations to repair or regenerate cartilage.

ECM Composition and Homeostasis

The ECM of the cartilage is maintained at levels that depend on synthesis and accumulation of structural molecules, as balanced by their degradation and loss. The composition and functional properties of cartilage change during maturation and with pathology and reflects several biologic and physical processes.

Collagen biosynthesis and assembly follows the normal pathway for a secreted protein. Many different types of collagen molecules are expressed in articular cartilage, but the backbone polymeric template during development is a copolymer of collagens II, IX, and XI. After skeletal growth has ceased, the rate of type II collagen synthesis by articular chondrocytes drops dramatically, with an estimated turnover time of 400 years for human femoral head cartilage.[20] The classic concept of collagen fibril degradation is through an initial cleavage of the collagen molecules (type I, II, or III) by collagenase into three-fourths-length and one-fourth-length fragments.[21]

Secreted aggrecan replaces those that are damaged by mechanical loading, removed by aggrecanases and/or proteases, or transported through the cartilage tissue via its migration down its concentration gradient, eventually exiting through the cartilage surface.[22-24] Other proteoglycans, including syndecans, glypican, small leucine-rich proteoglycans, decorin, biglycan, and perlecan, among others, are expressed during chondrogenesis and aid in assembly and maintenance of the cartilage ECM.[25]

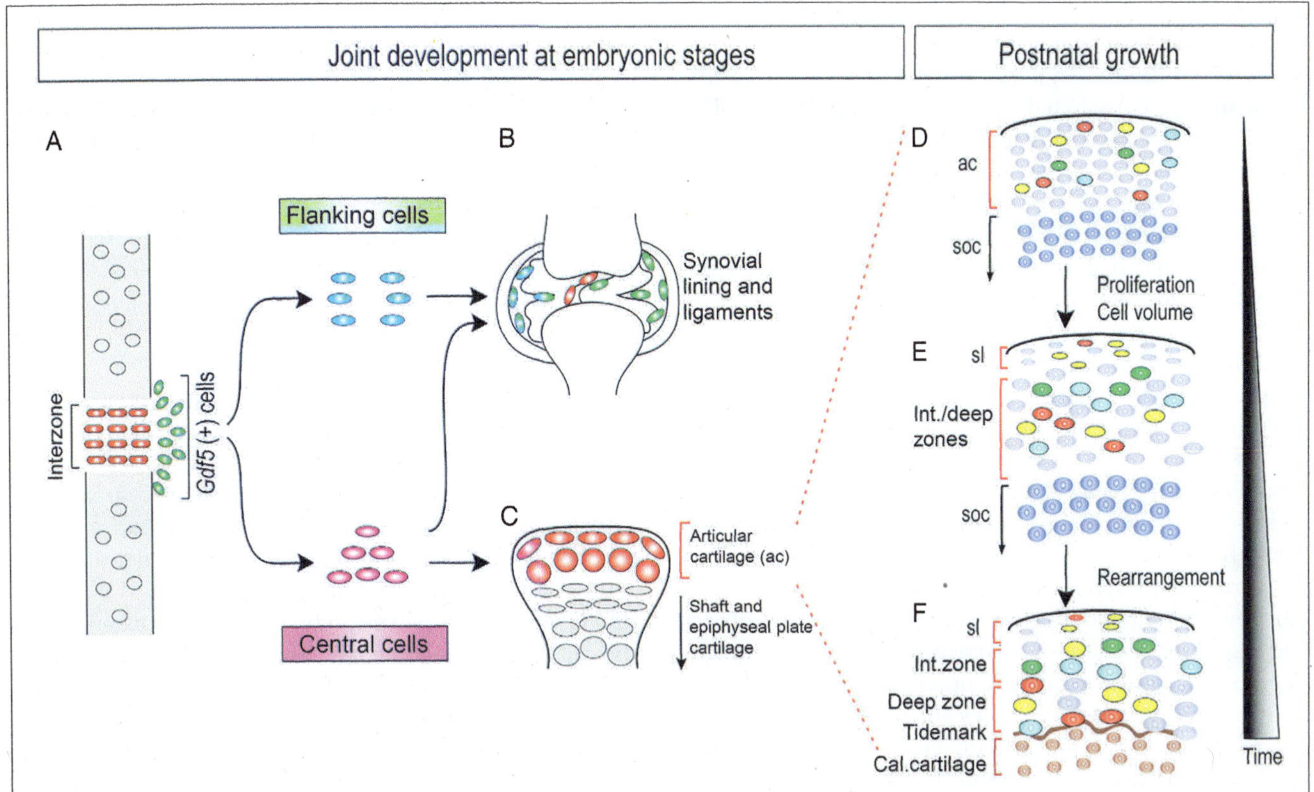

FIGURE 5 Model of synovial joint formation and postnatal growth and morphogenesis. **A**, Mesenchymal Gdf5+ cells constituting the interzone area at incipient joint sites in early embryonic limbs comprise centrally located descendants of chondrocytes (red color) and flanking cells recruited from surrounding tissues into the Gdf5 lineage (green color). **B** and **C**, Both populations increase in number, but do not migrate significantly over time and give rise to distinct local tissues, with the flanking cells largely producing synovial lining, capsule, and peripheral ligaments and central cells generating articular cartilage and intrajoint ligaments. **D** through **F**, Starting at neonatal stages and proceeding into adulthood, knee articular cartilage (ac) progressively acquires its functional organization and structure that include superficial layers (sl), intermediate (int) and deep zones, and a tidemark overlaying the calcified (cal) cartilage and secondary ossification center (soc). Growth in thickness is driven by limited proliferation at neonatal stages (**D**) and by cell volume increases at subsequent stages (**E** and **F**). The characteristic cell stacks perpendicular to the articular surface entail repositioning and intercalation of neighboring chondrocytes, producing stacks of nondaughter cells. (Reproduced with permission from Decker RS, Um HB, Dyment NA, et al: Cell origin, volume and arrangement are drivers of articular cartilage formation, morphogenesis and response to injury in mouse limbs. *Dev Biol* 2017;426[1]:56-68.)

The ECM contains a variety of matrix-degrading enzymes that are present in precursor and active forms. The activation of stress-induced and inflammation-induced signaling and transcriptional and posttranscriptional events results in the release of the chondrocytes from growth arrest, imbalanced homeostasis, and chondrocyte activation with aberrant expression of inflammation-related genes.[7] The ECM acts as a depot, storing growth factors and other signaling molecules. Changes in physiologic conditions can trigger protease activity that enables the release of such depots and activation of catabolism and inflammation, which can be modulated by targeted delivery of drugs and other signaling factors.[26]

Tissue Composition and Pathophysiology

The therapeutic effect of orthobiologic interventions depends on the residence time of the intervention within the joint space, if implemented by intra-articular injection, as well as penetration and residence time within the cartilage tissue itself. Soluble therapeutics (eg, growth factors and cytokines) are subject to convective and diffusive effects within the joint tissues.

Retention of solutes within the cartilage is affected by loading, ECM content, and integrity, as well as electrostatic interactions between the tissue and solute. Transport occurs relatively rapidly in areas of low matrix density, such as near the articular surface, but is also affected by mechanical loading and residence time within the synovial fluid and cartilage.[27]

Synovial fluid is an ultrafiltrate of plasma with additional molecules secreted by local cell populations. The composition of synovial fluid is normally in dynamic equilibrium and reflects a balance between cellular secretion and loss due to transport through the synovial capillaries, synovial interstitium, and the lymphatic drainage system.[28,29] The residence time of molecules within the synovial fluid depends on molecular mass and shape as well as joint state, including inflammation, vascular permeability, and synovial thickening.[29,30] The half-life of drugs in the synovial fluid after injection is as short as ~1 hour (eg, acetaminophen).[31] However, residence time can be higher with increased molecular size, increased viscous and aggregating properties, and enhanced interaction with joint tissues, including the synovium and cartilage.[32]

Turnover of synovial fluid constituents is driven, in part, by size-dependent clearance through the lymphatic and capillary systems. Clearance of particles from the joint may occur through the lymphatics for larger species, and through venous capillaries for smaller species.[33] In the rabbit model, after anterior cruciate ligament transection, the molecular weight distribution of injected hyaluronan within the knee shifted toward a predominance of low-molecular-weight species (<1,000 kDa) and a lower hyaluronan residence time.[34] Synovial permeability also depends on disease state. Increased synovial inflammation in patients with various forms of arthritis is associated with increases in vascular and lymphatic permeability, synovial hyperplasia, and cellular infiltration.[29,34,35] Thus, strategies to increase retention time of therapeutic solutes within the context of an inflammatory joint environment may be important for effective orthobiologic interventions.

Within the cartilage, fluid flows produced by mechanical loading induce convection of solutes.[27] Furthermore, as the cartilage degrades, the collagen network is disrupted, proteoglycans are lost from the tissue, and tissue permeability increases. Increased permeability of diseased cartilage enables enhanced transport of therapeutic agents within the cartilage, and allows for transport of large molecules, but can reduce retention times within the tissue.

The dense polyanionic ECM of articular cartilage not only provides the tissue with its essential load-bearing properties but also governs the regulation of chondrocytes by soluble factors. Because of the net negative fixed charge density within the cartilage, solute partitioning within the tissue is hindered, or enhanced, by the molecular size and charge of the solute.[36] According to effects of steric exclusion and Donnan equilibrium, the distribution as well as the diffusion coefficients of a particular solute decreases with increasing molecular weight and size and is sensitive to variations in fixed charge density.[37] These physicochemical principles affect the access of solutes to chondrocytes and may be the basis of biologic therapies. For instance, cationic carrier molecules may enhance the transport of biologically active molecules into the cartilage.[32] However, cationic molecules have the potential to neutralize tissue fixed charge, which could counteract the natural load-bearing mechanism of cartilage and affect chondrocyte behavior.[38]

OVERVIEW OF THERAPEUTIC OPTIONS: CELLS, SCAFFOLDS, AND SIGNALS

Therapeutic approaches and developments target particular forms and stages of articular cartilage damage. Focal chondral and osteochondral defects are injuries or areas of degeneration that are limited to a defined area. Focal defects may occur because of acute traumatic injury or may be idiopathic. Defects can present as (1) partial-thickness chondral defects where damage is restricted to the chondral layer, (2) full-thickness chondral defects extending to the calcified cartilage or subchondral bone, and (3) osteochondral defects that affect both the cartilage and underlying bone (**Figure 6**). Defects may present as softened or partially eroded tissue and are classified according to size and geometry.[39] Conversely, osteoarthritis is characterized by widespread joint degeneration due to progressive loss of articular cartilage and pathophysiologic bone and cartilage remodeling including fibrocartilage formation, sclerosis of subchondral bone, and osteophyte formation.[40,41] Repair of cartilage and osteochondral injuries involve not only replacement or regeneration of the bulk cartilage tissue but also integration with appropriate interfaces for the various types of defect repair.

Cartilage repair strategies can be classified according to the type of therapeutic modality, either mechanical or biologic, as well as the method in which the therapy is delivered (**Table 1**). Mechanically directed treatment strategies aim to correct abnormal joint loading and joint malalignment or provide tissues or tissue substitutes that promptly restore mechanical (ie, load bearing) function. Conversely, regenerative therapies enable a biologic response that aims to regenerate the tissue or establish a reparative microenvironment that restores normal structure and function, and which has a longer time horizon to achieve functional repair.

Therapeutic interventions, and their evaluation, can be delivered, or assessed, at the tissue, organ, and whole-body levels (**Figure 7**). Although most orthobiologic interventions are delivered directly to the joint by means of intra-articular injection or surgical procedures, soluble signals may be administered orally or intravenously. In addition, therapeutic efficacy may be assessed from a holistic perspective (ie, surveys and questionnaires regarding patient-reported measures of pain and function),[42] as well as locally at multiple scales by clinical

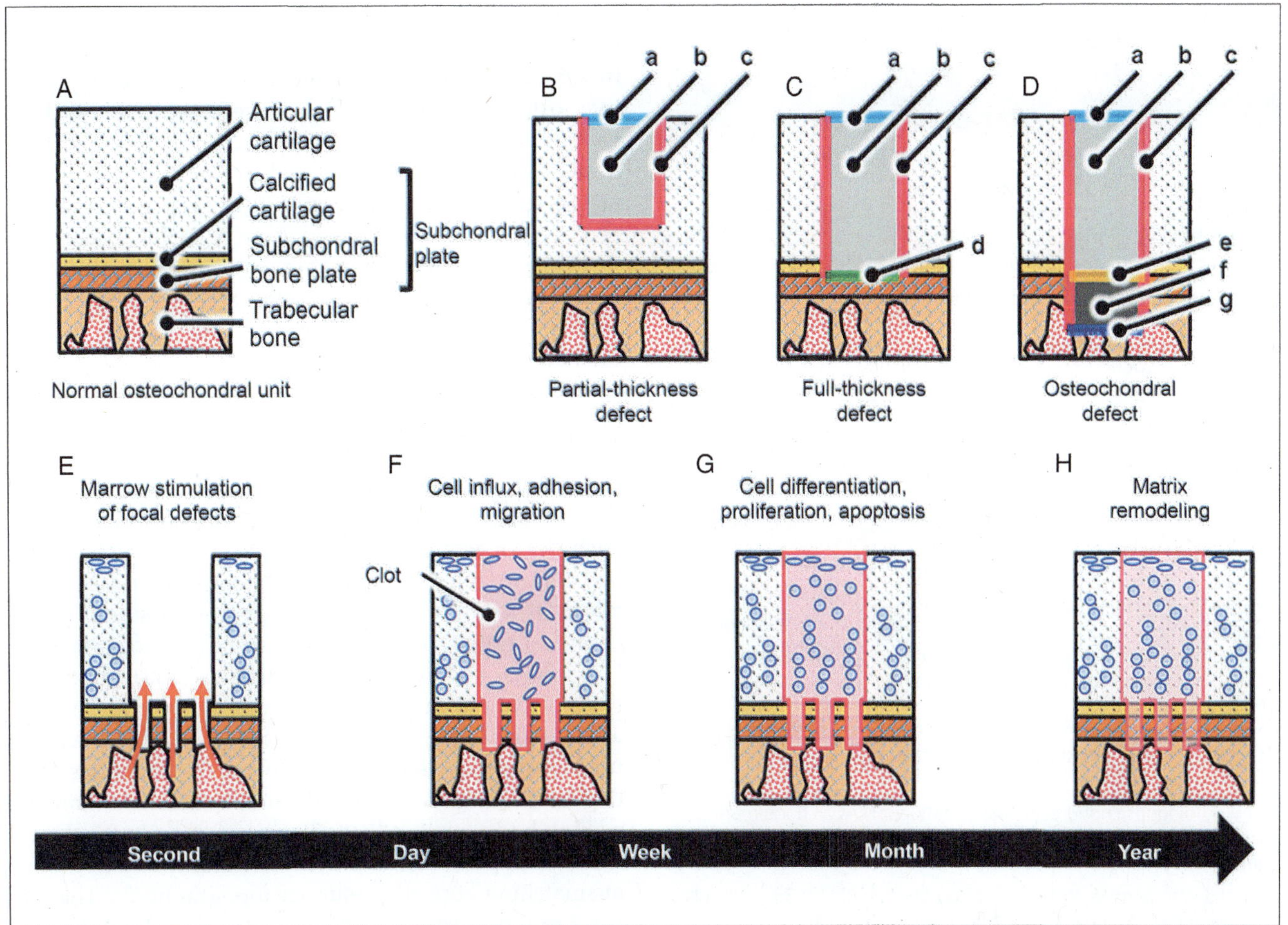

FIGURE 6 Schematic of normal osteochondral unit and spatiotemporal aspects of cartilage defect repair. **A**, Normal osteochondral unit. Defects that are partial thickness (**B**), full thickness (**C**), and osteochondral and spatial aspects of repair strategies (**D**). Specialized surfaces, tissues, and interfaces include the articular surface (a), bulk cartilage (b), interface of repair with host cartilage (c), interface of repair cartilage with subchondral plate (d), formation of a bone-cartilage interface (e), repair of trabecular bone (f), and interface of repair with host bone (g). In microfracture, penetration of the subchondral bone plate (**E**) leads to formation of a clot containing cells, growth factors, and matrix molecules (**F**). Over time, cells remain at the defect site, differentiate (**G**), and form and maintain the repair tissue (**H**). (Adapted with permission from Gacasan EG, Sah RL: Ch 33 – Articular cartilage repair: Augmentation, regeneration, replacement, and substitution, in Aaron R, ed: *Orthopaedic Basic Science*, ed 5. American Academy of Orthopaedic Surgeons, 2020, pp 415-432.)

imaging of the joint and biopsy of the joint tissues.[43] Biochemical analysis of fluids, including urine, blood, and synovial fluid, may also be used to identify by-products of joint degeneration and assess the metabolic state of the body or joint.

Orthobiologic substances can be categorized into three substances: (1) scaffolds, (2) signals, and (3) cells, which can be used individually, or in combination, to elicit a biologic response that aids in repair, regeneration, or restoration of injured tissue (**Figure 8**). Scaffolds, either natural or synthetic in nature, provide a supportive material to guide matrix synthesis and organization and can be manufactured with complex geometries and topography.[44] Signals, which regulate behavior of either endogenous or delivered cells, can either be biochemical or mechanical in nature. Biochemical signals include growth factors (transforming growth factor beta [TGF-β], platelet-derived growth factors [PDGFs], bone morphogenetic protein (BMP), etc), drugs, genes, and exosome therapies, as well as other agents that inhibit or activate specific enzymes and metabolic pathways.[45-48] Additionally, blood products such as platelet-rich plasma (PRP) and bone marrow aspirate concentrate (BMAC) contain a milieu of reparative factors that may influence cellular behavior.[49,50] Both autologous and allogeneic cells have been used in developing orthobiologic therapies and are often expanded in vitro, imbued within scaffolds, and preconditioned with mechanical and biomechanical stimulation. Allogeneic

TABLE 1 Repair Strategies to Treat Chondral and Osteochondral Lesions

		Therapy	
		Mechanical	**Biologic**
Mode of delivery	**Systemic** (oral, intravenous)	Exercise/physical therapy, weight loss, orthotics	NSAIDs, analgesics, nutritional supplements
	Local (intra-articular, topical)	Viscosupplements, CPM, braces	Corticosteroids, stem cells, PRP, BMAC, growth factors, extracellular vesicles, drugs
	Surgical	Osteotomy, allografts, autografts, total/partial joint replacement	Bone marrow stimulation, ACI, engineered grafts, joint distraction

Repair strategies can be classified according to their primary therapeutic mode of action, biomechanical or biologic, and also by mode of delivery (systemic, local, or surgical).

ACI = autologous chondrocyte implantation, BMAC = bone marrow aspirate concentrate, CPM = continuous passive motion, PRP = platelet-rich plasma

Adapted with permission from Gacasan EG, Sah RL: Ch 33 – Articular cartilage repair: Augmentation, regeneration, replacement, and substitution, in Aaron R, ed: *Orthopaedic Basic Science*, ed 5. American Academy of Orthopaedic Surgeons, 2020, pp 415-432.

cell sources, often cartilage stem or progenitor cells, have been derived from bone marrow, adipose, muscle, bone, synovium, periosteum, umbilical cord, and amniotic tissues.[51] Cells, particularly MSCs, can also be used as a paracrine signaling source that establishes a regenerative microenvironment by secreting factors that regulate the local immune response.[52] Biomechanical conditioning of cells and cellular scaffolds with regimens of compression, shear, and/or hydrostatic pressure modulates cellular phenotype and can enhance chondrogenesis and matrix biosynthesis.[46] Thus, many orthobiologic therapies for cartilage repair involve a combination of scaffolds, signals, and cells, which ideally form and maintain repair tissue (**Table 2**).

STANDARD APPROACHES TO CARTILAGE REPAIR

Functional Tissue Replacement: Osteochondral Grafting

Osteochondral grafting involves transfer of intact osteochondral units from autologous or allogeneic sources to replace damaged tissue and restore normal load-bearing function. Osteochondral grafts consist of full-thickness viable articular cartilage and a layer of attached devitalized subchondral bone to provide a (1) mechanically functional (a) hyaline cartilage tissue and (b) osteoinductive, osteoconductive, and osteogenic scaffold, and (2) viable chondrocytes in normal organization. In addition, implanted tissue may act as a depot of pro-regenerative factors that are retained in, and slowly released from, the graft.

Autologous grafts, either by single or multiple (mosaicplasty) plugs, are generally used to resurface focal defects of 1 to 4 cm^2 and can be accomplished arthroscopically or as an open procedure. Conversely, allogeneic grafting involves the transfer of size-matched osteochondral allograft tissue from a cadaver donor into chondral and osteochondral defects (>2 cm^2).[53] To ensure fit, the lesion location, size, and the overall shape and contour of the joint are assessed such that a size-matched graft can be harvested from the donor. Depending on the defect size and severity, allograft morphology may range from a single osteochondral plug to massive osteoarticular allografts.

Good 5- and 10-year survival rates (>80%) and high rates of patient satisfaction depend on selection of suitable patient populations, often with full-thickness nonkissing defects and who do not have lesions with degenerative etiology, uncorrectable joint malalignment, or high body mass index (>35 kg/m^2).[54-57] Graft survival rate also depends on chondrocyte viability and appropriate matching of cartilage surface topography.[58,59] The utility of mosaicplasty may also be constrained by donor-site availability and morbidity, and availability of appropriately matched osteochondral allograft donor tissue may be limited.

Autologous Chondrocyte Implantation

Autologous chondrocyte implantation (ACI), or autologous chondrocyte transplantation, was the first commercially marketed cell-based therapy for cartilage regeneration. ACI is a two-stage procedure involving arthroscopic biopsy of cartilage from a non–load-bearing area, isolation and in vitro expansion of chondrocytes, and implantation of the chondrocyte suspension into the defect site. The cartilage (200 to 300 mg) is harvested from healthy tissue and the sample is sent to a commercial good manufacturing practice facility to isolate and expand chondrocytes in vitro. The final product is a liquid suspension of cells,[60] or cell-laden scaffold,[61] which is extensively tested for chondrocyte morphology, sterility, viability, and endotoxins before it is shipped for implantation in the second stage. Indications for ACI are mixed and may be used for management of full-thickness injuries (>2 cm^2) as a primary intervention or in patients in whom another primary intervention has failed.[62]

First developed in the 1990s by Brittberg et al,[60] ACI evolved from successful preclinical studies in a

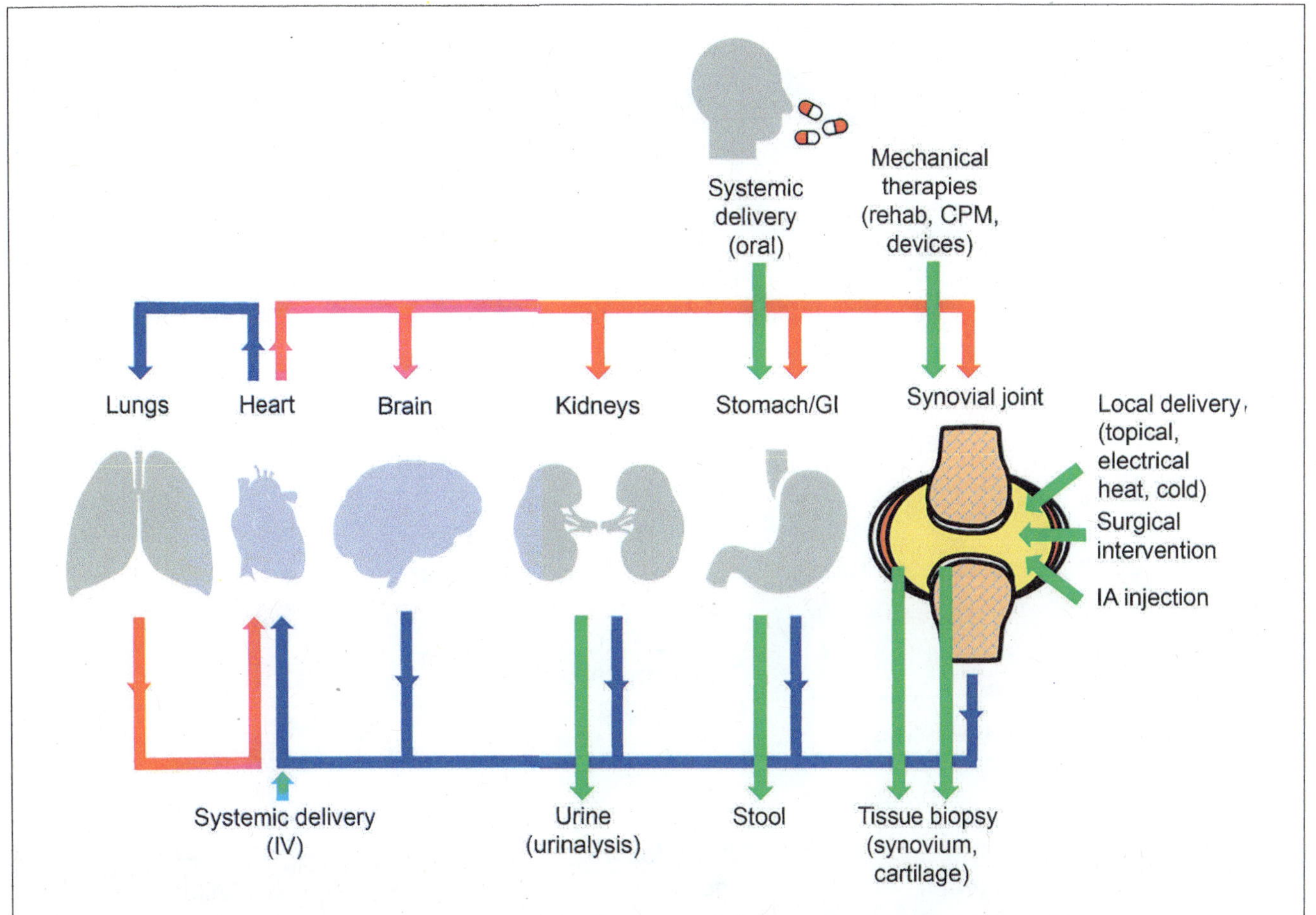

FIGURE 7 Organ system and whole-body model of transport to and from synovial joints. Systemic illustration shows different metrics and methodologies that can be used to assess cartilage and overall joint health, before and after therapeutic interventions. Monitoring and sampling can facilitate evaluation of the general state of the body as well as the condition of specific sites within the joint or repair tissue. Red: flow of oxygenated blood. Blue: flow of deoxygenated blood. Green: system or tissue where intervention or assessment is undertaken. CPM = continuous passive motion, GI = gastrointestinal, IA = intra-articular, IV = intravenous. (Adapted with permission from Gacasan EG, Sah RL: Ch 33 – Articular cartilage repair: Augmentation, regeneration, replacement, and substitution, in Aaron R, ed: *Orthopaedic Basic Science*, ed 5. American Academy of Orthopaedic Surgeons, 2020, pp 415-432.)

rabbit model.[63] ACI has undergone several generations of development wherein the method of in vitro expansion and anchorage to the defect site during the secondary procedure has varied.[62] First-generation ACI involved suturing of autologous periosteum over the defect and implantation of expanded chondrocytes by syringe through the periosteal flap. However, to reduce complexity and potential complications, second-generation ACI procedures used purpose-designed collagen membranes such as Chondro-Gide (Geistlich Pharma AG) instead of periosteum. Third-generation ACI techniques involve implantation of a chondrocyte-laden biomaterial scaffold. Matrix-assisted chondrocyte transplantation allows for culture of chondrocytes in a more physiologically relevant environment and facilitates a surgical procedure that is simpler, more rapid, and has less morbidity by removing the need for periosteal harvest or membrane suturing. Third-generation ACI procedures include MACI (Vericel Corporation) and NOVOCART 3D (TETEC AG), among others, which differ in their preparation and culture of autologous chondrocytes and choice of biomaterial scaffold.

Additional advances in bioreactor design and cell culture methodologies have resulted in the development of fourth-generation ACI techniques where culture conditions facilitate ECM production and preservation of chondrogenic phenotype. For instance, cell spheroid–based ACI techniques, including ChondroSphere (CO.DON AG) and CartiLife (Biosolution Co., Ltd.), use autologous chondrocytes that are cultivated into spheroids

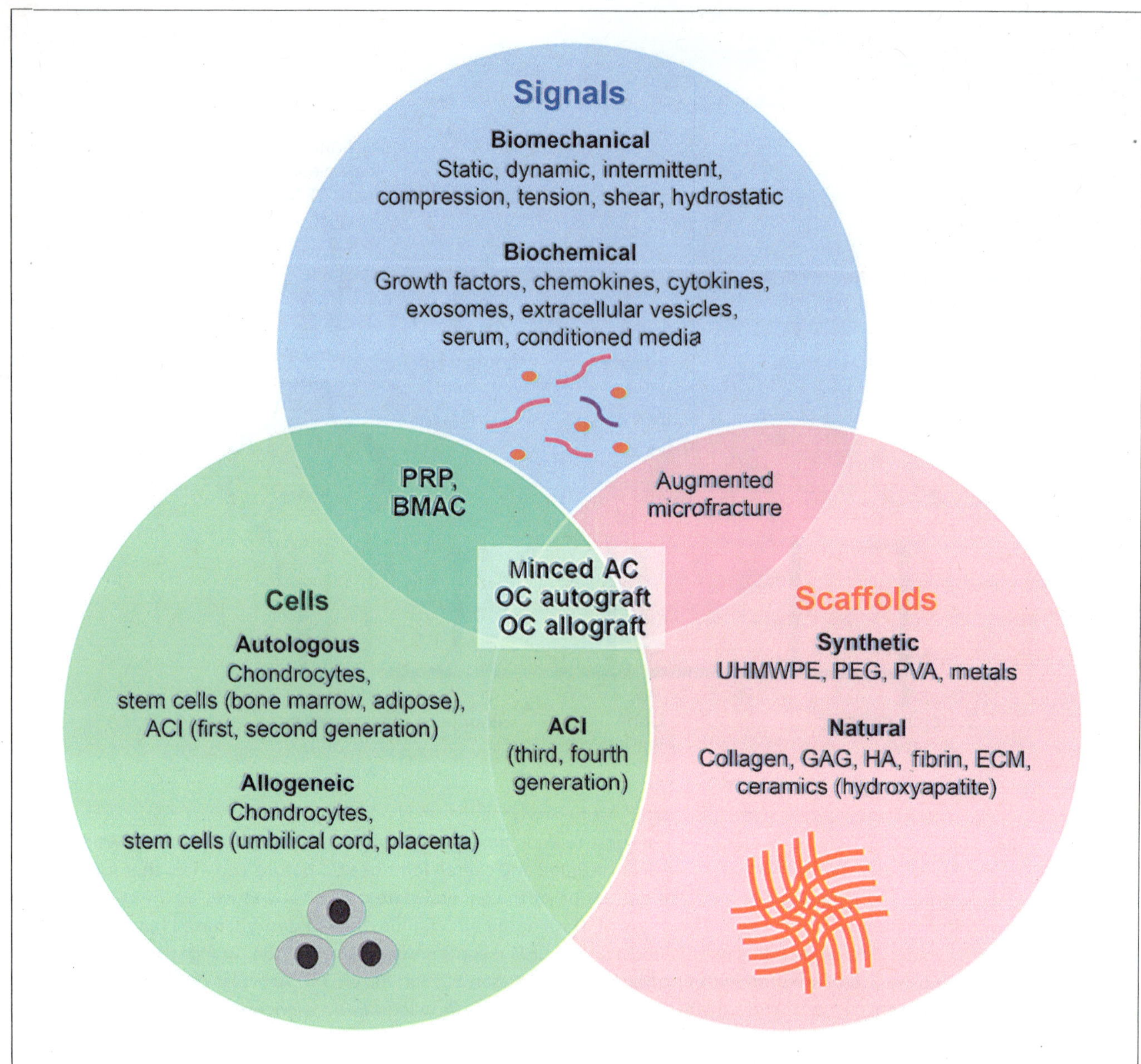

FIGURE 8 Engineered tissue components. Venn diagram shows that signals, cells, and scaffolds are the major elements of pharmacologic and tissue engineering approaches to cartilage repair. These elements may be used separately, or in combination, to treat symptomology or affect regeneration or restoration of tissue function. AC = articular cartilage, ACI = autologous chondrocyte implantation, BMAC = bone marrow aspirate concentrate, ECM = extracellular matrix, GAG = glycosaminoglycan, HA = hyaluronic acid, OC = osteochondral, PEG = polyethylene glycol, PRP = platelet-rich plasma, PVA = polyvinyl alcohol, UHMWPE = ultra-high–molecular-weight polyethylene. (Adapted with permission from Gacasan EG, Sah RL: Ch 33 – Articular cartilage repair: Augmentation, regeneration, replacement, and substitution, in Aaron R, ed: *Orthopaedic Basic Science*, ed 5. American Academy of Orthopaedic Surgeons, 2020, pp 415-432.)

containing cell aggregates and autologous cartilagelike ECM.[61] Although third-generation and fourth-generation products have shown promising results, limitations of all ACI methodologies include high cost due to the in vitro cell expansion in a commercial good manufacturing practice facility and the fragility of the initial repair tissue.

Augmentation of Intrinsic Repair: Bone Marrow Stimulation

For symptomatic defects of small size (<2 cm^2), bone marrow stimulation by breach of the subchondral bone through various means including microfracture, microdrilling, and other methods is typically a

TABLE 2 Orthobiologics for Cartilage Repair and Osteoarthritis

# (NCT)	Product/Trade Name	Company	Cell Type	Scaffold Material	Signal	Delivery	Market Status (USA)
1	Cartiform	Osiris Therapeutics	Allogeneic chondrocytes	Osteochondral allograft	—	Surgical	✔ (HCT/P)
2	CartiMax	MTF Biologics	Allogeneic chondrocytes	Lyophilized extracellular matrix	—	Surgical	✔ (HCT/P)
3 (01733186)	CARTISTEM	MEDIPOST	Allogeneic umbilical cord–derived MSCs	Hyaluronic acid–based	—	Surgical	—
4 (01329445)	DeNovo NT	Zimmer Biomet	Allogeneic chondrocytes	Minced juvenile cartilage allograft	—	Surgical	✔ (HCT/P)
5 (03588975)	MACI	Vericel Corporation	Autologous chondrocytes	Collagen membrane	—	Surgical	✔ (BLA)
6 (01957722)	NOVOCART 3D	Aesculap, Inc.	Autologous chondrocytes	Biphasic collagen scaffold with chondroitin sulfate	—	Surgical	—
7 (03319797)	NOVOCART inject plus	TETEC AG	Autologous chondrocytes	In situ polymerizable hydrogel (albumin, hyaluronic acid)	—	Surgical	—
8 (03873545)	ProChondrix CR	AlloSource	Allogeneic chondrocytes	Laser-etched, cryopreserved fresh osteochondral allograft	—	Surgical	✔ (HCT/P)
9 (02844751)	StroMed	VivaTech International, Inc.	Autologous adipose-derived MSCs	Adipose ECM	—	Intra-articular	—
10 (03383081)	19#iSCLife-OA	Sclnow Biotechnology Co., Ltd.	Allogeneic umbilical cord–derived MSCs	—	—	Intra-articular	—
11 (04208646)	AlloJoin	Cellular Biomedicine Group, Inc.	Allogeneic adipose-derived MSCs	—	—	Intra-articular	—
12 (04744402)	CartiLife	Biosolution Co., Ltd.	Autologous chondrocytes (cell spheroids)	—	—	Surgical	—
13 (04863183)	Cellistem OA	Cells for cells	Allogeneic umbilical cord–derived MSCs	—	—	Intra-articular	—

(Continued)

TABLE 2 Orthobiologics for Cartilage Repair and Osteoarthritis continued

# (NCT)	Product/Trade Name	Company	Cell Type	Scaffold Material	Signal	Delivery	Market Status (USA)
14 (04520945)	Chondrogen	Meluha Therapeutics Sdn Bhd	Allogeneic umbilical cord–derived MSCs	—	—	Intra-articular	—
15 (01222559)	ChondroSphere	Co.Don AG	Autologous chondrocytes (cell spheroids)	—	—	Surgical	—
16 (03203330)	TissueGene-C	Kolon TissueGene	Allogeneic nontransduced chondrocytes, irradiated transduced human GP2-293 cells expressing TGF-β1	—	—	Intra-articular	—
17 (03696394)	BioCartilage	Arthrex	—	Allogeneic micronized cartilage matrix	—	Surgical	✔ (HCT/P)
18 (01246895)	BST-CarGel	Smith & Nephew plc	—	Chitosan	—	Surgical	—
19 (01410136)	Chondrofix	Zimmer Biomet	—	Allogeneic decellularized osteochondral graft	—	Surgical	✔ (HCT/P)
20 (04537013)	Chondro-Gide	Geistlich Pharma	—	Bilayer collagen I/III membrane	—	Surgical	—
21 (02659215)	HYALOFAST	Anika Therapeutics	—	Hyaluronic acid–based	—	Surgical	—
22 (03968913)	KINERET	Sobi	—	—	Anakinra (IL-1β receptor antagonist)	Intra-articular	—
23 (03727022)	—	Biosplice Therapeutics	—	—	SM04690 (Wnt inhibitor)	Intra-articular	—
24 (03072147)	—	Eli Lilly and Company Corporate Center	—	—	Teriparatide (promotes bone formation)	Intra-muscular	—
25 (04875754)	—	ICM Biotech	—	—	ICM-203 (gene therapy)	Intra-articular	—
26 (01919164)	—	Merck KGaA	—	—	Sprifermin (rhFGF-18)	Intra-articular	—
27 (03275064)	—	Novartis	—	—	LNA043 (ANGPTL3 agonist)	Intra-articular	—
28 (04097379)	—	Novartis	—	—	LRX712 (pro-regenerative)	Intra-articular	—

TABLE 2 Orthobiologics for Cartilage Repair and Osteoarthritis continued

# (NCT)	Product/Trade Name	Company	Cell Type	Scaffold Material	Signal	Delivery	Market Status (USA)
29 (02837900)	—	OrthoTrophix, Inc.	—	—	TPX-100 (regulates hard tissue, phosphate metabolism)	Intra-articular	—
30 (04318041)	Artrodar	TRB Chemedica International SA	—	—	Diacerein (IL-1β inhibitor)	Oral	—
31 (03595618)	—	Galapagos NV	—	—	GLPG1972 (ADAMTS-5 inhibitor)	Oral	—
32 (02705625)	—	Medivir	—	—	MIV-711 (cathepsin K inhibitor)	Oral	—

The National Clinical Trial (NCT) number of recently registered studies are indicated as well as if the product is marketed in the United States for use in cartilage repair as minimally manipulated human cells, tissues, and cellular-based and tissue-based products (HCT/Ps) or under a Biologics License Application (BLA).

ECM = extracellular matrix, IL-1β = interleukin 1 beta, MSC = mesenchymal stem cell, TGF-β1 = transforming growth factor beta 1

first-line treatment because of the relatively low cost and straightforward technique compared with other surgical interventions (**Figure 6**). Marrow stimulation leverages the intrinsic cartilage repair response after subchondral bone penetration by releasing a milieu of marrow elements, including MSCs, growth factors, and other signals, into the injured site to promote formation of fibrocartilaginous repair tissue.[64,65] At the defect, the marrow clots and provides a structural framework, or scaffold, on which repair can occur. However, lack of control on the differentiation process often leads to variable formation of suboptimal fibrocartilage repair tissue with inferior biochemical and biomechanical properties having a higher proportion of type I collagen than hyaline cartilage.[65,66]

Recent advances in microfracture involve augmentation with biomaterial scaffolds to stabilize clot formation and promote chondrogenesis and formation of hyaline cartilage in a method often referred to as autologous matrix-induced chondrogenesis. This method may be achieved using micronized or particulated allogeneic cartilage (BioCartilage; Arthrex), as well as biomaterial scaffolds such as chitosan (BST-CarGel; Smith & Nephew) and hyaluronan (HYALOFAST; Anika Therapeutics). In addition to biomaterials scaffolds, marrow stimulation techniques are often paired with BMAC or PRP to enhance cartilage repair.

NOVEL ORTHOBIOLOGIC APPROACHES TO CARTILAGE REPAIR

Novel approaches to orthobiologic repair aim to modulate or activate the response of endogenous or exogenous cells as a stand-alone procedure or to augment cartilage restoration surgery, to promote formation of hyaline-like cartilaginous repair tissue. Many orthobiologic interventions aim to enhance matrix formation by promoting anabolic or suppressing catabolic pathways.

PRP and BMAC

PRP and BMAC have demonstrated promising results in the clinical application for repair of chondral defects as an adjuvant procedure (eg, to bone marrow stimulation) or as an independent management technique via intra-articular injection.[49,50] PRP and BMAC are cellular preparations of autologous blood and bone marrow aspirate, respectively, that have been concentrated, usually by centrifugation, and are often activated with thrombin. These autologous point-of-care cell therapies contain a high concentration of platelets, growth factors, chemokines, and cytokines as well as MSCs and a variety of hematopoietic cells that provide potentially beneficial anabolic and anti-inflammatory mediators.[67] Although translational studies have demonstrated good clinical efficacy of PRP and BMAC, methods of preparation are variable and there is inherent patient-to-patient variability in composition.[49]

Standardized, high-quality studies are needed to demonstrate efficacy.

Extracellular Vesicles

Treatment strategies using extracellular vesicles represent a novel class of therapeutics that act to modulate the inflammatory response and stimulate matrix production to restore and maintain cartilage homeostasis.[68] Extracellular vesicles, including exosomes and microvesicles, are secreted membrane-enclosed vesicles. Extracellular vesicles are isolated from extracellular fluids (conditioned cell culture media, body fluids) and may contain proteins, including growth factors and cytokines, functional nucleic acids (mRNA, miRNA, etc), and lipids, which function as intercellular communication vehicles.[69,70] Preclinical in vitro and in vivo studies have demonstrated that the immunomodulatory, chondroprotective, and regenerative effects of MSC-derived extracellular vesicles are equivalent or superior to MSCs alone.[68] Compared with cell-based therapies, extracellular vesicle–based treatment strategies minimize difficulties associated with living cell therapeutics (viability, potency, and differentiation).

Gene Therapy Strategies

Gene therapy strategies for cartilage repair often aim to reduce inflammation, inhibit matrix degradation, and increase matrix synthesis through the delivery of nucleic acids to target tissues or cells using viral (adenovirus, lentivirus, retroviruses, etc) or nonviral (siRNAs, miRNAs) vectors. Gene therapies targeting the interleukin 1 (IL-1), tumor necrosis factor alpha (TNF-α), interferon-beta (IFN-β), and hypoxia-inducible factor alpha (Hif-2α) pathways, which mediate chondrocyte catabolism, as well as insulinlike growth factor 1 (IGF-1), TGF-β, SOX9, and PRG4, which mediate anabolism and chondrogenesis, have been investigated preclinically, with some being evaluated in clinical trials.[71] TissueGene-C (Kolon TissueGene), a biologic drug product consisting allogeneic human chondrocytes virally transduced to express TGF-β1, promoted cartilage regeneration in rabbit preclinical studies and is considered safe and effective for improving pain and motor scores in patients with moderate to severe disease.[71] TissueGene-C was approved in Korea for the treatment of moderate knee osteoarthritis for which standard of care has failed, and is currently in phase 3 clinical trials in the United States (NCT03203330).

Additional Targets for Small-Molecule Therapies

Other biologic therapies target the inflammatory or biosynthetic pathways by interacting with cell receptors or providing growth factors. Anti-inflammatory agents such as bradykinin B_2 receptor agonists, which reduce osteoarthritic knee pain compared with placebo, anakinra, an IL-1β receptor antagonist that reduces pain and improves knee function 2 weeks after acute injury compared with placebo, and TNF inhibitors (infliximab, etanercept) have been proposed to manage knee osteoarthritis.[72,73] In addition, growth factor treatment strategies with recombinant human bone morphogenetic protein-7 (rhBMP7) and recombinant human fibroblast growth factor-18 (rhFGF18, sprifermin) have demonstrated positive outcomes (reduction in Western Ontario and McMaster Universities Osteoarthritis Index pain scores) compared with placebo but have not been evaluated in long-term clinical studies.[48] Therapeutic utility of these agents, typically delivered by intra-articular injection, is diminished by short retention times within the joint space as well as limited transport within the cartilage tissue. Such limitations may be ameliorated by coupling the therapeutic agent to positively charged carriers of optimal size and charge so that the cartilage can act as a reservoir for sustained intratissue delivery.[32]

Alternative Cell Sources

Investigations into the feasibility and clinical utility of alternative cell sources for cartilage repair are ongoing. Unfortunately, the use of autologous chondrocytes is limited by donor-site morbidity and complicated by the relatively low cellularity in adult articular cartilage, requiring in vitro expansion. Furthermore, repair tissue involving autologous chondrocytes is often fibrocartilaginous in nature and not characteristic of native hyaline cartilage.[51]

MSCs have been studied extensively in vitro and in vivo within the context of cartilage repair.[51,74] MSCs are capable of differentiating into bone and cartilage and have been derived from bone marrow, bone, synovium, periosteum, muscle, dermis, adipose, umbilical cord, and placental tissues. In particular, bone marrow–derived MSCs secrete a variety of synthetic, proliferative, and regenerative factors that, when introduced to the joint, interact with endogenous cells to modulate the repair response.[75] However, because the number of bone marrow–derived MSCs decreases significantly with age,[76] MSCs isolated from umbilical cord and adipose tissues, which are readily available and highly cellular, have been developed and are in clinical trials.[51,77] Additional cell sources that have been investigated include induced pluripotent stem cells, as well as stem cells from peripheral blood and amniotic tissue.[46,51,78]

Utilization of cell-based therapies is limited by the undefined dose, regimen, and mode of delivery of cells to the injured site. Cells may be preconditioned in vitro with biomechanical and biochemical stimuli to modulate phenotype and behavior, and subsequently used as a stand-alone drug or biologic, delivered by intra-articular injection, or as a component of a more complex intervention. Future studies are necessary to establish the long-term clinical benefit of cell-based therapeutics for cartilage repair and identify indications and criteria for their use.

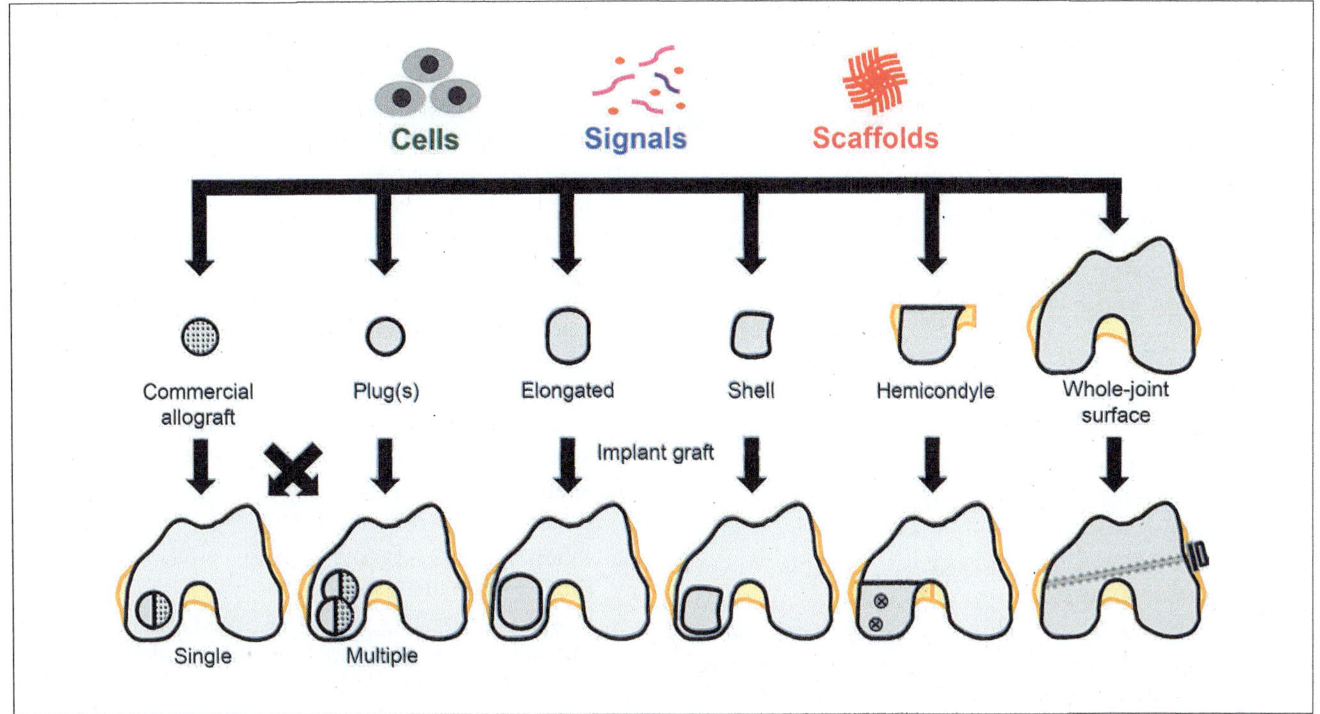

FIGURE 9 Chondral and osteochondral grafting techniques. Systemic illustration shows that depending on the size of the defect, cartilage and osteochondral lesions may be treated with allogeneic or autologous as well as tissue-engineered (osteo) chondral grafts. (Adapted with permission from Gacasan EG, Sah RL: Ch 33 – Articular cartilage repair: Augmentation, regeneration, replacement, and substitution, in Aaron R, ed: *Orthopaedic Basic Science*, ed 5. American Academy of Orthopaedic Surgeons, 2020, pp 415-432.)

Bioreactors are used in the development and production of orthobiologics to apply a combination of mechanical and biochemical signals. During development of engineered articular cartilage or osteochondral tissues, mechanical stimulation during culture regulates and improves the mechanical properties of the engineered tissue.[79,80] In addition, bioreactors are used to screen for drug candidates and evaluate cartilage repair strategies. Emerging microfluidic chip-based platforms enable high-throughput screening of drug candidates. Cartilage-on-a-chip and joint-on-a-chip models aim to mimic aspects of the joint and recapitulate physiologic responses in response to drug candidates.[81,82] Three-dimensional culture of chondrocytes within engineered constructs or in explanted osteochondral tissues is also used to evaluate drug candidates and cartilage repair strategies at the tissue and joint scales.[83,84] Bioreactor systems are also used in bioprocessing to produce therapeutic tissues, cells, and cellular derivatives, such as gene and extracellular vesicle therapies. Production of these biologics may require cellular expansion, cultivation on three-dimensional material scaffolds, and additional purification processes.[46,85,86]

SUMMARY

Repair of cartilage injuries, due to traumatic focal defects or chronic disease, aims to restore cartilage function and prevent, slow, or reverse cartilage degeneration. Conventional treatment strategies for cartilage repair, including osteochondral grafting and ACI, are limited by donor availability and donor-site morbidity and are difficult to scale and produce as off-the-shelf products. Ultimately, orthobiologic therapies may help to reduce the use of allogeneic or autologous tissue grafts for treatment of focal and widespread joint deterioration (**Figure 9**).

Emerging orthobiologic interventions provide a combination of cells, scaffolds, and signals that aim to establish a regenerative environment to facilitate repair. Local delivery of PRP, BMAC, and extracellular vesicles, which are enriched with growth factors and cytokines, as well as gene therapies and other small molecule therapeutics modulate matrix formation and cellular behavior by targeting anabolic and catabolic pathways. In addition, PRP and BMAC contain MSCs that aid in repair. Furthermore, cellular therapies using autologous and allogeneic MSC sources are being developed as an alternative to autologous chondrocytes. Therapeutic components should be engineered to maximize retention within the joint space and synovial fluid, if introduced via intra-articular injection, and within the cartilage itself by using the native physicochemical properties of the tissue.

REFERENCES

1. Hunter W: Of the structure and disease of articulating cartilages. *Philos Trans R Soc Lond* 1743;42:514-421.
2. Brannan SR, Jerrard DA: Synovial fluid analysis. *J Emerg Med* 2006;30:331-339.
3. Carlson CS, Cullins LD, Meuten DJ: Osteochondrosis of the articular-epiphyseal cartilage complex in young horses: evidence for a defect in cartilage canal blood supply. *Vet Pathol* 1995;32:641-647.
4. Carlson CS, Hilley HD, Henrikson CK: Ultrastructure of normal epiphyseal cartilage of the articular-epiphyseal cartilage complex in growing swine. *Am J Vet Res* 1985;46:306-313.
5. Aspden RM: Osteoarthritis: A problem of growth not decay? *Rheumatology* 2008;47:1452-1460.
6. Sun HB: Mechanical loading, cartilage degeneration, and arthritis. *Ann N Y Acad Sci* 2010;1211:37-50.
7. Goldring MB: Articular cartilage degradation in osteoarthritis. *HSS J* 2012;8:7-9.
8. Poole AR, Kojima T, Yasuda T, Mwale F, Kobayashi M, Laverty S: Composition and structure of articular cartilage: A template for tissue repair. *Clin Orthop Relat Res* 2001;391:S26-S33.
9. Han E, Chen SS, Klisch SM, Sah RL: Contribution of proteoglycan osmotic swelling pressure to the compressive properties of articular cartilage. *Biophys J* 2011;101:916-924.
10. Dudhia J: Aggrecan, aging and assembly in articular cartilage. *Cell Mol Life Sci* 2005;62:2241-2256.
11. Heinegard D, Saxne T: The role of the cartilage matrix in osteoarthritis. *Nat Rev Rheumatol* 2011;7:50-56.
12. Temple MM, Bae WC, Chen MQ, et al: Age- and site-associated biomechanical weakening of human articular cartilage of the femoral condyle. *Osteoarthritis Cartilage* 2007;15:1042-1052.
13. Aigner T, Zien A, Gehrsitz A, Gebhard PM, McKenna L: Anabolic and catabolic gene expression pattern analysis in normal versus osteoarthritic cartilage using complementary DNA-array technology. *Arthritis Rheum* 2001;44:2777-2789.
14. Grogan SP, Duffy SF, Pauli C, et al: Zone-specific gene expression patterns in articular cartilage. *Arthritis Rheum* 2013;65(2):418-428.
15. Darling EM, Hu JC, Athanasiou KA: Zonal and topographical differences in articular cartilage gene expression. *J Orthop Res* 2004;22:1182-1187.
16. Kozhemyakina E, Zhang M, Ionescu A, et al: Identification of a Prg4-positive articular cartilage progenitor cell population. *Arthritis Rheumatol* 2015;67(5):1261-1273.
17. Decker RS, Um H-B, Dyment NA, et al: Cell origin, volume and arrangement are drivers of articular cartilage formation, morphogenesis and response to injury in mouse limbs. *Dev Biol* 2017;426:56-68.
18. Lei L, Newton PT, Bouderlique T, et al: Superficial cells are self-renewing chondrocyte progenitors, which form the articular cartilage in juvenile mice. *FASEB J* 2016;31(3):1067-1084.
19. Karlsson C, Thornemo M, Henriksson HB, Lindahl A: Identification of a stem cell niche in the zone of Ranvier within the knee joint. *J Anat* 2009;215:355-363.
20. Maroudas A: Physicochemical properties of articular cartilage, in Freeman MAR, ed: *Adult Articular Cartilage*. 1979, pp 215-290.
21. Eyre DR, Weis MA, Wu J-J: Articular cartilage collagen: An irreplaceable framework? *Eur Cell Mater* 2006;12:57-63.
22. Belcher C, Yaqub R, Fawthrop F, Bayliss M, Doherty M: Synovial fluid chondroitin and keratan sulphate epitopes, glycosaminoglycans, and hyaluronan in arthritic and normal knees. *Ann Rheum Dis* 1997;56:299-307.
23. Bayliss MT, Howat S, Davidson C, Dudhia J: The organization of aggrecan in human articular cartilage. Evidence for age-related changes in the rate of aggregation of newly synthesized molecules. *J Biol Chem* 2000;275:6321-6327.
24. Smith DW, Gardiner BS, Zhang L, Grodzinsky AJ: *Articular Cartilage Dynamics*. Springer, 2019, pp 65-243.
25. Knudson CB, Knudson W: Cartilage proteoglycans. *Semin Cell Dev Biol* 2001;12:69-78.
26. Gao Y, Liu S, Huang J, et al: The ECM-cell interaction of cartilage extracellular matrix on chondrocytes. *Biomed Res Int* 2014;2014:648459.
27. DiDomenico CD, Lintz M, Bonassar LJ: Molecular transport in articular cartilage – What have we learned from the past 50 years? *Nat Rev Rheumatol* 2018;14:393-403.
28. Levick JR, McDonald JN: Fluid movement across synovium in healthy joints: Role of synovial fluid macromolecules. *Ann Rheum Dis* 1995;54:417-423.
29. Hui AY, McCarty WJ, Masuda K, Firestein GS, Sah RL: A systems biology approach to synovial joint lubrication in health, injury, and disease. *Wiley Interdiscip Rev Syst Biol Med* 2012;4:15-37.
30. Levick JR: A method for estimating macromolecular reflection by human synovium, using measurements of intra-articular half-lives. *Ann Rheum Dis* 1998;57:339-344.
31. Owen SG, Francis HW, Roberts MS: Disappearance kinetics of solutes from synovial fluid after intra-articular injection. *Br J Clin Pharmacol* 1994;38:349-355.
32. Bajpayee AG, Grodzinsky AJ: Cartilage-targeting drug delivery: Can electrostatic interactions help? *Nat Rev Rheumatol* 2017;13:183-193.
33. Doan TN, Bernard FC, McKinney JM, Dixon JB, Willett NJ: Endothelin-1 inhibits size dependent lymphatic clearance of PEG-based conjugates after intra-articular injection into the rat knee. *Acta Biomater* 2019;93:270-281.
34. McCarty WJ, Cheng JC, Hansen BC, et al: The biophysical mechanisms of altered hyaluronan concentration in synovial fluid after anterior cruciate ligament transection. *Arthritis Rheum* 2012;64:3993-4003.
35. Bouta EM, Bell RD, Rahimi H, et al: Targeting lymphatic function as a novel therapeutic intervention for rheumatoid arthritis. *Nat Rev Rheumatol* 2018;14(2):94-106.
36. Lesperance LM, Gray ML, Burstein D: Determination of fixed charge density in cartilage using nuclear magnetic resonance. *J Orthop Res* 1992;10:1-13.

37. Maroudas A: Distribution and diffusion of solutes in articular cartilage. *Biophys J* 1970;10:365-379.

38. Eisenberg SR, Grodzinsky AJ: Swelling of articular cartilage and other connective tissues: Electromechanochemical forces. *J Orthop Res* 1985;3:148-159.

39. Hjelle K, Solheim E, Strand T, Muri R, Brittberg M: Articular cartilage defects in 1,000 knee arthroscopies. *Arthroscopy* 2002;18:730-734.

40. Buckwalter JA, Saltzman C, Brown T: The impact of osteoarthritis: Implications for research. *Clin Orthop Relat Res* 2004;427:S6-S15.

41. Bijlsma JW, Berenbaum F, Lafeber FP: Osteoarthritis: An update with relevance for clinical practice. *Lancet* 2011;377:2115-2126.

42. Lotz M, Loeser RF: Effects of aging on articular cartilage homeostasis. *Bone* 2012;51:241-248.

43. Marlovits S, Singer P, Zeller P, Mandl I, Haller J, Trattnig S: Magnetic resonance observation of cartilage repair tissue (MOCART) for the evaluation of autologous chondrocyte transplantation: Determination of interobserver variability and correlation to clinical outcome after 2 years. *Eur J Radiol* 2006;57:16-23.

44. Smith BD, Grande DA: The current state of scaffolds for musculoskeletal regenerative applications. *Nat Rev Rheumatol* 2015;11:213-222.

45. Mastbergen SC, Saris DB, Lafeber FP: Functional articular cartilage repair: Here, near, or is the best approach not yet clear? *Nat Rev Rheumatol* 2013;9:277-290.

46. Kwon H, Brown WE, Lee CA, et al: Surgical and tissue engineering strategies for articular cartilage and meniscus repair. *Nat Rev Rheumatol* 2019;15(9):550-570.

47. Steinert AF, Noth U, Tuan RS: Concepts in gene therapy for cartilage repair. *Injury* 2008;39(suppl 1):S97-S113.

48. Jones IA, Togashi R, Wilson ML, Heckmann N, Vangsness CT Jr. Intra-articular treatment options for knee osteoarthritis. *Nat Rev Rheumatol* 2019;15:77-90.

49. Chahla J, Cinque ME, Piuzzi NS, et al: A call for standardization in platelet-rich plasma preparation protocols and composition reporting: A systematic review of the clinical orthopaedic literature. *J Bone Joint Surg Am* 2017;99:1769-1779.

50. Piuzzi NS, Hussain ZB, Chahla J, et al: Variability in the preparation, reporting, and use of bone marrow aspirate concentrate in musculoskeletal disorders: A systematic review of the clinical orthopaedic literature. *J Bone Joint Surg Am* 2018;100:517-525.

51. Makris EA, Gomoll AH, Malizos KN, Hu JC, Athanasiou KA: Repair and tissue engineering techniques for articular cartilage. *Nat Rev Rheumatol* 2015;11:21-34.

52. Caplan AI, Correa D: The MSC: An injury drugstore. *Cell Stem Cell* 2011;9:11-15.

53. Chahal J, Gross AE, Gross C, et al: Outcomes of osteochondral allograft transplantation in the knee. *Arthroscopy* 2013;29:575-588.

54. Frank RM, Lee S, Levy D, et al: Osteochondral allograft transplantation of the knee. Analysis of failures at 5 years. *Am J Sports Med* 2017;45:864-874.

55. Cavendish PA, Everhart JS, Peters NJ, Sommerfeldt MF, Flanigan DC: Osteochondral allograft transplantation for knee cartilage and osteochondral defects: A review of indications, technique, rehabilitation, and outcomes. *JBJS Rev* 2019;7:e7.

56. Wang D, Chang B, Coxe FR, et al: Clinically meaningful improvement after treatment of cartilage defects of the knee with osteochondral grafts. *Am J Sports Med* 2019;47:71-81.

57. Hangody L, Fules P: Autologous osteochondral mosaicplasty for the treatment of full-thickness defects of weight-bearing joints. Ten years of experimental and clinical experience. *J Bone Joint Surg Am* 2003;85-A(suppl 2):25-32.

58. Sherman SL, Garrity J, Bauer K, Cook J, Stannard J, Bugbee W: Fresh osteochondral allograft transplantation for the knee: Current concepts. *J Am Acad Orthop Surg* 2014;22:121-133.

59. Chahla J, Hinckel BB, Yanke AB, et al: An expert consensus statement on the management of large chondral and osteochondral defects in the patellofemoral joint. *Orthop J Sports Med* 2020;8:2325967120907343.

60. Brittberg M, Lindahl A, Nilsson A, Ohlsson C, Isaksson O, Peterson L: Treatment of deep cartilage defects in the knee with autologous chondrocyte transplantation. *N Engl J Med* 1994;331:889-895.

61. Huang BJ, Hu JC, Athanasiou KA: Cell-based tissue engineering strategies used in the clinical repair of articular cartilage. *Biomaterials* 2016;98:1-22.

62. Krill M, Early N, Everhart JS, Flanigan DC: Autologous Chondrocyte Implantation (ACI) for knee cartilage defects: A review of indications, technique, and outcomes. *JBJS Rev* 2018;6:e5.

63. Grande DA, Pitman MI, Peterson L, Menche D, Klein M: The repair of experimentally produced defects in rabbit articular cartilage by autologous chondrocyte transplantation. *J Orthop Res* 1989;7:208-218.

64. Rutgers M, van Pelt MJ, Dhert WJ, Creemers LB, Saris DB: Evaluation of histological scoring systems for tissue-engineered, repaired and osteoarthritic cartilage. *Osteoarthritis Cartilage* 2010;18:12-23.

65. Mithoefer K, McAdams T, Williams RJ, Kreuz PC, Mandelbaum BR: Clinical efficacy of the microfracture technique for articular cartilage repair in the knee: An evidence-based systematic analysis. *Am J Sports Med* 2009;37:2053-2063.

66. Steadman JR, Briggs KK, Rodrigo JJ, Kocher MS, Gill TJ, Rodkey WG: Outcomes of microfracture for traumatic chondral defects of the knee: Average 11-year follow-up. *Arthroscopy* 2003;19:477-484.

67. Kennedy MI, Whitney K, Evans T, LaPrade RF: Platelet-rich plasma and cartilage repair. *Curr Rev Musculoskelet Med* 2018;11:573-582.

68. Velot É, Madry H, Venkatesan JK, Bianchi A, Cucchiarini M: Is extracellular vesicle-based therapy the next answer for cartilage regeneration? *Front Bioeng Biotechnol* 2021;9:645039.

69. Lötvall J, Hill AF, Hochberg F, et al: Minimal experimental requirements for definition of extracellular vesicles and their functions: A position statement from the International Society for Extracellular Vesicles. *J Extracell Vesicles* 2014;3:26913.

70. Toh WS, Lai RC, Hui JHP, Lim SK: MSC exosome as a cell-free MSC therapy for cartilage regeneration: Implications for osteoarthritis treatment. *Semin Cell Dev Biol* 2017;67:56-64.
71. Grol MW, Lee BH: Gene therapy for repair and regeneration of bone and cartilage. *Curr Opin Pharmacol* 2018;40:59-66.
72. Kraus VB, Birmingham J, Stabler TV, et al: Effects of intraarticular IL1-Ra for acute anterior cruciate ligament knee injury: A randomized controlled pilot trial (NCT00332254). *Osteoarthritis Cartilage* 2012;20:271-278.
73. Hunter DJ: Are there promising biologic therapies for osteoarthritis? *Curr Rheumatol Rep* 2008;10:19-25.
74. Noth U, Steinert AF, Tuan RS: Technology insight: Adult mesenchymal stem cells for osteoarthritis therapy. *Nat Clin Pract Rheumatol* 2008;4:371-380.
75. Pittenger MF, Discher DE, Péault BM, Phinney DG, Hare JM, Caplan AI: Mesenchymal stem cell perspective: Cell biology to clinical progress. *NPJ Regen Med* 2019;4:22.
76. Rao MS, Mattson MP: Stem cells and aging: Expanding the possibilities. *Mech Ageing Dev* 2001;122:713-734.
77. Wang L, Tran I, Seshareddy K, Weiss ML, Detamore MS: A comparison of human bone marrow-derived mesenchymal stem cells and human umbilical cord-derived mesenchymal stromal cells for cartilage tissue engineering. *Tissue Eng Part A* 2009;15:2259-2266.
78. Gomoll AH, Farr J, Cole BJ, et al: Safety and efficacy of an amniotic suspension allograft injection over 12 Months in a single-blinded, randomized controlled trial for symptomatic osteoarthritis of the knee. *Arthroscopy* 2021;37:2246-2257.
79. Salinas EY, Hu JC, Athanasiou K: A guide for using mechanical stimulation to enhance tissue-engineered articular cartilage properties. *Tissue Eng Part B Rev* 2018;24:345-358.
80. Martin I, Smith T, Wendt D: Bioreactor-based roadmap for the translation of tissue engineering strategies into clinical products. *Trends Biotechnol* 2009;27:495-502.
81. Occhetta P, Mainardi A, Votta E, et al: Hyperphysiological compression of articular cartilage induces an osteoarthritic phenotype in a cartilage-on-a-chip model. *Nat Biomed Eng* 2019;3:545-557.
82. Paggi CA, Teixeira LM, Le Gac S, Karperien M: Joint-on-chip platforms: Entering a new era of in vitro models for arthritis. *Nat Rev Rheumatol* 2022;18:217-231.
83. Makarczyk MJ, Gao Q, He Y, et al: Current models for development of disease-modifying osteoarthritis drugs. *Tissue Eng Part C Methods* 2021;27:124-138.
84. Nugent-Derfus GE, Takara T, O'neill JK, et al: Continuous passive motion applied to whole joints stimulates chondrocyte biosynthesis of PRG4. *Osteoarthritis Cartilage* 2007;15:566-574.
85. Moutsatsou P, Ochs J, Schmitt RH, Hewitt CJ, Hanga MP: Automation in cell and gene therapy manufacturing: from past to future. *Biotechnol Lett* 2019;41:1245-1253.
86. Grangier A, Branchu J, Volatron J, et al: Technological advances towards extracellular vesicles mass production. *Adv Drug Deliv Rev* 2021;176:113843.

CHAPTER

7 Overview of Orthobiologics for Bone Repair

Mirtijn van Griensven, MD, PhD • Elizabeth Rosado Balmayor, PhD

INTRODUCTION

An overview of physiologic bone composition regarding cells and matrix as well as the anatomic features is provided. This natural information is the basis for describing the possible therapeutic options comprising biomaterials, cells, or a combination thereof. These orthobiologic approaches are discussed in detail, along with the importance of the different components for certain pathologies. Furthermore, the individual entities and the combinations have different legislative implications, such as the law on advanced therapy medicinal products.

BRIEF BIOLOGY OF BONE

The bone is a very specialized organ; its main function is to support the human body. Because of its composition, it is a hard material allowing the skeleton to protect the inner organs. In addition to the structural support, the bone contains bone marrow that is important for the production of blood and also contains other progenitor cells, including mesenchymal stem cells (MSCs). The bone plays an important role in calcium homeostasis as well as in the secretion and sequestration of growth factors and cytokines.[1]

Composition: Matrix and Cells

The bone is characterized as a connective tissue. The main component is mineralized extracellular matrix. In the extracellular matrix, different cell types are embedded. The extracellular matrix consists of an organic and an inorganic part. The organic extracellular matrix part together with the different bone cells comprises the organic mass. The organic bone mass consists of 90% of collagen type I and the other 10% of small proteins such as osteonectin and osteocalcin.[2] The inorganic bone mass, which is approximately 70% of the bone dry mass, consists of 99% of the alkaline mineral hydroxyapatite.

The bone consists of three major cell types: osteoblasts, osteoclasts, and osteocytes. Furthermore, osteoprogenitor cells being part of the MSCs are also present. Osteocytes are terminally differentiated cells in the bone. Osteoblasts, however, are able to build up new bone. In contrast, osteoclasts dissolve bone mass. The osteoblasts are derived from the MSCs, whereas osteoclasts are derived from hematopoietic stem cells.

Function: Structural and Biologic

The bone tissue has different functions that are structural and biologic. Structurally, bones provide protection to the inner organs from outside forces. Furthermore, bones allow humans to stand upright and maintain their posture. These functions depend on the strength of the bone and are related to its hardness. This is determined by the mineralized extracellular matrix. This results in the biologic function for calcium homeostasis. Bone tissue is a depot for calcium and is involved in the intricate homeostatic circle of calcium depending on resorption in the intestine, excretion in the kidney, and storage in the bone tissue. This homeostasis is closely regulated by hormones such as calcitonin, calcitriol, and parathyroid hormone (PTH). The amount of calcium also partially depends on estrogens, as can be seen that during menopause when estrogen levels are decreased, a decreased calcium content in bones is observed. Because certain bones, as outlined in the next section, contain bone marrow, bone also has an important function in the production of blood cells. Moreover, bone marrow hosts not only hematopoietic stem cells for blood production but also MSCs for the regeneration of other tissues.

HIERARCHY OF STRUCTURE, INCLUDING MORPHOLOGY AND HISTOLOGY

Macroanatomy

The human skeleton consists of 206 bones. The skeleton can be divided into an axial skeleton and an appendicular skeleton. The axial skeleton consists of cranial bones, spine, ribs, and sternum. The upper and lower extremities, the shoulder, and the pelvis belong to the appendicular skeleton. In total, five different bone types are present in the body: long, short, flat, irregular, and sesamoid bones. The long bones are characterized by a longer length than diameter. In the middle of the long bone, a hollow space mostly filled with bone marrow is available. This hollow space is absent in short bones, and the ratio between length and diameter is close to 1 and these bones are mostly cubic. Flat bones are extensive but flat as the

Dr. van Griensven or an immediate family member serves as a board member, owner, officer, or committee member of DGOU and TERMIS. Dr. Balmayor or an immediate family member serves as a board member, owner, officer, or committee member of DGOU, EORS, and TERMIS.

name indicates. These are, for instance, the cranium, pelvis, scapula, and ribs. Bones that cannot be characterized by the previously described forms are called irregular bones such as vertebra and bones of the face. Sesamoid bones are the smallest bones in the body, and they have a special role where tendon is entering other type of bones. The sesamoid bones serve as a type of force reductor.

Long Bones

Long bones as stated previously have a medullary canal. This is in the middle two-thirds of the length of the long bone, which is called the diaphysis. The wall of the diaphysis is the cortex and consists of compact bone. On both ends of the diaphysis, the epiphysis is present. The transition from diaphysis to epiphysis is the metaphysis, which is the area of the long bone where growth occurs before having reached the final length. The epiphysis has an irregular structure and is part of the joints. Therefore, the epiphysis is covered with cartilage. The inside of the epiphysis is spongy bone and here bone marrow is also present. The entire long bone is surrounded by periosteum. The periosteum consists of two layers and is connected to the cortical bone by very strong collagen fibers that are called Sharpey fibers. The periosteum is important because it comprises bone progenitor cells, blood vessels, and nerves. When the periosteum is not present, fracture healing is more difficult and often delayed. In the metaphysis during the growth phase, hypertrophic cartilage is present. The cartilage columns proliferate and lead to length growth of the long bones. The cartilage cells are then mineralizing and change into osteoblasts. This is the so-called enchondral ossification. Examples of long bones are femur, tibia, humerus, radius, and ulna.

Flat Bones

Flat bones are broad plates consisting of two layers of compact bone and in between a variable thickness layer of cancellous bone. In this spongy part, bone marrow is present and is one of the most prominent spaces where erythrocytes are formed. Flat bones have periosteum on both sides. Flat bones typically have a protective function; for instance, they surround the brain, lungs, and heart. Furthermore, they are insertion points for muscles. Flat bones can have different shapes such as a concave shape for the skull, a triangular shape for the scapulae, and a long flat shape for the sternum for instance. Flat bones typically develop via mesenchymal ossification, meaning directly ossified from stem cells. The osteoblasts that are present in the flat bones produce the calcium phosphate for mineralizing the flat bones. After having reached the final shape, many osteoblasts retract their extensions and thereby small channels, known as canaliculi, remain empty. Nutrients and fluid are transported via the canaliculi to the resting osteoblasts that are then called osteocytes because they are much less active, resting cells. In addition to the bone-building cells, there are also osteoclasts present that are important for bone remodeling and for calcium homeostasis.

Cancellous Bone

Cancellous bone is a porous bone and is also called spongy bone or even trabecular bone. Trabecular bone originates from the presence of the trabeculae in the cancellous bone. These trabeculae are bridges of bone on the inside of the bone (mainly in the epiphysis of the long bones and in between the compact bone plates of the flat bones). These trabeculae are aligned according to the load they carry. They are also closer together in areas where the bone encounters more force such as the femoral neck. In between the trabeculae, open spaces are present and are mostly filled with red bone marrow. Because of its structure, cancellous bone has less weight compared with the same volume of compact bone. It also provides structural support and flexibility along the lines of stress. Approximately 20% of the human skeleton is formed by cancellous bone. Because cancellous bone is important for diverting the stress and taking up load, it has a high level of metabolic activity and can be easily remodeled by osteoblasts and osteoclasts. The smallest unit in cancellous bone is called the spongy osteon. Here, bone cells form a unit together with vessels and nerves.

Compact Bone

Eighty percent of the skeleton consists of compact bone. Compact bone is also built up by bone lamellae that are, however, much denser and closer together than in cancellous bone. Thus, the structure per se is similar to cancellous bone, but the density is higher. In compact bone, these lamellae are mostly ordered in a parallel manner. This ordering is also in the direction of the load. Compact bone is found in the cortex of long bones and is also called cortical bone. It forms the outer part of both the long bones and the flat bones. Because of its compact nature, this bone is very strong, is not very flexible, and provides a high degree of protection. The smallest bone structures in compact bones are also called osteons, and they are called haversian channels. These are concentric circles of lamellae with blood vessels in the middle and bone cells concentrically arranged around them. The canaliculi are perpendicular to the circles. These haversian channels comprise approximately 45% of compact bone. These channels are also important in sensing load or movement stresses. Haversian channels are perpendicularly connected by Volkmann channels. Immature compact bone is often referred to as woven bone. Compact bone mainly consists of a very solid hydroxyapatite matrix.

Haversian Channels and Blood Supply

As stated previously, blood vessels are at the center of haversian osteons. Bone is indeed a richly vascularized organ. This is important for the exchange of oxygen and carbon dioxide as well as nutrients and waste material. Furthermore, the blood cells that are produced in the bone marrow are transported from the bone marrow and inner parts of the bones via this vascular system. Approximately 10% to 20% of the cardiac output is reverted to the bones.[3,4] Many blood vessels are present in the area with red bone marrow.[5] Long bones receive blood via external vascular systems. In general, intraosseous and extraosseous blood supply by the blood vessels can be distinguished. In long bones, a systemic artery is present parallel to the longitudinal axis of the long bone. From this longitudinal artery, an artery is derived entering the diaphysis. Myoperiosteal vessels build transversal anastomoses around the diaphysis and the epiphysis. From those, additional blood vessels are derived that nurture the epiphysis and metaphysis.[6] Because of this network of blood vessels, a typical structure occurs in the bone tissue. Affluent blood vessels are perpendicular to the central channel from the osteons and are also perpendicular to the Volkmann channels. Therefore, a connection between the Volkmann channels and the periosteal vasculature exists. The nutrient arteries enter the cortex via the nutrient canals to supply the diaphysis with blood. These are the strongest vessels supplying the bone tissue and clearly visible in macerated bone. The vessels are mostly paired and branch further into the medullary cavity, going up and down and further branching into. a fine capillary net. Those vessels are responsible for approximately half of the circulation in the long bones.[7] Per long bone, two or more of such diaphyseal arteries are present.[8]

As stated previously, the periosteum contains many blood vessels as well. Because the periosteum is surrounding the entire bone, the compact bone is mainly nurtured via perfusion because of periosteal vessels. However, as already mentioned, the periosteal vessels have a connection with haversian and Volkmann channels.[9] It is also still not clear how much both supply routes fulfill the metabolic needs of the bones.

The blood flow inside the bone occurs under unique circumstances. It is a closed cavity system, in which the pressure needs to stay constant. This occurs by changing the flow rate of the blood or via angiogenesis and/or vasculogenesis.[10] In adult bone, the blood flow occurs centrifugal, meaning from the medullary cavity in the direction of the periosteum. This is due to the high blood pressure in the nutrient arteries and the lower pressure in the periosteal system.[11-13] The venous blood flow is local in the epiphysis and metaphysis via a sinusoidal capillary system.[8] The sinusoids drain into a central venous channel. Collecting veins flow to an emissary vein, and in the diaphysis, this vein joins the nutrient artery through the bone cortex.[14] The venous system of the periosteum has connections with this collecting vein as well as with intramuscular and interfascicular veins. The venous blood flow is centripetal, meaning from the outside to the inside and mostly parallel to the arterial vessels of the bones.[15]

Enchondral and Mesenchymal Regeneration

Bone defects can regenerate in two different ways. This is also according to normal embryonic development. When bone regeneration occurs directly via the activity of MSCs, mesenchymal regeneration is present. Homing of stem cells to the bone defect occurs, and they differentiate into bone cells that induce mineralization of the matrix and bone tissue is formed. The MSCs can also produce messenger molecules that attract other cells that are also important for bone regeneration.

Indirect regeneration occurs when the defect starts to show chondrocytes. These chondrocytes are mostly hypertrophic as in the metaphysis; they proliferate and fill up the defect. On the guidance of other growth factors, the hypertrophic chondrocytes start to mineralize and differentiate in osteoblasts (enchondral ossification). During enchondral regeneration in the cartilage phase, the defect is softer and more flexible than normal bone.

CELL BIOLOGY AND LINEAGE DESCRIPTION

Osteoblasts

Osteoblasts are the bone-building cells derived from MSCs. Osteoprogenitor cells develop as a result of differentiation of MSCs, and they are essential for maintaining the osteoblastic cell population.[16] The Wnt/β–catenin signal pathway plays an important role in the differentiation from osteoprogenitor cells to osteoblasts.[17] Osteoprogenitor cells have a spindlelike morphology, whereas osteoblasts have a more quadratic morphology. Differentiated osteoblasts are approximately 20-μm mononuclear cells and are the only cell population in the human body capable of producing unmineralized bone matrix.[16]

The production of this new bone matrix is only possible when several osteoblasts work together. This can be seen in the histology where the osteoblasts are arranged similar to a pearl necklace on the surface of new bone. These structures are also called osteoids. While building new bone, osteoblasts produce unmineralized bone matrix, which mainly consists of cross-linked collagen and some highly specialized proteins such as osteocalcin and osteopontin. Osteoblasts highly express alkaline phosphatase. This enzyme is important to prepare the secreted proteins for the later mineralization.[18]

The organic matrix that has been produced by the osteoblasts is subsequently mineralized by the deposition of hydroxyapatite. This starts to occur especially in the grooves of the collagen. Because of the mineralization of the bone matrix, a connective tissue arises, which is typical for the structural strength of the bone. During mineralization of the bone matrix, singular osteoblasts are closed up by the minerals. Then the osteoblasts are differentiated further into osteocytes that cannot produce any bone matrix anymore. In addition, osteoblasts can differentiate into so-called bone lining cells after the bone matrix has been materialized and they are localized at the surface of the bone. The activity of osteoblasts is regulated by different hormones and growth factors.[16] They also play an important role by the activation of osteoclast progenitor cells.

Osteoclasts

Osteoclasts are derived from mononuclear progenitor cells in the bone marrow. They are approximately 50 to 100 µm in size and are localized at the surface of the bone.[19] Osteoclasts are polyploid, and they are the only known cell type to be able to resorb bone. This polyploidy is based on the development of the osteoclasts because they are derived from a fusion of several mononuclear osteoclast progenitor cells. Osteoclasts are able to resorb mineralized bone matrix because of the presence of highly active ion channels (H^+-ATPase) in their plasma membranes. With the help of these channels, the osteoclasts can pump protons in the extracellular space and locally massively decrease the pH. The protons stay local because when the osteoclasts have close contact with the bone matrix, the actin skeleton reorganizes and a sealing zone with the contact border occurs. The interaction between osteoclasts and the surface of the bone is mainly organized via integrins. The resorption spaces are called Howship lacunae. The highly acidic environment dissolves the bone mineral.

In addition to the secretion of protons, osteoclasts also produce hydrolytic enzymes and procollagenases. Those enzymes digest the organic bone matrix. Osteoclasts are activated by two main soluble proteins, receptor activator of nuclear factor kappa B ligand and macrophage colony-stimulating factor.[20]

Osteocytes

Osteocytes are the main cell type in the mineralized bone matrix. Osteocytes are connected to each other through protrusions of the plasma membrane. Via these protrusions, the osteocytes communicate both with each other and with the surrounding microenvironment. Osteocytes are the mechanosensory cells in the bone. Depending on the mechanical environment, they regulate when and where resorption or bone construction will take place.

Osteoprogenitor Cells Including MSCs

As stated previously, osteoprogenitor cells are derived from MSCs. MSCs can be found in almost all tissues of the body. In bone tissue, MSCs are found in the bone marrow. Adult bone marrow MSCs can differentiate into various cell types and form new tissue including bone. Because they are located in the bone niche, it is claimed that this is the most optimal source for the regeneration of bone. There are approximately 30 MSCs/mL of bone marrow. They belong to the nucleated cells present in the bone marrow, which are approximately 25×10^3/µL. MSCs are characterized by the markers CD73, CD90, and CD105. They lack the markers CD45 and CD34.[21]

MSCs can be isolated from the bone marrow and used for therapeutic purposes as explained later. Depending on the environment including the mechanical stresses and the humoral factors present, MSCs differentiate in a certain cell type among other osteoblasts. Interestingly, it could be shown that MSCs from older patients can be earlier and more pronounced and be differentiated to osteoblasts in vitro than the ones obtained from younger patients. However, over time, MSCs from older patients lose activity and become senescent.

In addition to the regenerative capacity of MSCs, they also play an important role in immunomodulation. MSCs are able to modulate the activity of immune cells. They have the ability to suppress T-cell activity both in a cellular and humoral-dependent way.[22]

EXTRACELLULAR MATRIX COMPOSITION AND HOMEOSTASIS

Collagen Composition and Calcium Deposition

As stated previously, approximately 90% of the organic bone matrix consists of collagen.[16] The main collagen type in the bone is collagen type I. Collagen consists of a triple helix of different alpha helices. In bone, mainly two alpha-1 helices and one alpha-2 helix are combined. Collagen is produced as a pre-procollagen, and one of the main features is the presence of hydroxylated proline and lysine. This hydroxylation is vitamin C dependent. Selected hydroxylysines can then be glycosylated. A procollagen triple helix is formed and subsequently secreted to the extracellular space where the propeptides are cleaved. There they are self-assembled into a fibril of approximately 10 to 300 nm in diameter. These collagen fibrils are then aggregated to form a collagen fiber with a diameter of approximately 0.5 to 3 µm. Collagen type I is the so-called fibrillar collagen.[23]

The amino acid sequence of collagen shows typical triplets of glycine–proline–amino acid or glycine–amino acid–hydroxyproline. The glycine in the collagen is important for the stabilization of the collagen fibers so that the single fibril can be brought closer together because it allows for intermolecular cross-linking. Hydroxyproline is important for the thermal stability of the triple helices. This may be partially based on hydrogen bonds.

The presence of these amino acids also enables the formation of curves in the fibrils. This leads to the presence of minor and major grooves. Together with the charge of the specific amino acids, these are the exact localizations where calcium and phosphate can be deposited. The collagen fibril diameter is probably also important for the calcium-to-phosphate ratio. This is important for the bone strength and is also related to pathologic circumstances such as osteoporosis and osteogenesis imperfecta.

Calcium Homeostasis

As mentioned previously, one of the main inorganic components of the bone is hydroxyapatite. This is a combination of calcium and phosphate. Approximately 99% of the calcium in the human body is stored in bone. The rest of the calcium can be found intracellularly and in the serum. There, it is highly important to be regulated in a very strict range. Therefore, calcium homeostasis is important. The term calcium homeostasis is mainly indicating the hormonal regulation of the serum calcium levels.

There are three important hormones that play a role: PTH (from the parathyroid gland), calcitriol (1,25-dihydroxyvitamin D), and calcitonin from the thyroid gland. In case the serum calcium levels are diminished, the thyroid gland starts to secrete PTH. PTH induces the production of calcitriol. In bone tissue, PTH induces bone resorption because of the activation of osteoclasts and the inhibition of osteoblasts. The secreted calcitriol stimulates calcium absorption in the gut and kidneys. In the bone, it further activates osteoclasts. Nevertheless, calcitriol also stimulates the mineralization of the osteoid. Calcitonin induces opposite reactions and thus more calcium deposition in bone tissue.

It is clear from the aforementioned information that the calcium balance is highly important for the amount of calcium in bone tissue. When people get older and especially in postmenopausal women due to a shortage of estrogen, this balance is disturbed and the calcium deposition in the bone is gradually reduced. This leads to a reduction in bone mass and bone strength. This is of course also dependent on the nutritional state.

OVERVIEW OF THERAPEUTIC OPTIONS

As previously described, it is clear that bone is an intricate tissue composed of several components. In pathologic situations in the orthopaedic and trauma field, bone can be lost, bone defects can occur, and then it needs to be regenerated. The components as described previously are taken into account, meaning that for treatment, the matrix can be considered in the form of biomaterials. In addition, cells can be used, and finally stimulatory molecules, the so-called morphogens, can be included in therapeutic approaches. Thereby, these components can be used separately or in combination (**Figure 1**).

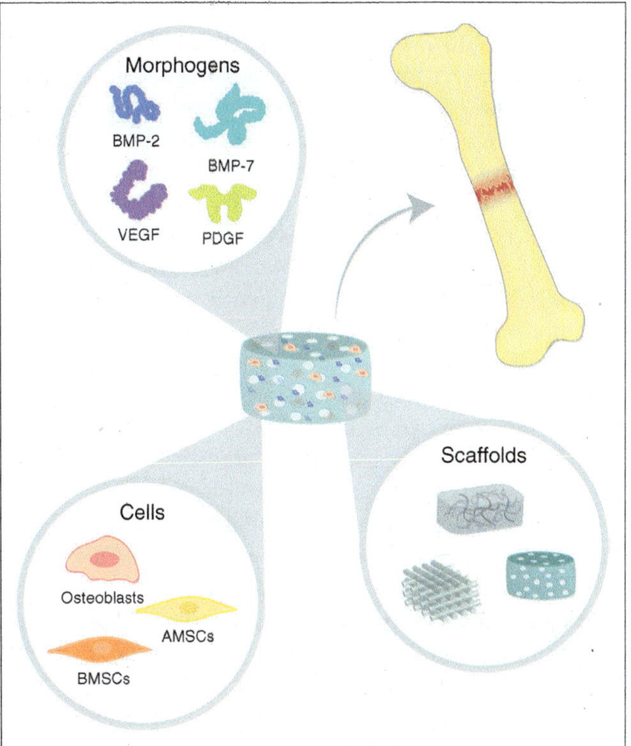

FIGURE 1 Schematic illustration shows the orthobiologic approach for bone regeneration using biomaterials as scaffolding material, cells (bone marrow–derived mesenchymal stem cells [BMSCs] or adipose tissue–derived mesenchymal stromal cells [AMSCs] or differentiated osteoblasts), and morphogens to induce osteogenesis (bone morphogenetic protein [BMP]-2 and BMP-7) and/or angiogenesis (vascular endothelial growth factor [VEGF] and/or platelet-derived growth factor [PDGF]).

Biomaterials

Biomaterials are materials used for biologic applications and can be of different origin, namely, natural, inorganic, and synthetic. They can be applied in different forms such as gels, powder, blocks, and using biofabrication techniques.

Natural Materials

Autologous bone grafts are still the gold standard for bone replacement therapy. The osteogenic properties are associated with the osteogenic progenitor cells and osteoblasts found in the graft. However, graft removal techniques and graft preparation can affect osteogenic properties. This is problematic mainly because of the risk of osteonecrosis. Therefore, it is necessary to carefully remove the grafts and use the correct implantation techniques. Furthermore, the osteoconductive properties are associated with the occurrence of growth factors in the graft. Some growth factors are known to exist in fresh autologous grafts.[24] Notably, bone morphogenetic protein (BMP)-2 and BMP-4, fibroblast growth factor, vascular endothelial growth factor, platelet-derived growth factor, and insulinlike growth factor I can be found. In addition, the osteoconductive properties depend on the three-dimensional structure of the graft. These determine the speed of bone integration.[25] For example, spongiosa grafts are usually incorporated much faster than cortical grafts because of their porous structure.[26]

Another form of the autologous bone graft is the so-called reamer–irrigator–aspirator (RIA). This system is derived from the normal reamer system for reaming of long bones to insert an intramedullary nail. Because this procedure could lead to pulmonary embolism, an additional suction was installed. The suction material contains bone marrow and bone dust from the cortex. By inserting a sieve system with a container, both the bone marrow and bone dust can be collected. That means a mixture of osteoprogenitor cells, growth factors, and bone extracellular matrix is obtained. Removing it from the container, a type of putty material is obtained with a volume of approximately 25 to 90 cm^3. When it was implanted in an ovine bone healing model, accelerated regeneration was observed. Therefore, this RIA material is an excellent material to fill bone defects because of osteotomy or during the second stage of the Masquelet procedure.

Allogeneic bone replacement grafts can come from a deceased or a living donor. For example, patients in whom a total hip endoprosthesis is implanted may be a good source of allogeneic grafts because the femoral head is resected and discarded. In this case, the allogeneic grafts are processed to remove the living cellular component so that no immunologic reaction can occur in the recipient. However, this resulted in allogeneic grafts no longer possessing osteogenic properties. This is an important limitation compared with autologous bone grafts.

A further disadvantage of allogeneic bone grafts is the possible risk of disease transmission. This risk is, however, rather low with 1:1,500,000 for HIV, 1:60,000 for hepatitis C, and 1:100,000 for hepatitis B. Allografts are largely used to fill voids during revision arthroplasty. The allografts add stability to the newly implanted prosthesis and allow a good bone regeneration. Allografts are widely used to fill bone defects after tumor resection. Because of tumor therapy, infections may occur in the transplant. Furthermore, the allograft itself may also fracture. Large critical defects or nonunion defects caused by trauma can be managed with allografts as well. The allograft biomaterial results in complete union of the defects after approximately 6 months. The allografts can be inserted as a block, granules, or chips. It can also be filled in the space after the Masquelet technique or use of a titanium mesh cage.

One of the best-known allogeneic bone grafts is demineralized bone matrix. This is commercially available in many different preparations, including spongiosa chips, gels, putty, or cement. One problem with demineralized bone matrix is the high batch-to-batch variability. BMP-2 concentrations were from 22 to 110 pg/mg when different lots of demineralized bone matrix were compared.[27] Similar results were obtained for BMP-7 concentrations. A general problem with allogeneic transplants is the risk of disease transmission and possible immunologic reactions.

Xenografts are a specific type of allograft but not from another human individual but from another species. Xenografts used for bone regeneration are almost exclusively derived from bovine tissue. These grafts are also provided as granules, chips, or complete blocks after a sintering process. Bovine xenografts have outcome characteristics similar to allografts. Bovine xenografts have been used in the area of maxillofacial surgery, pelvis surgery, and open wedge osteotomies as well as in bone defects in the tibia. The typical time of healing ranges from 4 to 9 months. No immunologic reactions are observed. Incorporation of the xenografts occurred, although at a slow pace as is seen for synthetic hydroxyapatite grafts.

Inorganic Materials

Inorganic bone replacement materials can serve as an alternative to autologous and allogeneic bone grafts to account for all the limitations associated with autologous and allogeneic grafts. Inorganic bone materials can be obtained directly (off the shelf) and are available as chips, granules, putty, and are paste shaped. Some can be injected into the patient. This is a great advantage because there is then the possibility of minimally invasive application or easy adaptation to irregular bone defects.

Different materials have been developed and are further modified to imitate the structure as well as chemical composition of natural bone. The most used materials are hydroxyapatite and tricalcium phosphate (TCP). Seventy percent of the dry weight of natural bone consists of hydroxyapatite.[28] Synthetic hydroxyapatite has been used as an inorganic bone substitute for many years. It is characterized by a very slow absorption time. Therefore, it can be detected for years in the implantation site,[29] which could be problematic. TCP is absorbed faster than hydroxyapatite. Its beta-crystalline form (ie, βTCP) has been successfully used in vertebral body fusions and dental procedures.[30,31] Mixtures of hydroxyapatite and βTCP aim to combine the good biomechanical properties and optimal absorption rates. These combinations are very popular among surgeons. They have been used in various areas, such as during spinal,[32] dental,[33] and hip[34] surgeries.

Synthetics

Polymers such as polylactic acid, polyglycolic acid, polycaprolactone (PCL) and their copolymers have also been presented as possible synthetic bone substitutes.[35] Polymers are mostly soft and not as rigid as ceramics. In addition, they have a high degree of flexibility. In addition, they can be processed much more easily than ceramic materials because they have viscous properties under elevated temperatures. They are biodegradable and biocompatible. Furthermore, these materials can be loaded with different growth factors to provide additional osteoconductive properties. However, the absence of mechanical properties can be an obstacle to use in bone replacement therapy. Therefore, it may be advantageous to use these materials in combinations with ceramic materials such as the abovementioned hydroxyapatite or βTCP. A combination of PCL and TCP was used to perform a large craniofacial reconstruction, which produced a very satisfactory result.[36] A 2014 study was completed at the National University Hospital in Singapore, recruiting 80 patients to undergo reconstruction of orbital fractures using either PCL/TCP matrices or titanium meshes.[37] The PCL/TCP matrices showed very good results. There are many examples of polymers and polymer/ceramic compositions that have been successfully used for bone reconstructions.

Despite many clinically satisfactory results, only a few polymer-based, synthetic bone replacement materials are still used in clinical practice for bone reconstruction. There is also little commercialization of these products.

Biofabrication Modalities

In addition to providing blocks, putty, granules, etc., biomaterials can also be shaped using additive manufacturing techniques. Biofabrication has a great potential to radically disrupt the area of medical devices and implants.[38] Biofabrication modalities are currently translated into the regenerative medicine field to induce the regeneration of tissues and organs.[39] This holds especially true for bone regeneration.[40] Many different techniques exist for biofabrication of scaffolds composed of different materials. Ceramics can be printed[41] as well as titanium[42] and other materials.[43,44] With biofabrication techniques, not only the macrostructure can be recapitulated but also on the microscale, pore optimizations are important and improve cell migration and osteogenesis.[45,46] Using shape memory biomaterials, four-dimensional printed scaffolds can be realized in the near future.[47]

Cells

There is increased interest in the application of cells as key factors for bone healing strategies. Cells naturally organize themselves to form tissues. Therefore, it can be assumed that they also possess this property to regenerate injured tissue if the right biologic stimulus is present. Therefore, it can be very important, especially for bone tissue, to transfer bone-forming cells to a bone defect to accelerate the healing process (**Figure 2**). The type of cell to use may be osteoblasts or osteoprogenitor cells.[48] However, some also recommend using MSCs from different sources. MSC can also differentiate into adult cells that produce different tissues. In addition, they have an immune-privileged status, which makes them attractive for cell transplants. MSCs from bone marrow or adipose tissue are mainly used in everyday clinical practice. This is due to the initial growth rate of these MSCs, which is much higher than that from other sources such as umbilical cord blood.[49]

Autologous Cells: Types, Sources, and Feasible Isolation in the Operating Room

It is very important for clinical use that both adipose tissue–derived MSCs and bone marrow–derived MSCs can be harvested directly in the operating room without external manipulation (ie, manipulation outside the operating room). Such manipulation outside the operating room would mean the need for good manufacturing practice (GMP) facilities with a concomitant increase in logistic burden.

Bone marrow–derived MSCs are concentrated from a bone marrow aspirate by means of a centrifuge, which can be placed directly in the operating room. Several different concepts exist in the market. Some use separating materials making use of cell density (eg, Harvest, Heraeus). Others analyze the flow out after centrifugation by means of ultraviolet spectroscopy and steer thereby separation of MSCs (eg, Arthrex). This approach has already been successfully applied in the management of nonunions and bone cysts.[50,51]

An automatic and standardized machine, Cellution (Cytori Therapeutics, Inc.), has been developed to isolate adipose tissue–derived MSC directly from the patient's own adipose tissue. The use of this technology is part of various clinical trials for orthopaedic applications.[52]

The ability to isolate cells directly from the same patient within the operating room using a standardized machine is an important step toward the clinical applicability of MSCs. In this way, regulatory aspects of cell expansion and ex vivo manipulation are not an issue.

Allogeneic Cells

For various reasons, autologous cells may not be a feasible option and therefore allogeneic cells could be used. Some in vivo studies explored this possibility. MSCs derived from umbilical cord or bone marrow were used. Allogeneic MSCs stimulated bone regeneration in an ovine and rabbit osteonecrosis model.[53,54] These cells were able to heal bone defects in a rat periodontitis model.[55] Umbilical cord MSCs showed bone formation in a murine intramuscular implantation model.[56]

A recent published study administered in vitro differentiated, allogeneic MSCs to delayed union fractures.[57] This study in 22 patients showed a safe approach with an improvement in radiologic union in 76% of the patients. The overall well-being and pain reduction improved as well. No immune reaction against the allogeneic MSCs was measured although there was a slight increase in donor-specific anti-HLA antibodies. The same product is used in clinical studies for tibial fracture (actively recruiting, NCT04432389), lumbar spine fusion (NCT02205138), and interbody fusion (NCT02328287).

Morphogens

Morphogens are important molecules that direct differentiation of the tissue, inducing differentiation or retaining cells in a certain state. However, they may also prohibit development of certain cells into another cell type. The characteristics of the morphogens are useful for

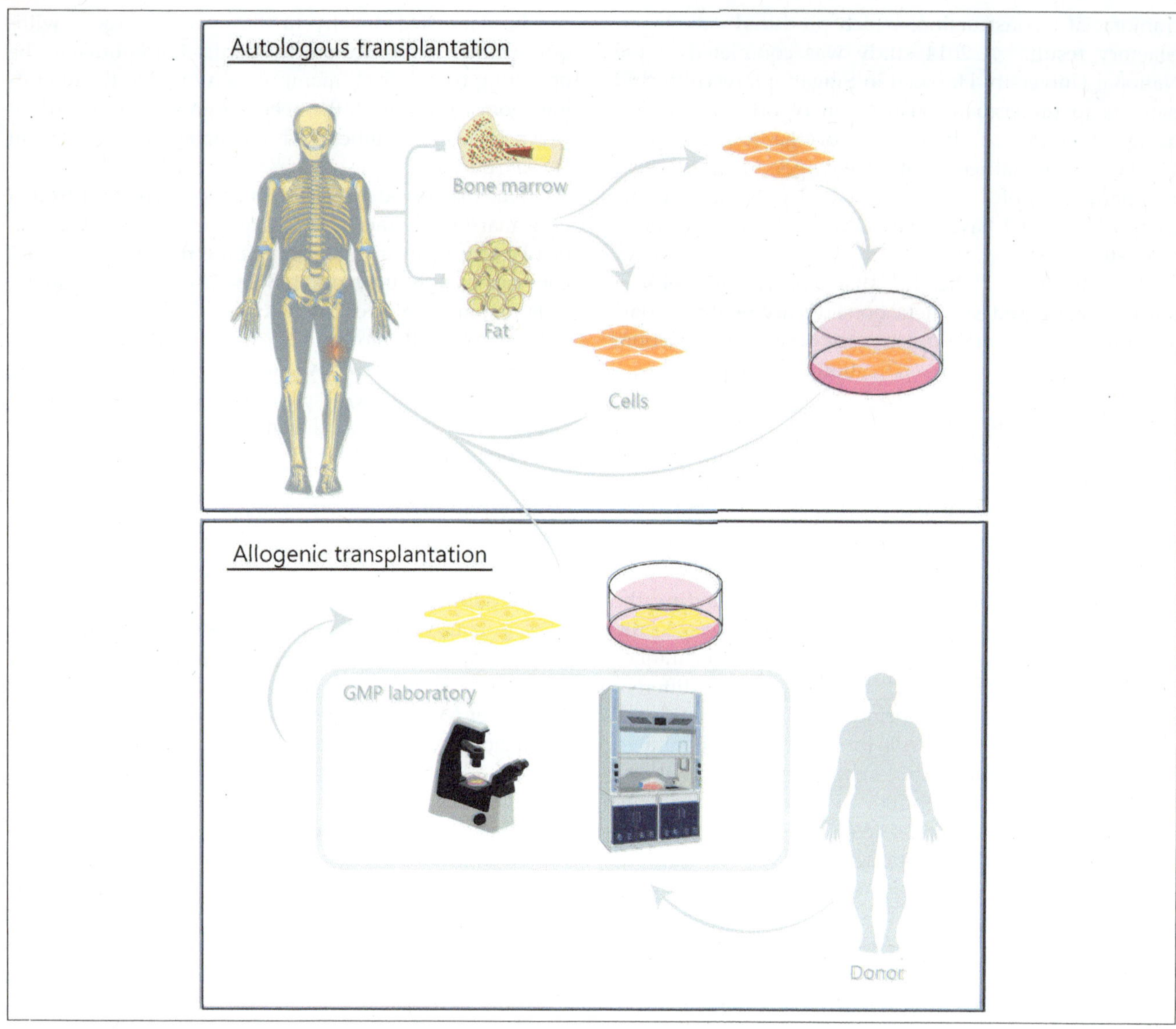

FIGURE 2 Schematic illustration shows the autologous or allogenic approaches. Mesenchymal stem cells can be derived from bone marrow or adipose tissue using operating room–based machines. They can be implanted directly to the bone defect or combined with biomaterials and/or morphogens before implantation in the patient. In the allogenic approach, these cells are derived from donors. The cells need to be treated in a good manufacturing practice (GMP) laboratory and can be packed, differentiated, combined with a biomaterial, etc., before being shipped to the hospital and implanted in the bone defect of the patient.

regenerative therapies to develop bone cells and bone tissue. Thereby, different morphogens are needed. For bone tissue, the main morphogens belong to the transforming growth factor beta superfamily and are BMPs. They are naturally secreted after a fracture has occurred. There is a temporal sequence of secretion related to their main function. Morphogens are not only proteins but also genetic codes that be considered for therapy (**Figure 3**).

Proteins

Many growth factors are said to have a stimulating effect on bone formation. In addition, there are claims that combinations, such as BMP-2 with vascular endothelial growth factor, can induce completely vascularized, new bone formation.[58] It is proven that BMP-2 and BMP-7 have excellent osteoinductive properties. These proteins act as potential regulators during bone and cartilage formation and their repair.[59] Of all BMPs identified thus far, only BMP-2, BMP-4, and BMP-7 have real osteogenic potential. Of these three, only BMP-2 and BMP-7 are approved for clinical use. BMP-2 is FDA approved for spinal cages and acute open tibial fractures. Some oromaxillofacial bone reconstructions are also approved. BMP-7 can be used for nonunion fractures of the tibia and for posterolateral

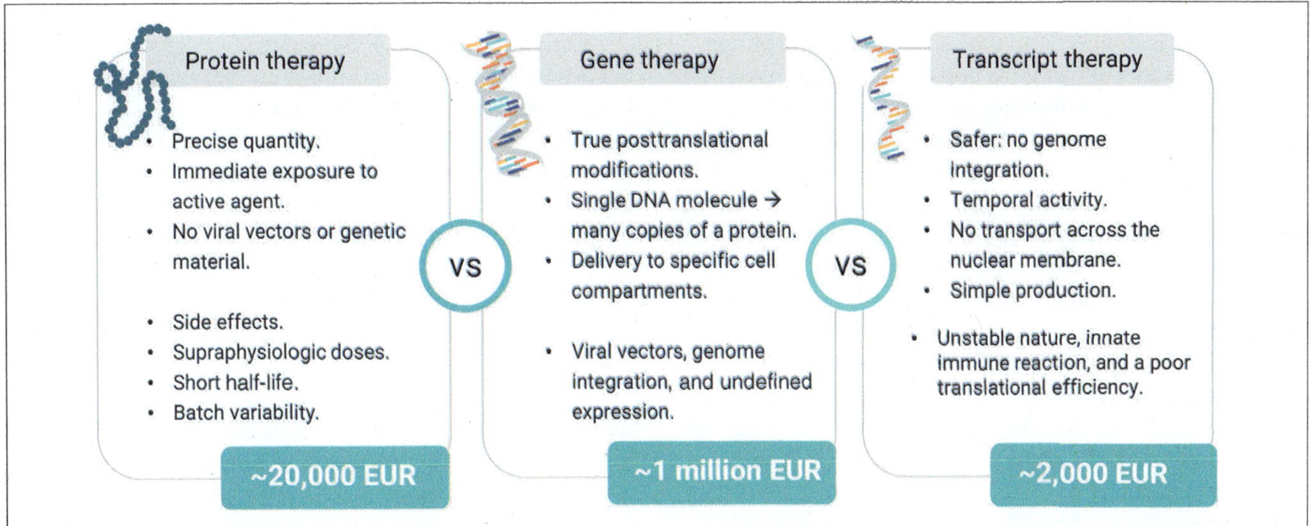

FIGURE 3 Morphogen usage in orthobiologic approaches using protein, DNA, or messenger RNA. The schematic shows the different features and the estimated costs per treatment.

lumbar spinal fusions. Unfortunately, the only BMP-7 product is no longer on the market. The reasons for this are not known.

Although modern genetic techniques allow the production of large quantities of recombinant BMP-2 and BMP-7, production costs are still very high. In addition, they have a very short half-life when they come into contact with fluids and tissues in the human body. Therefore, they are broken down relatively quickly after they have been inserted in a bone defect. Thus, high supraphysiologic doses are necessary to achieve a good therapeutic effect. These high doses (approximately 40 mg in some BMP products[59]) may cause undesirable adverse effects. Several studies show adverse effects of BMPs, such as swelling and seroma formation at low doses[60] and dose-dependent cancer risks.[59,61] Other possible adverse effects include anaphylaxis and an increased risk of infection, as well as osteolysis of the bone before the bone is completely healed.[62]

One way to address these issues is to develop drug delivery systems for BMPs. There is a lot of research activity to develop such systems for BMPs so that they can be released in a controlled manner, whereby their biologic activity can be maximized. Collagen type I, calcium phosphate ceramics, and some biodegradable polymers are some of the biomaterials used for this purpose. However, the existing systems are still inefficient and better systems are currently in the development stage. Therefore, there is an important focus on autologous products that inherently possess growth factors. An example of this is platelet-rich plasma (PRP). This product is derived from the plasma fraction of the blood, which has an increased platelet concentration over the baseline. It contains more than 30 proteins, including platelet-derived growth factor, transforming growth factor beta, platelet-derived angiogenesis factor, epidermal growth factor, platelet-derived endothelial growth factor, epithelial cell growth factor, insulinlike growth factor, and vascular endothelial growth factor.[63] These factors are produced and released after the platelets have been activated. Clinical application of PRP may occur after platelet activation or with an inactivated product. During surgical procedures, calcium chloride is often added to the PRP (platelet-activating step). After that, it is often mixed with thrombin to induce coagulation. This leads to the formation of a gel that can be applied very easily during the surgical procedure. Thus, it is clear that PRP products are present in either liquid (ie, inactivated) or gel form (eg, calcium chloride or thrombin activated).[64] In addition, they can be incorporated into materials such as gelatin or collagen to form hydrogels or sponges. Advanced material science findings show that it is even possible to develop self-aggregating systems for PRP nanofiber products.[64,65] Likewise, mixtures of PRP with ceramics and polymer materials for matrix development are investigated.[66,67]

Liquid PRP products are rarely used clinically in the field of bone healing[64] but have been used for managing nonunion of bones.[68] PRP gels have antibacterial properties and can be loaded with cells (MSCs) to enhance their therapeutic effect.[64]

Gene Therapy

The production of morphogens as protein is cumbersome, and the posttranslational modifications are difficult to obtain in vitro. Moreover, morphogens administered as protein need supraphysiologic concentrations that make the therapy more costly and result in detrimental adverse effects as indicated previously. To have a more physiologic therapy, gene therapy can be considered.[69,70] Thereby, the genetic code is delivered to the cells and the morphogens are produced in situ using the body's own machinery. The production is also controlled by natural feedback mechanisms. Gene therapy can be applied in many different forms. DNA can be used as a template for mRNA and finally protein production. Because this requires entering the DNA into the nucleus with several steps in between the protein production, mRNA therapy may be a feasible and more efficient alternative. The mRNA only needs to cross the cell membrane and the translation process to protein can immediately start in the cytosol.

mRNA, however, is instable and immunogenic. Therefore, the mRNA needs to be modified by nucleotides that prevent enzymatic digestion and evoke a less immune response. This has been successfully used for chemically modified mRNA for BMP-2.[71,72] This chemically modified mRNA induces osteogenesis and, when administered to a rat critical-size defect, a dose-dependent healing could be observed.[73] Implant coating can also be considered.[74]

Another possible gene therapy lies in the entity of microRNA (miRNA). miRNAs inhibit certain mRNAs. It has been shown that miRNAs are upregulated, for instance, in osteoporotic fractures,[75] and correlate with bone mineral density.[76] Counteracting those miRNAs would lead to increased osteogenesis. This counteracting can be performed by antagomirs. This is an antisense nucleotide sequence of a certain miRNA. The beauty of miRNAs lies in the fact that one miRNA can inhibit several mRNAs and one mRNA can be inhibited by several miRNAs. Therefore, this seems to be a very versatile therapeutic possibility.

PREFERRED ORTHOBIOLOGIC PRODUCT APPROACHES FOR EACH TISSUE

Single Component Versus Combination Approaches

As discussed previously, biomaterials, cells, and morphogens may be needed for bone regeneration. Each of these components has its own advantages and disadvantages. The components also have different characteristics and thereby different roles for bone regeneration. Each of these entities represents a part of natural bone, whereby biomaterials represent the extracellular matrix, the cells, the cellular component, the morphogens, the growth factors, and other inducing molecules present after a fracture has occurred. Depending on the patient circumstances, it may be necessary to use all three components at the same time for bone regeneration. However, it may also be sufficient to only apply one of the components where there may be a lack of.

Is a Biomaterial Needed?

A biomaterial is needed as a void filler and can also be used as a means to trap morphogens and to guide cells into the defect area. The biomaterial itself may also provide mechanical stability. However, this is often overestimated because the fracture needs to be stabilized with osteosynthesis material that will take over the load-bearing necessities. In that case, the biomaterial is really used for filling the defect to prevent connective tissue from entering and to provide the niche for regenerative components such as the cells and growth factors to be spatially contained.

Using biofabrication techniques as described previously, the shape of the tissue as it was before the defect occurred can be regained. This may be important for later function and for esthetic reasons.

The biomaterial by itself may also have osteoconductive properties. Thereby, after implantation of the biomaterial, cells from the edges of the bone defect are in close contact with the biomaterial. The cells enter the biomaterial and disperse in it. The biomaterial is then slowly remodeled and the components of the biomaterial can be used for building up neotissues.

In conclusion, a biomaterial is a necessary component. Depending on the exact function that is necessary, the composition and shape of the biomaterial can vary.

Are Cells Needed?

Cells are of utmost importance for the regeneration of bone. However, the cells may be recruited from the remaining host bone, bone marrow, or surrounding muscle tissue. In case the defect is not too large and the patient is in a healthy condition except for the fracture, it may be sufficient to provide time for recruiting the surrounding cells.

In case the local situation does not allow sufficient recruitment of cells, for instance, due to poor vasculature or compromised soft tissue, exogenous cells may be needed. This may also be the case when systemic comorbidities such as diabetes mellitus and osteoporosis are present. As stated previously, cells are of utmost importance for osteogenesis. Thus, they are always needed. It is difficult to determine whether or not cells need to be administered during the surgical procedure. Certainly, fracture scores may help in determining the viability of the tissue and thus the ability to recruit cells. However, this is not standardized and very much dependent on the experience of the surgeon.

The determination whether autologous or allogeneic cells are used is dependent on the circumstances whether autologous cells can be harvested. When the patient, for instance, is experiencing bone marrow–related cancer or any other cancer, harvesting autologous cells may not be the perfect solution. Under such circumstances, allogenic cells may be the better alternative. In both cases, the number of cells to be transplanted is still a matter of debate. Furthermore, it is important to realize that when transplanting cells, a healthy nutritional and oxygenation environment needs to be present.

Are Morphogens Needed?

When transplanting biomaterials and/or cells, morphogens may be needed to steer the entire process in the right direction of bone regeneration. Again, this is very much dependent on the local fracture situation as well as the overall condition of the patient. Several biomaterials are able to start certain differentiation of cells. Locally recruited cells may produce morphogens themselves that in an autocrine or in a paracrine way stimulate osteogenesis. Furthermore, after a fracture has occurred, the body itself starts to produce morphogens in a spatiotemporal manner. Thus, autologously produced morphogens may be trapped by, for instance, a biomaterial locally in the defect and this may suffice for optimal bone regeneration.

As previously discussed for the cells, in case morphogens are not present in the right concentration or in the right space or time, exogenous addition of morphogens may be necessary. This is again important for an optimal bone regeneration. Determining whether cells need to be exogenously administered is difficult, and it is even more difficult to determine the autologous morphogen situation. This is partially dependent on the local vascularization and soft-tissue environment. However, systemic conditions may negatively affect the production of morphogens. Until now, no real diagnostic tests are available to determine intrinsic morphogen production. Again, surgeon experience will dictate whether or not morphogens should be administered.

Currently, morphogens are administered as protein that is mainly BMP-2 (in the past, this included BMP-7, which is no longer on the market). In the future, other morphogens may be administered. Moreover, gene therapy is a viable option, especially taking into account therapies using chemically modified mRNA encoding morphogens.

When to Combine Which Entities?

As already discussed earlier, there are no hard criteria to determine which entities to combine and when. The prerequisites of bone regeneration in the area of delayed or nonunion are certainly biomaterials. They need to be administered to fill the void and to allow regeneration of this space. Cells and morphogens can be recruited from the patient. However, if that is possible, it is dependent on multiple factors such as the local condition of the tissue as well as comorbidities influencing vascularization, cell migration ability, cell functioning, and morphogen production. Until there are no longer real measures for intrinsic cell functioning, cell migration, or morphogen production, it remains up to the surgeon whether to add cells and/or morphogens to the biomaterial during reconstructive surgery.

What Is Currently Possible and What Is Feasible From an Approval Standpoint?

The orthobiologic approaches described previously with biomaterials, cells, and/or morphogens have been extensively studied in vitro and in vivo. Many different animal models in small and large animals have been used. Even models with more relevant clinical conditions such as diabetes, osteoporosis, or infection have been included in the analyses. Thus, it seems that this type of orthobiologic therapy is indeed feasible and can lead to advantageous results. To translate these therapies to human patients, however, has some hurdles related to human physiology (patients may have several comorbidities and are typically older than laboratory animals, etc.) and in the legal framework. This legal framework varies by region. The European Medicines Agency and the US FDA are the main institutions responsible for approving such therapies. Asian and Latin American countries have their own set of rules. Therefore, generally valid standpoints considering orthobiologics and combinations of biomaterials, cells, and morphogens are not possible. Nevertheless, the most basic ideas can be reflected here.

Autologous Approaches

The autologous setting is advantageous because the material is derived from and implanted in the same patient. The easiest approach is when autologous implantation is performed during the same surgical intervention without using a multistep procedure. MSC isolation is possible to perform intraoperatively. Several devices exist in the market for concentrating MSCs, which along with adipose tissue can be isolated from bone marrow samples. Bone marrow samples are typically concentrated using density centrifugation with or without subsequent separation for size and granularity. MSCs from adipose tissue can be processed in a one-step machine with digestion of the adipose tissue and subsequent separation of the MSCs from the debris. It has been shown that increasing the concentration of MSCs is effective intraoperatively and the cell suspension can be administered to the bone defect.

Another autologous approach intraoperatively is the use of RIA. The long bone is reamed and material containing MSCs as well as extracellular matrix is collected and applied to the defect. The RIA is therefore a combination of cells and scaffold. There are other ways of intraoperatively producing autologous scaffolds, by drawing blood and producing fibrin, for instance. In the field of biofabrication, research is conducted to manufacture a handheld three-dimensional printer for in situ printing of a scaffold. However, this is still very much in the preclinical experimental phase.

Autologous cells may also be used in a multistep procedure, where in the first step, the cells are harvested and brought to a GMP-compliant laboratory. There the cells are expanded and partially differentiated including cultivation on scaffolds before replanting them in the same patient in the next surgery. This multistep approach requires many administrative, legal, and logistic hurdles.

Allogenic Approaches

The issues identified concerning autologous cells used in a multistep procedure also apply to the allogeneic approach. Stem cells are harvested from a patient/volunteer, brought to a GMP facility, and after preparation, they are implanted in a patient different from the individual from whom the material was harvested. This allogenic approach is mainly used with cells, and several clinical studies are performed using bone marrow–derived MSCs. The MSCs are harvested and differentiated into early osteoblasts. These osteoblasts are then implanted or percutaneously injected in the bone defect of the patient. This allogenic transplantation must conform to the transplantation laws and there is always a risk of transmitting diseases.

In addition to the use of allogenic cells, allogenic biomaterials are on the market, for instance, in the form of the mineralized bone matrices. The manufacturing process must ensure that no disease entities remain in the final product.

Advanced Therapy Medicinal Product Approaches and Hurdles

The single approaches with biomaterials and cells need to adhere to many different laws and certain restrictions as identified for multistep procedures with cells for instance. It is possible to combine the different products such as a biomaterial, intraoperatively isolated MSCs, and morphogens in a single surgical procedure by one surgeon. Each of the administrations is regarded as single entity by itself during the entire surgical process. Each entity of course needs to adhere to the previously outlined requirements, but mostly it is irrelevant from a legal point of view whether they are combined intraoperatively or not.

This changes when the combination of the different entities is performed outside of surgery. Such combining must again be performed in a GMP facility. Furthermore, the advanced therapeutic medicinal product laws state that cells can only be minimally manipulated for self-transplantation. Moreover, nonhomologous transplantation is in some countries also regarded as an advanced therapy medicinal product.

In the case that two or more components are combined at a place and time other than during implantation in the patient, it is a legal requirement to state the exact mechanism of regeneration for each of the components. Such a question can be partially answered by preclinical studies. However, the combination may be synergistic and such a componential separation cannot be performed.

FUTURE CONSIDERATIONS

Currently, bone regeneration in the operating room can be performed with biomaterials, cells, and morphogens alone or in combination. However, this needs to be refined using a more personalized and precision medicine approach. Vascularization needs to be considered as well.

Personalized Medicine Approach

Biomaterials can also be shaped using biofabrication techniques with optimal pore sizes and interconnectivity. In the future, this will be further developed by material combinations and more refined printing techniques. For instance, it is known that the shape of the pores determines the migration distance of cells and also their differentiation.[77] Furthermore, bone regeneration will require a personalized medicine approach for larger bone defects. As already discussed, the surgeon determines which components to use without hard facts. Therefore, it would be helpful to have diagnostic tools to determine the patient-specific local necessity for the different components. Thereby, genetic approaches with determining certain miRNA signatures as have been determined for osteoporotic fractures, for instance, may aid the surgeon in the decision. It would also be helpful to measure morphogen concentrations in the fracture and also be able to determine the ability to produce such morphogens in a timely manner. Thereby, this approach would rely on typical procedures known from other specialties in medicine where on measurement of certain markers the therapy is determined.

Imaging modalities also play an important role not only for shaping the implants to the defect but also to determine the viability of the tissue and the vascularization density. Therefore, imaging modalities such as CT, MRI, and positron emission tomography should be combined.

Combination With Vascularization Approaches

Vascularization of the defect is one of the main issues. Vascularization is important for occupying a biomaterial scaffold with cells, when cells are transplanted to keep them alive with oxygen and nutrients, and also for distribution of morphogens. Therefore, it is also important to take vascularization approaches into account. These can be performed not only using cells and morphogens for vascular structures but also using another type of biomaterials that can be formed and shaped in a tubular manner to provide a platform for vascular regeneration.

FUTURE DIRECTIONS

Personalized medicine is the future for using orthobiologics in bone regeneration. The biology of the patient as well as the characteristics of the injury/defect will determine which type of material needs to be used. It also determines whether this needs to be combined with cells and/or growth factors. Research should aim to identify markers (molecular markers, imaging, etc.) that guide the surgeon to choose the correct orthobiologic regenerative therapy. This will result in more optimal results and will thereby benefit not only the patient but also society.

SUMMARY

It can be appreciated that this interdisciplinary field uses different entities for the optimal patient treatment. A personalized approach is to be favored.

REFERENCES

1. Taichman RS: Blood and bone: Two tissues whose fates are intertwined to create the hematopoietic stem-cell niche. *Blood* 2005;105(7):2631-2639.
2. Kini U, Nandeesh BN: Physiology of bone formation, remodeling, and metabolism, in Fogelman I, Gnanasegaran G, van der Wall H, eds: *Radionuclide and Hybrid Bone Imaging*. Springer, 2012, pp 29-57.
3. Shim S, Patterson FP: A direct method of qualitative study of bone blood circulation. *Surg Gynec Obstet* 1967;125:261-268.
4. Aalto K, Slätis P: Blood flow in rabbit osteotomies studied with radioactive microspheres. *Acta Orthop* 1984;55(6):637-639.
5. Khurana JS: *Bone Pathology*. Humana press a part of Springer science+business, 2009.
6. Barkow J: *Comparative Morphologie des Menschen und der Thiere*, Theil 6. Hirt, 1868.
7. Trueta J: The role of the vessels in osteogenesis. *J Bone Joint Surg Br* 1963;45(2):402-418.
8. Murray B, Revell WJ: *Blood Supply of Bone, Scientific Aspects*. Springer, 1998.
9. Frick H, Leonhardt H, Starck D: *Allgemeine und spezielle Anatomie*, in *Taschenlehrbuch der gesamten Anatomie*, Bd. 1 und 2. Thieme, 1992.
10. Laroche M: Intraosseous circulation from physiology to disease. *Joint Bone Spine* 2002;69(3):262-269.
11. Brookes M, Harrison R: The vascularization of the rabbit femur and tibiofibula. *J Anat* 1957;91(pt 1):61.
12. Gothman L: Venous transport of Na22 from healing fractures in the rabbit tibia. *Acta Radiol* 1960;54(6):469-482.
13. Brookes M, Elkin A, Harrison R, Heald C: A new concept of capillary circulation in bone cortex: Some clinical applications. *Lancet* 1961;277(7186):1078-1081.
14. De Bruyn PP, Breen PC, Thomas TB: The microcirculation of the bone marrow. *Anat Rec* 1970;168(1):55-68.
15. Brånemark P-I: Experimental investigation of microcirculation in bone marrow. *Angiology* 1961;12(7):293-305.
16. Ducy P, Schinke T, Karsenty G: The osteoblast: A sophisticated fibroblast under central surveillance. *Science* 2000;289(5484):1501-1504.
17. Logan CY, Nusse R: The Wnt signaling pathway in development and disease. *Annu Rev Cell Dev Biol* 2004;20:781-810.
18. Whyte MP: Hypophosphatasia and the role of alkaline phosphatase in skeletal mineralization. *Endocr Rev* 1994;15(4):439-461.
19. Boyle WJ, Simonet WS, Lacey DL: Osteoclast differentiation and activation. *Nature* 2003;423(6937):337-342.
20. Teitelbaum SL: Osteoclasts: What do they do and how do they do it? *Am J Pathol* 2007;170(2):427-435.
21. Dominici M, Le Blanc K, Mueller I, et al: Minimal criteria for defining multipotent mesenchymal stromal cells. The International Society for Cellular Therapy position statement. *Cytotherapy* 2006;8(4):315-317.
22. Kronsteiner B, Wolbank S, Peterbauer A, et al: Human mesenchymal stem cells from adipose tissue and amnion influence T-cells depending on stimulation method and presence of other immune cells. *Stem Cell Dev* 2011;20(12):2115-2126.
23. Georgiadis M, Muller R, Schneider P: Techniques to assess bone ultrastructure organization: Orientation and arrangement of mineralized collagen fibrils. *J R Soc Interface* 2016;13(119):20160088.
24. Schmidmaier G, Herrmann S, Green J, et al: Quantitative assessment of growth factors in reaming aspirate, iliac crest, and platelet preparation. *Bone* 2006;39(5):1156-1163.
25. Pape HC, Evans A, Kobbe P: Autologous bone graft: Properties and techniques. *J Orthop Trauma* 2010;24(suppl 1):S36-S40.
26. Burchardt H: Biology of bone transplantation. *Orthop Clin N Am* 1987;18(2):187-196.
27. Bae H, Zhao L, Zhu D, Kanim LE, Wang JC, Delamarter RB: Variability across ten production lots of a single demineralized bone matrix product. *J Bone Joint Surg Am* 2010;92(2):427-435.
28. Brydone AS, Meek D, Maclaine S: Bone grafting, orthopaedic biomaterials, and the clinical need for bone engineering. *Proc Inst Mech Eng H* 2010;224(12):1329-1343.
29. Khan SN, Tomin E, Lane JM: Clinical applications of bone graft substitutes. *Orthop Clin N Am* 2000;31(3):389-398.
30. Epstein NE: Beta tricalcium phosphate: Observation of use in 100 posterolateral lumbar instrumented fusions. *Spine J* 2009;9(8):630-638.
31. Ogose A, Hotta T, Kawashima H, et al: Comparison of hydroxyapatite and beta tricalcium phosphate as bone Substitutes after excision of bone tumors. *J Biomed Mater Res B Appl Biomater* 2005;72(1):94-101.
32. Moro-Barrero L, Acebal-Cortina G, Suarez-Suarez M, Perez-Redondo J, Murcia-Mazon A, Lopez-Muniz A: Radiographic analysis of fusion mass using fresh autologous bone marrow with ceramic composites as an alternative to autologous bone graft. *J Spinal Disord Tech* 2007;20(6):409-415.
33. Friedmann A, Dard M, Kleber BM, Bernimoulin JP, Bosshardt DD: Ridge augmentation and maxillary sinus grafting with a biphasic calcium phosphate: Histologic and histomorphometric observations. *Clin Oral Implants Res* 2009;20(7):708-714.
34. Blom AW, Wylde V, Livesey C, et al: Impaction bone grafting of the acetabulum at hip revision using a mix of bone chips and a biphasic porous ceramic bone graft substitute. *Acta Orthop* 2009;80(2):150-154.
35. Polo-Corrales L, Latorre-Esteves M, Ramirez-Vick JE: Scaffold design for bone regeneration. *J Nanosci Nanotechnol* 2014;14(1):15-56.
36. Probst FA, Hutmacher DW, Muller DF, Machens HG, Schantz JT: [Calvarial reconstruction by customized bioactive implant]. *Handchir Mikrochir Plast Chir* 2010;42(6):369-373.

37. National University Hospital Singapore: *Polycaprolactone/Tricalcium Phosphate (PCL/TCP) v Titanium Orbital Implant: Randomised Trial*. ClinicalTrial.gov Identifier: NCT01119144, 2014.
38. Lyons B: Additive manufacturing in aerospace: Examples and research outlook. *Bridge* 2014;44(3):13-19.
39. Melchels FPW, Domingos MAN, Klein TJ, Malda J, Bartolo PJ, Hutmacher DW: Additive manufacturing of tissues and organs. *Prog Polym Sci* 2012;37(8):1079-1104.
40. Ghayor C, Weber FE: Osteoconductive microarchitecture of bone substitutes for bone regeneration revisited. *Front Physiol* 2018;9:960.
41. Lin K, Sheikh R, Romanazzo S, Roohani I: 3D printing of bioceramic scaffolds-barriers to the clinical translation: From promise to reality, and future perspectives. *Materials (Basel)* 2019;12(17):2660.
42. Mani N, Sola A, Trinchi A, Fox K: Is there a future for additive manufactured titanium bioglass composites in biomedical application? A perspective. *Biointerphases* 2020;15(6):068501.
43. Poh PSP, Chhaya MP, Wunner FM, et al: Polylactides in additive biomanufacturing. *Adv Drug Deliv Rev* 2016;107:228-246.
44. Calore AR, Sinha R, Harings J, Bernaerts KV, Mota C, Moroni L: Additive manufacturing using melt extruded thermoplastics for tissue engineering. *Methods Mol Biol* 2021;2147:75-99.
45. Lehder EF, Ashcroft IA, Wildman RD, Ruiz-Cantu LA, Maskery I: A multiscale optimisation method for bone growth scaffolds based on triply periodic minimal surfaces. *Biomech Model Mechanobiol* 2021;20(6):2085-2096.
46. Poh PSP, Valainis D, Bhattacharya K, van Griensven M, Dondl P: Optimization of bone scaffold porosity distributions. *Sci Rep* 2019;9(1):9170.
47. Hendrikson WJ, Rouwkema J, Clementi F, van Blitterswijk CA, Fare S, Moroni L: Towards 4D printed scaffolds for tissue engineering: Exploiting 3D shape memory polymers to deliver time-controlled stimulus on cultured cells. *Biofabrication* 2017;9(3):031001.
48. Rupani A, Balint R, Cartmell SH: Osteoblasts and their applications in bone tissue engineering. *Cell Health Cytoskelet* 2012;4:49-61.
49. Rebelatto CK, Aguiar AM, Moretao MP, et al: Dissimilar differentiation of mesenchymal stem cells from bone marrow, umbilical cord blood, and adipose tissue. *Exp Biol Med (Maywood)* 2008;233(7):901-913.
50. Docquier PL, Delloye C: Treatment of simple bone cysts with aspiration and a single bone marrow injection. *J Pediatr Orthop* 2003;23(6):766-773.
51. Hernigou P, Poignard A, Manicom O, Mathieu G, Rouard H: The use of percutaneous autologous bone marrow transplantation in nonunion and avascular necrosis of bone. *J Bone Joint Surg Br* 2005;87(7):896-902.
52. Cytori Therapeutics: *Safety and Feasibility of ADRCs (Adipose Derived Regenerative Cells) in Patients With Grade II Hamstring Tears (RECOVER)*. ClinicalTrial.gov Identifier: NCT02045888, 2014.
53. López-Fernández A, Barro V, Ortiz-Hernández M, et al: Effect of allogeneic cell-based tissue-engineered treatments in a sheep osteonecrosis model. *Tissue Eng Part A* 2020;26(17-18):993-1004.
54. Li Z, Liao W, Zhao Q, et al: Angiogenesis and bone regeneration by allogeneic mesenchymal stem cell intravenous transplantation in rabbit model of avascular necrotic femoral head. *J Surg Res* 2013;183(1):193-203.
55. Du J, Shan Z, Ma P, Wang S, Fan Z: Allogeneic bone marrow mesenchymal stem cell transplantation for periodontal regeneration. *J Dent Res* 2014;93(2):183-188.
56. Lim J, Razi ZRM, Law JX, et al: Mesenchymal stromal cells from the maternal segment of human umbilical cord is ideal for bone regeneration in allogenic setting. *Tissue Eng Regen Med* 2018;15(1):75-87.
57. Jayankura M, Schulz AP, Delahaut O, et al: Percutaneous administration of allogeneic bone-forming cells for the treatment of delayed unions of fractures: A pilot study. *Stem Cell Res Ther* 2021;12(1):363.
58. Hernandez A, Reyes R, Sanchez E, Rodriguez-Evora M, Delgado A, Evora C: In vivo osteogenic response to different ratios of BMP-2 and VEGF released from a biodegradable porous system. *J Biomed Mater Res A* 2012;100(9):2382-2391.
59. Carreira AC, Lojudice FH, Halcsik E, Navarro RD, Sogayar MC, Granjeiro JM: Bone morphogenetic proteins: facts, challenges, and future perspectives. *J Dent Res* 2014;93(4):335-345.
60. Leknes KN, Yang J, Qahash M, Polimeni G, Susin C, Wikesjo UM: Alveolar ridge augmentation using implants coated with recombinant human bone morphogenetic protein-2: Radiographic observations. *Clin Oral Implants Res* 2008;19(10):1027-1033.
61. Devine JG, Dettori JR, France JC, Brodt E, McGuire RA: The use of rhBMP in spine surgery: Is there a cancer risk? *Evid Base Spine Care J* 2012;3(2):35-41.
62. Sonnet C, Simpson CL, Olabisi RM, et al: Rapid healing of femoral defects in rats with low dose sustained BMP2 expression from PEGDA hydrogel microspheres. *J Orthop Res* 2013;31(10):1597-1604.
63. Dhillon MS, Behera P, Patel S, Shetty V: Orthobiologics and platelet rich plasma. *Indian J Orthop* 2014;48(1):1-9.
64. Rodriguez IA, Growney Kalaf EA, Bowlin GL, Sell SA: Platelet-rich plasma in bone regeneration: Engineering the delivery for improved clinical efficacy. *BioMed Res Int* 2014;2014:392398.
65. Yoshimi R, Yamada Y, Ito K, et al: Self-assembling peptide nanofiber scaffolds, platelet-rich plasma, and mesenchymal stem cells for injectable bone regeneration with tissue engineering. *J Craniofac Surg* 2009;20(5):1523-1530.
66. Chen JC, Ko CL, Shih CJ, Tien YC, Chen WC: Calcium phosphate bone cement with 10 wt% platelet-rich plasma in vitro and in vivo. *J Dent* 2012;40(2):114-122.
67. Rai B, Oest ME, Dupont KM, Ho KH, Teoh SH, Guldberg RE: Combination of platelet-rich plasma with polycaprolactone-tricalcium phosphate scaffolds for segmental bone defect repair. *J Biomed Mater Res A* 2007;81(4):888-899.

68. Taylor DW, Petrera M, Hendry M, Theodoropoulos JS: A systematic review of the use of platelet-rich plasma in sports medicine as a new treatment for tendon and ligament injuries. *Clin J Sport Med* 2011;21(4):344-352.

69. Balmayor ER, van Griensven M: Gene therapy for bone engineering. *Front Bioeng Biotechnol* 2015;3:9.

70. De la Vega RE, Atasoy-Zeybek A, Panos JA, Griensven MV, Evans CH, Balmayor ER: Gene therapy for bone healing: Lessons learned and new approaches. *Transl Res* 2021;236:1-16.

71. Balmayor ER, Geiger JP, Koch C, et al: Modified mRNA for BMP-2 in combination with biomaterials serves as a transcript-activated matrix for effectively inducing osteogenic pathways in stem cells. *Stem Cell Dev* 2017;26(1):25-34.

72. Zhang W, De La Vega RE, Coenen MJ, et al: An improved, chemically modified RNA encoding BMP-2 enhances osteogenesis in vitro and in vivo. *Tissue Eng* 2019;25(1-2):131-144.

73. Balmayor ER, Geiger JP, Aneja MK, et al: Chemically modified RNA induces osteogenesis of stem cells and human tissue explants as well as accelerates bone healing in rats. *Biomaterials* 2016;87:131-146.

74. Fayed O, van Griensven M, Tahmasebi Birgani Z, Plank C, Balmayor ER: Transcript-activated coatings on titanium mediate cellular osteogenesis for enhanced osteointegration. *Mol Pharm* 2021;18(3):1121-1137.

75. Seeliger C, Karpinski K, Haug AT, et al: Five freely circulating miRNAs and bone tissue miRNAs are associated with osteoporotic fractures. *J Bone Miner Res* 2014;29(8):1718-1728.

76. Kelch S, Balmayor ER, Seeliger C, Vester H, Kirschke JS, van Griensven M: miRNAs in bone tissue correlate to bone mineral density and circulating miRNAs are gender independent in osteoporotic patients. *Sci Rep* 2017;7(1):15861.

77. Valainis D, Dondl P, Foehr P, et al: Integrated additive design and manufacturing approach for the bioengineering of bone scaffolds for favorable mechanical and biological properties. *Biomed Mater* 2019;14(6):065002.

CHAPTER

8

Orthobiologics for Tendon and Ligament Repair

Hani Awad, PhD • Rahul Alenchery, MSc • Raquel Ajalik, MSc • Victor Z. Zhang, BSc

INTRODUCTION

Surgery to repair soft musculoskeletal tissues, including tendon and ligament, represents more than 20% (approximately 2.5 million) of major orthopaedic procedures.[1] Minor procedures such as the injection of a therapeutic agent (eg, steroids or platelet-rich plasma [PRP]) into a joint or a tendon represent an additional approximately six million procedures annually.[1] Injuries to tendons and ligaments resulting from work, sport, or trauma can be acute or chronic. Acute injuries include strains/sprains and partial or full tissue rupture, whereas chronic injuries constitute a spectrum of painful degenerative injuries known as tendinopathy, which result from the repetitive accumulation of microdamage due to overuse or aging. The most frequent injuries typically involve the Achilles, patellar, quadriceps, hamstring, supraspinatus (rotator cuff), hand and wrist flexor tendons, the anterior cruciate ligament (ACL), ankle ligaments, and the collateral ligaments in the elbow and knee joints. Innovations in orthobiologics that target molecular underpinnings in scar-mediated repair and chronic injuries of tendon and ligament promise to transform the management of these injuries. It is important to provide a concise review of the basics of tendon and ligament injury and repair to define principles that could guide the development of orthobiologic therapies. In addition, various orthobiologics in preclinical and clinical testing are also reviewed and clinical evidence about their efficacy in treating tendon and ligament injuries is evaluated.

ANATOMY, STRUCTURE, AND FUNCTION

Tendons and ligaments share similar biologic and structural attributes but have distinct mechanical demands and functions. Tendons transfer forces generated by muscle contraction to the skeleton, facilitating joint flexion and storage and dissipation of energy.[2] Ligaments traverse joints connecting bone to bone, and in doing so stabilize the joint and constrain motion in various degrees of freedom depending on their anatomic positions. Tendons and ligaments exhibit diversity based on structural (fascia-like to cordlike), anatomic (axial or appendicular), and functional (positional or energy storing) criteria. Both tissues are composed predominantly of type I collagen, organized across several hierarchical scales to form fascicles of highly aligned fibers that give the tissue its characteristic tensile resilience (**Figure 1, A**). Other fibrillar, fibril-associated, and nonfibrillar collagens constitute a minor fraction of the tendon and ligament extracellular matrix (ECM) and play important biologic, structural, and mechanical roles. Noncollagenous proteins and proteoglycans also contribute to the tissue's elastic and viscoelastic properties.

Tendons and ligaments are viscoelastic materials, with characteristic time-dependent creep, stress relaxation, and energy dissipation responses. When tendons and ligaments are monotonically loaded at relatively fast rates, they exhibit a quasi-elastic behavior that defines their tensile stiffness, strength, and resilience. In general, tendons tend to be stronger and stiffer than ligaments because of increased alignment of the collagen fibers along the tissue's loading axis[3] (**Figure 1, B**).

The cellular and structural complexity at interface regions connecting muscle to tendon (myotendinous junction) or tendon to bone (enthesis) represent important functional adaptations and are key to regenerative repair of common injuries at these sites (**Figure 2**). The myotendinous junction's main function is to store and release mechanical energy, and as such it is mechanoresponsive, susceptible to high rates of turnover and remodeling of muscle fibers, and vulnerable to overload strain injuries.[4] The enthesis is a common feature of both tendon and ligament insertion into bone. It is typically described as four successive zones: dense fibrous tendon, uncalcified fibrocartilage, calcified fibrocartilage, and bone.[5] The fibrocartilage intermediate between the elastic tendon and rigid mineralized bone is designed to buffer strain mismatches and reduce stress concentrations to protect the interface.

Victor Zhang or an immediate family member serves as a paid consultant to or is an employee of Black Diamond Therapeutics and has stock or stock options held in Black Diamond Therapeutics. None of the following authors or any immediate family member has received anything of value from or has stock or stock options held in a commercial company or institution related directly or indirectly to the subject of this chapter: Dr. Awad, Rahul Alenchery, and Raquel Ajalik.

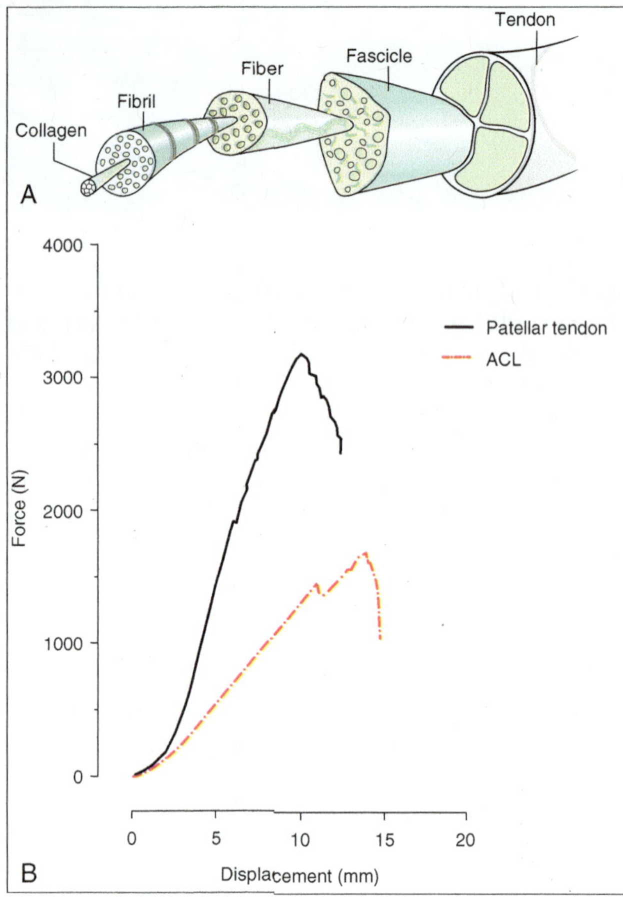

FIGURE 1 **A**, Diagrammatic representation of structural hierarchy and organization in tendon and ligament. **B**, Representative tensile force-displacement plot depicting the higher strength and stiffness of tendons compared with ligaments. ACL = anterior cruciate ligament. (Plot created based on data from Noyes FR, Butler DL, Grood ES, Zernicke RF, Hefzy MS: Biomechanical analysis of human ligament grafts used in knee-ligament repairs and reconstructions. *J Bone Joint Surg Am* 1984;66[3]:344-352.)

TRANSCRIPTIONAL REGULATION IN DEVELOPMENT AND REPAIR

The cellular interactions, signaling pathways, and transcription factors involved in tendon and ligament development can be key to discovering regenerative therapies. Tendons and ligaments derive from mesodermal progenitor aggregates under mitogenic and morphogenic programs that ultimately activate phenotypic transcription factors to generate the cells fated to form the tissue and produce its abundant ECM. The molecular regulation of tendon specification during vertebrate development has been extensively studied using genetically manipulated mouse models as well as chick and zebrafish models, but the molecular programs involved in ligament specification are less studied. The literature identifies Scleraxis (*Scx*),[6] Mohawk (*Mkx*),[7] and Early Growth Response 1 (*Egr1*)[8] as putative transcription factors critical for tendon development, induction of tenogenesis in stem cells, and orchestrating the response to tendon injury in animal models. However, these transcription factors are not exclusively specific to tendon and ligament because they are expressed in numerous tissues in development and throughout life and are involved in numerous biologic functions. Furthermore, despite the plethora of data in rodents and other animal models, the evidence linking them to tendon and ligament pathology in humans is scarce.

CELLULAR BIOLOGY: NEW INSIGHTS

Recent studies have challenged the historical dogma about the uniformity of tendon and ligament cells, typically referred to as tenocytes or ligamentocytes, respectively. In addition to these fibrocytes that reside in the tissue's midsubstance and in the epitendon and endotenon sheaths, tendons and ligaments contain tissue-resident stem cells,[9] endothelial and perivascular cells,[10] and tissue-resident macrophages (tenophages).[11] The mature tenocytes and ligamentocytes express the antiangiogenic type II transmembrane glycoprotein tenomodulin (*Tnmd*) under the direct control of *Scx* and *Mkx* transcription factors.[12] In rodents, *Tnmd* has been shown to be critical for the postnatal tendon and ligament growth, proliferation of tenocytes and ligamentocytes and the maintenance of the tissue's progenitors, and the maturation of the collagenous ECM and its adaptation to mechanical loading. Interestingly, recent advances using single-cell RNA sequencing and spatial transcriptomics have led to the discovery of a previously unrecognized diversity of subtypes of fibroblasts in a variety of tissues including tendon and ligament in rodents[13] and humans.[14] This discovery adds to the complexity of cellular and molecular interactions in tendon and ligament injury and repair but could ultimately enhance understanding of key cell subtypes and pathways that could be therapeutic targets.

ACUTE TENDON AND LIGAMENT INJURIES

Connective tissue repair is classically described in terms of sequential and overlapping phases, each of which is orchestrated by distinctive cellular and molecular cascades. The first phase is characterized by coagulation and inflammation.[15] This is soon followed by proliferation and repair, during which growth factors and other cytokines secreted by inflammatory cells stimulate the migration and proliferation of fibroblasts and ECM synthesis.[15] These factors also modulate the synthesis and activation of matrix metalloproteinases that act to degrade and turnover the ECM in the final remodeling stage of healing (**Figure 3**). The balance between ECM synthesis and turnover determines the extent of tissue remodeling into a mature fibrous tissue, which represents the last stage

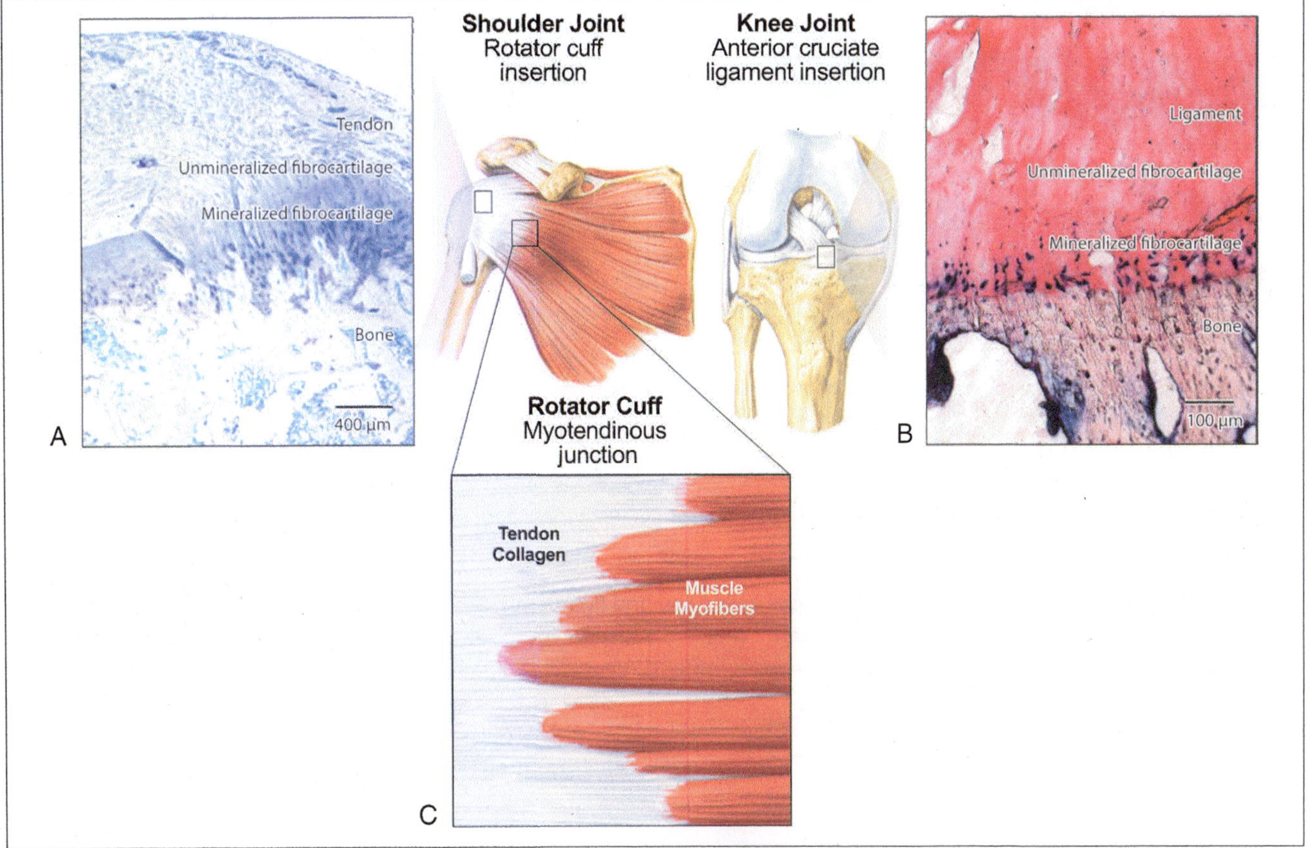

FIGURE 2 Histologic and illustrative representation of specialized interface tissues in tendons and ligaments. **A** and **B**, The tendon-to-bone insertion (enthesis). **C**, The myotendinous junction. (Reproduced with modification from Lu HH, Thomopoulos S: Functional attachment of soft tissues to bone: development, healing, and tissue engineering. *Annu Rev Biomed Eng* 2013;15:201-226.)

of repair. As such, the outcome of the repair can be variable and could lead to a chronic fibrovascular scar.

The role of innate immunity has been extensively studied in the context of tendon and ligament response to acute injury (**Figure 4**). Neutrophils dominate the early stages of inflammation within hours and set the stage for repair of tissue damage by macrophages, which could last for weeks. The functional consequences of activation of circulating monocytes to macrophages depend on their phenotypic polarization, with M1 macrophages effecting phagocytosis and proinflammatory cytokines secretion and M2 macrophages typically credited with anti-inflammatory cytokine and growth factor secretion to initiate tissue repair.[16] Therefore, macrophages are an important orthobiologics target in tendon and ligament injury. The role of adaptive immunity in tendon and ligament healing is largely unexplored, although recent studies have begun to investigate it.[17-19] Recent reports implicate macrophagedendritic cell interactions in (lung) fibrosis.[20] In addition, dendritic cells and macrophages have been reported to interact to stimulate naive $CD8^+$ T cells to proliferate, develop effector function, and differentiate.[21] Not surprisingly, pharmacologic immune modulators including NSAIDs and corticosteroids are routinely used in the treatment of tendon injury with mixed results.

During the proliferation and repair phase of healing, a variety of growth factors are temporally and spatially regulated to stimulate fibroblasts and other cells to migrate to the site of injury and proliferate, and consequently repair the damaged tissue by secreting ECM proteins to form a hypercellular and highly vascular tissue known as granulation tissue. The matrix in this phase of healing is composed of a provisional disorganized mixture of collagens I, III, V, and XII and other ECM components, including fibronectin, glycosaminoglycans, and proteoglycans.[15]

The remodeling and scar resolution or maturation phase is characterized by elevated collagen I production, while the expression of other ECM proteins declines. Type I collagen fibers gradually replace the provisional matrix formed earlier, which is turned over by matrix metalloproteinases, and the collagen fibers are organized and remodeled along the axis of the tendon, allowing the tendon to regain some of its mechanical strength. The key

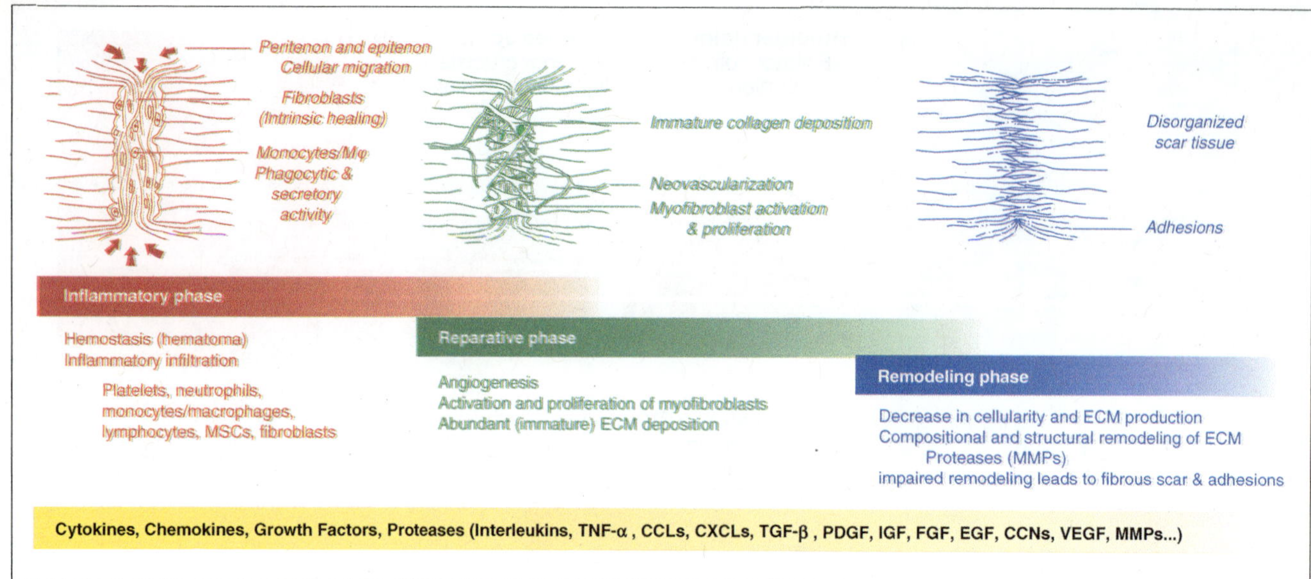

FIGURE 3 A simplified representation of the phases of tendon and ligament healing. ECM = extracellular matrix; MMP = matrix metalloproteinase; MSC = mesenchymal stem cell. (Reproduced with modification from Beredjiklian PK: Biologic aspects of flexor tendon laceration and repair. *J Bone Joint Surg Am* 2003;85[3]:539-550.)

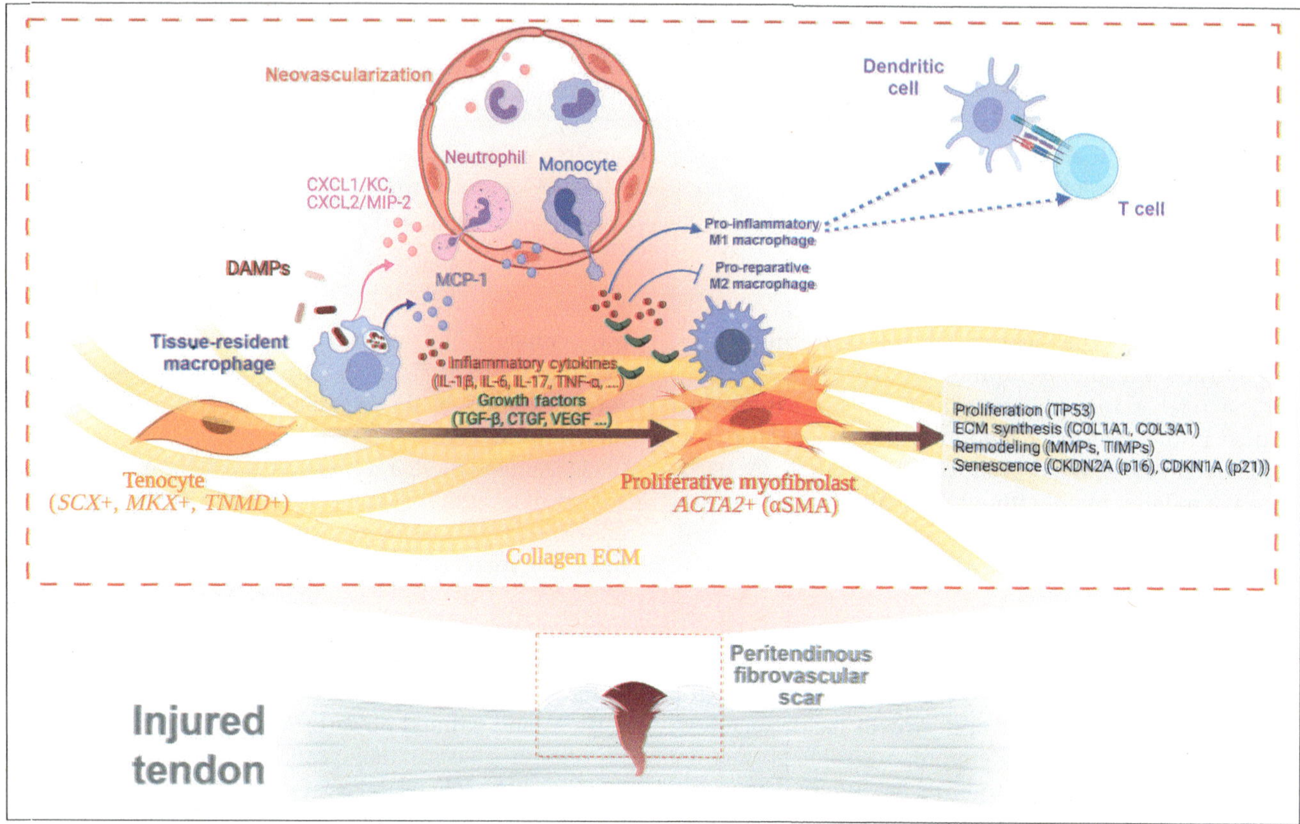

FIGURE 4 Schematic representation of the inflammatory-fibrotic cellular and molecular interactions in peritendinous fibrovascular scarring. CTGF = connective tissue growth factor; CXCL1/KC = chemokine (C-X-C motif) ligand 1; DAMPs = damage-associated molecular patterns; ECM = extracellular matrix; IL = interleukin; MCP-1 = monocyte chemoattractant protein 1; MIP-2 = macrophage inflammatory protein 2; MMP = matrix metalloproteinase; SMA = smooth muscle actin; TGF-β = transforming growth factor beta; TIMP = tissue inhibitor of metalloproteinase; TNF-α = tumor necrosis factor alpha; VEGF = vascular endothelial growth factor

cellular mediators of collagen I expression and ECM remodeling during scar maturation are myofibroblasts. Myofibroblasts likely originate from tissue-resident fibroblasts that have converted into a proliferative, contractile phenotype, in response to transforming growth factor beta 1 (TGF-β1), which is one of the key inflammatory growth factors released during the earlier stages of healing. One of the characteristics that differentiates normal fibroblasts from myofibroblasts is the high expression of alpha-smooth muscle actin (α-SMA) in myofibroblasts.[22] The expression and incorporation of α-SMA into the stress fibers of the myofibroblast cytoskeleton corresponds with an increase in their contractile ability and their ability to drive fibrosis. TGF-β1 is considered to be the most potent cause of myofibroblast differentiation. After becoming activated, myofibroblasts also produce TGF-β1, activating an autocrine loop and eventually resulting in the excess deposition of collagen into scar tissue over a long period of healing. Therefore, α-SMA-expressing myofibroblasts have emerged as a therapeutic target in numerous recent animal studies, but the mechanisms of their activation are yet to be fully understood.

CHRONIC INJURIES—TENDINOPATHY

Although there is a lack of basic science literature on chronic ligament injury, chronic painful degeneration of tendons and the associated decline in their function are well documented and studied. These chronic pathologies, generally referred to as tendinopathy, are attributed to multiple factors, including strenuous overuse and repetitive activity, metabolic dysregulation such as in obesity and diabetes, adverse effects of drugs such as statins and fluoroquinolones, or aging. Regardless of the etiology, tendinopathy manifests with common features, including disorganization of its ECM, an increase in cellularity, vascularization, and sensory innervation, and inflammation (**Table 1**). The management of these chronic injuries, which are interchangeably referred to as tendinopathy, tendinitis, or tendinosis in the literature, is often ineffective, motivating continued research of their pathophysiology.[23] The lack of agreement on terminology associated with these chronic conditions and the absence of a consistent definition of whether tendinopathy is a single disease or a spectrum of degenerative pathologies

TABLE 1 Mechanisms of Pathogenesis in Tendinopathy

Mechanism	Details
ECM/collagen disruption	ECM remodeling homeostasis disrupted Abundance of type III collagen that is not replaced by type I collagen Other ECM components disrupted leading to reduced biomechanical properties of tendon Activation of MMPs Regulated by a variety of factors including mechanical stress/stimulation, transcriptional and molecular signaling, and inflammation
MicroRNA	Angiogenesis is normal during injury response Vascular growth may compromise the structure of tendon Regulators of vascular growth have also been associated with type III collagen production
Neuronal ingrowth	May contribute to increased pain experienced by patients Increased signaling by various neuropeptides and the glutamatergic system Acetylcholine signaling also increased, which may be tied to inflammation
Inflammatory/immune response	Complex responses that contribute to tendinopathy Both proinflammatory and anti-inflammatory responses are seen Major cytokines including TNF, IFN-γ, IL-1β, IL-4, and IL-6 Responses from tenocytes as well as immune cells (macrophages, mast cells) Contribute to regenerative processes and structural remodeling of the tendon
Oxidative damage	ROS produced during stress responses Not unique to tendinopathy but contributes to damage of many tissues Apoptotic activation also seen (caspases and BCL2)
Adaptive responses	Fibroblasts are activated and adopt pro-inflammatory phenotype Common feature among different tendons TSPC loss in tendinopathy leading to reduced regenerative capacity of important cell populations

ECM = extracellular matrix, IFN = interferon, IL = interleukin, MMPs = matrix metalloproteinases, ROS = reactive oxygen species, TNF = tumor necrosis factor, TSPC = tendon stem/progenitor cell contribute to the incomplete understanding and lack of effective orthobiologics treatments.

One prominent feature of tendinopathy is the disruption of ECM components in the tendon, including collagen. Tendinopathic tissues exhibit an abundance of type III collagen, which is disorganized and has poor mechanical strength when compared with type I collagen. Tendinopathy also exhibits disruption of noncollagenous ECM components including elastin, proteoglycans, and others, possibly reflecting aberrant differentiation of tenocytes and tendon-resident progenitors. Although healthy tendon is sparsely vascularized, tendinopathy can be associated with angiogenesis and aberrant neovascularization, which could have detrimental effects on tendon structure leading to chronic degeneration accompanied by pain.[24] This may be associated with imbalance or dysregulation of proangiogenic and antiangiogenic factors. Vascular endothelial growth factor is highly expressed in injured tendon. In addition to vascular growth, tendinopathy biopsies have also shown neural proliferation. This neural proliferation could lead to the increased pain experienced by many patients; however, this mechanism is poorly understood. Several studies have shown increased signaling by some neuropeptides (eg, substance P) as well as the glutamatergic system.[23] These systems likely lead to the neuropathies experienced by patients; however, it is possible that these neuropeptides may have a direct role in structural remodeling as well. Tenocytes have also been shown to produce acetylcholine, which potentially implicates a cholinergic signaling system contribution to neuropathy.[25] Studies have also shown a role for microRNAs in regulating tendon's response to injury.

Inflammatory and immune processes contribute significantly to the pathogenesis of tendinopathy and possibly to the pain experienced by patients.[25] Research has also shown that these processes may in turn regulate ECM remodeling by way of nuclear factor kappa B, extracellular signal-regulated kinase, mitogen-activated protein kinase, Wnt, and TGF-β signaling.[26] The major inflammatory cytokines and chemokines involved are tumor necrosis factor alpha, interferon gamma, interleukin (IL)-1β, IL-4, IL-6, and IL-17, among many others secreted by the tenocytes themselves as well as native immune cells such as macrophages and mast cells.[27]

SIGNALING IN TENDON AND LIGAMENT INJURY AND REPAIR

The temporal and spatial patterns of expression of growth factors, which regulate gene transcription of cell proliferation and matrix synthesis during tendon and ligament healing, are dynamic and can contribute to the regenerative or fibrotic healing outcome. Despite a plethora of preclinical data, no growth factor treatments have been adopted clinically, arguably because the mechanisms of action and interactions of the various signaling pathways remain incompletely understood in the context of human tissue repair.

Transforming Growth Factor Beta

Members of the TGF-β family of proteins are critical to tendon and ligament development and healing. In response to injury, TGF-β1 expression is autoinductive and is initially produced by inflammatory cells.[28] TGF-β1 stimulates fibroblast proliferation and migration, synthesis of collagen and fibronectin, and inactivation of metalloproteinases.[29] Increased expression of TGF-β1 in both tenocytes and infiltrating fibroblasts and inflammatory cells from the tendon sheath has been reported in a rabbit zone II flexor tendon healing model.[30] The inflammatory cells stimulate synovial and epitenon fibroblasts, partly through TGF-β1, to produce scar matrix. Although fetal cutaneous wound healing and tendon repair are scar free, the in utero administration of TGF-β1 to fetal rabbit wounds results in fibrotic scarring similar to that observed in adult rabbits.[31] These observations motivated the development of experimental anti-TGF-β1 therapies for flexor tendon adhesions, for example. Neutralizing antibodies to TGF-β1 reduced flexor tendon adhesions following transection in a rat model[32] and treatment with TGF-β1 inhibitors such as decorin or mannose-6-phosphate improved the postoperative range of motion in rabbit zone II flexor tendon repair, but unfortunately reduced the mechanical properties,[33] suggesting that directly targeting TGF-β1 might not be a tenable therapeutic approach in load-bearing tissues such as tendon and ligament.

Growth and Differentiation Factors

The growth and differentiation factors (GDFs) or cartilage-derived morphogenetic proteins are members of the bone morphogenetic protein (BMP) superfamily, which have been shown to induce the production of tendonlike tissue in vitro and in vivo and improve tendon repair.[34] This subfamily of proteins, which includes GDF-5, GDF-6, and GDF-7 (cartilage-derived morphogenetic proteins 1, 2, and 3 or BMP-14, BMP-13, and BMP-12, respectively), is important for skeletal development in general and for tendon formation and repair in particular.[35] GDF-5 deficiency in mice leads to disruption of tail tendon form and function and altered ultrastructure, mechanical properties, and composition of the Achilles tendon, causing delayed tendon healing.[36] GDF-5 regulates cell migration, adhesion, differentiation, proliferation, and angiogenesis in vitro and in vivo. Therefore, a number of therapeutic and tissue engineering strategies in tendon repair have focused on GDF-5. For example, GDF-5 and GDF-6 soaked collagen scaffolds stimulated healing of injured rat Achilles tendon.[37]

Platelet-Derived Growth Factors

Platelet-derived growth factors (PDGFs) are growth factors secreted by human activated platelets as well as other cells including endothelial and epithelial cells. Of the five known isoforms, which typically form homodimer or heterodimer ligands, PDGF AA, BB, and AB have been shown to have potent mitogenic effects on numerous skeletal cells including ligament and tendon fibroblasts and stem cells. PDGF signaling is initiated when the dimer ligand binds to its homodimer platelet-derived growth factor receptors alpha and beta (PDGFRα and β) or the heterodimer PDGFRαβ receptor. Studies have shown that sustained delivery of PDGF-BB from a fibrin matrix enhances canine flexor tendon repair by increasing cell proliferation and ECM remodeling.[38] A dose escalation of bolus injections in a rat model of collagenase-induced tendinopathy reported dose-dependent, transient increases in cell proliferation and long-lasting enhancements in the tendon's biomechanical properties. Furthermore, PDGFs are highly concentrated in PRP and correlate positively with ECM gene expression in tendon and ligament.

Cellular Communication Network Factors

This family of the matricellular cellular communication network (CCN) factors are nonstructural proteins that act as signaling molecules. With six currently known family members, these factors have wide-ranging and often overlapping or opposite effects.[39] Perhaps most relevant to skeletal repair is CCN2, also known as connective tissue growth factor or CTGF, which is widely recognized for its profibrotic effects. However, CCN2/CTGF has pleiotropic effects on numerous skeletal cells, including effects on chondrogenesis and angiogenesis.[40] Therefore, pharmacologic inhibitors of CCN2/CTGF, such as Pamrevlumab, currently in advanced clinical trials for idiopathic pulmonary fibrosis, can be promising candidates for fibrovascular pathologies in tendon and ligaments. Interestingly, in animal models both CCN1 and CCN2 are expressed in tendon and reportedly mediate mechanotransduction and Hippo pathway signaling.[41] Interestingly, CCN1, also known as cysteine-rich angiogenic inducer 61 (Cyr61), is reported to have antifibrotic effects by inducing fibroblast senescence and restricting fibrosis in cutaneous wounds.[42] In humans, however, the data associating CCNs in general, and CCN2/CTGF, in particular, are scarce.[43]

Fibroblast Growth Factors

Fibroblast growth factors (FGFs) are a large family of potent morphogens and signaling factors, which play important roles in limb specification, growth, and patterning. Coordinated TGF-β/FGF signaling is critical for proper tendon and ligament development.[44] In rats, FGF-2 delivery through a gelatin hydrogel promoted proliferation and growth of the tenogenic progenitor cell and increased the expression of tenogenic markers *Scx* and *Tnmd* in injured supraspinatus tendons, which were associated with improvements in mechanical properties.[45] Adeno-associated viral type-2 mediated gene delivery of bFGF increased expression of type I collagen, cellular proliferation, and tendon strength in injured flexor tendons in chicken.[46] These animal studies suggest a therapeutic effect for FGFs in surgical repair of acute tendon injuries. However, although genetic polymorphisms in FGF3 and FGF10 were associated with increased risk of overuse tendinopathy in male volleyball athletes,[47] there appears to be no preclinical or clinical evidence of therapeutic effects for FGFs in the treatment of tendinopathy.

Insulinlike Growth Factors

Insulinlike growth factor 1 (IGF-1) is an endocrine hormone secreted primarily by the liver but can be secreted by different cell types where it induces a range of anabolic effects. Because of its molecular homology to insulin, it is able to bind not only to its own receptor tyrosine kinase (IGF1R) but also to the insulin receptor, activating several signaling cascades, most notably the PI3K/AKT/mTOR pathway. Therefore, IGF-1, which is induced by mechanical signals and interacts with other growth hormones and factors, plays a critical role in cell metabolism and the regulation of important processes in muscle, tendon, and ligament response to injury including proliferation, senescence, and apoptosis. In injured canine flexor tendon, repair stump tissue showed high expression of various growth factors including IGF-1, which were associated with a densely cellular, disorganized collagenous ECM.[48] Mouse experiments involving ablation injuries of the Achilles tendon reported a role for IGF-1 in regulating cell cycle and ECM synthesis through PI3K/AKT and other kinases.[49] Gene delivery of IGF-1 into injured rat Achilles tendon enhanced tendon repair and reduced scarring, especially when combined with short hairpin RNA targeting TGF-β1.[50] Furthermore, a veterinary clinical study investigating the effects of intralesional (tendinitis) injections of IGF-1 into superficial digital flexor tendons of racehorses showed reduced lesion severity by ultrasonography and moderate functional improvements allowing for return to competitive racing.[51] However, a study in sheep demonstrated that although mechanical tension slowed degeneration of injured musculotendinous junction of the rotator cuff, additional pharmacologic treatment with IGF-1 did not have significant effects on the degeneration of the injury site.[52] A randomized, double-blind, placebo-controlled clinical trial investigated whether IGF-1 injections combined with heavy slow resistance training enhanced matrix synthesis and structure, and patient-reported outcomes in patellar tendinopathy. The study reported that within 3 weeks, the combination of heavy slow resistance training and IGF-1 injections significantly improved patient-reported pain scores (Victorian Institute of Sports Assessment-Patellar and visual analog scale) with no discernible differences in tissue size and structure. However, a 1-year follow-up analysis failed to identify any long-term benefits for intralesional IGF-1 injections.[53]

Hedgehog Proteins

The hedgehog (Hh) family of proteins, first identified and studied extensively in *Drosophila*, includes three homologs in mammals, which act as important signaling morphogens that control cell growth, survival, and phenotype. Hh proteins are critical during development and regulate patterning of various tissues and organs including the limbs through concentration gradientsensitive responses. Hh binding to its receptor initiates activation of downstream proteins (smoothened or *Smo*), which in turn inactivate transcriptional repressors and trigger transcriptional activators of the Gli family of transcription factors. In tendon and ligament, Indian hedgehog (Ihh) gradients and the downstream regulation of Gli transcription factors are critical for the proper establishment of the entheses.[54] Mouse studies have demonstrated that Ihh continues to exert important regulatory roles in adult patellar tendon enthesis. In particular, genetic deletion of *Smo* in tendon cells during development resulted in inferior adult patellar tendon mechanics and abnormalities in mineralized enthesis formation.[55] The responses to mechanical loading in the enthesis depend on Hh signaling through the mechanosensory cellular structures known as cilia.[56] Not surprisingly, ACL graft pretensioning resulted in increased Ihh signaling at the interface between the tendon graft and the bony tunnel.[57] Furthermore, Ihh signaling in the enthesis is upregulated in mesenchymal stem cell–augmented repair of injured rat rotator cuff.[58] Thus, the preclinical data suggest that pharmacologic modulation of Hh signaling, potentially through engineered gradients within biomaterial scaffolds, could be a viable strategy for orthobiologic reconstruction of injured entheses in tendon and ACL repair procedures.

Wnt Proteins

In the canonical Wnt signaling pathway, the binding of the Wnt protein to its G-protein-coupled receptors frees up the transcription factor β-catenin from a ubiquitination complex, allowing it to accumulate in the cytosol and activate its transcriptional activity. The role of Wnt/β-catenin in tendon and ligament injury has only recently been described. Wnt/β-catenin signaling was activated at sites of puncture injuries in rat Achilles tendon. Furthermore, the in vitro activation of Wnt/β-catenin signaling in tenocytes suppresses gene expressions of *Scx*, *Mkx*, and *Tnmd* via inhibition of TGF-β/Smad signaling.[59] It was also reported that inhibition of WNT/β-catenin is necessary and sufficient to induce *Scx* expression in developing tendons of chicken limbs.[60] Pharmacologic inhibition of Wnt signaling in vitro promoted tenocyte differentiation and inhibited pro-inflammatory and catabolic pathways in human marrow stem cells and tendon progenitors. Topical application of Wnt inhibitor reduced tendon inflammation and promoted tendon regeneration, decreased pain, and improved function in a rat collagenase-induced tendinopathy model.[61] Baicalein, an extract of Chinese herbs, has been reported to enhance tendon-to-bone healing in a rat model via activation of Wnt/β-catenin signaling, suggesting potential benefits in ACL reconstructions.[62] Thus, the emerging role of Wnt/β-catenin in the treatment of acute or chronic tendon and ligament injuries merits further investigation.

ORTHOBIOLOGICS—STATE OF THE ART

Overview

Interventional clinical studies of tendon or ligament injuries investigate a wide range of treatment options that are typically classified as conservative behavioral and physical therapy, surgical procedures, devices, drugs, and biologics. Most of these studies typically investigate (1) interventions that target pain using analgesics, nerve block, NSAIDs, steroids, or homeopathic treatments including acupuncture, dry needling, massage, and psychological biomodulation; (2) functional rehabilitation (physical therapy or exercise); (3) surgical repair; or (4) traditional graft reconstruction. However, orthobiologics are increasingly being investigated in clinical studies based on principles of tissue engineering and regenerative medicine (**Figure 5**). Orthobiologics include cells or cell

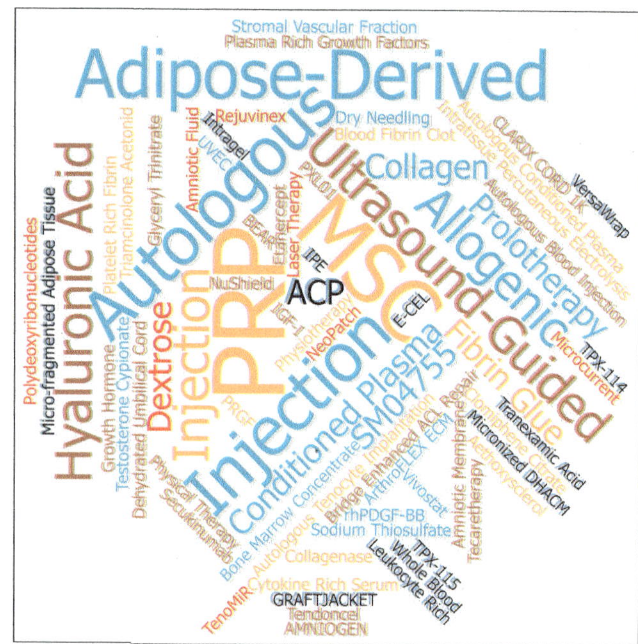

FIGURE 5 Word cloud representation of orthobiologics currently in clinical trials.

products delivered via transplanted scaffolds or intralesional injection to augment healing, disease-modifying genes, proteins or molecules, and bioactive material scaffolds or hydrogels. The major classes of orthobiologics for tendon and ligament injury are cell therapy, PRP, extracellular vesicles, gene therapy, and bioactive scaffolds.

Cell Therapy

Cell therapy involves the implantation of cells in vivo, either alone or in combination with a carrier scaffold to treat tissue injury and promote its regeneration. Over the past 3 decades, a plethora of animal studies investigated the efficacy of cell-based therapies, with special focus on marrow or adipose stem cells in the treatment of tendon and ligament injuries. Stem cells have been touted in regenerative medicine applications because of their immunomodulatory effects, ability to migrate to injury sites, and secrete growth factors, cytokines, and chemokines to recruit other cells.[63] The lack of standardization in animal models, approaches, outcomes, and, in some instances, scientific rigor confounds the ability to make conclusive statements on treatment efficacy. A recent report commissioned by the American Society for Bone and Mineral Research and the Orthopaedic Research Society critically evaluated the preclinical literature on cell-based therapies in the treatment of a range of musculoskeletal pathologies. For tendons and ligaments, studies generally investigated cell therapies for repair and reconstruction of experimentally injured tendons and ligaments, modulating inflammation in models of chronic tendinopathies, and development of cell-seeded scaffolds for tendon or ligament grafting.[64,65] Although rodents (mouse and rat) and rabbits were commonly used in the literature, larger animal models, particularly athlete horses in clinical veterinary studies, may better meet FDA guidelines for demonstrating preclinical efficacy. Furthermore, the functional and radiographic reporting in the preclinical literature varies widely and lacks standardization in semiquantitative scoring, pain outcomes are almost never included, and the evaluation of the fate of implanted cells and their contribution to the repair are rarely reported.

Clinically, cell therapy products intended for human use are regulated by the Center for Biologics Evaluation and Research at the FDA as human cells, tissues, and cellular and tissue-based products (HCT/P). The HCT/P classification imposes enforceable restrictions on unapproved off-label uses and preapproval commercialization of such products. Based on FDA guidance, cell therapy products must apply for investigational new drug designation to be approved for clinical studies. In most cases, cell therapy products will be regulated as a drug or biologic product unless they meet several exceptions. Specifically, these products (1) must be minimally manipulated products, (2) must be intended for homologous use only, (3) must not be combined with other articles that raise clinical safety concerns, (4) do not induce systemic effects, and (5) do not depend on the cells' metabolism for the primary function of the product (with exceptions in cases of autologous use or allogeneic use in close relatives). Despite these regulatory restrictions, there are several clinical studies investigating the use of fibroblasts and stem cells, either derived from bone marrow or adipose tissues, in the treatment of Achilles tendon ruptures and rotator cuff tears and refractory tendinopathies, tendinitis, and epicondylitis. Published randomized clinical trials with level I evidence (**Table 2**), which investigated the safety and efficacy of marrow-derived or adipose-derived stem/stromal cells or skin-derived collagen-producing tendonlike cells in the management of tendinopathy, reported significant clinical improvement with virtually no adverse events.[66-69] Most studies reported clinical outcomes based on measures of functional improvement such as the Victorian Institute of Sports Assessment score as primary outcomes. Other commonly used outcomes include pain measurements such as the visual analog scale score. However, the small number of studies and patient cohorts along with variabilities in cell source and application strategy negatively affect the reliability of evidence that would be required for clinical adoption and FDA approval. In summary, although the limited randomized clinical trials show evidence of safety and efficacy, cell therapy for musculoskeletal conditions remains experimental. At this time, there are no FDA-approved cell therapies for the treatment of acute or chronic tendon and ligament injuries. None of the cell therapy products reported in the reviewed clinical studies meets the exception criteria that would exempt them from investigational new drug designation and extensive testing of safety and efficacy in clinical trials, making them costly options in terms of product development and commercialization.

Platelet-Rich Plasma

The theory behind the therapeutic potential of PRP, derived from centrifuged whole blood extract obtained autologously from the patient, is that the resulting injectable product is replete with very high concentrations of platelets and growth factors, believed to enhance the body's own regenerative capabilities and accelerate the healing process.[70] PRP is not approved by the FDA as a drug or HCT/P. Rather, the devices that produce PRP intraoperatively are cleared through the 510(k) pathway to produce PRP preparations intended to be mixed with bone graft materials to enhance their handling properties. Therapeutic applications of PRP, such as in intralesional injections for the treatment of tendinopathy, are considered off-label uses. Although these are becoming increasingly widespread, their safety and efficacy have not been well established. This is likely due to the varied nature of PRP and its different preparations. A classification of different PRP

TABLE 2 Summary of Randomized Human Clinical Trials Investigating Cell Therapy for the Treatment of Tendinopathy

Reference	Study Design/Size	Condition	Treatment/Control	Outcomes
Clarke et al (2011)[69]	RCT/60 patellar tendons in 46 patients (age 20-51 yr)	Refractory patellar tendinopathy	US-guided injections of laboratory-prepared, collagen-producing cells derived from dermal fibroblasts and suspended in autologous plasma from centrifuged autologous whole blood/ autologous plasma alone	improvement in VISA score relative to plasma control Faster response of treatment and significantly greater improvement in pain and function relative to plasma controls
Lee et al (2015)[68]	RCT/12 patients (age 51.8 ± 9.5 yr)	Chronic lateral epicondylosis	US-guided injections of allogeneic adipose-derived mesenchymal stem cells (allo-ASC) at 10^6 or 10^7 cells/mL concentrations	No adverse effects through 52 wk of follow-up VAS scores progressively decreased Elbow performance scores improved. Tendon lesions decreased by ultrasonography
Rodas et al (2021)[67]	Prospective, double-blinded, randomized, two-arm parallel group, active controlled, phase 1/2 single-center clinical study/20 participants (age 18-48 yr)	Refractory proximal patellar tendinopathy	US-guided intratendinous and peritendinous injections of autologous BM-MSCs/Lp-PRP	VAS scores improved in both groups at all time points Significant reduction in pain during sporting activities VISA-P scores progressively increased compared with baseline in both groups Statistically significant improvements in tendon structure on ultrasonography and MRI in the BM-MSC group compared with the Lp-PRP group at 6 mo No significant adverse events in either group
Usuelli et al (2018)[66]	RCT/44 patients (age 18-55 yr)	Achilles tendinopathy	SVF injection/PRP injection	VAS, AOFAS, and VISA-A scored significantly better at 15 and 30 d in the SVF in comparison with PRP group Both treatments were safe and induced significant improvement with respect to baseline at later time points No correlation reported between clinical and radiologic findings

AOFAS = American Orthopaedic Foot and Ankle Society Hindfoot Score, BM = bone marrow, Lp-PRP = leukocyte-poor platelet-rich plasma, MSC = mesenchymal stem/stromal cell, PRP = platelet-rich plasma, RCT = randomized controlled trial, SVF = stromal vascular fraction, VAS = visual analog scale scores, VISA-A = Victorian Institute of Sports Assessment-Achilles, VISA-P = Victorian Institute of Sports Assessment-Patellar, US = ultrasound preparations was proposed in 2009: (1) pure PRP, (2) leukocyte and PRP, (3) pure platelet-rich fibrin, and (4) leukocyte and platelet-rich fibrin.[71] Each of the preparations of PRP may be useful for different therapeutic applications because of their varied compositions, but this remains an open question. Currently, PRP is being investigated for the treatment of tendon and ligament injuries either as a stand-alone nonsurgical treatment or in conjunction with more invasive interventions such as surgery.

With increasing interest in the therapeutic potential of PRP, there are numerous clinical trials attempting to elucidate its effectiveness. **Table 3** summarizes several meta-analyses that reviewed clinical trials investigating PRP's effectiveness for the treatment of several musculoskeletal injures, including tendinopathy. In general, results of these meta-analyses range from inconclusive to demonstrating the benefit of using PRP for the treatment of various injuries. Several studies demonstrated improvement in clinical outcomes after the administration of PRP when compared with controls.[70,72-76] Other studies were unable to draw conclusions because of lack of reliable study results.[70,75,76] However, another major

TABLE 3 Summary of Meta-analyses Investigating Platelet-Rich Plasma for Tendon Injury

Author (Year)	Injury	# of Studies	Treatment	Outcome Measures	Conclusions
Andia et al (2014)[75]	Tendinopathy	13 studies (12 RCTs) with 636 participants	L-PRP injection	Varied functional assessments, most included VAS	Reduction of pain in participants; however, study heterogeneity limits ability to make recommendation
Chen et al (2017)[72]	Tendon and ligament injury	21 RCTs with 1,031 participants	PRP injection	Pain measured with VAS	PRP may reduce pain
Fitzpatrick et al (2016)[73]	Tendinopathy	18 RCTs with 1,066 participants	L-PRP or autologous blood injection	Varied functional assessments	L-PRP provides clinically significant benefit in the management of tendinopathy
Hamid et al (2021)[74]	Rotator cuff tendinopathy	8 RCTs with 552 participants	PRP injection, some with exercise/rehab	Varied functional assessments	Safe and effective for long-term pain control and shoulder function
Moraes (2014)[70]	MSK soft-tissue injuries	19 studies (RCT or quasi-RCT) with 1,088 participants	PRP injection	Functional evaluations, pain, local and adverse effects of PRP (primary); recovery time, nonreturn to previous activity, QOL, recurrence, need for secondary treatment, participant satisfaction (secondary)	Insufficient evidence to support the use of platelet-rich therapies. Further study is needed in addition to standardization of preparation methods
Zhang et al (2018)[76]	Chronic Achilles tendinopathy	4 RCTs with 170 participants	PRP injection with subsequent rehabilitation	VISA-A score (primary); tendon thickness, color Doppler activity, functional measures (secondary)	No significant improvement in outcomes, more study is needed, not recommended as first-line treatment

L-PRP = leukocyte and platelet-rich plasma; MSK = musculoskeletal; PRP = platelet-rich plasma; QOL = quality of life; RCT = randomized controlled trial; VAS = visual analog scale scores; VISA-A = Victorian Institute of Sports Assessment-Achilles issue is the lack of standardization in the preparation and use of platelet-based therapies,[70,75] and it remains unclear if PRP practices are becoming more consistent as it is becoming increasingly adopted as standard practice. In summary, PRP has great potential as a therapeutic tool and is likely already helping patients experiencing certain musculoskeletal ailments including tendon and ligament injury. Further research is needed to better understand the precise mechanisms by which PRP works, and more clinical trials are needed to concretely establish its benefit.

Extracellular Vesicles and Exosomes

Extracellular vesicles may have functional similarities to PRP. Exosomes are a type of small (approximately 100 nm in diameter) extracellular vesicles secreted by all cells. Their contents are varied and may include DNA, RNA, lipids, proteins, and other bioactive substances.[77] Because exosomes are naturally involved with different signaling and developmental processes, they have potential for use as a therapeutic tool. Exosomes may be isolated from different types of cells, or may even be engineered to deliver specific contents.[77] This flexibility lends them to many clinical applications; however, research is in the early stages to truly understand this potential. The current understanding of how exosomes work is limited and the technology for isolating and storing them is not optimized or standardized. Despite this, there is considerable interest in the therapeutic potential of exosome-based therapies, including in tendon and ligament repair. That said, clinical applications of exosome products intended to treat diseases or conditions in humans await FDA approval. There are currently no FDA-approved exosome products.

Table 4 summarizes several animal studies that investigated extracellular vesicle–based therapies including exosomes in tendon and ligament healing.[82-84,86-89] The extracellular vesicles were derived from different sources including bone marrow stromal cells, tendon-derived stem cells (TDSCs), and adipose stem cells. All of the studies demonstrated promising results for the treatment of tendon and ligament injuries with varying degrees of improvement in lesion resolution, collagen organization, and inflammation modulation. It seems the primary effects of exosome therapy are modulation of postinjury inflammation and regulation of collagen production. Additionally, some of the results suggest exosome

TABLE 4 Mesenchymal Stem/Stromal Cell-Extracellular Vesicle Therapeutic Effect on Tendon Repair in Animal Models

Author (Year)	Animal Model	Extracellular Vesicle	Results
Chamberlain et al (2019)[82]	Nude mouse Achilles tendon transection	Exosome-educated macrophages (EEMs) (M2 phenotype)	EEM treatment improved biomechanical properties of healing tendon and reduced expression of type I collagen with no improvement in collagen fiber organization
Kornicka-Garbowska et al (2019)[83]	Case study of horse with suspensory ligament injury	Allogeneic microvesicles	Improved lesion filling, angiogenesis, and elasticity of tissue
Shi et al (2019)[84]	Rat patellar tendon injury	Rat BMSC-EV	Improved tendon healing with reduced inflammation and apoptotic cells and increased tendon progenitor cells at healing site
Wang et al (2019)[86]	Rat Achilles tendon tendinopathy model	Rat Achilles tendon TDSC-derived exosomes	Improved tendon repair comparable to TDSC treatment
Shi et al (2020)[87]	Mouse Achilles tendon-bone reconstruction	Mouse BMSC-derived exosomes in hydrogel	Exosome treatment led to more fibrocartilage and improved biomechanical properties
Wang et al (2020)[88]	Rabbit rotator cuff repair	ASC-derived exosomes	Improved biomechanical properties and other markers compared with control
Yu et al (2020)[89]	Rat patellar tendon injury	Rat BMSC-derived exosomes in fibrin glue	Exosomes improved healing and biomechanical properties with proliferation of resident stem cells and increased expression of tenomodulin and type I collagen

ASC = adipose stem cell, BMSC = bone marrow stromal cell, EV = extracellular vesicle, TDSC = tendon-derived stem cell

Adapted with permission from Lee DK: A preliminary study on the effects of acellular tissue graft augmentation in acute Achilles tendon ruptures. *J Foot Ankle Surg* 2008;47(1):8-12..

therapies may be as effective as other stem cell–based therapies in achieving similar results. An advantage of exosomes would be fewer safety concerns that are associated with stem cells such as tumorgenicity, infection transmission, and immune incompatibility. The research conducted in animal models is promising and points to therapeutic utility for exosomes in the treatment of tendon and ligament injuries. However, much research is needed before this becomes a reality. This includes investigation into how exosomes work as well as techniques for harvesting and storing them efficiently. Eventually, exosome therapies could become a helpful tool for treatment of tendon and ligament injuries.

Gene Therapy

Pharmacologic delivery of recombinant proteins can be nonspecific and limited by therapeutic window limitations and failure to target the underlying condition. Alternatively, systemic or targeted delivery of genes that express the relevant healing factors may mediate sustained expression of these factors. Gene therapy holds potential to treat numerous musculoskeletal conditions, including tendinopathy. However, the delivery of therapeutic genes is hindered by the body's protective mechanisms. The genetic package must evade the body's immune response, home to the target cells, traverse the negatively charged cellular membrane, and successfully express the target gene.[90] Gene delivery can currently be accomplished by viral or nonviral vectors or direct gene transfer through physical or chemical transfection techniques.

The considerations for the vector of choice include efficacy, safety, and cost. Adenovirus, adeno-associated virus, retrovirus, and lentivirus are the principal viral vectors. Although viral vectors are generally most efficient, they carry several concerns including disrupting normal genes, activation of proto-oncogenes, and insertional mutagenesis. Nonviral vectors have several advantages over viral delivery, including their lower immunogenicity and toxicity, enhanced cell specificity, and cost-effective production. Nonviral vectors are primarily composed of the two classes, organic and inorganic vectors. Organic vectors include lipids, natural and synthetic polymers, or peptides. Liposome vectors have garnered great interest in research because of their long circulation times, low uptake by off-target cells such as macrophages, and slow clearance from the bloodstream.[91] Furthermore, liposomal surfaces can be modified with fluorescent tags for traceability in vivo.

The ability of viral and nonviral vectors to successfully modulate gene expression in the tendon and ligament healing environment are typically first investigated by forced expression of reporters such as β-galactosidase with a *LacZ* gene transfection to demonstrate proof of concept. Over the past number of years, gene therapy has been used to deliver various growth factors and cytokines for the treatment of tendon and ligament injuries in animals. In general, these studies demonstrated that the therapy modulated proliferation and matrix synthesis leading to improved tendon and ligament repair, as detailed in **Table 5**.[46,92-96] Despite these encouraging preclinical data, there have been no randomized clinical trials to establish the safety and efficacy of gene therapy in the treatment of acute or chronic tendon and ligament injuries. Like cell therapy, gene therapy is regulated by the FDA, and currently there are no FDA-approved products or applications of gene therapy in the treatment of tendon and ligament pathologies.

Biomaterial Scaffolds

The tissue engineering and regenerative medicine fields have pressed for design strategies to optimize regenerative healing of ligament and tendon tissues based three main pillars: (1) reparative cells that can modulate the repair environment, (2) bioactive molecules, such as cytokines and growth factors that support and regulate the cells, and (3) an appropriate scaffold for transplantation and structural and biologic support. Biomaterial scaffolds are critical for tendon and ligament repair as artificial grafts because of the load-bearing nature of these tissues, and must be designed to favorably influence the proliferation, chemotaxis, and differentiation of cells while inducing a tolerable immune response. They are derived from biologic, synthetic, or composites thereof. Scaffolds can be designed and fabricated to mimic the ECM in composition and architecture. Also critical is the presence of void spaces within the scaffold structure to promote uniform cell delivery and allow for sufficient nutrient supply and tissue ingrowth.[97] Biodegradability following implantation is essential as the controlled resorption of the scaffold orchestrates replacement by newly regenerated tissue. The degradation products should be nontoxic and metabolized by the body without invoking a systemic response.

Synthetic soft-tissue scaffolds to augment tendon and ligament injuries, such as expanded polytetrafluoroethylene patches such as Gore-Tex, have been used in human patients with large rotator cuff tears since the early 2000s with mixed results.[98] Polycarbonate polyurethane patches have also been used to augment rotator cuff repair with 90% of patients maintaining intact repair at 12 months with no adverse events reported.[99] Similar results have also been reported for polyethylene terephthalate (Dacron) patches.[100] Nevertheless, there are concerns for risk of infection and long-term cytotoxicity associated with these nondegradable scaffolds. A 30-year follow-up study of a randomized controlled trial of ACL reconstruction surgery reported long-term outcomes of 150 patients with acute ACL ruptures who were randomly treated with primary repair, repair with a synthetic polypropylene ligament augmentation device, or reconstruction

TABLE 5 Selected Experimental Studies on Gene Therapy for Tendon and Ligament Injuries

Author	Vector	Gene	Target	Result
Lou et al[92]	Adenovirus	BMP-12	Chicken flexor profundus tendon laceration	Twofold increase of tensile strength and stiffness of repaired tendons
Bolt et al[93]	Adenovirus	BMP-14	Achilles tendon of 90 male Sprague-Dawley rats	Less visible gapping, a greater number of neotenocytes at the site of healing, and 70% greater tensile strength
Delalande et al[94]	Imidazole cationic liposomes or linear PEI nanoparticles	Fibromodulin or PDGF	Adult Wistar rats Achilles tendon repair	Stiffer tendons, improved collagen matrix organization, hypercellularity
Suwalski et al[95]	Silica nanoparticles (MSN)	PDGF-B	Adult Wistar rats Achilles tendon repair	Increased maximal load to failure, maximum stress and Young modulus. Improved structural organization
Zhou et al[96]	Nanoparticle/plasmid complex-coated sutures	bFGF and VEGFA	Adult white Leghorn chicken flexor tendon and mature male Wistar rat Achilles tendon	Increasing tendon healing strengths, enhancing gliding function, and inhibiting adhesion formation
Tang et al[46]	AAV2	bFGF and VEGF	Chicken flexor tendons	Enhanced collagen production, ECM molecules, proliferation, tendon strength

AAV2 = adeno-associated viral type-2, bFGF = basic fibroblast growth factor, BMP = bone morphogenetic protein, ECM = extracellular matrix, MSN = mesoporous silica nanoparticle, PDGF = platelet-derived growth factor, PEI = polyethyleneimine, VEGFA = vascular endothelial growth factor A

with an autologous bone-patellar tendon-bone graft with retention of the ACL remnants. The results indicated superior outcomes for the bone-patellar tendon-bone group with respect to revisions outcomes, yet no significant differences were found in range of motion, laxity, activity, function, radiographic evidence of osteoarthritis, and knee arthroplasties.[101] Therefore, synthetic scaffolds demonstrate the greatest promise, when applied to augment tendon or ligament repair.

Biologic scaffolds are derived from mammalian (human, porcine, bovine, and equine) tissues and undergo extensive decellularization processing to minimize host rejection while maintaining the structural and mechanical properties of the ECM. There are currently more than 80 commercially available products composed of intact ECM derived from a variety of tissues and organs and are typically regulated as devices by the FDA to allow for use in a wide variety of clinical applications. A partial list of products available for tendon and ligament are listed in **Table 6**. Decellularized tissue scaffolds, such as ArthroFLEX and GRAFTJACKET, have been successfully used in both preclinical animal studies and human clinical studies. The tissues are processed to remove immunogenic cellular materials while retaining the ECM proteins, proteoglycans, and growth factors and then freeze-dried to retain the native architecture. These natural scaffolds are packaged prehydrated for simpler handling[102] and can be rehydrated before surgical implantation. Certain limitations to biologic tissue-derived scaffolds include tissue availability, immunogenic responses, and compromised mechanical strength of the scaffolds due to extensive processing. Although patients report improved pain and mobility scores as early as 4 to 6 weeks after injury with many of the commercially available scaffolds,[85] long-term data on the safety and efficacy of these scaffolds typically are not available.

Purified ECM proteins have also been developed as natural polymer scaffolds or hydrogels, including collagen, silk, chitosan, and hyaluronic acid. These natural polymer scaffolds typically have challenging physical and handling properties. To address this, natural polymers can be combined with synthetic biodegradable polymers such as polylactic acid, polyglycolic acid, poly(lactic-co-glycolic acid), and poly(ε-caprolactone). This strategy produces bioactive scaffolds for tendon and ligament, in the form of gels, membranes, or three-dimensional fibrous scaffolds. These composite scaffolds address the poor mechanical properties[78] and processing reproducibility of stand-alone natural polymer scaffolds. An example of an FDA-cleared composite scaffold is the BioBrace, which is composed of a highly porous collagen sponge reinforced with resorbable polylactic acid microfilaments to increase its mechanical properties and promote tissue regenerative functions while slowly reabsorbing in approximately 2 years. A new device, Bridge-Enhanced ACL Repair (BEAR), has recently been approved by the FDA. BEAR is composed of a bovine collagen scaffold placed in the

TABLE 6 Selected Commercially Available Biologic Scaffolds Sold as Patches for Tendon or Ligament Augmentation

Scaffold	Trade Name—Manufacturer	Clinical Applications	FDA Standing
Human dermis	GraftJacket—Wright Medical Arthroflex—LifeNet Health AlloDerm—BioHorizons Dermaspan—Zimmer Biomet	Achilles tendon, rotator cuff, posterior tibial tendon, peroneal tendon, quadriceps tendon, hip bone graft, total joint arthroplasties, mooring ligaments, lateral ankle stabilization, root coverage, gingival augmentation	FDA regulated
Human amniotic membrane	Clarix Surgical Allograft—Amniox	Joint, ligament and tendon repair, nerve decompression, trauma, arthroplasty urology, gynecology, and general surgery	FDA regulated
Porcine dermis	CollaMend FM—Bard Permacol—Medtronic XenMatrix—BD Biosciences	Hernia reinforcement, surgical repair of damage or ruptured soft tissues such as tendons and ligaments	510(K) cleared
Fetal bovine dermis	TissueMend—Stryker	Soft-tissue repair during tendon repair surgery, including reinforcement of the rotator cuff, patellar, Achilles, biceps, quadriceps, or other tendons	510(K) cleared
Porcine small intestinal submucosa	Restore—DePuy Synthes CuffPatch—Arthrotek Oasis—Smith and Nephew Restore—DePuy Biodesign—Cook Medical MatriStem—ACell	Rotator cuff repair and augmentation, diabetic foot ulcers, traumatic wounds, and soft-tissue lacerations, and necrotizing soft-tissue infections	510(K) cleared
Bovine dermis	Bio-Blanket—Kensey Nash Corp	Rotator cuff, neurologic repairs, spine dura repairs, and bone graft containment	510(K) cleared
Equine pericardium	OrthoADAPT—Synovis	Rotator cuff, patellar, Achilles, biceps, quadriceps, hernias, suture-line reinforcement, muscle flap reinforcement	510(K) cleared
Poly(urethane urea)	Sportmesh—Zimmer Biomet	Rotator cuff, patellar, Achilles, biceps, quadriceps	510(K) cleared
Expanded polytetrafluoroethylene (ePTFE)	Gore-Tex patch—WL Gore & Associates	Laparoscopic hernia repair, inguinal herniorrhaphy, bridging facial defects, tendon, and ligament repairs	510(K) cleared
Polyethylene (PET)	Poly-tape—Neoligaments	Ligament, tendon, and soft-tissue injuries	510(K) cleared
Type I collagen and poly(L-lactide) (PLLA) microfilaments	BioBrace—Biorez	Tendon and ligament repair	510(K) cleared
Type I collagen and poly D(L-lactide) (PDLLA)	Tapestry—Embody	Tendon and ligament repair	510(K) cleared

gap between recently torn ACL ends in combination with suture repair and infusion with patient's blood to promote hematoma formation and stimulate the biologic healing response. A prospective, randomized clinical trial reported 2-year results that indicate comparable patient-reported outcomes, knee stability, muscle strength improvements, and reinjury rates to standard autograft ACL reconstruction in young patients.[79]

In summary, biomaterial scaffolds represent the largest sector of orthobiologics currently used in the management of tendon and ligament injuries. With the exception of BEAR, these devices have been designed to mechanically and structurally augment or replace injured tendons and ligaments. As the success of BEAR has shown, there are opportunities to use these devices in combination with blood, cells, and cell products to stimulate the biologic response of the tissue to injury. Such strategies should take into account regulatory guidance to avoid protracted FDA approvals and capitalize on predicate devices through the 510(k) pathway.

BARRIERS AND OPPORTUNITIES

Over the past few decades, despite encouraging preclinical and clinical evidence, clinical adoption and commercialization of orthobiologics for the treatment of acute and chronic tendon and ligament injuries have stagnated, perhaps with the exception of biomaterial scaffolds. This is partly attributed to:

1. Incomplete understanding of the mechanisms of action and the lack of biomarkers to define biologic efficacy criteria that can complement current patient-reported and functional outcomes.
2. Poor translation from preclinical animal studies to human clinical applications, which relates to the aforementioned inconsistencies but also to fundamental species differences in anatomy, pathophysiology, and biology.
3. Inconsistencies in preclinical and clinical studies with respect to use indications, preparation protocols, dosing, delivery vehicles and routes, and scientific rigor and reproducibility.
4. Regulatory hurdles related to classifying most orthobiologics as biologic drugs, HCT/P, or combination devices, which require extensive testing of safety and efficacy in multiphase clinical trials.

The emerging technology of human microphysiological systems (hMPS) might offer transformative opportunities to cost-effectively address the aforementioned barriers (**Figure 6**). hMPS is a wide-encompassing term for sophisticated in vitro human models, also known as tissue-on-chip and organ-on-chip, carefully designed to offer standardized predictive models by mimicking physiologically relevant aspects of living tissues

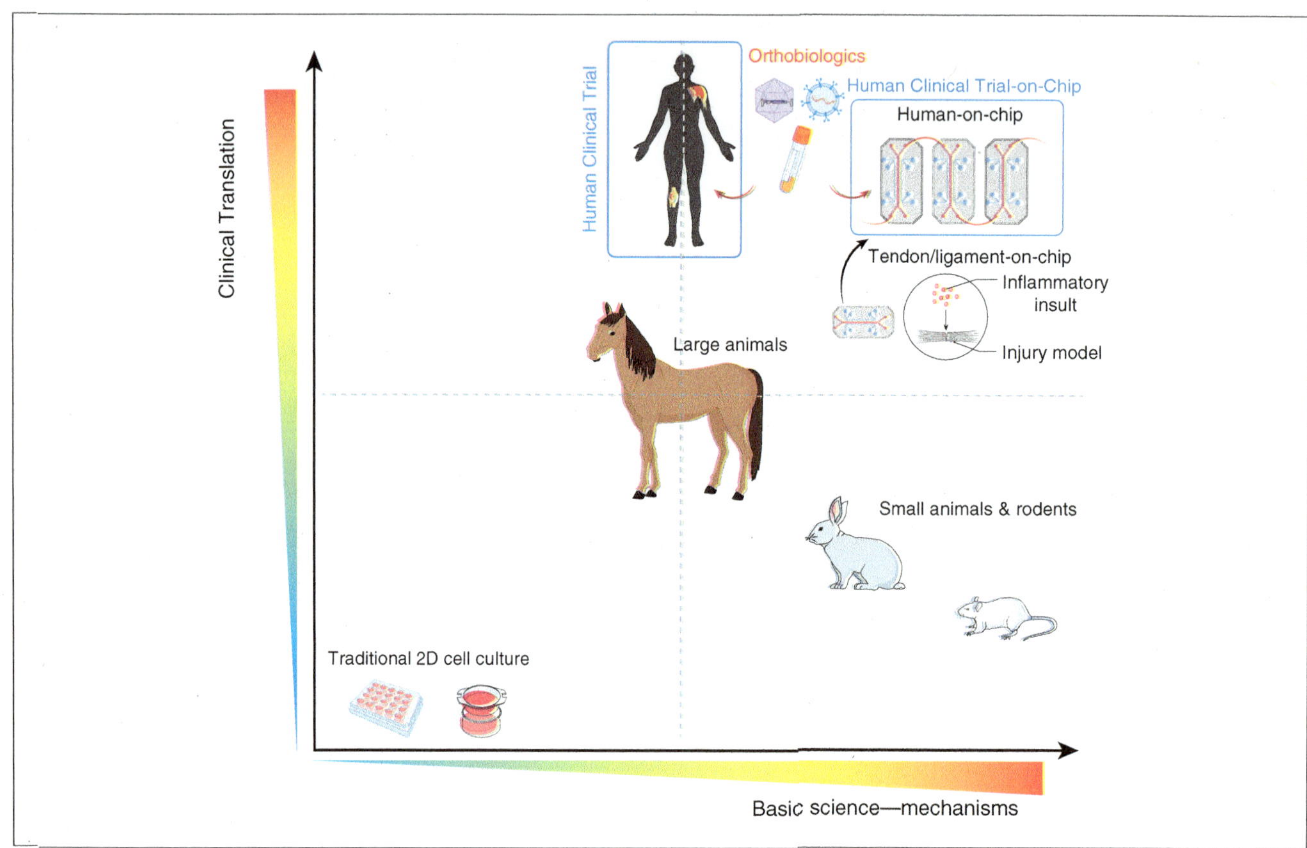

FIGURE 6 A Pasteur quadrant representation of current and prospective models for the development and evaluation of orthobiologics. Traditional in vitro systems involving two-dimensional (2D) monocultures or co-cultures are least informative on both the basic science and clinical translation scales. Rodents can be powerful basic science models to uncover mechanisms of pathologies. Larger animals are more valuable on the translation scale, but their basic science value and cost effectiveness are diminished. Clinical trials in humans are the gold standard for clinical translation but not for early scientific experimentation. Human microphysiological systems provide clinically relevant, advanced understanding of musculoskeletal pathologies and a platform for virtual clinical trials to de-risk orthobiologics before they are tested in humans.

and organ systems.[80] hMPS are designed to incorporate the tissue's multicellular microenvironment including immune system components from primary donor sources or isogenic human stem cell derivatives, a relevant three-dimensional ECM, and physical aspects of the tissue microenvironment including stretch and vascular flow. The technology's greatest potential as more advanced in vitro human models was identified early on by the science community to reduce inefficiencies and high costs associated with drug discovery, development, and testing. Although in vivo animal experiments have been vital tools to study mechanisms of tissue development and disease, they are not reliable models of drug pharmacokinetics and pharmacodynamics studies, and as discussed throughout this chapter, their results do not translate well to humans. Numerous multicellular hMPS have been developed for skeletal and cardiac muscle, lung, kidney, liver, gastrointestinal tract, blood-brain barrier, bone marrow, and articular joints. hMPS simulate physiologically relevant aspects of the pathologies that afflict these tissues, demonstrate predictable responses to clinically used drugs, and are already proving to be promising platforms for new drug candidate discovery and testing. With the proliferation and refinement of various hMPS to model the vital organs of the human body, integrated patient-specific hMPS chips are closer than ever to model absorbance, distribution, metabolism, excretion, and toxicity and pharmacokinetics and pharmacodynamics in a human-on-chip platform. Several groups are working on tendon-on-chip models, and these should be embraced by the tendon and ligament community and the regulatory agencies as standard tools that promote scientific rigor and reproducibility to de-risk, optimize, and establish mechanisms of actions and biomarkers for orthobiologics in clinically challenging models of fibrovascular scar, tendinopathy, and enthesopathy.

SUMMARY

Injuries to tendons and ligaments represent a large segment of musculoskeletal pathologies with rates rising because of increasing sport activities, overwork, and an aging population. Although current treatments including surgery, physical therapy, and anti-inflammatory or pain-suppressing drugs can restore function and address symptoms, they have several shortcomings. Improved understanding of the cellular interactions and signaling pathways involved may lead to novel regenerative therapies. Injury induces an inflammatory response that activates innate and adaptive cellular and humoral immunity responses in sequential and overlapping stages, which involves numerous cytokines and growth factors that regulate the pathobiology of tendon and ligament healing. Therefore, inflammation has been a target of preclinical investigations and clinical interventions. However, no cytokines or growth factors have been established as a clinical treatment. The inflammatory response, while indispensable as a protective mechanism, can result in activating a proliferative and ECM-synthetic myofibroblast phenotype, which has been linked to fibrovascular scar formation and, therefore, identified as a target for biologic therapies. Bioactive scaffolds represent the most advanced technology in the translational pipeline, exemplified by the recent BEAR device for ACL reconstruction and numerous other biomaterial scaffolds used to augment tendon and ligament tears. Numerous orthobiologic interventions including cell therapy, PRP, extracellular vesicles, and gene therapy are in various stages of preclinical and clinical development and testing. Despite promising preclinical evidence, these therapies have yet to translate to the clinic. Several barriers have slowed the translation including lack of a thorough understanding of pathology mechanisms and biomarkers, inconsistent protocols using poor models of the human pathobiology, and regulatory hurdles. Recent advances in microphysiological systems have the potential to overcome these barriers by creating faithful human models of tendon and ligament pathobiology that could elucidate cellular and molecular mechanisms and therapeutic targets, accelerate the discovery of disease-modifying therapies, and de-risk them before they can be tested in clinical trials.

REFERENCES

1. United States Bone and Joint Initiative: *The Burden of Musculoskeletal Diseases in the United States (BMUS)*, ed 3, 2014. Accessed August 9, 2021. Available at: http://www.boneandjointburden.org.
2. Thorpe CT, Screen HR: Tendon Structure and Composition. *Adv Exp Med Biol* 2016;920:3-10.
3. Noyes FR, Butler DL, Grood ES, Zernicke RF, Hefzy MS: Biomechanical analysis of human ligament grafts used in knee-ligament repairs and reconstructions. *J Bone Joint Surg Am* 1984;66(3):344-352.
4. Jakobsen JR, Krogsgaard MR: The myotendinous junction-a vulnerable companion in sports. A narrative review. *Front Physiol* 2021;12:635561.
5. Lu HH, Thomopoulos HH: Functional attachment of soft tissues to bone: Development, healing, and tissue engineering. *Annu Rev Biomed Eng* 2013;15:201-226.
6. Murchison ND, Price BA, Conner DA, et al: Regulation of tendon differentiation by scleraxis distinguishes force-transmitting tendons from muscle-anchoring tendons. *Development* 2007;134(14):2697-2708.
7. Nakamichi R, Kataoka K, Asahara H: Essential role of Mohawk for tenogenic tissue homeostasis including spinal disc and periodontal ligament. *Mod Rheumatol* 2018;28(6):933-940.
8. Havis E, Duprez D: EGR1 transcription factor is a multifaceted regulator of matrix production in tendons and other connective tissues. *Int J Mol Sci* 2020;21(5):1664.

9. Bi Y, Ehirchiou D, Kilts TM, et al: Identification of tendon stem/progenitor cells and the role of the extracellular matrix in their niche. *Nat Med* 2007;13(10):1219-1227.
10. Tempfer H, Traweger A: Tendon vasculature in health and disease. *Front Physiol* 2015;6:330.
11. Lehner C, Spitzer G, Gehwolf R, et al: Tenophages: A novel macrophage-like tendon cell population expressing CX3CL1 and CX3CR1. *Dis Model Mech* 2019;12(12):dmm041384.
12. Shukunami C, Takimoto A, Nishizaki Y, et al: Scleraxis is a transcriptional activator that regulates the expression of tenomodulin, a marker of mature tenocytes and ligamentocytes. *Sci Rep* 2018;8(1):3155.
13. Harvey T, Flamenco T, Fan CM: A Tppp3+Pdgfra+ tendon stem cell population contributes to regeneration and reveals a shared role for PDGF signalling in regeneration and fibrosis. *Nat Cell Biol* 2019;21(12):1490-1503.
14. Kendal AR, Layton T, Al-Mossawi H, et al: Multi-omic single cell analysis resolves novel stromal cell populations in healthy and diseased human tendon. *Sci Rep* 2020;10(1):13939.
15. Kumar V, Abbas AK, Fausto N: *Tissue repair: Cellular growth, fibrosis, and wound healing*, in *Robbins & Cotran Pathologic Basis of Disease*, Elsevier, 2005.
16. Sunwoo JY, Eliasberg CD, Carballo CB, Rodeo SA: The role of the macrophage in tendinopathy and tendon healing. *J Orthop Res* 2020;38(8):1666-1675.
17. Arvind V, Huang AH: Reparative and maladaptive inflammation in tendon healing. *Front Bioeng Biotechnol* 2021;9:719047.
18. Crosio G, Huang AH: Innate and adaptive immune system cells implicated in tendon healing and disease. *Eur Cell Mater* 2022;43:39-52.
19. Noah AC: Adaptive and innate immune cell responses in tendons and lymph nodes after tendon injury and repair. *J Appl Physiol (1985)* 2020;128(3):473-482.
20. Paplinska-Goryca M, Misiukiewicz-Stepien P, Nejman-Gryz P, Proboszcz M, et al: Epithelial-macrophage-dendritic cell interactions impact alarmins expression in asthma and COPD. *Clin Immunol* 2020;215:108421.
21. Pozzi LAM, Maciaszek JW, Rock KL: Both dendritic cells and macrophages can stimulate naive CD8 T cells in vivo to proliferate, develop effector function, and differentiate into memory cells. *J Immunol* 2005;175(4):2071.
22. Hinz B, Formation and function of the myofibroblast during tissue repair. *J Invest Dermatol* 2007;127(3):526-537.
23. Millar NL: Tendinopathy. *Nat Rev Dis Prim* 2021;7(1):1.
24. Pufe T, Petersen WJ, Mentlein R, Tillmann BN: The role of vasculature and angiogenesis for the pathogenesis of degenerative tendons disease. *Scand J Med Sci Sports* 2005;15(4):211-222.
25. Fredberg U, Stengaard-Pedersen K: Chronic tendinopathy tissue pathology, pain mechanisms, and etiology with a special focus on inflammation. *Scand J Med Sci Sports* 2008;18(1):3-15.
26. Millar NL, Akbar M, Campbell AL, et al: IL-17A mediates inflammatory and tissue remodelling events in early human tendinopathy. *Sci Rep* 2016;6(1):27149.
27. Dakin SG, Newton J, Martinez FO, et al: Chronic inflammation is a feature of Achilles tendinopathy and rupture. *Br J Sports Med* 2018;52(6):359-367.
28. Wojciak B, Crossan JF: The accumulation of inflammatory cells in synovial sheath and epitenon during adhesion formation in healing rat flexor tendons. *Clin Exp Immunol* 1993;93(1):108-114.
29. Farhat YM, Al-Maliki AA, Easa A, O'Keefe RJ, Schwarz EM, Awad HA: TGF-beta1 suppresses plasmin and MMP activity in flexor tendon cells via PAI-1: Implications for scarless flexor tendon repair. *J Cell Physiol* 2015;230(2):318-326.
30. Chang J, Most D, Stelnicki E, et al: Gene expression of transforming growth factor beta-1 in rabbit zone II flexor tendon wound healing: evidence for dual mechanisms of repair. *Plast Reconstr Surg* 1997;100(4):937-944.
31. Krummel TM, Michna BA, Thomas BL, et al: Transforming growth factor beta (TGF-beta) induces fibrosis in a fetal wound model. *J Pediatr Surg* 1988;23(7):647-652.
32. Jorgensen HG, Mclellan S, Crossan J, Curtis A: Neutralisation of TGF beta or binding of VLA-4 to fibronectin prevents rat tendon adhesion following transection. *Cytokine* 2005;30(4):195-202.
33. Bates SJ, Morrow E, Zhang AY, Pham H, Longaker MT, Chang J: Mannose-6-phosphate, an inhibitor of transforming growth factor-beta, improves range of motion after flexor tendon repair. *J Bone Joint Surg Am* 2006;88(11):2465-2472.
34. Wolfman NM, Hattersley G, Cox K, et al: Ectopic induction of tendon and ligament in rats by growth and differentiation factors 5, 6, and 7, members of the TGF-beta gene family. *J Clin Invest* 1997;100(2):321-330.
35. Mikic B: Multiple effects of GDF-5 deficiency on skeletal tissues: implications for therapeutic bioengineering. *Ann Biomed Eng* 2004;32(3):466-476.
36. Clark RT, Johnson TL, Schalet BJ, et al: GDF-5 deficiency in mice leads to disruption of tail tendon form and function. *Connect Tissue Res* 2001. 42(3):175-186.
37. Aspenberg P, Forslund C: Enhanced tendon healing with GDF 5 and 6. *Acta Orthop Scand* 1999;70(1):51-54.
38. Thomopoulos S, Zaegel M, Das R, et al: PDGF-BB released in tendon repair using a novel delivery system promotes cell proliferation and collagen remodeling. *J Orthop Res* 2007;25(10):1358-1368.
39. Jun JI, Lau LF: Taking aim at the extracellular matrix: CCN proteins as emerging therapeutic targets. *Nat Rev Drug Discov* 2011;10(12):945-963.
40. Hall-Glenn F, Lyons KM: Roles for CCN2 in normal physiological processes. *Cell Mol Life Sci* 2011;68(19):3209-3217.
41. Park MH, Kim AK, Manandhar S, et al: CCN1 interlinks integrin and hippo pathway to autoregulate tip cell activity. *Elife* 2019;8:e46012.
42. Jun JI, Lau LF: The matricellular protein CCN1 induces fibroblast senescence and restricts fibrosis in cutaneous wound healing. *Nat Cell Biol* 2010;12(7):676-685.

43. Morita W, Snelling SJB, Dakin SG, Carr AJ: Profibrotic mediators in tendon disease: a systematic review. *Arthritis Res Ther* 2016;18(1):269.

44. Havis E, Bonnin MA, Esteves de Lima J, Charvet B, Milet C, Duprez D: TGFβ and FGF promote tendon progenitor fate and act downstream of muscle contraction to regulate tendon differentiation during chick limb development. *Development* 2016;143(20):3839-3851.

45. Tokunaga T, Shukunami C, Okamoto N, et al: FGF-2 stimulates the growth of tenogenic progenitor cells to facilitate the generation of tenomodulin-positive tenocytes in a rat rotator cuff healing model. *Am J Sports Med* 2015;43(10):2411-2422.

46. Tang JB, Wu YF, Cao Y, et al: Basic FGF or VEGF gene therapy corrects insufficiency in the intrinsic healing capacity of tendons. *Sci Rep* 2016;6(1):20643.

47. Salles JI, Amaral MV, Aguiar DP, et al: BMP4 and FGF3 haplotypes increase the risk of tendinopathy in volleyball athletes. *J Sci Med Sport* 2015;18(2):150-155.

48. Lu CC, Zhang T, Reisdorf RL, et al: Biological analysis of flexor tendon repair-failure stump tissue: A potential recycling of tissue for tendon regeneration. *Bone Joint Res* 2019;8(6):232-245.

49. Disser NP, Sugg KB, Talarek JR, Sarver DC, Rourke BJ, Mendias CL: Insulin-like growth factor 1 signaling in tenocytes is required for adult tendon growth. *Faseb J* 2019;33(11):12680-12695.

50. Xiang X, Leng Q, Tang Y, et al: Ultrasound-targeted microbubble destruction delivery of insulin-like growth factor 1 cDNA and transforming growth factor beta short hairpin RNA enhances tendon regeneration and inhibits scar formation in vivo. *Hum Gene Ther Clin Dev* 2018;29(4):198-213.

51. Witte TH, Yeager AE, Nixon AJ: Intralesional injection of insulin-like growth factor-I for treatment of superficial digital flexor tendonitis in thoroughbred racehorses: 40 cases (2000-2004). *J Am Vet Med Assoc* 2011;239(7): 992-997.

52. Wieser K, Farshad M, Meyer DC, Conze P, von Rechenberg B, Gerber C: Tendon response to pharmacomechanical stimulation of the chronically retracted rotator cuff in sheep. *Knee Surg Sports Traumatol Arthrosc* 2015;23(2):577-584.

53. Olesen JL, Hansen M, Turtumoygard IF, et al: No treatment benefits of local administration of insulin-like growth factor-1 in addition to heavy slow resistance training in tendinopathic human patellar tendons: a randomized, double-blind, placebo-controlled trial with 1-year follow-up. *Am J Sports Med* 2021;49(9):2361-2370.

54. Liu CF, Breidenbach A, Aschbacher-Smith L, Butler D, Wylie C: A role for hedgehog signaling in the differentiation of the insertion site of the patellar tendon in the mouse. *PLoS One* 2013;8(6):e65411.

55. Breidenbach AP, Aschbacher-Smith L, Lu Y, et al: Ablating hedgehog signaling in tenocytes during development impairs biomechanics and matrix organization of the adult murine patellar tendon enthesis. *J Orthop Res* 2015;33(8):1142-1151.

56. Fang F, Schwartz AG, Moore ER, Sup ME, Thomopoulos S: Primary cilia as the nexus of biophysical and hedgehog signaling at the tendon enthesis. *Sci Adv* 2020. 6(44):eabc1799.

57. Carbone A, Carballo C, Ma R, et al: Indian hedgehog signaling and the role of graft tension in tendon-to-bone healing: Evaluation in a rat ACL reconstruction model. *J Orthop Res* 2016;34(4):641-649.

58. Zong JC, Mosca MJ, Degen RM, et al: Involvement of Indian hedgehog signaling in mesenchymal stem cell-augmented rotator cuff tendon repair in an athymic rat model. *J Shoulder Elbow Surg* 2017;26(4):580-588.

59. Kishimoto Y, Ohkawara B, Sakai T, et al: Wnt/β-catenin signaling suppresses expressions of Scx, Mkx, and Tnmd in tendon-derived cells. *PLoS One* 2017;12(7):e0182051.

60. Garcia-Lee V, Díaz-Hernandez ME, Chimal-Monroy J: Inhibition of WNT/β-catenin is necessary and sufficient to induce Scx expression in developing tendons of chicken limb. *Int J Dev Biol* 2021;65(4-6):395-401.

61. Deshmukh V, Seo T, O'Green AL, et al: SM04755, a small-molecule inhibitor of the Wnt pathway, as a potential topical treatment for tendinopathy. *J Orthop Res* 2021;39(9):2048-2061.

62. Tian X, Jiang H, Chen Y, et al: Baicalein accelerates tendon-bone healing via activation of Wnt/β-catenin signaling pathway in rats. *BioMed Res Int* 2018;2018:3849760.

63. Malekpour K, Hazrati A, Zahar M, et al: The potential use of mesenchymal stem cells and their derived exosomes for orthopedic diseases treatment. *Stem Cell Rev Rep* 2022;18(3):933-951.

64. O'Keefe RJ, Tuan RS, Lane NE, et al: American society for bone and mineral research-orthopaedic research society joint task force report on cell-based therapies. *J Bone Miner Res* 2020;35(1):3-17.

65. O'Keefe RJ, Tuan RS, Lane NE, et al: American society for bone and mineral research-orthopaedic research society joint task force report on cell-based therapies - secondary publication. *J Orthop Res* 2020;38(3):485-502.

66. Usuelli FG, Grassi M, Maccario C, et al: Intratendinous adipose-derived stromal vascular fraction (SVF) injection provides a safe, efficacious treatment for Achilles tendinopathy: results of a randomized controlled clinical trial at a 6-month follow-up. *Knee Surg Sports Traumatol Arthrosc* 2018;26(7):2000-2010.

67. Rodas G, Soler-Rich R, Rius-Tarruella J, et al: Effect of autologous expanded bone marrow mesenchymal stem cells or leukocyte-poor platelet-rich plasma in chronic patellar tendinopathy (with gap >3 mm): Preliminary outcomes after 6 months of a double-blind, randomized, prospective study. *Am J Sports Med* 2021;49(6):1492-1504.

68. Lee SY, Kim W, Lim C, Chung SG: Treatment of lateral epicondylosis by using allogeneic adipose-derived mesenchymal stem cells: A pilot study. *Stem Cell* 2015;33(10): 2995-3005.

69. Clarke AW, Alyas F, Morris T, Robertson CJ, Bell J, Connell DA: Skin-derived tenocyte-like cells for the treatment of patellar tendinopathy. *Am J Sports Med* 2011;39(3): 614-623.
70. Moraes VY: Platelet-rich therapies for musculoskeletal soft tissue injuries. *Cochrane Database Syst Rev* 2014;2014(4): CD010071.
71. Dohan Ehrenfest DM, Rasmusson L, Albrektsson T: Classification of platelet concentrates: From pure platelet-rich plasma (P-PRP) to leucocyte- and platelet-rich fibrin (L-PRF). *Trends Biotechnol* 2009;27(3):158-167.
72. Chen X, Jones IA, Park C, Vangsness CT: The efficacy of platelet-rich plasma on tendon and ligament healing: A systematic review and meta-analysis with bias assessment. *Am J Sports Med* 2018;46(8):2020-2032.
73. Fitzpatrick J, Bulsara M, Zheng MH: The effectiveness of platelet-rich plasma in the treatment of tendinopathy: A meta-analysis of randomized controlled clinical trials. *Am J Sports Med* 2017;45(1):226-233.
74. Hamid MSA, Sazlina SG: Platelet-rich plasma for rotator cuff tendinopathy: A systematic review and meta-analysis. *PLoS One* 2021;16(5):e0251111.
75. Andia I, Latorre PM, Gomez MC, Burgos-Alonso N, Abate M, Maffulli N: Platelet-rich plasma in the conservative treatment of painful tendinopathy: a systematic review and meta-analysis of controlled studies. *Br Med Bull* 2014;110(1):99-115.
76. Zhang YJ, Xu SZ, Gu PC, et al: Is platelet-rich plasma injection effective for chronic Achilles tendinopathy? A meta-analysis. *Clin Orthop Relat Res* 2018;476(8):1633-1641.
77. Kalluri R, Lebleu VS: The biology, function, and biomedical applications of exosomes. *Science* 2020;367(6478): eaau6977.
78. Baldwin M, Snelling S, Dakin S, Carr A: Augmenting endogenous repair of soft tissues with nanofibre scaffolds. *J R Soc Interface* 2018;15(141):20180019.
79. Murray MM, Fleming BC, Badger GJ, et al: Bridge-enhanced anterior cruciate ligament repair is not inferior to autograft anterior cruciate ligament reconstruction at 2 years: Results of a prospective randomized clinical trial. *Am J Sports Med* 2020;48(6):1305-1315.
80. Kopec AK, Yokokawa R, Khan N, et al: Microphysiological systems in early stage drug development: Perspectives on current applications and future impact. *J Toxicol Sci* 2021;46(3):99-114.
81. Beredjiklian PK: Biologic aspects of flexor tendon laceration and repair. *J Bone Joint Surg Am* 2003;85(3):539-550.
82. Chamberlain CS, Clements AEB, Kink JA, et al: Extracellular vesicle-educated macrophages promote early Achilles tendon healing. *Stem Cell* 2019;37(5):652-662.
83. Kornicka-Garbowska K, Pędziwiatr R, Woźniak P, Kucharczyk K, Marycz K: Microvesicles isolated from 5-azacytid ine-and-resveratrol-treated mesenchymal stem cells for the treatment of suspensory ligament injury in horse – A case report. *Stem Cell Res Ther* 2019;10(1):394.
84. Shi Z, Wang Q, Jiang D: Extracellular vesicles from bone marrow-derived multipotent mesenchymal stromal cells regulate inflammation and enhance tendon healing. *J Transl Med* 2019;17(1):211.
85. Lee DK: A preliminary study on the effects of acellular tissue graft augmentation in acute Achilles tendon ruptures. *J Foot Ankle Surg* 2008;47(1):8-12.
86. Wang Y, He G, Guo Y, et al: Exosomes from tendon stem cells promote injury tendon healing through balancing synthesis and degradation of the tendon extracellular matrix. *J Cell Mol Med* 2019;23(8):5475-5485.
87. Shi Y, Kang X, Wang Y, et al: Exosomes derived from Bone Marrow Stromal Cells (BMSCs) enhance tendon-bone healing by regulating macrophage polarization. *Med Sci Mon Int Med J Exp Clin Res* 2020;26:e923328.
88. Wang C, Hu Q, Song W, Yu W, He Y: Adipose stem cell–derived exosomes decrease fatty infiltration and enhance rotator cuff healing in a rabbit model of chronic tears. *Am J Sports Med* 2020;48(6):1456-1464.
89. Yu H, Cheng J, Shi W, et al: Bone marrow mesenchymal stem cell-derived exosomes promote tendon regeneration by facilitating the proliferation and migration of endogenous tendon stem/progenitor cells. *Acta Biomater* 2020;106:328-341.
90. Docheva D, Müller SA, Majewski M, Evans CH: Biologics for tendon repair. *Adv Drug Deliv Rev* 2015;84:222-239.
91. Immordino ML, Dosio F, Cattel L: Stealth liposomes: review of the basic science, rationale, and clinical applications, existing and potential. *Int J Nanomed* 2006;1(3):297-315.
92. Lou J, Tu Y, Burns M, Silva MJ, Manske P: BMP-12 gene transfer augmentation of lacerated tendon repair. *J Orthop Res* 2001;19(6):1199-1202.
93. Bolt P, Clerk AN, Luu HH, et al: BMP-14 gene therapy increases tendon tensile strength in a rat model of Achilles tendon injury. *J Bone Joint Surg Am* 2007;89(6):1315-1320.
94. Delalande A, Gosselin MP, Suwalski A, et al: Enhanced Achilles tendon healing by fibromodulin gene transfer. *Nanomed Nanotechnol Biol Med* 2015;11(7):1735-1744.
95. Suwalski A, Dabboue H, Delalande A, et al: Accelerated Achilles tendon healing by PDGF gene delivery with mesoporous silica nanoparticles. *Biomaterials* 2010:31(19):5237-5245.
96. Zhou YL, Yang QQ, Yan YY, et al: Gene-loaded nanoparticle-coated sutures provide effective gene delivery to enhance tendon healing. *Mol Ther* 2019;27(9):1534-1546.
97. Cámara-Torres M, Sinha R, Mota C, Moroni L: Improving cell distribution on 3D additive manufactured scaffolds through engineered seeding media density and viscosity. *Acta Biomater* 2020;101:183-195.

98. Hirooka A, Yoneda M, Wakaitani S, et al: Augmentation with a Gore-Tex patch for repair of large rotator cuff tears that cannot be sutured. *J Orthop Sci* 2002;7(4):451-456.

99. Encalada-Diaz I, Cole BJ, MacGillivray JD, et al: Rotator cuff repair augmentation using a novel polycarbonate polyurethane patch: preliminary results at 12 months' follow-up. *J Shoulder Elbow Surg* 2011. 20(5):788-794.

100. Nada AN, Debnath UK, Robinson DA, Jordan C: Treatment of massive rotator-cuff tears with a polyester ligament (Dacron) augmentation: clinical outcome. *J Bone Joint Surg Br* 2010;92(10):1397-1402.

101. Sporsheim AN, Gifstad T, Lundemo TO, et al: Autologous BPTB ACL reconstruction results in lower failure rates than ACL repair with and without synthetic augmentation at 30 years of follow-up: A prospective randomized study. *J Bone Joint Surg Am* 2019;101(23):2074-2081.

102. Nicholson GP, Breur GJ, Van Sickle D, Yao JQ, Kim J, Blanchard CR: Evaluation of a cross-linked acellular porcine dermal patch for rotator cuff repair augmentation in an ovine model. *J Shoulder Elbow Surg* 2007;16(5 suppl):S184-S190.

CHAPTER

9 Summary and Perspectives

Edward M. Schwarz, PhD • Christopher H. Evans, PhD • Robert E. Guldberg, PhD

INTRODUCTION

The field of orthobiologics has reached its third decade and remains focused on the development of amalgamated products that combine cells, growth factors, and scaffolds into tissue engineering solutions for the treatment of musculoskeletal injury and disease. The significance of orthobiologics continues to be evident in the great demand for treatment strategies that can ameliorate illnesses that range from birth defects to degenerative changes caused by injuries and aging, for which standards of care remain unproven and offer limited benefit. Although there have been several advances in the field, transformative orthobiologic solutions for the most challenging musculoskeletal problems remain elusive because of the lack of understanding of disease pathogenesis, the absence of predictive models and translational outcome measures, the limitations of tissue engineering approaches, and the demands for regulatory approval and cost-effectiveness in the era of health. It has also been argued that the broad use of unproven orthobiologic products in clinical practice has set the field back. Thus, various subfields of orthobiologics have emerged to facilitate focus on problems specific to a particular musculoskeletal tissue or disease, which often involves novel tools of discovery.

KEY THEMES AND PERSPECTIVES WITHIN ORTHOBIOLOGICS

Research studies on stem/progenitor cell therapies have been transformed by single-cell mRNA sequencing, spatial transcriptomics, and in vivo lineage tracing technologies that allow for rigorous characterization of the starting material and assessment of in vivo functional potential. The chapters in this section highlight these advances in the authors' understanding of how stem/progenitor cells participate in autologous and paracrine roles to mediate musculoskeletal tissue development, repair, and regeneration and how their absence and dysfunction from chronic inflammation and aging lead to a lack of healing and fibrosis. Additionally, with these technologies, there may finally be a way to derive a dose for stem/progenitor cell therapy, which is critical for rigor, reproducibility, regulatory approval, and addressing the demands of evidence-based medicine.

In addition to studies with new proteins, research on growth factors for orthobiologics has markedly expanded in recent years based on the clinical success of novel delivery methods. As described in the chapters in this section, these new approaches include the same recombinant viral vectors and mRNA lipid nanoparticles used as vaccines for coronavirus disease 2019 (COVID-19). Another approach to provide signals for biologic tissue repair and regeneration that is becoming more common is the use of endosomes generated from mesenchymal stem cells (MSCs). There is also a new appreciation that tissue growth and differentiation can be stimulated by the inhibition of endogenous inhibitors (eg, sclerostin, noggin, dickkopf) with antibodies, receptor antagonists, and small interfering RNA.

Because nanotechnologies have matured, advances in orthobiologic biomaterials have extended well beyond toxicity, biocompatibility, and durability. Current research now focuses on hypotaxis, durotaxis, osteoinduction, and biointegration of various composite biomaterials. There have also been breakthroughs in personalized three-dimensional printing of metals and cells. The chapters in this section describe these current technologies as well as scaffold coatings to well-established biomaterials, to engender them with antimicrobial properties and improve biointegration.

Because in vivo proof of concept is a critical step toward clinical translation of orthobiologics, there have been major advances in animal models for specific orthopaedic indications. Indeed, the importance of this work is evidenced by the establishment of subresearch groups

Dr. Schwarz or an immediate family member is a member of a speakers' bureau or has made paid presentations on behalf of Asahi KASEI Pharma Corporation; serves as a paid consultant to or is an employee of Asahi KASEI Pharma Corporation, DePuy, A Johnson & Johnson Company, Integrated Biotechnology, MedImmune, Musculoskeletal Transplant Foundation, and Regeneron; has stock or stock options held in Parvizi Surgical Innovations, LLC and Telephus Biosciences; has received research or institutional support from DePuy, A Johnson & Johnson Company, Eli Lilly, and Telephus; and has received nonincome support (such as equipment or services), commercially derived honoraria, or other non–research-related funding (such as paid travel) from Telephus Biosciences. Dr. Evans or an immediate family member serves as a paid consultant to or is an employee of Cellastra Inc., L&J Inc., and Orthogen AG and has stock or stock options held in Cellastra Inc., Genascence Inc., Orthogen AG, and TissueGene. Dr. Guldberg or an immediate family member serves as a board member, owner, officer, or committee member of Restor3D, MiMedx, Penderia Technologies, Huxley Medical, and the Knight Cancer Institute.

within international societies (eg, the Preclinical Models Section of the Orthopaedic Research Society) and evolving requirements to comply with new regulations on the ethical use of animals for research. As such, each chapter of this text articulates the state-of-the-art in vivo model for a particular orthobiologic, and their intended purpose from initial proof of concept in small animal models (mice, rats), through Investigational New Drug/Investigational Device Exemption enabling large animal studies (dogs, sheep, horses).

Randomized controlled clinical trials are the only level I evidence to support the safety and efficacy of orthobiologics. Because the costs in time, money, labor, and numbers of human subjects needed for prospective statistical outcomes are prohibitive for many desired treatment strategies, a subfield of research has emerged on the biomarkers of clinical outcomes. The chapters in this section describe some of these surrogate outcome measures of pain, function, and musculoskeletal repair obtained from real-world experience (eg, clinical registries) and prospective clinical pilots, which serve to better understand clinical response to treatment and reduce risk in new orthobiologics. Most notable is the use of at-home wearable devices that connect to electronic medical records from personal smartphones, which now allow for 24-hour data collection in real time, and the potential to introduce telehealth interventions as an adjuvant to orthobiologic therapy.

Delivery is a major challenge when using proteins such as growth factors and morphogens to regenerate damaged tissues or modulate pathophysiologic processes. Because most proteins of interest in the orthobiologic context are rapidly cleared from the site of application, they often do not persist long enough to have a meaningful beneficial effect. Gene transfer has been suggested as a means of overcoming this limitation. Under this strategy, genes, usually as their cDNA equivalents encoding the gene product of interest, are transferred to the site of disease or tissue damage. Here the encoded protein is synthesized endogenously for an extended period. In addition to enabling long-term persistence, gene transfer delivers a product that has undergone posttranslational modification and is presented by the genetically modified cells in a biologically authentic manner, thereby enhancing its potency. If the mode of gene delivery is ex vivo, gene therapy can be combined with cell therapy. In this context, the use of genetically modified MSCs is being evaluated in preclinical models. A variety of different viral and nonviral vectors are available for gene transfer, each with its own idiosyncratic properties. In general, viral vectors are more efficient, but nonviral vectors are considered to be safer and less expensive.

In recent years, the FDA has given marketing approval to the first gene therapies. None of these addresses orthopaedic conditions, but progress in preclinical research suggests that gene-based orthobiologics will become available within the next 5 years or so. Several clinical trials targeting osteoarthritis have been initiated and industry involvement is growing. Although gene therapy has made considerable progress in overcoming earlier safety and expression issues that impeded its path to the clinic, viral vector manufacture and cost have emerged as more recent bottlenecks that slow progress.

The scope of gene therapy can be expanded to include the use of RNA to enhance or inhibit the synthesis of specific gene products, and the first experimental applications using RNA in an orthopaedic context have been reported. Gene editing also holds enormous potential, but its orthopaedic applications are just beginning to be investigated.

Regardless of the modality, novel orthobiologics need to be evaluated for safety and efficacy in animal models before they can receive marketing approval from the FDA. The choice of animal model is crucial and often rate limiting for the development of the product. Murine models are very appealing in terms of cost, availability, housing, and, importantly, the existence of a wide range of genetically modified animals. Because it is possible to perform experiments involving large numbers of animals, considerable statistical power can be obtained. However, mice are too small for certain surgical procedures, their growth plates never close, and, in the context of regenerative orthopaedics, they heal much better than humans, resulting in false optimism. It is highly probable that a novel orthobiologic will need to be tested in a large animal at some stage during its development. A variety of such animals are available, each with their idiosyncratic advantages and disadvantages. Because they are companion animals, dogs are used less and less frequently. Certain anatomic and physiologic properties of pigs have much in common with those of humans, and the development of minipigs to address size issues has led to their increasing use in preclinical testing. Sheep and goats are also popular for studies of surgically induced osteoarthritis or the regeneration of the bone, tendon, ligament, cartilage, and meniscus. Horses, although expensive and cumbersome, are of particular use for studies of cartilage repair and osteoarthritis because the thickness of the articular cartilage is similar to that of humans and horses develop osteoarthritis idiopathically, as occurs clinically. Many procedures used in human medicine, such as arthroscopy, can be performed in horses. Moreover, horses are often athletes, an advantage for studies in a sports medicine context.

Cartilage has a deceptively complex microarchitecture that presents challenges for the regeneration of authentic repair tissue. Nevertheless, many procedures are used clinically with successful outcomes; some are strictly surgical. For instance, osteochondral autografting or allografting, analogous in many ways to bone grafting, is usually performed for large defects. Smaller defects are frequently treated by using marrow stimulation techniques, such as microfracture and microdrilling, that facilitate entry of marrow elements into the damaged area. The marrow forms a clot within the lesion, thereby trapping marrow chondroprogenitor cells that differentiate into chondrocytes in situ and help form a cartilaginous repair tissue. Microfracture involves technically straightforward arthroscopic surgery and gives good short-term to medium-term results. However, the repair tissue is not authentic articular cartilage and it eventually fails in many patients. Experimental approaches to improving the quality of the repair cartilage include the use of scaffolds and the addition of platelet-rich plasma or bone marrow concentrate. As an alternative, small pieces of living, juvenile cartilage isolated from transplant donors are commercially available as allograft material for the repair of chondral lesions.

Chondral defects can also be treated with autologous chondrocyte implantation, the first cell therapy approved for use in regenerative orthopaedics. Although successful, it requires two invasive procedures, one to harvest cartilage and the other to implant the autologous chondrocytes grown from it, and the rehabilitation time is long. The use of allogeneic chondrocytes reduces the procedure to a single surgery and the protocol has been simplified by growing the chondrocytes on a scaffold for implantation during matrix-assisted chondrocyte implantation. The use of MSCs instead of chondrocytes is also being explored, in conjunction with various morphogens that direct MSCs into the chondrogenic lineage. Further refinements are under preclinical development, including the implantation of cell spheroids, the use of improved scaffolds, and the inclusion of small molecules to improve outcomes. Gene therapy approaches are also being explored.

Current options for promoting bone regeneration with orthobiologics include the use of a wide range of biomaterials, cells, and growth factors. Although approved for certain applications, delivery of bone-inducing morphogens such as bone morphogenetic protein 2 can produce adverse effects often associated with the use of supraphysiologic doses. Extensive work developing novel biomaterial-mediated sustained delivery systems has shown promise for functional bone regeneration using lower and presumably safer doses; however, these next-generation delivery systems have not yet been translated into clinical use. Patient-specific fabrication of bone repair scaffold biomaterials via three-dimensional printing has been translated into clinical use and may represent a possible future of medical device manufacturing. Other patient-specific factors such as age, diabetes, local vascularization, and immune status should also be considered when selecting treatment options for promoting bone regeneration.

This section also includes an in-depth overview of the basic biology and current state of orthobiologic treatment strategies for both acute and chronic tendon and ligament injuries. Nonsurgical injections of therapeutics to address pain and dysfunction associated with the most commonly injured tendons and ligaments are prevalent in the clinical setting and increasingly guided by rapid advancements in the understanding of cellular and molecular interactions during tendon and ligament development and repair. The long-standing misconception that tendons and ligaments are composed of a uniform population of fibrocytes has been dispelled by recent work identifying a complex mix of cells, including tissue-resident stem cells and macrophages, revealing a rich set of new potential therapeutic targets. Following detailed descriptions of the structure and function of tendons and ligaments, a thorough review of the key regulatory signals during tendon and ligament injury and repair is provided, including insights on current evidence of the efficacy of delivering various growth factors on functional restoration following injury. A comprehensive update on the current status of each of the major classes of orthobiologics (cells, platelet-rich plasma, extracellular vesicles, gene therapy, and bioactive scaffolds) follows. Despite a preponderance of encouraging preclinical and limited clinical data supporting the use of orthobiologics for tendon and ligament repair, commercialization and clinical adoption have been slowed by a combination of regulatory and scientific factors. The difficulty in using animal models that have limited relevance to human patients is highlighted as a key factor and the emergence of human microphysiologic systems proposed as a potential transformative opportunity to more effectively and efficiently translate orthobiologic treatment strategies.

CONCLUSION AND FUTURE OPPORTUNITIES

The "Biologic Options for Tissue Repair and Regeneration" section includes nine chapters covering the primary orthobiologic product classes, animal model considerations, and overviews of the current state-of-the-art applications in cartilage, bone, tendon, and ligament. Recent advances have been enabled by the explosive growth in new fundamental knowledge related to how tissue repair and regeneration processes are regulated and depend on patient-specific factors such as the immune response to injury. Even so, level I evidence to support the safety and efficacy of orthobiologics has remained elusive because of a host of factors, including the high cost of rigorously designed clinical trials. Identification of circulating biomarkers and other surrogate outcome measures may be a key strategy toward truly evidence-based clinical application of orthobiologics. Robust recent federal investments in biomanufacturing offer additional hope for progress through defining critical quality attributes of stem cell and other biologic therapies that are predictive of clinical efficacy. Understanding how batch-to-batch variations in orthobiologic products affect potency may explain inconsistent patient responses and suggest improved biomanufacturing processes to enhance therapeutic efficacy. Innovations in human microphysiologic system testbeds may accelerate the development and testing of orthobiologic treatment strategies by augmenting or, in some cases, replacing animal models known to produce results that are not always translatable to human patients. Although much work remains to be done, efforts to develop and validate effective orthobiologic treatment strategies will continue because of the high prevalence of musculoskeletal pain and disability, the lack of effective treatment options, and patient demands to live life at their peak functional potential.

SECTION

2

Technology Development, Regulation, and the Commercialization Pathway

Section Editors
Scott P. Bruder, MD, PhD, FORS
Anthony Ratcliffe, PhD

CHAPTER 10

Pitfalls in the Assessment of Outcomes in Randomized Clinical Trials

Joseph Harrington, BS • Jennifer Racine-Avila, MBA • Roy K. Aaron, MD, FAAOS, FORS

INTRODUCTION

The progress of a new orthobiologic material or construct through clinical trials and the regulatory process into clinical use requires rigorous testing and high-confidence data. Selected features of the experimental process, describing points of vulnerability that compromise the generation of high-confidence data, are examined. Randomized clinical trials (RCTs), the intention-to-treat (ITT) method of analysis, data acquisition, the selection of scales and scores, and the use of the minimal clinically important difference (MCID) indicating points of vulnerability to bias that can be avoided by good experimental design and protocol adherence are considered.

RANDOMIZED CLINICAL TRIALS

The RCT has, from its inception, been the best-accepted experimental method with which to demonstrate causality and efficacy by resisting biases that can confound conclusions. The structure of the RCT incorporates several techniques to minimize bias. Following good experimental design within the RCT increases confidence that data are unbiased[1,2] (**Figure 1**).

The structure of an RCT offers opportunities for the development of a research plan that is resistant to bias. However, points of vulnerability to the intrusion of bias must be recognized and good protocol construction and adherence are necessary to take best advantage of the RCT structure. Several points of vulnerability and techniques to reinforce the RCT structure are as follows:

1. The creation of the initial state can be a complicated business and the value of the study depends on several considerations. First, there are some clinical circumstances in which it would be unethical or clinically dangerous for the control cohort to be untreated or treated with placebo: for example, venous thromboembolism after joint replacement, where the risk of thromboembolic disease is well established and it would be inappropriate to have an untreated control group. In these circumstances, the experimental treatment would have to be compared with an established treatment. However, it needs to be justified that equipoise prevents a placebo-treated control group. Second, internal validity of a study depends, to a degree, on the homogeneity and comparability of the experimental and control (or comparison) cohorts. Tighter, more cohesive, cohort composition can result in data with less variability and greater statistical significance. However, homogeneous composition can often limit generalizability of the results to populations with different clinical characteristics than those in the study cohorts. In terms of an orthobiologic, this can limit the label claim. Internal validity and generalizability can be at variance with one another and careful consideration has to be given to the balance between them in designing eligibility criteria and cohort composition. Third, the initial state and randomization must demonstrate equivalence of cohorts. Randomization by itself, although useful, does not guarantee equal distribution of risk if known risk factors exist, and stratified randomization that would ensure equal distribution of risk to the study groups could be considered. Ideally, consecutive, or at least a high percentage of, eligible patients would be enrolled in the research study.
2. The relationship of sample size to structural errors needs to be appreciated. A type I, or alpha, error is due to a false-positive result, that is, finding a positive result where none exists. A type II, or beta, error is due to a false-negative result, finding a negative result from positive data. Appropriate sample sizes will minimize both type I and type II errors. Sample size has a well-known relationship to type II errors.[3] A large-enough sample size will minimize type II errors and ensure that negative results are valid. Negative observations can be very meaningful if sample size prevents a type II error. Sample size also has a less commonly considered relationship to type I errors. Statistical significance, in terms of P values, can result in a type I error if the sample size is inappropriately large given the expected effect size and variance. Given enough subjects, any difference can have statistical significance even if the effect size is clinically unimportant[4] (**Table 1**).

None of the following authors or any immediate family member has received anything of value from or has stock or stock options held in a commercial company or institution related directly or indirectly to the subject of this chapter: Joseph Harrington, Jennifer Racine-Avila, and Dr. Aaron.

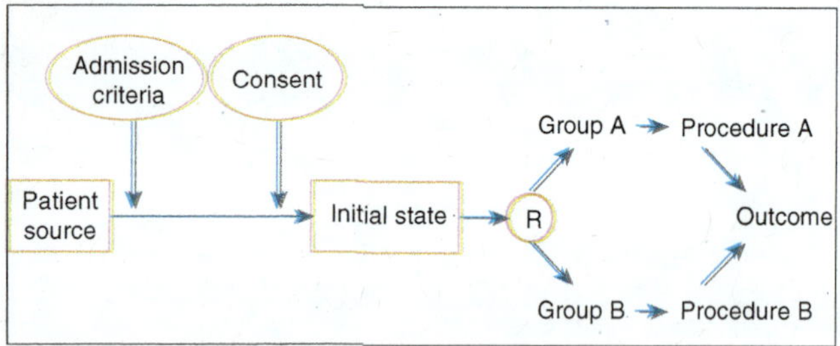

FIGURE 1 Schematic diagram showing the structure of a randomized clinical trial. R = randomization point. (Redrawn with permission from Rudicel S, Esdaile J: The randomized clinical trial in orthopaedics: Obligation or option? *J Bone Joint Surg Am* 1985;67:1284-1293.)

3. Adequate randomization and allocation concealment are often flawed in surgical trials. Subjects crossing over from control to experimental groups must be guarded against and techniques for allocation concealment need to be creative, such as the use of limb stockings to conceal incisions or other visible signs of interventions.
4. Accurate, unbiased assessment of outcomes by blinded, disinterested observers is essential, and treating physicians, including residents, are often not able to provide this. Research nurses or technicians should be considered as evaluators of outcome.
5. Precise assessment of outcomes requires validated, sensitive, and responsive outcome instruments, and a hierarchy of outcomes to avoid multiple assessments or data torturing, that make statistical assessment and clinical relevance difficult.
6. Equal follow-up of control and experimental groups is essential. Missing data are to be avoided. Most importantly, crossovers from the allocated group to another group will confound the ITT analysis.

The structure of an RCT is resistant but not impervious to bias, and RCTs can exhibit susceptibility to the intrusion of inadvertent bias if adherence to the experimental design is flawed.[5] Because the structure of an RCT is susceptible to the intrusion of biases, a biased RCT is particularly pernicious because it can give the appearance of accuracy yet actually convey inaccurate or false information. An RCT depends on adherence to its inherent structural and procedural strengths and good experimental procedures, which can be summarized as protocol adherence. If protocol adherence is high, confidence in results is maintained. Vulnerabilities to bias can be exhibited at several points in the RCT process (**Figure 2**).

FIGURE 2 Schematic diagram shows the points of vulnerability to intrusion of biases. (Redrawn with permission from Rudicel S, Esdaile J: The randomized clinical trial in orthopaedics: Obligation or option? *J Bone Joint Surg Am* 1985;67:1284-1293.)

In this context, bias can be defined as systematic errors in data acquisition or management that degrade confidence in results and decrease internal validity. Bias can be, and often is, unrecognized and inadvertent and can consist of unknown confounding variables. Therefore, avoidance of bias consists of recognizing points of vulnerability of the RCT structure as well as design of, and adherence to, experimental procedures to resist bias (**Table 2**).

Susceptibility or selection bias can occur when the initial cohorts are not equivalent. Attention should be given

TABLE 1 Relationship of Sample Size and *P* Value

Sample Size	*P* Value
20	0.33
200	0.24
2000	0.01
20,000	0.00001

Adapted from Olak J, Chiu R: A surgeon's guide to biostatistical inferences: How to avoid pitfalls, in Troidl H, ed: *Surgical Research*, ed 3. Springer, 1997, p 329.

TABLE 2 Trial Design Elements to Minimize Bias

1. Randomized prospective design with allocation concealment
2. Demonstration of group comparability
3. Adequate sample size, sampling interval, and follow-up with minimal losses
4. Measurement of outcome variables appropriate to the study by blinded, disinterested observers who are unaware of the subjects' treatment
5. Appropriate statistical techniques to demonstrate significance

to characteristics that may influence outcome. However, because biases may not be recognized, ideally consecutive enrollment of eligible subjects, demonstration of cohort equivalency, robust randomization and allocation concealment, and consideration of stratified randomization when risk factors are known should be described. Performance bias can occur when dissimilar skill levels exist in the performance of a procedure or the application of an intervention. In orthobiologics, all investigators should have equal training and comparable skill levels in the management of the intervention and the assessment of outcomes. Detection bias can occur when the methods of measurement of outcomes are dissimilar among experimental groups. This can occur if different observers use subjective criteria, if different criteria are being used, or if the observers are not blinded to the treatment or are not disinterested (ie, they have a stake in the outcome). Transfer bias can occur when there is a differential loss to follow-up among experimental groups. Transfer bias may also be suspected if the loss to follow-up is greater than expected. Are those subjects whose outcomes are not being measured more or less successfully treated than those being assessed? To demonstrate minimal transfer bias in differential or exaggerated loss to follow-up, it is advisable to report the relevant characteristics of subjects whose outcomes are and are not available for analysis.

ITT METHOD OF DATA ANALYSIS

The ITT method of data analysis is most often used to assess the results of RCTs. It analyzes outcomes of subjects according to the group to which they were randomized regardless of whether they underwent the intervention of the randomized group or that of a comparison or control group. Under ideal experimental conditions, the ITT method preserves the randomization scheme. However, under circumstances of poor protocol adherence, especially a substantial number of subjects being treated in a group other than the one to which they were randomized (crossovers), the ITT method actually measures allocation or *assignment* to interventions but indicates little about the efficacy of the intervention.[6,7]

The problem of research subjects not receiving the treatment to which they were randomized is a problem for ITT analysis and is common in orthopaedic RCTs; for example, they may cross over to another group. The problem of crossovers has been encountered in 26% of total knee arthroplasties, 43% to 57% of spine surgeries, 39% of anterior cruciate ligament reconstructions, and 25% to 30% of meniscectomies.[8]

The ITT method preserves randomization and minimizes false-positive (type I) errors, preventing overestimation of clinical efficacy. However, the ITT method tends to minimize differences in the effects of interventions, which tends to make two interventions appear similar and dilutes the intervention difference of interest. Objections to the ITT method arise when there is a lack of protocol adherence because the ITT method ignores noncompliance and protocol deviations that occur after randomization. First, considering a subject to have undergone treatment when in fact they did not indicates very little about the efficacy of treatment; second, outcome data can differ markedly among compliant and noncompliant subjects, and among subjects who withdraw; and third, the problems in analysis are compounded by subjects crossing over into another intervention.[7,9]

In a 2013 study of knee arthroscopy study with 29% crossovers, the ITT analysis showed no difference between surgically and nonsurgically treated groups, but an as-treated analysis of the same data showed superiority of the surgical treatment.[10] Other analytic methods, including the as-treated and per-protocol methods, may provide more relevant information about treatment efficacy but compromise randomization, allowing greater selection bias, because crossovers may have different characteristics from the randomized cohort and usually overestimate the value of treatment (**Figure 3**).

If protocol adherence is high, the ITT method is considered the most accurate largely because it preserves

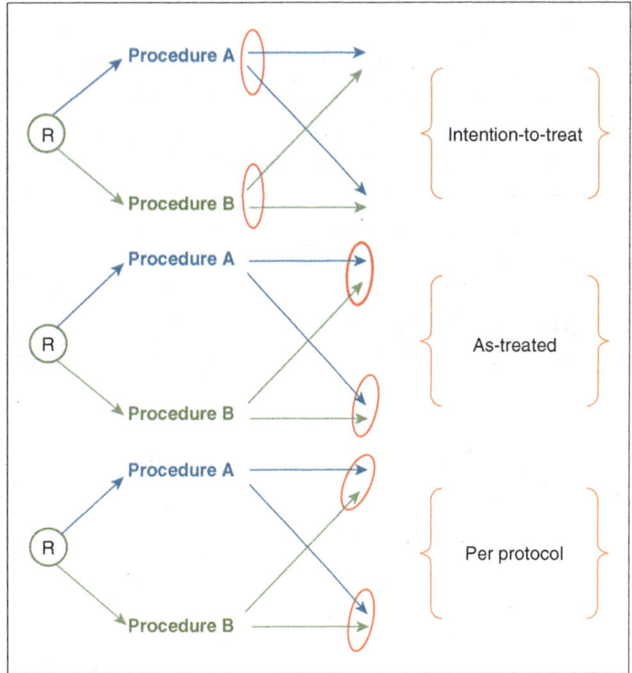

FIGURE 3 Schematic diagram shows the alternative methods of outcome assessment. Ovals indicate points of analysis. Intention-to-treat method: Analysis is according to randomization. As-treated method: Assesses data from subjects according to treatment actually received and assumes comparability between compliers and noncompliers. Per protocol method: Assesses data from subjects who complete the trial as originally randomized and may introduce selection bias because the randomization scheme is violated.

randomization and, therefore, the equivalency of the cohorts. However, the utility of the ITT method also depends on good protocol adherence, especially compliance with the basic assumption of ITT, and that subjects remain in their assigned groups and undergo the intervention to which they are randomized. The fidelity of the investigator to maintaining the randomized cohorts as constructed is essential.

In summary, the responsibilities of investigators performing RCTs with good protocol adherence are as follows: (1) Create relevant eligibility criteria and enroll a high percentage of subjects who meet those criteria in the study. The numbers of eligible subjects and the number enrolled should be specified. (2) Equivalency of the initial cohorts should be ensured and reported. (3) Sample sizes should be appropriate to avoid both type I and II errors. (4) Subjects should be treated equally except for the experimental variable and performance bias should be avoided. (5) Ensure blinding of outcome assessment as described. (6) Maintain adherence to group assignment and robust and equal follow-up between, or among, experimental groups. Rigorously avoid subjects crossing from the assigned group to another.

PLANNING THE ACQUISITION AND MANAGEMENT OF DATA

A data analysis plan should be part of the experimental protocol and statistical consultation should be sought at the writing of the protocol. An appropriate hierarchy of outcome measures should be planned considering the interests of regulatory agencies. A data hierarchy will prevent multiple outcomes that will present conceptual and statistical problems at the end of the study. However, it is important to also consider that outcome instruments can represent differing outcome domains such as pain and function. In addition, although patient-reported outcomes (PROs) are desirable, biologic or mechanical outcomes may add important objective information to the assessment of outcome. For example, in studies of arthritis of the knee, the Knee injury and Osteoarthritis Outcome Score may be a primary outcome measure, but there are also PROs of function that represent complementary information. Objectively measured functional domains of importance such as range of motion or strength, and biologic measurements such as joint fluid cytokine concentration or cartilage scores, also yield important information. Therefore, a data hierarchy must be carefully considered, planned, and specified. The influence of multiple analyses without a data hierarchy[11] is shown in **Table 3**. Multiple nonhierarchical analyses will result in the possibility of false-positive results that have to be dealt with statistically as with the Bonferroni correction but can be avoided by recognizing that different outcome domains can be analyzed and reported separately.

TABLE 3 Independent Analysis and False-Positive Results[a]

Number of Analyses	Likelihood of One False-Positive Result[a]
1	0.05
2	0.10
3	0.14
5	0.23
10	0.40
15	0.54

[a]Each analysis is done with a *P* value of 0.05. The formula used to calculate the likelihood of a false-positive result is $1 - (0.95)^n$, where n is the number of analyses.

Reproduced with permission from Laupacis A, Rorabeck CH, Bourne RB, Feeny D, Tugwell P, Sim DA: Randomized trials in orthopaedics: Why, how, and when? *J Bone Joint Surg Am* 1989;71(4):535-543.

The investigator should anticipate whether the data will be continuous or categorical (binary) and plan statistical tests accordingly. Continuous data are easily managed by tests such as the Student *t*-test, whereas categorical data are best tested by the chi-square or Fisher exact test. Other more sophisticated statistical tests such as regression analysis, multivariate analysis, and analysis of variance are available for complex data. Once data are produced, it should be tested for normality with one of the several equations such as the Kolmogorov-Smirnov equation. Statistical tests should be appropriate to parametric (normal) or nonparametric data. Consultation with a statistician at the writing of the research protocol is strongly advised.

The data analysis plan must consider clinical versus statistical significance. Statistical significance is a function of effect size, variability, and sample size and can be influenced by each. An apparent effect, such as differences in serum electrolyte concentration, can be made to appear statistically significant with large sample sizes and small variability, but may be clinically insignificant. However, clinical significance may vary by perceptions of the patient and the observer.

SCALES AND SCORES

It is essential that clinical measurement instruments appropriate to the hypothesis posed, and the data generated, be used to assess the outcome of clinical trials. Using an inappropriate measurement instrument can bias the outcome, yield spurious results, and compromise the true assessment of an intervention. Discussed here are general universal characteristics of measurement instruments by their structure (anatomy) and function (physiology).

Reporting the key characteristics of a measuring instrument increases the confidence that the results being reported have been appropriately measured by responsive, reliable, and valid techniques.

Scale Anatomy

Clinical scales are designed to measure specific aspects of health status. Some scales measure general health assessment (Medical Outcomes Study 36-Item Short Form); others measure specific disease status (Western Ontario and McMaster Universities Osteoarthritis Index for arthritis); and others assess anatomic function (Knee injury and Osteoarthritis Outcome Score). Although there are some shared assessments (eg, pain scores), each type of scoring system gives complementary overall information and, although several types may be used in assessing outcome, the hierarchy of assessment is advantageous to focus assessment on the most important features yet capture other health information as secondary outcomes.

A scale can serve several functions, with the three most common being prediction, description, or evaluation.[12] Predictive scales assess prognosis and describe disease stages. They are useful for categorizing treatment effects according to the severity of disease. Descriptive scales measure differences in populations at a fixed period. Evaluative scales measure change over time and are useful for assessing the effects of treatment interventions. All scales must have appropriate range to encompass status and change. A scale attenuation effect occurs when the scale measurement range is inappropriate to the status or effects being measured. Two types of attenuation effects can occur: ceiling and floor effects. Ceiling effects limit the ability of a scale to accurately detect high values. Floor effects occur when a measuring scale has a lower limit to the data values it can reliably measure. The range of a scale must be permissive to detect both improvement or deterioration. If subjects cluster at the upper or lower limits of a scale before intervention, the scale may not be able to detect improvement or deterioration, respectively.

Scale Physiology

Clinical measuring instruments have functional characteristics that are important to understand so that the range of available measurements, the increments of measurement, and the reproducibility of the measurement are appropriate to the quantity (data element) being measured. Data can easily be lost or misrepresented if the measuring scale is inappropriate in these ways. Several definitions are important to consider in the selection of outcome instruments. Reliability and repeatability are concepts that reflect the measurement of an outcome to predictable and reproducible degrees. Three features of scale function are reproducibility, responsiveness, and validity.[13,14] Reproducibility denotes that measurements should be the same on repeated tests in nonchanging subjects. Reproducible scales have minimal interobserver and intraobserver variability. Reliable scales exhibit high test–retest reproducibility. Responsiveness is the degree to which a scale is able to detect a change in the outcome parameters. The scale should measure change in changing subjects and no change in stable subjects. Validity expresses the property of a scale to measure what it is designed to measure. Some key features of validity that are important to note are as follows:[14]

- Content validity indicates that the measurement reflects the content domain of what is being measured.
- Construct validity indicates that empirical tests confirm theoretical concepts (constructs).
- Face validity is an assessment of whether a measurement appears to be appropriate.
- Criterion validity indicates that the measurement reflects other, related assessments.

Scale Confidence

Confidence in a scale encompasses reliability and repeatability, properties of measuring outcomes in a reproducible metric.[14] Confidence is described in **Figure 4** as the precision of tests. **Table 4** contains a glossary of terms related to scale confidence.

THE MINIMAL CLINICALLY IMPORTANT DIFFERENCE

For research and development applications, it can be advantageous to report outcomes in binary or categorical terms that represent the success or failure of an experimental intervention. To be most useful on a patient level, the outcomes should reflect clinically meaningful changes that are reported by the patient to represent a successful or unsuccessful intervention. PRO measures express clinically meaningful outcomes usually as continuous scales

	Disease Present	Disease Absent
Test positive (abnormal)	True positive	False positive
Test negative (normal)	False negative	True negative

$$\text{Sensitivity} = \frac{TP}{TP + FN} \qquad \text{PPV} = \frac{TP}{TP + FP}$$

$$\text{Specificity} = \frac{TN}{TN + FP} \qquad \text{NPV} = \frac{TN}{TN + FN}$$

FIGURE 4 Schematic diagram shows the precision of tests. FN = false negative, FP = false positive, NPV = negative predictive value, PPV = positive predictive value, TN = true negative, TP = true positive

TABLE 4 Confidence Descriptors

Assessment	Definitions
Precision	Similar to test–retest reliability, precision is the property of a scale to have the same or very similar result on repeated measurements.
Accuracy	This is the ability of a measurement to represent the quantity under evaluation.
Sensitivity	The degree to which a measuring instrument is able to detect an event under evaluation (true positive). A sensitive test will cast a wide net and detect an event at the cost of inclusion of nonevents (false positive). Sensitive tests are useful as screening instruments because they are likely to detect the events being screened for.
Specificity	The ability of a measuring instrument to detect and exclude negative events (true negative). A measurement of high specificity will detect a high percentage of events at the cost of excluding a few (false negative).
ROC curve	Developed during World War II to assess the precision of radar operators to detect true events (aircraft) from false events (birds), receiver operating characteristic (ROC) curves relate sensitivity versus specificity and create a graph in which the area under the curve (concordance or, C-index) is a representation of the accuracy of a measurement.
Positive predictive value	This is the value of a positive finding on a measurement instrument. It expresses the likelihood that a positive event is accurately detected.
Negative predictive value	This is the value of a negative finding on a measurement and expresses the likelihood that a negative result accurately reflects the absence of an event.

with no definitive criteria for success/failure. One way of transforming PRO measures to binary or categorical scales is with the MCID, which reflects important clinical changes and can indicate success or failure of an experimental intervention.[15]

The concept of MCID was first proposed in 1989 and defined as "the smallest difference in score, within the domain of interest, which patients perceive as beneficial and which would mandate, in the absence of troublesome side effects and excessive costs, a change in a patient's management."[16] Three general methods have been used to calculate MCID: (1) distribution-based methods, which rely on the variability of the data; (2) anchor-based methods, which compare changes in scores with an anchor reference question; and (3) the consensus method, which relies on experts to reach a consensus regarding the MCID value.

Distribution-based methods are statistical methods that measure the variability of an element within a sample. Standard error of measurement, minimal detectable difference (MDD), 0.5 SD, and effect size are a few of the elements within the distribution-based approaches. Although distribution-based methods ensure statistical significance of an MCID value, they do not address clinical importance. Distribution-based methods are additionally limited by their ability to define only a minimal value below which a change in outcome score for a given measure may be due to measurement error. Conceptual frameworks require that the MDD be less than the MCID. An MCID that is smaller than an MDD should not be considered a valid estimate.[17] Distribution-based MCIDs and MDDs tend to be lower than anchor-based MCIDs and only anchor-based MCIDs represent clinical relevance.

Anchor-based methods compare changes in the outcome from baseline to an external criterion standard, or anchor, that represents the subject's perspective. Types of anchors are (1) patient's global impression of change that reflects a patient's rating of overall improvement, (2) patient global assessment, and (3) transition questions.[18] The two primary variations of anchor-based approaches are (1) the within-patients score change and (2) the between-patients score change. Within-patients score change defines MCID as the change in PRO scores of a group of patients selected according to their answers to an assessment scale.[19] Between-patients score change compares the scores or the PRO chance scores of groups of patients with different responses to an assessment scale. The application of different anchors may produce different values of the MCID. Whether data collection of the anchor was prospective, retrospective, or how well the anchor captures a patient's true response, all produce various MCID values.

The consensus method, similar to a Delphi method, uses a panel of experts to provide independent assessments of what constitutes a clinically relevant change.[10] Assessments are revised until the panel reaches a consensus for the MCID value. The consensus method uses clinical experts, rather than patients, to define the MCID. Expert opinions may not be a valid way to determine what the patients perceive as important.

Integrative methods add mathematical rigor to the anchor-based method using a receiver operating characteristic curve and have the advantage of maintaining clinical representation but using the receiver operating characteristic curve to enhance precision. They have the advantage over anchor only–based methods by accounting for the variability of the sample and have the advantage over distribution-based methods of having clinical relevance.

Early studies suggested that the MCID was a singular quantity. However, subsequent studies demonstrated differences among reported MCID values for the same outcomes and showed that MCIDs are, in fact, not singular values and are not necessarily comparable among studies.[17,20-22] Comparisons of MCIDs among studies are difficult because (1) there are many methods of calculating the MCID; (2) the MCID calculations depend on factors extrinsic to the calculation such as subject characteristics, including socioeconomic status, mental health, and social support, and disease type and severity; and (3) the estimates of the MCID depend on a variety of methodologic factors intrinsic to the calculations that affect both the magnitude and the precision of the estimate. These observations indicate the need for caution when interpreting the MCID, especially when it is used to compare studies or populations because of the variety of factors that can influence the MCID. It is advisable for clinical studies to calculate and present their individual MCIDs and not rely on published values.

SUMMARY: STUDY ARCHITECTURE TO MAXIMIZE CONFIDENCE AND MINIMIZE BIAS

The purpose of clinical research and its presentation is to convince the readers to alter their clinical practice patterns, in the case of orthobiologics, to use a new or different approach or device. This conviction is based on the appreciation by the reader of high-confidence data and evidence-based conclusions. Systematic errors, confounding elements, and methodologic flaws introduce bias that degrades confidence in the data and weakens the commitment to change. For the investigator, important data require a suitable study structure and adherence to protocol. Some characteristics of clinical studies that result in high-confidence data are as follows:

1. Creation of a hierarchy of outcomes based on preclinical data and intended label claims.
2. Selection of appropriate outcome instruments with documentation of their relevant characteristics—range, responsiveness, etc.
3. Design of entry study elements including eligibility criteria, appropriate sample size, and suitable criteria for success/failure.
4. Formation of study cohorts and tactics for randomization and allocation concealment. Documentation of equivalence of initial control and experimental cohorts is essential to avoiding selection bias. Other attributes of the initial cohort state include an appropriate control group and enrollment of a suitable percentage of eligible, consenting subjects—ideally consecutive—to minimize selection bias.
5. Application of experimental intervention without performance bias.
6. Maintenance of adherence to the experimental protocol. Subject retention and follow-up are essential to prevent data loss and transfer bias. Crossovers from one initial cohort to another group must be prevented to permit high-confidence data analysis.
7. Blinded assessment of results by disinterested observers will minimize detection bias.
8. Data analysis by appropriate statistical tests can be enhanced by understanding the characteristics of the outcome data and by the consultation with a knowledgeable statistician.
9. Conclusions must be based on the evidence generated, highlighting the importance of experimental design and protocol adherence.

REFERENCES

1. Rudicel S, Esdaile J: The randomized clinical trial in orthopaedics: Obligation or option? *J Bone Joint Surg Am* 1985;67(8):1284-1293.
2. Aaron J, Racine-Avila J: *Randomized Controlled Trials: Structure and Management of Bias. Principles of Clinical Research Learn ORS Module*, Orthopaedic Research Society, 2020. https://www.ors.org/learnors-clinical-research/.
3. Freedman KB, Bernstein J: Sample size and statistical power in clinical orthopaedic research. *J Bone Joint Surg Am* 1999;81(10):1454-1460.
4. Olak J, Chiu R: A surgeon's guide to biostatistical inferences: How to avoid pitfalls, in Troidl H, ed: *Surgical Research*, ed 3. Springer, 2007, p 329.
5. Cowan J, Lozano-Calderón S, Ring D: Quality of prospective controlled randomized trials. Analysis of trials of treatment for lateral epicondylitis as an example. *J Bone Joint Surg Am* 2007;89(8):1693-1699.
6. Bang H, Davis CE: On estimating treatment effects under non-compliance in randomized clinical trials: Are intent-to-treat or instrumental variables analyses perfect solutions? *Stat Med* 2007;26(5):954-964.
7. Forbes SP, Aaron RK, Trikalinos TA: Bounding the implications of noncompliance in randomized controlled trials in orthopaedics: An example in arthroscopic surgery. *J Am Acad Orthop Surg* 2022;30(1):e25-e33.
8. Katz JN, Wright J, Spindler KP, et al: Predictors and outcomes of crossover to surgery from physical therapy for meniscal tear and osteoarthritis: A randomized trial comparing physical therapy and surgery. *J Bone Joint Surg Am* 2016;98(22):1890-1896. Erratum in: *J Bone Joint Surg Am* 2018;100(14):e100.
9. Gupta SK: ntention-to-treat concept: A review. *Perspect Clin Res* 2011;2(3):109-112.
10. Katz JN, Brophy RH, Chaisson CE, et al: Surgery versus physical therapy for a meniscal tear and osteoarthritis. *N Engl J Med* 2013;368(18):1675-1684.
11. Laupacis A, Rorabeck CH, Bourne RB, Feeny D, Tugwell P, Sim DA: Randomized trials in orthopaedics: Why, how, and when? *J Bone Joint Surg Am* 1989;71(4):535-543.

12. Schechter M: Sensitivity specificity and predictive value, in Troidl H, McKneally M, Mulder D, et al, ed: *Surgical Research*, ed 3. Springer, 1998, pp 258-276.
13. Charlson M, Johnson N, Williams P, et al: Scaling, scoring and staging, in Troídl H, McKneally M, Mulder D, et al, ed: *Surgical Research*, ed 3. Springer, 1998, pp 271-281.
14. Gagnier J: Principles of Clinical Studies, in Aaron R, ed: *Orthopedic Basic Science*, ed 5. Wolters Kluwer, 2021, pp 512-513.
15. Molino J, Harrington J, Racine-Avila J, Aaron R: Deconstructing the Minimum Clinically Important Difference (MCID). *Orthop Res Rev* 2022;14:35-42.
16. Jaeschke R, Singer J, Guyatt GH: Measurement of health status. Ascertaining the minimal clinically important difference. *Control Clin Trials* 1989;10(4):407-415.
17. Lyman S, Lee YY, McLawhorn AS, Islam W, MacLean CH: What are the minimal and substantial improvements in the HOOS and KOOS and JR versions after total joint replacement? *Clin Orthop Relat Res* 2018;476(12):2432-2441.
18. Katz NP, Paillard FC, Ekman E: Determining the clinical importance of treatment benefits for interventions for painful orthopedic conditions. *J Orthop Surg Res* 2015;10:24.
19. Copay AG, Glassman SD, Subach BR, Berven S, Schuler TC, Carreon LY: Minimum clinically important difference in lumbar spine surgery patients: A choice of methods using the Oswestry Disability Index, Medical Outcomes Study questionnaire Short Form 36, and pain scales. *Spine J* 2008;8(6):968-974.
20. Monticone M, Ferrante S, Salvaderi S, Motta L, Cerri C: Responsiveness and minimal important changes for the Knee Injury and Osteoarthritis Outcome Score in subjects undergoing rehabilitation after total knee arthroplasty. *Am J Phys Med Rehabil* 2013;92(10):864-870.
21. Paulsen A, Roos EM, Pedersen AB, Overgaard S: Minimal clinically important improvement (MCII) and patient-acceptable symptom state (PASS) in total hip arthroplasty (THA) patients 1 year postoperatively. *Acta Orthop* 2014;85(1):39-48.
22. Kuo AC, Giori NJ, Bowe TR, et al: Comparing methods to determine the minimal clinically important differences in patient-reported outcome measures for veterans undergoing elective total hip or knee arthroplasty in veterans health administration hospitals. *JAMA Surg* 2020;155(5):404-411.

CHAPTER 11

Measuring and Reporting Outcomes

Joel J. Gagnier, ND, MSc, PhD • Matthew J. Hadad, MD • Nicolas S. Piuzzi, MD • Evangeline Fumina Kobayashi, MD

INTRODUCTION

Orthobiologics, including cell-based therapies, stem and progenitor cells, growth factors, plasma-derived products, and bone graft, are used in orthopaedic surgery to promote bone and soft-tissue healing. Both experimental and observational studies are used to evaluate orthobiologic products. Key structural, physiologic, and functional outcomes from various studies are summarized. An updated summary of the study designs, measurement of outcomes, and outcome reporting methodology used in orthobiologics research is presented.

OVERVIEW OF STUDY DESIGN IN ORTHOBIOLOGICS RESEARCH

Orthobiologics research refers to the investigation of the efficacy and safety of materials of biologic origin that are intended to address musculoskeletal pathology. Examples of orthobiologics include cell-based therapies, stem and progenitor cells, growth factors, plasma-derived products, and bone graft. A common reason to use orthobiologics within orthopaedic surgery is to promote bone healing, specifically to supplement a deficient aspect of the bone healing process, which comprises osteogenic cells, osteoconductive scaffolds, growth factors, and the mechanical environment, collectively described as the "Diamond Concept."[1] Orthobiologics may also be used to promote the healing of cartilage, ligaments, tendons, and muscles within a variety of degenerative or traumatic conditions.

In the United States, the FDA regulates the use of orthobiologics. It is important for clinicians to understand the processes by which the FDA evaluates and approves orthobiologics for clinical applications. The FDA's authority over biologics is nested in Section 351 of the Public Health Service Act (PHSA) of 1944, with specific regulations delineated in Part 1271 of Title 21 of the Code of Federal Regulations. Section 351 of the PHSA states that a product has a biologic mode of action if "it acts by means of a virus, therapeutic serum, toxin, antitoxin, vaccine, blood, blood component or derivative, allergenic product, or analogous product."[2] An orthobiologic product may or may not be considered a biologic product under Section 351 of the PHSA, depending on its contents and mechanism of action. In addition, Section 361 of the PHSA authorizes the FDA to prevent the transmission and spread of communicable diseases.

If an orthobiologic is not considered to have a biologic mode of action, the orthobiologic is not regulated by Section 351 of the PHSA, and thus it may be regulated under Section 361 of the PHSA alone. To qualify for regulation under Section 361 alone, the product must be minimally manipulated, intended for homologous use only, not combined with another article, and have no systemic effects, with some exceptions.[3] Examples of orthobiologics that may be regulated under Section 361 alone include bone graft, fascia, ligament, and tendon. These products are still regulated in several FDA domains, but formal clinical studies are typically not needed.[4]

Orthobiologics that are deemed to have a biologic mechanism of action under Section 351 of the PHSA are required to undergo the more rigorous FDA premarket and postmarket evaluation. This process begins with laboratory and animal testing to evaluate for the product's safety profile. If determined safe, the orthobiologic may be authorized as an Investigational New Drug (IND). Part 312 of Title 21 of the Code of Federal Regulations delineates the requirements for an IND and the phases of investigation.[5] In brief, phase 1 trials are the first introduction of the IND in healthy humans or patients with the disease of interest in small trials and primarily evaluate for safety and side effects. If phase 1 suggests the IND is safe, phase 2 trials are conducted to evaluate the IND's efficacy to treat a particular condition. If phase 2 trials are suggestive that the IND is effective, the IND may move to phase 3,

Dr. Gagnier or an immediate family member serves as a paid consultant to or is an employee of Bartimus Frickleton Robertson Rader P.C. and Rubin Anders Scientific and serves as a board member, owner, officer, or committee member of the Orthopaedic Research Society. Dr. Piuzzi or an immediate family member serves as a paid consultant to or is an employee of Regeneron and Stryker; has received research or institutional support from RegenLab and Zimmer; and serves as a board member, owner, officer, or committee member of the American Association of Hip and Knee Surgeons, ISCT, and the Orthopaedic Research Society. Neither of the following authors nor any immediate family member has received anything of value from or has stock or stock options held in a commercial company or institution related directly or indirectly to the subject of this chapter: Dr. Hadad and Dr. Kobayashi.

in which expanded controlled and uncontrolled trials are used to gather more data on the effectiveness and safety of the IND in comparison to the current standard of care. An IND with demonstrated safety and efficacy may qualify for approval through a Biologics License Application, regulated under Parts 600 to 680 of Title 21 of the Code of Federal Regulations. Phase 4 postmarket studies are conducted after the product is approved to monitor the efficacy and safety of a treatment or intervention.

The FDA provides some flexibility in the study designs used in the evaluation of orthobiologics, because some products may not fall into the traditional phases of trials.[4] Likewise, much of the literature on orthobiologics is conducted outside the FDA approval process or occurs internationally and beyond the governance of the FDA. Clinicians and researchers will be increasingly tasked to design and interpret studies in the evaluation of orthobiologics to guide clinical decision making. It is important to provide an updated summary of the study designs, measurement of outcomes, and outcome reporting methodology used in orthobiologics research.

Both experimental and observational studies may be used in the evaluation of orthobiologic products. Experimental studies, typically in the form of randomized controlled trials (RCTs), assign the orthobiologic intervention of interest to a group of patients in the study and compare select outcome measures against a placebo group or standard of care. Experimental studies, in comparison to observational studies, allow for randomization and more control over the participants in the study, but they are often more expensive and time consuming. Matching may help control for confounding variables in the sample and blinding the patient and/or the evaluator may decrease the risk of bias. Both types of studies may have strong external validity if the studies are properly conducted and appropriately powered.[6] However, RCTs often lack the possibility of finding associations between risk factors, interventions, and outcomes for specific subgroups of patients. Observational studies investigate the association of an intervention (ie, an orthobiologic) with outcomes, but without affecting which patients are exposed to the intervention. Cohort studies, a type of comparative observational study, involve the identification of a sample of people that was exposed to a particular variable and another sample that was not exposed, and a subsequent outcome of interest is compared between the groups. Hence, large prospective cohort studies have the capacity to address the gap left by RCTs by providing tailored recommendations on an individual patient basis by developing multivariate analysis.[7] In contrast, case-control studies, another type of comparative observational study, involve identifying samples of people with and without a particular condition, and the frequency of a past exposure of interest is compared between the groups. For example, Chauhan et al[8] presented a retrospective matched cohort study investigating whether the use of platelet-rich plasma (PRP) injections before starting nonsurgical management of elbow ulnar collateral ligament injuries in professional baseball players affects time to return to throwing, return to play, and MRI findings. In this study, the authors did not influence which players received or did not receive a PRP injection.

Overall, orthobiologics in musculoskeletal medicine remain a source of great promise and opportunity, and a source of public controversy, confusion, and misinformation.[9,10] Further high-quality multicenter clinical trials will be required in addition to physicians and institutions offering biologic therapies establishing high-quality patient registries and biorepository-linked registries that can be used for postmarket surveillance, quality, and efficacy assessments.[9,10]

KEY STRUCTURAL OUTCOMES IN STUDIES OF ORTHOBIOLOGIC PRODUCTS

Local biologic enhancement therapies with orthobiologic products include the addition of scaffolds, growth factors, and cell therapies. The purpose of these materials is to promote tendon, ligament, muscle, and bone healing.

Growth factors and stem cells, such as mesenchymal stem cells (MSCs), are the foundation of orthobiologics. Growth factors are a set of proteins essential in stimulating biologic activity, including bone morphogenetic proteins (BMPs), vascular endothelial growth factor, fibroblast growth factors, insulinlike growth factor, and platelet-derived growth factor. MSCs are important because it can differentiate toward cartilage, tendon, or bone cells. Cell therapies have been used to enhance healing, which include bone marrow aspirate concentrate and PRP. Bone marrow aspirate concentrate contains red bone marrow and MSCs, which have the potential capability to trigger repair. PRP is an autologous concentrate of platelets containing and releasing cytokines to enhance the healing process of injured tissues.[11] PRP has been used in diverse musculoskeletal conditions including tendinopathy, rotator cuff tears, osteoarthritis, ligament reconstruction, plantar fasciitis, and nonunion.

Tendons have limited blood supply and are notorious for inadequate healing and lingering issues. Injuries to the musculotendinous junction may be acute or chronic, and chronicity tends to be more problematic. Microtrauma to the tendon over time causes disruption of the internal structure leading to degeneration and pain. Multiple studies have investigated injection of cell therapies including PRP and bone marrow aspirate concentrate into the tendon to induce healing. Ultrasonographic techniques have been used to characterize the tendon tissue before and after orthobiologic intervention to analyze the uniformity and organization of tendon bundles as well as the cross-sectional area of the pathologic area.[12] MRI has been used to assess improvement in percentage of tendinopathy and degree of tendon involvement after therapies.[13] Animal studies have investigated the histologic analysis of tendons after intervention with an orthobiologic with variable outcomes. Results ranged from reduction of tendon fiber disorganization and histologic lesions to no significant difference when compared with a control group.[14]

Articular cartilage undergoes extensive and repetitive physical stress and can become damaged by a variety of mechanical, chemical, and microbiologic agents. Cartilage is also avascular, thus it cannot receive the necessary inflammatory and reparative cells when injured. MRI has been used to determine changes in total volume of articular cartilage at various time points after intervention with an orthobiologic.[15] Some studies have used the Koshino staging system, which evaluates the status of regenerated cartilage on a macroscopic scale ranging from no regenerative change to total cartilage regeneration with white, even, smooth cartilage.[16]

The process of bone formation is dependent on a multitude of events, including the differentiation of mesenchymal precursor cells into osteogenic cells (osteogenesis), stimulation of the function of required bone-forming cells (osteoinduction), a scaffold for the bone to form (osteoconduction), and continued remodeling. Orthobiologics are used to target one or more of these essential components to improve outcomes.

Bone grafts have been used in several orthopaedic and trauma procedures in which bone augmentation and regeneration is needed. The types of bone grafts include autologous, allogeneic, synthetic, and xenogeneic synthetic. Autografts combine all properties required for biologic graft including osteogenic, osteoconductive, and osteoinductive properties. The subtypes of autografts include cortical and cancellous grafts. Cortical grafts act as biologic structures or intramedullary support in combination with other internal fixation deices. Cancellous grafts can be obtained from the medullary canal of long bones via a reamer-irrigator-aspirator, which has less structural support, but with more rapid incorporation. Allografts are available in various shapes and subtypes including cortical, cancellous, osteochondral, and whole-bone segments. They can be fresh, fresh frozen, or freeze dried. Freeze-dried and fresh-frozen allografts induce better vascularization and integration, but it takes longer to achieve these results compared with autografts. Demineralized bone matrix is a bone-substitute allograft that contains the organic matrix, such as collagenous peptides and growth factors, and the inorganic mineral is removed.

Synthetic bone substitutes are used more often and include calcium sulfate, calcium phosphate, hydroxyapatite, and bioactive glass. These bone substitutes lack structural integrity and are used primarily for filling voids of bone defects. The organic matrix stimulates MSCs to differentiate into osteoblasts and initiate endochondral ossification. Furthermore, the use of BMP has been widely used in the orthopaedic field because of its role in stimulating healing.[17,18] BMP-2 and BMP-7 enhance the production of cartilage and woven bone within the hard callus to allow for remodeling.[19,20]

The simplest and most preferred imaging modality assessing bone graft integration includes orthogonal radiographic imaging demonstrating bridging callus as evidence for fracture union. The Radiographic Union Score[21] was developed to aid in quantitative evaluation of fracture healing using radiographs that showed high correlation to physical properties of healing and distinguished healed versus nonhealed fractures.[22] However, CT is considered the gold standard to assess bone healing because the sensitivity to detect nonunion is reportedly up to 100%.[23] Total bone callus volume has also been studied with CT along with measurements of mineralized bone volume and density.[16]

KEY PHYSIOLOGIC OR FUNCTIONAL OUTCOMES IN STUDIES OF ORTHOBIOLOGIC PRODUCTS

The biologic effects after intra-articular injection of PRP and stem cells have been examined via synovial fluid analysis at specific time points after the intervention. Markers that have been tested include interleukin 1 beta, tumor necrosis factor alpha 6, and prostaglandin E2 in animal and human clinical studies.

Biomechanical testing on animal models has been performed after orthobiologic intervention on tendons and bone. When testing tendons, samples are preloaded at a predefined distance and then loaded to failure at a constant speed. Measurements of elongation at ultimate tensile load and cross-sectional area are then performed.[24] The bone of interest has been tested for bending stiffness and ultimate force applied before a fracture is measured.[15]

Return to sport or work is a common functional outcome obtained after intervention with orthobiologics. This includes level of activity, time to return to activity, and to what degree of disability is secondary to the injury. Clinical healing also has been arbitrarily defined as having achieved full weight bearing with a low visual analog scale pain score during walking.

PATIENT-REPORTED OUTCOME MEASURES IN STUDIES OF ORTHOBIOLOGIC PRODUCTS

Patient-reported outcome measures (PROMs) have emerged as useful measures of patient health and satisfaction after orthopaedic interventions. This is especially important because value-based outcomes, in which high-quality centers and surgeons are rewarded for value over volume, may be measured in part by PROMs.[25,26] PROMs are administered in a standardized manner, and consequently allow for the comparison of outcomes between populations and studies. Because PROMs are increasingly being reported to measure outcomes across subspecialties within orthopaedics,[27-30] PROMs may also be useful tools to measure outcomes after orthobiologic interventions.

The measurement of patient traits through PROMs is rooted in the field of psychometrics. Item response theory (IRT) and classical test theory (CTT) are two paradigms within psychometrics that are used to create and score assessments. In IRT, assessments are developed with a focus on item-level information. Respondent traits are determined based on their response to individual question items, and each question item is validated to determine that it measures the trait that it is expected to measure.[31] In contrast, CTT is focused on the respondent's overall performance on the assessment. In CTT, each question item is not individually validated, and thus, items cannot be compared between assessments. Within IRT, the unidimensionality, local independence, and differential item functioning of each question item are interrogated to validate each item. Unidimensionality refers to the item's measurement of a single respondent trait, local independence refers to the item's unique contribution to measuring a trait, and differential item functioning refers to deviations in responses to an item from respondents in different subgroups but with the same underlying trait of interest.[32,33] IRT is generally preferred over CTT because it allows for more flexibility in assessment administration and permits item-level comparisons between assessments.

Assessments can be administered using static or adaptive methodology. In static examinations, respondent responses do not affect the sequence of subsequent items, and all items are presented to the examinee. In computerized adaptive testing, the respondent's responses to items affect the sequence and number of items presented. The software may be programmed to assess each respondent's traits of interest in real time and it can potentially conclude the assessment early if the traits of interest are determined with preset precision.[31] Computerized adaptive testing is enabled by IRT, and PROM measures have been described with IRT and computerized adaptive testing methodology in the evaluation of orthopaedic outcomes, including in literature on the upper extremity,[27] foot and ankle,[28] spine,[29] and total knee arthroplasty.[30]

PROM data in orthopaedics are largely collected in the clinic setting. The collection of PROMs from patients and orthopaedic surgeons in outpatient clinics has been shown to be cost effective and scalable within a large hospital system,[34] and therefore, it may be feasible to routinely collect PROMs from patients before and after surgery with orthobiologics. The collection of PROMs for the purpose of measuring clinical outcomes naturally translates to their use in clinical research; however, there is inconsistency in PROM selection and outcome reporting methodology.[35] For example, Vajapey et al[36] found that 35 unique PROMs were used in the reporting of hip function after total hip arthroplasty in their meta-analysis of 159 RCTs. Likewise, Lloyd-Hughes et al[37] found that 21 unique PROMs were reported in the hand literature in their meta-analysis of 854 studies. Such variety highlights the number of different domains available to measure patient outcomes, but the inconsistency in selection limits comparisons between studies.

The variety in PROM selection extends to the orthobiologic literature as well. PROMs including the Knee Injury and Osteoarthritis Outcome Score, Lysholm score, and Western Ontario and McMaster Universities Osteoarthritis score have been reported in the evaluation of orthobiologic interventions for knee osteoarthritis.[9,38-41] The Oswestry Disability Index, Short Form 36 North American Spine Society Outcome Questionnaire, and the Functional Rating Index have been used to evaluate orthobiologics in patients with spine conditions.[42,43] In the shoulder literature, Snow et al[44] selected the following PROMs in their evaluation of delayed leukocyte-rich PRP injections after arthroscopic rotator cuff repair: American Shoulder and Elbow Score; Constant score; Western Ontario Rotator Cuff Index; and the Disabilities of the Arm, Shoulder and Hand score. In contrast, in the foot and ankle literature, the American Orthopaedic Foot and Ankle Society Ankle-Hindfoot score has been well adopted.[45,46] This list is not meant to be exhaustive, and it is beyond the scope of this chapter to delineate the specific traits or benefits of each PROM; rather, the intention is to illustrate the variety of PROMs across and within the orthopaedic subspecialties. This information should encourage the thoughtful selection of PROMs in future studies on orthobiologics, because the use of the same PROMs in different studies may assist in meaningful comparisons between studies.

The methodology of PROM reporting, specifically in the determination of clinically important outcome values (CIOVs), is also variable. CIOVs include, but are not limited to, the Minimum Clinically Important Difference (MCID) and the Patient Acceptable Symptom State (PASS). MCID refers to the smallest difference needed for a patient to perceive a change in the outcome of interest, and PASS refers to the minimum threshold of the outcome of interest beyond which the patient is satisfied.[47,48] Both MCID and PASS have been used in the orthobiologic literature to demonstrate clinically meaningful changes in PROMs.[38,49] An important limitation of CIOV reporting in clinical research is patient loss to follow-up. Imam et al[50] found that patients who were nonresponders to postoperative outcome questionnaires after total hip arthroplasty were more likely to have lower satisfaction. Although more data are needed to determine the satisfaction of nonresponders after other orthopaedic interventions, Imam et al's findings suggest that nonresponders after orthopaedic interventions may be less satisfied. Therefore, reporting MCID or PASS as a measure of clinically significant change in PROMs in a scenario of high patient loss to follow-up may overestimate the true outcomes in the sample. A possible solution to this problem, as described by Orr et al,[48] is the robustness ratio. The robustness ratio is determined by the ratio of the number of individuals with a clinically significant outcome to the number of individuals at the beginning of the study period. No studies to date have reported a robustness ratio for PROM outcomes, but from a theoretical standpoint, reporting the robustness ratio may reduce response bias and better represent a postoperative plateau of PROMs, if one exists. Of note, no clinically meaningful difference in 1-year postoperative PROMs has been reported in patients who were followed up by automated methods compared with those who required contact by manual methods after hip, knee, or shoulder procedures.[51] These data are reassuring that manually contacting patients to improve the PROM response rate from a sample may not bias the study to finding decreased PROMs.

With the increasing focus on PROMs as measures of outcomes in orthopaedic surgery, it is beneficial to assess PROMs against other objective measurements of outcomes. In patients who underwent total ankle arthroplasty, better postoperative range of motion of the surgical ankle has been positively correlated with PROMs.[52] Likewise, the arc of elbow flexion-extension after surgical fixation for distal humerus fractures has been associated with improved PROMs.[53] In the orthobiologic literature, Jo et al[54] found that high-dose MSC injections for knee osteoarthritis was associated with improved PROMs and a significant decrease in the size of cartilage defects of the medial femoral and lateral tibial condyles on MRI at 2-year follow-up; however, the authors did not determine CIOVs, such as MCID or PASS, for their selected PROMs. It is reassuring that physical examination and radiographic findings are associated with PROMs in these select studies. Given the lack of standardization of PROM selection and reporting methodology, study outcomes may be strengthened with additional objective data, if available.

KEY CONCEPTS TO CONSIDER WHEN USING PROMS IN CLINICAL RESEARCH

Causation, Association, and Correlation

There are several ways to conceptualize how variables within a study may relate to each other. Three such ways are a causative relationship, an association, or a correlation, or no relationship at all. A causative relationship between variables means that some variable (X) is a necessary component in the existence or level of some other variable (Y). That is, X is a causative factor for Y. If there is a causal relationship, X causes Y, then X and Y are also associated. However, X and Y may appear to be associated, for instance, when a third variable A causes both X and Y. That is, X and Y have a common cause. Association means that one variable provides some sort of information about another variable, but it does not infer causation. It is important to remember that spurious associations are likely when many variables are examined in complex systems, which arise simply by chance. Correlation is a type of association, where variables show some common trend, either increasing or decreasing or more complex bimodal or other trend. However, correlations should not infer causation, though correlated variables can be causally related. "Correlated" is a word frequently used as a term for any association, but this is incorrect because correlation does not mean causation. Also, when there is in fact a causative association, calling this correlated downplays the relationship between variables and misleads the reader. Generally, use of the terms correlated or correlated with should be avoided when intending to infer causation. High/strong correlations can arise in random data. Interpretation of associations of any kind should be done with caution because biases can make it seem as though there is an association when in reality there is not.

Biases in Outcomes Research

Bias is generally defined as a systematic deviation from the truth and can arise at any stage in clinical research. There are many forms of bias that have been reported in the literature. Generally, the classes of bias are as follows: selection bias, performance bias, detection bias, attrition bias, reporting bias, and biases due to conflicts of interest (eg, funding source, intellectual property) (**Table 1**). Selection bias arises when participant inclusion and

TABLE 1 Categories of Bias in Clinical Research

Categories of Bias in Clinical Research	Definition
Selection bias	Systematic differences between baseline characteristics of the groups that are compared
Performance bias	Systematic differences between groups in the care that is provided, or in exposure to factors other than the interventions of interest
Detection bias	Systematic differences between groups in how outcomes are determined
Attrition bias	Systematic differences between groups in withdrawals from a study
Reporting bias	Systematic differences between reported and unreported findings
Other biases	Other sources of bias that are relevant only in certain circumstances

allocation procedures result in unequal characteristics (eg, age, disease severity, comorbidities) in the groups being compared. These characteristics can be identified by examining baseline and demographic variables in each group, typically in any clinical study (experimental or observational). Observational studies are at a particular risk of selection bias. In an observational study (eg, a cohort study), patients are not allocated to interventions/exposures (eg, PRP injection versus corticosteroid injection) by the investigators, they are self-chosen, or the choice of exposure is codetermined by patient and physician. Thus, patients in each arm of a cohort study may differ because of factors other than the exposure. For example, those with less severe osteoarthritis may receive one intervention more often than the other. Therefore, the sampling procedure and any related matching methods must be done very carefully to ensure similarity of the groups, and if not, subgroup analyses or adjustments must be made in the statistical procedures. In RCTs, the allocation methods, random assignment, and allocation concealment (methods to prevent foreknowledge of the forthcoming treatment allocations) dictate group similarity, if the sample size is large enough.

Performance bias refers to systematic differences between groups in the care provided (eg, how physical therapy was done) or in exposures (eg, cointerventions) other than the interventions related to the research questions and hypotheses (ie, confounders or effect modifiers). In RCTs, blinding procedures of study participants and study personnel reduce the risk that any knowledge of the intervention received can affect the outcomes. In observational studies (eg, a cohort study), performance bias may arise because of subtle differences in the interventions received, such that in a comparative effectiveness study, group A, for example, has varying cointerventions that are distinct from those in group B. Therefore, the groups are being differentially exposed to cointerventions that could potentially influence the measured outcomes. Careful patient selection and allocation as well as the measurement of all known confounders and cointerventions can mitigate performance bias.

Detection bias refers to systematic differences in how outcomes are being measured between the groups. For example, a study comparing an orthobiologic therapy with a placebo has an outcome of range of motion at the shoulder, and suppose the outcome assessor knows which group a particular patient is in. The bias, even unconscious, of the unblind outcome assessor may affect range of motion measurements, to the extent that these are done in systematically different ways in each group, biases comparisons. In all prospective clinical research studies, blinding of outcome assessors can mitigate this as can careful attention to outcomes assessments being performed in the same manner in each group.

Attrition bias refers to systematic differences in the withdrawals from a study or from incomplete data (eg, missing data points for multiple follow-ups). Withdrawals or incomplete data arise because of attrition (where patients are lost to follow-up for a variety of reasons) and exclusions (where patients are withdrawn from the study after initial inclusion and participation in the study). With both scenarios, the loss of outcome data can systematically alter the data and bias the comparisons. There are several methods to reduce the risk of bias due to attrition such as imputation methods for missing data (filling in the missing data) and sensitivity analyses (eg, doing separate analyses for those with missing data verses those with no missing data, to examine the influence of this missingness). This is not the same as intention-to-treat analyses. The intention to treat in RCTs preserves the randomization process, such that patients are analyzed in the groups to which they were originally allocated, even if they did not actually receive that intervention (at all or in part). The problem is that if many patients are either noncompliant with the active intervention or are seeking out other related treatments, and these patients are treated as if they are in a treatment group other than to what they were originally assigned, then it is possible that the original randomization process (which should equally distribute all uncontrolled variables between allocation groups) is undermined and the participant groups may vary on some important characteristics related to them being noncompliant (eg, adverse effects of the intervention they were assigned to originally). Intention-to-treat analyses protect against this bias.

Reporting bias refers to systematic differences between reported and unreported findings, or when outcome priority is changed from the protocol to the published report (eg, secondary outcomes are switched to primary outcomes). Generally, statistically significant differences are more likely to be reported than nonsignificant ones, and outcome priority, when changed, is changed in favor of statistically significant findings. This is also called outcome reporting bias or selective reporting bias. To mitigate reporting biases, it is important not to change outcome priority or to selectively publish particular findings; if there is a legitimate reason to do either, it must be reported in full because transparency is key. Depending on the question, hypotheses and study design, or implementation, other biases may be relevant. Some biases may specifically relate to particular study designs. For example, when performing cluster-randomized studies, relevant grouping variables must be carefully accounted for analytically (eg, recruitment site) and when performing crossover studies, carryout effects must also be examined and considered.

When planning clinical research, care should be taken to control for these biases up front or attempt to account for or control for them in the data analysis. When reading and interpreting research, the risk of bias of that research should be carefully and comprehensively considered. There are several accepted tools to assess risks of bias that can be used to determine the potential for bias in a study.[55]

Using PROMs to Establish Sample Sizes for Clinical Research

Sample size calculations must be done for all clinical research. In some cases, pilot and feasibility clinical research can go without an a priori sample size calculation when designed to test the feasibility of study methods (eg, recruitment, follow-up) or to collect data to be used for a sample size calculation for a larger follow-up study. In most cases, even for a pilot study, a sample size calculation can be done, but when absolutely no other data are available for the question under study, and no data for closely related questions are available, then a sample size calculation is simply not possible and tangential findings applied to such a calculation would be misleading. To calculate the sample size, data from related research are required, and the exact type of data will depend on the type of primary outcome data to be collected. The focus will be on PROM data that are dichotomous (eg, meet some cutoff or not) and continuous data (eg, a score on a PROM), though sample size calculations are possible for any type of data (nominal, ordinal, dichotomous, ratio, continuous).

For continuous data (eg, PROM score change from baseline or difference between groups), the following are required: alpha (typically set at $P = 0.05$ in biomedical research) or risk of type I error; beta (typically set at 0.20), which is risk of type II error (making your power 0.80 or 80%); some expected mean difference (delta) between comparison groups on primary outcome (eg, range of motion of 20°); and a measure of the variance for this difference, either a standard error or standard deviation (SD) is typical. With these numbers, the sample size required to detect a particular difference can be determined.

With dichotomous data (eg, meeting the minimally important difference for a PROM within 1 year or not: Yes or No), to perform a sample size calculation the following are required: the total number of events in the exposure group A (eg, those getting knee injection A) and the total number of participants exposed in this group, and the number of event events in the exposure group B (eg, knee injection B) and the total number of participants exposed in the this group. There will be two values, one for group A and one for group B. These could be risk ratios (RR) or odds ratios or some other ratio value. These values can then be used with any statistical program to calculate the sample size required.

It is important to account for potential dropouts or loss-to-follow-up data, especially if prospective research is performed. Typically, 15% to 20% dropouts should be accounted for, but of course the exact expectation may be different depending on the details of the project being implemented. That is, the exact amount will be dictated by the type of interventions and outcomes and can be found from pilot data or from related published research. Potential dropouts must be accounted for to avoid being underpowered to detect a difference in outcomes if there are not enough patients at some follow-up point. So, if the sample size yielded 50 patients in total, and 15% of the sample is expected to drop out, then the following equation needs to be solved for X: $X/100\% = 50/80\%$ which results in $50/0.80 = 62.5$ patients total, which in a two-group study results in 31.25 patients per group, with rounding up to 32 patients per group, resulting in a total of 64 patients required.

There are two main types of errors to be concerned with in clinical research (**Figure 1**). A type I error is the probability

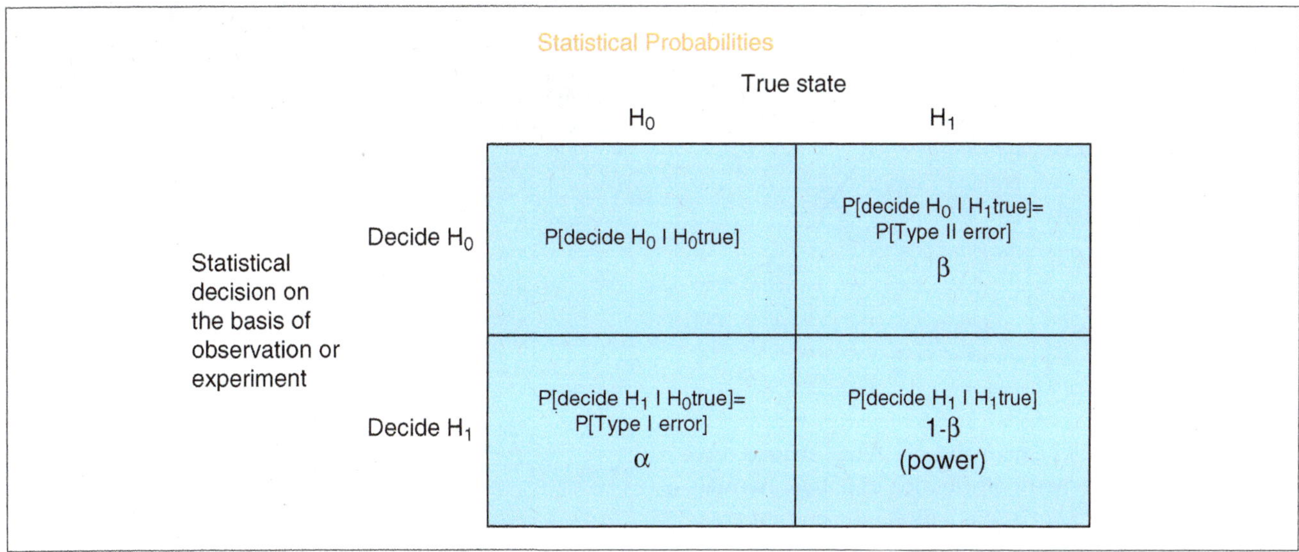

FIGURE 1 Graph shows statistical errors and the two main types of errors: type I and type II.

of rejecting the null hypothesis in favor of the alternative hypothesis when in fact the null hypothesis is true. Conversely, a type II error is the probability of failing to reject the null hypothesis when the truth is that the null hypothesis should be rejected in favor of the alternative hypothesis.

Parametric Versus Nonparametric Findings/Data

It is important when looking at summaries of the continuous data to determine whether the data are parametric or nonparametric. That is, are the data normally distributed (**Figure 2**)? When plotted in a line graph, there should be a relatively obvious grouping of observations in the center of the graph and less moving away from the center. The bell-shaped curve is a classic example of a parametric distribution of data or a normal distribution, though such a symmetric plot of real data will not likely be seen from a sample. Moving away from the center of the bell (marked as 0), the frequency of observations decreases. SDs are marked on this figure, indicating the percentage of the area under the curve or percentage of observations in each shaded area. Within the area between −1 and +1 SD there is approximately 68% of the sample of observations. The SD is a measure of the distance from the center of the sample (eg, mean). When using descriptive statistics to summarize parametric continuous data, a mean and a measure of variance (SD or a confidence interval [CI]) are sufficient. SD is essentially the average deviation from the mean of all observations, and it is in the same units as the mean. CI is another measure of the spread of the observations and gives some idea of the precision of an estimate. Generally, a 95% CI means that there is 95% confidence that the values between the lower and upper limit contain the true parameter value that this data set is attempting to explain. More specifically, a 95% CI means that if 100 random samples are taken from the same population and 100 different CIs calculated, approximately 95 would cover the true population mean and 5 would not. Thus, a 95% CI is an estimate of these 100 CIs. Several parametric inferential statistical tests for continuous data include t tests, repeated-measures t tests, analysis of variance, and repeated-measures analysis of variance.

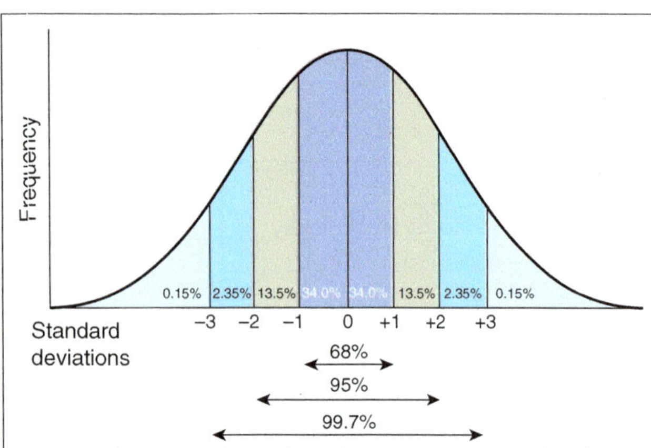

FIGURE 2 Graph shows a normal curve. A bell-shaped curve is an example of parametric distribution of data or normal distribution. Standard deviations indicate the percent area under the curve and are a measure of the distance from the center of the sample.

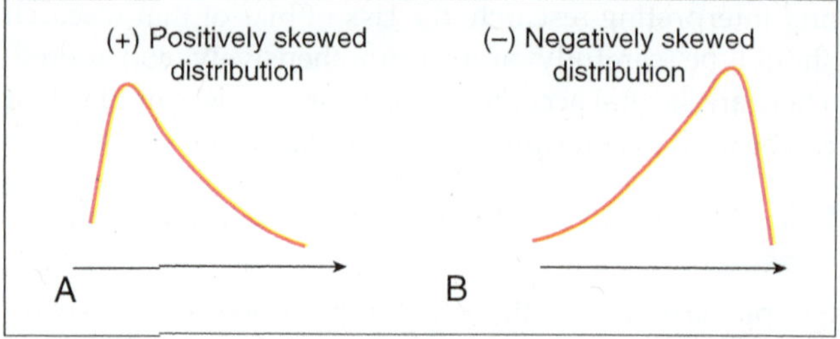

FIGURE 3 Graph shows skewed distributions. Two examples of nonparametric curves demonstrating positively **(A)** and negatively **(B)** skewed curves.

The distribution or curve may not be symmetric and may not approximate a normal/parametric curve. **Figure 3** illustrates two nonparametric curves, the one on the left positively skewed (meaning there is a long tail of observations to the right of the center of the curve) in the direction of positive values. The curve on the right is negatively skewed (with a long tail of observations to the left of the center of the curve) in the direction of negative values. In the case of nonparametric continuous data, nonparametric statistical tests including the sign test, Wilcoxon signed-rank test, Mann-Whitney U test, Kolmogorov-Smirnov test, Kruskal-Wallis test, and Friedman test will need to be used. **Table 2** compares parametric and nonparametric tests for different forms of parametric and nonparametric data.

TABLE 2 Parametric and Nonparametric Statistical Tests

Number of Samples Being Compared	Parametric Tests	Nonparametric Tests
One	One-sample t test	Sign test Wilcoxon signed-rank test
Two	Paired t test Unpaired t test (Student t test)	Sign test Wilcoxon signed-rank test Mann-Whitney U test Kolmogorov-Smirnov test
K-samples	Analysis of variance Two-way analysis of variance	Kruskal-Wallis test Jonckheere test Friedman test

To determine whether or not a sample of data is normal, the distribution of data can be visually examined as previously suggested (the so-called eyeball test). In addition, there are several formal statistical tests that can be run, including the Kolmogorov-Smirnov test and Shapiro-Wilk test, which are both available in most statistical packages.

P-values

Finally, after all descriptive analyses and inferential testing have been completed, effect estimates and *P*-value for these effect estimates can be calculated. A *P*-value is the probability of obtaining a more extreme test statistic than what was observed if the null hypothesis is true. It is not the probability that the null hypothesis is true or that the result is due to chance. A *P*-value reflects the extent to which the hypothesis being tested is compatible with the observed results. The smaller the *P*-value, the less compatible the null hypothesis is with the observed results. In most applications, the hypothesis being tested is the null hypothesis of no association between the exposure or treatment of interest and the outcome. An important caveat is that the accuracy of the *P*-value is only as good as the underlying statistical model and the related assumptions used to arrive at it. If the model is appropriate, a small *P*-value casts doubt on the null hypothesis. In contrast to common belief, statistical findings never reveal whether or not there is a treatment or exposure effect. Rather, statistical results—estimated associations—convey a continuum of information used, along with other information, to make inferences about hypothesized effects. CIs are recommended to complement the interpretation of findings because they convey information about the magnitude and direction of the association as well as the precision with which the parameter has been estimated.[56]

Statistical Significance Versus Clinical Significance

A smaller *P*-value does not indicate a larger effect. The *P*-value tells nothing about the magnitude of the association. A very small absolute risk reduction of surgical site infection, when comparing interventions, may yield a small *P*-value (eg, <0.05) but not be clinically meaningful at all. That is, a study with a large sample size or high precision of measurement (eg, a small standard deviation, or standard error and a narrow confidence interval) can produce small *P*-values in the presence of weak associations, especially in the era of big data. The converse is true as well; a strong association in studies with small sample sizes or low precision may produce large *P*-values. If this is the case, the effect estimate may be clinically meaningful even in the presence of a large *P*-value. Relying on a single study's result to guide clinical decision making is fraught with problems. It has been shown repeatedly that initial research findings are frequently contradicted later by larger, more precise studies.[57]

The main issue is the confusion of statistical significance with clinical significance relative to research findings. Statistical significance refers to the *P*-value for testing the null hypothesis being below or above a designated value (typically 0.05), corresponding to the accepted probability of a type I error (falsely rejecting the null hypothesis). As noted previously, the *P*-value depends on both the magnitude of the association and the sample size. Clinical significance conveys how important a finding is for a given outcome and its relevance to the patient or clinician.[58,59] This importance depends on not only on the magnitude and direction of the association, but also on estimation precision (confidence interval width), the type, severity, and prognostic implication of the outcome, and social context, age, and other relevant characteristics.

ESTABLISHING A HIERARCHY OF OUTCOMES FOR SUCCESS

There are several ways to identify how an outcome was measured, which generally should start with the knowledge gained from a review of the relevant literature. The surgeon should have a good idea of how an outcome has been measured, but this does not mean this is exactly the next step. For example, the surgeon may be interested in measuring patient-reported shoulder function following a type of surgical repair for a full-thickness rotator cuff tear, and may note that a particular PROM is used and reported frequently in the literature. These measures and their quality must be comprehensively vetted before they are blindly applied. They may not have good measurement properties, meaning they may not be reliable, valid, or responsive. That is, a rational and logical decision must be made regarding what to measure and how to measure it. This goes for any other measures (eg, a laboratory measure using a serum marker). It must be confirmed that the measure squarely focuses on, or at least partly focuses on, the phenomenon to be measured and tracked. If this is the case, how good are the measurement properties of it? For example, if a PROM is found that proposes to measure the phenomena of interest (eg, rotator cuff physical function), then there must be evidence of its psychometric/measurement properties.

Just like any other type of outcome, a PROM should be valid, reliable, responsive, and interpretable. A measurement tool is considered valid when it actually measures what it proposes to measure. There are several types of validity, including content, construct, and criterion validity. Reliability is the property of measuring some phenomenon in a predictable manner (repeatability). Some forms of reliability include internal consistency, test-retest or intrarater, and interrater reliability. Responsiveness is the ability to detect change in the underlying construct over time, even if the changes are small. Finally, interpretability refers to the ability to derive meaning from the scores of the PROM; that is, is it clear what high or low scores mean, clinically or for the patient, or are there cutoffs or important values on the measure, etc? **Table 3** describes the psychometric properties that should be considered. A systematic review of measurement properties can sometimes help guide the surgeon on how good a measure is, but in some cases additional evidence will need to be gathered to make a determination. Simply using an outcome measure because it appears in the literature with high frequency is not justification for using it in research. Using a poor measure severely biases the outcome measurement and can, as a result, harm patients to which such incorrect findings are applied or waste resources. Another consideration is the ease of use of a measure. That is, the surgeon should have the ability to implement the measurement tool for the types of patients, for the particular question of interest, for the timing needed; in some cases, funds will need to be allocated to cover the cost of the measure. In particular, the timing or staging of an outcome measure is very important. In some cases, only one time point is being looked at, but in many cases there will be multiple time points—for example, when performing longitudinal research. The exact timing depends on the measure being used, what phenomenon is being measured, and the research participants' ability to complete the measure.

Thus, when attempting to choose a PROM for use clinically or for research in orthopaedics, and any other area, an appropriate instrument must identified for a specific purpose and then data collected on the quality of that instrument. Frequent use of an instrument in the published literature does not guarantee its quality. In fact, there is extensive evidence that PROMs used in many areas of orthopaedics are significantly flawed or, at the very least, lack data on their psychometric properties.[60-62] The use of poor quality instruments will result in biased or unreliable effect estimates and can potentially mislead decision makers relying on this evidence as well as harm patients and waste resources.

There is some empirical evidence that clinical trials that use poor or unknown quality PROMs are more likely to report that a particular treatment was superior to a control treatment, by up to 89% (RR 1.89, 95% CI 1.40 to 2.56), and the effect was even greater in nonpharmacologic trials, 168% (RR 2.68, 95% CI 1.86 to 3.84).[63] Furthermore, a recent rigorous assessment of the magnitude of bias associated with varying quality PROMs found that PROMs with poor or unknown psychometric properties overestimate treatment effects in clinical research of rotator cuff disease by 68.4%.[64] Therefore, researchers and clinicians using data from PROMs must be cautious to explore the quality of that measure so as to not mislead decision making resulting from biased outcomes.

TABLE 3 Psychometric Properties of Patient-Reported Outcome Measures

Property	Description
Reliability	
Internal consistency	The extent to which items in a questionnaire (sub)scale are correlated (homogeneous), thus measuring the same concept
Reliability	The extent to which patients can be distinguished from each other, despite measurement error (relative measurement error)
Measurement error	The extent to which the scores on repeated measures are close to each other (absolute measurement error)
Validity	
Content validity	The extent to which the domain of interest is comprehensively sampled by the items in the questionnaire
Structural validity	The extent to which the scores of an instrument are an adequate reflection of the dimensionality of the construct to be measured
Hypothesis testing	The extent to which scores on a particular instrument relate to other measures in a manner that is consistent with theoretically derived hypotheses concerning the concepts that are being measured
Criterion validity	The extent to which scores on a particular instrument relate to a gold standard
Responsiveness	
Responsiveness	Responsiveness is a measure of longitudinal validity. In analogy to construct validity, longitudinal validity should be assessed by testing predefined hypotheses, for example, about expected correlations between changes in measures, or expected differences in changes between known groups.

SUMMARY

Orthobiologics are used in orthopaedic surgery to promote bone, cartilage, and soft-tissue healing with the use of osteogenic cells, osteoconductive scaffolds, and growth factors. Although orthobiologics are regulated by the FDA, the flexibility in study designs and studies performed outside the FDA approval process occurs. Experimental and observational studies, when properly conducted and appropriately powered, have strong external validity. The proper study of choice is determined by the proposed patient population and projected outcome measurements. Key outcomes measured include structural, physiologic, and functional outcomes. An important functional outcome includes PROMs and is useful to assess patient health and satisfaction after orthobiologic interventions. When conducting clinical studies, the methodology of PROM reporting is variable and the relationship between causation, association, and correlation must be considered. The validity, reliability, and interpretability of a PROM should be confirmed before its use in clinical studies because the quality of the outcome measured may suffer resulting in biased or unreliable evidence.

REFERENCES

1. Giannoudis PV, Einhorn TA, Marsh D: Fracture healing: the diamond concept. *Injury* 2007;38(suppl 4):S3-S6.
2. Code of Federal Regulations Title 21 Section 3.2. Available at: https://www.accessdata.fda.gov/scripts/cdrh/cfdocs/cfcfr/cfrsearch.cfm?fr=3.2. Accessed May 31, 2021.
3. Guidance for Industry Regulation of Human Cells, Tissues, and Cellular and Tissue-Based Products (HCT/Ps): Small Entity Compliance Guide. Available at: https://www.fda.gov/files/vaccines,%20blood%20&%20biologics/published/Regulation-of-Human-Cells--Tissues--and-Cellula. Accessed May 31, 2021.
4. Christensen K, Cox B, Anz A: Emerging orthobiologic techniques and the future. *Clin Sports Med* 2019;38(1):143-161.
5. Code of Federal Regulations Title 21 Section 312. Available at: https://www.ecfr.gov/cgi-bin/text-idx?SID=8a3ae221bc1231ccc50d763b61d4a922&mc=true&node=pt21.5.312&rgn=div5. Accessed May 31, 2021.
6. Concato J: Observational versus experimental studies: What's the evidence for a hierarchy? *NeuroRx* 2004;1(3):341-347.
7. Emara AK, Klika AK, Piuzzi NS: Evidence-based orthopedic surgery-from synthesis to practice. *JAMA Surg* 2020;155(11):1009-1010.
8. Chauhan A, McQueen P, Chalmers PN, et al: Nonoperative treatment of elbow ulnar collateral ligament injuries with and without platelet-rich plasma in professional baseball players: A comparative and matched cohort analysis. *Am J Sports Med* 2019;47(13):3107-3119.
9. Chu CR, Rodeo S, Bhutani N, et al: Optimizing clinical use of biologics in orthopaedic surgery: Consensus recommendations from the 2018 AAOS/NIH U-13 conference. *J Am Acad Orthop Surg* 2019;27(2):e50-e63.
10. Piuzzi NS, Dominici M, Long M, et al: Proceedings of the signature series symposium "cellular therapies for orthopaedics and musculoskeletal disease proven and unproven therapies—promise, facts and fantasy," international society for cellular therapies, Montreal, Canada, May 2, 2018. *Cytotherapy* 2018;20(11):1381-1400.
11. Oh JH, Kim W, Park KU, Roh YH: Comparison of the cellular composition and cytokine-release kinetics of various platelet-rich plasma preparations. *Am J Sports Med* 2015;43(12):3062-3070.
12. de Vos RJ, Weir A, Tol JL, Verhaar JA, Weinans H, van Schie HT: No effects of PRP on ultrasonographic tendon structure and neovascularisation in chronic midportion Achilles tendinopathy. *Br J Sports Med* 2011;45(5):387-392.
13. Owens RF Jr. Ginnetti J, Conti SF, Latona C: Clinical and magnetic resonance imaging outcomes following platelet rich plasma injection for chronic midsubstance Achilles tendinopathy. *Foot Ankle Int* 2011;32(11):1032-1039.
14. Darrieutort-Laffite C, Soslowsky LJ, Le Goff B: Molecular and structural effects of percutaneous interventions in chronic achilles tendinopathy. *Int J Mol Sci* 2020;21(19):7000.
15. Lu L, Dai C, Zhang Z, et al: Treatment of knee osteoarthritis with intra-articular injection of autologous adipose-derived mesenchymal progenitor cells: A prospective, randomized, double-blind, active-controlled, phase IIb clinical trial. *Stem Cell Res Ther* 2019;10(1):143.
16. Bosemark P, Isaksson H, McDonald MM, Little DG, Tagil M: Augmentation of autologous bone graft by a combination of bone morphogenic protein and bisphosphonate increased both callus volume and strength. *Acta Orthop* 2013;84(1):106-111.
17. Cho TJ, Gerstenfeld LC, Einhorn TA: Differential temporal expression of members of the transforming growth factor beta superfamily during murine fracture healing. *J Bone Miner Res* 2002;17(3):513-520.
18. Dimitriou R, Dahabreh Z, Katsoulis E, Matthews SJ, Branfoot T, Giannoudis PV: Application of recombinant BMP-7 on persistent upper and lower limb non-unions. *Injury* 2005;36(suppl 4):S51-S59.
19. Kawaguchi H, Oka H, Jingushi S, et al: A local application of recombinant human fibroblast growth factor 2 for tibial shaft fractures: A randomized, placebo-controlled trial. *J Bone Miner Res* 2010;25(12):2735-2743.
20. Yu YY, Lieu S, Lu C, Colnot C: Bone morphogenetic protein 2 stimulates endochondral ossification by regulating periosteal cell fate during bone repair. *Bone* 2010;47(1):65-73.
21. Leow JM, Clement ND, Tawonsawatruk T, Simpson CJ, Simpson AH: The radiographic union scale in tibial (RUST) fractures: Reliability of the outcome measure at an independent centre. *Bone Joint Res* 2016;5(4):116-121.
22. Cooke ME, Hussein AI, Lybrand KE, et al: Correlation between RUST assessments of fracture healing to structural and biomechanical properties. *J Orthop Res* 2018;36(3):945-953.
23. Bhattacharyya T, Bouchard KA, Phadke A, Meigs JB, Kassarjian A, Salamipour H: The accuracy of computed tomography for the diagnosis of tibial nonunion. *J Bone Joint Surg Am* 2006;88(4):692-697.

24. de Lima Santos A, Silva CGD, de Sa Barretto LS, et al: Biomechanical evaluation of tendon regeneration with adipose-derived stem cell. *J Orthop Res* 2019;37(6):1281-1286.
25. Franklin PD, Harrold L, Ayers DC: Incorporating patient-reported outcomes in total joint arthroplasty registries: Challenges and opportunities. *Clin Orthop Relat Res* 2013;471(11):3482-3488.
26. Sambare TD, Bozic KJ: Preparing for an era of episode-based care in total joint arthroplasty. *J Arthroplasty* 2021;36(3):810-815.
27. Kaat AJ, Buckenmaier CT III, Cook KF, et al: The expansion and validation of a new upper extremity item bank for the Patient-Reported Outcomes Measurement Information System® (PROMIS). *J Patient Rep Outcomes* 2019;3(1):69.
28. O'Neil JT, Plummer OR, Raikin SM: Application of computerized adaptive testing to the foot and ankle ability measure. *Foot Ankle Int* 2021;42(1):2-7.
29. Boody BS, Bhatt S, Mazmudar AS, Hsu WK, Rothrock NE, Patel AA: Validation of Patient-Reported Outcomes Measurement Information System (PROMIS) computerized adaptive tests in cervical spine surgery. *J Neurosurg Spine* 2018;28(3):268-279.
30. Banerjee S, Deirmengian GK, Levicoff E, Abboud JA, Plummer O, Courtney PM: Accuracy and validity of computer adaptive testing for outcome assessment in patients undergoing total knee arthroplasty. *J Arthroplasty* 2020;35(7):1819-1825.
31. Brodke DJ, Hung M, Bozic KJ: Item response theory and computerized adaptive testing for orthopaedic outcomes measures. *J Am Acad Orthop Surg* 2016;24(11):750-754.
32. Scott NW, Fayers PM, Aaronson NK, et al: Differential item functioning (DIF) analyses of health-related quality of life instruments using logistic regression. *Health Qual Life Outcomes* 2010;8:81.
33. Reeve BB, Fayers P: Applying item response theory modeling for evaluating questionnaire item and scale properties. *Assess Qual Life Clin Trials Methods Pract* 2005;2:55-73.
34. OME Cleveland Clinic Orthopaedics: Implementing a scientifically valid, cost-effective, and scalable data collection system at point of care: The Cleveland Clinic OME Cohort. *J Bone Joint Surg Am* 2019;101(5):458-464.
35. Orr M, Klika A, Piuzzi N: Patient reported outcome measures: Challenges in the reporting! *Ann Surg Open* 2021;2(3):e070.
36. Vajapey SP, Morris J, Li D, Greco NG, Li M, Spitzer AI: Outcome reporting patterns in total hip arthroplasty: A systematic review of randomized clinical trials. *JBJS Rev* 2020;8(4):e0197.
37. Lloyd-Hughes H, Geoghegan L, Rodrigues J, et al: Systematic review of the use of patient reported outcome measures in studies of electively-managed hand conditions. *J Hand Surg Asian Pac Vol* 2019;24(3):329-341.
38. Zahir H, Dehghani B, Yuan X, et al: In vitro responses to platelet-rich-plasma are associated with variable clinical outcomes in patients with knee osteoarthritis. *Sci Rep* 2021;11(1):11493.
39. Smith PA: Intra-articular autologous conditioned plasma injections provide safe and efficacious treatment for knee osteoarthritis: An FDA-sanctioned, randomized, double-blind, placebo-controlled clinical trial. *Am J Sports Med* 2016;44(4):884-891.
40. Lee W-S, Kim HJ, Kim K-I, Kim GB, Jin W: Intra-articular injection of autologous adipose tissue-derived mesenchymal stem cells for the treatment of knee osteoarthritis: A Phase IIb, randomized, placebo-controlled clinical trial. *Stem Cells Transl Med* 2019;8(6):504-511.
41. Kim SH, Ha C-W, Park Y-B, Nam E, Lee J-E, Lee H-J: Intra-articular injection of mesenchymal stem cells for clinical outcomes and cartilage repair in osteoarthritis of the knee: A meta-analysis of randomized controlled trials. *Arch Orthop Trauma Surg* 2019;139(7):971-980.
42. García de Frutos A, González-Tartière P, Coll Bonet R, et al: Randomized clinical trial: Expanded autologous bone marrow mesenchymal cells combined with allogeneic bone tissue, compared with autologous iliac crest graft in lumbar fusion surgery. *Spine J* 2020;20(12):1899-1910.
43. Tuakli-Wosornu YA, Terry A, Boachie-Adjei K, et al: Lumbar intradiskal Platelet-Rich Plasma (PRP) injections: A prospective, double-blind, randomized controlled study. *PM R* 2016;8(1):1-10.
44. Snow M, Hussain F, Pagkalos J, et al: The effect of delayed injection of leukocyte-rich platelet-rich plasma following rotator cuff repair on patient function: A randomized double-blind controlled trial. *Arthroscopy* 2020;36(3):648-657.
45. Plaass C, Knupp M, Barg A, Hintermann B: Anterior double plating for rigid fixation of isolated tibiotalar arthrodesis. *Foot Ankle Int* 2009;30(7):631-639.
46. Easley ME, Trnka HJ, Schon LC, Myerson MS: Isolated subtalar arthrodesis. *J Bone Joint Surg Am* 2000;82(5):613-624.
47. Cepeda NA, Polascik BA, Ling DI: A primer on clinically important outcome values: Going beyond relying on P values alone. *J Bone Joint Surg Am* 2020;102(3):262-268.
48. Orr M, Klika A, Gagnier J, Bhandari M, Piuzzi N: A call for a standardized approach to reporting patient reported outcome measures: Robustness ratio. *J Bone Joint Surg Am* 2021;103(22):e91.
49. Fitzpatrick J, Bulsara MK, O'Donnell J, McCrory PR, Zheng MH: The effectiveness of platelet-rich plasma injections in gluteal tendinopathy: A randomized, double-blind controlled trial comparing a single platelet-rich plasma injection with a single corticosteroid injection. *Am J Sports Med* 2018;46(4):933-939.
50. Imam MA, Barke S, Stafford GH, Parkin D, Field RE: Loss to follow-up after total hip replacement: A source of bias in patient reported outcome measures and registry datasets? *Hip Int* 2014;24(5):465-472.
51. OME Cleveland Clinic Orthopaedics: Value in research: Achieving validated outcome measurements while mitigating follow-up cost. *J Bone Joint Surg Am* 2020;102(5):419-427.

52. Dekker TJ, Hamid KS, Federer AE, et al: The value of motion: patient-reported outcome measures are correlated with range of motion in total ankle replacement. *Foot Ankle Spec* 2018;11(5):451-456.

53. Bhashyam AR, Ochen Y, van der Vliet QMJ, et al: Association of patient-reported outcomes with clinical outcomes after distal humerus fracture treatment. *J Am Acad Orthop Surg Glob Res Rev* 2020;4(2):e19.00122.

54. Jo CH, Chai JW, Jeong EC, et al: Intra-articular injection of mesenchymal stem cells for the treatment of osteoarthritis of the knee: A 2-year follow-up study. *Am J Sports Med* 2017;45(12):2774-2783.

55. Centre for Evidence-Based Medicine. Critical Appraisal Tools. Available at: https://www.cebm.net/2014/06/critical-appraisal/. Accessed September 25, 2021.

56. Gagnier JJ, Morgenstern H: Misconceptions, misuses, and misinterpretations of P values and significance testing. *J Bone Joint Surg Am* 2017;99(18):1598-1603.

57. Ioannidis JPA: Contradicted and initially stronger effects in highly cited clinical research. *J Am Med Assoc* 2005;294:218-228.

58. Oltean H, Gagnier JJ: Use of clustering analysis in randomized controlled trials in orthopaedic surgery. *BMC Med Res Methodol* 2015;15:17.

59. Jevsevar DS, Sanders J, Bozic KJ, et al: An introduction to clinical significance in orthopaedic outcomes research. *JBJS Rev* 2015;3(5):e2.

60. Huang H, Grant JA, Miller BS, et al: A systematic review of the psychometric properties of patient-reported outcome instruments for use in patients with rotator cuff disease. *Am J Sports Med* 2015;43(10):2572.

61. Gagnier JJ, Mullins M, Huang H, et al: A systematic review of measurement properties of patient-reported outcome measures used in patients undergoing total knee arthroplasty. *J Arthroplasty* 2017;32(5):1688-1697.e7.

62. Jia Y, Huang H, Gagnier JJ: A systematic review of measurement properties of patient-reported outcome measures for use in patients with foot or ankle diseases. *Qual Life Res* 2017;26(8):1969-2010.

63. Marshall M, Lockwood A, Bradley C, Adams C, Joy C, Fenton M: Unpublished rating scales: A major source of bias in randomized controlled trials of treatments for schizophrenia. *Br J Psychiatry* 2000;176:249-252.

64. Gagnier JJ, Johnston BC: Poor quality patient reported outcome measures bias effect estimates in orthopaedic randomized studies. *J Clin Epidemiol* 2019;116:36-38.

CHAPTER 12 The US FDA Regulatory Landscape and Compliance

Aric Kaiser, MS

INTRODUCTION

To protect the public health, the US FDA provides regulatory oversight to the manufacturing, sale, distribution, and clinical study of human and veterinary drugs, biological products, medical devices and radiation-emitting products, human and animal food, tobacco products, and cosmetics. The Agency also promotes the development of these products through its interactions with the regulated industries. As the types of regulated products change, for example, by the introduction of orthobiologics in the management of orthopaedic diseases, the laws, regulations, and interactions with the Agency are also modified to maintain an appropriate regulatory environment and speed the introduction of safe, effective, and innovative treatments and products to the American public.

REGULATORY AUTHORITY

Although a number of activities took place starting as early as the early 1800s to address concerns related to medicines and foods, the predecessor of the current US FDA was not formally brought into existence until passage of the Pure Food and Drugs Act in 1906. From this initial attempt to address misbranding and adulteration of food and drugs, the FDA's role has expanded to protecting and promoting the development of human and veterinary drugs, biological products, medical devices and radiation-emitting products, human and animal food, tobacco products, and cosmetics.

Before being available for the treatment, management, or diagnosis of disease or impaired function, all medical products subject to premarket review requirements are assessed for safety and effectiveness by the FDA. The FDA's authority to regulate drugs, biological products, and devices is defined by different laws and regulations. The laws governing drugs and devices are defined in the Federal Food Drug and Cosmetics Act (also referred to as the Act)—Title 21 Chapter 9. The laws corresponding to biological products are contained in the Public Health Service Act—Title 42 Chapter 6A.

The corresponding regulations (interpretations of the respective laws) for these entities are located in the Code of Federal Regulations (CFR) Title 21, for example:

- Biological products: 21 CFR Parts 600–680
- Human cells, tissues, and cellular and tissue-based products: 21 CFR Parts 1270/1271
- Drugs: 21 CFR Parts 200–299 and 300–369
- Devices: 21 CFR Parts 800–898

In addition to the laws (written by Congress) and the regulations (written by the FDA), a third source of information related to medical product regulation is guidance documents. These nonbinding documents written by the FDA are intended to provide the Agency's current thinking on a topic. Guidance documents may be written to cover general topics applicable to a variety of products (horizontal), for example, interpretation of the ISO 10993 biocompatibility standard or to address the requirements of a specific regulated product (vertical), for example, cartilage repair products. In each case, guidance documents are governed by Good Guidance Practices and generally require posting of a draft version that is available for a period of public comment followed by a subsequent publication of a final version that takes into account all of the public comments that were received.

REGULATED PRODUCTS: DEFINITIONS

Each of the types of regulated products—biological products, drugs, devices, and combination products—is defined in the statutes and/or regulations. **Table 1** contains the legal definitions for these regulated products.[1-6] Fortunately, biological products, drugs, and devices can be described in simpler terms:

- Biological products: vaccines, human blood, or blood-derived products, monoclonal and polyclonal immunoglobulins, products containing cells, tissues or micro-organisms, and gene therapy.
- Drugs: generally, products that achieve their primary intended purposes through chemical action within or on the body or are dependent on being metabolized. They include peptides or carbohydrates produced

Neither Aric Kaiser nor any immediate family member has received anything of value from or has stock or stock options held in a commercial company or institution related directly or indirectly to the subject of this chapter.

TABLE 1 Regulatory/Statutory Definitions of Biological Products, Drugs, Devices, and Combination Products

Biological product	"…a virus, therapeutic serum, toxin, antitoxin, vaccine, blood, blood component or derivative, allergenic product, protein, or analogous product, or arsphenamine or derivative of arsphenamine (or any other trivalent organic arsenic compound), applicable to the prevention, treatment, or cure of a disease or condition of human beings. 1. A virus is interpreted to be a product containing the minute living cause of an infectious disease and includes but is not limited to filterable viruses, bacteria, rickettsia, fungi, and protozoa; 2. A therapeutic serum is a product obtained from blood by removing the clot or clot components and the blood cells; 3. A toxin is a product containing a soluble substance poisonous to laboratory animals or to man in doses of 1 mL or less (or equivalent in weight) of the product, and having the property, following the injection of nonfatal doses into an animal, of causing to be produced therein another soluble substance which specifically neutralizes the poisonous substance and which is demonstrable in the serum of the animal thus immunized; 4. An antitoxin is a product containing the soluble substance in serum or other body fluid of an immunized animal which specifically neutralizes the toxin against which the animal is immune; 5. A product is analogous: (i) To a virus if prepared from or with a virus or agent actually or potentially infectious, without regard to the degree of virulence or toxicogenicity of the specific strain used; (ii) To a therapeutic serum, if composed of whole blood or plasma or containing some organic constituent or product other than a hormone or an amino acid, derived from whole blood, plasma, or serum; (iii) To a toxin or antitoxin, if intended, irrespective of its source of origin, to be applicable to the prevention, treatment, or cure of disease or injuries of man through a specific immune process; 6. A protein is any alpha amino acid polymer with a specific, defined sequence ie, greater than 40 amino acids in size. When two or more amino acid chains in an amino acid polymer are associated with each other in a manner that occurs in nature, the size of the amino acid polymer for purposes of this paragraph (h)(6) will be based on the total number of amino acids in those chains, and will not be limited to the number of amino acids in a contiguous sequence…"
Drug	"…(A) Articles recognized in the official US Pharmacopeia, official Homeopathic Pharmacopeia of the USA, or official National Formulary, or any supplement to any of them; and (B) articles intended for use in the diagnosis, cure, mitigation, treatment, or prevention of disease in man or other animals; and (C) articles (other than food) intended to affect the structure or any function of the body of man or other animals; and (D) articles intended for use as a component of any articles specified in clause (A), (B), or (C)…"
Device	"…An instrument, apparatus, implement, machine, contrivance, implant, in vitro reagent, or other similar or related article, including any component, part, or accessory, which is (1) recognized in the official National Formulary, or the United States Pharmacopeia, or any supplement to them, (2) intended for use in the diagnosis of disease or other conditions, or in the cure, mitigation, treatment, or prevention of disease, in man or other animals, or (3) intended to affect the structure or any function of the body of man or other animals, and which does not achieve its primary intended purposes through chemical action within or on the body of man or other animals and which is not dependent upon being metabolized for the achievement of its primary intended purposes…"
Combination product	"…(1) A product composed of two or more regulated components, ie, drug/device, biologic/device, drug/biologic, or drug/device/biologic, that are physically, chemically, or otherwise combined or mixed and produced as a single-entity, (2) two or more separate products packaged together in a single package or as a unit and composed of drug and device products, device and biological products, or biological and drug products, (3) a drug, device, or biological product packaged separately that according to its investigational plan or proposed labeling is intended for use only with an approved individually specified drug, device, or biological product where both are required to achieve the intended use, indication, or effect and where upon approval of the proposed product the labeling of the approved product would need to be changed, eg, to reflect a change in intended use, dosage form, strength, route of administration, or significant change in dose, or (4) any investigational drug, device, or biological product packaged separately that according to its proposed labeling is for use only with another individually specified investigational drug, device, or biological product where both are required to achieve the intended use, indication, or effect…"

synthetically or from cell culture or in animal fluids by genetic alteration.
- Devices: entities whose primary intended purposes are not achieved through chemical action within or on the body or by being metabolized.

The definition of human cells, tissues, and cellular and tissue-based products (HCT/Ps) is more complicated. HCT/Ps are defined as human cells or tissues intended for implantation, transplantation, infusion, or transfer into a human recipient.[2] These are best defined by examples, which include bone (intact and demineralized), skin, corneas, ligaments, tendons, dura mater, heart valves, vascular grafts (arteries and veins, excluding preserved umbilical cord veins), pericardium, hematopoietic stem/progenitor cells derived from peripheral and cord blood, oocytes and semen, cultured cartilage and nerve cells, lymphocyte immune therapy, gene therapy products, and collagen. Vascularized human organ transplants such as the kidney, liver, heart, lung, or pancreas are not considered to be HCT/Ps.

Section 351 of the Public Health Service Act identifies the types of products that would be regulated as biological products, referred to as 351 products. Section 361 of the Public Health Service Act does not identify specific products, but provides the FDA's authority to regulate certain products to prevent disease introduction and transmission. 21 CFR 1271.10(a) outlines criteria for a risk-based approach to regulating HCT/Ps. HCT/Ps that meet these criteria are regulated as 361 products. 361 products do not require submission of a marketing application before being made available to the public. Manufacturers of these types of products are allowed to self-designate those products that meet the criteria. A key component of this analysis is the assessment of whether the HCT/P is "more than minimally manipulated" or "intended for homologous use". 351 products must be evaluated in a marketing application and receive FDA permission before being legally marketed. **Table 2** identifies the criteria that must be met for an HCT/P to be considered a 361 product, as well as examples of 351 products.

Until recently, medical management consisted of the use of these products that were readily categorized into one of three groups: biological products, drugs, or devices. This practice has changed over the years because of an increase in the number of combination products available to physicians. Combination products are medical products that comprise two or more different products listed previously, that is, drug/device, biological product/device, drug/biological product, or drug/device/biological product. These different products are referred to as constituent parts of the combination product. Combination products can include two or more single-entity products that are chemically or physically combined into a single product or may comprise two or more single-entity products that are copackaged or cross-labeled and intended to be used together. Importantly, a combination product should not be confused with medical products that include two or more components from a single category of the single-entity products noted previously, that is, device/device, drug/drug, biological product/biological product. Combination products have distinct regulations and require cross-discipline review and assessment by the components of the FDA that are responsible for the regulation of each type of constituent part of the combination product.

TABLE 2 361 Product Requirements (All Must be Present) and Examples of 351 Products

361 Product Requirements
Minimally manipulated
Intended for homologous use
Not combined with other components, except for water or components intended for sterilization, preservation, or storage
No systemic effect and not dependent on metabolic activity of living cells for primary function; or has a systemic effect or is dependent on activity living cells for its primary function and is for autologous use, allogeneic use in first-degree or second-degree blood relatives, or for reproductive use
351 Product Examples
Cultured cartilage cells
Cultured nerve cells
Lymphocyte immune therapy
Gene therapy products
Human cloning
Human cells used in therapy involving the transfer of genetic material (cell nuclei, oocyte nuclei, mitochondrial genetic material in ooplasm, genetic material contained in a genetic vector)
Unrelated allogeneic hematopoietic stem cells
Unrelated donor lymphocytes for infusion

STRUCTURE AND ORGANIZATION OF THE FDA

The FDA is one of the Agencies located within the Department of Health and Human Services. The FDA includes multiple Centers that are each responsible for the regulation of a specific type of medical product. These Centers are the Center for Biologics Evaluation and Research (CBER), the Center for Drug Evaluation and Research (CDER), the Center for Devices and Radiological Health (CDRH), the Center for Veterinary Medicine, the Center for Tobacco Products, and the Center for Food Safety and Nutrition. Although nonregulatory, the National Center for Toxicological Research is also located within the FDA. For the medical products typically in the orthobiologics category, regulation would occur in CBER, CDER, or CDRH. **Figure 1** summarizes the FDA's structure.

Biological products are primarily regulated within CBER; drugs are primarily regulated within CDER; and devices are primarily regulated within CDRH (CBER also has the authority to regulate certain devices and drugs that are determined to be under CBER jurisdiction). Depending on a number of factors, HCT/Ps may be regulated as either 361 products under the authority of CBER if the HCT/P meets the eligibility criteria outlined in 21 CFR 1271.10 or as 351 products which are further classified as biological products, drugs, or devices, under the authority of CBER, CDER, or CDRH, respectively. Because of its regulation of transgenic animals, the Center for Veterinary Medicine may also provide support to the regulation of products intended for humans.

The organizational differences between the Centers result in practical review and regulatory differences. CBER and CDER are organized similarly with separations along diseases or intended uses. Within a CBER or CDER Division, review staff are organized in parallel branches by discipline. Physicians are grouped with other physicians, chemists with other chemists, and so on. Each of these discipline groups within the review Division is managed independently. Input related to different disciplines must come from interactions between different groups. CDRH is generally organized along medical disciplines. Groups within a review Division are not organized by discipline, but by medical specialty or product type. In this arrangement, engineers, physicians, and other scientists are within the same group and managed together. Because of this mixing of staff with varied backgrounds, input related to different disciplines can often emanate from within a single group.

Contact with review staff differs across the Centers as well. In CBER and CDER, all submissions are assigned to a regulatory project manager (RPM). The RPM is not responsible for providing any review input, but is responsible for the administrative activities associated with the project and for confirming that the appropriate regulations are followed. All information for the various review teams is funneled through the RPM. In most cases, this information is then passed along to a lead reviewer who is typically a medical officer. Communication between manufacturers and the FDA occurs through the RPM. In contrast, each submission under the jurisdiction of CDRH is assigned to a lead reviewer who is generally not a medical officer, but who is the primary engineering or scientific contact for the submission. The lead reviewer is responsible for coordination and delegation of the internal and administrative activities, as well as serving as the main point of contact internally and with industry.

Each of the Centers has access to personnel and expertise associated with managing the regulatory life cycles of its assigned regulated products. In the case of combination products, a single Center is typically not sufficient to address all of the legal, regulatory, and scientific concerns and any one Center was not intended to address

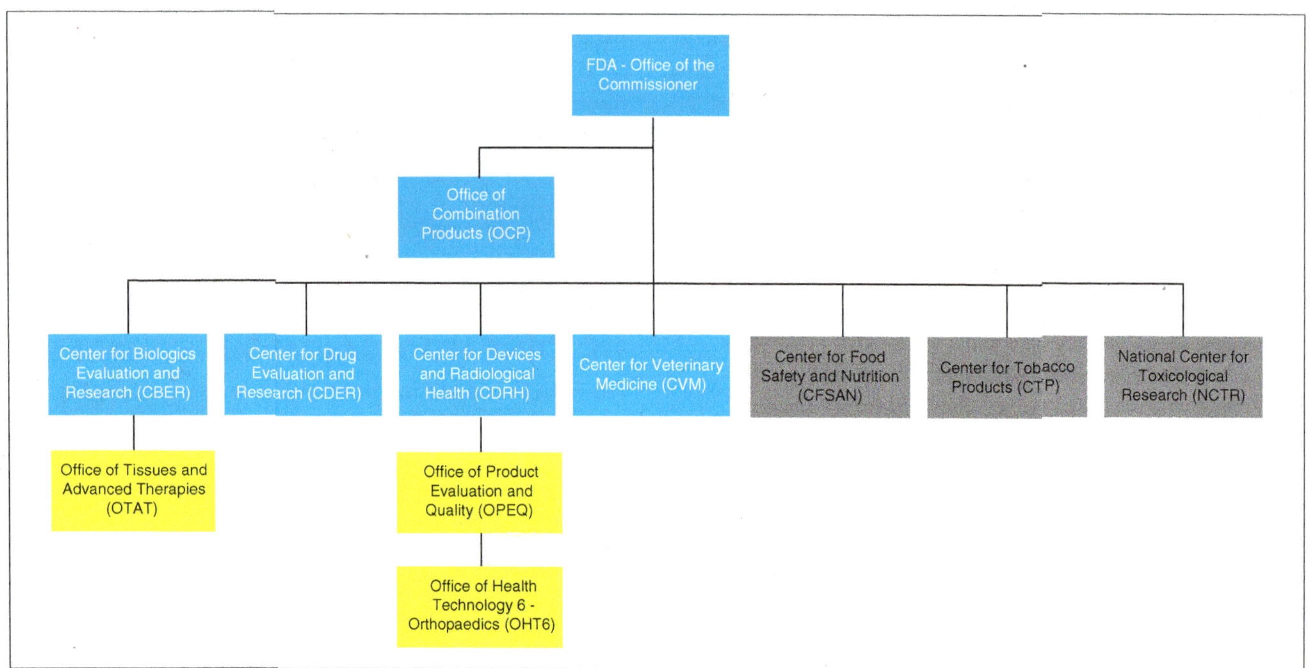

FIGURE 1 Organizational chart shows the FDA's structure. Groups that could be involved in regulation of orthobiologics are identified in blue, with the specific staff within the relevant Center identified in yellow. Centers identified in gray would generally not be involved in the regulation of orthobiologics.

the classification and jurisdiction of medical products that include biological products, drugs, and/or devices. In other words, the issues associated with combination products cross the regulatory and scientific boundaries between Centers. To address the types of complex issues associated with combination products, Congress and the Agency determined that it was necessary to establish a group who would be responsible for addressing the unique challenges associated with combination products.

In accordance with Section 204 of the Medical Device User Fee and Modernization Act of 2002, the Office of Combination Products (OCP) was established within the Commissioner's Office of FDA. OCP is responsible for the coordination of all combination product activities across the FDA. The Office also serves as a focal point for queries from industry, consumers, and FDA staff. As part of these efforts, OCP does the following:

- Develops guidance and regulations as an aid to the appropriate regulation of combination products
- Classifies products as drugs, devices, biological products, or combination products and assigns a Center to have primary jurisdiction over the product if jurisdiction is unclear
- Resolves disputes regarding the timeliness of premarket review of combination products
- Ensures timely and effective premarket review by overseeing the timeliness of reviews and coordinating reviews involving more than one Center
- Ensures consistency and appropriateness of postmarket regulation of combination products

This legislation also required that OCP submit annual reports to Congress outlining their activities and their effect on the regulatory process. OCP also provides outreach to the medical products community via participation in internal and external workshops and meetings throughout the year. As part of the 21st Century Cures Act, OCP was given additional responsibilities. These include the ability to address disputes related to combination products, determine the relevance of a chemical action of a combination product, and meet with manufacturers to discuss issues related to combination product marketing, postmarket modifications, and good manufacturing practices.

SUBMISSIONS AND INTERACTIONS

Request for Designation, Determination of the Primary Mode of Action, and Jurisdiction Assignment

Before regulation of a medical product can occur, the Center with jurisdiction must be identified. For single-entity products, that is, drugs, devices, or biological products, this is typically an easy and obvious process. For single-entity products, a manufacturer works closely with a single Center. The statutory and regulatory provisions governing that Center's products would apply. Because only a single Center is involved in the review process, it is relatively straightforward for a manufacturer to determine which rules apply to their product and how to comply with them. It is also relatively simple to determine which group within a particular Center is responsible for the product's regulation.

For combination products, this can be less straightforward and the regulation of combination products requires that all constituent parts of the combination product be taken into consideration. In some cases, it may be necessary to interact with OCP to determine which Center has jurisdiction. Initial interaction with the incorrect Center would be counterproductive to the efficient and timely evaluation and introduction of new medical treatments. To ensure that a manufacturer is working with the appropriate Center, it is necessary first to determine the appropriate jurisdiction of the combination product. A method of assigning jurisdiction is the Request for Designation (RFD) process.

The RFD process serves two functions. The first function allows for the Agency to officially classify the product as a biological product, device, drug, or combination product when the status is in question. The second function provides a means for clearly identifying which Center within the Agency would have primary responsibility for regulation of the identified product.

Although the FDA makes the final determinations, manufacturers are responsible for providing the information that allows the Agency to make these decisions. In general terms, the RFD process requires that manufacturers describe their product and how they think it works, categorize which type of regulated product they believe it to be (biological product, device, drug, or combination product), and propose a Center for lead regulatory jurisdiction. The Agency has published a guidance document titled "How to Write a Request for Designation" that describes this process in more detail.[6]

An RFD can take one of two forms: a pre-RFD or a formal RFD. The pre-RFD[7] allows for more interaction between the manufacturer and OCP. In a pre-RFD, a manufacturer is also able to provide more information to describe their product and support their rationale for designation of the type of product they have and which Center should have jurisdiction. There is an ongoing dialogue between the manufacturer and OCP. In the pre-RFD process, OCP provides nonbinding informal feedback. A formal RFD has a 15-page limit and does not allow for interaction between the manufacturer and OCP while the submission is under review. The benefit for this trade-off is a statutorily defined limited review period (60 days) and receipt of a binding decision with respect to the type of product and the Center assigned jurisdiction.

Aside from describing the various components of the product, the RFD also needs to include a discussion of the product's primary mode of action (PMOA). The individual components of the combination product are each responsible for acting in specific ways. In many cases, one of these actions usually takes precedence over the others and provides the most important therapeutic action of the combination product. This is the PMOA.

Identification of the PMOA as it relates to assignment of jurisdiction is the cornerstone of the RFD submission. A product's modes of action are often critical to the FDA's determination of the regulatory identity of a single-entity product, and a combination product's PMOA determines its assignment. The regulation requires that manufacturers provide a description of all known modes of action and, in the case of combination products, identify the single mode of action that provides the most important therapeutic action of the product, and identify the basis for that determination. Although the manufacturer is required to identify what they believe to be the PMOA, as well as the lead Center, it is up to the Agency to make these final determinations. It is important that manufacturers provide as much relevant information as possible concerning their understanding of the PMOA. The Agency will use this, as well and any other publicly available information, for example, literature, patents, etc, in establishing the PMOA.

The mode of action as defined in 21 CFR 3.2.(k) is the means by which a product achieves an intended therapeutic effect or action. In this context, therapeutic action or effect includes any effect or action of the product intended to diagnose, cure, mitigate, treat, or prevent disease, or affect the structure or any function of the body. Products may have a drug, biological product, or device mode of action. Because combination products are composed of more than one type of regulated article and each constituent part contributes its own mode of action, combination products will have more than one mode of action.

The PMOA is defined in 21 CFR 3.2(m) as "...the single mode of action of a combination product that provides the most important therapeutic action of the combination product. The most important therapeutic action is the mode of action that is expected to make the greatest contribution to the overall intended therapeutic effects of the combination product..."[8] When describing the mode of action believed to be the PMOA, it is necessary to include the reasons why that mode of action would be expected to be the most important and why the other mode(s) of action would be secondary.

Under ideal conditions, there is a readily identifiable PMOA resulting from the actions of a single component of the combination product. For some products, however, it may not be possible for a manufacturer or the FDA to determine, at the time the RFD is submitted, which single mode of action of a combination product provides the most important therapeutic action. Determining the PMOA of a combination product is also complicated for products where the product has two completely different modes of action, neither of which is subordinate to the other. To address this dilemma, the FDA has devised an algorithm (defined in 21 CFR 3.4(b)) to assign jurisdiction of these types of products with as much consistency, predictability, and transparency as possible. Manufacturers are required to follow the same algorithm in their analysis of their product if a PMOA is not readily identifiable.

In those cases where the PMOA cannot be readily determined, the combination product would be assigned to the Center that regulates other combination products that present similar questions of safety and effectiveness with regard to the combination product as a whole. When there are no other combination products that present similar questions of safety and effectiveness with regard to the combination product as a whole, for example, it is the first such combination product, or differences in its intended use, design, formulation, etc, present different safety and effectiveness questions, the combination product would be assigned to the Center with the most expertise related to the most significant safety and effectiveness questions presented by the combination product.

Presubmissions

To receive feedback before submission of a marketing application or request to initiate a clinical study, a manufacturer may seek feedback from the FDA. For simple questions, this may be accomplished informally by contacting the FDA by telephone or e-mail. In most cases, however, manufacturers are seeking more extensive feedback. This is handled through a formal presubmission process. The processes differ between the Centers.

In CBER and CDER, a pre-Investigational New Drug (pre-IND) meeting may be requested by a manufacturer to discuss the drug development plan and future clinical trials for a specific product.[9] The purpose of pre-IND meetings is to discuss safety issues related to the proper identification, strength, quality, purity, or potency of the investigational drug and to identify potential clinical hold issues before the submission of an IND. A pre-IND meeting is a formal interaction with the FDA in which discussions are nonbinding.[10]

To support the development of innovative CBER-regulated products, manufacturers may request an Initial Targeted Engagement for Regulatory Advice on CBER Products meeting. An Initial Targeted Engagement for Regulatory Advice on CBER Products meeting enables a manufacturer to obtain preliminary consultation for innovative investigational products at an early stage of development, before the pre-IND meeting phase. In general, the Initial Targeted Engagement for Regulatory Advice on CBER Products program consists of a single, informal, nonbinding consultation on products that introduce unique challenges because of unknown safety profiles resulting from the use of complex manufacturing technologies, development of innovative devices, or cutting-edge testing methodologies.

In CDRH, the Q-Submission program handles these types of requests. The types of interactions and processes are described in detail in the guidance document titled "Requests for Feedback and Meetings for Medical Device Submissions: The Q-Submission Program".[11] A presubmission is the most common type of Q-submission. The presubmission process allows a manufacturer to request FDA feedback to specific questions. In response, CDRH will provide written feedback to the manufacturer's questions, as well as other comments related to the submission that are determined to be appropriate and potentially helpful. If the manufacturer wants to have a follow-up discussion related to their original questions and CDRH's feedback, a mutually agreeable meeting date is identified at the beginning of the review process. Currently, written feedback is issued within 70 days of receipt of the presubmission or 5 calendar days before a scheduled meeting, whichever is sooner.

Presubmissions can contain questions related to any topic, for example, regulatory approach, nonclinical testing requirements and protocols, and clinical testing requirements and protocols. The questions should be of sufficient detail as to allow CDRH to provide useful feedback. To allow for adequate review time, the number of questions should be limited. Splitting nonclinical and clinical questions between different presubmissions is recommended to allow sufficient time for useful discussions at scheduled meetings.

In CBER and CDER, there is a limit to the number of presubmissions related to a specific product—one for nonclinical issues and one for clinical issues. There are currently no limits on the number of presubmissions that a manufacturer can submit to CDRH related to a specific product. This is an important factor for manufacturers to keep in mind when they are devising their regulatory strategy.

Meetings

The ability of manufacturers to meet with Agency staff is crucial to the proper regulation of all medical products, including combination products. In order for these interactions to run smoothly and be productive, each Center has devised certain requirements. Some of these are mandated by statute and some have come about through evolution of Center policies. Requests for meetings regarding a combination product should generally be submitted to the lead Center for the product, in accordance with that Center's corresponding processes.

In CBER and CDER, manufacturers may request formal meetings to discuss product development. There are three meeting types that are subject to different procedures and timelines defined in the Prescription Drug User Fee Act. Type A meetings are held to address stalled product development and are scheduled within 30 days of FDA receipt of a written request. Type B meetings include pre-IND meetings, certain end-of-phase 1 meetings, end-of-phase 2 and pre-phase 3 meetings, and pre–new drug applications or prebiological license application meetings. Type B meetings are scheduled to occur within 60 days of request. Type C meetings are meetings are those other than Type A and B and are scheduled 75 days of request.[12]

For the most part, CDRH follows a more informal meeting structure. Presubmission meetings are generally held within 75 days of receipt of the presubmission packet. Agreement meetings and appeal meetings are formal meetings described by regulation and used for a very specific purpose. These meeting descriptions and their timeframes are described by statue. Because of regulatory limitations, they are requested and held very infrequently.

Clinical Trials

Before initiating a clinical study in the United States, it is necessary to receive permission to initiate the study from the designated Center. Aside from the general types of regulations associated with subject protection that apply to all clinical studies, for example, informed consent and institutional review boards (IRBs), there are two sets of regulations that are Center dependent. For new biological products or drugs (or old versions of these products being evaluated for new uses or target populations), CBER and CDER follow the IND regulations (21 CFR Part 312). Devices regulated by CDRH and CBER are governed by the Investigational Device Exemptions (IDEs) regulations (21 CFR Part 812). The exemptions that are outlined in these regulations are those related to aspects of the product manufacturing and compliance with the device Quality System Regulations (QSRs). **Figure 2** summarizes the various types of clinical study submissions described in more detail in the following text.

CBER and CDER recognize three types of studies, referred to as phase 1, 2, and 3. In general, each of these phases is required for each investigational product. It is not uncommon, however, for a manufacturer to combine two phases into a single study: for example, a phase 1/2 or 2/3 study. With each subsequent phase, the number of enrolled subjects in the clinical studies increases. The goal of each phase is different. Phase 1 studies are usually performed to gather initial safety data. Phase 2 studies are larger than phase 1 studies and provide the initial data from use of the investigational product in the target population. Phase 3 studies are large-scale, multicenter, randomized trials designed to collect safety and effectiveness data in the target population. Phase 3 drug trials may enroll thousands of subjects. For clinical studies regulated under the IND regulations, there is a requirement for at least two phase 3 studies.

CDRH does not have a formal phased study approach to clinical trials. Although different types of studies are recognized, they do not map directly to the three phases of IND studies. In addition, each type of study is not required for every investigational device. The number of studies is dependent on the device type and its associated questions.

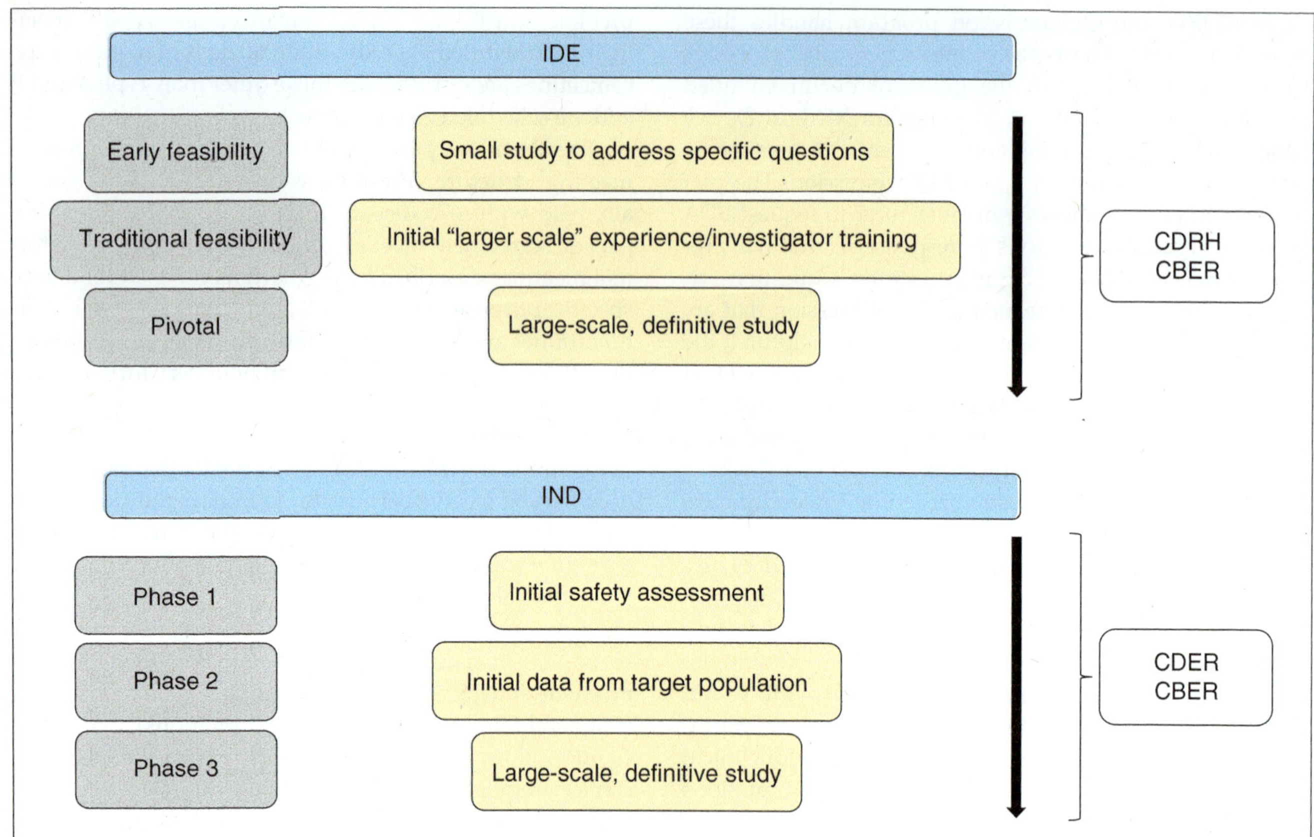

FIGURE 2 Chart summarizing clinical study types and Center that uses them. Arrows indicate increasing sample size and study duration. Two Investigational New Drug (IND) phase 3 studies are generally required to support marketing. CBER = Center for Biologics Evauation and Research; CDER = Center for Drug Evaluation and Research; CDRH = Center for Devices and Radiological Health; IDE = Investigational Device Exemption

There are three main study types: early feasibility (previously referred to as feasibility studies), traditional feasibility (previously referred to as pilot studies), and pivotal. Early feasibility studies are small studies (often fewer than 20 patients enrolled across fewer than five investigational sites). They are usually designed to evaluate specific aspects associated with a device, for example, different surgical techniques or implant design features, or evaluation instruments. Because of their small size, they cannot be used to support marketing applications or make statistical assessments. Traditional feasibility studies are larger than early feasibility studies, but not as large as pivotal studies. They are often used to collect more detailed data from a larger group of subjects. Because of the larger sample sizes, statistical assessments may be possible. Pivotal studies are often large-scale, multicenter, randomized trials designed to collect safety and effectiveness data in support of a marketing application. In contrast to phase 3 drug and biological product trials, pivotal studies of devices are generally smaller, often enrolling several hundred subjects in each group (investigational and control). In addition, there is no requirement for multiple clinical studies, and if clinical data are necessary, only a single IDE pivotal study could be adequate to support marketing.

Although the ultimate goal of a clinical trial in CBER, CDER, and CDRH is the same, that is, the collection of data to determine the safety and effectiveness of a particular product for a particular use in a particular target population, differences in the IND and IDE regulations warrant differences in clinical study review. Not unexpectedly, the details of the internal review process also differ between the INDs under the jurisdiction of CBER and CDER and the IDEs under the jurisdiction of CBER and CDRH.

INDs are reviewed, but they are not approved. Within 30 days after an IND is received by the Agency, a safety review is performed and the review team determines whether a study is reasonably safe to proceed or will be placed on clinical hold. A clinical hold is an order issued by the Agency to delay initiation of a proposed IND or suspend an ongoing IND. Each aspect of the IND is reviewed somewhat independently and separate determinations can be made for the clinical and nonclinical aspects of the proposal. The grounds for imposing a clinical hold differ between phase 1, phase 2, and phase 3 trials. For phase 1 trials, a clinical hold would be imposed if patients would be exposed to an unreasonable and significant risk of illness or injury; investigators are determined to be unqualified;

the Investigator Brochure is found to be misleading, erroneous, or incomplete; there is insufficient information to assess the potential risks; or there is an exclusion by sex for life-threatening disease. In the case of phase 2 or 3 trials, a clinical hold would be imposed for any of the reasons outlined for phase 1 trials, as well as if the proposed protocol is found to have design deficiencies that would prevent it from meeting its stated objectives. If a clinical hold is issued, it is not necessary for the manufacturer to respond to the clinical hold. If a response is submitted, the FDA will respond to the manufacturer within 30 days. The FDA's response will either be to remove or maintain the clinical hold. The manufacturer may not proceed with the clinical study until the FDA has lifted the clinical hold, at such time the study may proceed.

Once an IDE submission is received, a 30-day review clock is started and the Agency initiates a complete review of all submitted material. The Agency is required to provide a written response by the 30th calendar day by approving, disapproving, or conditionally approving the submission. An IDE is approved (or conditionally approved) only if the complete submission contains no issues that raise concerns related to the "relative safety" of the investigational product. If no written response is issued by the 30th day, the IDE submission is automatically deemed approved and the manufacturer is allowed to proceed with the contents of the proposal unless the Agency overturns the deemed approval. There is no current provision for extending the review process beyond 30 days. Based on the 2012 amendments to the Act (the Food and Drug Administration Safety and Innovation Act, referred to as FDASIA), an IDE can only be disapproved if there are aspects of the study that directly affect subject safety. Proposed studies that lack scientific soundness can no longer be disapproved. The nonbinding study design concerns are issued as part of the approval or conditional approval letter and are referred to as Study Design Considerations. Although FDASIA also gave CDRH the authority to issue a clinical hold for IDEs, this would only apply to ongoing studies and has not been implemented.

Although the specific types of nonclinical data that must be submitted in support of initiating a clinical trial under an IND or IDE are dependent on the nature of the product, the actual data being submitted would be identical regardless of the Center that has been assigned jurisdiction. The only differences between the Centers are those associated with the timing of the submission of the various types of data and the conditions for initiating the trial. In CBER and CDER, it is not necessary to submit all the data before initiation of the trial. These Centers allow manufacturers to commit to submitting certain types of data during the trial. This is partially related to the fact that each phase of an IND is designed to address specific sets of questions. In CDRH any data that are determined to be necessary for demonstrating the relative safety of the product must be submitted before initiation of the trial. In general, nonclinical data are not submitted to an IDE after it has been approved. The only exceptions to this are the submission of additional nonclinical data intended to supplement data that already support an adequate determination of relative safety or new data to address problems that have been identified during the course of the trial, for example, failure of a specific aspect of the device component.

Marketing Applications

Before initiating sales of a product, it is necessary for manufacturers to notify the FDA of their intent and obtain permission. The types of marketing applications available are defined in the laws and regulations. Just as each Center has different laws and regulations, each Center has access to use different types of marketing applications.

Products assigned to CDER are marketed using either a New Drug Application (or an Abbreviated New Drug Application or ANDA) for products where assignment was associated with the drug constituent part or a Biologics License Application for products where assignment was associated with a therapeutic protein constituent part. There are two review time frames associated with these submissions. A standard submission is reviewed using a 10-month review cycle, whereas a priority submission is reviewed using a 6-month review cycle. Although they could be a component of a combination product, the presence of an over-the-counter drug monograph product in a combination product would not alter the type of marketing application available for that particular combination product.

Products assigned to CDRH are primarily marketed using either the premarket notification (510(k)) or the Premarket Approval (PMA) route. The review timeframe for 510(k)s and PMAs is 90 and 180 days, respectively. The risk associated with the products marketed under each of these routes is different. In general, products marketed using the 510(k) route are associated with low to medium risk, whereas those marketed using the PMA route are associated with the highest risk. In a 510(k) submission, a manufacturer provides a demonstration that its device or combination product is substantially equivalent either to another device or combination product cleared for marketing via the 510(k) route or to a device(s) already on the market before May 28, 1976. In the case of a PMA, a manufacturer must demonstrate a reasonable assurance of safety and effectiveness of its product, which in most cases will entail an assessment of safety and effectiveness in comparison to a control treatment.

Another marketing application in CDRH is the De Novo classification process. This process is used for low to moderate risk products that are associated with a new intended use or whose technologic characteristics raise different questions of safety and effectiveness and, therefore, do not have a predicate. As a result, they are ineligible for using the 510(k) pathway and would automatically be designated postamendments class III. Although class III devices would ordinarily follow the PMA route, those that are associated with low to moderate risk can petition for classification through the De Novo pathway. For these products, a reasonable assurance of safety and effectiveness for the identified intended use can be provided by application of appropriate general or general and special controls. They are assigned a classification through the De Novo classification process and can serve as predicate devices for subsequent 510(k) submissions. The FDA review timeframe for a De Novo submission is 150 days.

Most products assigned to CBER use the Biologics License Application route. Biological product devices may also be marketed using the same routes that CDRH uses, that is, the PMA, De Novo, and 510(k). CBER also uses the New Drug Application process where appropriate. A summary of the various submission types and the Centers that use them is outlined in **Figure 3**. **Figure 4** describes the theoretical FDA interaction flow based on Center jurisdiction assignment.

Tissue Reference Group

The Tissue Reference Group (TRG) was created in 1997 as part of the FDA's approach to regulating HCT/Ps. This group is primarily made up of staff from CBER and CDRH, each providing three permanent members to the group. Each Center's Product Jurisdiction Officer counts as one of its members. Additional attendees from each Center or other parts of the FDA who possess particular expertise related to the topics being discussed are also invited to attend as needed. The purpose of the TRG is to serve as a single point within the FDA for questions related to the regulation and jurisdiction of HCT/Ps. These questions may be submitted directly to the TRG or referred to the group from the Centers themselves. Manufacturers can also request OCP review of the informal feedback from the TRG.

One of the primary activities of the TRG is performing analyses of the description of products in an effort to determine their regulatory status, that is, as 361 products or 351 products The regulations (21 CFR 1271.10) identify the criteria that must be met for an HCT/P to be regulated as a 361 product. Given the variety of HCT/P sources, processing approaches, and uses, this is often not a straightforward process. Although a goal of the TRG is to identify groups of products that can be regulated similarly, the subtle differences between different products often make this difficult. The process for evaluating minimal manipulation and homologous use is described in more detail in the guidance document titled "Regulatory Considerations

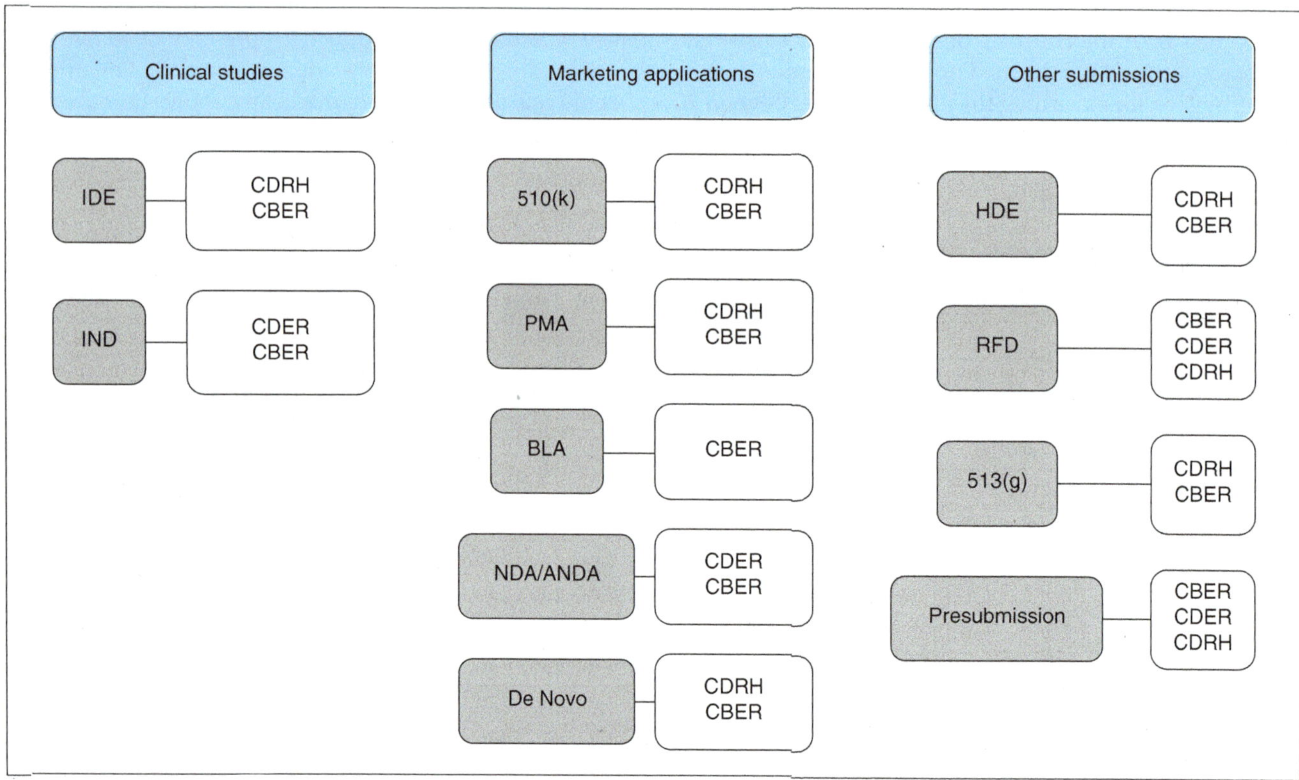

FIGURE 3 Chart showing a summary of select submission types by category and Center that uses them. BLA = biologics license application; CBER = Center for Biologics Evauation and Research; CDER = Center for Drug Evaluation and Research; CDRH = Center for Devices and Radiological Health; HDE = Humanitarian Device Exemption; IDE = Investigational Device Exemption; IND = Investigational New Drug; NDA/ANDA = New Drug Application/Abbreviated New Drug Application; PMA = Premarket Approval; RFD = Request for Designation

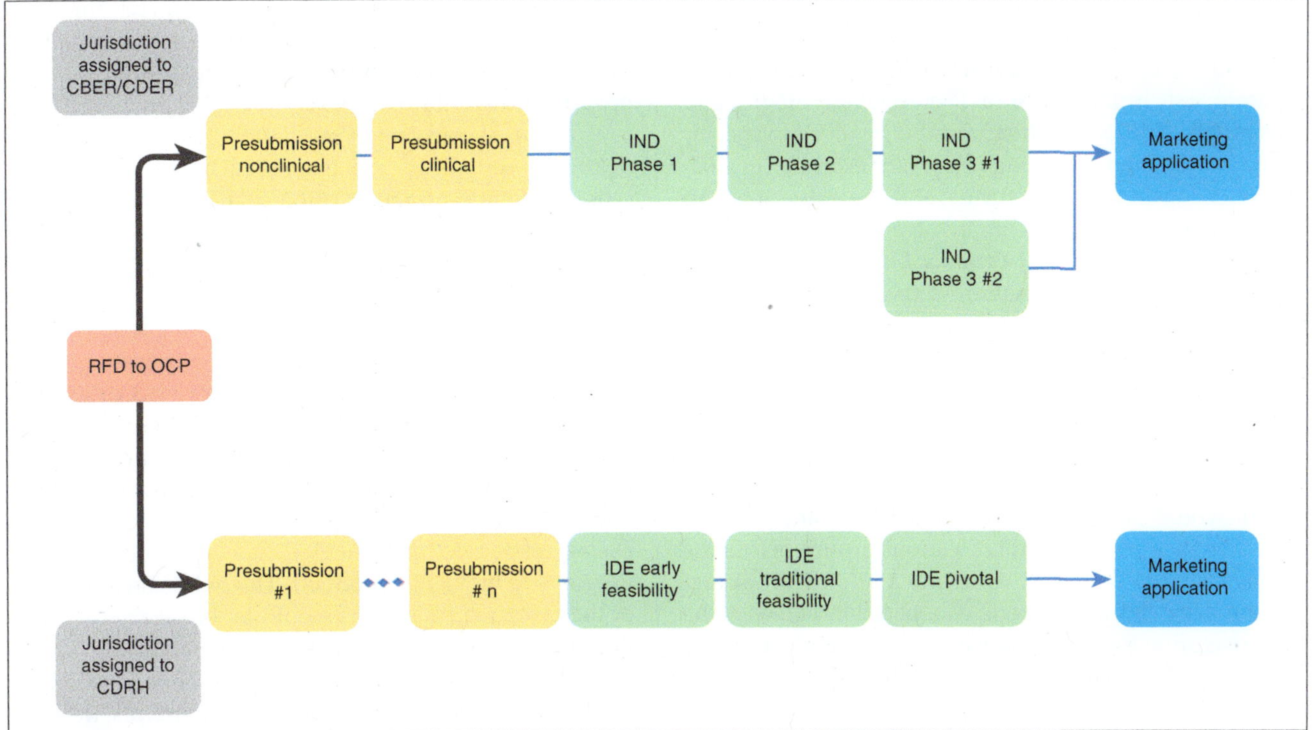

FIGURE 4 Chart showing the theoretical FDA interaction based on assignment of jurisdiction. Under certain circumstances, Investigational New Drug (IND) phases may be combined. Two phase 3 IND studies are generally required prior to marketing. The Center for Devices and Radiological Health (CDRH) does not limit the number of presubmissions. Depending on the product type and safety concerns, all Investigational Device Exemption study types are not required prior to marketing. CBER = Center for Biologics Evauation and Research; CDER = Center for Drug Evaluation and Research; IDE = Investigational Device Exemption; OCP = Office of Combination Products; RFD = Request for Designation

for Human Cells, Tissues, and Cellular and Tissue-Based Products: Minimal Manipulation and Homologous Use."[13]

Dispute Resolution

Under normal circumstances, all communication between a manufacturer and the FDA concerning a particular submission is addressed by working directly with the review group assigned to the project. In most cases, any conflicts can be addressed with the review team or their management. In the rare cases where this is not possible, manufacturers have the right to seek assistance from an Ombudsman. Each Center, as well as the Commissioner's Office, has an Ombudsman's Office that is available to aid manufacturers in resolving disputes that could not be addressed through other means.

MANUFACTURING, COMPLIANCE, AND POSTMARKET REPORTING

Quality System Regulation, Current Good Manufacturing Practice, and Current Good Tissue Practice

Because of the differences between the different product types, the type of manufacturing and compliance data submitted to the Agency differs by Center. CDER applies the current Good Manufacturing Practices (21 CFR Parts 210 and 211). CDRH applies the QSRs (21 CFR Part 820) and is in the process of incorporating aspects of ISO 13485:2016 into the QSRs. As has been described previously for other processes, CBER applies both the current Good Manufacturing Practices and QSRs as appropriate.

Products that incorporate an HCT/P component must also comply with the current Good Tissue Practices and donor eligibility rules (both found in 21 CFR Part 1271). The biological product regulations (21 CFR Parts 600–680) also contain relevant information. In the case of combination products, the specific configuration of the combination product would determine how these various sets of regulations are actually applied.

The differences in these regulations result in differences in the types of manufacturing data that must be collected and maintained by the manufacturer, as well as differences in the timing and types of regulatory submissions. Differences in the organizational structure of each of the Centers also contribute to differences in the number and type of Agency interactions. In CBER, most of these activities are handled by the Office of Compliance and Biologics Quality. The product review staff in the appropriate review Office are also involved in some of these activities, particularly with respect to facility inspections and review of data relating to release specifications. In CDER, manufacturing and compliance issues are handled by the Office of Pharmaceutical Quality. Similar to CBER, separate staff in the Office of Therapeutic Biologics and Biosimilars (a different Office) are also involved in specific aspects of the manufacturing review, for example, evaluation of chemistry, manufacturing, and controls data. Staff from both of these groups are involved in facility inspections. In CDRH, the Total Product Lifecycle reorganization resulted in the elimination of the separate Office of Compliance. All postmarket activities related to manufacturing and compliance, with the exception of inspections, have been moved to the new Office of Product Evaluation and Quality, which is responsible for the regulation of all premarket and postmarket activities. Inspections are handled by a separate Office within CDRH.

As would be expected, manufacturing and compliance activities occurring in the various groups across the Agency need to be coordinated into a unified set of regulatory activities and actions. Cooperation between the manufacturing and compliance reviewers and the product reviewers is extremely important. In CBER and CDER, these activities are coordinated by the project managers. In CDRH, the lead reviewer is ultimately responsible; however, staff with more extensive manufacturing and compliance experience may also be included as part of the product review team.

A more detailed discussion of how the FDA addresses manufacturing requirements for combination products is provided in the guidance document titled "Current Good Manufacturing Practice Requirements for Combination Products".[14]

Reporting

Like the current Good Manufacturing Practice and QSR requirements, postmarket reporting requirements differ across the Centers. For single-entity products, the reporting requirements are those outlined in the regulations associated with that Center. These are described in 21 CFR Parts 310 and 314 for drugs, 21 CFR Parts 600 and 606 for biological products, and 21 CFR Part 803 for devices. Each constituent part of a combination product is governed by one of three differing sets of provisions for postmarket safety reporting. Although these requirements share many similarities and have a common underlying purpose, protection of the public health by ensuring a product's continued safety and effectiveness, each set of regulations has certain reporting standards and time frames with unique requirements based on the characteristics of the products for which the regulations were designed.

Without development of processes specific to combination products, an adverse event reporter would have followed the safety reporting regulations associated with the type of marketing application used to approve or clear the combination product. Because this could become complicated for combination products and result in potential overreporting or underreporting, a regulation was developed to address this situation—21 CFR 4, Subpart B.

In general, each set of regulations requires reports of death and serious adverse events, each provides for periodic and follow-up reports, and each provides a method to signal certain types of safety events that warrant expedited reporting. Because of these similarities, it is possible to consolidate the requirements so that the combination product is subject primarily to the reporting requirements associated with the type of marketing application under which the combination product is approved or cleared. However, there are certain significant differences in the three sets of regulations. These differences are designed to facilitate adverse experience reporting that adequately addresses the distinct characteristics and potential safety issues related to a particular type of product (drug, device, and biological product). The public health benefit of these unique provisions would be lost if the combination products were subject solely to the reporting requirements associated with the type of marketing application. To account for these specific, limited differences, the common reporting requirements would be supplemented by the preservation of certain reports.

A detailed discussion of how this regulation is applied and the rationale behind the Agency's approach is beyond the scope of this chapter. Details are provided in the guidance document titled "Postmarketing Safety Reporting for Combination Products Guidance for Industry and FDA Staff".[15]

Although most reports are submitted by manufacturers, reports describing problems with medical products or adverse events resulting from their use may be submitted by physicians, other health care providers, health care facilities, and consumers. This type of reporting is voluntary. These reports serve as an extremely useful source of information on the actual use and performance of medical products. These types of reports are submitted through the MedWatch Program.[16,17]

Compliance Activities

Under ideal circumstances, a manufacturer will follow all applicable laws and regulations and there will be no concerns that they have been implemented improperly. In addition, every product will be manufactured perfectly and never malfunction. Practically, this is not the case. At some point, every manufacturer will encounter a situation where there is a question or problem related to compliance with the manufacturing regulations and/or their product will not be manufactured in such a way as to meet all of its design requirements. When these situations occur, the FDA will become of aware of them either because the manufacturer has reported it voluntarily or the FDA has identified the problem during an inspection.

The response to these situations can range from issuance of various types of letters requiring action on the part of the manufacturer, for example, untitled or warning letters, issuance of cease and desist orders, to product seizure, fines, or incarceration of personnel.

One area of particular concern in the regulation of orthobiologics is the different way that laws and regulations apply to a manufacturer and a physician. Manufacturers must comply with all of the relevant laws and regulations. For example, manufacturers cannot promote off-label uses of products. Physicians, based on their knowledge of the product, a particular patient, and the disease state of that patient, are free to use any legally marketed medical product in a manner they consider medically appropriate. This is covered under the practice of medicine. The FDA does not regulate physicians and their use of marketed medical products. This is left to each state's medical board. Under certain circumstances, however, physicians may no longer be covered by the practice of medicine. For example, if a physician harvests cells or tissues and processes them onsite for reimplantation, the physician could be considered to be acting as a manufacturer and the harvested cells or tissues could be considered more than minimally manipulated and/or used for a nonhomologous purpose. In this situation, the physician would be subject to the same laws and regulations as a manufacturer.

SPECIAL REGULATORY OPPORTUNITIES AND CONSIDERATIONS

Orphan Product Designation

Under certain specific conditions, provisions are available for marketing biological products, devices, and drugs that are intended to treat rare conditions. These products are known as orphan drugs[18] or humanitarian devices.[19] They are intended for populations where the number of individuals affected by the disease or condition in the United States is less than 200,000 per year in the case of orphan drugs or biological products, or 8,000 per year in the case of humanitarian devices. In the case of orphan drugs reviewed as a New Drug Application or Biologics License Application, the review is generally a priority review with a 6-month cycle. In the case of humanitarian devices, the overall review cycle is 75 days. These programs allow for market access based on submission of less information than would generally be required for a regular marketing application. The trade-off is that there are limitations, for example, humanitarian devices are restricted with respect to the need for an institutional review board approval before use and limitations on the types of expenses that can be recovered as part of the price charged for the device. In the case of orphan drugs and biological products, there are also incentives associated with tax credits and regulatory exclusivity if certain conditions are met. The Office of Orphan Products Development in the Commissioner's Office oversees these programs and should be contacted for details.

Breakthrough Designation

Each of the Centers has developed programs to foster development of new technologies. These are referred to as the Breakthrough Therapy designation (CDER), the Breakthrough Devices Program (CDRH), the Safer Technologies Program (STeP) (CDRH), and the Regenerative Medicine Advanced Therapy (RMAT) designation (CBER). Although the details of each program differ, the intent of all of them is to identify products that have the potential to offer improvements in patient treatment. The Breakthrough Therapy designation is intended to "... expedite the development and review of drugs that are intended to treat a serious condition and preliminary clinical evidence indicates that the drug may demonstrate substantial improvement over available therapy on a clinically significant end point(s)..."[20] The Breakthrough Devices Program is intended to identify "...products that have the potential to provide for more effective treatment or diagnosis of life-threatening or irreversibly debilitating diseases or conditions..."[21] Safer Technologies Program is for devices or combination products under the jurisdiction of CDRH that are "...reasonably expected to significantly improve the safety of currently available treatments..." for that are not as serious as those eligible for Breakthrough designation, including conditions that are nonlife threatening or reasonably reversible.[22] The RMAT designation is intended only for regenerative therapy products where "...preliminary clinical evidence indicates that the [product] has the potential to address unmet medical needs..."[23] To gain the most benefit from these programs, the requests should be submitted relatively early in the development process—no later than the phase 1 or 2 studies for a Breakthrough Therapy designation, at any point before submission of the marketing application for the Breakthrough Devices Program or Safer Technologies Program and either concurrently with submission of a new IND or as an amendment to an existing IND for the RMAT designation.

As stated, the intent of each of these programs is to identify medical products that have the potential to significantly advance clinical care. Product development may be enhanced by the earlier and more frequent interactions with the FDA. The result may be that these products enter clinical studies and reach the market earlier than products that do not meet the program requirements. The specific number of interactions and the FDA review time is dependent on the program and the availability of FDA resources. To take advantage of any of these benefits, however, it is critical that manufacturers expend the effort to prepare detailed and complete submissions and be willing to work closely with and heed the FDA's recommendations.

21st Century Cures Act and Additional Legislation

In December 2016, the 21st Century Cures Act[24] was enacted as an amendment to the Act. This set of amendments was designed to accelerate the development and delivery of new medical treatments. In addition to legislation related to the Breakthrough Devices and RMAT programs described previously, it also contains other provisions that would be expected to have an effect on the regulation of orthobiologics, including the following: (1) creation of intercenter institutes that would coordinate activities associated with major diseases across the Centers and improve the regulation of combination products, for example, the Oncology Center for Excellence; (2) increase in the use of real-world evidence and patient-reported outcome measures in the assessment of product safety and effectiveness; (3) development of standards for regenerative and advanced therapies; (4) creation of additional guidance documents specific to the regulation of combination products; (5) implementation of processes that would facilitate development of regenerative and advanced therapies; and (6) creation of additional provisions specific to the regulation of combination products, including additional guidance documents.

Because of the large number of initiatives that were identified in the 21st Century Cures Act, as well as the need to coordinate activities across multiple Centers and components of FDA, implementation is a complicated, ongoing process. The 21st Century Cures Act should not be viewed as the final legislation related to orthobiologics, however. There will be future legislation affecting these types of products both directly and indirectly. The benefit to the development of orthobiologics and their ability to treat the debilitation attributed to orthopaedic disorders, however, is expected to be significant.

SUMMARY

The FDA is responsible for protecting the public health as it relates to medical products, food, tobacco products, and cosmetics. This is accomplished by the use of appropriate levels of regulatory oversight, as well as interactions with the regulated industries. Compliance and enforcement activities are designed to ensure that unsafe or ineffective products are kept out of circulation. To keep pace with new technologies, the FDA introduces new regulations or modifies existing regulations. Programs that encourage development of novel treatments are also created. All of these activities allow the FDA to meet its regulatory responsibilities, protect the public health, and encourage the introduction of innovative products to improve the health of the US population.

REFERENCES

1. 21 CFR 600.3(h), see also Section 351(a) of the Public Health Service Act. Available at: https://www.ecfr.gov/current/title-21/chapter-I/subchapter-F/part-600. Accessed June 14, 2022.
2. Section 201(g) of the Federal Food, Drug and Cosmetic Act. Available at: https://www.govinfo.gov/content/pkg/COMPS-973/pdf/COMPS-973.pdf. Accessed June 14, 2022.
3. Section 201(h) of the Federal Food, Drug and Cosmetic Act. Available at: https://www.govinfo.gov/content/pkg/COMPS-973/pdf/COMPS-973.pdf. Accessed June 14, 2022.
4. Section 503(g) of the Federal Food, Drug and Cosmetic Act and 21 CFR 3.2(e). Available at: http://uscode.house.gov/view.xhtml?req=granuleid:USC-prelim-title21-section353&num=0&edition=prelim and https://www.ecfr.gov/current/title-21/chapter-I/subchapter-A/part-3/subpart-A/section-3.2. Accessed June 14, 2022.
5. Section 1271.3(d) of the Federal Food, Drug and Cosmetic Act. Available at: https://www.govinfo.gov/content/pkg/CFR-2012-title21-vol8/pdf/CFR-2012-title21-vol8-part1271.pdf. Accessed June 14, 2022.
6. US Food & Drug Administration - How to Write a Request for Designation (RFD). Available at: https://www.fda.gov/regulatory-information/search-fda-guidance-documents/how-write-request-designation-rfd. Accessed June 29, 2021.
7. US Food & Drug Administration - How to Prepare a Pre-Request for Designation (Pre-RFD). Available at: https://www.fda.gov/media/102706/download. Accessed August 30, 2021.
8. 21 CFR 3.2(m).
9. US Food & Drug Administration - FAQs on pre-IND process. Available at: https://www.fda.gov/drugs/cder-small-business-industry-assistance-sbia/small-business-and-industry-assistance-frequently-asked-questions-pre-investigational-new-drug-ind. Accessed June 29, 2021.
10. US Food & Drug Administration - Guidance for Industry: IND Meetings for Human Drugs and Biologics. Available at: https://www.fda.gov/files/Guidance-for-Industry---IND-Meetings-for-Human-Drugs-and-Biologics---Chemistry–Manufacturing--and-Controls-Information-%28PDF%29.pdf. Accessed June 29, 2021.
11. US Food & Drug Administration - Requests for Feedback and Meetings for Medical Device Submissions: The Q-Submission Program. Available at: https://www.fda.gov/media/114034/download. Accessed June 29, 2021.
12. US Food & Drug Administration - FDA Guidance for Industry: Formal Meetings Between FDA and Manufacturers or Applicants. Available at: https://www.fda.gov/media/72253/download. Accessed June 29, 2021.
13. US Food and Drug Administration - Regulatory Considerations for Human Cells, Tissues, and Cellular and Tissue-Based Products: Minimal Manipulation and Homologous Use. Available at: https://www.fda.gov/media/109176/download. Accessed September 2, 2021.
14. US Food & Drug Administration - Current Good Manufacturing Practice Requirements for Combination Products. Available at: https://www.fda.gov/media/90425/download. Accessed June 29, 2021.
15. US Food & Drug Administration - Postmarketing Safety Reporting for Combination Products Guidance for Industry and FDA Staff. Available at: https://www.fda.gov/media/111788/download. Accessed June 29, 2021.

16. US Food & Drug Administration - MedWatch: The FDA Safety Information and Adverse Event Reporting Program. Available at: https://www.fda.gov/safety/medwatch-fda-safety-information-and-adverse-event-reporting-program. Accessed September 2, 2021.
17. US Food & Drug Administration - MedWatch Form 3500. Available at: https://www.fda.gov/media/76299/download. Accessed September 2, 2021.
18. US Food & Drug Administration - Orphan Drugs and Biological Products. Available at: https://www.fda.gov/industry/developing-products-rare-diseases-conditions/designating-orphan-product-drugs-and-biological-products. Accessed June 29, 2021.
19. US Food & Drug Administration - Humanitarian Device Exemption. Available at: https://www.fda.gov/medical-devices/premarket-submissions/humanitarian-device-exemption. Accessed June 29, 2021.
20. US Food & Drug Administration - Breakthrough Therapy Designation. Available at: https://www.fda.gov/patients/fast-track-breakthrough-therapy-accelerated-approval-priority-review/breakthrough-therapy. Accessed June 29, 2021.
21. US Food & Drug Administration - Breakthrough Devices Program. Available at: https://www.fda.gov/medical-devices/how-study-and-market-your-device/breakthrough-devices-program. Accessed June 29, 2021.
22. US Food & Drug Administration - Safer Technologies Program (STeP). Available at: https://www.fda.gov/medical-devices/how-study-and-market-your-device/safer-technologies-program-step-medical-devices. Accessed June 29, 2021.
23. US Food & Drug Administration - Regenerative Medicine Advanced Therapy Designation. Available at: https://www.fda.gov/vaccines-blood-biologics/cellular-gene-therapy-products/regenerative-medicine-advanced-therapy-designation. Accessed June 29, 2021.
24. US Food & Drug Administration - 21st Century Cures Act. Available at: https://www.fda.gov/regulatory-information/selected-amendments-fdc-act/21st-century-cures-act. Accessed June 29, 2021.

RELEVANT/USEFUL WEBSITES

1. US Food & Drug Administration main webpage. Available at: http://www.fda.gov. Accessed June 29, 2021.
2. US Food & Drug Administration Organizational Structure. Available at: https://www.fda.gov/about-fda/fda-organization. Accessed June 29, 2021.
3. US Government Publishing Office - Federal Food Drug & Cosmetic Act. Available at: https://www.govinfo.gov/content/pkg/COMPS-973/pdf/COMPS-973.pdf. Accessed June 29, 2021.
4. US Government Publishing Office - Public Health Service Act. Available at: https://www.govinfo.gov/content/pkg/COMPS-8773/pdf/COMPS-8773.pdf. Accessed June 29, 2021.
5. US Food & Drug Administration - Code of Federal Regulations Title 21 (21 CFR). Available at: http://www.accessdata.fda.gov/scripts/cdrh/cfdocs/cfcfr/cfrsearch.cfm. Accessed June 29, 2021.

CHAPTER 13

Product Development

Lara Ionescu Silverman, PhD • Daniel Rodriguez-Granrose, PhD • Niloofar Farhang, PhD • Angelica Adrian Highsmith, MS

INTRODUCTION

Product development of orthobiologics is a complex process that involves regulatory interactions, quality compliance, preclinical and clinical studies, and manufacturing development. Broadly, product development can be organized into three major phases (**Figure 1**). The development of a product in orthobiologics is specifically outlined, but it can be applied to other products as well. The first phase is development justification, which includes analyzing a broad range of topics that frame, describe, and define the novel product. The second phase is data generation, where the bulk of experimentation, documentation, and manufacturing setup occur. The third phase is human use, where a particular product is being used in humans routinely and additional activities still occur. Phases 1 and 2 are generally performed in a linear manner, and phase 3 contains a number of iterative steps that occur repeatedly throughout human use.

PHASE 1: DEVELOPMENT JUSTIFICATION

The first phase of product development is to evaluate the many facets that will affect the potential success of the idea. The opportunity must be evaluated for medical, scientific, and business merit. In addition, the product must be defined at a high level and vetted for feasibility with key stakeholders to identify any shortcomings early and mitigate risks. Changes to a product in later stages of development can be expensive and time consuming. In addition, the product must have suitable protection to maintain a competitive edge. Finally, the regulatory categorization and pathway must be defined, which is extremely diverse in the field of orthobiologics.

Opportunity Identification

A brand-new approach may be uncovered to fix a problem that is considered to be very serious, expensive, or inconvenient. However, before forging ahead with expensive development efforts, the merits of such an idea must be vetted in an objective way (**Table 1**). This exercise requires involvement from a diverse array of people to ensure that differing voices are included and the opportunities are suitably understood. In addition, a general plan for staffing and facilities should occur during this step.

First, the medical merit of the product must be identified and described. This exercise is best vetted by the end user of the product, which is typically a doctor or nurse. These medical professionals have a keen eye for the gaps and needs that are present. They also understand how a new product might fit into an existing practice and surgical armamentarium. The practical aspects of logistics, storage, and day-to-day product usage must also be considered.

Another important aspect is that the story resonates with doctors. During the very early stages of defining the product and fleshing out the details, it is important to ensure that over the long term, the idea has potential for adoption. Research can occur during reading of peer-reviewed papers or reviews, attendance at medical association meetings or trade shows, or performance of direct interviews or focus groups with the future end user. These discussions can also shape what will be presented to the regulatory agencies as the product makes its way through development stages and into approval.

The medical merit is tied closely to the scientific merit of the new idea. Preliminary research is needed to point toward some mechanisms of action or functional benefits that the novel product will provide. Sometimes, a novel product will have very few scientific data, whereas in other cases, there could be a decade of published literature describing the idea. It is possible that both types of ideas ultimately possess scientific merit and are suitable for further development. Scientific studies, both in vitro and in vivo, will be critical in early conversations with doctors, funding resources, and regulatory agencies. Over time, many studies will likely be performed to answer questions from these three distinct groups of stakeholders. But to begin, at least some scientific data must justify the larger investment that will be required with development.

Dr. Silverman or an immediate family member serves as a paid consultant to or is an employee of LIS BioConsulting and serves as a board member, owner, officer, or committee member of the Orthopaedic Research Society. Dr. Rodriguez-Granrose or an immediate family member serves as a paid consultant to or is an employee of DiscGenics Inc. and has stock or stock options held in DiscGenics Inc. Dr. Farhang or an immediate family member serves as a paid consultant to or is an employee of ARUP Laboratories. Neither Angelica Highsmith nor any immediate family member has received anything of value from or has stock or stock options held in a commercial company or institution related directly or indirectly to the subject of this chapter.

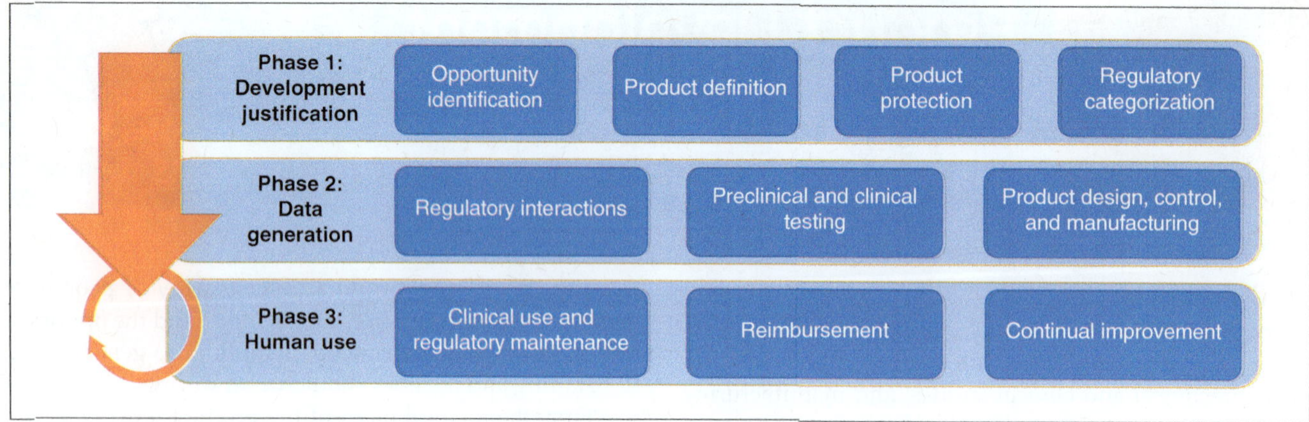

FIGURE 1 Schematic representation of the three-phase approach to product development in orthobiologics. Phase 1 justifies the upcoming development efforts, phase 2 generates the required data and information required for safe and effective human use, and phase 3 includes iterative activities to support and sustain long-term human use, allowing for revenue generation to recover funds spent in phases 1 and 2.

In addition, a scientific understanding of how the product will be made must be established, including evaluating whether the process can be reproducible, what equipment might be needed, and if the process can be automated or scaled up for efficient production.

Finally, once the medical and scientific merits are established, the business merit of the idea must be thoroughly vetted. A good place to start is to establish the prevalence and incidence of the disease state or injury. A disease state or injury that has high prevalence can justify high development costs even if a low adoption rate is expected. In contrast, a disease state or injury with low prevalence requires higher adoption to recover the development costs. For example, if a disease has a relatively high incidence rate of 15 million annually and has a low target market capture of 1%, that would still be 150,000 units of the product sold annually. If a pathology has a relatively low incidence rate of 300,000 annually, it would need a 50% target market capture to achieve the same sales rate as the pathology with the higher incidence. One caveat to this logic is that regulatory agencies, including the FDA, have specialized approval pathways for low-incidence disease states or injuries to increase the likelihood of product development for these conditions.

With an understanding of prevalence and incidence, then revenue and profit estimates can be made. Using the pathology prevalence, estimated product sale price, and estimated percent of target market that will be captured,

TABLE 1 Questions to Ask During Opportunity Identification

Questions	Resources Involved
Does this idea have medical merit? How will it be used in the clinic? Does the story/idea resonate with medical personnel and patients?	End users such as doctors and nurses (perform individual interviews, host panel discussions, attend conferences, etc) Administrators and logistics providers
Does this idea have scientific merit? Is a mechanism of action or functional benefit known? How will the product be made?	Scientists Review of existing literature Preliminary benchtop and animal studies Manufacturing professionals
Does the idea have business merit? What is the prevalence and incidence of the disease state or injury? (If small, are there specialized regulatory pathways to incentivize development?) What is the revenue/profit potential? What resources will be needed to staff, execute development, and market this idea? What is the competitive landscape, and how will this idea fit in?	Scientists, medical personnel, and experts Business, finance, and fundraising professionals Market research (interview experts in field, perform Internet research, hire specialized firm, etc)

the product revenue is estimated. The estimated profit is then calculated by subtracting product development and manufacturing costs from the estimated revenue. Financial models that allow for shifting of development costs versus future revenue based on different market shares can be made. These types of exercises are useful to estimate fundraising needs beforedevelopment efforts begin.

Understanding the competitive landscape is also a critical step in assessing a new product's business merit because an area too crowded may not have room for a new competitor, but a space completely empty may signal a lack of market need. A competitive landscape assessment is divided into two categories: marketed products and products in development (with estimated launch dates). Each product or concept in development is described briefly, with key differentiating technical features succinctly summarized. A high-level comment on safety or efficacy data, intellectual property (and expiry dates), regulatory classification and status, and price/reimbursement status is identified. In addition, the company itself must be evaluated, including size, longevity, market cap, reputation, and track record of other products. The company assessment is especially relevant for small companies or first-time leadership teams, where their executional prowess is not yet proven. This type of exercise provides a quick snapshot of the market and can help promote market differentiation early in development.

The activities previously described allow for the assessment of business merit. It is important to note, though, that regulatory agencies have special designations for extremely rare conditions that expedite approval, thereby reducing overall cost to developers and making a product that had limited business potential a worthwhile endeavor. An orphan drug is one that treats a medical condition that is so rare; it would not be possible to develop without government assistance and is designed to treat a condition that affects fewer than 200,000 patients in the United States, fewer than 5 in 10,000 patients in the European Union, and fewer than 50,000 patients in Japan. For drugs that treat rare or serious conditions, fast-track, breakthrough, accelerated approval and priority review designations are available to accelerate FDA approval.

Another exception is that certain orthobiologic products may fall within a regulatory category known as 361 products. These products are categorized as human cells, tissues, and cellular and tissue-based products (HCT/Ps) that must meet a strict set of rules, including that the product was minimally manipulated, is intended for homologous use, and is not combined with other products, among other requirements. The FDA has recently issued additional guidance documents clarifying the requirements for 361 products and intent to enforce the regulation.[1] If a product falls into this category,[2] significantly less development effort is needed, although basic infrastructure similar to highly regulated products must still be implemented such as training, documentation, and quality review.[3]

A last consideration is resource assessment. Taking a new medical idea from concept to clinic requires many different people with different specialties. During both the preclinical and clinical development stages, the developer must determine the level of in-house versus external resources that are used. Preclinical studies, both in vitro and in vivo, can be performed using internal company staff and equipment or outsourced to an external laboratory. Common external resources include contract research organization and university laboratories with expertise in the area. University laboratories typically lack quality systems or standard operating procedures needed for regulatory filings (although that has been improving in recent years), and the time lines can be longer. However, such laboratories often possess credibility, expertise, and experience, particularly with animal models that can be tricky to implement and evaluate. Typically, a combination of laboratories is used. In addition, the manufacturing can be performed internally or externally using a contract manufacturing organization. The infrastructure required to manufacture may be cost prohibitive for smaller companies but in the end may result in a more bespoke facility that suits the needs of the specific technology.

Product Definition

Once the merits of a novel orthobiologic product are known and there is a desire to move forward, the next step is to define the product. A useful tool is a target product profile (TPP), which is a succinct written summary of all aspects of the product. It often includes aspirational features of the product, which allows for alignment across teams and clarity on the product characteristics as development occurs. Through development, the TPP becomes more specific to reflect new data or changes to product strategy.

A TPP is a critical document to guide both internal and external communication regarding a new product. For the developer, it is a useful tool to align desired characteristics, communicate between groups, and identify known gaps. For regulators, a TPP is a valuable snapshot of a product in development, allowing for quick reference and clear answers.[4] In addition, it can be used to highlight changes that require regulator's attention.

The format of a TPP can vary based on the business need, people involved, and stage of development. However, all TPPs include certain general topics such as definition of the users and patients, use descriptions, summary of findings, and safety/efficacy profile. Early in development, some of these categories are still unknown (eg, the dosing profile cannot be determined until after testing has occurred). Therefore, it is useful to include both base-case and best-case ranges or descriptions for each category. Over time, these can be updated as more information is available.

The contents of the TPP should focus on medical and scientific facts. In some instances, an addendum to the TPP can be included, which includes aspects such as price and project sales volumes, but this type of financial information should not be provided to the regulatory agencies, which are primarily interested in safety and efficacy of the product.

Every product must have an intended use for a target population. If clinical trials are required, the patient population will closely match the clinical population included in trials. Sometimes, the patient population may shift as clinical data are generated or the competitive landscape changes in such a way that a new target population is needed for commercial viability. If useful, the TPP can include information on incidence and prevalence of the disease or injury. In addition, it may be helpful to identify the type of medical professional (eg, orthopaedic surgeon) who will administer, deliver, or use the product.

The product description includes the form (pill, liquid, medical device, etc) and the routine or mode of delivery. If a procedure is required, a brief overview can be provided. In addition, dose information is important, which typically becomes more specific as development progresses and the human dose that is both safe and efficacious is identified. For a medical device, the product should be physically described with relevant information such as shape, size, and material composition. Another aspect of use is the storage conditions (such as temperature) and shelf life for the product. In some instances, fast shipping is required because of extremely short product shelf life, and this process can be described as well.

In addition, the proposed efficacy profile is provided in the TPP. Results from human clinical testing are briefly summarized, when available. Any safety risks or warnings are identified. References to both preclinical and clinical data can be made, which elucidate the safety profile of the product. Sometimes it is helpful to include the lot release criteria as part of the TPP. This can be a general list of the tests being used or a specific list of the tests and allowable ranges for lot release.

When defining a novel product, it is critical to articulate the mode of action or the way in which the product will cause its intended effect or action. In some cases, the mode of action is straightforward (eg, a tendon allograft replaces a damaged native tendon), but in other cases, the mode of action may take time to fully understand. It is important to identify a mode of action because it will guide what measurements are taken in preclinical and clinical studies. In addition, the mode of action will likely be involved in verification, validation, or lot release testing of the product before human use. It is possible for combination products to have multiple modes of action, which may either be separate or synergistic. In this case, a primary mode of action must be identified to identify which regulatory agency will lead review and approval.

Product Protection

Once the product is well defined, a strategy to protect it must be established. Protection comes in many forms, including legal forms such as intellectual property and trade secrets, as well as general barriers to entry.

A novel idea, device, or method can be legally protected as intellectual property. Intellectual property includes patents, copyrights, industrial design rights, trademarks, and trade secrets. For a new product, a patent is a very useful (and often necessary) tool to ensure that competitors will not directly mimic the invention. A patent is a right granted by the government that gives the owner the ability to exclude others from making, using, selling, offering to sell, and importing an invention for a limited period, in exchange for the public disclosure of the invention. To be granted a patent, a product must meet three criteria: novelty, nonobviousness, and usefulness. Patents are issued on a country-by-country basis, which often results in an expensive and labor-intensive effort. However, owning intellectual property is critical to protect individual ideas and avoid direct replicates of them.

In the field of orthobiologics, some products are actually products of nature, meaning they are found in nature and cannot be patented. For example, cells or tissues that are removed from the body and replaced back into the body in an unaltered form cannot be patented.[5] Instead, developers may find another aspect of harvesting, processing, storage, or delivery that is unique so that some legal protection from competition exists.

Although patent law provides strong protections for proprietary inventions and creations, they do not last forever. A patent is good for 20 years. In contrast, a company can choose to identify trade secrets that possess the following characteristics: they are not known or readily accessible by competitors, have commercial value or provide a competitive advantage in the marketplace, and are protected from disclosure through reasonable efforts to maintain secrecy. This type of intellectual property can be maintained indefinitely and can be protected in a court of law. However, misappropriation of trade secrecy information risk has increased with an increase in networking and storage of data on web servers. Physical security, digital or network security, and legal measures, such as confidentiality, noncompete, and nondisclosure agreements, are all measures by which trade secret information remains secret.[6]

In addition to intellectual property rights, financial and regulatory impediments can also help protect innovators and creators in the medical field. The capital requirements for developing a new drug or medical technology can prohibit those seeking to replicate the same or similar product. Refined knowledge that can only be developed through the use of costly equipment, clinical

TABLE 2 Regulatory Categorization for Orthobiologics in the United States

Biologics (human blood–derived products, vaccines, monoclonal antibodies, etc)	**Drugs** (achieve intended purpose through metabolization)	**Medical devices** (do not use chemical or metabolism mechanisms)
Combination products (two or more of the above)		

The group of products known as human cells, tissues, and cellular and tissue-based products (HCT/Ps) can fall into any category depending on the identified mode of action.

data collection, and the building of manufacturing sites for such products indirectly provide additional forms of product protection as well.

Regulatory Categorization

The primary mode of action will determine what department of a government regulatory agency will oversee development and approval of a novel product. Orthobiologics can be grouped into a number of departments in the United States. They could be regulated as a biologic, drug, medical device, or combination (**Table 2**). Orthobiologics can also be grouped into a special category known as HCT/Ps, which can be biologics, drugs, or devices, depending on their mode of action, which includes the less rigorously reviewed 361 products previously described. The different regulatory departments that oversee each type of product have unique premarket review requirements and testing needs. In addition, manufacturing requirements vary, with drugs and biologics requiring adherence to current good manufacturing practices and devices to quality system regulations. HCT/Ps must also adhere to current good tissue practices and donor eligibility rules.

PHASE 2: GENERATE DATA

The next phase of process development is the lengthiest and most expensive. This is where cross-functional teams must work in parallel to turn the idea into a usable human product. This includes preclinical studies, clinical studies (when required), and manufacturing (which includes design, process development, and analytics).

Regulatory Interactions

Product development is largely guided by the requirements set forth by regulatory agencies. This can include preclinical requirements, clinical requirements, and marketing applications. Because each regulatory agency and department varies in their requirements, the pathway must be defined and understood carefully at the beginning of product development. Recent changes to the FDA pathway for 361 products, which include clarification for designations that were previously vaguely defined, have resulted in some products to shift pathways during development.

In the United States, for products that have a main mode of action categorized as a drug (led by the Center for Drug Evaluation and Research [CDER]) or biologics (led by the Center for Biologics Evaluation and Research [CBER]), pre–Investigational New Drug (IND) meetings can be requested with the FDA to discuss topics related to preclinical testing, manufacturing, and future clinical testing. CBER also allows for meetings before the pre-IND called INTERACT meetings, which allow for more information and strategic discussions. For products that have a main mode of action categorized as a device (led by the Center for Devices and Radiological Health [CDRH]), presubmission meetings are handled through the Q-Submission program[7] (**Figure 2**).

To begin human testing, the sponsor will need to submit an IND application (for drugs and some biologics[8]) or an Investigational Device Exemption application (for devices and some biologics[9]). The IND and IDE application includes a comprehensive report on all the preclinical data collected on the proposed product, including animal and toxicologic studies, manufacturing information such as drug composition and controls, and a detailed proposal of the study design for clinical trials (if needed) (**Figure 2**).

During process development, products being reviewed by CDER and CBER can request various types of meetings with the FDA to discuss urgent matters (type A meeting), routine meetings that are needed before and after clinical studies and before marketing applications (type B meetings), and other needs that do not fall into the first two categories (type C meetings). Products reviewed by CDRH have a more informal meeting structure and process. These types of meetings are critical to ensure that the data presented in marketing applications will meet the regulators' requirements so that commercial use can commence.

After testing but before routine human use, a marketing application must be reviewed and approved by regulatory agencies (except for HCT/Ps that qualify as 361s). In the United States, for low- to medium-risk devices, a 510k notification or de novo classification must be completed. For medium- to high-risk products, a Premarket Approval application must be completed. For biologics not classified as having a primary function of a device, a Biologics License Application must be completed. Drugs must be approved using a New Drug Application (**Figure 2**). For drugs with extremely low populations, a Humanitarian Device Exemption categorization may be obtained.

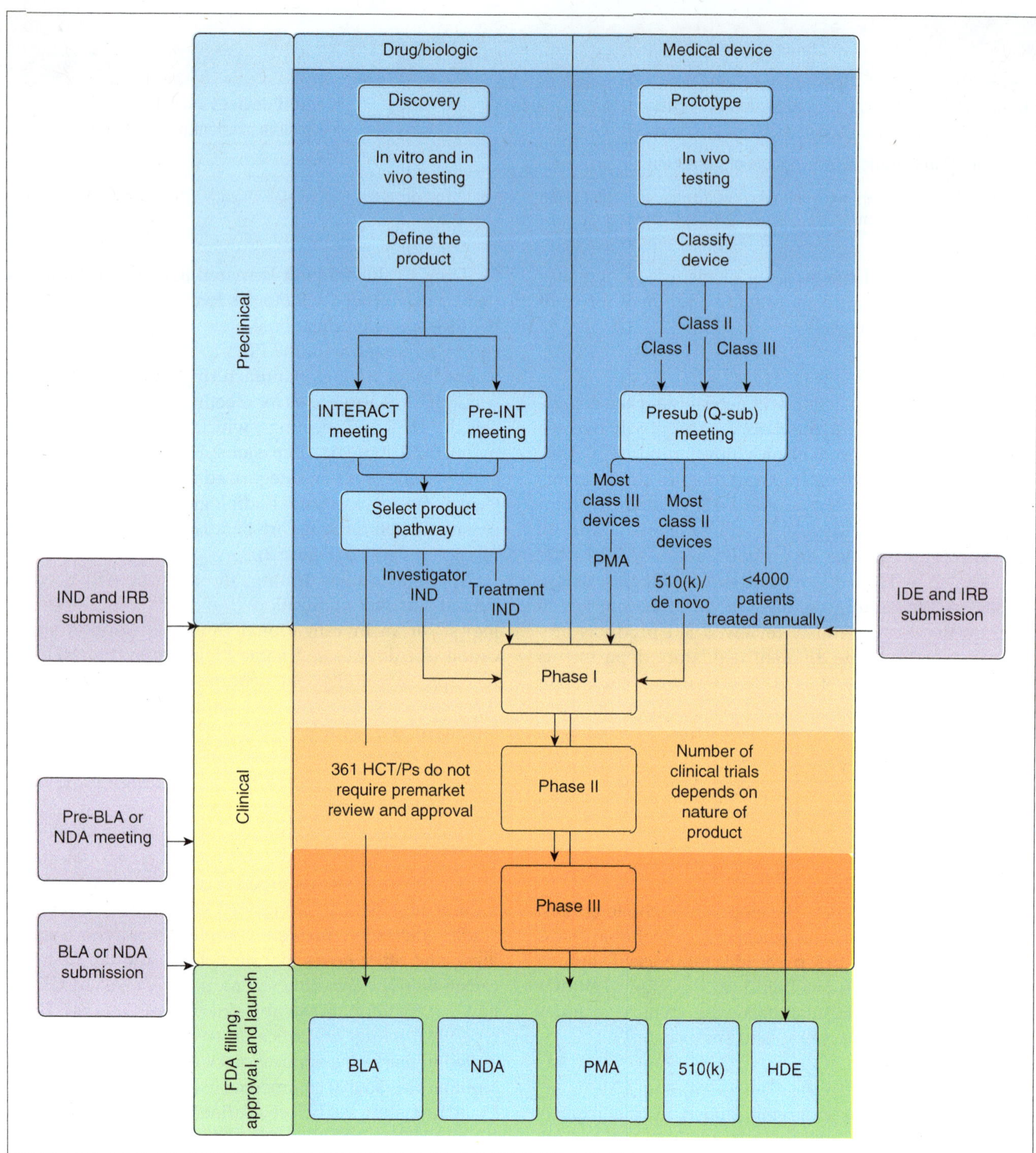

FIGURE 2 Schematic representation of an overview of the regulatory pathway for orthobiologic products, which includes a preclinical phase, clinical phase, and finally filing, approval, and launch. Note that human cells, tissues, and cellular and tissue-based products (HCT/Ps) that fall into the 361 category do not require premarket approval by the FDA. BLA = biologics license application, HDE = humanitarian device exemption, IDE = investigational device exemption, IND = investigational new drug, IRB = institutional review board, NDA = new drug application, PMA = premarket approval

Preclinical and Clinical Testing

For all orthobiologic products, some level of preclinical scientific work must occur before human use. A proposed benefit or mode of action must be established through benchtop studies and sometimes animal studies. Various studies may be required by regulators to suitably assess safety, bioactivity, and mode of delivery/implantation. Such studies are also critical in providing scientific information to medical professionals who will eventually use the product. In vitro studies may be a suitable and sufficient way to evaluate the potential efficacy of a product. In many cases, however, animal models must also be used to assess safety and efficacy. The decision to perform animal studies is dependent on the requirements set forth by the regulator as well as case-by-case requests made during consultations and meetings. Ethically, a sponsor should always strive to reduce the frequency and size of animal studies. It is challenging to identify animals with a suitable injury or disease or consistently generate a model that recapitulates or simulates the intended injury or disease for purposes of testing.[10] Organizations such as the Orthopaedic Research Society are championing the optimization and minimization of animal testing, which is recognized as being at times necessary for human translation.

Animal testing can be a lengthy period of development for orthobiologic products. Testing begins in the discovery phase, which includes establishing a reproducible and appropriate injury/disease model in one or multiple animal species and performing proof-of-concept studies with low sample sizes often in small animals. These data are key in establishing future studies and also beginning conversations with regulators. Next, the preclinical phase of testing can include small animal testing with larger sample sizes as well as specific evaluations that include pharmacokinetics, toxicity, and biocompatibility. Often, a large animal model is needed because it more closely recapitulates the size of humans. Finally, pivotal animal studies are used to justify human clinical trials. These studies must be performed in a testing laboratory that complies with good laboratory practices, which ensures thorough documentation, quality assurance, and controlled laboratory spaces that allow regulators to suitably evaluate the data.[11] Although discovery phase and some preclinical phase animal studies can be performed in academic settings, the final preclinical phase and pivotal animal studies are typically performed with a contract research organization that can meet documentation, facility, and audit requirements and is used to generating reports for regulatory review purposes.

When clinical testing is desired or required, the time line to commercial use can be significantly longer. The benefits of clinical testing, beyond regulatory approval, are that the product can command a higher price and there will likely be wider adoption by the medical community. Clinical testing seeks understanding of safety and efficacy of a product in a specific patient population with a certain delivery or mode of use. Proper design of the trials is key. The designs are based on precedent clinical trials for similar products, the findings from preclinical testing, and input from doctors. These clinical trials can be led by a company or they can be an Investigator-Initiated Trial led by a physician in partnership with a sponsor. Most clinical trials are listed on the website www.clinicaltrial.gov (there are rules on what trials must be included).[12]

Any product that seeks to make efficacy claims must perform clinical trials. Such human testing requires an informed consent process and documentation, as well as institutional review board review and approval. These requirements are on top of regulatory oversight and adherence to good clinical practices. Typically, multiple human studies are performed, which increase in size and also yet decrease in scope, with two or three trials being standard. Although early-stage studies may be small (approximately 10 to 50 patients) and will explore a broad range of doses and end points, late-stage studies are typically much larger (approximately 100 to 1,000 patients) with very narrow enrollment criteria, set doses, and specific end points. Statistical and clinical significance against placebo or standard of care is needed to demonstrate efficacy before approval. Although most products reviewed by CBER and CDER require multiple clinical trials, some products that are reviewed by CDRH may only require one study, although more typically multiple studies are performed.

For biologic products, a mechanism of action that is used to define the potency assay for lot release must be identified. Although ideally the potency assay is clearly tied to a robust mechanism of action, in some instances, the FDA will allow potency assays to be based on a reasonable hypothesis, because of the known challenges of proving mode of action for regenerative medicine products.[13] In some other instances, clinical performance can be used to demonstrate potency if the manufacturing process is well controlled, and the mode of action is not fully known. In either case, the potency will play a key role ensuring manufacturing consistency over time.

Product Design, Control, and Manufacturing

Because product development is a complex process, the industry has galvanized together to establish standard frameworks for development. For devices, the framework is design control, and for biologics and drugs, the framework is quality by design (QbD). Both frameworks are recognized by regulators worldwide because it allows for harmonization of efforts between sponsors.

A core tenet of both frameworks is that quality should be built into the product, meaning a proactive approach to ensuring quality must be taken. In addition, testing alone is not sufficient to ensure product quality;[14] the process used to create the product is equally important. A quality system must be established by a manufacturer, which includes clear documentation, responsibilities, and reviews. Many aspects of compliance associated with future marketing authorizations are captured within a quality system, such as control of facilities and equipment, control of outsourced operations, labeling, addressing nonconformities, analyzing data for trends, internal audits, documentation, and stability monitoring.[15] On average, 25% of product development efforts are spent on quality compliance.[16]

Design control begins by defining user needs, which can include elements of the TPP. From this, design inputs are defined. Once the production process is designed and units are made, the design outputs are measured and verified against the original design inputs. The device is then validated against the original user needs. Between each step, a documented review is performed[17,18] (**Figure 3**). To tie everything together, a traceability matrix should be made to show the linkages and relationship between each activity. Design control activities must be compiled into a design history file and made available for regulatory audit.[19]

The development process for drugs and biologics should follow a framework known as QbD. The goal of QbD is to link process inputs to quality outputs defined in the quality TPP and measured by validated analytical methods.[20] QbD uses risk assessments, mechanistic models, design of experiments, and data analysis to build an understanding of the effect and severity of process variation on quality outputs.[21] The process includes three phases, which are process design, process qualification, and process monitoring (**Figure 3**).

The first phase, process design, is a multistep activity used to establish the method for generating the product. A TPP (previously described) is established and then the process is described by process parameters (eg, the temperature setting) and resulting attributes (eg, the sterility). Attribute measurements can be in-process tests or final lot release tests and must be defined and qualified; a subset of attributes are selected as critical to defining the product. In addition, raw materials must be chosen and their attributes defined. Then, risk factors are identified and risk assessments are performed, which allow for the prioritization of optimization and eventual reduction of variability. Next, a design space is created, which creates relationships between input variables (eg, material attributes) and process parameters that have been demonstrated to provide assurance of quality.[20] For areas that remain higher risk, a control strategy is established to minimize risk, followed by continuous improvement of the process to further decrease risk and variability. An important consideration is comparability of the process throughout the product life cycle because typically the process changes over time as more information is known and more sophisticated manufacturing is implemented. Although some amount of change is allowable, any changes must be well understood and documented.

The second phase in QbD, process performance qualification, demonstrates that the process and associated

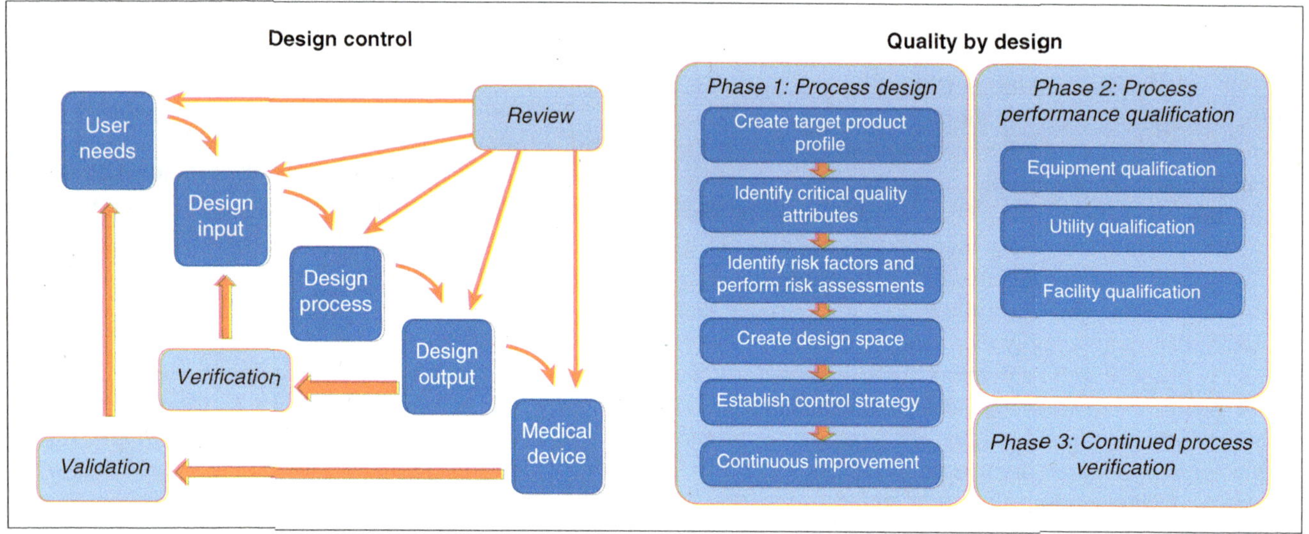

FIGURE 3 Schematic representation of industry frameworks for process development. The design control process follows five steps beginning with user needs and ending with the medical device, with verification, validation, and reviews between each step (based on FDA guidance document). Design inputs describe the exact specifications of the product, including what it will do and how it will perform, as mandated by user needs. Design outputs document the exact materials, components, subassemblies, and configurations needed to build the device. In the case of a combination product, the biologic agent or drug quality attributes should be considered a design input for the combination product. Quality by design follows three steps including process design, process qualification, and process monitoring (based on FDA guidance document).

equipment are robust and validated. The purpose of process performance qualification is to confirm that the design space delivers appropriate results at the manufacturing production scale. This is generally done by running the process multiple times to demonstrate consistency and prove that it can be maintained over time. Along with validating the process, this phase includes qualification of equipment, utilities, and facilities to ensure they are performing to the needed standards. These activities are costly and time consuming, but critical to ensure that reproducible manufacturing will occur.

Finally, the third phase, continued process verification, is an activity performed after product approval to ensure that continued control of manufacturing is maintained.[22] In this stage, data are constantly generated and analyzed to build on the design space and identify areas for improvement or further refine control of manufacturing. This activity, called change control, focuses on managing change to prevent unintended consequences.

PHASE 3: HUMAN USE

Now the product is ready for human use. Although this is a milestone to be celebrated, it is important to note that the role of the sponsor remains extremely active with additional activities.

Clinical Use and Regulatory Maintenance

Each regulatory agency has a specific requirement for annual or repetitive reporting during commercial use to ensure continued safety and efficacy of the product. A manufacturer may report issues directly to the regulators during the annual report, or they may be uncovered during a routine inspection. Regulatory agencies then have oversight to ensure that the deficiency is rectified quickly to limit patient harm.

Once the product is on the market, additional clinical trials could identify new indications for the product, new routes of administration, or new doses. These studies could be initiated by the product developer or by medical staff who are using the product and see another opportunity during use. The label change requires a supplemental New Drug Application or supplemental Biologics License Application and can increase overall sales potential for a given product.

Medical devices in Europe now require postmarket surveillance (PMS) according to the Medical Device Regulation, to proactively identify risks during the practical use of the product that could change how the product is used or administered. The type of PMS required is based on the risk class and type of device. This builds on the requirements by most regulators to monitor and report on known serious safety issues related to their product during routine use.

For drugs, the FDA requires PMS of adverse events to augment the data collected during clinical evaluation. The information can be used to update labeling or, on rare occasion, change approval decisions. The FDA Adverse Event Reporting System is designed to be used by all drugs and therapeutic biologic products. In addition, an annual report must be submitted to the FDA, which includes any changes (application supplements or 30-day notices or filing changes), additional scientific information, and statistics on products shipped or sold. PMS data should be included.[23]

Reimbursement

Although reimbursement becomes an obvious priority during commercial use, preparing for reimbursement should occur during all phases of product development. Reimbursement strategy can be particularly important for a product intended to be launched globally, where payer systems vary significantly by country.

The current price for competitive products will likely create a window of pricing for future sales that can affect decisions around development and execution. Early discussions with payers can provide key insights into reimbursement opportunities, as well as advise on what specific aspects of preclinical and clinical studies could contribute to a favorable decision for payment by a payer. In some cases, the clinical data requested by regulars are different than what are requested by payers. To receive reimbursement for a device, a suitable coding of the service using current procedural terminology must exist, a suitable coding using International Classification of Diseases, Ninth Revision, of the diagnosis must exist, and the associated fee according to the Centers for Medicare & Medicaid Services should be determined.[24] For products in a well-established space, this is straightforward, but for products in an underservice indication, this could require some preliminary activities and efforts to establish novel codes.

Continued Process Verification and Sustaining Engineering

For products that follow QbD, phase 3 must be executed continuously to ensure constant process monitoring and improvement. For medical device manufacturing, sustaining engineering must occur continuously, which includes fixing manufacturing glitches, obsolescence management, feature enhancements, and addressing custom complaints. So, this effort can work to drive down cost, which may come in handy as additional competitors enter the market or the reimbursement market shifts.

SUMMARY

A well-designed new orthobiologic product has the potential to help address unmet medical needs in the field of orthopaedics. The process begins by determining if a new idea is suitable for development. This includes factors such as the opportunity size, the competitive landscape, the product protection strategy, and the regulatory categorization. Next, data from preclinical, clinical, and manufacturing activities must be generated and assembled for regulatory oversight and approval. Finally, during human use, repetitive activities such as regulatory notifications, reimbursement maintenance, and manufacturing activities must constantly occur. With proper planning, a strong team with diverse backgrounds, and suitable funding, new products in orthobiologics will continue to be developed for human use, significantly improving outcomes for patients.

REFERENCES

1. *Questions and Answers Regarding the End of the Compliance and Enforcement Policy for Certain Human Cells, Tissues, or Cellular or Tissue-based Products (HCT/Ps)*. Food and Drug Administration. 2021. Available at: https://www.fda.gov/vaccines-blood-biologics/cellular-gene-therapy-products/questions-and-answers-regarding-end-compliance-and-enforcement-policy-certain-human-cells-tissues-or. Accessed September 14, 2021.
2. Bruder S, Allen K, Bailey S, Petricek J: The product development process from discovery, through the FDA, and into the clinic, in Aaron R, ed: *Orthopaedic Basic Science: Foundations of Clinical Practice*, ed 5. American Academy of Orthopaedic Surgeons, 2020.
3. Silverman LI, Flanagan F, Rodriguez-Granrose D, Simpson K, Saxon LH, Foley KT: Identifying and managing sources of variability in cell therapy manufacturing and clinical trials. *Regen Eng Transl Med* 2019;5(4):354-361.
4. Tyndall A, Du W, Breder CD: The target product profile as a tool for regulatory communication: Advantageous but underused. *Nat Rev Drug Discov* 2017;16(3):156.
5. Aaron R, Aaron D, Racine-Avila J, Menikoff J: The use of human biospecimens for research. *J Orthop Res* 2021;39(8):1603-1610.
6. Kasdan M, Smith KM, Daniels B: Trade secrets: What you need to know. *Natl Law Rev* 2019;XII:255.
7. Food and Drug Administration: Requests for Feedback and Meetings for Medical Device Submissions: The Q-Submission Program Guidance for Industry and Food and Drug Administration Staff. 2021. Available at: https://www.fda.gov/media/114034/download. Accessed September 14, 2021.
8. Food and Drug Administration: Guidance for Industry IND Meetings for Human Drugs and Biologics. 2001. Available at: https://www.fda.gov/files/Guidance-for-Industry---IND-Meetings-for-Human-Drugs-and-Biologics---Chemistry--Manufacturing--and-Controls-Information-%28PDF%29.pdf. Accessed September 14, 2021.
9. Food and Drug Administration: Investigational Device Exemptions (IDEs) for Early Feasibility Medical Device Clinical Studies, Including Certain First in Human (FIH) Studies Guidance for Industry and Food and Drug Administration Staff. 2013. Available at: https://www.fda.gov/regulatory-information/search-fda-guidance-documents/investigational-device-exemptions-ides-early-feasibility-medical-device-clinical-studies-including. Accessed September 14, 2021.
10. Allen MJ, Hankenson KD, Goodrich L, Boivin GP, von Rechenberg B: Ethical use of animal models in musculoskeletal research. *J Orthop Res* 2017;35(4):740-751.
11. Food and Drug Administration: Guidance for Industry Good Laboratory Practices Questions and Answers. 2007. Available at: https://www.fda.gov/media/75866/download. Accessed September 14, 2021.
12. FDAAA 801 and the Final Rule. clinicaltrials.gov. Available at: https://clinicaltrials.gov/ct2/manage-recs/fdaaa. Accessed September 14, 2021.
13. Food and Drug Administration: FDA Briefing Document Oncologic Drugs Advisory Committee (ODAC) Meeting Session on Product Characterization (AM Session). 2020. Available at: https://www.fda.gov/media/140988/download. Accessed September 12, 2021.
14. Food and Drug Administration: Guidance for Industry Quality Systems Approach to Pharmaceutical CGMP Regulations. 2006. Available at: https://www.fda.gov/media/71023/download. Accessed September 11, 2021.
15. Rathore AS, Mhatre R, eds: *Quality by Design for Biopharmaceuticals: Principles and Case Studies*. Wiley, 2009.
16. Niazi S, Brown JL: *Fundamentals of Modern Bioprocessing*. CRC Press, Taylor & Francis Group, CRC Press is an imprint of the Taylor & Francis Group, an Informa business, 2016.
17. Food and Drug Administration: Design Control Guidance For Medical Device Manufacturers Guidance for Industry. 1997. Available at: https://www.fda.gov/regulatory-information/search-fda-guidance-documents/design-control-guidance-medical-device-manufacturers. Accessed September 11, 2021
18. Food and Drug Administration: Guidance for Industry Process Validation: General Principles and Practices. 2011. Available at: https://www.fda.gov/files/drugs/published/Process-Validation--General-Principles-and-Practices.pdf. Accessed September 11, 2021.
19. Teixeira MB, Teixeira M, Bradley R: *Design Controls for the Medical Device Industry*. CRC Press, 2013.
20. Pharmaceutical development q8(r2), in *ICH Harmonised Tripartate Guideline*. International Conference on Harmonisation of Technical Requirements for Registration of Pharmaceuticals for Human Use (ICH). 2009.
21. Lipsitz YY, Timmins NE, Zandstra PW: Quality cell therapy manufacturing by design. *Nat Biotechnol* 2016;34(4):393-400.
22. Ostrove SA: *How to Validate a Pharmaceutical Process*. Elsevier, 2016.
23. Food and Drug Administration: *Annual Reports for Approved Premarket Approval Applications (PMA) Guidance for Industry and Food and Drug Administration Staff*. 2019. Available at: https://www.fda.gov/media/73391/download. Accessed September 12, 2021
24. Beck DE, Margolin DA: Physician coding and reimbursement. *Ochsner J* 2007;7(1):8-15.

CHAPTER 14

Allograft and Xenograft Tissue Technology

Stephen F. Badylak, DVM, PhD, MD • Emily Dianne Henderson, BS

INTRODUCTION

Although skeletal muscle and bone have robust regenerative potential, volumetric tissue loss overwhelms this innate regenerative capacity. Tendons, ligaments, and cartilage have limited regenerative potential, and the repair of these tissues following injury can be challenging.[1] The United States Bone and Joint Initiative estimates that for nearly one in two Americans older than 18 years, movement is restricted by a musculoskeletal disorder such as arthritis, back pain, fracture, osteoporosis, sports trauma, and other ailments that affect function and mobility. Regardless of the cause, musculoskeletal injuries represent a major cause of disability and burden to the health care system.[2] Strategies that can improve the restoration of functional tissue beyond that possible with current treatment methods are welcome and needed.

In the broadest sense, orthobiologics can be defined as those available naturally occurring products that have the potential to influence the behavior of cells and tissues. The targeted purpose of orthobiologic products is the repair of injured musculoskeletal tissues beyond a functional outcome that would otherwise be possible without their presence or influence. Orthobiologic products may include cells such as mesenchymal stromal cells (MSCs), isolated signaling molecules including bone morphogenetic protein, platelet products such as platelet-rich plasma, bioscaffold materials such as XenMatrix (porcine dermal surgical mesh), and demineralized bone matrix.

Autografts and allografts have not generally been considered as an orthobiologic and have generally been regulated as a human cells, tissues, and cellular and tissue-based product (HCT/P), but if the aforementioned definition is accepted, then such harvested tissues should also be considered as orthobiologics. It is recognized that these definitions and labels represent arbitrary semantics; however, these semantics are important in the discussion of autografts, allografts, and xenografts.

AUTOGRAFTS, ALLOGRAFTS, AND XENOGRAFTS

The use of tissue grafts in knee surgery, including the repair of cruciate and collateral ligament and meniscal injuries, is commonplace. Therefore, a brief historical review of such grafts at this anatomic site is relevant to the concept of orthobiologics. The use of autologous or allogeneic tissue to facilitate musculotendinous tissue repair has more than a century of reported use. Similarly, Lexer reported articular cartilage transplant during a span of almost 2 decades beginning in 1908.[3] In 1913, Giertz[4] described the use of autologous fascia lata for medial collateral ligament repair, and another study reported the use of fascia lata for anterior cruciate ligament (ACL) repair in 1917.[5] The use of hamstring grafts for ACL repair was first reported by Galeazzi in 1924,[6] and Franke[7] was the first to describe the use of free bone–patellar tendon–bone grafts in 1969 for the same application. The use of allografts became more commonplace in the early 1980s when Curtis et al[8] described the use of freeze-dried fascia lata for ACL repair. The process is referred to as fibrovascular creeping substitution, that is, the cellular, vascular, and connective tissue changes that occurred within the graft over time. The very concept of graft remodeling at the cellular level provided the stimulus for interventional strategies that could promote desirable tissue remodeling events and inhibit undesirable events.

THE CONCEPT OF GRAFT REMODELING

In 1987, Jackson et al[9] presented disappointing findings of ACL freeze-dried bone–patellar tendon–bone allografts in an experimental study in goats, but in 1991, more favorable findings were reported when a more thorough freeze/thaw process was used to remove cellular elements, that is, decellularization. In retrospect, the likely explanation between these disparate outcomes involves the fate of the cells in non-decellularized tissue grafts.

Free graft tissue is, by definition, devascularized and injured. As with all injured tissue, the initial response

Dr. Badylak or an immediate family member is a member of a speakers' bureau or has made paid presentations on behalf of BD/Bard, DiFusion Technology, and Triad; serves as a paid consultant to or is an employee of Biostage and ECM Therapeutics; has stock or stock options held in ECM Therapeutics; and has received research or institutional support from BD/Bard, Difusion Technology, ECM Therapeutics, Triad, and Xeltis. Neither Emily Henderson nor any immediate family member has received anything of value from or has stock or stock options held in a commercial company or institution related directly or indirectly to the subject of this chapter.

of the recipient to such a graft involves activation of the innate immune system by cell debris and the associated damage-associated molecular patterns.[10] An infiltration of neutrophils is quickly followed by mononuclear macrophages, the secretome of which largely determines downstream remodeling events. These downstream events include neovascularization, graft matrix degradation, fibroblast infiltration, and the formation of scar tissue. The cellular and extracellular components of every tissue and organ are repeatedly replaced (ie, turnover), albeit at different rates, as part of normal, healthy homeostatic processes. It is not surprising, therefore, that the same phenomenon occurs following surgical placement of decellularized autologous, allogeneic, and xenogeneic tissue and that it may occur at an accelerated rate compared with native healthy tissue. In the absence of cellular debris and other proinflammatory stimuli (eg, bacteria), the proinflammatory response is mitigated and the constructive replacement of native tissue occurs.

In contrast to default wound healing that typically results in scar tissue formation and absence of new functional tissue, the presence of an (acellular) extracellular matrix (ECM)-based bioscaffold provides not only a structural template but also biologically relevant signaling molecules that contribute to a functional, three-dimensional tissue replacement structure. It should be noted that the early stages of bioscaffold remodeling involve many of the same biologic processes that characterize inflammation, that is, cell infiltration and neovascularization that manifest as swelling, redness, and heat. The relevance of these events is the potential effect on the clinical evaluation and interpretation of normal graft remodeling versus an adverse inflammatory response or the presence of an infectious process. Both processes will manifest as swelling with possible redness in the early phase, but the downstream outcome will differ. An understanding of the biology of autografts, allografts, and xenografts will avoid misinterpretation of otherwise desirable events.

ALLOGRAFTS, XENOGRAFTS, AND DECELLULARIZED TISSUE PRODUCTS

Xenotransplantation, or transplantation of organs or tissues across species boundaries, marked the earliest attempt at functional organ transplantation in the early 1900s. Although the clinical outcome was unsuccessful, these initial attempts identified the presence of a humoral substance that mediated rejection.[11,12] Owen[13] suggested a genetic component to allogeneic and xenograft rejection when a kidney from one calf was successfully transplanted into its identical twin. Although transplantation of xenogeneic organs is still not feasible, the use of decellularized tissue (ie, the remaining ECM) products is commonplace.

Acellular xenogeneic and allogeneic ECM scaffold materials do not elicit an adverse immune response; rather, these materials activate the immune system toward a prohealing, restorative immune response.[14-18] Such materials are available as surgical meshes,[19-21] topical powders and hydrogels, and hybrid forms as inductive scaffolds for wound healing.[22,23] The reservoir of cytokines, chemokines, and matrix-bound nanovesicles released from ECM bioscaffolds facilitate events that promote not only the development but also the maintenance and repair of tissues when such bioscaffolds are placed at the site of injury. These processes facilitate the inherent restorative capacity of the human body to the extent possible in adult mammals.[16,24-28]

The use of biologic materials to support and promote tissue healing, specifically allogeneic and xenogeneic tissues, has become commonplace in a variety of surgical applications, including orthopaedic surgery. Although autologous and allogeneic donor tissue has been used to replace damaged or missing tissue/organs for at least 80 years, the value of removing cells from these donor tissues and using the remaining ECM was not fully recognized until the 1990s.[29] Just as the antigenic epitopes of allogeneic and xenogeneic cells elicit an acute rejection response, the effect of cytoplasmic and nuclear cell debris present within poorly decellularized tissue products elicits an inflammatory response that typically leads to scar tissue formation. In contrast, the thorough removal of cells and cell debris from harvested donor tissues tends to promote a constructive and functional tissue remodeling response. The message here is that not all bioscaffolds are created equal, and a working knowledge of their manufacturing considerations and the biology of graft remodeling will markedly improve the chances for a favorable clinical outcome.

Allografts and Xenografts: Manufacturing Considerations

The manufacturing of allografts and xenografts, whether they are classified as an HCT/P or as a device, is highly regulated. The reagents used in the manufacturing process must meet rigorous standards,[30,31] and the biocompatibility testing that medical devices must pass is comprehensive.

One major consideration for ECM-based allografts and xenografts is the thoroughness of decellularization. As discussed previously, the amount of cell debris remaining in the final product has a strong influence on the local tissue response of the recipient and the clinical outcome. There are currently no uniform standards by which to quantify decellularization; therefore, there is wide disparity among available products. Suggested guidelines for decellularization have been proposed,[32] and products that meet these guidelines have been well received.

A second important manufacturing consideration for xenografts is the source tissue. Because biologic variability is unavoidable, every effort should be made to minimize structural and compositional differences that are present because of age, breed, diet, and processing methods. Numerous suppliers of animal tissues now provide documentation that guarantees that certain standards are met.

Finally, all medical devices must be terminally sterilized. Common methods of sterilization include ethylene oxide, electron-beam irradiation, and gamma irradiation. Each of these methods has the potential to alter ECM structure and the integrity of the bioactive signaling molecules. Although not a complete list, consideration of the aforementioned three variables will go a long way toward improved clinical outcomes when bioscaffolds are used for tissue repair.

Regulatory Considerations

A wide range of regulatory pathways determine the processes by which implants derived from animal and human tissue sources become available on the market. A review of these regulatory guidelines is provided as they relate to bioscaffolds.

American Association of Tissue Banks Standards

Human tissue products and tissue banks that supply allografts are regulated by the FDA. Industry standards regarding tissue retrieval, processing, packaging, labeling, storage, and distribution are developed by the American Association of Tissue Banks (AATB), the premier standard-setting body promoting the safety and use of donated human tissue. The AATB Standards for Tissue Banking are recognized in both the United States and around the world as the definitive guide for tissue banking. These standards include guidance on records management, authorization and consent practices, donor screening, parameters surrounding tissue recovery surgeries, and the establishment of a quality program. The AATB estimates that there are 58,000 tissue donors annually, with approximately 3,300,000 allografts being distributed annually.[33]

Human Cell and Tissue Products

Tissue products that are harvested from a donor and are minimally processed or manipulated can be marketed as HCT/Ps. For a tissue to be considered manufactured with minimal manipulation and processing, the biologic properties of the tissue or its cells must not be altered. Stated differently, the processing of the structural tissue must not alter its original characteristics because they relate to the tissue's utility for reconstruction, repair, or replacement (21 Code of Federal Regulations [CFR] 1271.3). Grafts manufactured with complex additives or processes that affect the characteristics of human cells or tissues disqualify them from this classification. HCT/P must also be labeled for homologous use; that is, the HCT/P must be placed in the same anatomic region of the recipient from where it was recovered from the donor and perform the same basic function or functions in the recipient as in the donor (21 CFR 1271.3).

The HCT/P classification covers a broad range of applications including blood transfusions and organ transplantation. The specific types of orthopaedic products that fall under this distinction include ligaments, tendons, fascia, cartilage, and bone, including demineralized bone matrix in powder form.[34] A partial list of orthobiologic products that are regulated as HCT/P is provided in **Table 1**.

HCT/Ps marketed under Section 361 are not required to obtain FDA Premarket Approval or clearance. Instead, manufacturers of these products are allowed to self-designate the tissue products as having met the criteria outlined under 21 CFR 1271.3(d)(1). Distributors and marketers of HCT/Ps must register their establishment with the FDA, submit a list of each HCT/P manufactured, and comply with any other applicable requirements set forth in 21 CFR 1271. In accordance with 21 CFR 1270 and 1271, a Tissue Establishment and Registration (Form FDA 3356) is required to be completed and updated annually.

Current Good Tissue Practices

The methods and facilities used to manufacture HCT/Ps are governed by Current Good Tissue Practices (cGTPs) established by the FDA. The details of these can be found in 21 CFR § 1271.150. cGTP requirements are established to prevent the introduction, transmission, and spread of communicable diseases or other adverse events.[35] All steps in tissue recovery, donor screening and testing, processing, storage, labeling, packing, and distribution are governed by cGTPs. Supplies and reagents, facility and equipment requirements, and environmental controls are also regulated by cGTPs.[36] Manufacturers of medical devices are required to retain records for their products for the lifetime of a device (21 CFR part 820). Because allografts must be able to be traced to specific donors in case of disease transmission and because grafts integrate into host tissue unlike some other implants, manufacturers maintain these records indefinitely.

Biologics License Application

Biologics, which differ from Drugs and Devices and exist outside of Section 361 criteria, require FDA approval of a Biologics License Application (BLA). A BLA is submitted by an entity that accepts responsibility for compliance with product and establishment standards. Issuance of a biologics license by the FDA is dependent on the demonstration of product safety and efficacy through extensive preclinical work for its intended use. A biologics license

TABLE 1 Partial List of Commercially Available Allografts and Xenografts That are Used for Soft-Tissue and Bone Repair

Product	Manufacturer	Source Tissue	Application Focus	Form	Cross-linking Agent	Terminal Sterilization	Regulatory
AlloDerm RTM	BioHorizons	Human dermis	Soft tissue, dentistry	Dry	—	—	HCT/P
AlloMax	BD Bard	Human dermis	Soft tissue	Dry	—	Gamma	HCT/P
AlloPatch HD	ConMed	Human dermis	Tendon	Dry	—	—	HCT/P
Biodesign Hernia Graft	Cook Biotech	Porcine small intestine	Soft tissue	Dry	—	Ethylene oxide	510(k) device
DermaSpan	Zimmer Biomet	Human dermis	Soft tissue, tendon	Dry	—	Gamma	HCT/P
FlexHD Pliable	Mentor	Human dermis	Breast	Hydrated	—	—	HCT/P
Fortiva	RTI Surgical	Porcine dermis	Soft tissue	Hydrated	—	Gamma	510(k) device
Gentrix Surgical Matrix	ACell	Porcine urinary bladder	Soft tissue	6 Layer	—	E-beam	510(k) device
GraftJacket	Wright Medical	Human dermis	Soft tissue	Dry	—	—	HCT/P
Grafton DBM	Medtronic	Human bone	Bone	Powder	—	—	510(k) device
MicroMatrix	ACell	Porcine urinary bladder	Wound care	Powder	—	E-beam	510(k) device
MiroDerm	Reprise Biomedical	Porcine liver	Soft tissue	Hydrated	—	E-beam	510(k) device
Peri-Guard Repair Patch	Baxter International	Bovine pericardium	Soft tissue	Hydrated	Glu	Liquid chemical	510(k) device
Permacol	Medtronic	Porcine dermis	Soft tissue	Hydrated	HMDI	Gamma	510(k) device
ProLayer	Stryker Corporation	Human dermis	Soft tissue	Hydrated	—	E-beam	HCT/P
Strattice	LifeCell Corporation	Porcine dermis	Soft tissue	Hydrated	—	E-beam	510(k) device
XenMatrix	BD Bard	Porcine dermis	Soft tissue	Hydrated	—	E-beam	510(k) device

DBM = demineralized bone matrix, E-beam = electron-beam irradiation, Gamma = gamma irradiation, Glu = glutaraldehyde, HCT/P = human cells, tissues, and cellular and tissue-based product, HMDI = hexamethylene diisocyanate

Adapted with permission from Madeline C,Cramer SFB: Extracellular matrix-based biomaterials and their influence upon cell behavior. *Ann Biomed Eng* 2020;48:2132-2153.

indicates that the product, its manufacturing process, and the facilities in which it is manufactured all meet requirements established to guarantee safety, purity, and potency of the product.

The FDA created the Tissue Reference Group, a multicenter forum established to determine appropriate regulatory classifications for human tissue products. If the Tissue Reference Group decides a product should not be regulated under Section 361, the Office of Combination Products and FDA centers intervene to determine the appropriate regulatory pathway based on the product's primary mode of action. Examples of combination products that are regulated as devices rather than the BLA route include demineralized bone combined with handling agents (glycerol, sodium hyaluronate, calcium sulfate, gelatin, and collagen) and bone-suture-tendon allografts.[34]

510(k)

Human cells and tissues that have been more than minimally manipulated cannot be considered HCT/Ps under Section 361 and are instead often classified as medical devices and marketed under a different set of guidelines. Along with xenografts, these devices are marketed in accordance with the 510(k) designation. Under the 510(k) designation, a new device can be cleared for the market if found to be substantially equivalent to a device marketed before April 28, 1976, the date when 510(k) regulations were put into effect. If a predicate device or one that is substantially equivalent exists, the new implant is regulated as a 510(k) device. Acellular products derived from human tissue that are not HCT/Ps and the acellular products manufactured with animal tissue for which there are predicate devices are generally considered as BLAs or medical devices that require 510(k) designation.

Beyond the HCT/P and 510(k) regulatory guidelines, more complex devices that contain living cells for which there is no predicate device are referred to as a biologic and require a BLA. To ensure product safety and efficacy after a product is approved and released on the market, postmarketing activities are also required. These postregulatory obligations include adverse event reporting and additional phase IV studies.

Clinical Applications

Examples of Musculoskeletal Applications

Surgical techniques for musculoskeletal repair often depend on the availability, quality, and quantity of graft materials. Although autografts have a long history of use for managing musculoskeletal injuries because of their inherent compatibility, donor-site morbidity can contribute to extended recovery times.[1] Thus, the potential use of allografts and xenografts poses an attractive alternative. Current efforts in regenerative medicine aim to provide solutions through the development of off-the-shelf allogeneic and xenogeneic bioscaffolds for use in meniscal injury repair, ACL repair, rotator cuff repair, bone grafting, cartilage repair, and Achilles tendon repair, among others.

Although bone and skeletal muscle have robust regenerative capacity, volumetric tissue loss overwhelms these regenerative properties. Cartilage, tendon, and ligamentous tissue have limited innate regenerative properties. Injury to these tissues can benefit markedly from the inductive properties of autografts, allografts, and xenografts. When possible, autografts are preferable because of the potential contribution of autologous cells, whereas allografts and xenografts require decellularization to avoid an adverse immune response. However, as stated previously, autografts are associated with donor-site morbidity. Regardless of the source, tissue grafts provide an abundance of signaling molecules that favorably affect stem and progenitor cell recruitment, proliferation and differentiation, antimicrobial activity, angiogenesis, and the immunobiology of wound healing.[37]

Ideally, the bioscaffold would possess the structural and biologic properties of the injured tissue; however, this rarely occurs. Cumulative findings of preclinical and clinical studies show that favorable outcomes are the result of the biocompatible microenvironment provided by these bioscaffolds and the site-appropriate remodeling that occurs as these grafts degrade and release their constructive signaling molecules.

Examples

Bone Grafts

Bone grafts are the second most common tissue transplanted in the United States, and attempts to stimulate bone healing make up a major proportion of clinical orthopaedic surgery. Although surgeons typically achieve good results in fracture repair and reconstructive surgery, complications that require surgeons to use bone graft do occur.[38]

- **Autologous bone grafts**: The term autograft refers to bone tissue harvested from and implanted in the same individual. Preparations of these autogenous grafts include aspirated bone marrow or processed osteogenic cells, cancellous bone, neovascularized cortical bone, and vascularized grafts.
- **Allografts**: Allografts are composed of tissue that has been harvested from one individual and implanted into another individual of the same species. Allograft bone is readily available and avoids the risks associated with harvesting autologous tissue.[39] Unlike most solid organ transplants, human bone allograft preparations involve the intentional removal of cells to minimize host immunologic rejection. The removal of cellular debris also decreases the risk of transplanting viral particles into the recipient. Bone allografts

TABLE 2 Terminology Used to Describe Bone Graft Materials Based on the Mechanism by Which New Bone is Formed

Material Properties	Definition
Osteogenic	Contains living cells that are capable of differentiation into bone
Osteoconductive	Promotes bone apposition to its surface; facilitates enhanced bone formation
Osteoinductive	Provides a biologic stimulus that induces local or transplanted cells to differentiate into mature osteoblasts

are classified based on the graft anatomy (ie, cortical, cancellous, osteochondral), methods of processing (ie, fresh, frozen, freeze-dried, demineralized), methods of sterilization (ie, irradiated, ethylene oxide), and how the final product is packaged (ie, powder, gel, paste, strips).

- Bone graft materials promote a bone healing response by providing osteogenic, osteoconductive, or osteoinductive activity to a local site, either alone or in combination with other materials[40,41] (**Table 2**).
- Because allografts lack viable cells, they may not provide the same osteogenic properties of autografts. Based on the methods of graft processing, the osteoconductive and osteoinductive properties of allografts vary.
- **Xenografts**: A robust immune response to bone xenografts (not decellularized), which are harvested from a different species, precludes their widespread use in clinical applications. Bovine collagen can be prepared as a gel, powder, sponge, paper, or mesh depending on preparation method and cross-linking. Studies evaluating the efficacy of bovine-based bone xenografts are limited but may indicate that xenografts incorporate more slowly than autografts or allografts.[42,43] Although bovine xenografts seem to be biocompatible, high rates of failure to achieve successful incorporation and poor clinical outcomes indicate that this may not be a viable alternative.

Rotator Cuff Repair

The recurrence of rotator cuff tears following primary repair remains unacceptably high, in large part because of the poor quality of remaining tendon tissue. Recurrence is particularly common with two and three tendon cuff tears. The use of bioscaffolds for cuff repair has greatly expanded the number of surgeries because of the increased chance of a favorable outcome. The use of a porcine-derived graft composed of small intestinal submucosa in the early 2000s showed limited success because of the lack of understanding of the biology associated with such materials. The robust cellular infiltration and angiogenesis that resulted following implantation of the small intestinal submucosa graft were interpreted as a rejection phenomenon instead of what is now known to be part of the tissue rebuilding process. Current bioscaffolds have clearly contributed to improved outcomes.

ACL Repair

One of the most frequently performed orthopaedic procedures is the reconstruction of the ACL. More than 250,000 people experience a torn ACL in the United States, with approximately 175,000 opting for reconstructive surgery.[44] Without surgical reconstruction, morbidity is significant. In addition, osteoarthritis will develop within 10 years in as many as 50% of individuals who sustain ACL tears.[45,46] During the past 30 years, treatment options for ACL injuries have advanced greatly. There is general consensus that ACL reconstruction involves the use of a tissue graft, but the processes for graft selection, the method of graft harvest, the positioning of tibial and femoral tunnels, and the method of graft fixation are debated.

- **Autografts**: ACL reconstruction often uses autografts originating from the patient's patellar tendon or hamstring tendon. Studies have been unable to find significant differences between the two types of grafts as related to long-term functional outcome;[47] therefore, patient-specific factors and surgeon preference may guide the selection of graft tissue. An obvious advantage of autografts is the decreased risk for host rejection and disease transmission, but postoperative pain at the graft harvest site can affect postsurgical rehabilitation efforts.
- **Allografts**: A major advantage of using allografts is the lack of donor-site morbidity; however, disadvantages include higher cost and possible increased time to complete healing.[48] Although the recovery and processing of human tissue from donors has improved and become safer, irradiation to sterilize the harvested tissues can affect the biomechanical properties and therefore influence clinical outcome.
- **Xenografts**: Clinical evaluations of ACL reconstruction with xenografts have shown comparable clinical outcomes to reconstruction using allografts but with high infection rates. A recent study that compared ACL reconstruction with immunochemically modified porcine patellar tendon xenograft against human Achilles tendon allograft found that harvesting and processing treatment strategies of xenograft tissue must be improved to reduce the infection rate.[49] It should be noted that the infections were associated with graft processing methods and not as a result of zoonotic origin.

- **Alternative biologic techniques**: Biologic treatment for ACL ruptures aims to optimize the ligamentous healing process through modulation of the inflammatory response and maximize the regenerative potential of cells within the native ACL by downregulating matrix degradative enzymes.[50] Biologic agents such as platelet-rich plasma and MSCs may be used to promote ACL healing. An approach that uses both a traditional ACL reconstruction procedure with a newer biologic method is the bridge-enhanced ACL repair technique. A collagen-based bioscaffold is soaked in autologous blood and placed near the torn ends of the ACL that are then tensioned with sutures.[51] The scaffold is used to bridge the gap between the two torn ends of the ligament. Preclinical models of this technique found similar mechanical properties between repairs with the bridge-enhanced ACL repair technique compared with those with traditional ACL reconstruction.[51,52]

Ethical Considerations

Sourcing and Harvesting of Human and Animal Tissues

The advantages and disadvantages of autografts, allografts, and xenografts have been identified previously. However, the process of graft harvesting deserves further discussion.

Allograft Tissue Collection

A potential human donor (or a family member) must voluntarily make the decision to donate tissue(s) for medical applications. The donor selection process then immediately moves into a detailed survey of an individual's medical and social history, including a close look into an individual's behavior that may categorize the potential donor in subpopulations with increased risks of disease transmission (eg, an individual who used intravenous drugs) and therefore put recipients of the tissue at increased risk. This process must start immediately so as to preserve the integrity of the tissues to be harvested. This first round of vigorous screening, which identifies health issues and high-risk behaviors, typically disqualifies a large percentage of donors. Deceased human donors deemed eligible after initial screening enter a donor pool where bodily fluids are tested for specific pathogens (21 CFR Part 1270). Blood samples are evaluated for infectious agents such as HIV, hepatitis B and C viruses, and the syphilis bacterium.

Human tissue must be retrieved quickly following death and by strict aseptic procedures. The tissue harvest is typically performed in a hospital operating room or facility specifically built for tissue retrieval, to minimize the risk of contamination. Tissues are excised and immediately placed in sterile containers to be sent for further processing and preparation. Additional pathogenic testing or specific evaluations for certain tissues and donor sites are also typically completed at this stage. All implants derived from human tissue must be meticulously tracked and able to be traced back to the donor. Tissue banks typically provide tracking labels with the tissue to be implanted, which are then transferred to the recipient's medical record. In the unlikely event of disease transmission to an implant recipient, clinicians must be able to track to a specific donor and treat other patients who may have also received a tissue derived from this individual. There are several risks and limitations associated with allografts as have already been mentioned but are worthy of repetition. Allografts are subject to a limited availability of donors, potential disease transmission, variable consistency due to innate diversity of human donors, host rejection, handling/storage and transportation of tissue, and ethical considerations.

Xenograft Tissue Collection

The typical source of animal tissue for xenografts is the commercial slaughterhouse or abattoir. It is common for commercial abattoirs to work with device manufacturers to provide animal tissue for medical use. These institutions are highly regulated by the US Department of Agriculture. It imposes cleanliness and sanitation standards referred to as hazard analysis and critical control point (Hazard Analysis Critical Control Point) guidelines. Some companies have evolved to specialize in the supply of animal tissue specifically for medical devices. These operations can carefully control all aspects of raising the animals, such as breeding/husbandry, genetics, and specific food supply, which ultimately grant the device manufacturers the ability to deliver a product with tighter specifications.

Implants derived from animal sources must also conform to a strict regimen of tests and screenings. Manufacturers of xenografts must have a known and reliable source of disease-free animals, that is, a closed herd. If importing animals from outside of the United States, herd records of the animals that include the design of the facility and conditions in which animals are kept are required.[53] Monitoring of the animals' genetic profile and health status, comprehensive microbiology, and serology evaluations for pathogens and isolating the herd from other sources all help to reduce the risk of disease transmission.

Factors that affect the variability of animal tissue used in the medical industry include but are not limited to species, age of the animal, the animal's diet, and geographic location of the herd. It is likely that regulatory bodies will continue to endorse strict controls over the sourcing of animal tissue for medical devices in the future.

SUMMARY

The field of orthobiologics comprises a diverse accumulation of cells, signaling molecules, blood products, and ECM-based bioscaffolds as well as a variety of clinical applications. The clinical use of these products appears to be steadily increasing and the long-term benefits are yet to be determined. It is important to shed light on variables that contribute to the ability of ECM-based scaffolds to facilitate constructive and functional tissue repair. An overview of the tissue source and manufacturing considerations, regulatory pathways, and biologic events that affect product performance has been presented in an attempt to provide the orthopaedic surgeon with the tools necessary to make informed decisions regarding the most appropriate product for each patient.

REFERENCES

1. Kalaskar D: 3D bioprinting for musculoskeletal applications. *J 3D Print Med* 2017;1(3):191-211.
2. Cherian M: The global burden of musculoskeletal injuries: Challenges and solutions. *Clin Orthop Relat Res* 2008; 466:2306.
3. Lexer E: Substitution of whole or half joints from freshly amputated extremities by free plastic operation. *Surg Gynecol Obstet* 1908;6:601-607.
4. Giertz KH: Über freie Transplantation der Fascia lata als Ersatz für Sehnen und Bänder. *Deutsche Zeitschrift für Chirurgie* 1913;125(5):480-496.
5. The classic. Operation for repair of the crucial ligaments Ernest W. Hey Groves, MD., F.R.C.S. *Clin Orthop Relat Res* 1980;147:4-6.
6. Galleazzi R: La ricostituzione dei ligamenti cociati del ginocchio, Atti e Memorie della Società. *Lombarda di Chirurgia* 1924;13:302-317.
7. Franke K: Clinical experience in 130 cruciate ligament reconstructions. *Orthop Clin N Am* 1976;7(1):191-193.
8. Curtis RJ, Delee JC, Drez DJ Jr: Reconstruction of the anterior cruciate ligament with freeze dried fascia lata allografts in dogs. A preliminary report. *Am J Sports Med* 1985;13(6): 408-414.
9. Jackson DW, Grood ES, Cohn BT, Arnoczky SP, Simon TM, Cummings JF: The effects of in situ freezing on the anterior cruciate ligament. An experimental study in goats. *J Bone Joint Surg* 1991;73(2):201-213.
10. Venereau EC, Ceriotti C, Bianchi ME: DAMPs from cell death to new life. *Front Immunol* 2015;6:422.
11. Deschamps J-Y, Roux FA, Pierre S, Gouin E: History of xenotransplantation. *Xenotransplantation* 2005;12(2):91-109.
12. Billingham RE, Brent L, Medawar PB: Quantitative studies on tissue transplantation immunity. III. Actively acquired tolerance. *Philos Trans R Soc Lond Ser B Biol Sci* 1956;239(666): 357-414.
13. Owen RD: Immunogenetic consequences of vascular anastomoses between bovine twins. *Science* 1945;102(2651):400-401.
14. Allman AJ, McPherson TB, Merrill LC, Badylak SF, Metzger DW: The Th2-restricted immune response to xenogeneic small intestinal submucosa does not influence systemic protective immunity to viral and bacterial pathogens. *Tissue Eng* 2004;8(1):53-62.
15. Brown BN, Londono R, Tottey S, et al: Macrophage phenotype as a predictor of constructive remodeling following the implantation of biologically derived surgical mesh materials. *Acta Biomater* 2012;8(3):978-987.
16. Brown BN, Valentin JE, Stewart-Akers AM, McCabe GP, Badylak SF: Macrophage phenotype and remodeling outcomes in response to biologic scaffolds with and without a cellular component. *Biomaterials* 2009;30(8):1482-1491.
17. Badylak SF, Valentin JE, Ravindra AK, McCabe GP, Stewart-Akers AM: Macrophage phenotype as a determinant of biologic scaffold remodeling. *Tissue Eng Part A* 2008;14(11):1835-1842.
18. Dziki JL, Huleihel L, Scarritt ME, Badylak SF: Extracellular matrix bioscaffolds as immunomodulatory biomaterials. *Tissue Eng Part A* 2017;23(19-20): 1152-1159.
19. Kulig BN, Luo X, Finkelstein EB, et al: Biologic properties of surgical scaffold materials derived from dermal ECM. *Biomaterials* 2013;34(23):5776-5784.
20. Young DA, McGilvray KC, Ehrhart N, Gilbert TW: Comparison of in vivo remodeling of urinary bladder matrix and acellular dermal matrix in an ovine model. *Regen Med* 2018;13(7):759-773.
21. Hood J, Hiles M: Constructive soft tissue remodelling with a biologic extracellular matrix graft: Overview and review of the clinical literature. *Acta Chir Belg* 2007;107(6): 641-647.
22. Bracaglia LG, Fisher JP: Extracellular matrix-based biohybrid materials for engineering compliant, matrix-dense tissues. *Adv Healthc Mater* 2015;4(16):2475-2487.
23. Sawyer M, Ferzoco S, DeNoto G: A polymer-biologic hybrid hernia construct: review of data and early experiences. *Polymers* 2021;13(12):1928.
24. Valentin JE, Turner NJ, Gilbert TW, Badylak SF: Functional skeletal muscle formation with a biologic scaffold. *Biomaterials* 2010;31(29):7475-7484.
25. Dziki J, Badylak S, Yabroudi M, et al: An acellular biologic scaffold treatment for volumetric muscle loss: Results of a 13-patient cohort study. *NPJ Regen Med* 2016;1:16008.
26. Badylak SF, Hoppo T, Nieponice A, Gilbert TW, Davison JM, Jobe BA: Esophageal preservation in five male patients after endoscopic inner-layer circumferential resection in the setting of superficial cancer: A regenerative medicine approach with a biologic scaffold. *Tissue Eng Part A* 2011;17(11-12):1643-1650.
27. Badylak SF: The extracellular matrix as a biologic scaffold material. *Biomaterials* 2007;28(25):3587-3593.
28. Mase VJ Jr. Hsu JR, Wolf SE, et al: Clinical application of an acellular biologic scaffold for surgical repair of a large, traumatic quadriceps femoris muscle defect. *Orthopedics* 2011;33(7):511.
29. Londono R, Dziki JL, Haljasmaa E, Turner NJ, Leifer C, Badylak SF: The effect of cell debris within biologic scaffolds upon the host response. *J Biomed Mater Res A* 2017;105(8):2109-2118.

30. Food and Drug Administration, HHS: Current good tissue practice for human cell, tissue, and cellular and tissue-based product establishments; inspection and enforcement. Final rule. *Fed Regist* 2004;69(226):68611-68688.

31. § 1271.210 Supplies and reagents. US Food and Drug Administration Code of Federal Regulations. Available at: https://www.accessdata.fda.gov/scripts/cdrh/cfdocs/cfcfr/CFRSearch.cfm?fr=1271.210. Accessed September 28, 2022.

32. Crapo PM, Gilbert TW, Badylak SF: An overview of tissue and whole organ decellularization processes. *Biomaterials* 2011;32(12):3233-3243.

33. The 2012 and 2015 National Tissue Recovery through Utilization Survey Report. Available at: https://www.hhs.gov/sites/default/files/ntrus-report-2015.pdf. Accessed September 28, 2022.

34. FDA Regulation of Human Cells, Tissues, and Cellular and Tissue-Based Products (HCT/P's) Product List. 2018. Available at: https://www.fda.gov/vaccines-blood-biologics/tissue-tissue-products/fda-regulation-human-cells-tissues-and-cellular-and-tissue-based-products-hctps-product-list. Accessed September 28, 2022.

35. Lindblad R, Fiky EA, Wood D, Armstrong G: Regulatory pathway for mesenchymal stromal cell-based therapy in the united states, in Viswanathan S, Hematti P, eds: *Mesenchymal Stromal Cells*. Academic Press, 2017, pp 227-242.

36. Hatcher HC, Atala A, Allickson JG: Landscape of cell banking, in Atala A, Allickson JG, eds: *Translational Regenerative Medicine*. Academic Press, 2015, pp 13-19.

37. Roberts SJ, Howard D, Buttery LD, Shakesheff KM: Clinical applications of musculoskeletal tissue engineering. *Br Med Bull* 2008;86(1):7-22.

38. Baldwin P, Li DJ, Auston DA, Mir HS, Yoon RS, Koval KJ: Autograft, allograft, and bone graft substitutes: clinical evidence and indications for use in the setting of orthopaedic trauma surgery. *J Orthop Trauma* 2019;33(4):203-213.

39. Vining NC, Warme WJ, Mosca VS: Comparison of structural bone autografts and allografts in pediatric foot surgery. *J Pediatr Orthop* 2012;32(7):19-23.

40. Gruskin E, Doll BA, Futrell FW, Schmitz JP, Hoolimger JO: Demineralized bone matrix in bone repair: History and use. *Adv Drug Deliv Rev* 2012;64(12):1063-1077.

41. Bauer TW, Muschler GF: Bone graft materials: An overview of the basic science. *Clin Orthop Relat Res* 2000;371:10-27.

42. Shibuya N, Jupiter DC, Clawson LD, La Fontaine J: Incorporation of bovine-based structural bone grafts used in reconstructive foot surgery. *J Foot Ankle Surg* 2012;51(1):30-33.

43. Ledford CK, Nunley JA II, Viens NA, Lark RK: Bovine xenograft failures in pediatric foot reconstructive surgery. *J Pediatr Orthop* 2013;33(4):458-463.

44. Kon E, Matteo BD, Altomare D, et al: Biologic agents to optimize outcomes following ACL repair and reconstruction: A systematic review of clinical evidence. *J Orthop Res* 2021;40(1):10-28.

45. Maffulli N, Lungo UG, Gougoulias N, Loppini N, Denaro V: Long-term health outcomes of youth sports injuries. *Br J Sports Med* 2010;44(1):21-25.

46. Schilaty ND, Nagelli C, Bates NA, et al: Incidence of second anterior cruciate ligament tears and identification of associated risk factors from 2001 to 2010 using a geographic database. *Orthop J Sports Med* 2017;5(8):2325967117724196.

47. Filbay SR, Grindem H: Evidence-based recommendations for the management of anterior cruciate ligament (ACL) rupture. *Best Pract Res Clin Rheumatol* 2019;33(1):33-47.

48. McGuire DA, Hendricks SD: Allograft tissue in ACL reconstruction. *Sports Med Arthrosc Rev* 2009;17(4):224-233.

49. Van Der Merwe W, Lind M, Faunø P, et al: Xenograft for anterior cruciate ligament reconstruction was associated with high graft processing infection. *J Exp Orthop* 2020;7(1):79.

50. Di Matteo B, Loibl M, Andriolo L, et al: Biologic agents for anterior cruciate ligament healing: A systematic review. *World J Orthop* 2016;7(9):592-603.

51. Murray MM, Kalish LA, Fleming BC, et al: Bridge-enhanced anterior cruciate ligament repair: Two-year results of a first-in-human study. *Orthop J Sports Med* 2019;7(3):2325967118824356.

52. Murray MM, Fleming BC: Use of a bioactive scaffold to stimulate anterior cruciate ligament healing also minimizes posttraumatic osteoarthritis after surgery. *Am J Sports Med* 2013;41(8):1762-1770.

53. US Food and Drug Administration: Medical Devices Containing Materials Derived from Animal Sources (Except for In Vitro Diagnostic Devices). Available at https://www.fda.gov/regulatory-information/search-fda-guidance-documents/medical-devices-containing-materials-derived-animal-sources-except-in-vitro-diagnostic-devices. Accessed November 18, 2022.

CHAPTER 15

Product and Provider Reimbursement in the Field of Orthobiologics

Spencer B. Bailey, MBA, CPC

INTRODUCTION

Because innovation in the field of orthobiologics influences medical practice, a key question that must be answered is, "Who will ultimately pay for a new therapy?", otherwise known as the concept of reimbursement. In the most simplistic sense, reimbursement is the financial compensation to a health care provider for delivering care to a patient, typically from a third-party insurer. An understanding of how novel orthobiologic interventions will be reimbursed is critical to driving adoption. Physicians and health care administrators must decipher the reimbursement landscape for new treatment strategies and make a dollars-and-cents evaluation of their effect on the budget. New therapies that lack sufficient reimbursement in general practice and are not financially sustainable will not achieve adoption over the long term. Clearly, reimbursement is a key ingredient for success of new therapy.

At the time of FDA market authorization (or 361 human cells, tissues, and cellular and tissue-based product [HCT/P] exemption), few truly novel therapies have the enablers for adequate reimbursement. In these cases, therapies face considerable barriers to clinical use and broad adoption. But how should reimbursement be evaluated for new therapies and what are the steps to obtain good reimbursement? It is important to introduce orthopaedic surgeons to the key features of the reimbursement systems in the United States and the processes to secure reimbursement for new, innovative orthobiologic interventions.

WHAT IS REIMBURSEMENT AND WHY IS IT IMPORTANT?

Reimbursement is how and under what circumstances medical services, devices, and drugs are paid for in the United States. Although the specific mechanisms can be quite complex, reimbursement can be summarized into three distinct and independent features—coding, coverage, and payment. Reimbursement is best thought of as the interaction of these three variables for each medical service or procedure provided to a patient (**Table 1**). In this way, a new orthobiologic therapy is reimbursed when there is a convergence of coding mechanisms, associated payment levels, and the willingness of insurers to cover the new therapy in its intended indication.

Established treatment strategies, for which reimbursement already exists, will typically have each of the three elements of reimbursement already in place. Billing codes will likely exist to describe the procedures, devices, or drugs used. Payment rates will typically already be established that reflect the cost of the care provided. Insurance coverage policies will already be in force that stipulate the terms of when and under what circumstances payment will be made. As a result, most orthopaedic interventions are already reimbursed.

New and emerging therapies, by contrast, may be lacking one or more of the necessary components of reimbursement. Emerging therapies in the field of orthobiologics are particularly susceptible to lacking one or more elements necessary for adequate reimbursement. New codes may need to be secured to accurately describe a new delivery procedure (eg, injection or implantation) or the biologic product itself. Payment rates that adequately reimburse for the cost of a new therapy may need to be established. Insurers may have coverage policies that limit the use of a new therapy or limit the patients eligible for such treatment strategies. Securing reimbursement for new therapies can be quite complex and may take years of engagement with various stakeholders.

The orthopaedic surgeon should have a foundational understanding of the reimbursement landscape for orthobiologics in the United States as well as an overview of the processes and strategies that may be used to secure reimbursement for new therapies.

TABLE 1 Coding, Coverage, and Payment

Coverage	Have payers evaluated the service or device? In what circumstances are they willing to pay?
Coding	Are procedure and/or device codes in place to describe the service or technology?
Payment	What are the payment terms for the venue of care? What are the payment amounts for the applicable procedure?

Spencer Bailey or an immediate family member serves as a paid consultant to or is an employee of MicroTransponder, Inc., Cook Biotech, Inc. Miach Orthopedics Regeneus, Ltd., and RTI Medical Systems, Inc. and has stock or stock options held in AgNovos, Inc.

INSURERS IN THE UNITED STATES

Insurers in the United States are the organizations that pay for almost all medical care provided to patients. From a process standpoint, hospitals, physicians, and other health care providers submit medical claims to the company that insures each patient and receive a corresponding payment amount based on the care provided. In practice, the process is far from simple—each insurer has its own set of policies and coverage rules and will remit payment at varying amounts. New orthobiologic therapies that are reimbursed well by one insurer may not be paid at all by another. Insurance companies use disparate methods to verify that care is provided appropriately, including prior authorization for treatment, claim audits, and requests for documentation. Therefore, an awareness of the insurance landscape is critical to anticipate the reimbursement of new and established interventions.

Most Americans are covered by governmental insurance plans (eg, payers) such as Medicare, Medicaid, and Tricare. Medicare is a federal plan generally for individuals older than 65 years or those with long-term disabilities. Medicaid plans are managed at the state level with federal oversight and are for individuals with lower incomes. Tricare is generally for active duty and retired military and families. In general, governmental payers have publicly available coverage terms and published payment rates that facilitate transparency in the reimbursement process.

Nongovernmental insurers, often referred to as commercial or private payers, are typically employer-sponsored plans or purchased on a health insurance exchange. Many of these plans are large, nationwide insurers that are authorized to cover patients at the state level. Although commercial insurance coverage rules are often publicly available, the negotiated payment amounts are not. Commercial insurers negotiate individually with hospitals, physicians, and other providers, and although the payment terms of these independent contracts are not public, they vary considerably from one provider to the next. As a result, it is difficult to precisely anticipate the payment amount or coverage terms for a new, innovative orthobiologic therapy.

Developing a framework to anticipate the payment for a new therapy first requires an analysis of which insurers are likely to cover the intended patient population. The relative percentage of insured lives can be a proxy for the coverage of new therapy (**Figure 1**), but there is significant variation in the mix of insurers based on geography and patient characteristics. For example, patients with osteoporotic spinal compression fractures are disproportionately covered by Medicare because of their age, whereas patients receiving novel treatment for osteoarthritis of the knee tend to be younger and are more likely to be covered by private insurance.

Each insurer will pay different amounts for the same therapy, complicating any analysis of whether or not a new therapy is financially advantageous for a provider. As a result, developing an understanding of insurance

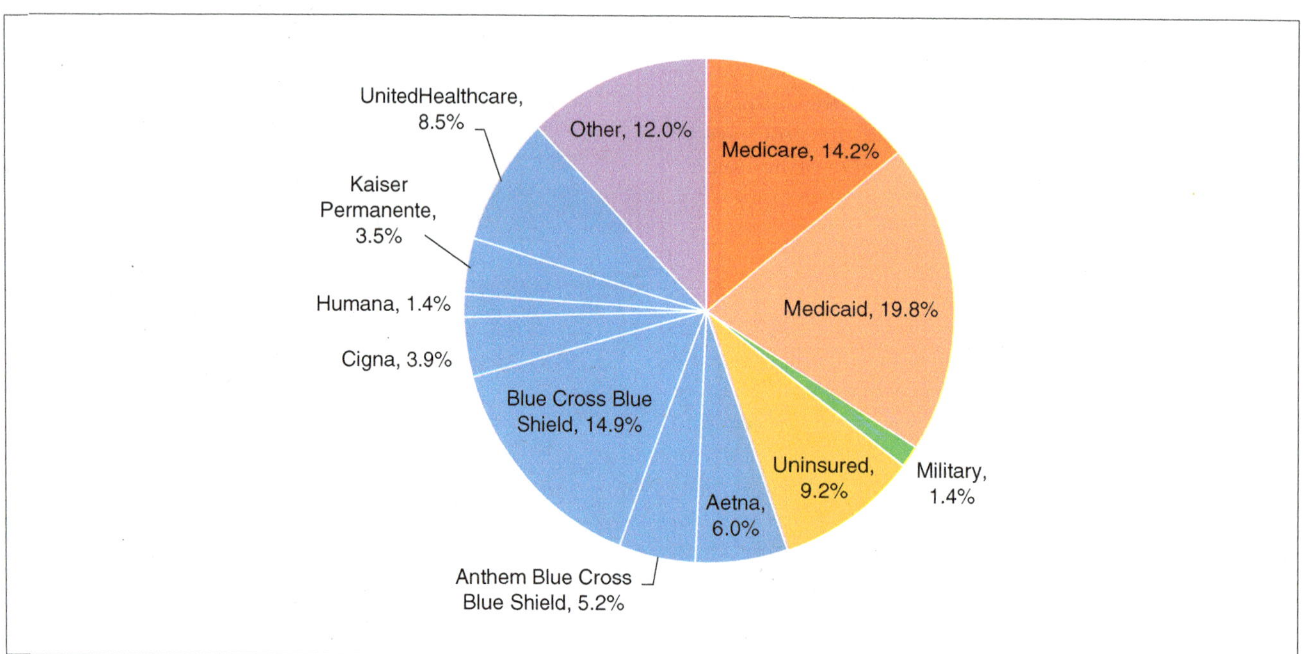

FIGURE 1 Pie chart shows 2020 primary insurance coverage in the United States. (With permission from Keisler-Starkey K, Bunch LN: *Health Insurance Coverage in the United States: 2020. Current Population Reports.* https://www.census.gov/library/publications/2021/demo/p60-274.html. Accessed September 14, 2021.)

landscape for a new therapy will inform whether the payment terms and payment levels are sufficient to make a compelling argument for adoption.

OVERVIEW OF CODING SYSTEMS IN THE UNITED STATES

Coding is the language of reimbursement and facilitates the reporting and reimbursement, with code sets that describe patient conditions, procedures, devices, biologics, and drugs. Each patient encounter is distilled into billing codes that are aggregated on a claim form, which is then sent to insurance companies for payment. Therefore, the various codes that are reported on claims are the essential enablers for complete and accurate reimbursement.

There are several coding systems that are used in the United States, which are maintained by either the Centers for Medicare & Medicaid Services (CMS) or the American Medical Association (AMA). An overview of each code set is provided in **Table 2**. The diagnosis coding set or International Classification of Diseases (ICD) was established by the World Health Organization and then adopted by nations around the world. The United States and many other countries use the 10th edition or ICD-10.

Coding for a typical patient encounter requires at least one diagnosis code (ICD-10 Clinical Modification) and at least one procedure code describing a service that was performed (Current Procedural Terminology [CPT]). Orthopaedic surgical procedures using orthobiologic injections or implants are described by CPT codes. The CPT code set for orthopaedic procedures is maintained by the AMA with input from the CPT Editorial Panel and the AMA CPT Advisory Committee. Codes are generally organized based on the following schema: musculoskeletal anatomy, type of surgical intervention, surgical approach, and other features of the procedure, such as whether an autograft is used.

It is important to note that the use of orthobiologic materials is frequently not included in the descriptor for musculoskeletal procedures. Therefore, the use of an orthobiologic implant is adjunctive to the procedure steps described by existing codes. Codes are reported based on the procedure(s) documented in the medical record and should be reviewed by a certified processional coder.

As described in **Table 2**, surgical procedures are described by CPT codes and the implantable devices, biologics, and drugs are reported using Healthcare Common Procedure Coding System (HCPCS) codes. HCPCS codes are maintained by CMS and describe categories of devices, biologics, drugs, durable medical equipment, and certain temporary codes.

Coding for new medical procedures can be challenging because surgical steps and approaches may not be adequately described by existing codes. Often, the CPT code description is supplemented with parenthetical references (ie, CPT Assistant), which contain additional details and specifics for how and when a particular CPT code should be used. In cases where an orthopaedic procedure is not described by an existing code, an unlisted procedure code may be reported.

Unlisted CPT codes are reserved for interventions that are performed infrequently, are not well established in the medical community, and are supported by limited published clinical evidence. As a result, billing for interventions using unlisted codes often poses reimbursement challenges to providers—because the procedure must often be billed with supporting medical record

TABLE 2 Coding Systems in the United States

Scope	Code Set	Description	Governing/ Oversight Body
Diagnosis coding	ICD-10-CM	Describe patients' diseases and/or conditions (69,000+ codes)	CDC
Physician procedure coding	CPT	Describe physician services and procedures (7,000+ codes)	AMA
Device/drug codes/ miscellaneous use codes	HCPCS	Describe drugs, biologics, devices, and temporary codes (5,000+ codes)	CMS
Procedure coding (hospital inpatient only)	ICD-10-PCS	Describe hospital services/procedures (72,000+ codes)	CMS
Inpatient DRG reimbursement code	MS-DRG	List of payment groups applicable to hospital inpatient encounters (1,000 codes)	CMS

AMA = American Medical Association, CDC = Centers for Disease Control and Prevention, CMS = Centers for Medicare & Medicaid Services, CPT = Current Procedural Terminology, HCPCS = Healthcare Common Procedure Coding System, ICD-10-CM = International Classification of Diseases, Clinical Modification, ICD-10-PCS = International Classification of Diseases, Procedure Coding System, MS-DRG = Medicare Severity Diagnosis Related Group documentation and is reimbursed at each insurer's discretion.

Securing a new CPT code can take several years and requires that new procedures be supported by clinical evidence and be performed broadly in the orthopaedic community. The process to obtain a CPT code begins with an unlisted code, then a Category II temporary code, and then a Category I CPT code, as described in **Figure 2**.

New procedures must also be supported by published literature. The published literature must be of sufficient quality and quantity—typically requiring at least five publications.[1]

In contrast to procedures, which are described by CPT codes, coding for devices, biologics, and drugs is described in the HCPCS. The HCPCS code set is maintained by CMS and contains categories of devices, biologics, and drugs. Similar to unlisted procedure codes, new devices, biologics, and drugs that are not described within the existing HCPCS code set may be reported using not otherwise classified HCPCS codes. Some examples of not otherwise classified HCPCS codes are shown in **Table 3**.

The process to secure a new category of HCPCS code for novel biologics requires an application to CMS.[2] There are several pathways to apply for a new HCPCS code, and to qualify for a new code, the biologic product must be truly new, meaning that it is not described by existing HCPCS codes. In some cases, new biologics that qualify for a new HCPCS code may also meet the criteria for transitional pass-through payment. In these cases, CMS will similarly assign an HCPCS code to describe the biologic product.

Recently, a new class of biologics has emerged with an FDA designation as HCT/Ps. These products are human derived and are reserved for homologous use only. In some cases, HCT/Ps are used in orthopaedic applications, such as intra-articular injection, or for tendon repair. As a general rule, HCT/Ps used exclusively in orthopaedic indications are reported under existing, general HCPCS codes and are not eligible to receive brand-specific HCPCS codes (ie, Q-codes), which are reserved for dermatologic treatment of wounds. Additionally, HCT/Ps may be subject to payer-specific coverage and reporting rules. The American Academy of Orthopaedic Surgeons maintains a list of orthobiologic products, which can assist surgeons in navigating the FDA approval status of biologics.[3]

TABLE 3 Not Otherwise Classified Devices, Biologics, and Drugs

HCPCS Code	HCPCS Code Description
C1899	Implantable/insertable device, not otherwise classified
C9399	Unclassified drugs or biologicals
J3490	Unclassified drugs
J3590	Unclassified biologics
L8699	Prosthetic implant, not otherwise specified
Q4100	Skin substitute, not otherwise specified

HCPCS = healthcare common procedure coding system

Date from Centers for Medicare & Medicaid Services (CMS), Healthcare Common Procedure Coding System (HCPCS). Released January 1, 2021.

INSURANCE PAYMENT SYSTEMS FOR MEDICAL SERVICES

Payment systems vary considerably based on the insurer, the venue of care (eg, hospital, office, and Ambulatory Surgery Center [ASC]), and the procedures performed. Surgical interventions that involve the use of orthobiologics typically take place in a hospital or ASC. In these settings of care, payment for surgical encounters consists of a facility payment to the hospital or ASC and a separate professional payment to the performing surgeon. Payment methodologies for each payer type and venue of care for facility and professional components are discussed in the next paragraphs.

Medicare Payment

Payment terms differ based on the venue of care where the patient is treated. For example, payment for a surgical procedure performed on a hospital outpatient basis (eg, no overnight stay) is vastly different than for the same procedure performed on a hospital inpatient basis.

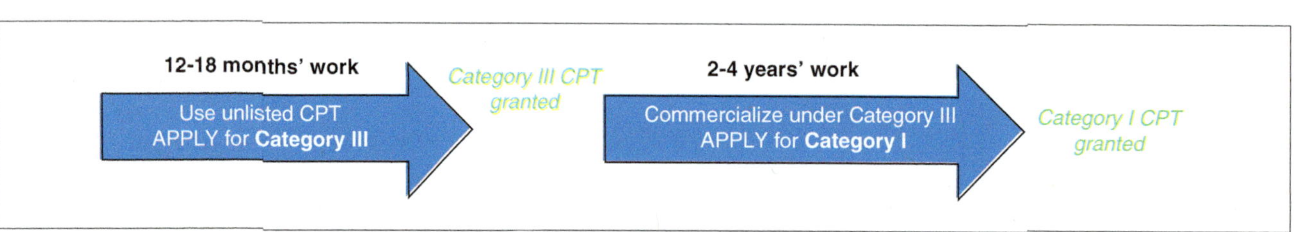

FIGURE 2 Schematic representation shows the process and requirements to secure a Current Procedural Terminology (CPT) code.[8]

The reimbursement implication of the venue of care is critical to understanding the payment terms and amounts for a new therapy.

Medicare Facility Payment

Medicare payments increasingly rely on what is called packaging, whereby facilities receive a single, lump-sum payment for all services, devices, drugs, and biologics used in a hospital stay.[2] For hospital outpatient and ASC surgeries, the payment is attached to the primary procedure performed and typically no separate payment is made for devices, drugs, or biologics used—these costs are packaged into the payment for the associated procedure.

Packaged payment schemes can disincentivize the use of new, more expensive orthobiologics where the incremental cost is not captured in the existing payment level. Some new drugs, biologics, and devices can apply for a Medicare pass-through payment to increase the payment amount to the hospital or ASC. More details on Medicare pass-through payment programs are presented in the next paragraphs.

Medicare pass-through programs are intended to provide Medicare beneficiaries access to technologies that are new, more costly, and have shown a substantial clinical improvement over standard of care treatment. These programs generally reimburse hospitals more for procedures involving new, pass-through eligible technologies for a period of 2 to 3 years. The 2- to 3-year period allows for Medicare reimbursement rates to incorporate the cost of the new therapy. An overview of the hospital inpatient and outpatient Medicare pass-through programs is provided in **Table 4**.

Unlike Medicare (CMS), which follows consistent payment methodologies, commercial insurances rely on individual contract terms to set hospital payments. Each contract is different and disparate contract terms often result in significant variability in payment amounts from one hospital or ASC to another for the same procedure. The payment variability among insurance providers can be significant. Therefore, it is important to understand the terms of commercial insurance contracts before initiating a new therapy.

Professional/Physician Payment

Professional or physician services are reimbursed separately by insurers for the surgeon or physician providing care. Professional services are paid under a different payment methodology than hospital or facility claims. Regardless of where a procedure is performed—hospital outpatient, hospital inpatient, or ASC—the professional/physician claim is paid as well. A comparison of Medicare reimbursement methodologies is presented in **Table 5** for each facility venue of care with comparison with the professional/physician component.

Unlike facility payments, which reimburse hospitals and surgery centers for the cost of performing a procedure, professional payments are intended to reimburse for the physician's time and expertise. Medicare calculates physician payment rates by multiplying a procedure's relative intensity by a payment rate conversion factor. Each procedure is assigned a relative intensity, called the relative value unit (RVU), which establishes how intensive a procedure is relative to other procedures. RVUs are created by the AMA and may be modified by Medicare for the purposes of payment.

The other variable in the payment of physician services—the payment rate conversion factor, or simply conversion factor—is published annually by CMS. Medicare payment rates for physician services are calculated by multiplying the RVU by the annual Medicare conversion factor, which has fluctuated at approximately $35 for the past several years (**Table 6**).

Medicare maintains the list of all CPT codes, corresponding RVU values, and payment rates in the Medicare Physician Fee Schedule. Most surgical interventions that involve the use of orthobiologics have an established

TABLE 4 Pass-Through Payment Programs

Program Name	New Technology Add-On Payment	Transitional Pass-Through Payment Program
Venue of care	Hospital inpatient	Hospital outpatient and ASC
Criterion overview	More costly (cost not reflected in existing MS-DRG payments)	More costly (cost not reflected in existing APC payments)
	Demonstrate substantial clinical improvement	Demonstrate substantial clinical improvement or be designated as an FDA Breakthrough Therapy
	Intervention must be new	Intervention must not be new and not described by existing HCPCS codes

APC = ambulatory payment classification, ASC = ambulatory surgery center, HCPCS = healthcare common procedure coding system, MS-DRG = Medicare severity diagnosis related group

With permission from CMS New Medical Services and New Technologies: Acute Inpatient PPS 42 CFR 412.87 and § 412.87(b). FY 2008 Final Rule.

TABLE 5 Comparison of Medicare Payment Programs by Venue of Care

	Facility			
	Hospital Outpatient	Hospital Inpatient	Ambulatory Surgery Center	Professional/Physician
Medicare payment program	Hospital outpatient prospective payment system	Hospital inpatient prospective payment system	Ambulatory surgery center fee schedule	Medicare physician fee schedule
Medicare payment methodology	Ambulatory payment classifications tied to reported CPT and HCPCS codes	Medicare severity diagnosis related groups tied to reported ICD-10-CM diagnoses and ICD-10-PCS procedures	Fee schedule amounts derived from Medicare Outpatient Prospective Payment System payments (with modifications) and tied to reported CPT and HCPCS codes	Fee schedule based on relative value units and a payment factor and tied to reported CPT and HCPCS codes

CPT = Current Procedural Terminology, HCPCS = Healthcare Common Procedure Coding System, ICD-10-CM = International Classification of Diseases, 10th Revision, Clinical Modification, PCS = Procedure Coding System

RVU value and are therefore paid under the Medicare Physician Fee Schedule. Note that Medicare allows for geographic variation in payment rates that correspond to higher and lower cost areas of the country. The national average payment rate is modified using the wage index of each country to arrive at a final payment rate to the physician/performing surgeon.

Commercial Insurance Payment for Physician Services

Commercial insurances follow a payment structure that is similar to Medicare for physician services, typically based on a fee schedule, albeit with differing payment amounts. Similar to facility reimbursements, commercial plans contract individually with physicians or physician groups to set payment rates. Therefore, physician payment amounts for the same procedure will differ from one commercial insurer to another. But in general, commercial insurers typically have higher payment levels than Medicare for physician services and follow a fee schedule–based payment structure.

Payment for New Medical Services

As described in the overview of coding systems in the United States, novel interventions and new surgical approaches are not yet included in the existing coding CPT code set. These services may be described by unlisted CPT codes (typically ending in -99) or by temporary CPT Category III codes (typically ending in the letter T). Both unlisted codes and CPT Category III codes are not yet assigned an RVU and are paid by Medicare and commercial insurances on a case-by-case basis.

For Medicare, unlisted CPT codes and CPT Category III codes are carrier priced, which means that these physician services are paid at the discretion of each individual Medicare Administrative Contractor (MAC) on a case-by-case basis. Physician claims for these services are typically submitted with medical record documentation and/or cross-references to existing, analogous CPT codes to facilitate payment. Commercial insurers follow a similar payment methodology and will pay claims for unlisted CPT and CPT Category III codes on a case-by-case basis.

COVERAGE OF MEDICAL SERVICES

Coverage is a separate and distinct facet of reimbursement and is based on published clinical evidence and accepted standards of practice. Coverage is simply defined as whether and under what circumstances insurers are willing to pay for a specific intervention. All insurers,

TABLE 6 Physician Payment Rate Calculation

CPT Code	CPT Description	Relative Value Unit (RVU)	Medicare Conversion Factor (CF)	National Average Payment Rate (RVU × CF)
29834	Arthroscopy, elbow, surgical; with removal of loose body or foreign body	14.61	$32.4085	$473.49

CF = conversion factor, CPT = current procedural terminology, RVU = relative value unit
With permission from CMS CY: Medicare Physician Fee Schedule Addendum B. 2021.

including Medicare, Medicaid, and commercial plans, establish coverage policies for surgical interventions.

Medicare establishes coverage for procedures either at a national level or a local level. National coverage policies, called national coverage determinations, apply to all Medicare jurisdictions, whereas local coverage determinations are established by MACs in each region. The MACs and regions are shown in **Figure 3**.

All Medicare coverage policies are accessible on the CMS website and may also include coverage articles that assist facility and physician providers in billing for certain services. Medicare has no prior authorization process or prior approval process to establish coverage before a procedure is performed. As a result, it is important for surgeons and hospital administrators to understand the Medicare coverage landscape before performing a procedure.

For new interventions, such as those described by unlisted CPT codes or CPT Category III codes, Medicare and other payers frequently deny payment for unlisted services, deeming them investigational or experimental. These denials are appealable to the local MAC. There are multiple appeal levels, whereby providers have the opportunity to establish coverage for new procedures on a case-by-case basis using supportive medical records and appeal letters. The Medicare appeal process is outlined in **Figure 4**.

Commercial insurance coverage is established by each insurer's medical policies, which typically specify the covered surgical interventions for a specific condition and any patient qualifying criteria. In the case of orthobiologics, medical policies for certain types of therapies, such as sacroiliac joint fusion or podiatric wound care, are highly detailed and list the named product and manufacturer of each covered products in an indication. Some insurers may cover classes of therapy or classes of products but are silent on the specific brands or manufacturers of products that may be used. As a result of the disparity in coverage policies across commercial insurers, it is necessary to review each patient's insurance coverage before initiating treatment.

Unlike Medicare, most commercial insurers require prior authorization for elective (ie, nonemergent) surgical interventions, such as orthopaedic surgery involving the use of orthobiologics. The prior authorization process provides documentation that the patient meets the criteria in the coverage policy and that a procedure will be covered. The prior authorization process also allows for a prospective appeal for coverage in the absence of such a policy, such as in the case mentioned earlier where a new product is specifically not covered or there is no medical policy at all for a new therapy. Therefore, it is necessary to check each insurer's medical policies to identify whether a new therapy is likely to be covered, whether

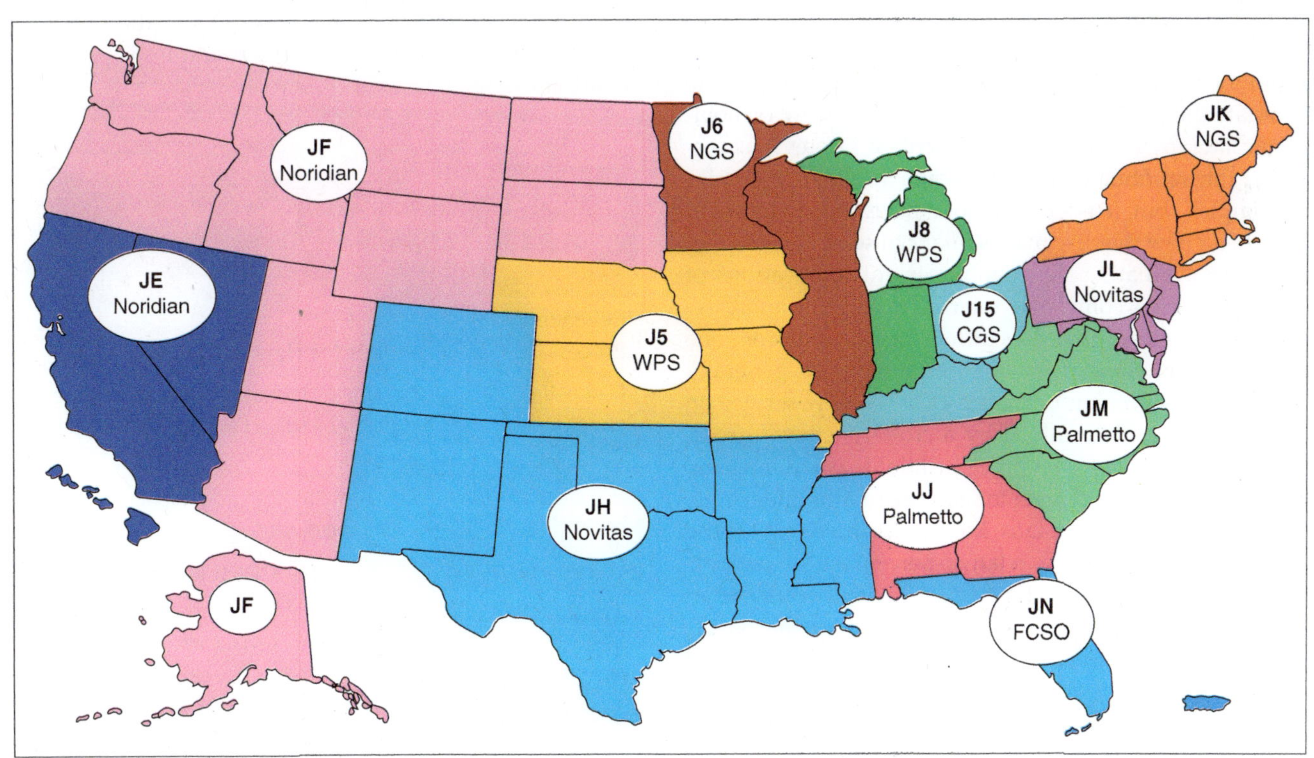

FIGURE 3 Map shows the Medicare Administrative Contractors. (With permission from CMS: Part A/B MAC Map December 2020. https://www.cms.gov/files/document/ab-jurisdiction-map-dec-2020.pdf.)

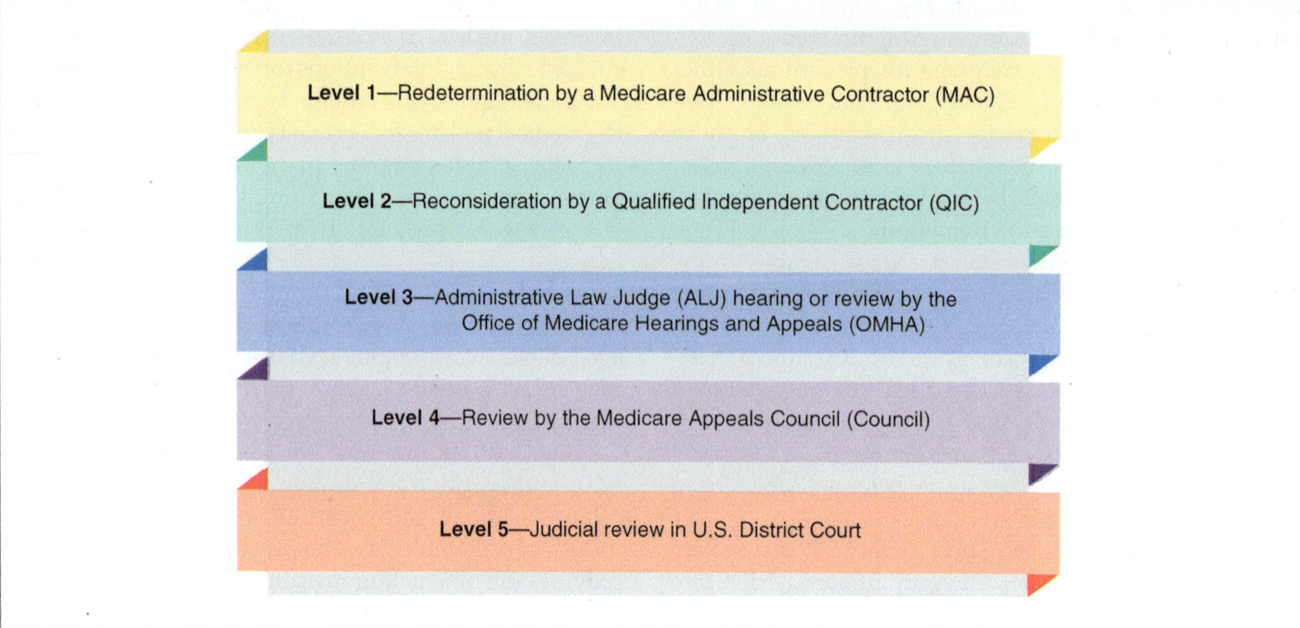

FIGURE 4 A simplified representation shows the Medicare Parts A and B appeals process. (With permission from CMS MedLearn (MLN006562): Parts A & B Appeal Process. 2021.)

an authorization is required, and to appeal for coverage for truly novel therapies. If products that are specifically noncovered are used on the patient and are not appropriately authorized through appeals, a claim may be denied for payment and could be uncollectible.

PRACTICE MANAGEMENT CONSIDERATIONS

From a practice management perspective, it is critical to evaluate the potential budgetary effect of a new orthobiologic therapy or product. As described in previous sections, the reimbursement landscape for new therapies is complex, but it is critical nonetheless to understand whether a new therapy makes financial sense. The framework for evaluating the reimbursement implications of new therapies is commonly referred to as value analysis.

Value analysis processes differ considerably from one hospital or physician practice to the next but generally include an estimation of the effect of the new service on the budget—as determined by a cross-functional group of decision makers. This process should, at a minimum, estimate the payment level for each insurer of interest (ie, Medicare, commercial plans, Medicaid) and weight those payments based on the relative percentage of patients covered by each plan. In this way, a hospital or physician practice can have a better understanding of the payer-weighted payment across all patients eligible for a new therapy and make an informed decision whether that weighted payment covers the cost of the therapy.

In addition to the value analysis process and estimating the effect on the budget, new therapies often require additional administrative support to facilitate reimbursement, such as appeals for prior authorization or payment denials. The process by which hospitals and physicians bill for and collect payment from insurers is commonly referred to as the revenue cycle. Each step in the revenue cycle can be problematic for new therapies. A list of revenue cycle process and the potential friction points for new, innovative therapies is provided in **Table 7**.

TABLE 7 Revenue Cycle Pitfalls for New Therapies

Revenue Cycle Process	Pitfalls for New Therapies
Prior authorization/ preservice clearance	New therapies may not readily be covered and may be subject to prior authorization appeals.
Documentation and coding	Administrative staff may not report accurate billing codes, causing claim denials.
Billable services and pricing	Prices billed to insurers may not reflect the actual cost of care.
Claim denial management	New therapies, particularly those described by unlisted codes, may result in claim denials and require claim appeals.
Patient collections	Collecting coinsurance amounts and deductibles may present challenges for new therapies.

Evaluating whether a new therapy is cost effective for the hospital or physician practice is time consuming and requires an understanding of the reimbursement landscape and the potential administrative hurdles. Nonfinancial considerations, such as referral strategy, quality metrics, and market dynamics, can come into play as well. A robust value analysis process should analyze new therapies holistically to ensure that all of the benefits and costs are identified, quantified, and acceptable to the organization as a whole.

REIMBURSEMENT COMPLIANCE AND PENALTIES

Coding guidelines and billing rules for new orthobiologic therapies are complex and the cost of making mistakes can be high. In fact, most hospitals and large physician practices have designated coding and billing compliance officers to mitigate financial risk. Even accidental coding mistakes can result in recovery audits by CMS or refunds to commercial insurers. Complete and accurate medical record documentation and coding can go a long way in reducing billing errors and financial risk from overpayments.

Each insurer has its own waste fraud and abuse prevention procedures. Medicare uses a retrospective audit model executed by third parties called Recovery Audit Contractors.[4] Each Recovery Audit Contractor creates an annual work plan, targeting certain categories of services, and conducts sampling audits to determine the amount of money that must be refunded to CMS. Commercial insurers may perform retrospective audits as does Medicare and do so without notifying providers of the scope of their audits. It is therefore crucial to ensure coding and billing compliance when submitting claims and to validate any audit findings to help mitigate the financial risk.

SUMMARY

Reimbursement is a key ingredient for the success of any new, innovative orthobiologics therapy. Securing the enablers for optimal reimbursement can be time consuming, complicated, and costly to execute. Coding needs to be in place to describe the procedure and/or therapeutic product, payment amounts must be established with major insurers, and payers must have medical policies in place that cover the therapy. Seldom are all of these elements in place immediately at FDA market authorization; therefore, it is incumbent on manufacturers and providers to develop interim solutions while working toward optimal coding, coverage, and payment. As practitioners, new orthobiologic interventions can pose reimbursement challenges, but they also bring the promise of better outcomes in difficult-to-treat populations. With the right reimbursement strategy and good processes in place, there is plenty of room for clinical and financial success.

REFERENCES

1. American Medical Association: Coding Change Application. Revised February, 2019. https://www.ama-assn.org/practice-management/cpt/cpt-code-change-applications.
2. CMS HCPCS Application Form and Instructions: HCPCS Decision Tree For External Requests to Add or Revise Codes. Revised November, 2018. https://www.cms.gov/Medicare/Coding/MedHCPCSGenInfo/downloads/HCPCS_Decision_Tree_and_Definitions.pdf.
3. American Academy of Orthopeadic Surgeons Biologics Dashboard: https://www.aaos.org/quality/biologics/biologics-dashboard/biologics-dashboard-frequently-asked-questions/. Accessed September 2022.
4. CMS Recovery Audit Contractor Expansion Program: Section 1893(h) of the 42 U.S.C. 1395 of the Social Security Act. 2015.
5. Keisler-Starkey K, Bunch LN: *Health Insurance Coverage in the United States: 2020*. https://www.census.gov/library/publications/2021/demo/p60-274.html. 2021.
6. AMA CPT® Assistant: CPT® 29827, 27381, 27645. https://www.ama-assn.org/practice-management/cpt/cpt-coding-support-latest-guidance-and-best-practices. Accessed January, 2021.
7. AMA CPT® Assistant: Unlisted procedure categories. https://www.ama-assn.org/practice-management/cpt/cpt-coding-support-latest-guidance-and-best-practices. Accessed January, 2021.
8. Category I/III CPT Code Change Application Literature Requirements American Medical Association. https://www.ama-assn.org/system/files/2020-06/category-I-III-literature-requirements.pdf. Accessed January, 2021.
9. CMS HCPCS Release. https://www.cms.gov/Medicare/Coding/HCPCSReleaseCodeSets. Accessed January 1, 2021.
10. CMS New Medical Services and New Technologies: Acute Inpatient PPS 42 CFR 412.87 and § 412.87(b). FY 2008 Final Rule. https://www.cms.gov/Medicare/Medicare-Fee-for-Service-Payment/AcuteInpatientPPS/newtech. Accessed January 1, 2022.
11. CMS CY: Medicare Physician Fee Schedule Addendum B. 2021. https://www.cms.gov/medicare/medicare-fee-for-service-payment/physicianfeesched.
12. CMS: Part A/B MAC Map December 2020. https://www.cms.gov/files/document/ab-jurisdiction-map-dec-2020.pdf. Accessed January 1, 2022.
13. CMS Medicare Payment Systems: MedLearn 6922507 (MLN6922507). 2021. https://www.cms.gov/outreach-and-educationmedicare-learning-network-mlnmlnproductsmln-publications/mln6922507.

CHAPTER

16 Summary and Perspectives

Anthony Ratcliffe, PhD • Scott P. Bruder, MD, PhD, FORS

INTRODUCTION

The pathway of converting a therapeutic orthobiologic concept to a commercially available product is complex and requires input from a range of disciplines and expertise including research and development, management of the regulatory pathway, clinical study design and execution, adherence to a quality system, and eventually, reimbursement. There are now multiple products being used in clinical settings across a variety of musculoskeletal pathologies, with many addressing previously unmet clinical needs. Bringing these complex products to market can be laborious and very expensive, costing as much as several hundred million dollars before the first commercial unit is ever sold. Although the use of allograft tissues (primarily bone, tendons, ligaments, articular cartilage, and dermis) has served as a foundation to service many needs with only modest research and development expenses and regulatory oversight, cell therapy, recombinant growth factor technology, gene therapy, and combination products typically require a decade of development efforts before the first products are FDA approved and available for broad use. Understanding the key activities and hurdles to overcome as inventors and sponsor companies bring a concept through development and onto the commercial market will help clinicians and scientists make informed choices about where to invest their time and resources if they choose to participate in the introduction of new technologies.

SUMMARY AND PERSPECTIVES

The chapters in section 2 highlight the discipline, tenacity, and perseverance required by the product development process from scientific discovery through the FDA and into the clinic. In the field of orthopaedics, the pathways for demonstrating preclinical (as well as clinical) safety and efficacy are very well established and governed by a variety of clearly documented guidelines promulgated by the FDA and the US Code of Federal Regulations. Navigating these development hurdles is resource intensive, and at the very least requires several million dollars for a simple device cleared through the 510(k) pathway (eg, devices for soft-tissue reinforcement or bone void filling), but may require hundreds of millions of dollars for a novel biologic or combination product requiring a biologics license application or a premarket approval (eg, Carticel or Infuse BMP-2).

Even after successfully meeting the FDA's requirements for market launch, the reimbursement landscape and requirements for getting paid must be considered. Therefore, careful development planning, and the creation of a commercialization strategy early in the process, is essential to determine whether the investment will meet the revenue and profitability objectives of those underwriting the project. With that in mind, ensuring that developers have a robust understanding of the product development process, or that they engage with partners who themselves have a keen understanding of the journey from "bench to bedside" will increase the likelihood of both clinical and commercial success. When meaningful technologic advancements are properly shepherded through the FDA (and other regulatory bodies), it is possible to make both important clinical contributions to the field of orthopaedics and create significant value for those who invest the time and money to succeed.

If an orthobiologic concept is thought to be useful as a product, the first priority is to map out a regulatory plan and product development process together with a cost assessment and revenue projections. This will provide an estimate of a return on investment that ideally becomes positive over time. The cost of bringing a product to market is highly dependent on the regulatory pathway necessary, and this early activity will help define the technologies that can and cannot be used for any given pathology or injury. For example, a product concept for a particular application

Dr. Ratcliffe or an immediate family member serves as a paid consultant to or is an employee of Synthasome, Inc and has stock or stock options held in Synthasome Inc. Dr. Bruder or an immediate family member serves as a paid consultant to or is an employee of Aesculap/B. Braun, AgNovos Inc., Alexis Bio, Alma Lasers, AnGes Inc., Anika Therapeutics, Artelon, Arthrex, Inc., Axogen, Axolotl Biosciences, Bruder Consulting & Venture Group, LLC, Celularity, Collagen Matrix Inc, ControlRad, Conventus Flower Orthopedics, Cook Biotech, Embody, GreenBone SpA, Histogen, HTL Biotech, Integra Lifesciences, Integrum, Kolon Tissue Gene, Kuros BioSciences AG, Lipogems, Modern Meadow, Molecular Matrix, MTF Biologics, Nexillus AG, Organogenesis, Personal Stem Cells, Regeneus Ltd, RTI Surgical, and Terumo BCT; has stock or stock options held in Embody, Kuros BioSciences AG, Lipogems, Spinal Elements, and Stryker; and serves as a board member, owner, officer, or committee member of AAOS.

that requires a cell-based technology will require a substantial revenue stream to justify the high cost of product development, and if the projected revenue does not support a positive return on investment, then an alternative solution should be explored. The use of financial analysis for each product concept is an important component in determining the technologies appropriate for each envisioned clinical application. As a general rule, the simplest technical solution that meets the least rigorous but meaningful clinical outcome parameters serves as the target product profile rather than overcomplicating matters by attempting to develop a technically sophisticated solution. For example, if a simple scaffold material can support tissue repair adequately, but a genetically modified cell with a novel promoter construct that triggers a downstream signal cascade in the body can achieve a little better outcome, most seasoned product development experts would opt to pursue the simple scaffold.

The regulatory approval, clinical use and acceptance, and commercial success of orthobiologic products require rigorous testing and high confidence of the clinical data. The randomized clinical trial is accepted as the most appropriate method to assess causality and efficacy, and there are methods that can minimize the bias of experimental design, execution, and analysis. In the field of regenerative medicine where the technologies are addressing unmet clinical needs, the identification of ideal control groups for clinical trials can be difficult or impossible and can result in failure of the clinical trial if not selected properly. In addition, determination of the standard by which success can or should be measured has proven to be somewhat of a moving target as new technologies emerge, regulations change, and patients' demand for the latest and greatest technology must be managed.

The use of the gold standard outcome measures will naturally remain key to the assessment of clinical effects. For example, the use of MRI for cartilage repair and regeneration is an objective measurable outcome, although continuous improvement of surrogate molecular and biochemical markers that can demonstrate the clinical effect is likely to be more cost effective and less influenced by the bias introduced from patients who otherwise provide subjective reports of pain and function. Although standardized patient-reported outcome measures have become a useful tool in measuring patient health and satisfaction after orthopaedic interventions, they are also limited because of a lack of standardization in their use. Striking the optimal balance between the structural improvements observed through objective criteria such as tissue changes seen on radiographic imaging, with the patient experience of pain and function, will continue to be a matter of debate. That said, even in the best case where MRI shows perfect restoration of an articular cartilage defect, if the patient has no meaningful improvement in pain or function, the technology will not be approved by the FDA. The most salient example of this lies in the consideration of products aimed at claiming disease modification (DMOD) in the setting of knee osteoarthritis. Both the FDA and third-party payers have clearly articulated that claims of DMOD must correlate structural changes visible on MRI with improvement in pain and function measured using a validated instrument for patient-reported outcome measures, such as the Western Ontario and McMaster Universities Osteoarthritis Index tool, for at least 2 years' duration. Currently, there are no examples of products that fulfill the criteria for DMOD in the management of knee osteoarthritis, although some cell-based therapies are hoping their results can support a claim of DMOD during this decade.

A distillation of the myriad FDA rules regarding product development and requirements for market authorization is beyond the scope of this text; however, for those interested in developing products, most currently envisioned technologies may be neatly assigned to one of the existing pathways for devices: biologics, drugs, or combination products. For human cell and tissue products (HCT/Ps), the regulation of these materials has been challenging for the FDA and comprehensive guidance documents that expand on the fundamental criteria of minimal manipulation and homologous use have been developed. An HCT/P will be regulated as a tissue (ie, not considered a drug/biologic/device) if it meets certain criteria listed in 21 Code of Federal Regulations 1271 for minimal manipulation and homologous use. These tissue products are regulated solely under Section 361 of the Public Health Services Act, and therefore do not require premarket authorization from the FDA, which means that they are not required to demonstrate evidence of safety and efficacy before being sold in the marketplace. Examples of such HCT/Ps often used in orthopaedics include almost all allograft tissues and certain preparations from bone marrow, adipose tissue, blood, amnion, and dermis. To be considered a 361 HCT/P, the product must meet all of the criteria as outlined in the FDA Guidance, and HCT/Ps that do not are regulated as drugs, biologics, or devices, based primarily on the mechanism of action on the body to achieve its intended purpose.

By contrast, HCT/Ps subject to Section 351 of the Public Health Services Act and the applicable 21 Code of Federal Regulations must have premarket clearance or approval by the FDA, which typically requires long and arduous development, qualification, and human clinical trials. Examples of such 351 HCT/Ps include culture-expanded chondrocytes for cartilage repair; ground and lyophilized amniotic membrane for modulating inflammation such as in the case of osteoarthritis; any purified stem cell preparation from fat, marrow, blood, or other tissue; and any combination of a tissue with another material. Interpreting and applying these criteria can be challenging; therefore, it is important to communicate with the FDA early in the development process to verify a shared understanding of the regulatory requirements.

In recent years, however, there has been an increase in companies offering a variety of products they claim to be "361 exempt" but have no legitimate basis for that qualification. Further, many of the firms have made no effort to engage the FDA in a proper development path toward regulatory approval. The most egregious offenders are akin to the "snake oil salesman" of the 1800s but are currently promoting HCT/Ps claimed to function as effective mesenchymal stem cells, exosomes, stromal vascular fraction, micronized amnion, and more. To be clear, these products are not eligible for Section 361 exemption, and the FDA has not approved any stem cell, exosome, stromal vascular fraction, or micronized amnion product for any indication. Those HCT/Ps are considered adulterated and illegal products when sold in the United States.

Finally, in how clinicians govern themselves regarding the use of novel products, it is fundamental to recall that the AAOS Code of Professional Ethics, as well as laws from the Federal Trade Commission, require that when one's clinical practice is marketed and promoted through any medium, it must not be done in a misleading, untruthful, or deceptive manner. Ignorance of the law or use of unsubstantiated evidence is not a legitimate defense. It is the responsibility of the clinician to demand rigorous clinical and scientific evidence from sales representatives, as well as unambiguous, nonconfidential correspondence from the FDA indicating the regulatory status of the product in question. If those materials are not convincing, or made available at all, the product probably is not in compliance with FDA or Federal Trade Commission regulations. Using and/or promoting such products in a noncompliant manner can be associated with significant risks to one's practice, reputation, livelihood, and, most importantly, patients.

CONCLUSIONS

The pathway from product concept to successful commercialization is a complex multistep journey that requires the interaction of a wide variety of stakeholders across multiple disciplines. Failure to adequately address any one of the topics described in this text will severely hamper the successful introduction of new therapeutics. Although simple and long-standing allograft products will continue to be a mainstay solution for many physicians, the collective effect of biology's intersection with engineering is accelerating, resulting in new approaches that have the potential to deliver profound benefit to human health. As the cost for such technologies is reduced through improved scale-up and more efficient clinical study designs, a larger cross-section of patients will be eligible to benefit from these advances in healthcare.

PART 2

Clinical Applications

SECTION

3

Solutions for Upper Extremity Pathology

Section Editors
Kathleen A. Derwin, PhD
Adam Yanke, MD, PhD, FAAOS

CHAPTER

17 Rotator Cuff Repair

Scott A. Rodeo, MD, FAAOS • Janice Havasy, BS, MD •
Claire D. Eliasberg, MD • Camila B. Carballo, PhD, PT

INTRODUCTION

Rotator cuff disease comprises a spectrum of disorders ranging from impingement syndrome to tendinopathy to full-thickness rotator cuff tears. The pathophysiology of rotator cuff disease is complex and likely involves a mix of extrinsic factors, such as the presence of a subacromial bone spur or a hypertrophic coracoacromial ligament, as well as intrinsic factors including vascular compromise, age-related degeneration, and repetitive microtrauma. Although nonsurgical treatment may be the first-line approach for the management of rotator cuff disease, patients in whom nonsurgical treatment has failed may require surgical intervention for rotator cuff repair (RCR). Despite advances in surgical techniques, implants, and fixation constructs, incomplete or failed healing following RCR remains a clinically challenging problem. As a result, orthobiologics have become a topic of increasing scientific and clinical interest with regard to RCR.

PLATELET-RICH PLASMA

Platelet-rich plasma (PRP) has been studied as a possible treatment modality in many different orthopaedic pathologies, including both bone and soft tissues. PRP is a collection of autologous blood that has a high concentration of platelets. Although various classification systems have been proposed to describe PRP prepared by different processing techniques, most commonly, PRP can be described as leukocyte rich or leukocyte poor.[1] The rationale for use of PRP is due to the high concentrations of growth factors such as platelet-derived growth factor (PDGF), transforming growth factor beta 1 (TGF-β1), insulinlike growth factor 1, epidermal growth factor, basic fibroblast growth factor (bFGF), and vascular endothelial growth factor.[2] PRP has also been noted to activate fibroblasts and collagen remodeling, two processes that are relevant to tendon healing and RCR.[3] The clinical use of PRP in rotator cuff tendinopathy has been studied in both the nonsurgical and surgical management of rotator cuff tears of all sizes; however, these data are inconclusive on the efficacy of PRP in decreasing the failure rate and biomechanical strength of the repaired tendon.

Current data suggest that PRP lacks efficacy as a nonsurgical management of rotator cuff disease. Kesikburun et al[4] studied PRP in patients with chronic tendinopathy and found no difference between PRP and control patients in improvement of quality of life, pain, disability, or shoulder range of motion at 1-year follow-up. Similarly, Schwitzguebel et al[5] demonstrated no difference in tendon healing or clinical scores, when compared with placebo groups. Additionally, this study observed a significantly higher rate of adverse events (pain lasting longer than 48 hours, frozen shoulder, extension of lesion to bursal or articular surface) in the PRP group (54%) compared with control patients (26%).[5] A systematic review by Hurley et al[6] includes five randomized controlled trials, totaling 108 patients treated with PRP and 106 control patients and found no significant effect of PRP in the nonsurgical management of rotator cuff disease. However, because of the variability in different PRP formulations and the lack of a large clinical trial to improve external validity in these studies, further rigorous study is required to reach a definitive conclusion on the effectiveness of PRP.

Arthroscopic repair of torn rotator cuffs is a common surgical procedure performed to decrease pain and improve shoulder function. However, contemporary studies demonstrate that incomplete or failed healing occurs in approximately 15% to 20% of patients and can be affected by surgical repair technique and tear characteristics including tear size, degree of retraction, chronicity, and muscle atrophy.[7,8] Although the data are mixed, there are some early data to support the role of PRP in augmentation of rotator cuff tendon healing for small to medium tear sizes. Zhao et al[9] demonstrated through a meta-analysis involving 742 patients that leukocyte-poor PRP preparations can decrease the retear rates in any sized tear at medium-term and long-term time points. For medium to large rotator cuff tears, augmentation of arthroscopic RCR with leukocyte-poor PRP did correlate to a decrease in retear rate (3.0% in PRP group versus 20.0% of control group, $P = 0.032$) and a significant

Dr. Rodeo or an immediate family member serves as a paid consultant to or is an employee of Teladoc and has stock or stock options held in Ortho RTI. Neither of the following authors nor any immediate family member has received anything of value from or has stock or stock options held in a commercial company or institution related directly or indirectly to the subject of this chapter: Dr. Havasy, Dr. Eliasberg, and Dr. Carballo.

increase in the cross-sectional area of the supraspinatus muscle in the PRP group when compared with control group.[10] In contrast, Castricini et al were not able to show any benefits, with similar results reported by Malavolta et al in 2018.[11,12] Additionally, repeated PRP injections after RCR do not seem to have any effect on early tendon-bone healing.[13]

Three meta-analyses have conflicting recommendations regarding the use of PRP in RCR, but all cite heterogeneity of the studies as a potential problem and suggest that larger, multicenter studies are required to be able to draw conclusions about the efficacy of this treatment.[14-16] A principal limitation of PRP studies is the tremendous heterogeneity in different proprietary processes for PRP preparation. Currently used processing techniques produce PRP with widely differing concentration of platelets, ranging from 3 to 15 times higher than normal whole blood, but also differing levels of leukocytes, which potentially may change the inflammatory milieu in the treated tissue after injection.[17] Unfortunately, many studies on PRP use for arthroscopic RCR lack statistical power and have important sources of bias and heterogeneity, so results should be interpreted with caution and should not yet determine clinical practice. It is clear that further studies in the area need to rigorously characterize the biologic activity and composition of PRP to allow identification of the optimal PRP formulation(s) for augmentation of rotator cuff tendon healing.

PATCHES, GRAFTS, AND SCAFFOLDS

Patches and grafts are often used in an effort to augment RCR by supplying additional extracellular matrix as a structural scaffold for healing. Synthetic, allogeneic, and xenogeneic materials have been used. A summary of clinical evidence for the use of grafts for rotator cuff repair[18-29] is presented in **Table 1**. Bryant et al[18] used porcine small intestine submucosa as a graft extending over the repaired tendon and reported no statistically significant differences between the graft and no-graft arms of the study in regard to failure rate, Western Ontario Rotator Cuff Index, or postoperative narcotic use. Lederman et al[19] demonstrated an improvement in patient-reported outcomes in patients treated with RCR augmented with porcine dermal matrix; however, there was no control group used in this study. The authors reported a retear rate of 43.9%, which they described as being lower than historical controls.[19] Nicholson et al[21] found that failure loads were similar between porcine small intestine submucosa, porcine dermal patch, and normal repair of an infraspinatus tear in an ovine model. Xenografts, such as porcine tissues, have fallen out of favor because of high complication rates secondary to severe inflammatory responses, which may be due to the presence of foreign DNA.[30,31]

There has been some success with the use of dermal allografts for RCR augmentation. These materials are also a popular choice for superior capsular reconstruction in the setting of a massive, irreparable rotator cuff tear. Some studies have found functional improvements when dermal allografts are used.[32] One example of a commercially available acellular dermal matrix is GRAFTJACKET (Wright Medical Group N.V.).[32] Wong et al[22] augmented the repair of massive rotator cuff tears in 45 patients with GRAFTJACKET and found that after 2 years of follow-up, these patients improved with few adverse events. Barber et al[23] demonstrated improved American Shoulder and Elbow Surgeons scores and Constant scores, along with a decreased retear rate in patients treated with GRAFTJACKET-augmented RCR compared with RCR alone in a sample of 22 patients. A follow-up study conducted by Johnson et al[24] on 14 shoulders demonstrated that 13 of the 14 repaired tendons were intact by 35 months after surgery.

As noted previously, there has been concern over immunogenicity because of residual DNA content from xenografts, and the same concern exists for allografts as well. Many of the commercially available xenografts contain nonnegligible amounts of DNA, even if it is claimed to be acellularized.[33] In addition, it has been established that these grafts and scaffolds have significantly inferior biomechanical properties compared with the native rotator cuff tendon.[33] It also has been shown that there are differences in the graft structure that may affect the ability of progenitor cells to adhere to and proliferate within the graft.[34] More high-quality data are required to draw conclusions regarding whether augmentation of RCR with biologic grafts and patches can lead to superior shoulder function and decreased retear rates compared with RCR alone, without an increased immunologically mediated inflammatory response.

Synthetic grafts are made from polypropylene, polycarbonate polyurethane, and poly-L-lactic acid and are usually biomechanically superior to biologic grafts and carry a lower risk of generating an immunogenic reaction.[35] Polycarbonate polyurethane does not demonstrate any inflammatory reaction while supporting tissue ingrowth; however, tissue integration does not replicate native collagen fibril longitudinal orientation.[36] A retrospective study conducted by Ciampi et al[25] with 36-month follow-up reported on 152 patients in three groups (open RCR only, open RCR with collagen patch, and open repair with polypropylene patch) to determine the efficacy of biologic versus synthetic grafts. These authors found a significantly higher University of California, Los Angeles (UCLA) shoulder rating scale and lower retear rates in patients treated with synthetic grafts when compared with both control patients and biologic grafts.[25] Additionally, the authors reported significantly improved range of motion (elevation in the scapular plane) and abduction strength in the polypropylene patch group.[25] A 2014 study of 18 patients treated with RCR with augmentation with

TABLE 1 Summary of Clinical Evidence for the Use of Grafts in Rotator Cuff Repair

Reference	Year	Graft Type	Results
Xenografts			
Examples: porcine SIS, porcine dermal matrix			
Reference	**Year**	**Graft Type**	**Results**
Schlegel et al[20]	2021	Bovine Achilles tendon–derived collagen implant	New tissue fill-in on MRI in 100% of intermediate-grade tears and 95% of high-grade tears; no control group
Bryant et al[18]	2016	Porcine SIS	No differences in failure rate, WORC index scores, or postoperative narcotic use compared with nongraft control groups
Lederman et al[19]	2016	Porcine dermal matrix	Retear rates of 43.9%; no control group
Nicholson et al[21]	2007	Porcine dermal matrix; porcine SIS	No differences in failure loads at 24 weeks after ovine infraspinatus repair between suture repair, SIS, and dermal matrix groups
Conclusions: Porcine-derived xenografts have fallen out of favor because of little evidence of efficacy, high complication rates, and the potential for robust inflammatory/immunogenic responses due to the presence of porcine DNA. In contrast, relatively favorable results have been reported using a resorbable bovine Achilles tendon–derived collagen implant.			
Allografts			
Examples: Human dermal allografts			
Reference	**Year**	**Graft type**	**Results**
Wong et al[22]	2010	Acellular dermal matrix	Improved postoperative outcomes scores; no control group
Barber et al[23]	2012	Acellular dermal matrix	Improved ASES and Constant scores and decreased retear rate in patients with dermal allografts compared with nongraft controls
Johnson et al[24]	2020	Acellular dermal matrix	93% of tendons repaired with dermal allograft were intact 35 months postoperatively
Conclusions: Use of dermal allografts may result in some functional improvements and lower retear rates compared with rotator cuff repairs without dermal allograft. However, dermal allografts may have inferior biomechanical properties compared with the native rotator cuff tendon. Additionally, differences in graft structure may affect the ability of progenitor cells to adhere to/proliferate within the graft.			
Synthetic grafts			
Examples: Polypropylene, polycarbonate polyurethane, poly-L-lactic acid			
Reference	**Year**	**Graft type**	**Results**
Ciampi et al[25]	2014	Polypropylene patch	Lower retear rates (17% versus 41% in control) and improved functional outcomes in synthetic patch group
Proctor[26]	2014	Poly-L-lactic acid patch	78% of repairs intact at 42 months postoperatively; no control group
Encalada-Diaz et al[27]	2011	Polycarbonate polyurethane patch	10% retear rate at 12 months postoperatively; no control group
Audenaert et al[28]	2006	Polyester mesh	3 of 41 patients had new tear at latest follow-up; no control group
Nada et al[29]	2010	Polyester graft	90.5% of patients had intact repair at 36 months postoperatively; no control group
Conclusions: Synthetic grafts may be biomechanically stronger than biologic patches and carry a lower risk of generating an inflammatory or immunogenic reaction. Although there are some early promising results, most of the literature is composed of small case series without control groups.			

ASES = American Shoulder and Elbow Surgeons, SIS = small intestine submucosa, WORC = Western Ontario Rotator Cuff Index

a poly-L-lactic acid bioabsorbable patch reported intact repairs in 83% of patients at 12 months and 78% of patients at 42 months after surgery.[26] Ten patients treated with open RCR augmented with polycarbonate polyurethane patch had a 90% intact rate at 12 months with no adverse events recorded.[27] Audenaert et al[28] studied the use of polyester mesh to bridge gaps between rotator cuff insertion point and tendon in 41 patients and found that the

Constant and Murley scores improved and patients experienced pain relief, with 2 patients experiencing moderate to severe pain and 4 patients with structural failure. Nada et al[29] described a case series using polyester grafts for arthroscopic repair of massive rotator cuff tears in 21 individuals and found that 90.5% of individuals had intact repairs at 36 months, with a mean patient satisfaction score of 90%.[29] The authors also reported significant improvements in abduction strength and range of motion (flexion, abduction, external rotation, and internal rotation) when comparing patients' preoperative and postoperative scores; however, there was no control group in this study for comparison.[29] In summary, although there are a few small studies that suggest that synthetic grafts may have potential for improved outcomes and function in the setting of RCR, these studies are limited by their retrospective nature and midterm follow-up data. Prospective randomized controlled studies are necessary to improve clinical confidence in the efficacy of synthetic scaffolds for augmentation of massive RCRs.

CELLULAR THERAPIES

Tissue-Specific Activated Endothelial Cells

Tissue-specific endothelial cells are terminally differentiated cells that have the ability to stimulate the proliferation and differentiation of tissue-resident progenitor cells.[37] This interaction has the potential to re-create the microstructure and composition of the native tendon-bone interface, and therefore, theoretically improving the strength of the RCR site. Preliminary evaluation of tendon-derived activated endothelial cells in a mouse model demonstrated increased tendon-bone interface biomechanical strength, with increased cellularity, collagen organization, and neovascularization.[38] Similarly, muscle-derived activated endothelial cells also resulted in improved supraspinatus biomechanical strength and increased collagen organization compared with the control group in a murine RCR model.[39] Although this cell lineage has been studied for its regenerative potential in neural tissue, liver, and lung epithelium, research into its potential benefits in orthopaedic soft tissues is lacking within the literature.[40]

Bone Marrow–Derived Progenitor Cells

The application of bone marrow–derived mesenchymal progenitor cells (BM-MPCs) to a shoulder joint after RCR has been studied as adjunct therapy.[41-43] Exogenous cells may exert a positive effect via secretion of anti-inflammatory and immunomodulatory mediators, cytokines, and other signaling molecules such as TGF-β, allowing this population of cells to suppress the activation of important cellular lineages of the immune system, such as T cells, B cells, and dendritic cells, while also promoting the polarization of macrophages into the proreparative M2 phenotype.[44] In rodent models, allogeneic BM-MPCs did not significantly alter the healing process of RCRs compared with the control group.[45] Degen et al[46] found that in an athymic rat model, the BM-MPC-treated repairs had superior biomechanical strength and histologic scoring at 2 weeks, but this effect was not significant at 4 weeks after RCR. BM-MPCs transduced with a transcription factor important for tendon development, scleraxis, in the rat model improved stress to failure and stiffness compared with nontransduced BM-MPCs.[47] BM-MPCs transduced with membrane-type 1 matrix metalloproteinase significantly increased the biomechanical strength of the repaired tendon at the 4-week time point.[48]

Further preclinical studies are evaluating the potential for a synergistic effect when combining two treatment modalities. In a rat model, demineralized bone matrix combined with BM-MPCs demonstrated promising results that included a return of bone mineral density of the enthesis to preinjury levels.[49] Tornero-Esteban et al[50] tested the efficacy of BM-MCPs with a collagen type I scaffold in the management of rotator cuff tears in rats and found that this combined therapy improved the repaired tendon's maximum load over time. A 2020 study reported on the use of three-dimensional printed poly(lactic-co-glycolic acid) scaffolds loaded with BM-MPCs in a rabbit rotator cuff model and showed that this technique increased the expression of collagen I and III at 4 weeks after implant when compared with scaffolds alone, and collagen I expression continued to be elevated at 8 and 12 weeks.[51] This same technique in the same rabbit model was used with BM-MPCs transfected to overexpress bone morphogenetic protein (BMP)-12, and the authors again found that more collagen fibers, chondrocytes, and fibrocartilage were present in the tendon-bone interface compared with the BM-MPCs-only control group.[52] The use of an engineered tendon-fibrocartilage-bone composite with BM-MPCs in a canine model demonstrated better histologic scores, greater fibrocartilage formation, and more organized collagen fibrils at the tendon-bone interface when compared with control animals.[53]

In humans, autologous BM-MPCs have been shown to improve healing outcomes in patients after undergoing arthroscopic repair of their rotator cuff tendon, especially within the acute setting. Hernigou et al[54] augmented an RCR with concentrated BM-MPCs aspirated from the iliac crest and found that patients in the control group were four times more likely to have a poorer outcome than the treatment group. At 6 months, patients who received BM-MPCs demonstrated accelerated tendon healing, and at 10 years after the repair, the treatment group had a retear rate of 13%, whereas the control group had a retear rate of 56%.[54] Ellera Gomes et al[55] used nonconcentrated bone marrow mononuclear cells in conventional RCR in 14 patients and found an increase in UCLA scores and tendon integrity in all patients at the 12-month follow-up. However, there was no control group in this study. It is clear that further clinical trials are required to demonstrate if the promising results obtained in the animal models translate to human patients.

Adipose-Derived Progenitor Cells

When compared with BM-MPCs, adipose-derived progenitor cells (AD-PCs) can be isolated from a less invasive procedure and have been shown to be multipotent and have good viability and the potential to differentiate into chondrogenic and osteogenic lineages.[56,57] To date, there has been one cohort study by Kim et al[58] that compared 35 patients treated with arthroscopic surgery for RCR alone with a matched group of 35 patients treated with arthroscopic surgery for RCR augmented with AD-PCs in fibrin glue. This clinical study found that an injection of AD-PCs did not significantly improve visual analog scale, Constant score, or UCLA score when compared with RCR alone; however, the retear rate was found to be significantly decreased in the AD-PC group compared with the control group (14.3% versus 28.5%, $P < 0.001$).[58] Much of the evidence regarding AD-PCs has been performed in preclinical animal models, and more human trials are now required to demonstrate the efficacy of this cell lineage in the augmentation of RCRs.

AD-PC augmentation of subscapularis healing in a rabbit model showed lower proportions of fatty infiltration and improvement of biomechanical strength compared with saline controls.[59] Lu et al[60] used adipose-derived stromal vascular fraction in a rabbit model and demonstrated improved tissue maturity in MRI scanning (measured as signal-to-noise ratio) in the adipose-derived stromal vascular fraction group compared with control groups 12 weeks after RCR with greater biomechanical strength of the repaired tendon in the adipose-derived stromal vascular fraction compared with control groups at 8 weeks.

In rodent models, there are mixed data on the use of AD-PCs for augmentation of RCRs. Valencia Mora et al[61] used AD-PCs on a collagen carrier in a rat model and found lower levels of inflammation on histology, but no improvement in biomechanical properties between controls and AD-PCs. The use of adipose-derived stem cell–seeded hydrogel led to improvement of bone morphometry at the tendon-bone interface but did not improve the biomechanical strength or collagen organization of the repaired rotator cuff.[62] Rothrauff et al[63] used AD-PCs and TGF-β3 and found that the application of AD-PCs was correlated with increased bone mineral density of the proximal humerus; however, no histologic or structural properties of the tendon itself were improved. Conversely, the application of AD-PC-derived exosomes to the RCR site increased the expression of RUNX2, SOX9, tenascin C, and scleraxis and also improved the biomechanical strength of the repaired tendon in the rat model.[64] Additionally, a relatively new cell population of interest is the stromal vascular fraction of subcutaneous adipose tissue. Stromal vascular fraction cells consist of fibroblasts, hematopoietic cells, adipose-derived stromal cells, and pericytes. In an immunocompromised rat, human stromal vascular fraction cells injected into the supraspinatus muscle demonstrated an improvement in muscle healing after chronic rotator cuff tear.[65]

The use of cellular therapy for rotator cuff repair remains an area of significant clinical interest. A search of rotator cuff tear and cell therapy performed on the National Institutes of Health ClinicalTrials.gov website in September 2021 demonstrated a total of 14 studies investigating cell therapy for the management of rotator cuff tears (**Table 2**, **Figure 1**). The major limitation in the area of cell therapy, similar to other orthobiologic approaches, is the tremendous heterogeneity in the different cell therapy formulations that are in current clinical use. Currently available techniques using cells derived from bone marrow or adipose tissue sustain from lack of rigorous characterization of cell types and signaling molecules produced by these heterogeneous mixtures. Techniques are needed to measure the purity, potency, and biologic activity of various cell therapy formulations to better characterize these materials and to move this field forward.

CYTOKINES AND GROWTH FACTORS

Cytokines and growth factors are small signaling molecules that play an important role in immune modulation and other cellular functions such as cell growth and matrix synthesis. During the acute rotator cuff tear and the body's attempt to heal it, there are fluctuations in important cytokines and growth factors that regulate the different stages of healing, but also apoptosis and cell death within the injured tendon.[66] Increased levels of interleukin (IL)-18, IL-15, IL-6, macrophage migration inhibitory factor, tumor necrosis factor alpha, and caspases 3 and 8 were elevated in the torn supraspinatus.[67] The use of both cytokines and growth factors to augment RCR presents a challenge because of the short half-lives of cytokines in plasma. Because the biologic milieu in the healing tendon is highly complex with numerous different cytokines, exogenous application of a single factor will likely have limited effect. Growth factors also typically have more than one downstream effect and often only function when combined with other signaling molecules, making it hard to predict the outcome of their application on a repaired tendon. There are many cytokines and growth factors that may affect the healing of the tendon-bone interface. Herein, current data on several cytokines tested in RCR models are summarized.

In an acute tear of a rotator cuff tendon, there is an increase in the expression of IL-1β initially, which causes the expression of cyclooxygenase-2, leading to the production of prostaglandin E2, a mediator of shoulder pain.[68] Inhibition of 5-lipoxygenase, cyclooxygenase-1,

TABLE 2 Summary of Clinical Trials Investigating Cell Therapy for the Management of Rotator Cuff Tears

ClinicalTrials.gov Identifier	Study Title	Cell Therapy Used	Status	Location
NCT03332238	Stromal vascular fraction cell therapy to improve the repair of rotator cuff tears	Stromal vascular fraction of adipose tissue	Recruiting	New York City, NY
NCT04057833	E-CEL UVEC cells as an adjunct cell therapy for the arthroscopic rotator cuff repair in adults	E-CEL UVEC cells	Recruiting	New York City, NY
NCT03688308	Bone marrow derived stem cells for the treatment of rotator cuff tears	Bone marrow–derived cells	Withdrawn	Redwood City, CA
NCT02298023	Treatment of tendon injury using allogenic adipose-derived mesenchymal stem cells (rotator cuff tear)	Adipose-derived cells	Completed	Seoul, Republic of Korea
NCT03279796	Treatment of tendon disease using autologous adipose-derived mesenchymal stem cells	Adipose-derived cells	Not yet recruiting	Hangzhou, Zhejiang, China
NCT03838666	Utilization of AMSC to enhance rotator cuff repair—safety and efficacy	Autologous mesenchymal cells	Terminated	Prague, Czech Republic
NCT04077190	Safety and efficacy of adult adipose-derived stem cell injection into partial thickness rotator cuff tears	Adipose-derived cells	Enrolling by invitation	Fargo, ND Sioux Falls, SD
NCT01687777	Mesenchymal stem cell (MSC) included in OrthADAPT membrane for rotator cuff tears repair	Mesenchymal cells	Unknown	Madrid, Spain
NCT01788683	Regenexx™ SD versus exercise therapy for rotator cuff tears	Bone marrow–derived cells	Active, not recruiting	Broomfield, CO
NCT02783352	Efficacy of microfragmented lipoaspirate tissue in arthroscopic rotator cuff repair	Adipose-derived cells	Completed	Milan, Italy
NCT03752827	Autologous adult adipose-derived regenerative cell injection into chronic partial-thickness rotator cuff tears	Adipose-derived cells	Recruiting	Multicenter study
NCT03068988	Clinical study on mesenchymal stem cells used in the reconstruction surgery of the supraspinatus muscle lesions	Mesenchymal cells	Active, no recruiting	Znojmo, Czech Republic
NCT02484950	Mesenchymal stem cell augmentation in patients undergoing arthroscopic rotator cuff repair	Mesenchymal cells	Recruiting	Chicago, Illinois
NCT03362424	Mesenchymal stem cells in rotator cuff repair	Mesenchymal cells	Recruiting	São Paulo, Brazil

and cyclooxygenase-2 enzymes by the drug licofelone has been shown to reduce fibrosis and lipid content in supraspinatus muscles after RCR.[69] There is an increase in proinflammatory IL-6 within the ruptured rotator cuff, as well as the subacromial synovium.[70] IL-6 seems to have multifunctional roles in both inflammation in the acute rupture injury and recovery from RCR. Ling et al[71] found that individuals with polymorphisms in the IL-6 and matrix metallopeptidase 3 genes had increased incidence and severity of postoperative stiffness. IL-8 is a cytokine correlated with IL-6 and IL-1β and was also found to be associated with resting pain in individuals with rotator cuff tears.[72] Inhibition of tumor necrosis factor alpha was shown to improve the biomechanical strength of the tendon-bone interface during the first 4 weeks after an RCR in rats.[73]

Immediately after repair, there is an increased expression of bFGF, BMP-12, BMP-13, BMP-14, cartilage oligomeric matrix protein, PDGF-B, and TGF-β1 in the supraspinatus tendon-bone interface. All levels return to baseline by 4 weeks after repair in animal models; however, bFGF and BMP-12 remained increased in expression at 8 weeks during the remodeling phase of healing in a rat supraspinatus model.[74] A repaired rat rotator cuff with sustained exposure of TGF-β3 through a heparin/fibrin delivery system demonstrated improvements in

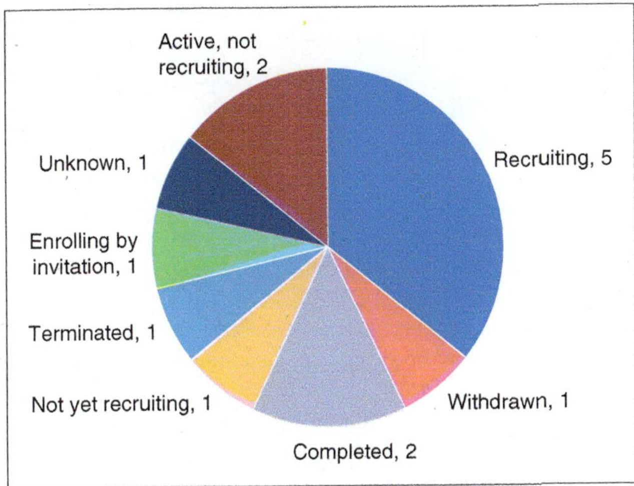

FIGURE 1 Pie chart shows the distribution of the status of clinical trials on the National Institutes of Health website pertaining to cell therapy for the management of rotator cuff tears.

biomechanical parameters, such as modulus and toughness at later time points compared with the control group.[75] Within a sheep model, recombinant human PDGF-BB was delivered using coated sutures, which did not show any difference compared with the control group, and interpositional graft, which demonstrated improved biomechanical strength and anatomic appearance.[76,77] Recombinant human PDGF-BB within a scaffold system used in RCR in rats demonstrated an early increase in cellular proliferation, but this did not change the strength of the healing tendon-bone interface.[78]

FGF2 has been studied in rotator cuff models because of its previously mentioned expression and assumed role during the remodeling phase. Application of FGF2-impregnated gelatin hydrogen sheet around the repair site increased the load to failure and stress to failure at 12 weeks after repair in rabbits.[79] FGF2 in a fibrin sealant placed under the repaired rotator cuff in rats demonstrated increased bone ingrowth in the tendon-bone interface seen on histology.[80] Rats treated with FGF2 in a fibrin sealant combined with an acellular dermal matrix graft demonstrated an acceleration of healing compared with acellular dermal matrix graft alone, as demonstrated by higher ultimate tensile failure load.[81] The major challenge with the use of single growth factor therapy is the requirement for the molecule to be present at the right time when a responding cell population is present and the environment is permissive. Further studies will be necessary to identify the temporal and spatial sequence of cytokine presence that is optimal for tendon healing because such information will guide development of materials that may permit appropriate timed release of cytokines and growth factors to improve tendon healing.

SUMMARY

Rotator cuff disease is a common shoulder pathology encountered in orthopaedics, and retear rates after RCR remain a challenging problem in the field of orthopaedic sports medicine. Many orthobiologics have been studied in the setting of RCR in an effort to improve the rate and quality of tendon-bone healing. Although PRP has demonstrated some promise in RCR augmentation, standardization of PRP formulations and rigorous clinical trials evaluating tendon healing and associated clinical outcomes of augmented repairs in comparison with standard repair approaches are necessary to better elucidate its efficacy. Additionally, both translational studies and prospective clinical trials exploring the role of grafts, novel scaffold materials, and cellular therapies are necessary to improve clinical confidence in the efficacy of these options for massive RCR. Finally, identification of the specific cytokines and growth factors that are effective in the management of rotator cuff disease must be elucidated to better define targeted treatment strategies.

REFERENCES

1. Rossi LA, Murray IR, Chu CR, Muschler GF, Rodeo SA, Piuzzi NS: Classification systems for platelet-rich plasma. *Bone Joint J* 2019;101-B:891-896.
2. El-Sharkawy H, Kantarci A, Deady J, et al: Platelet-rich plasma: Growth factors and pro- and anti-inflammatory properties. *J Periodontol* 2007;78:661-669.
3. Hudgens JL, Sugg KB, Grekin JA, Gumucio JP, Bedi A, Mendias CL: Platelet-rich plasma activates proinflammatory signaling pathways and induces oxidative stress in tendon fibroblasts. *Am J Sports Med* 2016;44:1931-1940.
4. Kesikburun S, Tan AK, Yilmaz B, Yasar E, Yazicioglu K: Platelet-rich plasma injections in the treatment of chronic rotator cuff tendinopathy: A randomized controlled trial with 1-year follow-up. *Am J Sports Med* 2013;41: 2609-2616.
5. Schwitzguebel AJ, Kolo FC, Tirefort J, et al: Efficacy of platelet-rich plasma for the treatment of interstitial supraspinatus tears: A double-blinded, randomized controlled trial. *Am J Sports Med* 2019;47:1885-1892.
6. Hurley ET, Hannon CP, Pauzenberger L, Fat DL, Moran CJ, Mullett H: Nonoperative treatment of rotator cuff disease with platelet-rich plasma: A systematic review of randomized controlled trials. *Arthroscopy* 2019;35:1584-1591.
7. Galatz LM, Ball CM, Teefey SA, Middleton WD, Yamaguchi K: The outcome and repair integrity of completely arthroscopically repaired large and massive rotator cuff tears. *J Bone Joint Surg Am* 2004;86:219-224.
8. Lafosse L, Brozska R, Toussaint B, Gobezie R: The outcome and structural integrity of arthroscopic rotator cuff repair with use of the double-row suture anchor technique. *J Bone Joint Surg Am* 2007;89:1533-1541.

9. Zhao D, Han YH, Pan JK, et al: The clinical efficacy of leukocyte-poor platelet-rich plasma in arthroscopic rotator cuff repair: A meta-analysis of randomized controlled trials. *J Shoulder Elbow Surg* 2021;30:918-928.
10. Jo CH, Shin JS, Shin WH, Lee SY, Yoon KS, Shin S: Platelet-rich plasma for arthroscopic repair of medium to large rotator cuff tears: A randomized controlled trial. *Am J Sports Med* 2015;43:2102-2110.
11. Malavolta EA, Gracitelli MEC, Assuncao JH, Ferreira Neto AA, Bordalo-Rodrigues M, de Camargo OP: Clinical and structural evaluations of rotator cuff repair with and without added platelet-rich plasma at 5-year follow-up: A prospective randomized study. *Am J Sports Med* 2018;46:3134-3141.
12. Castricini R, Longo UG, De Benedetto M, et al: Platelet-rich plasma augmentation for arthroscopic rotator cuff repair: A randomized controlled trial. *Am J Sports Med* 2011;39:258-265.
13. Wang A, McCann P, Colliver J, et al: Do postoperative platelet-rich plasma injections accelerate early tendon healing and functional recovery after arthroscopic supraspinatus repair? A randomized controlled trial. *Am J Sports Med* 2015;43:1430-1437.
14. Wang C, Xu M, Guo W, Wang Y, Zhao S, Zhong L: Clinical efficacy and safety of platelet-rich plasma in arthroscopic full-thickness rotator cuff repair: A meta-analysis. *PLoS One* 2019;14:e0220392.
15. Chahal J, Van Thiel GS, Mall N, et al: The role of platelet-rich plasma in arthroscopic rotator cuff repair: A systematic review with quantitative synthesis. *Arthroscopy* 2012;28:1718-1727.
16. Warth RJ, Dornan GJ, James EW, Horan MP, Millett PJ: Clinical and structural outcomes after arthroscopic repair of full-thickness rotator cuff tears with and without platelet-rich product supplementation: A meta-analysis and meta-regression. *Arthroscopy* 2015;31:306-320.
17. Wasserman A, Matthewson G, MacDonald P: Platelet-rich plasma and the knee-applications in orthopedic surgery. *Curr Rev Musculoskelet Med* 2018;11:607-615.
18. Bryant D, Holtby R, Willits K, et al: A randomized clinical trial to compare the effectiveness of rotator cuff repair with or without augmentation using porcine small intestine submucosa for patients with moderate to large rotator cuff tears: A pilot study. *J Shoulder Elbow Surg* 2016;25:1623-1633.
19. Lederman ES, Toth AP, Nicholson GP, et al: A prospective, multicenter study to evaluate clinical and radiographic outcomes in primary rotator cuff repair reinforced with a xenograft dermal matrix. *J Shoulder Elbow Surg* 2016;25:1961-1970.
20. Schlegel TF, Abrams JS, Angelo RL, Getelman MH, Ho CP, Bushnell BD: Isolated bioinductive repair of partial-thickness rotator cuff tears using a resorbable bovine collagen implant: Two-year radiologic and clinical outcomes from a prospective multicenter study. *J Shoulder Elbow Surg* 2021;30:1938-1948.
21. Nicholson GP, Breur GJ, Van Sickle D, Yao JQ, Kim J, Blanchard CR: Evaluation of a cross-linked acellular porcine dermal patch for rotator cuff repair augmentation in an ovine model. *J Shoulder Elbow Surg* 2007;16:S184-S190.
22. Wong I, Burns J, Snyder S: Arthroscopic GraftJacket repair of rotator cuff tears. *J Shoulder Elbow Surg* 2010;19:104-109.
23. Barber FA, Burns JP, Deutsch A, Labbe MR, Litchfield RB: A prospective, randomized evaluation of acellular human dermal matrix augmentation for arthroscopic rotator cuff repair. *Arthroscopy* 2012;28:8-15.
24. Johnson SM, Cherry JV, Thomas N, Jafri M, Jariwala A, McLeod GG: Clinical outcomes and ultrasonographic viability of GraftJacket® augmented rotator cuff repair: A prospective follow-up study with mean follow-up of forty-one months. *J Clin Orthop Trauma* 2020;11:S372-S377.
25. Ciampi P, Scotti C, Nonis A, et al: The benefit of synthetic versus biological patch augmentation in the repair of posterosuperior massive rotator cuff tears: A 3-year follow-up study. *Am J Sports Med* 2014;42:1169-1175.
26. Proctor CS: Long-term successful arthroscopic repair of large and massive rotator cuff tears with a functional and degradable reinforcement device. *J Shoulder Elbow Surg* 2014;23:1508-1513.
27. Encalada-Diaz I, Cole BJ, Macgillivray JD, et al: Rotator cuff repair augmentation using a novel polycarbonate polyurethane patch: Preliminary results at 12 months' follow-up. *J Shoulder Elbow Surg* 2011;20:788-794.
28. Audenaert E, Van Nuffel J, Schepens A, Verhelst M, Verdonk R: Reconstruction of massive rotator cuff lesions with a synthetic interposition graft: A prospective study of 41 patients. *Knee Surg Sports Traumatol Arthrosc* 2006;14:360-364.
29. Nada AN, Debnath UK, Robinson DA, Jordan C: Treatment of massive rotator-cuff tears with a polyester ligament (Dacron) augmentation: Clinical outcome. *J Bone Joint Surg Br* 2010;92:1397-1402.
30. Zheng MH, Chen J, Kirilak Y, Willers C, Xu J, Wood D: Porcine small intestine submucosa (SIS) is not an acellular collagenous matrix and contains porcine DNA: Possible implications in human implantation. *J Biomed Mater Res B Appl Biomater* 2005;73:61-67.
31. Derwin K, Androjna C, Spencer E, et al: Porcine small intestine submucosa as a flexor tendon graft. *Clin Orthop Relat Res* 2004;423:245-252.
32. Bond JL, Dopirak RM, Higgins J, Burns J, Snyder SJ: Arthroscopic replacement of massive, irreparable rotator cuff tears using a GraftJacket allograft: Technique and preliminary results. *Arthroscopy* 2008;24:403-409 e1.
33. Derwin KA, Baker AR, Spragg RK, Leigh DR, Iannotti JP: Commercial extracellular matrix scaffolds for rotator cuff tendon repair. Biomechanical, biochemical, and cellular properties. *J Bone Joint Surg Am* 2006;88:2665-2672.
34. Beitzel K, McCarthy MB, Cote MP, et al: Properties of biologic scaffolds and their response to mesenchymal stem cells. *Arthroscopy* 2014;30:289-298.
35. Charles MD, Christian DR, Cole BJ: The role of biologic therapy in rotator cuff tears and repairs. *Curr Rev Musculoskelet Med* 2018;11:150-161.

36. Cole BJ, Gomoll AH, Yanke A, et al: Biocompatibility of a polymer patch for rotator cuff repair. *Knee Surg Sports Traumatol Arthrosc* 2007;15:632-637.

37. Lebaschi A, Nakagawa Y, Wada S, Cong GT, Rodeo SA: Tissue-specific endothelial cells: A promising approach for augmentation of soft tissue repair in orthopedics. *Ann N Y Acad Sci* 2017;1410:44-56.

38. Lebaschi AH, Camp CL, Carballo C, et al: Murine supraspinatus tendon detachment and repair model augmented with tendon-derived, activated endothelial cells: A new concept in biologic enhancement of tendon-to-bone healing. *Orthop J Sports Med* 2017;5:2325967117S00444.

39. Wada S, Lebaschi A, Nakagawa Y, et al: Muscle-derived activated endothelial cells as a new cell source to enhance tendon-to-bone healing: In vivo study in a murine rotator cuff repair model. *J Shoulder Elbow Surg* 2019;28:e209-e210.

40. Rafii S, Butler JM, Ding BS: Angiocrine functions of organ-specific endothelial cells. *Nature* 2016;529:316-325.

41. Castro-Manrreza ME, Montesinos JJ: Immunoregulation by mesenchymal stem cells: Biological aspects and clinical applications. *J Immunol Res* 2015;2015:394917.

42. Piuzzi NS, Hussain ZB, Chahla J, et al: Variability in the preparation, reporting, and use of bone marrow aspirate concentrate in musculoskeletal disorders: A systematic review of the clinical orthopaedic literature. *J Bone Joint Surg Am* 2018;100:517-525.

43. Carballo CB, Lebaschi A, Rodeo SA: Cell-based approaches for augmentation of tendon repair. *Tech Shoulder Elbow Surg* 2017;18:e6-e14.

44. Li N, Hua J: Interactions between mesenchymal stem cells and the immune system. *Cell Mol Life Sci* 2017;74:2345-2360.

45. Gulotta LV, Kovacevic D, Ehteshami JR, Dagher E, Packer JD, Rodeo SA: Application of bone marrow-derived mesenchymal stem cells in a rotator cuff repair model. *Am J Sports Med* 2009;37:2126-2133.

46. Degen RM, Carbone A, Carballo C, et al: The effect of purified human bone marrow-derived mesenchymal stem cells on rotator cuff tendon healing in an athymic rat. *Arthroscopy* 2016;32:2435-2443.

47. Gulotta LV, Kovacevic D, Packer JD, Deng XH, Rodeo SA: Bone marrow-derived mesenchymal stem cells transduced with scleraxis improve rotator cuff healing in a rat model. *Am J Sports Med* 2011;39:1282-1289.

48. Gulotta LV, Kovacevic D, Montgomery S, Ehteshami JR, Packer JD, Rodeo SA: Stem cells genetically modified with the developmental gene MT1-MMP improve regeneration of the supraspinatus tendon-to-bone insertion site. *Am J Sports Med* 2010;38:1429-1437.

49. Thangarajah T, Sanghani-Kerai A, Henshaw F, Lambert SM, Pendegrass CJ, Blunn GW: Application of a demineralized cortical bone matrix and bone marrow-derived mesenchymal stem cells in a model of chronic rotator cuff degeneration. *Am J Sports Med* 2018;46:98-108.

50. Tornero-Esteban P, Hoyas JA, Villafuertes E, et al: Efficacy of supraspinatus tendon repair using mesenchymal stem cells along with a collagen I scaffold. *J Orthop Surg Res* 2015;10:124.

51. Chen P, Cui L, Fu SC, et al: The 3D-printed PLGA scaffolds loaded with bone marrow-derived mesenchymal stem cells augment the healing of rotator cuff repair in the rabbits. *Cell Transplant* 2020;29:963689720973647.

52. Chen P, Cui L, Chen G, et al: The application of BMP-12-overexpressing mesenchymal stem cells loaded 3D-printed PLGA scaffolds in rabbit rotator cuff repair. *Int J Biol Macromol* 2019;138:79-88.

53. Liu Q, Yu Y, Reisdorf RL, et al: Engineered tendon-fibrocartilage-bone composite and bone marrow-derived mesenchymal stem cell sheet augmentation promotes rotator cuff healing in a non-weight-bearing canine model. *Biomaterials* 2019;192:189-198.

54. Hernigou P, Flouzat Lachaniette CH, Delambre J, et al: Biologic augmentation of rotator cuff repair with mesenchymal stem cells during arthroscopy improves healing and prevents further tears: A case-controlled study. *Int Orthop* 2014;38:1811-1818.

55. Ellera Gomes JL, da Silva RC, Silla LM, Abreu MR, Pellanda R: Conventional rotator cuff repair complemented by the aid of mononuclear autologous stem cells. *Knee Surg Sports Traumatol Arthrosc* 2012;20:373-377.

56. Bunnell BA, Flaat M, Gagliardi C, Patel B, Ripoll C: Adipose-derived stem cells: Isolation, expansion and differentiation. *Methods* 2008;45:115-120.

57. Costa-Almeida R, Calejo I, Gomes ME: Mesenchymal stem cells empowering tendon regenerative therapies. *Int J Mol Sci* 2019;20:3002.

58. Kim YS, Sung CH, Chung SH, Kwak SJ, Koh YG: Does an injection of adipose-derived mesenchymal stem cells loaded in fibrin glue influence rotator cuff repair outcomes? A clinical and magnetic resonance imaging study. *Am J Sports Med* 2017;45:2010-2018.

59. Oh JH, Chung SW, Kim SH, Chung JY, Kim JY: 2013 Neer Award: Effect of the adipose-derived stem cell for the improvement of fatty degeneration and rotator cuff healing in rabbit model. *J Shoulder Elbow Surg* 2014;23:445-455.

60. Lu LY, Kuang CY, Yin F: Magnetic resonance imaging and biomechanical analysis of adipose-derived stromal vascular fraction applied on rotator cuff repair in rabbits. *Chin Med J (Engl)* 2018;131:69-74.

61. Valencia Mora M, Antuna Antuna S, Garcia Arranz M, Carrascal MT, Barco R: Application of adipose tissue-derived stem cells in a rat rotator cuff repair model. *Injury* 2014;45(suppl 4):S22-S27.

62. Kaizawa Y, Franklin A, Leyden J, et al: Augmentation of chronic rotator cuff healing using adipose-derived stem cell-seeded human tendon-derived hydrogel. *J Orthop Res* 2019;37:877-886.

63. Rothrauff BB, Smith CA, Ferrer GA, et al: The effect of adipose-derived stem cells on enthesis healing after repair of acute and chronic massive rotator cuff tears in rats. *J Shoulder Elbow Surg* 2019;28(4):654-664.

64. Fu G, Lu L, Pan Z, Fan A, Yin F: Adipose-derived stem cell exosomes facilitate rotator cuff repair by mediating tendon-derived stem cells. *Regen Med* 2021;16:359-372.

65. Gumucio JP, Flood MD, Roche SM, et al: Stromal vascular stem cell treatment decreases muscle fibrosis following chronic rotator cuff tear. *Int Orthop* 2016;40:759-764.

66. Bedi A, Maak T, Walsh C, et al: Cytokines in rotator cuff degeneration and repair. *J Shoulder Elbow Surg* 2012;21: 218-227.

67. Millar NL, Wei AQ, Molloy TJ, Bonar F, Murrell GA: Cytokines and apoptosis in supraspinatus tendinopathy. *J Bone Joint Surg Br* 2009;91:417-424.

68. Koshima H, Kondo S, Mishima S, et al: Expression of interleukin-1beta, cyclooxygenase-2, and prostaglandin E2 in a rotator cuff tear in rabbits. *J Orthop Res* 2007;25:92-97.

69. Oak NR, Gumucio JP, Flood MD, et al: Inhibition of 5-LOX, COX-1, and COX-2 increases tendon healing and reduces muscle fibrosis and lipid accumulation after rotator cuff repair. *Am J Sports Med* 2014;42:2860-2868.

70. Nakama K, Gotoh M, Yamada T, et al: Interleukin-6-induced activation of signal transducer and activator of transcription-3 in ruptured rotator cuff tendon. *J Int Med Res* 2006;34:624-631.

71. Ling Y, Peng C, Liu C, Zhang N, Yue S: Gene polymorphism of IL-6 and MMP-3 decreases passive range of motion after rotator cuff repair. *Int J Clin Exp Pathol* 2015;8:5709-5714.

72. Okamura K, Kobayashi T, Yamamoto A, et al: Shoulder pain and intra-articular interleukin-8 levels in patients with rotator cuff tears. *Int J Rheum Dis* 2017;20:177-181.

73. Gulotta LV, Kovacevic D, Cordasco F, Rodeo SA: Evaluation of tumor necrosis factor alpha blockade on early tendon-to-bone healing in a rat rotator cuff repair model. *Arthroscopy* 2011;27:1351-1357.

74. Wurgler-Hauri CC, Dourte LM, Baradet TC, Williams GR, Soslowsky LJ: Temporal expression of 8 growth factors in tendon-to-bone healing in a rat supraspinatus model. *J Shoulder Elbow Surg* 2007;16:S198-S203.

75. Manning CN, Kim HM, Sakiyama-Elbert S, Galatz LM, Havlioglu N, Thomopoulos S: Sustained delivery of transforming growth factor beta three enhances tendon-to-bone healing in a rat model. *J Orthop Res* 2011;29:1099-1105.

76. Hee CK, Dines JS, Dines DM, et al: Augmentation of a rotator cuff suture repair using rhPDGF-BB and a type I bovine collagen matrix in an ovine model. *Am J Sports Med* 2011;39:1630-1639.

77. Uggen C, Dines J, McGarry M, Grande D, Lee T, Limpisvasti O: The effect of recombinant human platelet-derived growth factor BB-coated sutures on rotator cuff healing in a sheep model. *Arthroscopy* 2010;26:1456-1462.

78. Kovacevic D, Gulotta LV, Ying L, Ehteshami JR, Deng XH, Rodeo SA: rhPDGF-BB promotes early healing in a rat rotator cuff repair model. *Clin Orthop Relat Res* 2015;473:1644-1654.

79. Tokunaga T, Karasugi T, Arimura H, et al: Enhancement of rotator cuff tendon-bone healing with fibroblast growth factor 2 impregnated in gelatin hydrogel sheets in a rabbit model. *J Shoulder Elbow Surg* 2017;26:1708-1717.

80. Ide J, Kikukawa K, Hirose J, et al: The effect of a local application of fibroblast growth factor-2 on tendon-to-bone remodeling in rats with acute injury and repair of the supraspinatus tendon. *J Shoulder Elbow Surg* 2009;18:391-398.

81. Ide J, Kikukawa K, Hirose J, Iyama K, Sakamoto H, Mizuta H: The effects of fibroblast growth factor-2 on rotator cuff reconstruction with acellular dermal matrix grafts. *Arthroscopy* 2009;25:608-616.

CHAPTER 18

Tendon Management, Protection, and Repair

Allan Mishra, MD, FAAOS • Michael W. Heffner, MD • Christopher Frey, MD

INTRODUCTION

Tendinopathy is a disorder characterized by variable pain and limb dysfunction. It is a common clinical problem with a prevalence that has been rising over the past century.[1] Of the various anatomic locations affected, the most common include rotator cuff tendons, epicondylar tendons, gluteal tendons, the patellar tendon, and the Achilles tendon. Each of these areas is characterized by specific pain patterns and disability. Lower extremity tendinopathy prevalence has been reported to be 10.52 to 16.6 per 1,000 person-years. This exceeds the incidence of osteoarthritis of 8.4 per 1,000 per person-years.[1,2] Upper extremity tendinopathy is quite prevalent as well, especially in the working population. A cross-sectional study performed in a primary care setting in the United Kingdom found that approximately 8% of this population was affected, with rotator cuff tendinopathy the most common at 5.2%, bicipital tendinopathy, 0.7%, lateral epicondylitis, 1.2%, and medial epicondylitis, 0.9%.[3] The rise of tendinopathy demands an improved understanding of its pathophysiology, better diagnostic tools, and more effective treatment options.

ECONOMIC EFFECT OF TENDINOPATHY

It is not surprising that, with its high prevalence and potential morbidity, tendinopathy is associated with a significant effect on society. A simple model of economic burden is summarized in the next paragraphs. There are some general assumptions such as no mortality or premature death from disease. Patients are also assumed to have a full recovery from the disease with complete reentry into the workforce. In addition, direct nonmedical costs such as the cost of any inpatient stays, outpatient visits, and transportation costs are assumed to be minimal. Morbidity is assumed to be limited to the cost of absenteeism and not a decline in work production while on the job. The productivity loss due to appointments includes office visits but not therapy sessions because this is assumed to be done outside of work hours. A one-half multiplying factor assumes that one-half of a standard workday productivity is lost.

Annual economic disease burden = Direct cost of disease + Indirect cost of disease

$$\text{Direct costs} = \text{medical cost}$$

$$\text{Medical cost} = \text{I}\big((\text{Rv} + \text{Ri} + \text{Rp}) + (\text{Ov} + \text{Oi} + \text{Op})\big)$$

$$\text{Indirect costs} = \text{I} * (\text{pm} + \text{pv} * 1/2)$$

$$\text{I} = \text{incidence},\ \text{R} = \text{reimbursement},\ \text{O} = \text{out-of-pocket},$$

$$\text{v} = \text{appointment},\ \text{i} = \text{intervention},\ \text{p} = \text{pharmaceuticals},$$

$$\text{P} = \text{productivity loss},\ \text{m} = \text{morbibdity}$$

An average personal income of $37,318.68 (2021 dollars) is based on data from the Federal Reserve Bank of St. Louis. Divided by 261 work days per calendar year, each day of absenteeism is anticipated to cost approximately $142.98. Thus, in this model, the primary driver of economic burden is anticipated to be the incidence of disease. The cost of missing work is significant, but likely to have less of an effect than surgery, which may cost approximately $4,400 based on reimbursement for open débridement of the lateral epicondyle.[4] This economic model can be useful to analyze the value of potential treatment interventions.

GENOMICS OF TENDINOPATHY

Emerging technology helps clinicians and researchers evaluate whole genomes, the exome, epigenetics, and the microbiome, among many others. This has helped uncover the role of genomics in tendinopathy. Polymorphisms within several genes including *COL5A1*, *TNC*, *MMP3*, and *ESSRA* have been associated with tendinopathy. Moreover, specific variants of the *PDFGB* gene have shown improved responses to treatment with platelet-rich plasma (PRP) in patients with chronic tennis elbow.[5] Many of the genes of interest are involved in collagen structure or inflammation, which is consistent with the underlying pathology. This knowledge has great potential for understanding risk factors and even guiding interventions. However, the combination of multiple complex genetic interactions and considerable heterogeneity in various populations make it difficult to pinpoint an exact genomic etiology.[1] In fact, one genome-wide association study found no significant correlation between any single nucleotide polymorphism and Achilles tendon tear or tendinopathy.[6]

Dr. Mishra or an immediate family member has received royalties from DePuy, a Johnson & Johnson Company and Zimmer. Neither of the following authors nor any immediate family member has received anything of value from or has stock or stock options held in a commercial company or institution related directly or indirectly to the subject of this chapter: Dr. Heffner and Dr. Frey.

Beyond the genome, posttranscriptional mechanisms allow for fine-tuning of genetic expression with mechanisms such as methylation, acetylation, and noncoding RNA. For example, small interfering RNA and micro RNA have been found to be intimately involved in standard cellular functioning as well as pathologic states. miRNA sequences involved in inflammation, such as interleukins and JAK2/STAT3, have been associated with tendinopathy, and many more are likely yet to be discovered.[7] This is an expanding field and there will likely be great innovation coming in the area of epigenetic regulation and tendon pathology as the technology becomes more prevalent.

In light of these discoveries, there has been recent interest in developing systems to deliver novel genetic-based therapies to treat tendinopathy.[8] Gene therapy using stem cells and viral or other small vectors have shown promise. Specifically, scleraxis gene delivery has been used to mimic its role in embryogenic tendon development using in vitro models. Growth factors such as bone morphogenetic proteins 12 and 14 have also had good early-stage results in treating tendinopathy models.[8] Regulatory or noncoding RNA has also been used with several miRNA injections expediting healing in animal models. Exosomes, which are small vesicles containing functional payloads, often derived from stem cells, have been shown to decrease inflammation to provide better healing environments in the extracellular matrix (ECM) and intracellularly with in vitro models. Although these early results illustrate the immense potential of genetic therapy, there is still much work to be done in the area before translating into human clinical trials.

FACTORS CONTRIBUTING TO THE DEVELOPMENT OF TENDINOPATHY

Multiple theories of the underlying pathophysiology of tendinopathy exist in the literature. The proposed pathways are not necessarily mutually exclusive and may actually be intertwined. Repetitive microtrauma via overuse or rapid macro-overload has been the primary suspect in the etiology of tendinopathy for many decades. Overuse may result in the release of oxidative compounds and subsequent tendon damage.[9] On a cellular level, this can lead to mucoid degeneration, a dysregulated ECM, and enhanced cellular apoptosis.[1] Lack of adequate tissue perfusion is another factor contributing to the development of tendinopathy. Inadequate blood flow in affected anatomic regions leads to mitochondrial dysfunction and induces apoptosis,[10] which is consistent with how tendinopathy most often occurs in hypoxic zones. Mitochondrial dysfunction then amplifies inflammation and nuclear factor kappa B, a known regulator of tissue inflammation. Mitochondrial transplantation–suppressed damage induced increases upregulation of nuclear factor kappa B, rescuing regular collagen production.[10] Angiofibroblastic dysplasia is thought to follow and ultimately result in tendinopathy with the development of disorganized hypervascular tissue (**Table 1**).

There may also exist a distinct neurogenic underpinning to the disease. Overexpression of glutamate and its receptors has been found in a variety of tendinopathies.[1] This upregulation can result in pain and also contribute to structural tendon abnormalities. Excessive neurostimulation of the glutamatergic and autonomic systems can also lead to release of neuropeptides such as substance P and calcitonin, thereby triggering mast cell degranulation.[1] This ultimately results in pain and inflammation. Neural causes of tendinopathy have not been fully explored and deserve more attention, especially in the context of emerging biologic treatment strategies.

Inflammation clearly plays a central role in the pathophysiology of tendinopathy. Injury can lead to the release of proinflammatory cytokines such as interleukin 6 and interleukin 1. Continued noxious stimuli may give rise to a complex cascade of cytokines, growth factors, and microRNAs, which may subsequently result in the development of tendinopathy. As a result, dysfunctional differentiation of tendon stem cells or progenitors into adipocytes, osteocytes, or chondrocytes further perpetuates the cycle.[1]

Through likely interrelated mechanisms, dysregulated immune homeostasis has recently been implicated in the development of tendinopathy. Akbar et al[11] found evidence of activated dendritic cells and subsequent activation of T cells. This study suggests that an unbalanced immune response to tendon microtrauma promotes a cycle of inflammation and aberrant tissue repair.[11] Dysfunction of the ECM may also play a role in the pathophysiology of tendinopathy via abnormal regulation of matrix metalloproteinases and tissue inhibitors of metalloproteinases.

TABLE 1 Factors Contributing to the Development of Tendinopathy

Macrotrauma or microtrauma	Tendon-muscle overloading leads to inflammation and degeneration
Vascular	Anatomic hypoxic zones lead to a poor healing response and mitochondrial dysfunction
Neurogenic	Imbalance of sympathetic and parasympathetic signaling results in increased levels of glutamate and substance P
Cellular and extracellular dysfunction	Increased apoptosis with dysregulated immune homeostasis in the extracellular matrix, impairment of stem cell, and perivascular cell function
Metabolic/endocrine	Connection to diabetes, obesity, hypothyroidism, and low vitamin D levels

This weakens the tendon-ECM construct, also contributing to the development of tendinopathy.[1]

Many studies have found an association between tendinopathy and metabolic derangement. Diabetes, hypercholesterolemia, and hypothyroidism were found to be associated with insertional calcific tendinopathy in one epidemiologic survey.[12] With regard to the upper extremity, body mass index and body fat percentage were correlated with higher incidence and severity of rotator cuff tears.[13] This was corroborated in a meta-analysis that found patients with diabetes had an odds ratio of 3.67 for development of tendinopathy compared with control patients without diabetes.[14] Although excess weight may simply cause more stress on tendons, this mechanism is not yet completely elucidated. The increased inflammatory state of these pathologies, however, may play a role. Weight reduction reduces systemic inflammation and may thereby reduce the risk of developing tendinopathy. This intervention strategy deserves more clinical attention and research evaluation.

Moreover, low vitamin D has been associated with tendinopathy and poor surgical outcomes.[15] O'Donnell et al[15] in a population study of more than 40,000 patients found that low vitamin D was associated with a higher risk of revision rotator cuff surgery. Age, male sex, smoking, obesity, and hyperlipidemia were other independent factors associated with the need for revision surgery in this study. Harada et al[16] also found a higher rate of complications in patients undergoing rotator cuff surgery when the level of vitamin D was less than 20 ng/mL, including an increased odds ratio of revision of 1.54 ($P < 0.001$).

Collectively, these five key factors represent an incomplete and/or inappropriate healing response within a tendon that has been acutely or chronically damaged. All of these factors contribute to the development of tendinopathy.

DIAGNOSIS AND PREVENTION OF TENDINOPATHY

Tendinopathy is a clinical disorder characterized by pain and dysfunction. There is no single definitive physical examination finding. Pain with palpation of a tendon near its origin or insertion is the most common finding. There is usually pain with resisted testing of the muscle unit as well. Tightness of the associated muscle is another important finding that contributes to the pain associated with tendinopathy. Activity-related pain is also almost universally reported by patients with tendinopathy. This combination of findings on history and physical examination is highly suggestive of a diagnosis of tendinopathy. Often, confirmatory imaging will then be performed to pinpoint the severity of the problem.

It is crucial, however, to focus on prevention of tendinopathy or simple noninvasive interventions before delving into the imaging modalities used to confirm the diagnosis. Too often, the health care system fails to correctly address and treat high-risk populations at a more easily treatable time point. This leads to presentation of the problem at later stages with increased severity and longer recovery. Stretching and exercise interventions have been investigated as possible tendinopathy prevention tools with variable success, although concrete data are still lacking.[17] Poor biomechanics and tight myotendinous tissue contribute to tendinopathy. Therefore, early detection is important.[18] For example, it is suggested that Achilles tendon stretching and posterior chain strengthening may be helpful in preventing Achilles tendinitis.[19] In a review of patellar tendinitis prevention, four of five studies yielded a decreased incidence with exercise intervention.[20] The four studies with positive results used progressively loaded isotonic strengthening, whereas the other study used unloaded exercise. However, methods to diminish stress on the tendon may also prove beneficial. Shock-absorbing shoe wear has been found to prevent Achilles tendinopathy in a 2016 study, but this has not been replicated with orthoses or basketball shoes.[17]

Risks may be compounded by physiologic states such as aging. It has been found that active postmenopausal women have a greater prevalence of Achilles tendon abnormalities than inactive women.[21] Hormone replacement was associated with decreased thickness and other tendon abnormalities in active postmenopausal women. Identifying specific risk factors such as vitamin deficiency or hormonal changes may augment prevention strategies and should be a high priority for clinicians and researchers.

In addition to these intrinsic causes, several modifiable external factors also play a role in disease development and progression. One commonly prescribed extrinsic risk factor is systemic fluoroquinolone use. A recent meta-analysis found that the use of this medication class was associated with an increase in Achilles tendinitis with an odds ratio of 3.95.[22] This effect was even more pronounced with age older than 60 years and concomitant use of oral corticosteroid. Although the mechanism of fluoroquinolone-induced tendon damage is not yet elucidated, it is thought to be a combination of direct toxicity and collagen degeneration.[22] Another iatrogenic cause of tendinitis is the use of statin treatment strategies. A recent cohort study found that statin use was associated with a hazard ratio of 1.5 for trigger finger and 1.43 for shoulder tendinopathy in men.[23] Women were also at elevated risk in this study. These extrinsic factors pose as possible modifiable risk factors that can help guide therapy for select patients or contribute to the cost-benefit analysis of prescribing them.

IMAGING

There are an increasing number of imaging modalities available to assist in evaluation, monitoring of treatment effect, and even prognostication.[24] More advanced technologies such as novel MRI techniques and ultrasound elastography are augmenting diagnostic accuracy, but ultimately clinical interpretation is intertwined with clinical symptomatology and physical examination. It is important to keep in mind that, as in osteoarthritis, there is not always a clear correlation between imaging findings and pain or disability. A detailed review of tendinopathy imaging is beyond the scope of this chapter.

ORTHOBIOLOGIC TREATMENT STRATEGIES FOR TENDINOPATHY

Exercise should be considered a biologic treatment for tendinopathy. Loading of tendons and their muscle units with specific exercise protocols has been shown to be an effective treatment for a variety of tendinopathies including Achilles, patellar, extensor, and rotator cuff tendinopathy. It is clear that isometric and eccentric exercise protocols have value and improve outcomes in the management of tendinopathy.[1] Although the exact mechanism has not been elucidated, several mechanisms have been proposed, including structural changes, changes in tendon length, neurovascular ingrowth, changes in intratendon fluid dynamics, and neuromuscular adaptation.[25] Although still in its infancy, blood flow restriction therapy is currently under investigation with some early positive results.[26]

Of note, steroid injections continue to be a popular treatment for tendinopathy, despite limited data supporting their long-term efficacy and data suggesting that they are detrimental. Dry needling without any steroid injection is preferred and has shown improvement in studies of chronic tendinopathy.[27] There is currently no pharmacologic intervention for tendinopathy that produces meaningful improvements in pain and function. Genomic and regenerative medicine approaches may eventually lead to specific small molecules with clinical value.

UPPER EXTREMITY PRP DATA

Lateral epicondylar tendinopathy was the first anatomic area to be treated using PRP. PRP is a component of whole blood that contains hundreds of bioactive growth factors and signaling molecules that can be prepared in a short period at the point of care. In a pilot study of 20 patients published in 2006, Mishra and Pavelko[28] found a 60% reduction in pain using leukocyte-rich PRP (LR-PRP) compared with 16% reduction in the control group at 8 weeks ($P = 0.001$). At final follow-up of an average of 25.6 months, the patient group treated with LR-PRP reported a 93% reduction in pain compared with before treatment ($P < 0.0001$). This study sparked worldwide interest in studying PRP for the treatment of tendinopathy.

Two prospective randomized trials were completed using the same protocol and type of PRP as this initial pilot study. The results were published in three separate studies. Initially, Peerbooms et al[29] published the results of a 100-patient prospective randomized trial of LR-PRP versus cortisone. This study found a 73% success rate for LR-PRP using visual analog scale pain scores versus 49% for cortisone at 1 year ($P < 0.001$). Gosens et al[30] published the 2-year results of this study and found that LR-PRP "reduces pain and increases function significantly, exceeding the effect of corticosteroid injection." Mishra et al[27] then published a prospective, double-blind, randomized controlled trial of 230 patients using the same protocol. This study found no differences in treatment outcomes at 12 weeks when comparing LR-PRP in a control group. At 24 weeks, however, clinically meaningful improvements were noted. The success rate for LR-PRP was 82.1% compared with 60.3% for the control group ($P = 0.008$) using the criteria of 50% or more improvement in pain scores.

These three studies represent 350 patients studied in controlled investigations. All of the studies favored the use of LR-PRP over control treatment. These collective data provide strong evidence supporting the use of this type of PRP and protocol for the management of chronic lateral epicondylar tendinopathy (**Figures 1** and **2**).

Surgery may be recommended for refractory cases in which nonsurgical interventions fail. It is important to understand the PRP literature in the context of surgical outcomes. PRP injection versus surgical intervention was investigated in a meta-analysis of five studies that included a total of 340 patients. This data set included 154 patients treated with surgery and 186 patients treated with PRP. The study concluded that the two treatment strategies were equivalent in pain scores and functional outcomes. They further concluded that PRP is a reasonable alternative to surgery.[31] Some meta-analysis studies have found limited value in using PRP for elbow tendinopathy. Unfortunately, these studies have lumped together a

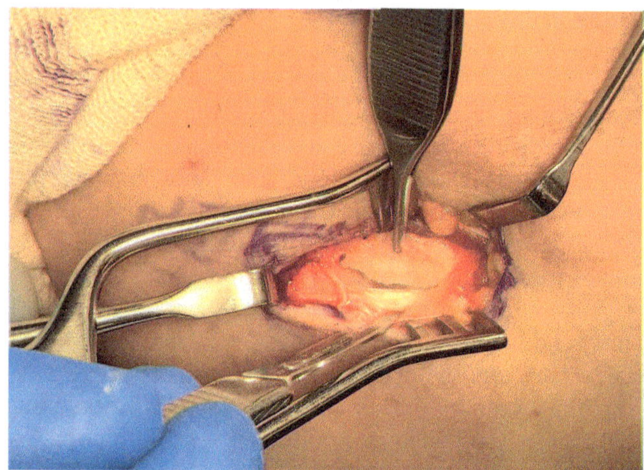

FIGURE 1 Clinical photograph obtained during surgical débridement of chronic lateral epicondylar tendinopathy shows an area of mucoid degeneration that is being surgically excised.

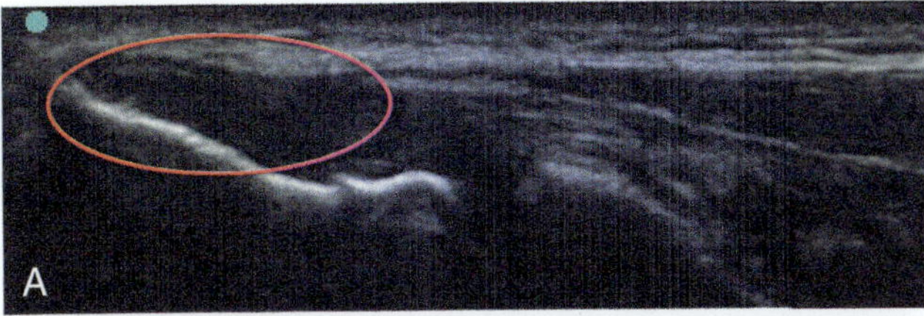

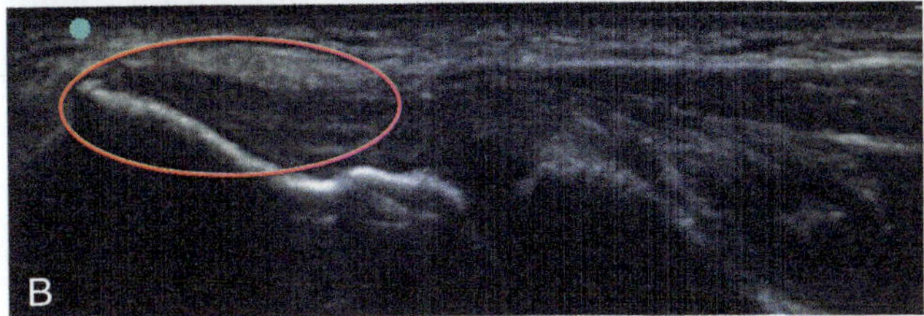

FIGURE 2 Ultrasonographic images of lateral epicondylar tendinopathy. **A**, Image obtained before treatment shows poor, disorganized tendon exotexture (circle). **B**, Image obtained 3 months after treatment with leukocyte-rich platelet-rich plasma shows increased fiber organization and echotexture of the common extensor tendon (circle).

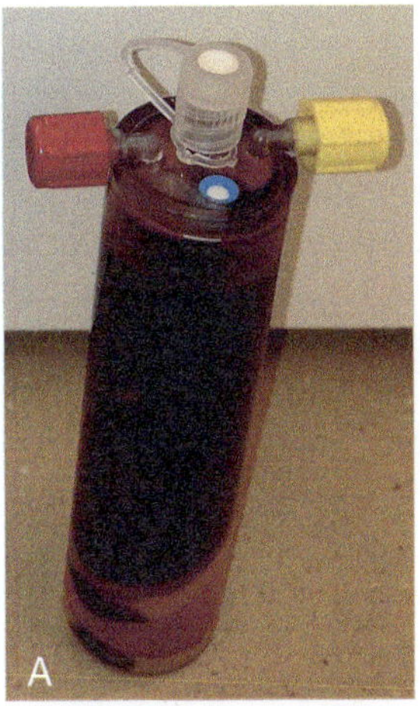

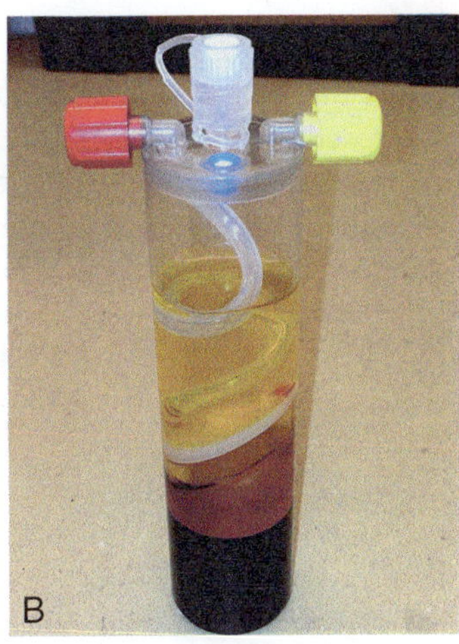

FIGURE 3 Photographs show whole blood (**A**) and blood following separation of components and leukocyte-rich platelet-rich plasma (**B**) after centrifugation for 15 minutes at 3,200 RPM. The process separates blood into the yellow plasma at the top of the tube, the red blood cells at the bottom of the tube, and the leukocyte-rich platelet-rich plasma in the middle.

variety of formulations and protocols. This undermines the conclusions of these studies and highlights the importance of uniformity in conducting trials on PRP.

Shoulder

The use of PRP in the shoulder has been controversial primarily because of the significant variation of protocols, formulations, and indications (**Figure 3**). Studies have used a variety of types of PRP for a multitude of variations of rotator cuff pathology. This makes it difficult to arrive at definitive conclusions about the utility of PRP in the context of rotator cuff tendinopathy.

One randomized controlled trial found a significant decrease in pain score for all time points when compared with nonaugmented surgery when used to augment arthroscopic rotator cuff repair.[32] Initial 3-month results demonstrated significantly higher Constant, Simple Shoulder Test, and the University of California, Los Angeles Shoulder Scores, as well as external rotation strength relative to the control group. Moreover, there was a shorter time (3 months versus 6 months) to improvement in postoperative Constant scores. By 10 years, these no longer significantly differed between the two arms.[33] These data imply that PRP augmentation may enhance the speed, but not the end outcome of rotator cuff repair.

Recent meta-analysis data present a positive but incomplete picture for PRP in the context of rotator cuff tendinopathy. Chen et al[34] concluded that "PRP may positively affect clinical outcomes, but limited data, study heterogeneity, and poor methodological quality hinder firm conclusions." Authors of a 2021 study[35] found that PRP injection was a safe and effective intervention for long-term pain control and shoulder function in patients with rotator cuff disorders. It was emphasized that there was no difference in short-term (3-week) outcomes, but it was found that PRP was significantly better at 6 and 12 months for pain and symptom control. A systematic analysis of meta-analyses found PRP to be effective in reducing retears after rotator cuff repair. PRP also improved functional outcome scores and reduced short-term pain.[36] A preclinical article found that LR-PRP induced more growth factor release and increased rotator cuff tenocyte proliferation compared with leukocyte-poor PRP (LP-PRP). This evidence suggests that LR-PRP may be the preferred formulation for tendinopathy.[37]

Overall, the PRP data for shoulder suggest that it has value to reduce retears and improve short-term outcomes. The indications, formulations, and specific protocols, however, are yet to be optimized.

Wrist and Hand

Uzun et al[38] compared the efficacy of corticosteroid with PRP injections in 40 patients with carpal tunnel syndrome. This was the first randomized controlled trial with PRP used for treatment of this condition. This work demonstrated better improvements in the symptom severity score and the functional capacity score of the PRP group when compared with the corticosteroid group at 3 months. The 6-month outcomes, however, were not significant. Wu et al[39] in a trial of 60 patients found that the LR-PRP group exhibited significant improvements in pain and function scores compared with those of the control group 6 months posttreatment. Chen et al[40] concluded that a single dose of ultrasound-guided perineural PRP provided therapeutic effect in a prospective, double-blind, randomized controlled trial.

Based on the limited studies conducted, PRP provides encouraging signs that it can potentially improve pain and function for patients in whom carpal tunnel syndrome is diagnosed. Larger studies using consistent protocols and PRP formulations are still needed to confirm the value of PRP for carpal tunnel syndrome.

OTHER ORTHOBIOLOGIC TREATMENTS IN THE UPPER EXTREMITY

PRP has by far the most data supporting its use as biologic treatment in upper extremity tendinopathy, but other biologic treatment strategies are also accumulating evidence. Baryeh et al[41] reviewed cellular treatment strategies for sports-related injuries of the upper extremity focusing on rotator cuff and epicondylar tendinopathy. This study discusses the many options including bone marrow concentrate, tenocytes, and mesenchymal stem cells. Mesenchymal stem cells are now recognized not to be stem cells per se, but rather progenitor cells with the potential to exert trophic, paracrine, and immunomodulatory effects when applied in vivo. Most cellular studies were found to be of low quality with a high level of heterogeneity.[41]

Di Matteo et al[9] also reviewed 13 studies using cell-based therapies such as bone and adipose-derived cells alone or in combination with PRP or bone marrow concentrate for shoulder and elbow tendinopathy. This study found cell-based approaches to be safe with some preliminary evidence of clinical value. Both of these reviews concluded that larger and more robust studies will be required to confirm or refute the value of specific cell-based approaches.

There are several novel injection and topical therapeutic modalities that are currently under investigation. Botulinum toxin or Botox has mostly been studied in the treatment of lateral epicondylitis. It has been found to significantly reduce pain compared with placebo but may slightly be less effective than corticosteroid injection in the early postinjection stage.[42] Topical glyceryl trinitrate generally has favorable short-term improvements in pain and function over placebo for rotator cuff tendinopathy but was associated with headaches in some patients.[43] The mild decrease in short-term to medium-term pain has been replicated in lateral epicondylitis studies as well.[43]

Prolotherapy, the injection of noxious compounds, typically hypertonic dextrose, has shown some promise with decreases in pain and improvement in Disabilities of the Arm, Shoulder and Hand scores compared with placebo for lateral epicondylitis.[44] Lhee and Park[45] found it to be associated with improvements in disability as well but was not significantly different than therapy alone. It has shown mixed results in rotator cuff pathology. These studies are limited in that there are no guidelines on the components of each injection and many included steroids and/or anesthetics that confound the outcomes. Few studies include proper controls to parse out the effect of individual intervention components, making it difficult to recommend prolotherapy at this time. Similarly, extracorporeal shock wave therapy and low-level laser therapy have been investigated as treatment strategies for tendinopathy with inconsistent methodology and results.[46,47]

LOWER EXTREMITY PRP DATA

Hip

Significant evidence supports the use of LR-PRP in the treatment of chronic gluteal tendinopathy. Fitzpatrick et al[48] studied 80 patients with this condition in a prospective, randomized, double-blind manner. These investigators found that the use of a single injection of LR-PRP resulted in more improvement in pain and functional scores than a single injection of corticosteroids. Modified Harris hip scores improved in patients treated with LR-PRP at an average of 54% at 2-year follow-up ($P < 0.001$). Conversely, the patients treated with corticosteroid showed maximal improvement at 6 weeks, which was not maintained beyond 24 weeks. This study represents level I data supporting the use of LR-PRP for chronic gluteal tendinopathy.

There have also been numerous trials examining PRP's effect on hamstring injuries, the first of which was performed in 2014 by Reurink et al.[49] This study of 80 athletes found that LP-PRP injection combined with a rehabilitation program was not significantly more effective in managing hamstring injuries than a rehabilitation program alone. A Hamid et al,[50] however, found that LR-PRP with a similar protocol did provide additional benefit. This theme of LR-PRP being better than LP-PRP for tendinopathy is consistent across many studies.

Davenport et al,[51] however, demonstrated no difference between LR-PRP and whole blood in patients with proximal hamstring tendinopathy. Hamilton et al conducted a three-arm study between LR-PRP, platelet-poor plasma, and placebo. This study found no benefit of a single PRP injection over intensive rehabilitation in athletes who sustained acute, MRI-positive hamstring injuries.[52] Rossi et al[53] investigated PRP's effect in hamstring injury recovery time. The results revealed that the PRP group achieved full recovery significantly earlier (21.1 days) compared with the control group (25 days). A recent meta-analysis confirmed that there may be some value when using PRP for this condition.[54]

Knee

Vetrano et al[55] published the first randomized controlled trial investigating the efficacy of PRP for patellar tendinopathy in 2013. This study randomized 46 athletes to receive either two PRP injections or three sessions of focused extracorporeal shock wave therapy. The patients treated with PRP had better clinical outcomes at 6 and 12 months. Dragoo et al[56] compared LR-PRP with dry needling for patients in whom nonsurgical treatment for patellar tendinopathy failed. This study of 23 patients found that LR-PRP injection combined with dry needling accelerated the recovery from patellar tendinopathy relative to exercise and dry needling alone. This study used the same LR-PRP device as in other tendinopathy studies.[27,30,48]

Scott et al[57] investigated whether LR-PRP or LP-PRP was effective compared with a saline control group for the improvement of patellar tendinopathy symptoms. Fifty-seven patients were randomized and given a single injection under ultrasound guidance using a PRP device that is marketed to produce both LR-PRP and LP-PRP. The authors found no differences between the three groups in terms of clinical outcomes. This study, however, is significantly flawed because of the type of PRP that was used. The platelet concentrations for the LR-PRP were 3.8 times higher than baseline. The platelet concentrations for the LP-PRP were 3.0 times higher than baseline. These are lower platelet concentrations than have been used in successful PRP tendinopathy trials. The leukocyte fold change for the LR-PRP was only 1.3 times higher than baseline. This is significantly lower than the approximately fivefold leukocyte change seen in studies that have shown significant patient improvements. It was also a single-blind study rather than double-blind study, which could have introduced bias into the conclusions.

The study by Scott et al[57] is an excellent example of the conclusions not being valid because of the type of PRP used in the study. It is simply not scientifically valid to claim LR-PRP was not effective when the leukocyte fold change was only 1.3 times higher than baseline. It also points to the value of leukocytes in the treatment of chronic tendinopathy. Clinicians must be cautioned to read the literature carefully and only use PRP systems and formulations that have proven to be effective. Importantly, preclinical data should also not be used to drive patient recommendations when human clinical trial data are available.

Published data suggested a trend toward PRP being useful for patellar tendinopathy over control, with LR-PRP being the preferred formulation. Not all patellar tendinopathy, however, can be effectively managed with PRP for reasons that are not clear. Larger and better trials are needed to answer these questions (**Figure 4**).

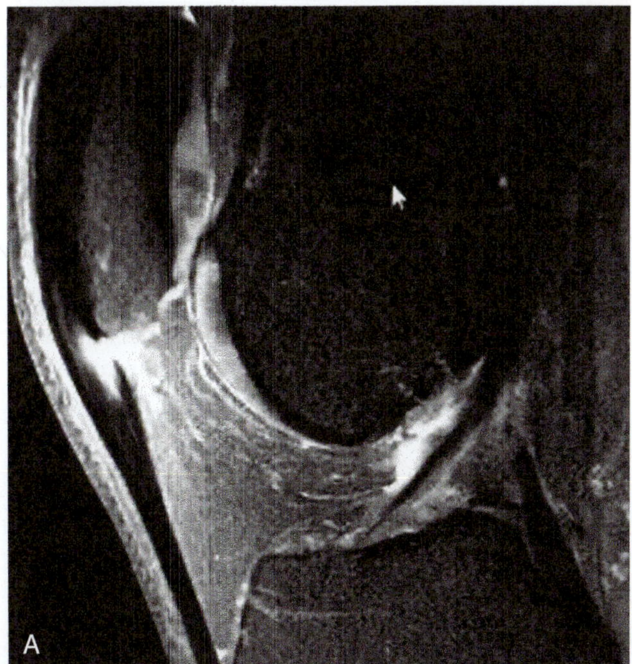

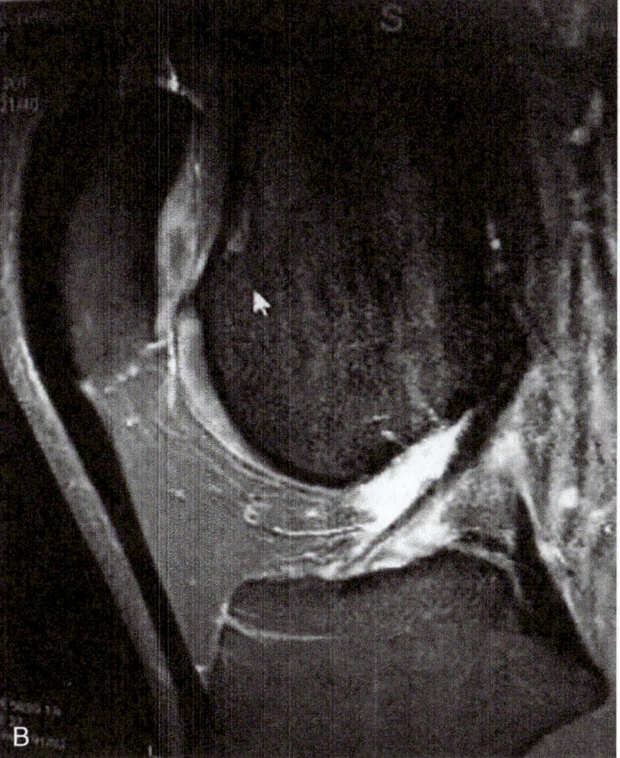

FIGURE 4 Lateral magnetic resonance images of proximal patellar tendinopathy before leukocyte-rich platelet-rich plasma treatment (**A**) and 5 years after treatment (**B**) showing sustained significant improvement.

Foot and Ankle

The first study to investigate the effect of PRP on Achilles tendinopathy was performed in 2010 by de Vos et al[58] (**Figure 4**). Fifty-four patients in this study were injected with either LR-PRP or saline in conjunction with a postinjection eccentric exercise program. At 24 weeks, the results demonstrated that a PRP injection did not result in greater improvement in pain and activity compared with saline. These results were further verified by a study performed by de Jonge et al[59] that examined 54 patients with chronic tendinopathy. These patients were randomized to receive either a LR-PRP or saline injection in addition to an eccentric training program. At 1-year follow-up, this trial showed no clinical or ultrasonographic superiority of PRP injection over placebo injection. Krogh et al[60] found similar results with LR-PRP at final 3-month follow-up.

A 2017 study performed by Boesen et al[61] investigated 57 patients with chronic midpoint Achilles tendinopathy who were given either a high-volume injection, LR-PRP, or eccentric training. This study found that at 24-week follow-up, treatment with a high-volume injection or PRP in combination with eccentric training in chronic Achilles tendinopathy was more effective in reducing pain, improving activity level, and reducing tendon thickness and intratendinous vascularity than eccentric training alone. However, it was also found that a high-volume injection was more effective in improving outcomes of chronic Achilles tendinopathy than PRP in the short term.

Nauwelaers et al[62] published a meta-analysis of PRP for the treatment of chronic midsubstance Achilles tendinopathy. They reviewed 367 studies and found "no clear additional value in management of chronic midsubstance Achilles tendinopathy."

PRP has also been investigated for the treatment of chronic plantar fasciitis in multiple studies.

Meta-analyses confirm that PRP is better than steroid injections for this condition. The best trial was performed by Peerbooms et al.[29] They investigated 115 patients in a prospective randomized trial comparing LR-PRP injection with corticosteroid injection. At 1-year follow-up, 84% of the LR-PRP group was at least 25% improved compared with 55.6% in the corticosteroid group (P = 0.003). Importantly, this study used the same protocol and LR-PRP device as the trials that showed positive results for lateral epicondylar tendinopathy and gluteal tendinopathy. LR-PRP based on the peer-reviewed published data is an effective treatment for chronic plantar fasciitis with superior outcomes compared with cortisone (**Table 2**).

Cellular or acellular preparations from concentrated bone marrow, adipose tissue, or allogeneic amniotic tissue have been applied to treat a variety of lower extremity tendinopathies. There is, however, no high-level evidence supporting the use of any of these approaches. Many of these therapies are touted to be stem cell treatment strategies without any supporting data. It is crucial for clinicians to avoid being duped by aggressive marketing of these treatment strategies until and unless there are enough level I data to support using these expensive interventions.

TABLE 2 Platelet-Rich Plasma Efficacy by Anatomic Area

Anatomic Area	Treatment Value
Elbow	LR-PRP has significant clinical value for lateral epicondylar tendinopathy
Shoulder	PRP has value in the management of rotator cuff tendinopathy. Protocols and formulations have not been optimized
Wrist/hand	Encouraging but not conclusive
Hip	LR-PRP has significant clinical value for gluteal tendinopathy
Knee	Encouraging but not conclusive
Foot/ankle	Not effective for midsubstance Achilles tendon LR-PRP works for plantar fasciitis

LR-PRP = leukocyte-rich platelet-rich plasma

FUTURE CONSIDERATIONS AND CONCLUSIONS

Tendinopathy is a complex, incompletely understood clinical disorder. Basic science data suggest the problem is related not just to microtrauma or macrotrauma but also to regional hypovascularity. Genomic variations, imbalance of neurogenic input, extracellular dysfunction, immune disturbances, and coexisting metabolic conditions all appear to contribute to the pathology of tendinopathy.

A breakthrough in the understanding of the exact mechanisms that cause chronic tendinopathy could lead to more precise and transformative solutions. Preventive strategies such as consistent stretching and vitamin D supplementation in at-risk populations are much less expensive than surgical or even biologic interventions. These interventions could lead to significant cost savings later.

Data supporting the use of orthobiologics for tendinopathy have existed for 15 years.[28] The use of LR-PRP has high-level evidence in the literature for three specific anatomic areas. Level I studies support the use of LR-PRP in the treatment of chronic epicondylar tendinopathy, gluteal tendinopathy, and plantar fasciitis, with clinically meaningful improvements in pain and function scores. More work needs to be done to confirm the value of LR-PRP or other formulations for other anatomic areas. Controversy will continue to exist surrounding the use of PRP until it is determined exactly when and why it works in the context of tendinopathy.

Other biologic treatment strategies do have value, but clarification is needed about how to best use them in the context of level I studies. It must be remembered that exercise is a biologic treatment. Better protocols and patient compliance may lead to improved outcomes when using this option. One possible option is the use of blood flow restriction to augment tendon training. Preliminary evidence suggests this approach has beneficial effects on tendon function, strength, and morphology.[26] Other cellular and acellular preparations such as bone marrow concentrate and tendon stem cells are being vigorously investigated but presently lack enough supporting data to recommend wide clinical use.

Tendinopathy is not a devastating disorder that leads to hospitalization or death. It is, however, a common clinical issue that leads to significant health care costs and disability. Therefore, cost-effective biologic strategies should be pursued and preventive measures emphasized to combat this problem. Matching the pathophysiology of tendinopathy with novel biologic treatment strategies could lead to transformative solutions.

REFERENCES

1. Millar NL, Silbernagel KG, Thorborg K, et al: Tendinopathy. *Nat Rev Dis Primers* 2021;7:1.
2. Riel H, Lindstrøm CF, Rathleff MS, Jensen MB, Olesen JL: Prevalence and incidence rate of lower-extremity tendinopathies in a Danish general practice: A registry-based study. *BMC Musculoskelet Disord* 2019;20:239.
3. Walker-Bone K, Palmer KT, Reading I, Coggon D, Cooper C: Prevalence and impact of musculoskeletal disorders of the upper limb in the general population. *Arthritis Rheum* 2004;51:642-651.
4. Degen RM, Conti MS, Camp CL, Altchek DW, Dines JS, Werner BC: Epidemiology and disease burden of lateral epicondylitis in the USA: Analysis of 85,318 patients. *HSS J* 2018;14:9-14.
5. Niemiec P, Szyluk K, Balcerzyk A, et al: Why PRP works only on certain patients with tennis elbow? Is PDGFB gene a key for PRP therapy effectiveness? A prospective cohort study. *BMC Musculoskelet Disord* 2021;22:710.
6. Kim SK, Roos TR, Roos AK, et al: Genome-wide association screens for Achilles tendon and ACL tears and tendinopathy. *PLoS One* 2017;12:e0170422.
7. Thankam FG, Boosani CS, Dilisio MF, Agrawal DK: Epigenetic mechanisms and implications in tendon inflammation (Review). *Int J Mol Med* 2019;43:3-14.
8. Ilaltdinov AW, Gong Y, Leong DJ, et al: Advances in the development of gene therapy, noncoding RNA, and exosome-based treatments for tendinopathy. *Ann N Y Acad Sci* 2021;1490:3-12.
9. Di Matteo B, Ranieri R, Manca A, et al: Cell-based therapies for the treatment of shoulder and elbow tendinopathies: A scoping review. *Stem Cells Int* 2021;2021:5558040.
10. Lee JM, Hwang JW, Kim MJ, et al: Mitochondrial transplantation modulates inflammation and apoptosis, alleviating tendinopathy both in vivo and in vitro. *Antioxidants (Basel)* 2021;10(5):696.
11. Akbar M, MacDonald L, Crowe LAN, et al: Single cell and spatial transcriptomics in human tendon disease indicate dysregulated immune homeostasis. *Ann Rheum Dis* 2021;80(11):1494-1497.
12. Giai Via A, Oliva F, Padulo J, Oliva G, Maffulli N: Insertional calcific tendinopathy of the Achilles tendon and Dysmetabolic diseases: An epidemiological Survey. *Clin J Sport Med* 2020;32(1):e68-e73.
13. Gumina S, Candela V, Passaretti D, et al: The association between body fat and rotator cuff tear: The influence on rotator cuff tear sizes. *J Shoulder Elbow Surg* 2014;23:1669-1674.
14. Ranger TA, Wong AMY, Cook JL, Gaida JE: Is there an association between tendinopathy and diabetes mellitus? A systematic review with meta-analysis. *Br J Sports Med* 2016;50:982-989.
15. O'Donnell EA, Fu MC, White AE, et al: The effect of patient characteristics and comorbidities on the rate of revision rotator cuff repair. *Arthroscopy* 2020;36:2380-2388.
16. Harada GK, Arshi A, Fretes N, et al: Preoperative vitamin D deficiency is associated with higher postoperative complications in arthroscopic rotator cuff repair. *J Am Acad Orthop Surg Glob Res Rev* 2019;3:e075.
17. Peters JA, Zwerver J, Diercks RL, Elferink-Gemser MT, van den Akker-Scheek I: Preventive interventions for tendinopathy: A systematic review. *J Sci Med Sport* 2016;19:205-211.
18. Beatty NR, Félix I, Hettler J, Moley PJ, Wyss JF: Rehabilitation and prevention of proximal hamstring tendinopathy. *Curr Sports Med Rep* 2017;16:162-171.
19. von Rickenbach KJ, Borgstrom H, Tenforde A, Borg-Stein J, McInnis KC: Achilles tendinopathy: Evaluation, rehabilitation, and prevention. *Curr Sports Med Rep* 2021;20:327-334.
20. Burton I: Interventions for prevention and in-season management of patellar tendinopathy in athletes: A scoping review. *Phys Ther Sport* 2022;55:80-89.
21. Cook JL, Bass SL, Black JE: Hormone therapy is associated with smaller Achilles tendon diameter in active post-menopausal women. *Scand J Med Sci Sports* 2007;17:128-132.
22. Alves C, Mendes D, Marques FB: Fluoroquinolones and the risk of tendon injury: A systematic review and meta-analysis. *Eur J Clin Pharmacol* 2019;75:1431-1443.
23. Eliasson P, Dietrich-Zagonel F, Lundin A-C, Aspenberg P, Wolk A, Michaëlsson K: Statin treatment increases the clinical risk of tendinopathy through matrix metalloproteinase release – A cohort study design combined with an experimental study. *Sci Rep* 2019;9:1-11.
24. Docking SI, Ooi CC, Connell D: Tendinopathy: Is imaging telling us the entire story? *J Orthop Sports Phys Ther* 2015;45:842-852.
25. O'Neill S, Watson PJ, Barry S: Why are eccentric exercises effective for achilles tendinopathy? *Int J Sports Phys Ther* 2015;10:552-562.
26. Burton I, McCormack A: Blood flow restriction resistance training in tendon rehabilitation: A scoping review on intervention parameters, physiological effects, and outcomes. *Front Sports Act Living* 2022;4:879860.
27. Mishra AK, Skrepnik NV, Edwards SG, et al: Efficacy of platelet-rich plasma for chronic tennis elbow: A double-blind, prospective, multicenter, randomized controlled trial of 230 patients. *Am J Sports Med* 2014;42:463-471.
28. Mishra A, Pavelko T: Treatment of chronic elbow tendinosis with buffered platelet-rich plasma. *Am J Sports Med* 2006;34:1774-1778.

29. Peerbooms JC, Lodder P, den Oudsten BL, Doorgeest K, Schuller HM, Gosens T: Positive effect of platelet-rich plasma on pain in plantar fasciitis: A double-blind multicenter randomized controlled trial. *Am J Sports Med* 2019;47:3238-3246.
30. Gosens T, Peerbooms JC, van Laar W, den Oudsten BL: Ongoing positive effect of platelet-rich plasma versus corticosteroid injection in lateral epicondylitis: A double-blind randomized controlled trial with 2-year follow-up. *Am J Sports Med* 2011;39:1200-1208.
31. Kim C-H, Park Y-B, Lee J-S, Jung H-S: Platelet-rich plasma injection vs. operative treatment for lateral elbow tendinosis: A systematic review and meta-analysis. *J Shoulder Elbow Surg* 2022;31:428-436.
32. Randelli P, Arrigoni P, Ragone V, Aliprandi A, Cabitza P: Platelet rich plasma in arthroscopic rotator cuff repair: A prospective RCT study, 2-year follow-up. *J Shoulder Elbow Surg* 2011;20:518-528.
33. Randelli PS, Stoppani CA, Santarsiero G, Nocerino E, Menon A: Platelet rich plasma in arthroscopic rotator cuff repair: Clinical and radiological results of a prospective RCT study at 10-year follow-up. *Arthroscopy* 2022;38(1):51-61.
34. Chen X, Jones IA, Togashi R, Park C, Vangsness CT Jr. Use of platelet-rich plasma for the improvement of pain and function in rotator cuff tears: A systematic review and meta-analysis with bias assessment. *Am J Sports Med* 2020;48:2028-2041.
35. A Hamid MS, Sazlina SG: Platelet-rich plasma for rotator cuff tendinopathy: A systematic review and meta-analysis. *PLoS One* 2021;16:e0251111.
36. Ahmad Z, Ang S, Rushton N, et al: Platelet-rich plasma augmentation of arthroscopic rotator cuff repair lowers retear rates and improves short-term postoperative functional outcome scores: A systematic review of meta-analyses. *Sports Med Arthrosc Rehabil Ther Technol* 2022;4:e823-e833.
37. Lin K-Y, Chen P, Chen AC-Y, Chan Y-S, Lei KF, Chiu C-H: Leukocyte-rich platelet-rich plasma has better stimulating effects on tenocyte proliferation compared with leukocyte-poor platelet-rich plasma. *Orthop J Sports Med* 2022;10:23259671221084706.
38. Uzun H, Bitik O, Uzun Ö, Ersoy US, Aktaş E: Platelet-rich plasma versus corticosteroid injections for carpal tunnel syndrome. *J Plast Surg Hand Surg* 2017;51:301-305.
39. Wu Y-T, Ho T-Y, Chou Y-C, et al: Six-month efficacy of platelet-rich plasma for carpal tunnel syndrome: A prospective randomized, single-blind controlled trial. *Sci Rep* 2017;7:94.
40. Chen S-R, Shen Y-P, Ho T-Y, et al: One-year efficacy of platelet-rich plasma for moderate-to-severe carpal tunnel syndrome: A prospective, randomized, double-blind, controlled trial. *Arch Phys Med Rehabil* 2021;102:951-958.
41. Baryeh K, Asopa V, Kader N, Caplan N, Maffulli N, Kader D: Cell-based therapies for the treatment of sports injuries of the upper limb. *Expert Opin Biol Ther* 2021;21(12):1561-1574.
42. Lin Y-C, Wu W-T, Hsu Y-C, Han D-S, Chang K-V: Comparative effectiveness of botulinum toxin versus non-surgical treatments for treating lateral epicondylitis: A systematic review and meta-analysis. *Clin Rehabil* 2018;32:131-145.
43. Challoumas D, Kirwan PD, Borysov D, Clifford C, McLean M, Millar NL: Topical glyceryl trinitrate for the treatment of tendinopathies: A systematic review. *Br J Sports Med* 2019;53:251-262.
44. Dwivedi S, Sobel AD, DaSilva MF, Akelman E: Utility of prolotherapy for upper extremity pathology. *J Hand Surg Am* 2019;44:236-239.
45. Lhee S-H, Park J-Y: Prospective randomized clinical study for the treatment of lateral epicondylitis: Comparison among PRP (Platelet-Rich Plasm), prolotherapy, Physiotherapy and ESWT. *J Shoulder Elbow Surg* 2013;22:e30-e31.
46. Okasha AE, El-Bahnasawy AS, Gharbia OM, Farrag SE: Comparison of platelet-rich plasma and laser therapy in treatment of chronic lateral epicondylitis. *Egyp Rheumatol Rehabil* 2019;46:202-207.
47. Testa G, Vescio A, Perez S, et al: Extracorporeal shockwave therapy treatment in upper limb diseases: A systematic review. *J Clin Med* 2020;9:453.
48. Fitzpatrick J, Bulsara MK, O'Donnell J, Zheng MH: Leucocyte-rich platelet-rich plasma treatment of gluteus medius and minimus tendinopathy: A double-blind randomized controlled trial with 2-year follow-up. *Am J Sports Med* 2019;47:1130-1137.
49. Reurink G, Goudswaard GJ, Moen MH, et al: Dutch hamstring injection therapy (HIT) study investigators: Platelet-rich plasma injections in acute muscle injury. *N Engl J Med* 2014;370:2546-2547.
50. A Hamid MS, Mohamed Ali MR, Yusof A, George J, Lee LPC: Platelet-rich plasma injections for the treatment of hamstring injuries: A randomized controlled trial. *Am J Sports Med* 2014;42:2410-2418.
51. Davenport KL, Campos JS, Nguyen J, Saboeiro G, Adler RS, Moley PJ: Ultrasound-guided intratendinous injections with platelet-rich plasma or autologous whole blood for treatment of proximal hamstring tendinopathy: A double-blind randomized controlled trial. *J Ultrasound Med* 2015;34:1455-1463.
52. Hamilton B, Tol JL, Almusa E, et al: Platelet-rich plasma does not enhance return to play in hamstring injuries: A randomised controlled trial. *Br J Sports Med* 2015;49:943-950.
53. Rossi LA, Molina Rómoli AR, Bertona Altieri BA, Burgos Flor JA, Scordo WE, Elizondo CM: Does platelet-rich plasma decrease time to return to sports in acute muscle tear? A randomized controlled trial. *Knee Surg Sports Traumatol Arthrosc* 2017;25:3319-3325.
54. Seow D, Shimozono Y, Tengku Yusof TNB, Yasui Y, Massey A, Kennedy JG: Platelet-rich plasma injection for the treatment of hamstring injuries: A systematic review and meta-analysis with best-Worst case analysis. *Am J Sports Med* 2021;49:529-537.
55. Vetrano M, Castorina A, Vulpiani MC, Baldini R, Pavan A, Ferretti A: Platelet-rich plasma versus focused shock waves in the treatment of jumper's knee in athletes. *Am J Sports Med* 2013;41:795-803.

56. Dragoo JL, Wasterlain AS, Braun HJ, Nead KT: Platelet-rich plasma as a treatment for patellar tendinopathy: A double-blind, randomized controlled trial. *Am J Sports Med* 2014;42:610-618.

57. Scott A, LaPrade RF, Harmon KG, et al: Platelet-rich plasma for patellar tendinopathy: A randomized controlled trial of leukocyte-rich PRP or leukocyte-poor PRP versus saline. *Am J Sports Med* 2019;47:1654-1661.

58. de Vos RJ, Weir A, van Schie HTM, et al: Platelet-rich plasma injection for chronic Achilles tendinopathy: A randomized controlled trial. *J Am Med Assoc* 2010;303:144-149.

59. de Jonge S, de Vos RJ, Weir A, et al: One-year follow-up of platelet-rich plasma treatment in chronic Achilles tendinopathy: A double-blind randomized placebo-controlled trial. *Am J Sports Med* 2011;39:1623-1629.

60. Krogh TP, Ellingsen T, Christensen R, Jensen P, Fredberg U: Ultrasound-guided injection therapy of Achilles tendinopathy with platelet-rich plasma or saline: A randomized, blinded, placebo-controlled trial. *Am J Sports Med* 2016;44:1990-1997.

61. Boesen AP, Hansen R, Boesen MI, Malliaras P, Langberg H: Effect of high-volume injection, platelet-rich plasma, and sham treatment in chronic midportion Achilles tendinopathy: A randomized double-blinded prospective study. *Am J Sports Med* 2017;45:2034-2043.

62. Nauwelaers A-K, Van Oost L, Peers K: Evidence for the use of PRP in chronic midsubstance Achilles tendinopathy: A systematic review with meta-analysis. *Foot Ankle Surg* 2020;27(5):486-495.

CHAPTER

19 Fresh Fracture, Challenging Bone Repair, and Nonunions

J. Tracy Watson, MD, FAAOS

INTRODUCTION

There are no well-defined indications for use of a specific type of bone graft substitute or use of bone growth adjuvants for the treatment of complex fractures or nonunion. With the widespread use of orthobiologics in everyday practice, attention must be directed to substantiate the evidence for their current use for the treatment of fractures or nonunions.

It is important to review the fracture healing cascade and where these materials have their locale of action. The available adjuvants and their indications for use are discussed with this context in mind.

FRACTURE HEALING CASCADE

Following initial trauma, the most common pathway for union is by endochondral bone formation. The inflammatory phase of fracture healing initiates this process via neovascular invasion. This response brings with it migrating pericytes that form undifferentiated mesenchymal stem cells (MSCs). Early callus formation is located adjacent to the fracture site and is initially a cartilage anlage developed from undifferentiated MSCs in the peripheral soft tissues that are recruited, proliferate, and differentiate into cartilage-forming cells.[1] These cells gradually become calcified and are replaced by bone (**Figure 1**).

Committed osteoprogenitor cells and undifferentiated MSCs derived from the periosteum contribute to the healing process via intramembranous bone formation that occurs on either side of the fracture.[2] Intramembranous ossification occurs at the periphery of the fracture ends and forms bone without an intervening cartilage phase, also referred to as hard callus (**Figure 2**).

Direct bone healing requires an anatomic reduction with absolute rigid stability limiting the strain at the fracture site. Direct healing allows the bone to immediately regenerate anatomic lamellar bone and new Haversian canals without any intervening remodeling steps.[3] Gaps at the point of contact will still be present and gap healing takes place by recapitulating the fracture healing pathway within these small gaps. Primary cortical healing occurs to reestablish cortical continuity with the aid of so-called cutting cones. Osteoclasts in these cutting cones tunnel directly across points of contact and ultimately provide stability via a resorption process that reestablishes new Haversian systems. Progenitor cells follow and differentiate into osteoblasts and secrete osteoid to bridge the fracture gap.[4] The callus is replaced by new osteons, requiring minimal participation from the periosteum, external soft tissues, and marrow elements.[5]

The inflammatory phase of fracture healing begins immediately after fracture with clot formation and hematoma development. This is accompanied by the invasion of macrophages, polymorphonuclear leukocytes, and lymphocytic cells.[6]

Platelets found in the hematoma degranulate, releasing various signaling molecules and cytokines involved in the processes of chemotaxis and angiogenesis. They also regulate cell proliferation and differentiation of the cells that have migrated to the site of the fracture.[7] The inflammatory phase is characterized by neovascularization and ingrowth of proliferative blood vessels. The attachment of undifferentiated MSCs to the extracellular matrix and conductive substrates occurs through the formation of cell adhesion complexes, which consist of integrins and many cytoplasmic proteins, such as alpha-actinin.[8] Cellular binding to conductive substrates is necessary for circulating inductive factors to stimulate the differentiation of these cells into an osteoblastic lineage[8] (**Figure 1**). Thus, any material that induces this process should be considered osteoinductive.

Cellular elements and conductive substrates require each other's presence to actively function as a viable adjunct for healing of skeletal tissues. Similarly, osteoconductive materials alone work well when filling non–critical-size defects in subchondral locations, but these materials require the migration osteoprogenitor cells into these matrices to incorporate and support the subchondral surfaces. For challenging critical-size defects, all three types of these materials are necessary to achieve efficacy equivalent to autograft.[9,10]

Dr. Watson or an immediate family member has received royalties from Arthrex, Inc., Biomet, NuVasive, and Smith & Nephew; is a member of a speakers' bureau or has made paid presentations on behalf of NuVasive, Zimmer, and Smith & Nephew; serves as a paid consultant to or is an employee of Bioventus, Radius, and Smith & Nephew; and serves as a board member, owner, officer, or committee member of the American Academy of Orthopaedic Surgeons and the Orthopaedic Trauma Association.

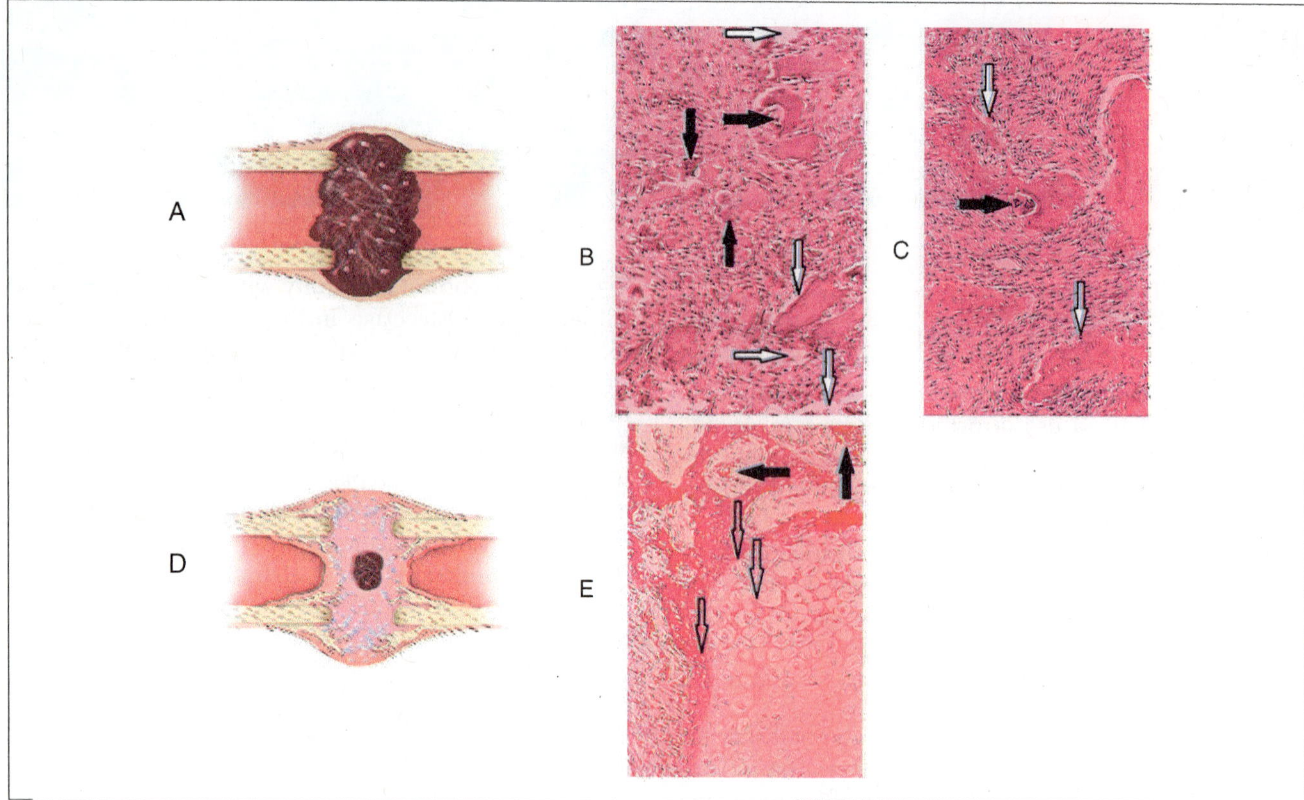

FIGURE 1 **A**, Image depicts the inflammatory phase and shows clot formation with platelet degranulation and initiation of neovascularization. **B**, Histologic slide (50×) from a fracture site demonstrating necrotic bone being resorbed and replaced by fibrous tissue. Empty lacunar spaces without osteocytes denote dead bone. Numerous multinucleate giant cell osteoclasts resorb dead bone spicules (black arrows) and small dark mononuclear inflammatory cells are present. Early vascular channels are developing with the early neovascularization process initiated (white arrows). **C**, The residual necrotic bone is resorbed and replaced by fibrous tissue and new vessel ingrowth. Fibrous tissue is undergoing early remodeling to early callus by osteolysis and orderly osteoblastic lining of the early collagen (white arrows). Osteoclast multinucleate giant cells can be seen (black arrow) in a receding osseous trabecula. **D**, Image depicts soft callus phase and shows proliferation of chondroprogenitor mesenchymal stem cells and differentiation into chondrocytes, with the expression of cartilage-specific matrix. Histologic slides show that at the fracture periphery, the cartilage cells have developed prominent nuclear and cytoplasmic vacuoles and appear as hypertrophic chondrocytes. The matrix between these swollen cells becomes calcified as the chondrocytes release calcium into the extracellular matrix. This forms a zone of provisional (preliminary) calcification (clear arrows). **E**, Soft callous phase (late): islands of young cellular cartilage (black arrows) have become mineralized with interlocking trabeculae of new woven bone rimmed by osteoblasts (black arrows). This intramembranous bone formation has intertrabecular stroma composed of cellular fibrocollagenous tissue (black arrows). Note the vascular channels (clear arrows) in this area of peripheral endochondral ossification.

FACTORS INFLUENCING THE INFLAMMATORY PHASE OF HEALING

Arachidonic Acid Metabolism

Arachidonic acid metabolism exerts complex control over many bodily systems, mainly involved in inflammation and immunity. The enzymes cyclooxygenase (COX)-1 and COX-2 metabolize arachidonic acid to prostaglandin G2 and prostaglandin H_2, which in turn may be converted to various prostaglandins. The classic COX inhibitors are the NSAIDs, which prevent the production of prostaglandin products. They are not selective and inhibit all phases of the inflammatory process, including fracture healing. Because COX-2 is specific to inflamed tissue, there is much less gastric irritation associated with COX-2 inhibitors. This selectivity of COX-2 does not seem to negate other fracture healing side effects of NSAIDs and should be avoided in patients at risk for delayed fracture healing.[11]

Wnt Pathway

Wnt signaling pathways are a group of signal transduction pathways made of proteins that pass signals from outside of a cell through cell surface receptors to the inside of the cell. These pathways are activated by the binding of a Wnt protein ligand to a Frizzled cell surface receptor. This leads to regulation of gene transcription and conversion of undifferentiated MSCs into an osteoblastic lineage.[12] Sclerostin

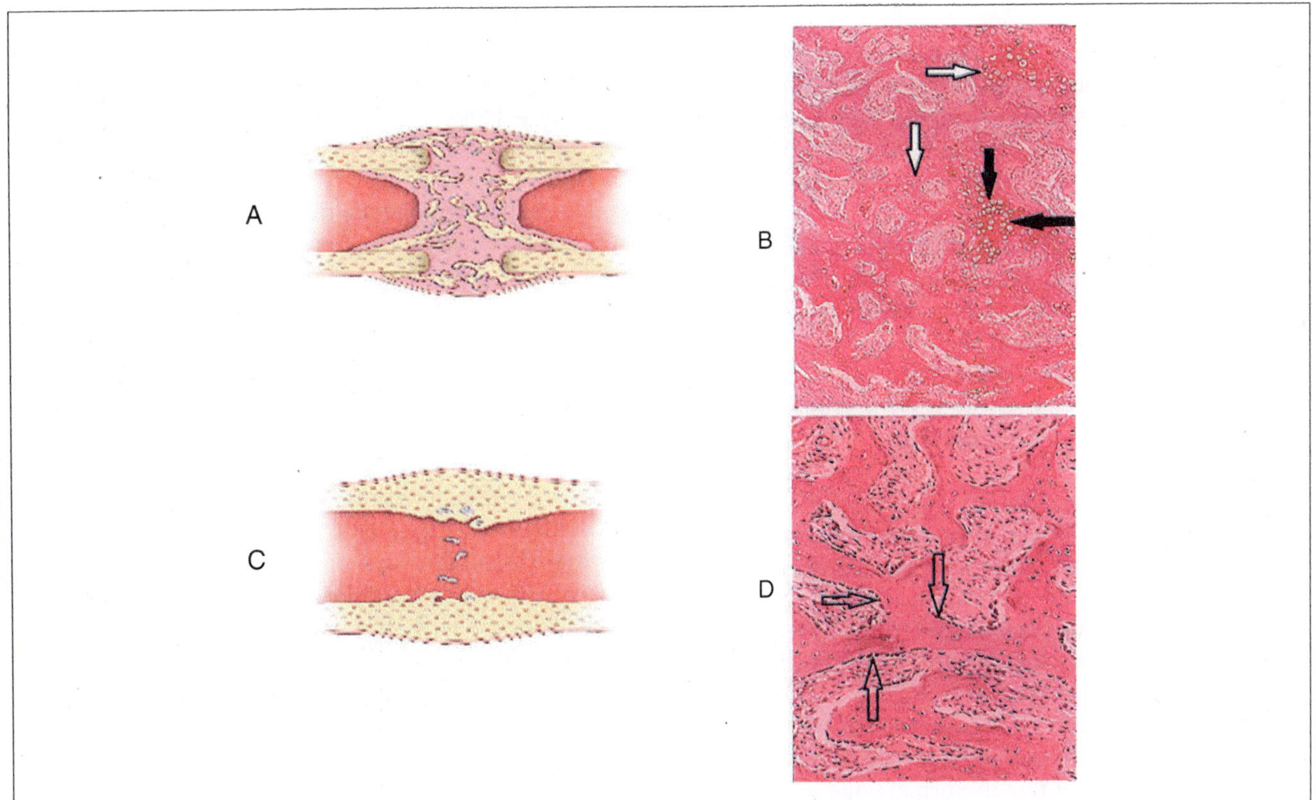

FIGURE 2 **A**, Image depicts mature callous phase and shows removal of calcified cartilage with remodeling of early calcified cartilage to secondary woven bone. **B**, Histologic image (magnification ×50) shows islands of young cellular cartilage (black arrows) have become mineralized with interlocking trabeculae of new woven bone rimmed by osteoblasts (white arrows). This intramembranous bone formation has intertrabecular stroma composed of cellular fibrocollagenous tissue (white arrows) **C**, Image depicts remodeling phase and shows formation of the woven bone with remodeling to form mature lamellar bone with cortical end plates and cortical structure. **D**, Histologic image (magnification x50) shows remodeling phase (mature callous). Osseous trabeculae reveal numerous lacunar spaces with prominent osteocyte characteristics of late woven bone in which the lining osteoblast population is prominent (clear arrows). The woven bone is being converted to mature lamellar bone with remodeling into cortical end plates and restoration of the marrow component.

is produced by the osteocyte and binds to a co-receptor group inhibiting the Wnt signaling pathway,[13] which leads to decreased bone formation. Antibodies against sclerostin have demonstrated promising results in promoting bone formation and increased callus size.[14] An antibody for sclerostin (romosozumab) is available and in clinical use (antisclerostin antibody). Its use has demonstrated increased bone growth and increased bone mineral density of the hip and spine,[15,16] but its effect on fresh fractures and nonunions is not known.

Early Callus Phase

The process of chondrogenesis begins as the early callus phase of healing approximately 7 to 10 days after injury. The migration and proliferation of chondroprogenitor MSCs and differentiation into chondrocytes with the expression of cartilage-specific matrix occur. The formation of a cartilage callus provides immediate mechanical stability to the fracture. Within 2 weeks, protein synthesis is complete and hypertrophic chondrocytes release calcium into the extracellular matrix to precipitate with phosphate ions[17] and calcification begins. Once enough cartilaginous callus is formed, mineralization occurs with the removal of the proteoglycan inhibitors,[18] which prevent mineralization (**Figure 1**).

Platelet concentrate contains alpha granules that contain more than 30 bioactive proteins, many of which have a fundamental role in hemostasis and/or tissue healing. Of these, platelet-derived growth factor (PDGF) and transforming growth factor beta (TGF-β) appear to have the most potent effect on the soft callus stage of healing.[19]

TGF-β activates fibroblasts to induce collagen formation, endothelial cells for angiogenesis, chondroprogenitor cells for cartilage, and MSCs in an effort to increase the population of factors all crucial to the propagation of the soft callus phase of healing. PDGF also activates macrophages, resulting in débridement of the traumatic site, which then triggers a second source of growth factors released from the host tissues.[19,20]

Mature Callus Phase

Calcification of the cartilaginous callus matrix occurs as hypertrophic chondrocytes develop budding of their membrane structures to form vesicularized bodies. These matrix vesicles migrate to the extracellular matrix. The chondrocytes then undergo apoptosis and mineral is laid down on the callus surfaces.[18]

Neovascularization brings in perivascular cells and osteoblast progenitors, which infiltrate the calcified matrix surfaces.[21] Chondroclasts invade along with bone-forming osteoblasts to begin the remodeling of the primary spongiosa (early calcified cartilage) to secondary spongiosa (woven bone), resulting in fracture union by approximately 4 to 5 weeks (**Figure 2**).

Remodeling Phase

As the formation of woven bone takes place, it remodels to mature lamellar bone and restores the original cortical end plates and cortical structure.[22] Osteoblastic cells secrete factors that induce fully differentiated osteoblasts to express ligands that regulate the activity of osteoclasts. Receptor activator of nuclear factor kappa B ligand (RANKL) is essential for the development of osteoclast precursors[22] because osteoclasts and osteoblasts play a vital role in normal bone remodeling. RANKL is strongly induced by fracture to increase its activity[22] and demonstrates a peak in expression just before calcified cartilage removal begins (remodeling phase) (**Figure 2**).

Estrogen inhibits the formation and activation of the bone-resorbing osteoclasts via suppression of RANKL signaling within the osteoclast. Selective estrogen receptor modulators are ligands for estrogen receptors that induce these receptors to affect intracellular transcriptional modulators. Raloxifene is such a class of selective estrogen receptor modulator, mimics estrogen's suppression of RANKL, and thus can also inhibit osteoclast formation. Denosumab is the first RANKL inhibitor to be approved by the FDA. Denosumab inhibits this maturation of osteoclasts by binding to and inhibiting RANKL, thus preventing the binding to RANK.

Parathyroid hormone (PTH) is a polypeptide involved in the regulation of calcium and phosphate metabolism. Bone resorption is caused by osteoclasts, which are indirectly stimulated by PTH. Because osteoclasts do not have a receptor for PTH, PTH binds to the osteoblasts, stimulating them to increase their expression of RANKL. PTH inhibits their expression of osteoprotegerin, which binds to RANKL and blocks it from interacting with RANK. The binding of RANKL to RANK stimulates these osteoclast precursors to fuse, forming new osteoclasts.[23] Although continual exposure to PTH leads to an increase in osteoclast activity and density, intermittent exposure stimulates osteoblasts more than osteoclasts and results in increased bone formation.

Teriparatide is a recombinant form of PTH identical to a portion of human PTH. It is an effective anabolic (ie, bone growing) agent[24] used in the treatment of some forms of osteoporosis. Clinically, recombinant PTH has been approved by the FDA for its use in the treatment of osteoporosis and several recent clinical trials have demonstrated that daily systemic treatment with PTH increases bone mineral density and reduces fracture risk in patients with osteoporosis. It is also used off-label to speed fracture healing and treat nonunions and has demonstrated increased fracture callus volume, enhanced mechanical properties, as well as increased bone mineral density, bone mineral content, and total osseous tissue volume.[25-29]

Diphosphonates are widely used for the treatment of osteoporosis and the prevention of fragility fractures and have two phosphonate [$PO(OH)_2$] groups. Diphosphonates inhibit the digestion of bone by encouraging osteoclasts to (1) undergo cell death or (2) inhibit the ruffled border with subsequent dysfunction of resorption. Both mechanisms thereby slow bone loss.[30-32]

There are concerns that long-term diphosphonate use can result in oversuppression of bone turnover. It is hypothesized that microfractures in the bone are unable to heal and eventually unite and propagate, resulting in atypical fractures. This phenomenon has been seen most prominently in the proximal femur, often in patients using biphosphates for prolonged periods of time.[33,34]

In cases where there is concern of such fractures, teriparatide is potentially an alternative because of reducing damage caused by suppression of bone turnover.[35]

In cases of atypical femur fracture where teriparatide has been shown to be effective in combination with surgical management, it is proposed that PTH increases bone remodeling resulting in the removal of more densely mineralized bone replaced with new, less-compact normal mineralized bone.[36,37]

Morphology for Acute Fractures and the Development of Nonunion

Many factors that can affect fracture healing are associated with the characteristics of the injury, including the pattern of bony injury, location of the fracture, status of the soft-tissue envelope, extent of bone loss, and the degree of stability (strain) afforded to the fracture site.[38]

Motion at the fracture site will allow callus to form and intermittent shear stresses are thought to encourage ossification.[39] The larger the stress, the greater the amount of callus formed up to an undefined limit of strain. Interfragmentary micromotion and low amounts of strain can stimulate both intramembranous and endochondral ossification.[40] If, however, the motion is excessive, a high-strain environment will result in fibrous tissue proliferation and damage the neovascularity, resulting in a deficient inflammatory phase of healing. The ideal degree of mechanical stability has yet to be determined.[41] Studies have shown that excessively rigid fixation may paradoxically impair fracture healing[42,43] via the inhibition of external callus formation, maintenance of a fracture gap aggravated by bone-end resorption, and excessive protection of the healing bone from normal stresses (stress shielding), all leading to adverse remodeling and nonunion. This has been clinically shown with the initial widespread use of locking plates and the overuse of locking screws, minimizing the micromotion and localizing the strain directed at the fracture site. Radiographs documented minimal callus formation and no cortical bridging. All these factors contributed to the high rate of plate failure and nonunion when this fixation montage was used.

Highly comminuted fractures with wide fracture gaps with increased strain fill these gaps with fibrous connective tissue, intervening areas of necrotic bone, and giant cells. This prevents neovascularization response and inhibits the chemotaxis and migration of MSCs. A wide diastasis makes any cellular interaction with circulating inductive factors very difficult (**Figure 3**).

Atrophic nonunion develops commonly under these circumstances and these types of nonunion have fracture gaps interspersed with dense avascular fibrous tissue, secondary to bone loss or infection. These nonunion types typically occur in concert with mechanical instability and thus both the biologic potential and mechanical stability must be restored. A stimulus to initiate the inflammatory phase of fracture healing and revascularization is necessary along with providing mechanical stability. Biologic adjuvants are then required and are delivered either through the direct application of viable osteoblasts (bone graft) or by providing inductive factors to initiate the chemotaxis and proliferation of MSCs.

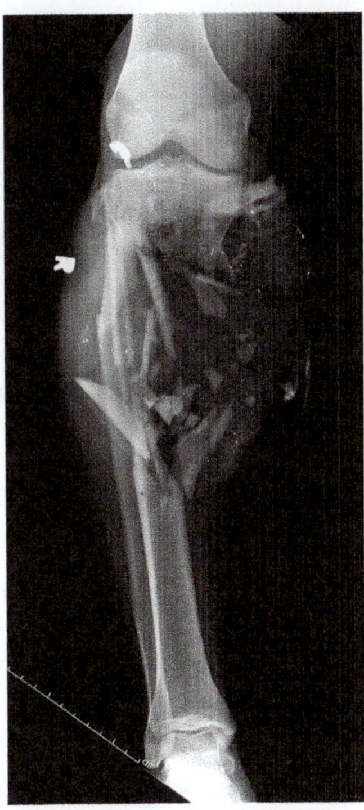

FIGURE 3 AP radiograph of the lower leg shows nonmodifiable factors of a fracture that went on to nonunion. Significant open soft-tissue injury, comminution, bone loss, and wide fragment diastasis are seen.

Basic principles of fracture fixation assert that comminuted fractures respond well to bridge plating and relative stability,[43] whereas simple fractures should be anatomically reduced, compressed, and rigidly stabilized.[41] Hypertrophic nonunion occurs when the biologic potential is intact and fracture callus is highly proliferative, but because of mechanical instability, large amounts of strain and excessive motion result in fibrous tissue at the fracture site. The treatment of this nonunion requires the augmentation of stability to allow fracture bridging to occur. No additional biologic stimulus is necessary.

CURRENT BIOLOGIC ADJUVANTS

Many of these materials have been shown to be efficacious when used for both the management of acute fracture and the augmentation of nonunion. The best use and indications for these materials will be outlined.

Autogenous Bone Graft

Fresh cancellous autograft provides the quickest and most reliable type of bone graft. These grafts depend on ingrowth of host vessels and perform best in well-vascularized beds. The large surface area of autograft allows for survival of numerous graft cells. Studies document success rates approaching 100% for sub–critical-size defects (1- to 2-cm defects) requiring 20 mL or less of autograft.[38,44,45] However, in many of these studies, multiple graft procedures were required to achieve solid union in defects larger than 3 to 4 cm.[46,47]

Iliac crest harvest volumes may limit the utility of this graft because crest volume averages 13 mL anteriorly and 30 mL posteriorly. The reamer-irrigator-aspirator (Synthes) offers a technique to achieve substantial amounts of graft volumes for the treatment of larger segmental defects for management of acute fractures as well as for chronic nonunion defects. The medullary canal of the femur or tibia is reamed with a device designed to collect the reamings and deliver them for grafting procedures.[48,49]

Varying amounts of harvested graft have been reported with this technique and range from 30 to 90 mL. Favorable union rates using RIA bone grafting versus autogenous iliac crest bone grafting (AICBG) have demonstrated its equivalency. Further study is required to demonstrate any superiority for larger defects versus the relative efficacy of AICBG.[48]

Investigators have documented elevated amounts of osteoinductive growth factors[50-54] and osteoprogenitor/endothelial progenitor cell types compared with standard iliac crest grafts. Cell viability and osteogenic potential are similar between bone grafts obtained from both the RIA system and the iliac crest.[9] Elevated levels of fibroblast growth factor alpha, PDGF, insulinlike growth factor-I, TGF-β1, and bone morphogenetic protein (BMP)-2 have been measured in the reaming debris as a rich source of growth factors with a content comparable with that from iliac crest.

In summary, both iliac crest bone graft and RIA are excellent sources for autogenous bone graft, the gold standard for augmentation of fracture healing as well as for the treatment of nonunion. RIA is an excellent harvest technique, especially when large volumes are needed, and data support that it supplies active, osteogenic tissue (**Tables 1** and **2**).

Bone Marrow Aspirate Concentrate

The critical component necessary to all bone formation is the ability to provide viable osteoprogenitor cells. Bone marrow is a plentiful source of musculoskeletal stem cells,[55] with a high concentration of connective tissue progenitors. One milliliter of iliac aspirate contains approximately 40 million nucleated cells, 1,500 of which are connective tissue progenitors.[56]

Bone marrow aspirate (BMA) has been used as a source of bone marrow–derived MSCs with its relative ease of harvest and low morbidity. The aspirate is typically concentrated by centrifugation to increase the number of MSCs. Concentrated bone marrow aspirate (cBMA) provides both stem cells and growth factors. Injection of cBMA into nonunion sites has had some limited success, but there are no good data showing its effectiveness for its solitary injection into an acute fracture site.

Current use relies on the development of a composite graft. Loading the cBMA onto a highly osteoconductive carrier with a specific three-dimensional architecture facilitates cellular attachment for graft delivery.[57,58] Common materials include cancellous allograft, demineralized bone matrix (DBM), and particulate calcium phosphate ceramics as porous carrier materials. Osseous regeneration is dependent on the number of cells available to participate in bone synthesis. However, the ultimate threshold concentration of cells necessary to promote osteogenesis is not known.[59,60]

Many commercially available systems have been developed that have the capability to concentrate progenitor cells three to four times and present them to the surgeon in a usable manner. These devices concentrate the cells via a fully automated closed-loop system for separating nucleated cells from bone marrow. These systems use either a centrifuge or a filtration type of mechanism to accomplish their goals.[61-63]

Current literature demonstrates perhaps faster healing times with similar union rates when using cBMA combined with cancellous allograft and or DBM compared with conventional autologous cancellous bone graft for treating nonunions with small defects.[64-69]

Currently, this technique appears to be as effective as AICBG for treating smaller acute fracture defects as well as nonunion defects, although no study has quantified the threshold defect size.[70] There continue to be discrepancies with regard to the method of centrifugation, variable cell count concentrations, and lack of standardized outcome measures. High-level, robust clinical evidence supporting these therapies is distinctly lacking, and an effective therapeutic range has yet to be established for nonunion treatment (**Tables 1** and **2**; **Figure 4**).

TABLE 1 Biologic Characteristics of Currently Available Biologic Adjuvants

	Potency of Available Biologic Adjuvants			
	Osteoconductive Scaffold	Osteopromotive Facilities Bone Formation	Osteoinductive Growth Factors	Osteogenic Living Cells
Synthetic materials	Ca Ceramics Collagen Degradable polymers	Electromagnetic stimulation Ultrasound stimulation	rBMP-2 rBMP-7 GDF-5	—
Allograft and autograft materials	Allograft struts, dowels, chips Autograft DBM Allograft stem cell prep	Platelet-rich plasma rPDGF	DBM Cancellous autograft RIA cBMA Allograft stem cell prep	Bone marrow elements (cBMA) Cancellous autograft RIA Allograft stem cell prep
Increasing Biologic Activity (ability to form bone) →				

cBMA = concentrated bone marrow aspirate, DBM = demineralized bone matrix, GDF = growth differentiation factor, rBMP = recombinant bone morphogenetic protein, RIA = reamer-irrigator-aspirator, rPDGF = recombinant platelet-derived growth factor

TABLE 2 Indications for Common Biologic Adjuvants

	Types of Graft Materials	Acute Fracture Management	Nonunion Augmentation	Segmental Bone Loss (Acute and Chronic)
Synthetic materials	Ca, Si Ceramics Collagen Degradable polymers	Periarticular defect augmentation	In combination with cBMA	–
Allograft materials	Allograft cortical struts, dowels chips DBM Allograft stem cell prep	Metaphyseal augmentation. Proximal humerus, distal femur Periprosthetic cortical defects ± –	Metaphyseal augmentation. Proximal humerus, distal femur Periprosthetic cortical defects In combination +	± – –
Autograft	Iliac Crest RIA cBMA Bone transport	+ + –	+ + +	+ + ± +
Growth factors	Platelet gel rhPDGF BMP-2	– – ±	– + Foot and ankle ±	– – +

BMP = bone morphogenetic protein, cBMA = concentrated bone marrow aspirate, DBM = demineralized bone matrix, rhPDGF = recombinant human platelet-derived growth factor, RIA = reamer-irrigator-aspirator

Allograft Bone Grafts

Allograft tissue is accessible, eliminates donor site morbidity, reduces operating time, and is advantageous when large defects are encountered.[71,72] Allografts can be used to augment repair of defects that produce construct instability, fill voids in osteoarticular regions, and serve as graft extenders. The use of cancellous allograft in treatment of nonunion may be necessitated when the defect is large, especially when used in concert with autograft as a graft extender. Results are variable, and limited studies have demonstrated prolonged time to union with higher rates of surgical revision in patients treated with allograft combined with autograft compared with autograft alone.[73]

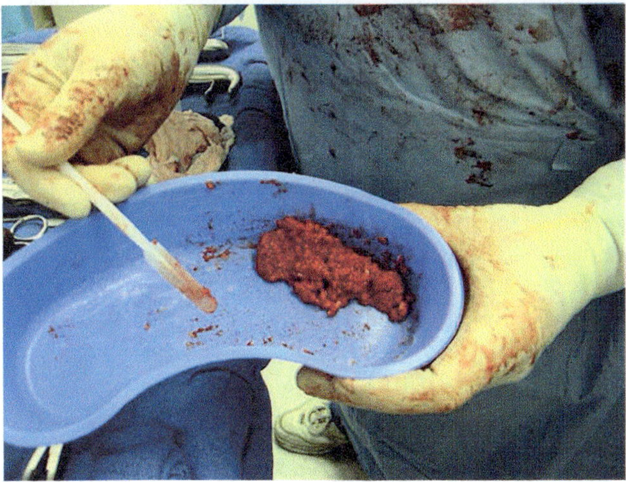

FIGURE 4 Clinical photograph shows composite bone graft consisting of concentrated bone marrow aspirate + cancellous allograft + demineralized bone matrix particulate. Consistency is that of autograft, which is handled in a similar manner.

Cortical allograft struts function to optimize mechanical stability of fracture sites. Periprosthetic fractures in the setting of a large canal-filling stem, transverse and short oblique fractures, fractures lacking medial contact, and atypical fractures may benefit from increased structural support afforded by allograft struts, particularly when treating proximal humerus and humeral shaft fractures.[54,74]

In the setting of atrophic nonunion with gross fracture site instability, the addition of an allograft strut adjunct functions to optimize stability. These grafts offer minimal biologic stimulus by themselves; however, for the treatment of nonunion with bone loss or poor bone quality, allograft struts are used in many locations and intramedullary allograft struts have demonstrated high rates of bony union, when treating diaphyseal and proximal humeral nonunion,[75-77] as well as distal femoral nonunion[78] (**Tables 1** and **2**).

Allograft Cellular Therapies

In an effort to avoid marrow harvest and provide a consistent graft material, allogeneic human stem cells harvested from cadavers are now available as a stem cell graft. Most technical information is proprietary and not readily available with regard to graft specifics in terms of harvesting, immunogenicity, and cell morphology. The grafts are composed of viable MSCs derived from cadaver donor tissue and are delivered on an osteoconductive substrate usually being DBM.

These grafts are preconcentrated, with a threshold concentration of cells present on arrival, without having to manipulate the cells before implantation. The grafts are delivered preadmixed with an osteoconductive substrate with a matrix designed for optimal cellular attachment. The matrix is designed to encourage rapid vascular ingrowth with maximal cellular viability. In theory, this type of graft has osteogenic, osteoinductive, and osteoconductive properties and is capable of directing new bone formation at the site of implantation.[79] Clinical data are lacking, limited to commercial white papers (level V), case reports (level V), and uncontrolled case series evaluating its use in foot and ankle fusions and spinal fusions (level IV).[80] There are currently no data on the use of this material for acute fractures (**Tables 1** and **2**).

Demineralized Bone Matrix

DBM is used widely as an osteoconductive substrate and is often used as an adjuvant to the fracture site when treating acute fractures. DBM is formed by acid extraction of the mineralized extracellular matrix of allograft bone. It contains type I collagen, noncollagenous proteins, and osteoinductive growth factors including the BMPs and other inductive factors found in the TGF-β group of proteins. DBM is highly osteoconductive because of its particulate nature and presents a large surface area and three-dimensional architecture to serve as a site of cellular attachment. Thus, using DBM as a carrier matrix is advantageous for delivering cellular materials.

In theory, the noncollagenous osteoinductive proteins such as the BMPs remain viable. The osteoinductive variability has been found not only across different DBM products but also among production lots from the same DBM formulation. This variability questions the reliability of DBM products, and possibly, the efficacy in providing consistent osteoinduction.[81-84] There is now evidence of differential potencies of DBM preparations based on the manufacturer and manufacturing process, and the carrier that is used to assist in the handling and delivery properties.[83]

If precise control of harvest, preparation, and sterilization conditions are not maintained, many proteins might be susceptible to chemical and physical degradation, which would render the proteins ineffective.[84] Most clinical series combine DBM with other adjuvants and the singular effectiveness of DBM alone is difficult to elucidate (**Tables 1** and **2**).

Ceramic Osteoconductive Scaffolds

There is considerable interest in creating osteoconductive matrices using nonbiologic porous structures that mimic the cancellous bony architecture that have specific surface kinetics to facilitate the migration, attachment, and proliferation of MSCs.[85]

Broad categories of these materials are available and in general are classified as calcium or silicone ceramics and are supplied as particulate or in injectable forms. These include the specific materials of calcium sulfate and phosphate, synthetic tricalcium phosphate as well as beta tricalcium phosphate, and coralline hydroxyapatite. These materials are used to augment and fill the metaphyseal defects that remain following the reduction of articular fractures. Hardware augmentation is also required as a fixation strategy. The superiority of these materials to maintain articular reductions in multiple metaphyseal locations has been clearly demonstrated in level I and level II studies comparing alloplastic ceramics with cancellous allograft[86-92] (**Figure 5**).

Additionally, all these materials have been used as carriers for composite bone graft materials, all with comparable results[92,93] in successful graft incorporation when used as substrates for cBMA (**Tables 1** and **2**).

Bone Morphogenetic Protein

BMPs promote bone healing by inducing MSCs to differentiate into osteoblasts. Currently, only recombinant human BMP-2 is available for clinical application. Despite the initial enthusiasm for the use of recombinant human BMPs for acute fracture and nonunion care, the evidence has not demonstrated the clinical superiority of these materials. Osteoinductive proteins still need to be considered as an alternative method in special cases, for patients with poor donor bone quality, poor surgical tolerance, or multiple failed surgeries. The results are comparable to those of autogenous bone graft for a variety of indications and locations for both acute fractures and nonunion care.[94-98] However, current evidence does not support the widespread use and application of BMP for improved outcomes in fracture and nonunion surgery[41] (**Tables 1** and **2**; **Figure 6**).

Platelet Concentrates

Platelet gels provide a rich source of growth factors that serve a critical function in wound and fracture healing and can stimulate the formation of blood vessels; the invasion of pluripotential MSCs, monocytes, and macrophages; and further aggregation of platelets.[99-102] These factors have direct chemotactic and mitogenic effects on osteoblasts and osteoblast precursors and act synergistically to help stimulate bone remodeling and healing.[19,103,104]

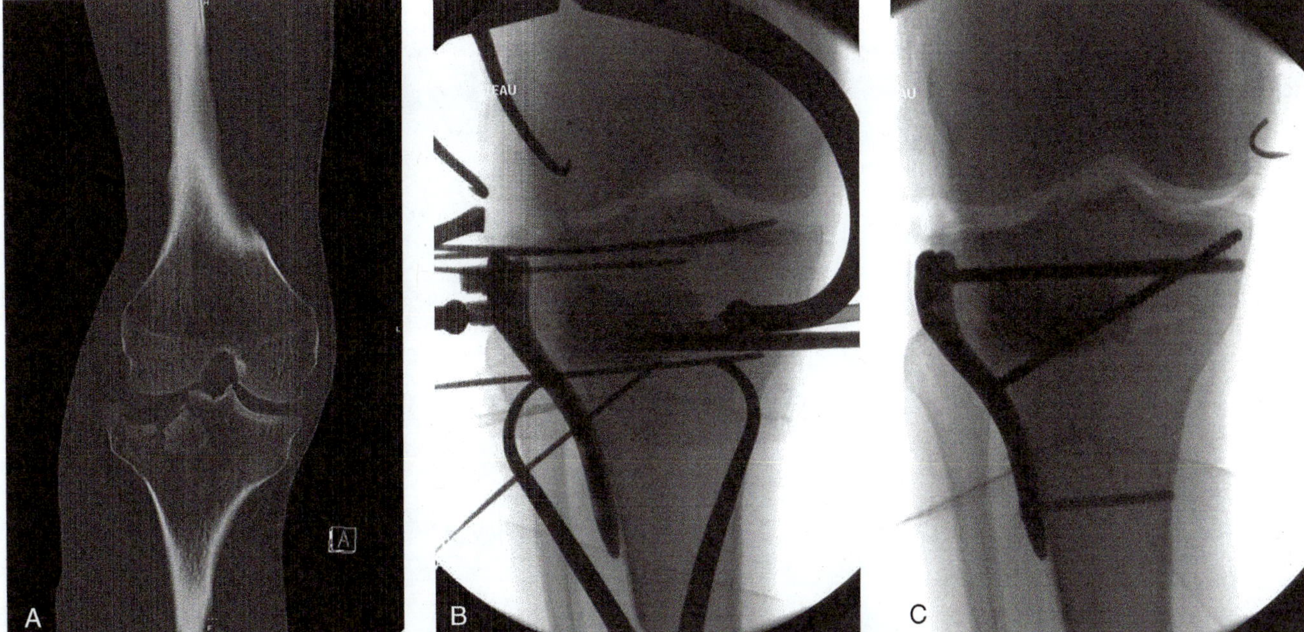

FIGURE 5 **A**, CT scan shows articular impaction. **B**, Intraoperative fluoroscopic image shows elevation of articular surface supported by Kirschner wires and the subchondral defect filled with a calcium ceramic alloplastic bone void filller. **C**, Intraoperative fluoroscopic image shows Kirschner wire removal, which demonstrates articular surface reduction has been maintained following the setting of the injectable material.

The clinical use of platelet-rich plasma has been reported for a wide variety of clinical applications, most predominately for the problematic wound, maxillofacial applications, and spine. It appears to have more consistent effects when used for soft-tissue modalities and when used as an adjuvant for the treatment of tendinopathies such as jumper's knee, tennis elbow, and Achilles tendinitis (**Table 1**).

Currently, there is no level I evidence to indicate using platelet-rich plasma alone or in combination with other materials has a substantial effect on fracture healing when used for acute fractures or for nonunion augmentation (**Table 2**). Overall, however, there is clearly a lack of scientific evidence to support the use of platelet-rich plasma in combination with bone grafts.[105,106]

Recombinant Human PDGF

AUGMENT, a fully synthetic bone graft material composed of recombinant human (rh)PDGF and a TCP matrix (rhPGDF/TCP), has been approved as a possible alternative to autogenous bone graft and has been used in many early preclinical and clinical studies.[107-109]

The data have consistently indicated that rhPDGF-BB treatment ameliorates the effects of diabetes on fracture healing by promoting early cellular proliferation that ultimately results in more bone formation.[108] Multiple randomized controlled trial (level I) studies have demonstrated efficacy in patients requiring hindfoot or ankle arthrodesis and repair of recalcitrant nonunions. Treatment with rhPDGF-BB/β-TCP resulted in comparable fusion rates and less pain, when compared with treatment with autograft[110-115] (**Tables 1** and **2**).

IMPAIRMENTS TO FRACTURE REPAIR

In the United States, delayed healing has been reported in approximately 600,000 fractures per year, 100,000 of which progress to nonunion.[38] Patient-dependent risk factors for nonunion include various medical comorbidities, age, sex, smoking, use of NSAIDs, genetic disorders (eg, neurofibromatosis, osteogenesis imperfecta, osteopetrosis), metabolic disease, and nutritional status.[116,117]

Bone regeneration depends on three essential elements: progenitor cells, growth factors (osteoinduction), and the appropriate biologic environment. This must include the presence of adequate vascularization, oxygen delivery, nutrient diffusion, and a competent osteoconductive surface to establish cellular attachment and differentiation. Delayed fracture repair and nonunion can result from a lack of osteoprogenitor cells, insufficient osteoinductive growth factors, defective local biologic environment, or a combination of these factors.

The epidemiology of fracture nonunions has been characterized in many prior studies. It is potentially possible to predict nonunion using patient-related risk factors. A nationwide claims database of approximately 90.1 million participants was used for a prediction model. Certain risk factors were important for predicting nonunion, which

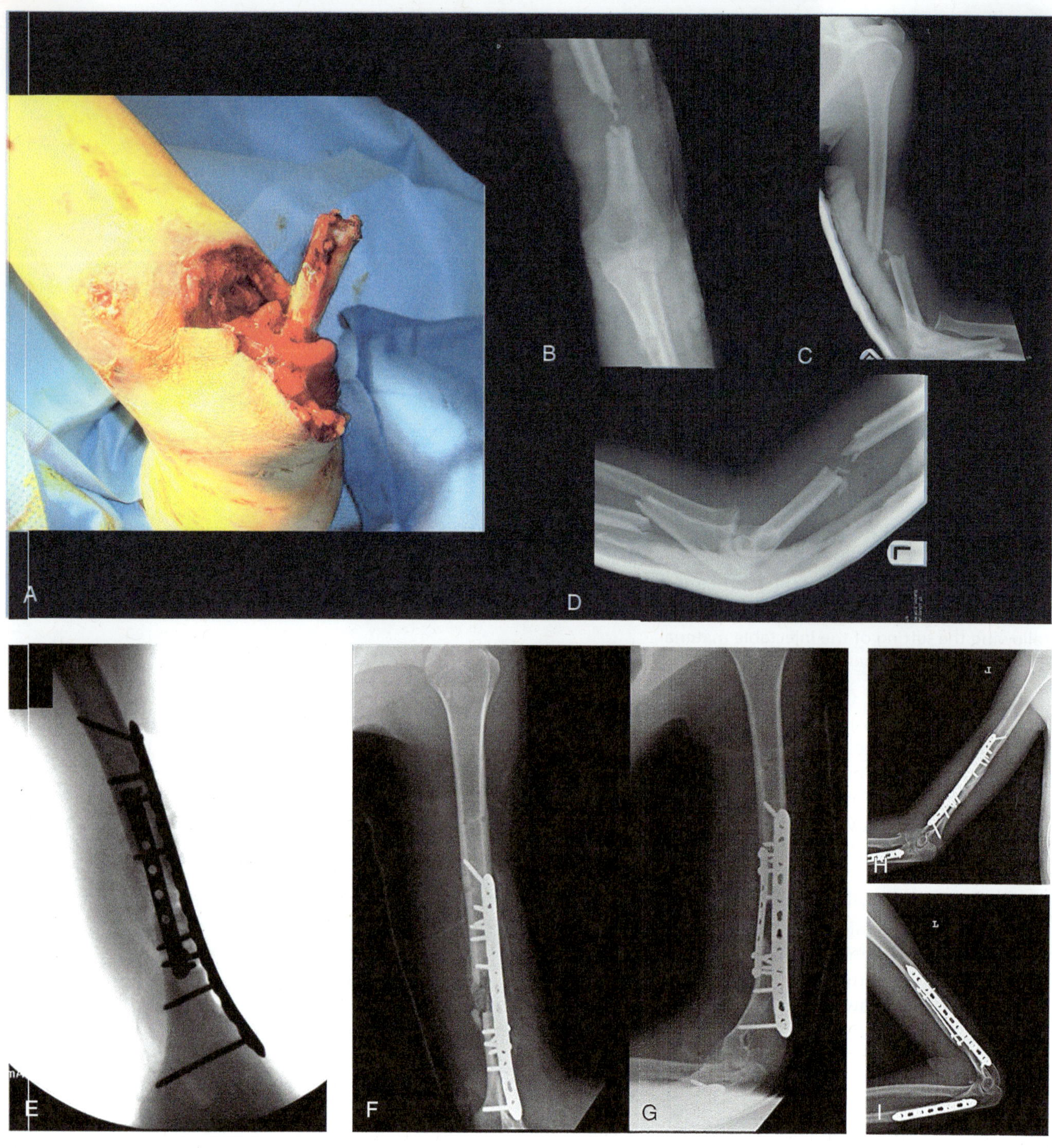

FIGURE 6 Images showing severe open fracture of the distal humerus with significant soft-tissue stripping and devascularization of the entire distal humerus. Bone loss is apparent at the fracture site. **A**, Intraoperative photograph. Preoperative AP (**B**) and lateral (**C** and **D**) radiographs show fractures of the humerus and ulna. **E**, Intraoperative fluoroscopic image shows dual plating with bone morphogenetic protein 2 and allograft augmentation, used for defect management. **F**, Radiograph obtained immediately postoperatively shows the graft and fixation. **G** through **I**, Radiographs obtained at 1-year follow-up show complete consolidation of a 2-cm segmental defect.

included the presence of open fractures, multiple fractures, osteoarthritis, surgical treatment for the fracture, and use of certain medications, including anticoagulants, anticonvulsants, or analgesics.[115,116] Comorbidities associated with increased risk of nonunion include past or current smoking, alcoholism, obesity or morbid obesity, osteoarthritis, rheumatoid arthritis, and type 2 diabetes.[117] Of these patient factors, smoking, diabetes, and alcohol are modifiable.

Modifiable Risk Factors

Smoking

Multiple studies have demonstrated that smoking and nicotine use are deleterious to several biochemical pathways important for fracture healing, with nicotine negatively affecting arteriolar blood flow.[118] Chronic hypoxia and hypercarbia increase arteriolar vasospastic activity, which has the added deleterious effect on the fragile neovascularization response. Hypoxia affects osteogenic differentiation of human MSCs by reducing the number of viable cells and altering the molecular signals produced.[119] Nicotine also has a negative effect on collagen synthesis and osteoblast formation and bone metabolism.[120-125]

Use of NSAIDs

Fracture healing is associated with inflammation and prostaglandin synthesis; NSAIDs that interfere with these processes should theoretically interfere with fracture healing, as well. A study by Giannoudis et al found a significant ($P = 0.000001$) association between femoral nonunion and the use of NSAIDs after injury.[122] Corticosteroids also inhibit fracture healing not only because of the potent anti-inflammatory response but also because of calcium homeostatic changes.

Metabolic Bone Disease

Metabolic bone disease has been reported to be highly prevalent in trauma patients who present with an unexplained nonunion. Many of these patients demonstrate a high incidence of previously undiagnosed metabolic or endocrine pathology.[126] The nutritional deficiencies including dietary calcium and vitamin D have been associated with nonunion and impaired fracture healing. Brinker noted that 68% of patients referred for nonunion were found to be vitamin D deficient. Numerous studies have shown the benefits of systemic administration of calcium and vitamin D on bone healing after fracture.[127]

Diabetes

Diabetes, with its associated peripheral neuropathy and peripheral vascular disease, directly affects fracture healing. However, the exact pathogenesis of impaired osseous healing has not been elucidated. Diabetes affects small and large vessels alike, leading to tissue hypoxia, a common secondary phenomenon. Regional and local ischemia with large-vessel arteriosclerosis, particularly of the lower extremities, and localized small-vessel angiopathy are noted in the diabetic population.[128]

Collagen synthesis is abnormal during the early stages of fracture healing in untreated diabetic animals. Spanheimer et al[129] reported that a decrease in type X collagen synthesis was in the fracture callus in this diabetic rat model. This is critical for endochondral ossification and vascular invasion during the inflammatory phase of fracture healing.[130]

Alcohol

Alcohol intoxication, present in up to 40% of trauma patients with orthopaedic injuries, has been shown to alter the immunoinflammatory pathway.[131-133] Acute and chronic alcohol intake independently influence aspects of the inflammatory response[134] and may cause different inflammatory profiles following serious injury.

Chronic alcohol intake likely causes a delay in the early fracture repair cascade rather than downstream at the time of remodeling. Thus, the effects of alcohol observed on early fracture repair may have important repercussions in determining the ultimate outcome of delayed healing or nonunion.[135,136]

TREATMENT OF NONUNION WITHOUT BONE DEFECT

Whether initial fracture treatment was nonsurgical or surgical, the final etiology of nonunion is mechanical or biologic and includes infection. Radiographic findings consistent with infection include failed implants, osteolysis, periosteal elevation, and wound issues consistent with erythema, tenderness, and drainage.

Prior to initiating any treatment plan, simple blood studies can help to further clarify the infection status. With the use of a combination of elevated white blood cell count, increased erythrocyte sedimentation rate, and C-reactive protein levels, the positive predictive values for three elevated risk factors were 100%.[137] Nuclear medicine studies were the least predictive method of revealing infection, are not cost effective, and are not routinely used.

For patients with hypertrophic nonunions, traditional nonunion principles suffice for effective nonunion treatment. If deformity coexists, particularly in the lower extremities, it is necessary to also realign the mechanical axis and restore normal axial forces.

Following the nonsurgical takedown of the nonunion to achieve mobility and yet maintain the biology, the deformity should be corrected with compression across the nonunion. Compression is an extremely effective method to achieve healing. For oblique nonunion, lag screws achieve excellent interfragmentary compression and are often all that is required to achieve union.

Lower extremity nonunion is primarily treated using intramedullary nails, which facilitate active weight bearing and achieve constant compression across the nonunion with the associated strain reduction and increased biomechanical stability. Most cases of diaphyseal noninfected nonunion of the femur and tibia that are well aligned are treated with conversion to a reamed nail. Simple exchange nailing results in high rates of union (up to 90% or more) for normotrophic and hypertrophic nonunion of both the tibia and femur that present without significant defect.

There is a distinct lack of consensus regarding both the definition and management of critical-size bone defects for acute traumatic and reconstruction nonunion deficiencies.[70] Most studies are difficult to stratify, as they include both infected and noninfected defects and may or may not have nonunion with associated soft-tissue defects.

For patients with nonunions without a defect that requires augmentation, the gold standard in this situation has clearly been iliac crest bone graft, and multiple case series have reported on its efficacy, with healing rates in the range of 85%. As noted previously, BMPs have since been used less commonly for fracture and nonunion treatment given the unknown factors around antibody production, heterotopic bone formation, and other concerns. cBMA and composite cBMA grafts are a promising therapy that deliver all the advantages of autogenous graft but without the issues related to iliac crest harvest[138] (**Figure 7**).

TREATMENT OF NONUNION WITH BONE DEFECT

Tibial defects of 2.5 cm or greater have a poor natural history when AICBG is being used, and the rates of union decrease significantly for larger defects.[139] The literature indicates that the maximum upper limit of success is 4 cm or less for one anterior iliac crest harvest.[140,141] The success rates approach almost 100% when smaller defects

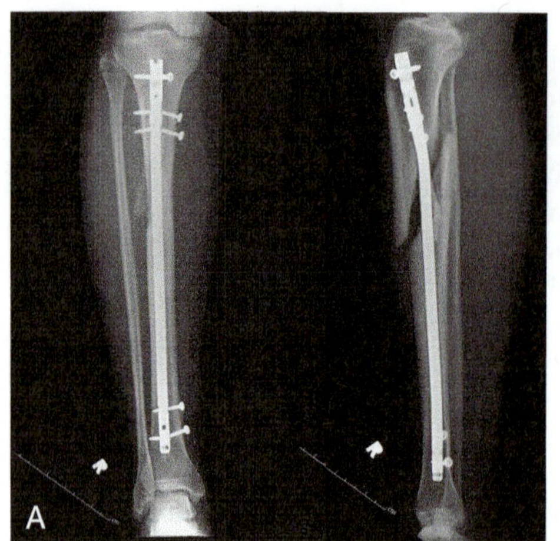

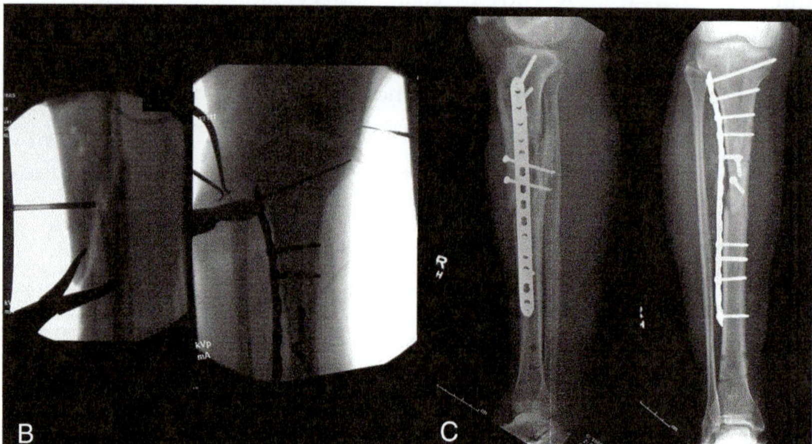

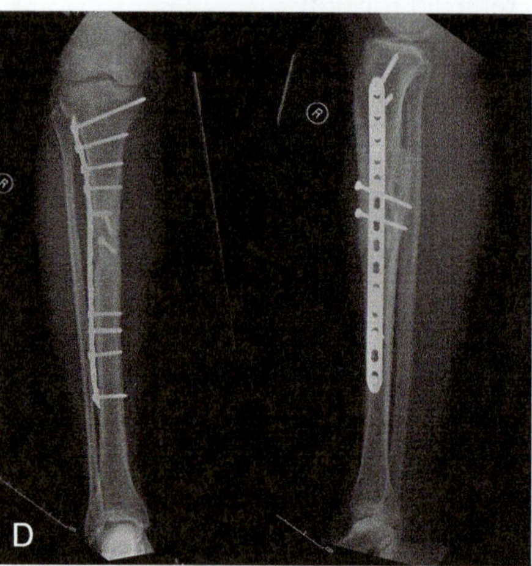

FIGURE 7 **A**, AP radiographs showing atrophic tibial nonunion with no reactive bone and mechanical instability (broken hardware). Intraoperative fluoroscopic images (**B**) and AP radiographs (**C**) showing application of composite bone graft (concentrated bone marrow aspirate + cancellous allograft + demineralized bone matrix) in concert with rigid internal fixation. **D**, AP radiographs showing complete healing with full weight bearing at 6 months.

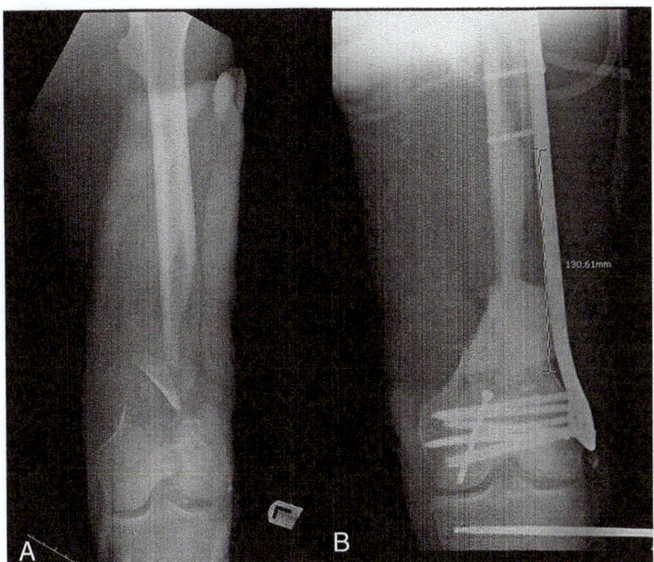

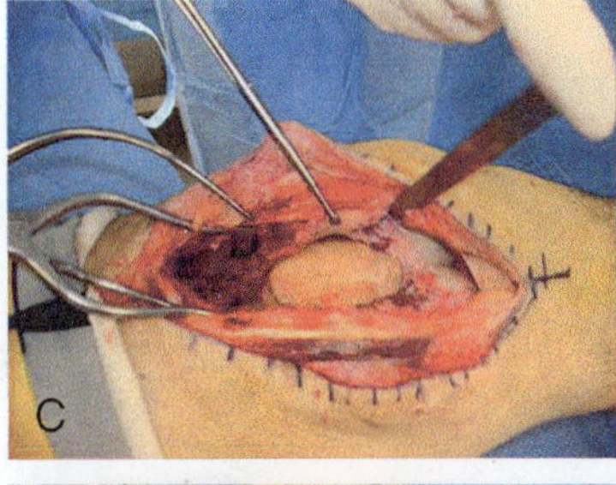

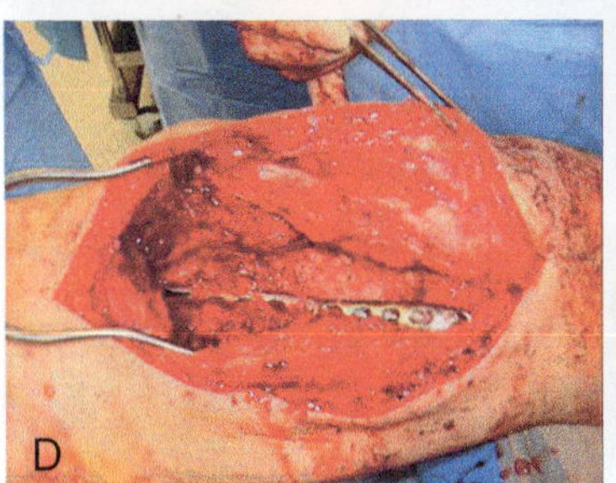

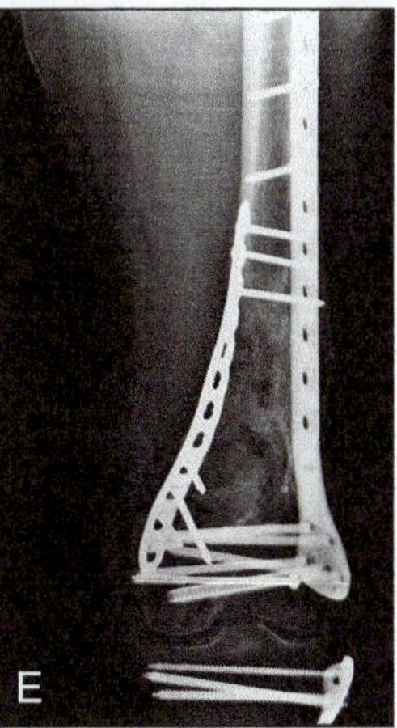

FIGURE 8 **A**, AP radiograph showing significant bone loss in an open distal femur fracture. **B**, AP radiograph showing stage 1 of the Masquelet technique with implantation of a large antibiotic spacer to develop a vascularized pseudoperiosteum to be utilized as a graft chamber in the second stage. **C** and **D**, Intraoperative photographs showing careful removal of the antibiotic spacer and preservation of the pseudoperiosteum (clamp on membrane). Reamer-irrigator-separator autografting into the defect with additional stabilization. **E**, Postoperative AP radiograph showing complete healing of the large segmental defect (approximately 14 cm).

requiring less than 20 mL of graft are treated for noninfected small nonunion gaps.

AICBG and cBMA composite grafts have a ceiling effect for success in the range of 3.5 cm for a single grafting episode.[60,142] With the knowledge of these limitations, defects larger than 3 to 4 cm are best treated using a two-step grafting procedure. The Masquelet or induced membrane technique consists of a planned two-stage procedure, with the first stage being débridement, bone stabilization, and placement of a polymethyl methacrylate cement spacer to develop a vascularized membrane for later grafting.

Residual open wounds or deep infection will negatively affect the outcome of this technique. An intramedullary device is preferred in comparison to a plate construct if a two-stage spacer technique is used. The primary graft material is the use of reamer-irrigator-aspirator harvested graft. Although less effective, allograft bone with osteogenic factors can be used for secondary grafting.[139] However, a ceiling effect has been noted for the consistent healing of defects in patients with defects in the range of 7 to 10 cm for patients undergoing induced membrane technique (grade C recommendations level IV or V evidence) (**Figure 8**).

Bone transport with distraction osteogenesis has proven to be a powerful tool for reconstruction and can eradicate infection, compensate bone defects, and promote bone union through progressive tissue histogenesis. Consistent results have been obtained for nonunion defects up to 10 cm. Traditional methods using ring fixation with wires or half-pin methodologies are supplanted by recent advancements in transport methodologies. This includes using hexapod frames with computer-assisted programs, internal cable transport of bone segments and transport over plates and nails, and a totally implantable bone transport nail (**Figure 9**) (grade C recommendations level IV or V evidence).

For extreme bone defects in the range of 10 cm or greater, very little evidence exists as to the best methodology of treatment. Free vascularized fibular grafting should be considered for patients with complicated soft-tissue defects, bone defects adjacent to joints, and large bone defects, and for patients able to tolerate microsurgery (grade C recommendations, level IV and V evidence). Often, a combination of these techniques is required to reconstruct these challenging defects.

When treating nonunion defects, the repair and reconstruction can be extremely challenging. Multiple reconstructive options are available, but it is difficult to reach consensus on treatment adjuvants especially when caring for extreme defects. Well-designed, randomized controlled trials are needed to obtain more substantial evidence for these conclusions.

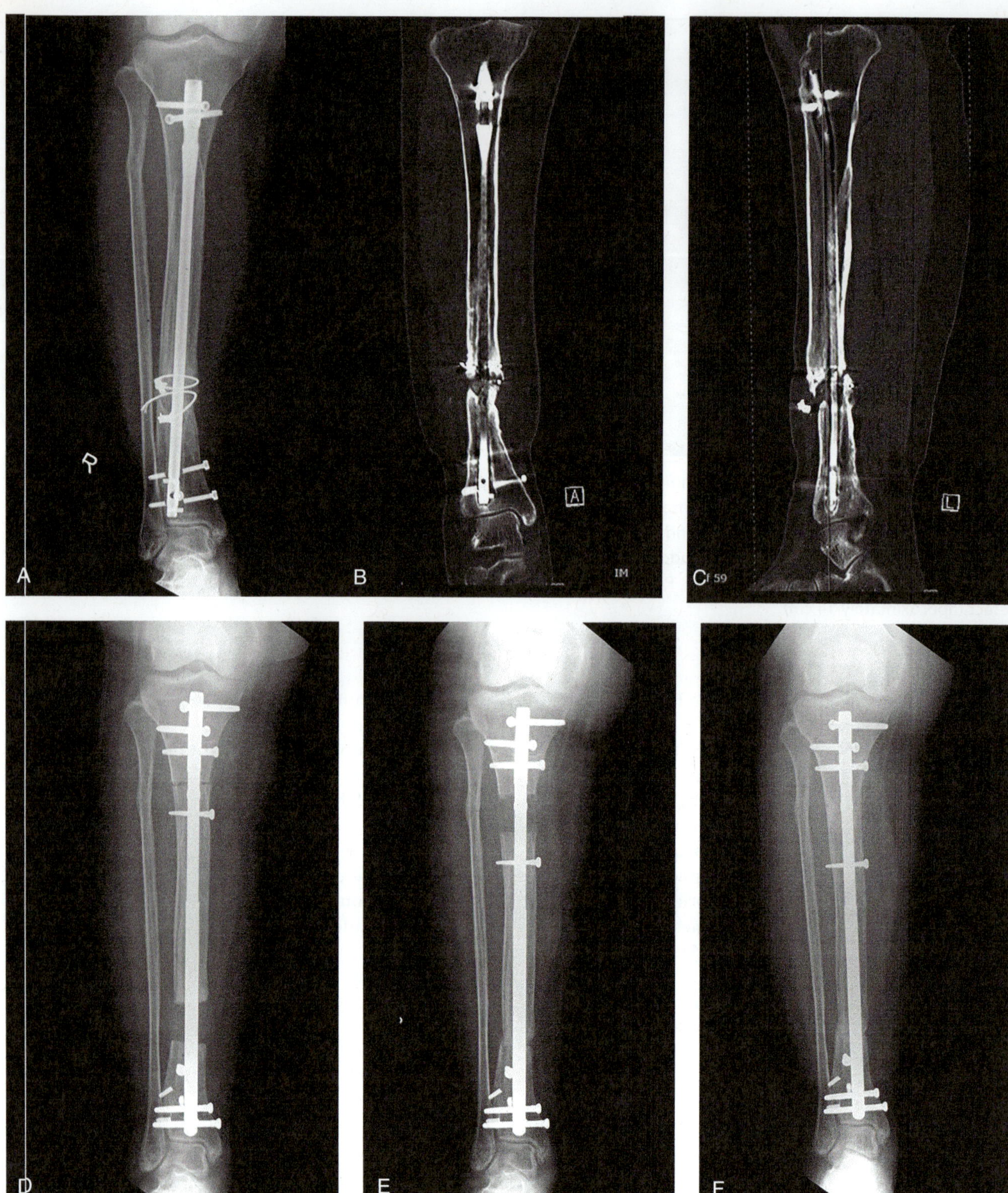

FIGURE 9 Preoperative AP radiograph (**A**) and coronal (**B**) and sagittal (**C**) CT scans show infected fracture with osteolysis at the fracture site and failed hardware. Inflammatory markers were all elevated, indicating probable deep infection. **D**, AP radiograph shows staged segmental resection to remove infected and dysvascular bone with implantation of an internal bone transport nail. **E**, AP radiograph shows proximal corticotomy with intercalary segmental transport achieving docking without the aid of an external fixator. The docking site was grafted to achieve solid union. **F**, AP radiograph obtained at 10-month final follow-up showing maturation of the proximal regenerate bone and solid healing of docking site.

SUMMARY

The biology of fracture healing is a complex biologic process that follows many specific regenerative patterns and involves changes in the expression of several gene pathways. The stages of fracture healing involve both anatomic and biochemical events, and these were reviewed to provide a general understanding of how fracture healing occurs. Within this context, the mechanisms of action and indications for use of the most commonly used categories of biologic adjuvants for the augmentation of fracture and nonunion repair are reviewed.

One of the key issues when initiating analysis of a nonunion is to attempt to determine why the fracture did not heal. There are many potential causes, but it is critical that the local environment should be the starting point when treating these patients. This is generally considered to be mainly either a mechanical or biologic failure. This assessment is an oversimplification, and many nonunions have elements of both, but it is generally a good starting point to determine what the next treatment will be and whether any biologics can be used at the nonunion site to stimulate healing. When choosing the ideal treatment when no defect exists, many cases of nonunion will respond favorably with deformity correction, compression, and stable internal fixation. There is little evidence and a distinct lack of consensus regarding both the definition and management of critical-size bone defects for acute traumatic and nonunion reconstructions. Given the heterogenous nature of cases of nonunion, the large number of confounding variables, and their relative rarity, there is a paucity of high-level evidence in the literature to guide decision making.

Developments in bone tissue engineering and bone biology have revealed the unique advantages of BMPs and other inductive factors for bone tissue repair, although current evidence does not support the widespread use and application of BMP for improved outcomes in fracture and nonunion surgery. However, alloplastic bone void fillers using calcium ceramics have been well established for the defect management of subchondral defects.

Cell-based therapies represent a promising therapy for the augmentation of fracture and nonunion repair. There is a robust body of preclinical evidence supporting their efficacy. Bone marrow aspirate has been used as a source of bone marrow–derived MSCs with its relative ease of harvest and low morbidity. There continue to be discrepancies between the literature with regard to the method of centrifugation, variable cell count concentrations, and lack of standardized outcome measures. The failures with unfractionated bone marrow reflected the paucity of osteoprogenitor cells present in the mature marrow aspirate. Although several studies have evaluated the effect of cell concentration on healing potential, an effective therapeutic range has yet to be established for nonunion treatment and should be an avenue for future research endeavors.

For the treatment of segmental bone loss, there are little data and a distinct lack of consensus regarding both the definition and management of critical-size bone defects for acute traumatic and reconstructive nonunion deficiencies. Issues with these studies begin with, what constitutes a critical-size defect? Most studies are difficult to stratify as they include both infected and noninfected defects and may or may not include nonunion with associated soft-tissue defects.

With the widespread use of orthobiologics in everyday practice, despite the limitations in the literature, attention must be directed to substantiate the evidence for their current use when treating fractures, nonunions, and bone defects. This chapter sought to provide the levels of evidence and indications for their correct use.

REFERENCES

1. Nakahara H, Bruder SP, Haynesworth SE, et al: Bone and cartilage formation in diffusion chambers by subcultured cells derived from the periosteum. *Bone* 1990;11:181-188.
2. Gerstenfeld LC, Cullinane DM, Barnes GL, et al: Fracture healing as a post-natal development process: Molecular, spatial and temporal aspects of its regulation. *J Cell Biochem* 2003;88:873-884.
3. Palomares KT, Gleason RE, Mason ZD, Cullinane DM, Einhorn TA: Mechanical stimulation alters tissue differentiation and molecular expression during bone healing. *J Orthop Res* 2009;27(9):1123-1132.
4. Schenck R, Willenegger H: On the histological picture of so-called primary healing of pressure osteosynthesis in experimental osteotomies in the dog. *Experientia* 1963;19:593-595.
5. McKibbin B: The biology of fracture healing in long bones. *J Bone Joint Surg Br* 1978;60:150-162.
6. Einhorn TA, Bonnarens F, Burnstein AH: The contributions of dietary protein and mineral to the healing of experimental fractures: A biomechanical study. *J Bone Joint Surg Am* 1986;68:1389-1395.
7. Casati L, Celotti F, Negri-Cesi P, Sacchi MC, Castano P, Colciago A: Platelet derived growth factor (PDGF) contained in Platelet Rich Plasma (PRP) stimulates migration of osteoblasts by reorganizing actin cytoskeleton. *Cell Adh Migr* 2014;8(6):595-602.
8. Triplett JW, Pavalko FM: Disruption of alpha-actinin-integrin interactions at focal adhesions renders osteoblasts susceptible to apoptosis. *J Physiol Cell Physiol* 2006;291(5):C909-C921.
9. Patterson TE, Kumagai K, Griffith L, Muschler GF: Cellular strategies for enhancement of fracture repair. *J Bone Joint Surg Am* 2008;90(suppl 1):111-119.
10. Goodman SB: Cell-based therapies for regenerating bone. *Minerva Ortop Traumatol* 2013;64(2):107-113.
11. Geusens P, Emans PJ, de Jong JJ, van den Bergh J: NSAIDs and fracture healing. *Curr Opin Rheumatol* 2013;25(4):524-531.
12. Kim JH, Liu X, Wang J, Chen X: Wnt signaling in bone formation and its therapeutic potential for bone diseases. *Ther Adv Musculoskelet Dis* 2013;5(1):13-31.

13. Li X, Zhang Y, Kang H, Liu W: Sclerostin binds to LRP5/6 and antagonizes canonical Wnt signaling. *J Biol Chem* 2005;280(20):19883-19887.
14. Bellido T, Saini V, Pajevic PD: Effects of PTH on osteocyte function. *Bone* 2013;54(2):250-257.
15. Ominsky MS, Vlasseros F, Jolette J, Smith SY: Two doses of sclerostin antibody in cynomolgus monkeys increases bone formation, bone mineral density, and bone strength. *J Bone Miner Res* 2010;25(5):948-959.
16. Recker RR, Benson CT, Matsumoto T, Bolognese MA: A randomized, double-blind phase 2 clinical trial of blosozumab, a sclerostin antibody, in postmenopausal women women with low bone mineral density. *J Bone Miner Res* 2015;30(2):216-224.
17. Einhorn TA: The cell and molecular biology of fracture healing. *Clin Orthop Relat Res* 1998;355:S7-S21.
18. Einhorn TA, Hirschman A, Kaplan C, et al: Neutral protein-degrading enzymes in experimental fracture callus: A preliminary report. *J Orthop Res* 1989;7:792-805.
19. Mehta S, Watson JT: Platelet rich concentrate: Basic science and current clinical applications. *J Orthop Trauma* 2008;22(6):432-438.
20. Cho T-J, Gerstenfeld LC, Einhorn TA: Differential temporal expression of members of the TGF-B superfamily during murine fracture healing. *J Bone Miner Res* 2002;17:513-520.
21. Goldring MB, Tsuchimochi K, Ijiri K: The control of chondrogenesis. *J Cell Biochem* 2006;97(1):33-44.
22. Einhorn TA, Gerstenfeld LC: Fracture healing: Mechanisms and Interventions. *Nat Rev Rheumatol* 2015;11(1):45-54.
23. Juppner H, Kronenberg HM: Parathyroid hormone, in Favus MJ, ed: *Primer on the Metabolic Bone Diseases and Disorders of Mineral Metabolism*, ed 5. American Society for Bone and Mineral Research, 2003, pp 117-124.77.
24. Riek AE, Towler DA: The pharmacological management of osteoporosis. *Mo Med* 2011;108(2):118-123.
25. Agholme F, Macias B, Hamang M, Lucchesi J, Adrian MD: Efficacy of a sclerostin antibody compared to a low dose of PTH on metaphyseal bone healing. *J Orthop Res* 2014;32(3):471-476.
26. Ellegaard M, Kringelbach T, Syberg S, Petersen S: The effect of PTH (1-34) on fracture healing during different loading conditions. *J Bone Miner Res* 2013;28(10):2145-2155.
27. Zhang D, Potty A, Vyas P, Lane J: The role of recombinant PTH in human fracture healing: A systematic review. *J Orthop Trauma* 2014;28(1):57-62.
28. Barnes GL, Kakar S, Vora S, Morgan EF, Gerstenfeld LC, Einhorn TA: Stimulation of fracture-healing with systemic intermittent parathyroid hormone treatment. *J Bone Joint Surg Am* 2008;90(suppl 1):120-127.
29. Li YF, Zhou CC, Li JH, Luo E, Zhu SS: The effects of combined human parathyroid hormone (1-34) and zoledronic acid treatment on fracture healing in osteoporotic rats. *Osteoporos Int* 2012;23(4):1463-1474.
30. Eriksen EF, Díez-Pérez A, Boonen S: Update on long-term treatment with bisphosphonates for postmenopausal osteoporosis: A systematic review. *Bone* 2014;58:126-135.
31. Weinstein RS, Roberson PK, Manolagas SC: Giant osteoclast formation and long-term oral bisphosphonate therapy. *N Engl J Med* 2009;360(1):53-62.
32. Frith J, Mönkkönen J, Blackburn G, Russell R, Rogers M: Clodronate and liposome-encapsulated clodronate are metabolized to a toxic ATP analog, adenosine 5′-(beta, gamma-dichloromethylene) triphosphate, by mammalian cells in vitro. *J Bone Miner Res* 1997;12(9):1358-1367.
33. Shane E: Evolving data about subtrochanteric fractures and bisphosphonates. *N Engl J Med* 2010;362(19):1825-1827.
34. Lenart BA, Lorich DG, Lane JM: Atypical fractures of the femoral diaphysis in postmenopausal women taking alendronate. *N Engl J Med* 2008;358(12):1304-1306.
35. Chiang CY, Zebaze RM, Ghasem-Zadeh A, Iuliano-Burns S, Hardidge A, Seeman E: Teriparatide improves bone quality and healing of atypical femoral fractures associated with bisphosphonate therapy. *Bone* 2013;52(1):360-365.
36. Yoon BH, Kim KC: Does teriparatide improve fracture union?: A systematic review. *J Bone Metab* 2020;27(3):167-174.
37. Im GI, Lee SH: Effect of teriparatide on healing of atypical femoral fractures: A systemic review. *J Bone Metab* 2015;22(4):183-189.
38. Urist MR, Strates BS: The classic: Bone morphogenetic protein. *Clin orthop Relat Res* 2009;467(12):3051-3062.
39. Christian EP, Bosse MJ, Robb G: Reconstruction of large diaphyseal defects, without free fibular transfer, in Grade-IIIB tibial fractures. *J Bone Joint Surg Am* 1989;71(7):994-1004.
40. Goulet JA, Senunas LE, DeSilva GL, Greenfield ML: Autogenous iliac crest bone graft. Complications and functional assessment. *Clin Orthop Relat Res* 1997;339:76-81.
41. Watson JT: Overview of biologics. *J Orthop Trauma* 2005;19(10 suppl):S14-S16.
42. Watson JT, Anders M, Moed BR: Management strategies for bone loss in tibial shaft fractures. *Clin Orthop Relat Res* 1995;315:138-152.
43. Belthur MV, Conway JD, Jindal G, Ranade A, Herzenberg JE: Bone graft harvest using a new intramedullary system. *Clin Orthop Relat Res* 2008;466(12):2973-2980.
44. Kobbe P, Tarkin IS, Frink M, Pape HC: Voluminous bone graft harvesting of the femoral marrow cavity for autologous transplantation. An indication for the "Reamer-Irrigator-Aspirator-" (RIA-)technique [German]. *Unfallchirurg* 2008;111(6):469-472.
45. Schmidmaier G, Herrmann S, Green J, et al: Quantitative assessment of growth factors in reaming aspirate, iliac crest, and platelet preparation. *Bone* 2006;39(5):1156-1163.
46. Cox G, McGonagle D, Boxall SA, Buckley CT, Jones E, Giannoudis PV: The use of the reamer-irrigator-aspirator to harvest mesenchymal stem cells. *J Bone Joint Surg Br* 2011;93(4):517-524.
47. Sagi HC, Young ML, Gerstenfeld L, Einhorn TA, Tornetta P: Qualitative and quantitative differences between bone graft obtained from the medullary canal (with a Reamer/Irrigator/Aspirator) and the iliac crest of the same patient. *J Bone Joint Surg Am* 2012;94(23):2128-2135.

48. Stannard JP, Sathy AK, Moeinpour F, Stewart RL, Volgas DA: Quantitative analysis of growth factors from a second filter using the reamer-irrigator-aspirator system: Description of a novel technique. *Orthop Clin North Am* 2010;41(1):95-98.
49. Hak DJ, Pittman JL: Biological rationale for the intramedullary canal as a source of autograft material. *Orthop Clin North Am* 2010;41(1):57-61.
50. Uppal HS, Peterson BE, Misfeldt ML, et al: The viability of cells obtained using the Reamer-Irrigator-Aspirator system and in bone graft from the iliac crest. *Bone Joint J* 2013;95-B(9):1269-1274.
51. Muschler GF, Boehm C, Easley K: Aspiration to obtain osteoblast progenitor cells from human bone marrow: The influence of aspiration volume. *J Bone Joint Surg Am* 1997;79(11):1699-1709.
52. Muschler GF, Midura RJ: Connective tissue progenitors: Practical concepts for clinical applications. *Clin Orthop Relat Res* 2002;395:66-80.
53. Hernigou P, Poignard A, Beaujean F, Rouard H: Percutaneous autologous bone-marrow grafting for nonunions. Influence of the number and concentration of progenitor cells. *J Bone Joint Surg Am* 2005;87(7):1430-1437.
54. Thua THL, Bui DP, Nguyen DT, et al: Autologous bone marrow stem cells combined with allograft cancellous bone in treatment of nonunion. *Biomed Res Ther* 2015;2:409-417.
55. Hernigou P, Homma Y, Flouzat Lachaniette CH, et al: Benefits of small volume and small syringe for bone marrow aspirations of mesenchymal stem cells. *Int Orthop* 2013;37(11):2279-2287.
56. Ridgway J, Butcher A, Chen PS, Horner A, Curran S: Novel technology to provide an enriched therapeutic cell concentrate from bone marrow aspirate. *Biotechnol Prog* 2010;26(6):1741-1748.
57. Dawson JI, Smith JO, Aarvold A, et al: Enhancing the osteogenic efficacy of human bone marrow aspirate: Concentrating osteoprogenitors using wave-assisted filtration. *Cytotherapy* 2013;15(2):242-252.
58. Bruder SP, Kraus KH, Goldberg VM, Kadiyala S: The effect of implants loaded with autologous mesenchymal stem cells on the healing of canine segmental bone defects. *J Bone Joint Surg Am* 1998;80(7):985-996.
59. Nauth A, Schemitsch E, Norris B, Nollin Z, Watson JT: Critical-size bone defects: Is there a consensus for diagnosis and treatment? *J Orthop Trauma* 2018;32(suppl 1):S7-S11.
60. Baldwin P, Li DJ, Auston DA, et al: Autograft, allograft, and bone graft substitutes: Clinical evidence and indications for use in the setting of orthopaedic trauma surgery. *J Orthop Trauma* 2019;33(4):203-213.
61. Rajan GP, Fornaro J, Trentz O, et al: Cancellous allograft versus autologous bone grafting for repair of comminuted distal radius fractures: A prospective, randomized trial. *J Trauma* 2006;60(6):1322-1329.
62. Flierl MA, Smith WR, Mauffrey C, et al: Outcomes and complication rates of different bone grafting modalities in long bone fracture nonunions: A retrospective cohort study in 182 patients. *J Orthop Surg Res* 2013;8:33.
63. Rollo G, Bonura EM, Huri G, et al: Standard plating vs. cortical strut and plating for periprosthetic knee fractures: A multicentre experience. *Med Glas (Zenica)* 2020;17(1):170-177.
64. Khashan M, Amar E, Drexler M, et al: Superior outcome of strut allograft-augmented plate fixation for the treatment of periprosthetic fractures around a stable femoral stem. *Injury* 2013;44(11):1556-1560.
65. Badman BL, Mighell M, Kalandiak SP, et al: Proximal humeral nonunions treated with fixed-angle locked plating and an intramedullary strut allograft. *J Orthop Trauma* 2009;23(3):173-179.
66. Van Houwelingen AP, McKee MD: Treatment of osteopenic humeral shaft nonunion with compression plating, humeral cortical allograft struts, and bone grafting. *J Orthop Trauma* 2005;19(1):36-42.
67. Willis MP, Brooks JP, Badman BL, et al: Treatment of atrophic diaphyseal humeral nonunions with compressive locked plating and augmented with an intramedullary strut allograft. *J Orthop Trauma* 2013;27(2):77-81.
68. Kanakeshwar RB, Jayaramaraju D, Agraharam D, et al: Management of resistant distal femur non-unions with allograft strut and autografts combined with osteosynthesis in a series of 22 patients. *Injury* 2017;48:S14-S17.
69. Rush SM, Hamilton GA, Ackerson LM: Mesenchymal stem cell allograft in revision foot and ankle surgery: A clinical and radiographic analysis. *J Foot Ankle Surg* 2009;48(2):163-169.
70. Scott RT, Hyer CF: Role of cellular allograft containing mesenchymal stem cells in high-risk foot and ankle reconstructions. *J Foot Ankle Surg* 2013;52(1):32-35.
71. Bormann N, Pruss A, Schmidmaier G, Wildemann B: In vitro testing of the osteoinductive potential of different bony allograft preparations. *Arch Orthop Trauma Surg* 2010;130(1):143-149.
72. Pietrzak WS, Woodell-May J, McDonald N: Assay of bone morphogenetic protein-2, -4, and -7 in human demineralized bone matrix. *J Craniofac Surg* 2006;17(1):84-90.
73. Bae HW, Zhao L, Kanim LE, Wong P, Delamarter RB, Dawson EG: Intervariability and intravariability of bone morphogenetic proteins in commercially available demineralized bone matrix products. *Spine* 2006;31(12):1299-1306.
74. Bae H, Zhao L, Zhu D, Kanim LE, Wang JC, Delamarter RB: Variability across ten production lots of a single demineralized bone matrix product. *J Bone Joint Surg Am* 2010;92(2):427-435.
75. Tiedeman JJ, Garvin KL, Kile TA, Connolly JF: The role of a composite, demineralized bone matrix and bone marrow in the treatment of osseous defects. *Orthopedics* 1995;18(12):1153-1158.
76. Lindsey RW, Wood GW, Sadasivian KK, Stubbs HA, Block JE: Grafting long bone fractures with demineralized bone matrix putty enriched with bone marrow: Pilot findings. *Orthopedics* 2006;29(10):939-941.
77. Braly HL, O'Connor DP, Brinker MR: Percutaneous autologous bone marrow injection in the treatment of distal metadiaphyseal tibial nonunions and delayed unions. *J Orthop Trauma* 2013;27(9):527-533.

78. Giannoudis PV, Gudipati S, Harwood P, Kanakaris NK: Long bone non-unions treated with the diamond concept: A case series of 64 patients. *Injury* 2015;46(suppl 8):S48-S54.

79. Jager M, Herten M, Fochtmann U, et al: Bridging the gap: Bone marrow aspiration concentrate reduces autologous bone grafting in osseous defects. *J Orthop Res* 2011;29(2):173-180.

80. Holmes RE, Bucholz RW, Mooney V: Porous hydroxyapatite as a bone-graft substitute in metaphyseal defects. A histometric study. *J Bone Joint Surg Am* 1986;68(6):904-911.

81. Mauffrey C, Fader R, Hammerberg EM, Hak DJ, Stahel PF: Incidence and pattern of technical complications in balloon-guided osteoplasty for depressed tibial plateau fractures: A pilot study in 20 consecutive patients. *Patient Saf Surg* 2013;7(1):8.

82. Szpalski M, Gunzburg R: Applications of calcium phosphate-based cancellous bone void fillers in trauma surgery. *Orthopedics* 2002;25(5 suppl):S601-S609.

83. McDonald E, Chu T, Tufaga M, et al: Tibial plateau fracture repairs augmented with calcium phosphate cement have higher in situ fatigue strength than those with autograft. *J Orthop Trauma* 2011;25(2):90-95.

84. McAndrew MP, Gorman PW, Lange TA: Tricalcium phosphate as a bone graft substitute in trauma: Preliminary report. *J Orthop Trauma* 1988;2(4):333-339.

85. Russell TA, Leighton RK: Comparison of autogenous bone graft and endothermic calcium phosphate cement for defect augmentation in tibial plateau fractures. A multicenter, prospective, randomized study. *J Bone Joint Surg Am* 2008;90(10):2057-2061.

86. Goff T, Kanakaris NK, Giannoudis PV: Use of bone graft substitutes in the management of tibial plateau fractures. *Injury* 2013;44(suppl 1):S86-S94.

87. Bajammal SS, Zlowodzki M, Lelwica A, et al: The use of calcium phosphate bone cement in fracture treatment. A meta-analysis of randomized trials. *J Bone Joint Surg Am* 2008;90(6):1186-1196.

88. Den Boer FC, Wippermann BW, Blokhuis TJ, Patka P, Bakker FC, Haarman HJ: Healing of segmental bone defects with granular porous hydroxyapatite augmented with recombinant human osteogenic protein-1 or autologous bone marrow. *J Orthop Res* 2003;21(3):521-528.

89. Govender S, Csimma C, Genant HK, et al: Recombinant human bone morphogenetic protein-2 for treatment of open tibial fractures: A prospective, controlled, randomized study of four hundred and fifty patients. *J Bone Joint Surg Am* 2002;84(12):2123-2134.

90. Carragee EJ, Hurwitz EL, Weiner BK: A critical review of recombinant human bone morphogenetic protein-2 trials in spinal surgery: Emerging safety concerns and lessons learned. *Spine J* 2011;11(6):471-491.

91. Swiontkowski MF, Aro HT, Donell S, et al: Recombinant human bone morphogenetic protein-2 in open tibial fractures. A subgroup analysis of data combined from two prospective randomized studies. *J Bone Joint Surg Am* 2006;88(6):1258-1265.

92. Chan DS, Garland J, Infante A, Sanders RW, Sagi HC: Wound complications associated with bone morphogenetic protein-2 in orthopaedic trauma surgery. *J Orthop Trauma* 2014;28(10):599-604.

93. Dumic-Cule I, Peric M, Kucko L, Grgurevic L, Pecina M, Vukicevic S: Bone morphogenetic proteins in fracture repair. *Int Orthop* 2018;42(11):2619-2626.

94. Zhou YQ, Tu HL, Duan YJ, Chen X: Comparison of bone morphogenetic protein and autologous grafting in the treatment of limb long bone nonunion: A systematic review and meta-analysis. *J Orthop Surg Res* 2020;15(1):288.

95. Marx RE: Platelet-rich plasma: Evidence to support its use. *J Oral Maxillofac Surg* 2004;62(4):489-496.

96. Marx RE, Carlson ER, Eichstaedt RM, Schimmele SR, Strauss JE, Georgeff KR: Platelet-rich plasma: Growth factor enhancement for bone grafts. *Oral Surg Oral Med Oral Pathol Oral Radiol Endod* 1998;85(6):638-646.

97. Grageda E: Platelet-rich plasma and bone graft materials: A review and a standardized research protocol. *Implant Dent* 2004;13(4):301-309.

98. Heldin CH, Westermark B: PDGF-like growth factors in autocrine stimulation of growth. *J Cell Physiol* 1987;133(suppl 5):31-34.

99. Watson JT: Chapter in skeletal trauma, in Jupiter JB, Browner BD, eds: *Biology and Enhancement of Skeletal Repair*. Lippincot, 2018.

100. Sanchez AR, Sheridan PJ, Kupp LI: Is platelet-rich plasma the perfect enhancement factor? A current review. *Int J Oral Maxill Implants* 2003;18(1):93-103.

101. Moraes VY, Lenza M, Tamaoki MJ, Faloppa F, Belloti JC: Platelet-rich therapies for musculoskeletal soft tissue injuries. *Cochrane Database Syst Rev* 2013;12:CD010071.

102. Hollinger JO, Hart CE, Hirsch SN, Lynch S, Friedlaender GE: Recombinant human platelet-derived growth factor: Biology and clinical applications. *J Bone Joint Surg Am* 2008;90(suppl 1):48-54.

103. Al-Zube L, Breitbart EA, O'Connor JP, et al: Recombinant human platelet-derived growth factor BB (rhPDGF-BB) and beta-tricalcium phosphate/collagen matrix enhance fracture healing in a diabetic rat model. *J Orthop Res* 2009;27(8):1074-1081.

104. Daniels T, DiGiovanni C, Lau JT, Wing K, Younger A: Prospective clinical pilot trial in a single cohort group of rhPDGF in foot arthrodeses. *Foot Ankle Int* 2010;31(6):473-479.

105. Daniels TR, Anderson J, Swords MP, et al: Recombinant human platelet-derived growth factor BB in combination with a beta-tricalcium phosphate (rhPDGF-BB/β-TCP)-Collagen matrix as an alternative to autograft. *Foot Ankle Int* 2019;40(9):1068-1078.

106. Loveland JD, McMillen RL, Cala MA: A multicenter, retrospective, case series of patients with charcot neuroarthropathy deformities undergoing arthrodesis utilizing recombinant human platelet-derived growth factor with beta-tricalcium phosphate. *J Foot Ankle Surg* 2021;60(1):74-79.

107. Sun H, Lu PP, Zhou PH, et al: Recombinant human platelet-derived growth factor-BB versus autologous bone graft in foot and ankle fusion: A systematic review and meta-analysis. *Foot Ankle Surg* 2017;23(1):32-39.

108. Digiovanni CW, Baumhauer J, Lin SS, et al: Prospective, randomized, multi-center feasibility trial of rhPDGF-BB versus autologous bone graft in a foot and ankle fusion model. *Foot Ankle Int* 2011;32(4):344-354.

109. Bishop JA, Palanca AA, Belino MJ, Lowenberg DW: Assesment of compromised fracture healing. *J Am Acad Orthop Surg* 2012;20(5):273-282.

110. Perlman MH, Thordarson DB: Ankle fusion in a high risk population: An assessment of nonunion risk factors. *Foot Ankle Int* 1999;20(8):491-496.

111. Frey C, Halikus NM, Vu-Rose T, Ebramzadeh E: A review of ankle arthrodesis: Predisposing factors to nonunion. *Foot Ankle Int* 1994;15(11):581-584.

112. Zura R, Braid-Forbes MJ, Jeray K, et al: Bone fracture nonunion rate decreases with increasing age: A prospective inception cohort study. *Bone* 2017;95:26-32.

113. Zura R, Watson JT, Einhorn T, et al: An inception cohort analysis to predict nonunion in tibia and 17 other fracture locations. *Injury* 2017;48(6):1194-1203.

114. El-Zawawy HB, Gill CS, Wright RW, Sandell LJ: Smoking delays chondrogenesis in a mouse model of closed tibial fracture healing. *J Orthop Res* 2006;24(12):2150-2158.

115. Potier E, Ferreira E, Meunier A, Sedel L, Logeart-Avramoglou D, Petite H: Prolonged hypoxia concomitant with serum deprivation induces massive human mesenchymal stem cell death. *Tissue Eng* 2007;13(6):1325-1331.

116. Rothem DE, Rothem L, Dahan A, Eliakim R, Soudry M: Nicotinic modulation of gene expression in osteoblast cells, MG-63. *Bone* 2011;48(4):903-909.

117. Porter SE, Hanley EN Jr: The musculoskeletal effects of smoking. *J Am Acad Orthop Surg* 2001;9(1):9-17.

118. Harvey EJ, Agel J, Selznick HS, Chapman JR, Henley MB: Deleterious effect of smoking on healing of open tibia-shaft fractures. *Am J Orthop (Belle Mead NJ)* 2002;31(9):518-521.

119. Nåsell H, Ottosson C, Törnqvist H, Lindé J, Ponzer S: The impact of smoking on complications after operatively treated ankle fractures--a follow-up study of 906 patients. *J Orthop Trauma* 2011;25(12):748-755.

120. Raikin SM, Landsman JC, Alexander VA, Froimson MI, Plaxton NA: Effect of nicotine on the rate and strength of long bone fracture healing. *Clin Orthop Relat Res* 1998;353:231-237.

121. Adams CI, Keating JF, Court-Brown CM: Cigarette smoking and open tibial fractures. *Injury* 2001;32(1):61-65.

122. Giannoudis PV, MacDonald DA, Matthews SJ, Smith RM, Furlong AJ, De Boer P: Nonunion of the femoral diaphysis: The influence of reaming and non-steroidal anti-inflammatory drugs. *J Bone Joint Surg Br* 2000;82:655-658.

123. Brinker MR, O'Connor DP, Monla YT, Earthman TP: Metabolic and endocrine abnormalities in patients with nonunions. *J Orthop Trauma* 2007;21(8):557-570.

124. Delgado-Martinez AD, Martinez ME, Carrascao MT, Rodriguez-Avial M, Munuera L: Effect of 25-OH vitamin D on fracture healing in elderly rats. *J Orthop Res* 1998;16(6):650-653.

125. Cotran R, Kumar V, Robbins S, eds: *Robbins Pathologic Basis of Disease*, ed 6. WB Saunders, 1999.

126. Topping RE, Bolander ME, Balian G: Type X collagen in fracture callus and the effects of experimental diabetes. *Clin Orthop Relat Res* 1994;308:220-228.

127. Blake RB, Brinker MR, Ursic CM, Clark JM, Cox DD: Alcohol and drug use in adult patients with musculoskeletal injuries. *Am J Orthop* 1997;26:704-709.

128. Levy RS, Hebert CK, Munn BG, Barrack RL: Drug and alcohol use in orthopedic trauma patients: A prospective study. *J Orthop Trauma* 1996;10:21-27.

129. Spanheimer RG, Umpierrez GE, Stumpf V: Decreased collagen production in diabetic rats. *Diabetes* 1988;37:371-376.

130. Natoli RM, Yu H, Meislin MC, et al: Alcohol exposure decreases osteopontin expression during fracture healing and osteopontin-mediated mesenchymal stem cell migration in vitro. *J Orthop Surg Res* 2018;13(1):101.

131. Imhof A, Froehlich M, Brenner H, Boeing H, Pepys MB, Koenig W: Effect of alcohol consumption on systemic markers of inflammation. *Lancet* 2001;357:763-767.

132. Bratton A, Eisenberg J, Vuchkovska A, Roper P, Callaci JJ: Effects of episodic alcohol exposure on BMP2 signaling during tibia fracture healing. *J Orthop Trauma* 2018;32(6):288-295.

133. Day M, Ostgrum R, Chao EY, Rubin CT, Aro HT, Einhorn TA: Bone injury, Regeneration and repair, in Buckwalter JA, Winhorn TA, Sikmon SR, eds: *Orthopaedic Basic Science*, ed 2. American Academy of Orthopaedic Surgeon, 2000.

134. Claes LE, Heigele CA, Neidlinger-Wilke C, et al: Effects of mechanical factors on the fracture healing process. *Clin Orthop Relat Res* 1998;355:S132-S147.

135. Ito K, Perren SM: Biology and biomechanics in bone healing, in Ruedi TP, Buckley RE, Moran CG, eds: *AO Principles of Fracture Management*, ed 2. Thieme, 2007, vol 1, pp 9-31.

136. Goodship AE, Kenwright J: The influence of induced micromovement upon the healing of experimental tibial fractures. *J Bone Joint Surg Br* 1985;67:650-655.

137. Bottlang M, Lesser M, Koerber J, et al: Far cortical locking can improve healing of fractures stabilized with locking plates. *J Bone Joint Surg Am* 2010;92(7):1652-1660.

138. Stucken C, Olszewski DC, Creevy WR, Murakami AM, Tornetta P: Preoperative diagnosis of infection in patients with nonunions. *J Bone Joint Surg Am* 2013;95(15):1409-1412.

139. Lin K, VandenBerg J, Putnam SM, et al: Bone marrow aspirate concentrate with cancellous allograft versus iliac crest bone graft in the treatment of long bone nonunions, *OTA Int* 2019: 2(1):e12.

140. Hoit G, Kain MS, Sparkman JW, Norris BL, Conway JD. Watson JT: The induced membrane technique for bone defects: Basic science, clinical evidence, and technical tips. *OTA Int* 2021;4(2 suppl):e106.

141. Watson JT, Anders M, Moed BR: Bone loss in tibial shaft fractures: Management strategies. *Clin Orthop Relat Res* 1995;316:1-17.

142. Moed BR, Thorderson N, Linden MD: Reharvest of iliac crest donor site cancellous bone. *Clin Orthop Relat Res* 1998;346:223-227.

CHAPTER 20

Peripheral Nerve Regeneration in the Hand

Minh Hoang Nguyen, MD • Amy M. Moore, MD • Ryan W. Schmucker, MD

INTRODUCTION

Peripheral nerve injuries are common and result in devastating functional outcomes. Fortunately, the peripheral nervous system (PNS) has the capability to regenerate. Nerve regeneration is a highly coordinated phenomenon and understanding the complexity is essential to diagnosis and treatment of patients with nerve injuries. It is important to review the basic principles of nerve injury and regeneration, and also explore innovations in surgical techniques and orthobiologic advances that have continued to move the field of nerve surgery forward.

ANATOMY, PHYSIOLOGY, AND BASIC CONCEPTS OF PERIPHERAL NERVE INJURIES

Normal Peripheral Nerve Anatomy and Physiology

Peripheral Nerve Fiber and Fascicular Anatomy

A fundamental understanding of nerve anatomy and physiology is essential to guide surgeons in the diagnosis and surgical management of peripheral nerve injuries. The PNS is a complex network that encompasses the nerves outside the brain and spinal cord and allows communication between the central nervous system and the body. The PNS is composed of afferent sensory nerve fibers, whose cell bodies are in the dorsal root ganglia, and efferent motor nerve fibers, whose cell bodies are in the anterior (ventral) horn of the spinal cord.

There are two basic types of cells within the nervous system: neurons and glial cells. Neurons are responsible for sending and receiving motor and sensory input throughout the body, whereas glial cells play a supportive role by maintaining homeostasis and forming the myelin sheath crucial to nerve function. There are two distinct types of axons: unmyelinated and myelinated. The myelin sheath of axons in the PNS is formed by Schwann cells (a type of glial cell) that wrap tightly around a single axon using multiple layers of plasma membrane. The gaps in the myelin sheath are called the nodes of Ranvier, which allow action potentials to pass rapidly between nodes in myelinated axons (saltatory conduction). Unmyelinated axons conduct action potentials slower and are mainly made up of C fibers that mediate nociception, temperature, and mechanical sensibilities.

The individual axon together with the surrounding Schwann cells is encased in a bilayered connective tissue structure called endoneurium (**Figure 1**). A bundle of several axons encased in endoneurium forms a fascicle and this is enveloped by perineurium composed of concentrically oriented layers of perineural cells. The functions of the perineurium are to protect the endoneurium from stretching forces, to maintain constant intrafascicular pressure and to serve as a blood-nerve barrier.[1,2] Epineurium, the outermost connective tissue layer, envelopes multiple fascicles and provides structural support. External to the epineurium is an areolar layer that contains extrinsic blood supply called mesoneurium, which is critical for nerve gliding.

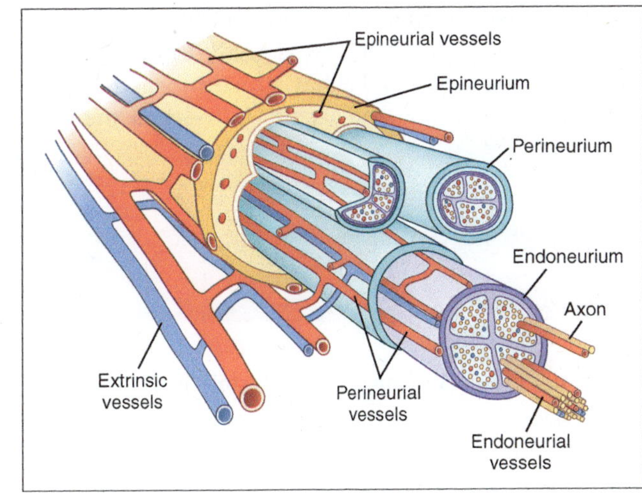

FIGURE 1 Illustration of the anatomy of the peripheral nerve. (Reproduced with permission from Power HA, Moore AM: Basic science of nerve compression, in Skirven TM, Osterman AL, Fedorczyck JM, Amadio PP, Feldscher SB, Shin EK, eds: *Rehabilitation of the Hand and Upper Extremity*, ed 7. Elsevier, 2019.)

Dr. Nguyen or an immediate family member has stock or stock options held in BioNTech. Dr. Moore or an immediate family member has received research or institutional support from Checkpoint Surgical, Inc. Neither Dr. Schmucker nor any immediate family member has received anything of value from or has stock or stock options held in a commercial company or institution related directly or indirectly to the subject of this chapter.

Nerve Blood Supply

Peripheral nerves are similar to any other tissue in the body in that they require adequate blood supply to maintain their integrity and function (**Figure 1**). Peripheral nerves rely on an intricate dual blood supply network, which consists of an extrinsic plexus that contains small vessels from major arteries running longitudinally in the epineural layer,[3] termed the vasa nervorum. The extrinsic plexus crosses the epineurium and perineurium to anastomose with the intrinsic system. Reduction or disruption of either extrinsic or intrinsic blood supply can contribute to nerve injury through local ischemia. The magnitude and duration of the insult dictates the severity of injury and its ability to recover.[4-8]

Basic Concepts of Peripheral Nerve Injury

Classification of Nerve Injury

When evaluating peripheral nerve injuries, it is important to understand the classification of nerve injuries as well as the mechanism of injury, level at which the injury occurred, chronicity, and patient-specific factors that can affect recovery. All these factors can guide surgeons in selecting the appropriate treatment in the setting of an acute or chronic nerve injury. The original classification of nerve injuries was first proposed by Seddon and Sunderland in 1947 and 1951, respectively.[3] In the original Seddon classification, the injuries are grouped as neurapraxia, axonotmesis, and neurotmesis. Sunderland categorized nerve injury as grade I to V based on the degree of injury and what structure was involved (**Table 1**). Mackinnon and Dellon introduced the sixth degree in 1988.

Wallerian Degeneration

After incurring traumatic injury, the peripheral nerve stump distal to the injury undergoes changes at the cellular level referred to as wallerian degeneration. Axon degeneration does not begin immediately after the injury, with axonal segments distal to the injury able to conduct action potentials for up to 3 days after the insult.[9,10] The hallmark of this degeneration process is the proteolysis and degeneration of the axonal cytoskeleton starting with sudden influx of mostly Ca^{+} ions.[11-13] This eventually leads to the fragmentation, disintegration, and removal of axons and their myelin sheath by both Schwann cells and macrophages.[9,14,15] In addition to changes at the distal nerve stump, there are also changes that happen at the proximal stump, which usually are limited to the first node of Ranvier.

NERVE REGENERATION

Nerve regeneration is complex. After injury, there is activation of many signaling pathways and transcription factors that promote cellular changes from the injury site to the soma allowing for regeneration. These complex coordinated events include membrane sealing, growth cone assembly, protein synthesis, and activation of signaling molecules and transcription factors. Neurotrophic factors also play a significant role in promoting a regenerative environment. There are three major groups of neurotrophic factors: neurotrophins, neuropoietic cytokines (ciliary neurotrophic factor and interleukin 6), and fibroblast growth factors.[16]

At a cellular level, macrophages are critical in the myelin degradation part of wallerian degeneration as

TABLE 1 Classification of Nerve Injury (Sunderland and Seddon)

Classification				
Sunderland	Seddon	Histologic Changes	Wallerian Degeneration	Spontaneous Recovery
I	Neurapraxia	Segmental demyelination without axonal injury	No wallerian degeneration	Fast Expect full recovery
II	Axonotmesis	Axonal injury	Wallerian degeneration of the nerve distal to the injury	Slow Expect full recovery
III	Axonotmesis	Axonal injury + endoneurium fibrosis	Same as second degree	Slow Partial recovery depending on severity
IV	Axonotmesis	Axonal injury + endoneurium and perineurium injury	No	None Surgery needed
V	Neurotmesis	Complete transection (damage to axon, endoneurium, perineurium, and epineurium)	No	None Surgery needed

Adapted with permission from Wood MD, Johnson PJ, Myckatyn TM: Anatomy and physiology for the peripheral nerve surgeon, in Mackinnon SE, ed: *Nerve Surgery*. Thieme, 2015.

well as in nerve regeneration. Nerve growth factor production is induced by the release of interleukin 1β by macrophages.[17,18] The production of nerve growth factor and other growth factors such as insulinlike growth factor 1, ciliary neurotrophic factor, and brain-derived neurotrophic factor are promoted by Schwann cells following nerve transection. In addition, nerve growth factor receptors are also upregulated on the surface of the Schwann cells[17] forming bands of Büngner.[19] Bands of Büngner are columns that serve as pathways for growing sprouts. At the end of each sprout, there is a growth cone that sends out filopodia. The growth cones are essential in determining the growth direction of the sprout.

CLASSIC AND ALTERNATIVE APPROACHES TO NERVE REPAIR

Principles of Nerve Repair

Decisions regarding timing of nerve repair are multifactorial and must consider mechanism of injury (sharp, crush, avulsion), closed or open nature of the injury, patient stability and comorbidities, and ability to determine zone of injury. Early nerve repair has the advantages of less nerve end retraction, an unscarred field, and the ability to stimulate the distal nerve stump up to 72 hours after injury, which can be useful for aligning fascicles and determining topography. Given the slow regeneration rate, early repairs allow for earlier, and potentially improved recovery as motor end plate viability is typically only maintained for 12 to 18 months after the initial injury.[20,21] Because nerves are estimated to grow approximately 1 to 3 mm per day,[22] earlier repair can help regenerating axons reach the muscle before muscle fibrosis occurs.

In general, open wounds with lack of nerve function should be explored for presumed nerve transection. Although often accompanied by an open wound, gunshot wounds are considered closed injuries as the blast mechanism allows the nerve to be moved out of the way. Thus, time for spontaneous recovery (6 months) should be allowed in the setting of gunshot wounds. In the setting of severely contaminated wounds or wounds with a large zone of injury, delayed repairs are beneficial to ensuring that the reconstruction is outside of the zone of injury.

For closed nerve injuries, such as with fractures and/or crush injuries, serial examinations are essential for monitoring recovery. Follow-up for patients with these injuries can begin with serial electromyography starting at approximately 10 weeks, which is the earliest time that motor unit action potentials would appear to indicate spontaneous recovery. If no recovery on electromyography or physical examination is detected by 3 to 6 months, surgical intervention is warranted.

Direct Nerve Repair

In 1972, Hanno Millesi introduced the technique of tension-free repair, which is now one of the basic tenets of nerve repair. Direct end-to-end tension-free nerve repair can be achieved in sharp transection injuries with minimal tissue loss. Loose epineurial repair is used most commonly as opposed to grouped fascicular repairs. Nerve ends are oriented visually by using visible fascicular matching and aligning any superficial vasa nervorum present in the epineurium for reference. If the topography of a mixed motor nerve is well known to the surgeon or able to be identified by distal nerve stump stimulation, then a fascicular repair can be performed. In situations where this is not possible, loose epineurial repair is preferable because of the principle of contact guidance whereby the nerves are guided by spatial cues and neurotrophic factors orient to their appropriate distal fascicles.

Nerve preparation is critical in achieving a successful nerve repair. Identifying and getting outside of the zone of injury is essential for success. Both nerve ends should be identified and débrided back to healthy bulging fascicles and evidence of intraneural blood flow. Nerve coaptation is achieved using 9-0 nylon sutures under microscopic or loupe magnification.[23] The extremity should be moved through full range of motion to ensure there is no tension on the repair and/or to assess the need for immobilization to protect the repair. Flexing joints to allow for primary repair is not recommended. If there is tension on the coaptation with range of motion, nerve grafting should be considered.

Management of Nerve Gap With Autologous Nerve Graft

When nerve gaps are encountered and nerves are not able to be coapted primarily, there are multiple options for bridging these gaps[24] (**Table 2**). Autologous nerve grafts are still currently considered the gold standard for nerve repair when gaps are present. Autologous nerves provide not only the essential scaffolding structure for nerve regeneration but also include endoneurial tubes, vascular bridges, and the critical cells that support regeneration, that is, Schwann cells. Small thin grafts and grafts that are shorter in length revascularize sooner and are often more reliable than long grafts and grafts with increasing diameter.

There are several factors that help determine the donor autograft, including donor nerve caliber and length, donor site morbidity, ease of harvest, and positioning. Two of the most commonly used donor nerves are sural nerve and medial antebrachial cutaneous nerve. Other expendable options include the lateral antebrachial cutaneous, the saphenous obturator branch to gracilis, and spare-part nerves from amputated digits or limbs. Potential drawbacks to nerve autograft include limited available nerve, donor site morbidity, loss of sensation in the donor distribution, scarring, and potential neuroma formation at the additional surgical site.[25]

TABLE 2 Options for Nerve Gap Fillers

Material	Pros	Cons	Usage
Autograft	Gold standard Retained nerve architecture Presence of Schwann cells	Donor site morbidities Donor site scar/healing Limited availability	Preferred for motor nerve and mixed nerve gap
Processed nerve allograft (PNA—Axogen Avance)	Readily available Retained nerve architecture	Additional cost Lack of Schwann cells Length limitation (further data needed)	Sensory nerve gap <3 cm Alternative for motor and mixed nerve when autograft not available
Conduit	Readily available	Lack of Schwann cells Lack of nerve architecture	Sensory nerve gap <3 cm

Adapted from Moore AM, Wagner IJ, Fox IK: Principles of nerve repair in complex wounds of the upper extremity. *Semin Plast Surg* 2015;29(1):40-47.

ORTHOBIOLOGICS

Nerve Allograft

Cadaver nerve allografts can provide similar advantages as autologous nerve graft while minimizing the donor site morbidity of nerve autograft. However, the use of cadaver nerve allograft requires temporary systemic immunosuppression, which can increase the risk of infection after surgery and has limited the use of these grafts clinically. The efforts to eliminate immunosuppression led to the development of processed (or acellular) nerve allografts (PNAs), which have gained popularity as an alternative to nerve autograft in the recent years. PNAs are processed cadaver nerves that remove immunogenic cellular components but retain the highly organized extracellular matrix to provide ideal scaffolding structure for nerve regeneration, thereby eliminating the need for immunosuppression.

Since the introduction of the PNAs, there are a few multicenter studies that have been published in the literature evaluating their efficacy. Notably, in 2008, a multicenter observational registry study (RANGER) was started; the first publication from this registry was released in 2012 by Brooks et al.[26] In this study, the nerve gap length was 5 to 50 mm and stratified into three different groups (5 to 14 mm, 15 to 29 mm, and 30 to 50 mm). The meaningful recovery was defined as S3-S4 or M3-M5 on the MacKinnon modification of the Medical Research Council grading system. In the 5- to 14-mm group, 100% had meaningful recovery, whereas the 15- to 29-mm group had a 76% meaningful recovery rate and the 30- to 50-mm group had a 91% meaningful recovery rate. When stratified by type of nerve repair, meaningful recovery was observed in 89% of sensory, 86% of motor, and 77% of mixed nerve repairs. When analyzed based on mechanism of injury, meaningful recovery was seen in 89% of the laceration group, 88% of the neuroma group, and 82% of the complex group (blast injury, avulsion, crush, compression, and gunshot wound). In 2020, a follow-up study by Safa et al[27] reported meaningful recovery of 82% for nerve gap up to 70 mm. This study showed similar findings in the repair of different nerve types when compared with the study by Brooks et al[26] (meaningful recovery 84%, 83%, and 71% for sensory, motor, and mixed nerve repairs, respectively). In the nerve gap subanalysis, the new study added another category of nerve gap, 50 to 70 mm. Meaningful recovery rates for less than 15 mm, 15 to 29 mm, and 30 to 49 mm were 91%, 85%, and 78%, respectively, and they were not significantly different. The meaningful recovery was significantly better in the less than 15-mm group when compared with the 50- to 70-mm group (91% versus 60%, $P = 0.011$). However, the 50- to 70-mm group had more complex injury than the less than 15-mm group. Of note, the RECON study, which is a multicenter prospective randomized subject and evaluator blinded comparative study of manufactured conduits and PNAs, has completed its enrollment and has met its primary end point required to officially apply for a biologics license application with the FDA.

Nerve Conduits

Nerve conduits are tubular structures used predominantly in the setting of short, noncritical sensory-only nerve gaps to guide the regenerating axons to the distal nerve stump. Multiple options for both autologous and synthetic conduits exist and are discussed in the following paragraphs; however, for many surgeons, the use of conduits has been largely replaced by acellular nerve allografts[28] (**Table 3**).

Autologous Nerve Conduits

In 1891, Büngner demonstrated sciatic nerve regeneration through a brachial artery.[29,30] However, this method of nerve conduit has become less popular because of high morbidity and lack of donor vessels. In 1980, Chiu introduced veins as an option for autologous nerve conduits.[31] In this study, successful nerve regeneration was done via

TABLE 3 Available Nerve Conduits

Product	Material	Degradation Time	Company
NeuroTube	Polyglycolic acid	3 months	Synovis Micro Companies
NeuraGen	Type I collagen	3-4 years	Integra LifeSciences Co.
NeuroFlex	Type I collagen	4-8 months	Collagen Matrix, Inc., Franklin
NeuroMatrix	Type I collagen	4-8 months	Collagen Matrix, Inc.
NeuraWrap	Type I collagen	36-48 months	Integra LifeSciences Co.
NeuroMend	Type I collagen	4-8 months	Collagen Matrix, Inc.
Neurolac	Poly-DL-lactide caprolactone	16 months	Polyganics BV
AxoGuard	Extracellular matrix derived from porcine small intestine submucosa	No data	AxoGen, Inc.

Adapted from Gaudin R, Knipfer C, Henningsen A, Smeets R, Heiland M, Hadlock T: Approaches to peripheral nerve repair: Generations of biomaterial conduits yielding to replacing autologous nerve grafts in craniomaxillofacial surgery. *Biomed Res Int* 2016;2016:3856262.

autologous vein nerve conduit with nerve gap of 1 cm in rat sciatic nerve. Suematsu et al and Chiu and Strauch validated this method of nerve conduit in their studies in 1988 and 1990, respectively.[32,33] Notably, Chiu and Strauch suggested that successful nerve repair can be achieved with vein conduits in nerve injury with nerve gap of 3 cm or less.

In addition to vein, muscle has also been used as a nerve conduit. It was thought that the longitudinal basal lamina in skeletal muscle with extracellular matrix can help direct the nerve growth.[34,35] The disadvantage of this method was the risk of axon loss due to nerve fiber growth into the muscle tissue during the regeneration and this method has been largely abandoned. Currently, autologous conduits are used infrequently because contemporary synthetic conduit options exist, which obviate the need for a donor site and often provide superior outcomes.

Nonautologous Biologic Conduits

Collagen is known to be a major component of the extracellular matrix that helps facilitate adhesion and survival of nonneuronal cells. Meaningful recovery with the use of collagen conduits in nerve gaps up to 20 mm has been reported by Bushnell et al, Wangensteen and Kalliainen, and Lohmeyer et al.[36-38] Although these studies showed some efficacy of collagen conduits to address sensory nerve gap up to 20 mm, they did not compare the effectiveness of these conduits to autograft or allograft.

Nonabsorbable Synthetic Conduits

Expanded polytetrafluoroethylene (Gore-Tex) was shown to have meaningful recovery in 79% of patients with ulnar and median nerve reconstructions with nerve gaps up to 40 mm in a study described by Stanec and Stanec in 1998.[39]

Another option for nonabsorbable synthetic conduit is silicone tube. Lungborg et al[40] described their use of silicone for gaps up to 5 mm as an alternative to direct suture repair. However, some patients required tube removal because of local tissue irritation, a complication that was also described in another study by Braga-Silva[41] and makes this a less desirable construct.

Absorbable Synthetic Conduits

The first FDA-approved bioabsorbable synthetic conduit on the market was composed of polyglycolic acid. The period of degradation for these conduits occurs 6 to 12 months after implantation. In 1990, MacKinnon and Dellon[42] showed 86% meaningful recovery in nerve gaps from 5 to 30 mm in 15 patients. In an attempt to address the efficacy of polyglycolic acid conduit in comparison with nerve autograft, Weber et al[43] performed a multicenter randomized controlled study in digital nerve repairs. Overall, no significant difference was recorded when comparing the rate of meaningful recovery between the conduit group and the autograft group ($P > 0.05$). However, when subanalysis was performed on different nerve gap groups, the conduit group performed better when the nerve gap was less than 4 mm and greater than 8 mm (9 to 30 mm). Given the positive result, Weber et al[43] favored the conduit because the conduit eliminated the need for harvesting a short nerve graft.

Bioengineered Nerve Scaffolds

The next evolution of conduit-assisted repair will be the development and utilization of three-dimensional nanoscaffolds within the conduit structure that guide axon growth across a gap. An increased understanding of the principle of contact guidance in nerve growth has allowed the development of nanoscaffolds that can optimize this process. Shakhbazau et al[44] were able to demonstrate in a rat model that a glycosaminoglycan matrix with appropriate microarchitecture was able to guide and facilitate Schwann cell migration and axon growth. Following this study, in a rat model, Lee et al[45] directly compared nerve gap repairs with hollow conduits versus conduits that were filled with a chondroitin-6-sulfate matrix and found superior recovery in motor function and axon counts compared with the hollow conduit alone. Building on this concept, there is now a clinically available product by Integra LifeSciences that uses this concept of a collagen conduit filled with a glycosaminoglycan scaffold to enhance nerve regeneration.

The next evolution of work being developed for scaffolds to augment nerve regeneration is using three-dimensional (3D) printing. In 2006, Goldner et al[46] showed that neurons will bridge across micropatterned grooves as long as the nanostructural parameters are optimized with regard to depth and width. Building on that, using newer techniques and technology available, many groups such as Du et al[47] are developing innovative scaffolds seeking to mimic the natural milieu the body creates to promote nerve regeneration in situ. They developed a 3D hierarchically aligned fibrin nanofiber hydrogel that is meant to resemble the architecture and biologic function of the native fibrin cables that the body produces to guide nerve repair. They found that this aligned fibrin nanofiber hydrogel supported Schwann cell cable formation and accelerated axon growth, which correlated with motor recovery. Going even further, Song et al[48] are developing innovative solutions such as their neural stem cell–laden 3D bioprinted electroconductive hydrogel scaffold, which they have shown is a viable substrate for neural stem cell growth and differentiation into neurons within that structure. Although these 3D printed hydrogels and nanoscaffolds are not yet clinically available, the future is bright for their use in augmenting and accelerating peripheral nerve repair and regeneration.

Nerve Transfer

Nerve transfers are defined as using a working, expendable nerve or fascicle and transferring it to a denervated nerve stump to restore function of that nerve (**Tables 4** and **5**). These transfers can be done closer to the denervated target muscle allowing for earlier reinnervation and ultimately a more expeditious return of function. Additional benefits include avoiding a nerve graft, operating out of a scarred field, and the ability to deliver more axons to the target organ. For these reasons, over the past 2 decades, there has been a paradigm shift from nerve grafting to nerve transfers.

Treatment Algorithm

The senior author's (AMM) preferred treatment algorithms are presented in **Figures 2** and **3**.

TABLE 4 Common Upper Extremity Nerve Injuries and Nerve Transfer

Nerve Injury	Nerve Transfer
Radial nerve	**Motor**: Median nerve branches (flexor digitorum superficialis to extensor carpi radialis brevis for wrist extension and flexor carpi radialis nerve is transferred to the posterior interosseous nerve for finger and thumb extension) **Sensory**: Lateral antebrachial cutaneous nerve transfer to the radial sensory nerve
Median nerve	**Motor**: Radial nerve branches, brachialis branches of the musculocutaneous nerve, and distal ulnar motor branches. **Sensory**: Distal digital branches of the radial, the dorsal cutaneous branch of the ulnar nerve, ulnar digital nerve of the ring finger
Ulnar nerve	**Motor**: Distal anterior interosseous nerve–to–ulnar motor nerve transfer (end to end or supercharged) **Sensory**: Palmar cutaneous branch of the median nerve, third web space nerve branch of the median nerve

ADDITIONAL THERAPIES

Electrical Stimulation

Nerve injuries in the PNS differ from those in the central nervous system in that there is regenerative potential of injured and transected axons with the support of the Schwann cells in the distal nerve stump. As discussed previously, regeneration proceeds at approximately 1 to 3 mm/d and thus proximal nerve injuries are often unable to reach their distal musculature in time for proper reinnervation and functional recovery.[22,49] Therapies aimed at

TABLE 5 Common Lower Extremity Nerve Injuries and Nerve Transfers

Nerve Injury	Nerve Transfer
Femoral nerve	**Motor**: Obturator nerve transfer to branches of the femoral nerve; sartorius nerve branches to branches of femoral nerve; sciatic fascicular transfers to femoral nerve branches
Gluteal nerves	**Motor**: Sciatic fascicular transfers to the inferior and/or superior gluteal nerves
Tibial nerve (of sciatic nerve)	**Motor**: Terminal femoral nerve branches to nerve to gastrocnemius muscle
Peroneal nerve (of sciatic nerve)	**Motor**: Partial tibial nerve transfers to peroneal nerve

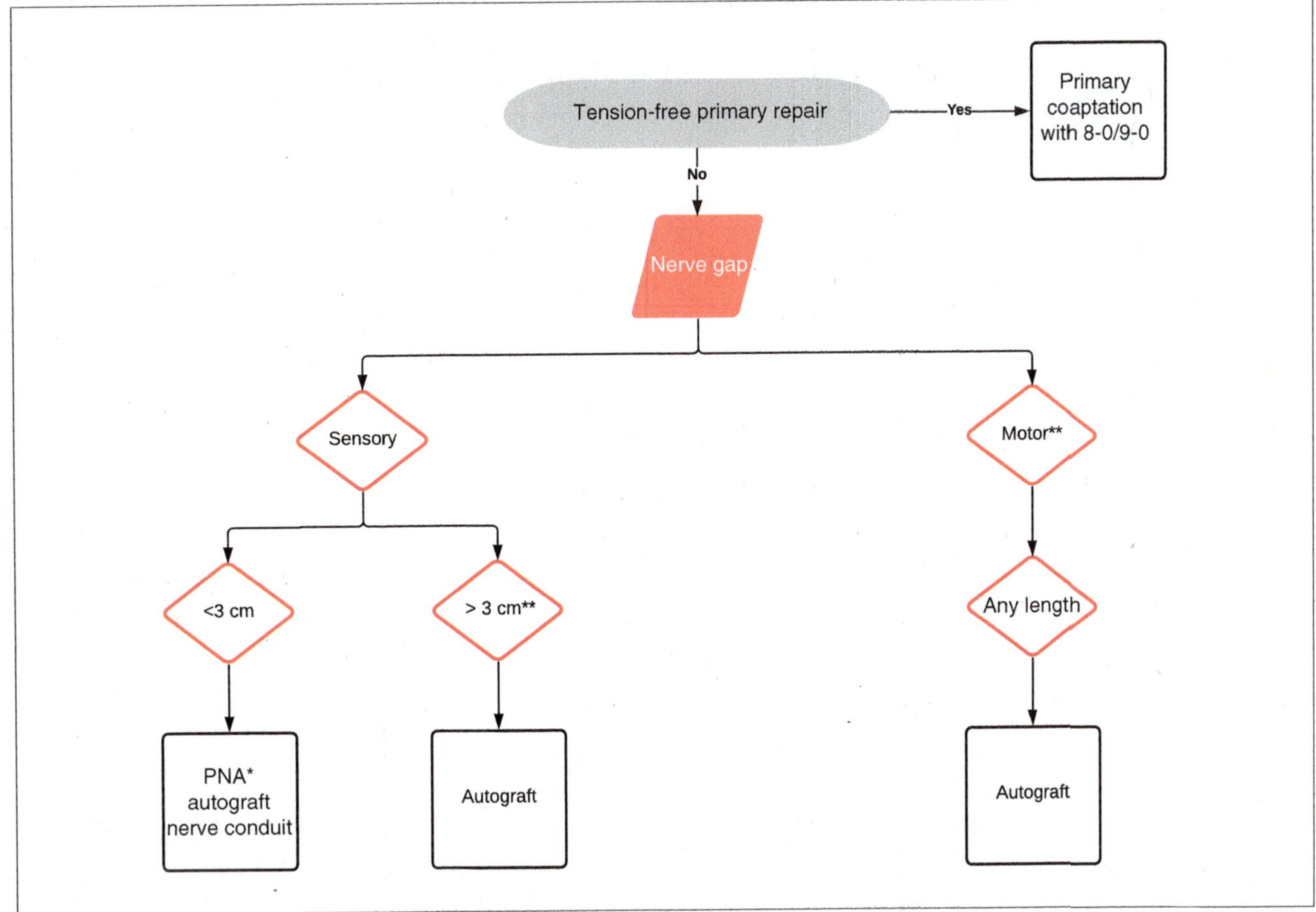

FIGURE 2 Flowchart shows the preferred algorithm for the treatment of nerve gaps. * Processed nerve allograft. ** Additional data are needed to determine length and efficacy of processed nerve allograft use for these categories.

accelerating axonal regeneration have been highly sought after, and work investigating electrical stimulation shows great promise in this arena.

The technique of electrical stimulation relies on brief low-frequency (≤20 mHz) stimulation applied directly after nerve repair for a variable duration of time. This has been shown in both animal and human studies to enhance functional recovery in both motor and sensory nerves.[50-54] The biologic basis of electrical stimulation was discovered by the finding that applying tetrodotoxin, which blocks proximal electrical impulses, to the proximal nerve negated the benefits of electrical stimulation on regenerating nerves.[55] Electrical stimulation exerts its influence through the retrograde conduction of action potentials to the neuronal cell bodies in the central nervous system. This stimulates cyclic adenosine monophosphate and upregulates other neurotrophic factors and genes that are expressed in the neuron and crucial to accelerating nerve regeneration. This leads to increased axonal regeneration across repair sites along with remyelination of regenerating axons, ultimately leading to increased functional recovery even after delayed surgical repair.[51,52,56-58]

In the clinical realm, recent prospective randomized controlled studies have shown the benefit of electrical stimulation on nerve regeneration in both the settings of chronic compression[59,60] and nerve injury.[61,62] In 2015, Wong et al[61] investigated the effects of electrical stimulation on recovery after digital nerve repair. Their double-blind, randomized controlled trial involved 31 patients who underwent digital nerve repair and were randomized into either 1 hour of electrical stimulation in a postanesthesia care unit through electrodes implanted before skin closure or sham stimulation. The electrical stimulation group showed statistically significantly more rapid recovery in all tested sensory modalities including Semmes-Weinstein monofilament testing, static two-point discrimination, and cold/warmth

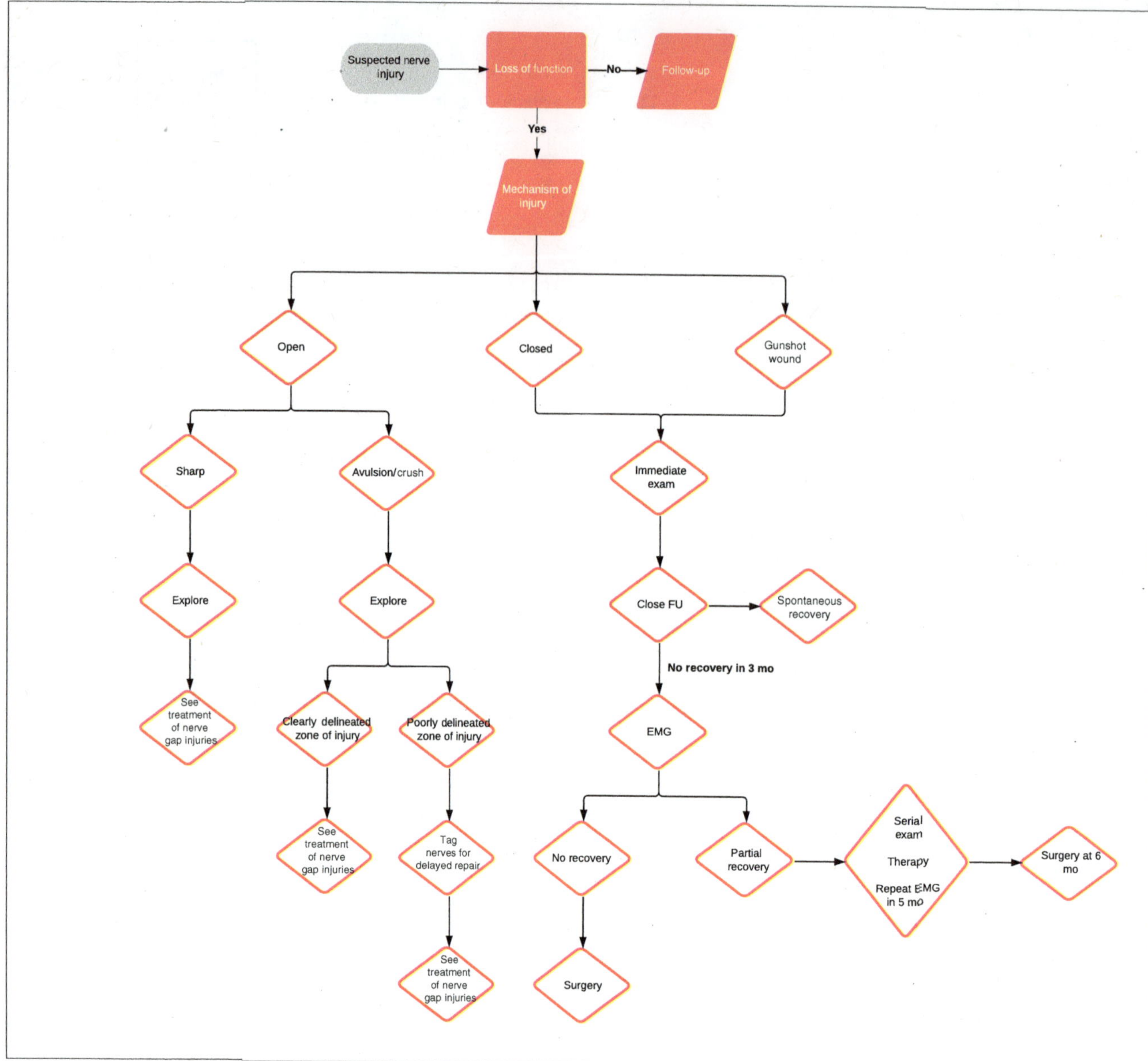

FIGURE 3 Flowchart shows the preferred algorithm for the timing of nerve diagnosis and repair. EMG = electromyography, FU = follow-up. * Decompression surgery + nerve transfer (end-to-side versus end-to-end).

detection thresholds, with each returning to near normal values.

Barber et al[62] conducted the first study that showed increased functional recovery with electrical stimulation compared with a control group. Their double-blind, randomized controlled trial evaluated electrical stimulation in 54 patients with head and neck cancer with spinal accessory nerve neurapraxia after neck dissections. Spinal accessory nerve injury was detected by intraoperative electromyography of the trapezius muscle and patients were then randomized to no stimulation or intraoperative stimulation of 1 hour at 20 mHz. At 1 year of follow-up, patients in the electrical stimulation group showed significantly better shoulder function scores and electrophysiologic studies demonstrated improved compound muscle action potentials compared with controls.

Although clinical details such as optimal delivery of stimulation, duration of stimulation needed, and timing of application (intraoperative versus postoperative) are still being worked out, the role of electrical stimulation in nerve recovery clearly has merit that may play a major role in clinical treatment of nerve injuries in the very near future.

Stem Cell Therapy

Another therapy currently being investigated to enhance peripheral nerve regeneration is stem cell transplantation. In the setting of nerve injury, Schwann cells secrete neurotropic factors and create a milieu that is favorable for axon regeneration; however, over the course of recovery after nerve transection, Schwann cells are not able to maintain a growth-conducive environment and therefore show a time-dependent decline in regenerative capacity.[21,63-65] Stem cells could be a potential source of Schwann-like cells that would, when applied to the nerve, cultivate and mature a proregenerative environment.

Stem cells are capable of differentiating into more specialized cell types and able to self-replicate. Possible sources that have been investigated for peripheral nerve regeneration include but are not limited to neural stem cells, embryonic stem cells, and mesenchymal stem cells (derived from bone marrow, adipose tissue, hair follicles, etc). Theoretically, stem cells that migrate to a site of nerve injury should be able to proliferate and differentiate into appropriate cell types to facilitate regeneration; however, the differentiation rate of precursor cells in the peripheral nerve is relatively low.[66] The process of predifferentiating stem cells toward the desired phenotype before implantation has been shown to be more effective than allowing the process to happen organically.[67] The optimal delivery system for stem cells is still under investigation and includes microinjection, cell-laden fibrin matrix for injection, injection or lamination into natural or synthetic conduits, and 3D printed scaffolds all of which have shown promise.[68-72]

Stem cells currently remain in the preclinical phase because of issues with optimization of differentiation and delivery, as well as concerns with cell instability and tumorigenesis. Despite this, stem cell therapy is an exciting frontier being explored with potential to enhance peripheral nerve regeneration in the future.

Tissue Engineering

Given the limited availability of nerve autograft donor site, tissue-engineered nerve graft can be a potential alternative to the gold standard of peripheral nerve repair. Yet, success in peripheral nerve tissue engineering has been limited despite the advancement in technologies in the past few decades. Tissue engineering is the new tissue creation by stimulation of target cells via a combination of molecular and mechanical signals[73] within a scaffold designed to assist the construction of the new desired tissue. Many available neural scaffolds exist, but nerve regeneration success with these scaffolds alone has been limited because of its lack of biochemical cues including supportive cells, cytokines, and growth factors, which are critical components of effective tissue-engineered nerve grafts.[74] Although important in peripheral nerve regeneration, obtaining a large number of autologous Schwann cells is difficult. There are some promising alternatives to autologous Schwann cells described in the literature, including bone marrow mesenchymal stem cells or bone marrow stromal cells[75,76] and induced pluripotent stem cells.[77,78]

In addition to support cells, growth factors play critical parts of the peripheral nerve regeneration. Although there are endogenous growth factors produced by the neural cells at the site of injury, the production may simply be not enough to support axonal regeneration. Hence, continuous supply of exogenous growth factors may be needed for successful tissue-engineered nerve graft. There are a few products that have been studied including fibrin gels loaded with glial cell line-derived neurotrophic factor–containing poly(lactic-co-glycolic) acid–based microspheres[79] or silicone-based nerve conduit seeded with fibroblast growth factor-2.[80] Despite ongoing publications on tissue-engineered nerve graft, there is much to learn and discover because there is no current optimal product on the market.

Polyethylene Glycol Fusion

As the frontiers of nerve surgery continue to expand, one of the most exciting new therapies being evaluated is the use of polyethylene glycol (PEG) in the setting of acute nerve repair. PEG is regarded as a fusogen in that it allows for the fusion of closely approximated cell membranes. This process occurs secondary to dehydration of membrane lipids by PEG, which causes instability and allows adjacent cells to fuse and then stabilize when they are rehydrated.[81] Since the concept of using PEG fusion in nerve repair was first introduced and refined by Bittner et al,[82] and Lore et al,[83] PEG has been studied extensively in mammalian models. Evidence of the drastic effects of PEG is best illustrated by the near-immediate restoration of compound action potentials in PEG-treated nerves,[84,85] as well as the use of the novel diffusion tensor imaging demonstrating axons crossing a repair site in PEG-treated nerves directly after repair.[86]

Protocols for PEG fusion vary, but the one demonstrated by Mikesh et al[87,88] in a rat sciatic nerve model has shown consistent results. It involves the irrigation of the cut nerve ends with a hypotonic calcium-free saline to open cut nerve ends, application of methylene blue as an antioxidant to keep the nerve ends open and prevent formation of vesicles, and then coaptation of the nerve endings with microsuture. After coaptation, the PEG solution is applied to the repaired nerve for 1 to 2 minutes and then irrigated with sterile lactated Ringer solution with calcium to facilitate axolemmal repair.[87,88] This protocol used in the rat sciatic nerve model has been shown to have multiple positive effects on nerve repair and regeneration; most notably it "(1) restores axonal continuity across coaptation site(s) within minutes, (2) prevents wallerian degeneration of many distal severed axons, (3) preserves neuromuscular junctions, (4) prevents target muscle atrophy, (5) produces rapid and improved recovery of voluntary behaviors compared with neurorrhaphy alone, and (6) PEG-fused allografts are not rejected, despite no tissue matching nor immunosuppression."[89] Given the incredible potential of PEG fusion to change the standard of care for nerve repair, this remains one of the most exciting interventions currently making its way from bench to bedside.

SUMMARY

The surgeon's toolkit for peripheral nerve repair continues to expand rapidly in the search for a reliable and reproducible way to restore sensation and motor function. Groundbreaking work in orthobiologics using 3D printing, nanoscaffolds, hydrogels, and stem cells continues to push the field of peripheral nerve regeneration forward. Considering the exciting advances in both biologic and synthetic technologies, it is important to look forward, as rigorous scientific evaluation of these and other emerging therapies must proceed carefully before a true paradigm shift can take place and transform the way peripheral nerve repair is approached.

REFERENCES

1. Hirasawa Y, Saiki T, Nakao Y, Katsumi Y: Regeneration of perineurium after nerve injury and autografting. An experimental study. *Int Orthop* 1994;18(4):229-235.
2. Piña-Oviedo S, Ortiz-Hidalgo C: The normal and neoplastic perineurium: A review. *Adv Anat Pathol* 2008;15(3):147-164.
3. Wood MD, Johnson PJ, Myckatyn TM: Anatomy and physiology for the peripheral nerve surgeon, in Mackinnon S, ed: *Nerve surgery*. Thieme, 2015, pp 1-40.
4. Lundborg G: Ischemic nerve injury. experimental studies on intraneural microvascular pathophysiology and nerve function in a limb subjected to temporary circulatory arrest. *Scand J Plast Reconstr Surg Suppl* 1970;6:3-113.
5. Gaspar MP, Pham PP, Kane PM: Basic science of peripheral nerve injury and repair, in Skirven TM, Osterman AL, Fedorczyck JM, Amadio PP, Feldscher SB, Shin EK, eds: *Rehabilitation of the Hand and Upper Extremity*. Elsevier, 2019, pp 569-579.
6. Lundborg G: The intrinsic vascularization of human peripheral nerves: Structural and functional aspects. *J Hand Surg Am* 1979;4(1):34-41.
7. Lundborg G: Structure and function of the intraneural microvessels as related to trauma, edema formation, and nerve function. *J Bone Joint Surg Am* 1975;57(7):938-948.
8. Power HA, Moore AM: Basic science of nerve compression, in Skirven TM, Osterman AL, Fedorczyck JM, Amadio PC, Feldscher SB, Shin EK, eds: *Rehabilitation of the Hand and Upper Extremity*. Elsevier, 2020, pp 677-684.
9. Gordon T: Peripheral nerve regeneration and muscle reinnervation. *Int J Mol Sci* 2020;21(22):8652.
10. Gaudet AD, Popovich PG, Ramer MS: Wallerian degeneration: Gaining perspective on inflammatory events after peripheral nerve injury. *J Neuroinflammation* 2011;8:110.
11. Vargas ME, Yamagishi Y, Tessier-Lavigne M, Sagasti A: Live imaging of calcium dynamics during axon degeneration reveals two functionally distinct phases of calcium influx. *J Neurosci* 2015;35(45):15026-15038.
12. Griffin JW, Thompson WJ: Biology and pathology of nonmyelinating schwann cells. *Glia* 2008;56(14):1518-1531.
13. George R, Griffin JW: The proximo-distal spread of axonal degeneration in the dorsal columns of the rat. *J Neurocytol* 1994;23(11):657-667.
14. Menorca RM, Fussell TS, Elfar JC: Nerve physiology: Mechanisms of injury and recovery. *Hand Clin* 2013;29(3):317-330.
15. Rotshenker S: Wallerian degeneration: The innate-immune response to traumatic nerve injury. *J Neuroinflammation* 2011;8:109.
16. Lundborg G: A 25-year perspective of peripheral nerve surgery: Evolving neuroscientific concepts and clinical significance. *J Hand Surg Am* 2000;25(3):391-414.
17. Lindholm D, Heumann R, Meyer M, Thoenen H: Interleukin-1 regulates synthesis of nerve growth factor in non-neuronal cells of rat sciatic nerve. *Nature* 1987;330(6149):658-659.
18. Nathan CF: Secretory products of macrophages. *J Clin Invest* 1987;79(2):319-326.
19. Taniuchi M, Clark HB, Schweitzer JB, Johnson EM Jr: Expression of nerve growth factor receptors by schwann cells of axotomized peripheral nerves: Ultrastructural location, suppression by axonal contact, and binding properties. *J Neurosci* 1988;8(2):664-681.
20. Kobayashi J, Mackinnon SE, Watanabe O, et al: The effect of duration of muscle denervation on functional recovery in the rat model. *Muscle Nerve* 1997;20(7):858-866.
21. Fu SY, Gordon T: Contributing factors to poor functional recovery after delayed nerve repair: Prolonged denervation. *J Neurosci* 1995;15(5 pt 2):3886-3895.
22. Seddon HJ, Medawar PB, Smith H: Rate of regeneration of peripheral nerves in man. *J Physiol* 1943;102(2):191-215.
23. Goldberg SH, Jobin CM, Hayes AG, Gardner T, Rosenwasser MP, Strauch RJ: Biomechanics and histology of intact and repaired digital nerves: An in vitro study. *J Hand Surg Am* 2007;32(4):474-482.
24. Moore AM, Wagner IJ, Fox IK: Principles of nerve repair in complex wounds of the upper extremity. *Semin Plast Surg* 2015;29(1):40-47.
25. Mackinnon SE: Surgical management of the peripheral nerve gap. *Clin Plast Surg* 1989;16(3):587-603.
26. Brooks DN, Weber RV, Chao JD, et al: Processed nerve allografts for peripheral nerve reconstruction: A multicenter study of utilization and outcomes in sensory, mixed, and motor nerve reconstructions. *Microsurgery* 2012;32(1):1-14.

27. Safa B, Jain S, Desai MJ, et al: Peripheral nerve repair throughout the body with processed nerve allografts: Results from a large multicenter study. *Microsurgery* 2020;40(5):527-537.
28. Gaudin R, Knipfer C, Henningsen A, Smeets R, Heiland M, Hadlock T: Approaches to peripheral nerve repair: Generations of biomaterial conduits yielding to replacing autologous nerve grafts in craniomaxillofacial surgery. *Biomed Res Int* 2016;2016:3856262
29. Lin MY, Manzano G, Gupta R: Nerve allografts and conduits in peripheral nerve repair. *Hand Clin* 2013;29(3):331-348.
30. Colen KL, Choi M, Chiu DTW: Nerve grafts and conduits. *Plast Reconstr Surg* 2009;124(6 suppl):e386-e394.
31. Tseng CY, Hu G, Ambron RT, Chiu DT: Histologic analysis of schwann cell migration and peripheral nerve regeneration in the autogenous venous nerve conduit (AVNC). *J Reconstr Microsurg* 2003;19(5):331-340.
32. Chiu DT, Strauch B: A prospective clinical evaluation of autogenous vein grafts used as a nerve conduit for distal sensory nerve defects of 3 cm or less. *Plast Reconstr Surg* 1990;86(5):928-934.
33. Suematsu N, Atsuta Y, Hirayama T: Vein graft for repair of peripheral nerve gap. *J Reconstr Microsurg* 1988;4(4):313-318.
34. Meek MF, Coert JH: Clinical use of nerve conduits in peripheral-nerve repair: Review of the literature. *J Reconstr Microsurg* 2002;18(2):97-109.
35. Meek MF, Varejão AS, Geuna S: Use of skeletal muscle tissue in peripheral nerve repair: Review of the literature. *Tissue Eng* 2004;10(7-8):1027-1036.
36. Bushnell BD, McWilliams AD, Whitener GB, Messer TM: Early clinical experience with collagen nerve tubes in digital nerve repair. *J Hand Surg Am* 2008;33(7):1081-1087.
37. Wangensteen KJ, Kalliainen LK: Collagen tube conduits in peripheral nerve repair: A retrospective analysis. *Hand (N Y)* 2010;5(3):273-277.
38. Lohmeyer JA, Siemers F, Machens HG, Mailänder P: The clinical use of artificial nerve conduits for digital nerve repair: A prospective cohort study and literature review. *J Reconstr Microsurg* 2009;25(1):55-61.
39. Stanec S, Stanec Z: Reconstruction of upper-extremity peripheral-nerve injuries with ePTFE conduits. *J Reconstr Microsurg* 1998;14(4):227-232.
40. Lundborg G, Rosén B, Abrahamson SO, Dahlin L, Danielsen N: Tubular repair of the median nerve in the human forearm. preliminary findings. *J Hand Surg Br* 1994;19(3):273-276.
41. Braga-Silva J: The use of silicone tubing in the late repair of the median and ulnar nerves in the forearm. *J Hand Surg Br* 1999;24(6):703-706.
42. Mackinnon SE, Dellon AL: Clinical nerve reconstruction with a bioabsorbable polyglycolic acid tube. *Plast Reconstr Surg* 1990;85(3):419-424.
43. Weber RA, Breidenbach WC, Brown RE, Jabaley ME, Mass DP: A randomized prospective study of polyglycolic acid conduits for digital nerve reconstruction in humans. *Plast Reconstr Surg* 2000;106(5):1036-1038.
44. Shakhbazau A, Archibald SJ, Shcharbin D, Bryszewska M, Midha R: Aligned collagen-GAG matrix as a 3D substrate for schwann cell migration and dendrimer-based gene delivery. *J Mater Sci Mater Med* 2014;25(8):1979-1989.
45. Lee JY, Giusti G, Friedrich PF, et al: The effect of collagen nerve conduits filled with collagen-glycosaminoglycan matrix on peripheral motor nerve regeneration in a rat model. *J Bone Joint Surg Am* 2012;94(22):2084-2091.
46. Goldner JS, Bruder JM, Li G, Gazzola D, Hoffman-Kim D: Neurite bridging across micropatterned grooves. *Biomaterials* 2006;27(3):460-472.
47. Du J, Liu J, Yao S, et al: Prompt peripheral nerve regeneration induced by a hierarchically aligned fibrin nanofiber hydrogel. *Acta Biomater* 2017;55:296-309.
48. Song S, Liu X, Huang J, Zhang Z: Neural stem cell-laden 3D bioprinting of polyphenol-doped electroconductive hydrogel scaffolds for enhanced neuronal differentiation. *Biomater Adv* 2022;133:112639.
49. Fu SY, Gordon T: The cellular and molecular basis of peripheral nerve regeneration. *Mol Neurobiol* 1997;14(1-2):67-116.
50. Gordon T: Electrical stimulation to enhance axon regeneration after peripheral nerve injuries in animal models and humans. *Neurotherapeutics* 2016;13(2):295-310.
51. Zuo KJ, Gordon T, Chan KM, Borschel GH: Electrical stimulation to enhance peripheral nerve regeneration: Update in molecular investigations and clinical translation. *Exp Neurol* 2020;332:113397.
52. Brushart TM, Hoffman PN, Royall RM, Murinson BB, Witzel C, Gordon T: Electrical stimulation promotes motoneuron regeneration without increasing its speed or conditioning the neuron. *J Neurosci* 2002;22(15):6631-6638.
53. Geremia NM, Gordon T, Brushart TM, Al-Majed AA, Verge VM: Electrical stimulation promotes sensory neuron regeneration and growth-associated gene expression. *Exp Neurol* 2007;205(2):347-359.
54. Willand MP, Nguyen MA, Borschel GH, Gordon T: Electrical stimulation to promote peripheral nerve regeneration. *Neurorehabil Neural Repair* 2016;30(5):490-496.
55. Al-Majed AA, Neumann CM, Brushart TM, Gordon T: Brief electrical stimulation promotes the speed and accuracy of motor axonal regeneration. *J Neurosci* 2000;20(7):2602-2608.
56. Al-Majed AA, Tam SL, Gordon T: Electrical stimulation accelerates and enhances expression of regeneration-associated genes in regenerating rat femoral motoneurons. *Cell Mol Neurobiol* 2004;24(3):379-402.
57. Gordon T, Udina E, Verge VM, de Chaves EI: Brief electrical stimulation accelerates axon regeneration in the peripheral nervous system and promotes sensory axon regeneration in the central nervous system. *Motor Control* 2009;13(4):412-441.
58. Elzinga K, Tyreman N, Ladak A, Savaryn B, Olson J, Gordon T: Brief electrical stimulation improves nerve regeneration after delayed repair in sprague dawley rats. *Exp Neurol* 2015;269:142-153.
59. Gordon T, Amirjani N, Edwards DC, Chan KM: Brief post-surgical electrical stimulation accelerates axon regeneration and muscle reinnervation without affecting the functional measures in carpal tunnel syndrome patients. *Exp Neurol* 2010;223(1):192-202.

60. Power HA, Morhart MJ, Olson JL, Chan KM: Postsurgical electrical stimulation enhances recovery following surgery for severe cubital tunnel syndrome: A double-blind randomized controlled trial. *Neurosurgery* 2020;86(6):769-777.
61. Wong JN, Olson JL, Morhart MJ, Chan KM: Electrical stimulation enhances sensory recovery: A randomized controlled trial. *Ann Neurol* 2015;77(6):996-1006.
62. Barber B, Seikaly H, Ming Chan K, et al: Intraoperative brief electrical stimulation of the spinal accessory nerve (BEST SPIN) for prevention of shoulder dysfunction after oncologic neck dissection: A double-blinded, randomized controlled trial. *J Otolaryngol Head Neck Surg* 2018;47(1):7-9.
63. Höke A, Gordon T, Zochodne DW, Sulaiman OA: A decline in glial cell-line-derived neurotrophic factor expression is associated with impaired regeneration after long-term schwann cell denervation. *Exp Neurol* 2002;173(1):77-85.
64. Höke A, Redett R, Hameed H, et al: Schwann cells express motor and sensory phenotypes that regulate axon regeneration. *J Neurosci* 2006;26(38):9646-9655.
65. Gordon T: Neurotrophic factor expression in denervated motor and sensory schwann cells: Relevance to specificity of peripheral nerve regeneration. *Exp Neurol* 2014;254:99-108.
66. Pan HC, Cheng FC, Chen CJ, et al: Post-injury regeneration in rat sciatic nerve facilitated by neurotrophic factors secreted by amniotic fluid mesenchymal stem cells. *J Clin Neurosci* 2007;14(11):1089-1098.
67. Jiang L, Jones S, Jia X: Stem cell transplantation for peripheral nerve regeneration: Current options and opportunities. *Int J Mol Sci* 2017;18(1):94.
68. Pang CJ, Tong L, Ji LL, et al: Synergistic effects of ultrashort wave and bone marrow stromal cells on nerve regeneration with acellular nerve allografts. *Synapse* 2013;67(10):637-647.
69. Costa HJ, Bento RF, Salomone R, et al: Mesenchymal bone marrow stem cells within polyglycolic acid tube observed in vivo after six weeks enhance facial nerve regeneration. *Brain Res* 2013;1510:10-21.
70. Yang Y, Yuan X, Ding F, et al: Repair of rat sciatic nerve gap by a silk fibroin-based scaffold added with bone marrow mesenchymal stem cells. *Tissue Eng Part A* 2011;17(17-18):2231-2244.
71. Pereira Lopes FR, Camargo de Moura Campos L, Dias Corrêa J Jr. et al: Bone marrow stromal cells and resorbable collagen guidance tubes enhance sciatic nerve regeneration in mice. *Exp Neurol* 2006;198(2):457-468.
72. Weightman A, Jenkins S, Pickard M, Chari D, Yang Y: Alignment of multiple glial cell populations in 3D nanofiber scaffolds: Toward the development of multicellular implantable scaffolds for repair of neural injury. *Nanomedicine* 2014;10(2):291-295.
73. Williams DF: To engineer is to create: The link between engineering and regeneration. *Trends Biotechnol* 2006;24(1):4-8.
74. Gu X, Ding F, Williams DF: Neural tissue engineering options for peripheral nerve regeneration. *Biomaterials* 2014;35(24):6143-6156.
75. Hu N, Wu H, Xue C, et al: Long-term outcome of the repair of 50 mm long median nerve defects in rhesus monkeys with marrow mesenchymal stem cells-containing, chitosan-based tissue engineered nerve grafts. *Biomaterials* 2013;34(1):100-111.
76. Ding F, Wu J, Yang Y, et al: Use of tissue-engineered nerve grafts consisting of a chitosan/poly(lactic-co-glycolic acid)-based scaffold included with bone marrow mesenchymal cells for bridging 50-mm dog sciatic nerve gaps. *Tissue Eng Part A* 2010;16(12):3779-3790.
77. Uemura T, Takamatsu K, Ikeda M, et al: Transplantation of induced pluripotent stem cell-derived neurospheres for peripheral nerve repair. *Biochem Biophys Res Commun* 2012;419(1):130-135.
78. Huang Z, Powell R, Phillips JB, Haastert-Talini K: Perspective on schwann cells derived from induced pluripotent stem cells in peripheral nerve tissue engineering. *Cells* 2020;9(11):2497.
79. Wood MD, Gordon T, Kemp SW, et al: Functional motor recovery is improved due to local placement of GDNF microspheres after delayed nerve repair. *Biotechnol Bioeng* 2013;110(5):1272-1281.
80. Timmer M, Robben S, Müller-Ostermeyer F, Nikkhah G, Grothe C: Axonal regeneration across long gaps in silicone chambers filled with schwann cells overexpressing high molecular weight FGF-2. *Cell Transplant* 2003;12(3):265-277.
81. Paskal AM, Paskal W, Pietruski P, Wlodarski PK: Polyethylene glycol: The future of posttraumatic nerve repair? Systemic review. *Int J Mol Sci* 2019;20(6):1478.
82. Bittner GD, Ballinger ML, Raymond MA: Reconnection of severed nerve axons with polyethylene glycol. *Brain Res* 1986;367(1-2):351-355.
83. Lore AB, Hubbell JA, Bobb DS Jr, et al: Rapid induction of functional and morphological continuity between severed ends of mammalian or earthworm myelinated axons. *J Neurosci* 1999;19(7):2442-2454.
84. Bittner GD, Keating CP, Kane JR, et al: Rapid, effective, and long-lasting behavioral recovery produced by microsutures, methylene blue, and polyethylene glycol after completely cutting rat sciatic nerves. *J Neurosci Res* 2012;90(5):967-980.
85. Bamba R, Riley DC, Kim JS, et al: Evaluation of a nerve fusion technique with polyethylene glycol in a delayed setting after nerve injury. *J Hand Surg Am* 2018;43(1):82.e1-82.e7.
86. Bamba R, Riley DC, Kelm ND, Does MD, Dortch RD, Thayer WP: A novel technique using hydrophilic polymers to promote axonal fusion. *Neural Regen Res* 2016;11(4):525-528.
87. Mikesh M, Ghergherehchi CL, Hastings RL, et al: Polyethylene glycol solutions rapidly restore and maintain axonal continuity, neuromuscular structures, and behaviors lost after sciatic nerve transections in female rats. *J Neurosci Res* 2018;96(7):1223-1242.
88. Mikesh M, Ghergherehchi CL, Rahesh S, et al: Corrigendum to "polyethylene glycol treated allografts not tissue matched nor immunosuppressed rapidly repair sciatic nerve gaps, maintain neuromuscular functions, and restore voluntary behaviors in female rats". *J Neurosci Res* 2018;96(9):1624.
89. Ghergherehchi CL, Mikesh M, Sengelaub DR, et al: Polyethylene glycol (PEG) and other bioactive solutions with neurorrhaphy for rapid and dramatic repair of peripheral nerve lesions by PEG-fusion. *J Neurosci Methods* 2019;314:1-12.

CHAPTER

21 Skeletal Muscle Regeneration

George J. Christ, PhD • Brian C. Werner, MD, FAAOS •
Sarah E. Dyer, BS • Shep Hurwitz, MD, FAAOS

INTRODUCTION

Skeletal muscle has a remarkable capacity for regeneration and repair following a variety of injuries. There are many recoverable muscle injuries, such as common sports injuries (strains or contusions) or injuries induced by myotoxins (notexin, cardiotoxin, and bupivacaine) or other chemical (barium chloride) or physical methods (freeze injury, crush, and irradiation), which can repair and remodel with minimal scar tissue formation and significant de novo regeneration within 1 month.[1-6] A high-level schematic depiction of the skeletal muscle repair process is shown in **Figure 1**. Although the degree of regeneration in the setting of extensive muscle ablation can be quite extraordinary, the robust nature and rate of functional recovery is largely dependent on the integrity of the existing extracellular matrix (ECM), blood vessel networks, and neuronal innervation to provide important guidance cues, as well as the structural and nutritional support required for productive wound healing and functional muscle regeneration, including the critical role of key growth factors.[2,6-8] Volumetric muscle loss (VML) is an irrecoverable skeletal muscle trauma/injury that stands in stark contrast to these requirements for more complete endogenous repair.[9]

PATHOLOGY AND NATURAL HISTORY OF VML EXTREMITY POLYTRAUMA

Traumatic injuries represent a significant health concern in both the military and civilian populations.[10,11] Although the battle mortality rate for US armed forces has decreased from 30% in World War II to less than 10% in Afghanistan and Iraq,[12] there has been a parallel increase in the number of seriously injured soldiers who survive with extraordinary injuries, especially complex and severe extremity and head/neck polytrauma.[13-16] Furthermore, of the approximately 7.9 million fractures that occur in the civilian population of the United States each year, approximately 10% are open fractures, which are characterized by concomitant soft-tissue damage.[17] Such composite tissue injuries present a major clinical challenge. In fact, both the treatment and wound healing response for complex limb trauma depend on both the severity and location of the injury, as well as relevant patient characteristics.[11,18-20] Therefore, open fractures/complex limb traumas require numerous treatment strategies/interventions and multiple surgeries and result in high direct and indirect health care costs,[21] all of which indicate the need for more individualized/personalized approaches to the therapeutics (eg, precision medicine).[18] Even so, almost two-thirds of patients remain significantly disabled over the long term (at 7 years postinjury, and likely beyond).[22]

Of note, simultaneous loss of surrounding muscle tissue is associated with poor wound healing in patients with open fracture.[20,23,24] This is important because orthopaedic injuries such as type III tibial fractures usually involve concomitant soft-tissue injury/loss. When the degree of skeletal muscle tissue loss is sufficient to result in permanent structural and functional deficits, it is referred to as a VML injury.[25] Despite the considerable regenerative capacity of skeletal muscle, VML injuries, by definition, exceed endogenous wound healing capacity and result in lasting functional and cosmetic deficits. In the setting of such complex limb trauma, the clinical focus is typically on bone healing, for which there are viable therapeutic options available, as opposed to managing the VML defect, for which there are few effective therapies.

Although the precise mechanism(s) responsible for impaired fracture healing in the presence of severe muscle trauma is unknown, impaired vasculature, loss of muscle-derived cells/stem cells, and/or concomitant growth factors and cytokines are all likely involved, and furthermore, thought to be critical for the creation of a more favorable regenerative microenvironment.[23] In addition, VML injury may have other downstream effects for the remaining native skeletal muscle that could, in turn,

Dr. Christ or an immediate family member has stock or stock options held in Ion Channel Innovations, LLC. Dr. Werner or an immediate family member is a member of a speakers' bureau or has made paid presentations on behalf of Arthrex, Inc.; serves as a paid consultant to or is an employee of Arthrex, Inc.; has received research or institutional support from Arthrex, Inc., Biomet, Exactech, Inc., and Flexion Therapeutics; and serves as a board member, owner, officer, or committee member of American Academy of Orthopaedic Surgeons, American Orthopaedic Society for Sports Medicine, and American Shoulder and Elbow Surgeons. Neither of the following authors nor any immediate family member has received anything of value from or has stock or stock options held in a commercial company or institution related directly or indirectly to the subject of this chapter: Sarah E. Dyer and Dr. Hurwitz.

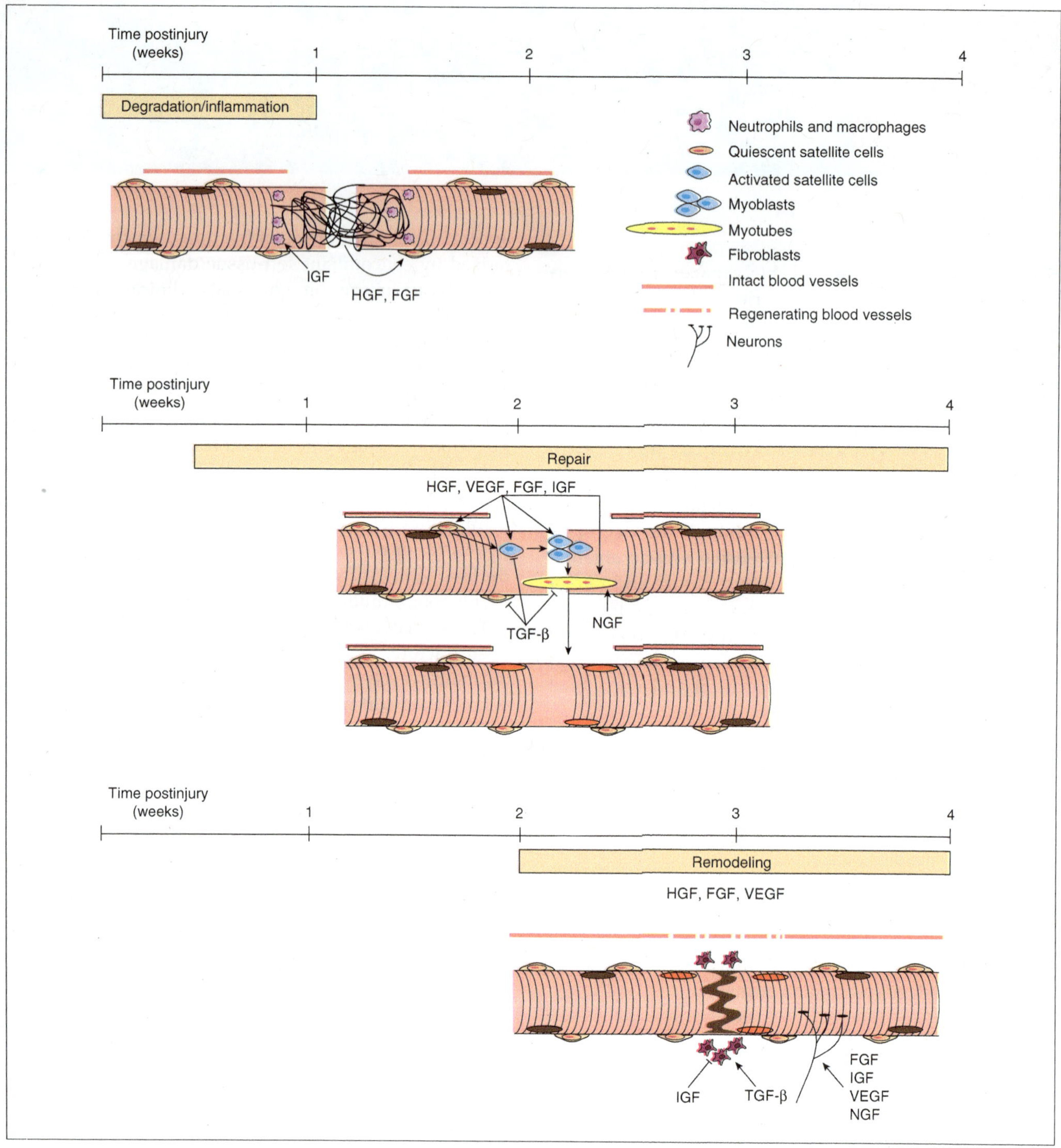

FIGURE 1 High-level schematic representation of the timeline of skeletal muscle repair and regeneration for recoverable injuries. This figure emphasizes the important role that cells and growth factors play during the three stages of muscle regeneration. As illustrated, insulinlike growth factor (IGF), fibroblast growth factor (FGF), and hepatocyte growth factor (HGF) play a crucial role in all stages of muscle regeneration, whereas transforming growth factor beta (TGF-β) is critical to establishing balance in the repair stage, but it has pronounced effect during the remodeling stage. Vascular endothelial growth factor (VEGF) and nerve growth factor (NGF) also play key roles during repair and remodeling stages of muscle regeneration. None of these features is present in the volumetric muscle loss injury space/setting, indicating the extreme challenges of this environment for promoting scarless wound healing and functional regeneration. (Reproduced with permission from Passipieri JA, Christ GJ: The potential of combination therapeutics for more complete repair of volumetric muscle loss injuries: The role of exogenous growth factors and/or progenitor cells in implantable skeletal muscle tissue engineering technologies. *Cells Tissues Organs* 2016;202[3-4]:202-213.)

limit recovery of the affected muscle/muscle group.[10,26] For example, VML injury is associated with significant fibrosis, which subsequently impairs range of motion, and could, in turn, result in reduced use and muscle atrophy. Furthermore, because physical rehabilitation of VML injuries does not significantly restore limb function or muscle strength of the injured musculature, it is not surprising that VML injuries are thought to represent a progressively deteriorating condition and/or disorder.[10,26]

Clearly, multicomposite tissue engineering/regenerative medicine solutions are ultimately required for more complete restoration of function following complex limb/extremity trauma. Improved therapeutics for skeletal muscle regeneration/repair are important to ensure more complete functional recovery following traumatic limb injury in the concomitant setting of VML injury. In this scenario, the importance of skeletal muscle regeneration and repair can be seen in the context of both improved fracture healing and improved limb function, and also (even when not completely restored, as noted previously) preserving range of motion, improving rehabilitation outcomes,[27] and thus, preventing further decline of function. The development of regenerative therapeutics for acceleration of more complete functional recovery of VML injury would address a major unmet medical need, and has been the subject of intensive recent investigations.

STRATEGIES FOR REPAIR OF VML INJURIES

As noted previously, the magnitude of the unmet medical need, in both the military and civilian populations, has stimulated significant research into development of novel and more effective therapeutic agents for addressing the permanent cosmetic and functional deficits associated with VML injury. The enormity of the technologic and biologic challenges presented by VML injuries is not surprising given the fact that they reflect a frank and simultaneous bulk loss of multiple tissue compartments, including the muscles, nerves, vessels, and ECM. Blood clotting, inflammation, and fibrosis/scarring are the default tissue response and create an environment that is not conducive to regeneration. In general, the preclinical approach has focused largely on the implantation of ECM in the presence[28-36] and absence[29,31,33,37] of therapeutic cells. **Figure 2** graphically summarizes the relative range of regenerative technologies currently being explored.

Certainly, implantation of commercially available decellularized ECM (dECM) alone (ie, without cells) provides the most straightforward path to clinical translation of regenerative therapeutics. However, preclinical results to date seem to favor the inclusion of a cellular component because this strategy leads to a greater degree of functional improvement.[29,31,33] Representative examples of the diversity of currently contemplated biomaterials approaches to VML repair are presented in the next paragraphs, accompanied by a high-level discussion of their potential to address this critical unmet medical need.

Implantation of dECM

The promise of dECM and other ECM-based biomaterials in tissue engineering has been recently reviewed.[38] The xenogeneic dECM approach being pioneered by Cramer and Badylak[38] for the treatment of VML injuries represents an example of the use of dECM alone. The rationale for this therapeutic strategy is related to the multiple putative mechanisms by which dECM is thought to support tissue remodeling and repair, including providing mechanical and structural support in the vacuous regenerative space, degradation and release of bioactive molecules, recruitment and/or differentiation of host cells, and immune modulation. Several clinical studies on the treatment of VML injury using implanted dECM scaffolds have shown modest functional recovery, but with little evidence of significant de novo muscle tissue regeneration at the injury site.[37,39-42] This line of effort bodes well for the utility of implantable dECM biomaterials, but there is still much room for therapeutic improvement. In short, these early clinical findings are largely congruent with the aforementioned preclinical results, further indicating the importance of a cellular component to more complete functional recovery, especially for larger, more complex VML injuries.

Implantation of Biofabricated Hydrogels, ECM, and Scaffolds

The importance of ECM for tissue repair in the setting of VML injury cannot be overstated. Prestwich and Healy[43] elegantly made the case for broad applications of ECM to regenerative medicine, but evaluation of biomaterial designs specific for utilization in skeletal muscle regeneration and repair is more recent and continues to grow. Several recent publications cover the spectrum of possibilities for VML therapeutics.[44-52]

In short, this newer cadre of biomaterials has been designed to provide a variety of desired features to enhance/restore the abrogated regenerative response characteristic of the VML injury environment. In this instance, material design features are created to optimize key aspects relevant to myogenesis and functional skeletal muscle regeneration, including cell/fiber alignment, conductivity, immune modulation, elastic modulus, cellular invasion and controlled degradation, and growth factor retention, as well as the potential for more physiologic delivery of therapeutic cells, drugs, and growth factors (functionalization). Although no biomaterial system currently provides a complete solution for functional recovery from VML injury, the lessons learned and knowledge derived from this spate of preclinical investigations should continue to drive the entire field forward

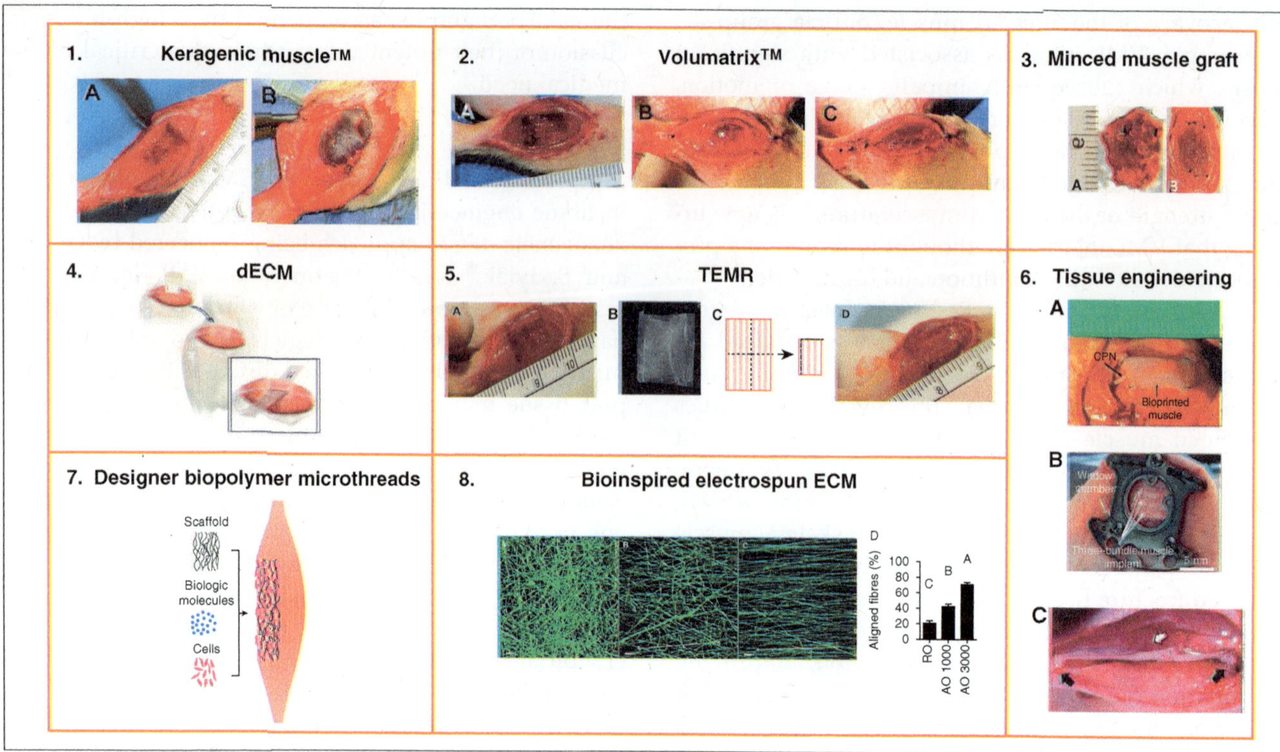

FIGURE 2 Schematic representation of the spectrum of regenerative technology for volumetric muscle loss (VML) muscle repair. VML muscle repair strategies. Frame **1**, Keratin-based hydrogels alone or with cells/growth factors can be injected into VML injuries. Frame **2**, Hyaluronic acid–based hydrogels have been implemented in tibialis anterior VML injury repair. Frame **3**, Minced muscle grafts deliver cells and tissue components into the injury site. Frame **4**, Decellularized extracellular matrices (dECM) support tissue during repair following VML injury. Frame **5**, Tissue-engineered muscle repair (TEMR) constructs are created by seeding acellular matrices with muscle progenitor cells, and this technology has been implemented in multiple VML injury models. Creation of a VML injury in the rat tibialis anterior (TA). (*A*) VML injury was created in the middle of the TA muscle measuring 1 × 0.7 × 0.5 cm and weighing no less than 20% of the TA. (*B*) An unfolded and trimmed TEMR scaffold with uniform cellularity. (*C*) Schematic depiction of TEMR construct folding before implantation. One-half of each construct was folded lengthwise, and then in half across the width. (*D*) The folded TEMR construct was carefully placed in the wound bed, sutured, and trimmed to remove excess material. Frame **6**, Biofabrication of tissue-engineered skeletal muscle includes hydrogel-based molding, fabrication of scaffold-free skeletal muscle units, and three-dimensional bioprinting. *A*, Structural maintenance and host nerve integration of the bioprinted muscle construct in in vivo study. The bioprinted muscle construct was subcutaneously implanted with the dissected CPN inserted into the printed muscle construct, and the harvested implants after 2 weeks of implantation showed the presence of organized muscle fibers and innervating capability (α-BTX-positive structures) within the implanted construct, as confirmed by immunostaining using skeletal muscle markers (desmin and MHC+ and α-BTX+ structure [arrows]). *B*, Vascular integration of implanted engineered muscle. Implanted muscle patch within the dorsal skin-fold window chamber. *C*, A pictorial representation of the VML and skeletal muscle unit (SMU) implantation procedure. A single SMU was implanted into the VML site, with one of its bone anchors inserted into a tibial bone tunnel and the other tendon end sutured to the distal TA tendon left from muscle volume removed. The tibial and distal TA tendon attachment sites (black arrows). A branch of the peroneal nerve with its vasculature was isolated and sutured to the mid-belly of the SMU (white arrows). Frame **7**, Biofabricated biomaterials combine scaffolds, such as biopolymer microthreads, with biologics and/or cells for implantation into VML injury. Frame **8**, Electrospinning can create highly aligned extracellular matrix (ECM) scaffolds for implantation. Tunable electrospun dECM fibers. (*A*) Confocal images of random (RO) fibers, (*B*) aligned fibers fabricated on a collector rotating at 1000 rpm (AO 1000), and (*C*) aligned fibers fabricated on a collector rotating at 3000 rpm (AO 3000). (*D*) Orientation graph of electrospun fibers aligned within 10° of the origin expressed as a percentage of all fibers. Scale bar represents 50 μm and is the same across images. The white arrow represents the direction of fiber alignment. Values represent mean ± SD (n = 5). Bars that share letters are not significantly different. Conversely, bars that do not share a letter are significantly different ($P < 0.05$). (Panel **1**, Reproduced with permission from Passipieri JA, Baker HB, Siriwardane M, et al: Keratin hydrogel enhances in vivo skeletal muscle function in a rat model of volumetric muscle loss. *Tissue Eng Part A* 2017;23[11-12]:556-571, Figure 1. Panel **2**, Reproduced with

(*Continued*)

FIGURE 2 *(Continued)*
permission from Dienes J, Browne S, Farjun B, et al: Semisynthetic hyaluronic acid-based hydrogel promotes recovery of the injured tibialis anterior skeletal muscle form and function. *ACS Biomater Sci Eng* 2021;7[4]:1587-1599. Copyright © 2021, American Chemical Society. Courtesy of Juliana Passipieri. Panel **3**, Reproduced with permission from Corona BT, Garg K Ward CL, McDaniel JS, Walters TJ, Rathbone CR: Autologous minced muscle grafts: A tissue engineering therapy for the volumetric loss of skeletal muscle. *Am J Physiol Cell Physiol* 2013;305[7]:C761-C775, Figure 1. Panel **4**, Dziki J, Badylak S, Yabroudi M, et al: An acellular biologic scaffold treatment for volumetric muscle loss: Results of a 13-patient cohort study. *NPJ Regen Med* 2016;1:16008. Reproduced with permission from Sicari BM, Rubin JP, Dearth CL, et al: An acellular biologic scaffold promotes skeletal muscle formation in mice and humans with volumetric muscle loss. *Sci Transl Med* 2014;6[234]:234ra58, Figure 2. Panel **5**, Reproduced with permission from Mintz EL, Passipieri JA, Franklin IR, et al: Long-term evaluation of functional outcomes following rat volumetric muscle loss injury and repair. *Tissue Eng Part A* 2020;26[3-4]:140-156, Figure 1. Panel **6**, Reproduced with permission from Kang HW, Lee SJ, Ko IK, Kengla C, Yoo JJ, Atala A: A 3D bioprinting system to produce human-scale tissue constructs with structural integrity. *Nat Biotechnol* 2016;34[3]:312-319, Figure 6 (top); Juhas M, Engelmayr GC Jr, Fontanella AN, Palmer GM, Bursac N: Biomimetic engineered muscle with capacity for vascular integration and functional maturation in vivo. *Proc Natl Acad Sci USA* 2014;111[15]:5508-5513, Figure 3 (middle); VanDusen KW, Syverud BC, Williams ML, Lee JD, Larkin LM: Engineered skeletal muscle units for repair of volumetric muscle loss in the tibialis anterior muscle of a rat. *Tissue Eng Part A* 2014;20[21-22]:2920-2930, Figure 1 (bottom). Panel **7**, O'Brien MP, Carnes ME, Page RL, Gaudette GR, Pins GD: Designing biopolymer microthreads for tissue engineering and regenerative medicine. *Curr Stem Cell Rep* 2016;2[2]:147-157. Reproduced with permission from Carnes ME, Pins GD: Skeletal muscle tissue engineering: biomaterials-based strategies for the treatment of volumetric muscle loss. *Bioengineering (Basel)* 2020;7[3]:85, Figure 4. Panel **8**, Reprinted with permission of AAAS from Smoak MM, Hogan KJ, Grande-Allen KJ, Mikos AG: Bioinspired electrospun dECM scaffolds guide cell growth and control the formation of myotubes. *Sci Adv* 2021;7[20]:eabg4123, Figure 1. © The Authors, some rights reserved; exclusive licensee AAAS. Distributed under a CC BY-NC 4.0 License (http://creativecommons.org/licenses/by-nc/4.0/.)

in a robust manner, and thus, accelerate the clinical application(s) of more rationally designed biomaterials for repair of increasing large musculoskeletal soft-tissue injuries, such as the complex polytraumatic composite tissue injuries that characterize VML.

IMPLANTATION OF BIOFABRICATED TISSUE-ENGINEERED SKELETAL MUSCLE

A limited number of investigators have pursued the development of implantable, biomimetic tissue-engineered skeletal muscle solutions for the treatment of VML injuries. Three general approaches have been taken.

Gel-Based Molding of Tissue-Engineered Skeletal Muscle

First, Juhas et al[53] from the Bursac group have described a hydrogel-based molding process for engineering highly functional, biomimetic skeletal muscle capable of vascular integration and further functional maturation after implantation in vivo in a murine model. They have also extended their biofabrication method(s) to include production of similar-scale bioengineered human myobundles that recapitulate key aspects of human skeletal muscle physiology (including contractility to both electric and chemical stimulation). As such, this platform also provides an important in vitro screening tool/model of human skeletal muscle physiology and disease (eg, Duchenne muscular dystrophy).[54,55]

Scaffold-Free Bioengineered Skeletal Muscle

A second tissue engineering approach is the scaffold-free bioengineering process that has been developed for creating skeletal muscle units (SMUs).[56-58] SMUs are tissue-engineered constructs composed of skeletal muscles with engineered bone-tendon ends, as well as incorporated myotendinous junctions and entheses. As with the approach described previously, tissue-engineered SMUs can generate contractile force; in this instance, both spontaneously and in response to electric stimulation. Although SMUs are phenotypically immature in vitro, they continue to mature when implanted in vivo, while also becoming vascularized and innervated. This functional maturation in vivo is reflected by the presence of an epimysiumlike outer layer of connective tissue, as well as increased formation of myofibers, and not surprisingly, increased contractile force. Importantly, these constructs were recently shown to be scalable to applications in more clinically relevant ovine VML injuries (eg, peroneus tertius[56]). Taken together, these findings suggest that SMUs appear to be a promising and evolving therapeutic strategy for improved management of VML injury.

Three-Dimensional Bioprinting of Tissue-Engineered Skeletal Muscle

Third, the continued evolution and enhanced capability and affordability of three-dimensional (3D) bioprinters is expected to have an important effect on further development of therapeutics for VML repair. In conjunction with the parallel development and availability of bioinks (ie, biomaterials developed for cell-based bioprinting applications), 3D bioprinting has provided another potentially exciting biofabrication platform for the creation of tissue-engineered skeletal muscle.[59-61] The potential application of bioprinted tissue-engineered constructs specifically designed for the management of VML injury has also been more recently described in the extant literature.[62-64] Preclinical studies have demonstrated that bioprinting clearly provides a huge opportunity for automated biomanufacturing of implantable tissue-engineered skeletal muscle. Nonetheless, despite this potential, eventually these constructs will need to be made at scale for applications to clinically relevant VML injury sizes. In this scenario, in vitro incorporation of vascularization and innervation of 3D bioprinted skeletal muscle will be a major rate-limiting step in the progression to clinical applications of this technology platform.

TISSUE-ENGINEERED MUSCLE REPAIR TECHNOLOGY FOR TREATMENT OF VML INJURIES

Tissue-engineered muscle repair (TEMR) is a flexible regenerative technology platform (both cell and biomaterial agnostic) that has been developed over at least the past 10 years as a potential therapeutic solution for VML[29,30,65] (**Figure 3**). The manually biomanufactured TEMR construct is created by seeding approximately one million muscle progenitor cells/cm^2 onto a decellularized bladder acellular matrix followed by bioreactor preconditioning in vitro (ie, 10% cyclic mechanical

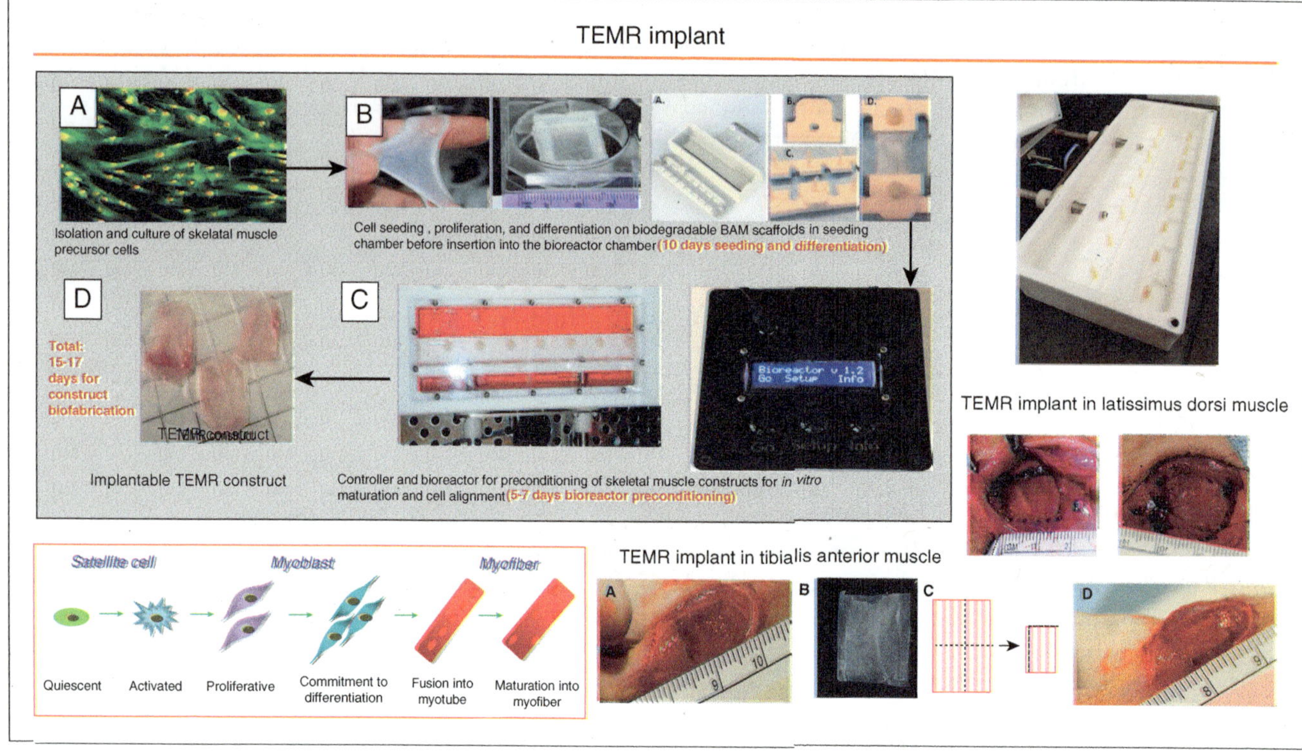

FIGURE 3 Illustration showing manual biomanufacturing process for tissue-engineered muscle repair (TEMR) for the treatment of sheetlike volumetric muscle loss injuries to hand and face. As illustrated, the entire process takes approximately 17 days postbiopsy and cell expansion—for a total of approximately 1 month. This process has been described in detail in several publications. BAM = bladder acellular matrix. (Corona BT, Ward CL, Baker HB, Walters TJ, Christ GJ: Implantation of in vitro tissue engineered muscle repair constructs and bladder acellular matrices partially restore in vivo skeletal muscle function in a rat model of volumetric muscle loss injury. *Tissue Eng Part A* 2014;20[3-4]:705-715. Reproduced with permission from Machingal MA, Corona BT, Walters TJ, et al: A tissue-engineered muscle repair construct for functional restoration of an irrecoverable muscle injury in a murine model. *Tissue Eng Part A* 2011;17[17-18]:2291-2303, Figure 1; Passipieri JA, Hu X, Mintz E, et al: In silico and in vivo studies detect functional repair mechanisms in a volumetric muscle loss injury. *Tissue Eng Part A* 2019;25[17-18]:1272-1288, Figure 1; Mintz EL, Passipieri JA, Franklin IR, et al: Long-term evaluation of functional outcomes following rat volumetric muscle loss injury and repair. *Tissue Eng Part A* 2020;26[3-4]:140-156, Figure 1; Zammit PS, Partridge TA, Yablonka-Reuveni Z: The skeletal muscle satellite cell: The stem cell that came in from the cold. *J Histochem Cytochem* 2006;54[11]:1177-1191; Figure 3.)

stretch; over 5 to 7 days). Implantation of TEMR at the site of VML injury increases the rate and magnitude of functional recovery (ie, contraction). Findings thus far have been quite encouraging, demonstrating an average of 60% to 70% functional recovery within 2 to 3 months of implantation in the mouse latissimus dorsi and rat tibialis anterior VML injury models.[29-31,65] These findings have been more recently confirmed and extended in the rat latissimus dorsi VML injury model, where the mean functional recovery was closer to 90%.[33] As described in more detail in the next paragraphs, attempts are being made to establish rigorous histologic and morphologic metrics for evaluating cell-level and tissue-level mechanisms of functional VML wound healing and repair (**Figure 4**).

The authors of this chapter have conducted a Pre-Investigational New Drug meeting with the FDA to discuss the application of a first-generation TEMR construct for the treatment of cleft lip as a first-in-human muscle-only defect. Moreover, the cleft lip indication scales well with the size of the current TEMR technology, as well as the biologic relevance of the rodent latissimus dorsi VML injury model. In addition, an Investigational New Drug application has been submitted to the FDA to support a pilot clinical trial for secondary revision of unilateral cleft lip—although the Investigational New Drug application is currently on clinical hold. From an orthopaedic perspective, the current TEMR technology also scales well to the repair of hand trauma (eg, gunshot wounds, table saw injuries, and lawn mower accidents). Clearly, further scaling and functionalization of the TEMR construct is both possible and necessary to accommodate the wider range of devastating orthopaedic extremity traumas.

STANDARDIZATION OF VML RESEARCH

In light of the aforementioned discussions, regardless of the exact tissue engineering or regenerative medicine approach taken, standardization of animal models and metrics is absolutely required to push the field of skeletal muscle regeneration forward with respect to development and evaluation of therapeutics for improved functional outcomes following management of diverse/distinct VML injuries, especially with respect to making comparisons across novel therapeutic platforms. Therefore, the experience of the chapter authors with respect to the utilization of some of the more established/biologically relevant small animal models of VML injury will be reviewed (**Figure 5**). The metrics and methods described should be applicable to the study of many, if not all, VML injury models. Both the models and measures are subject to change over time as more data come online, but several publications[28,29,32,33,66,67] and the work of others have established a firm foundation for current these efforts.

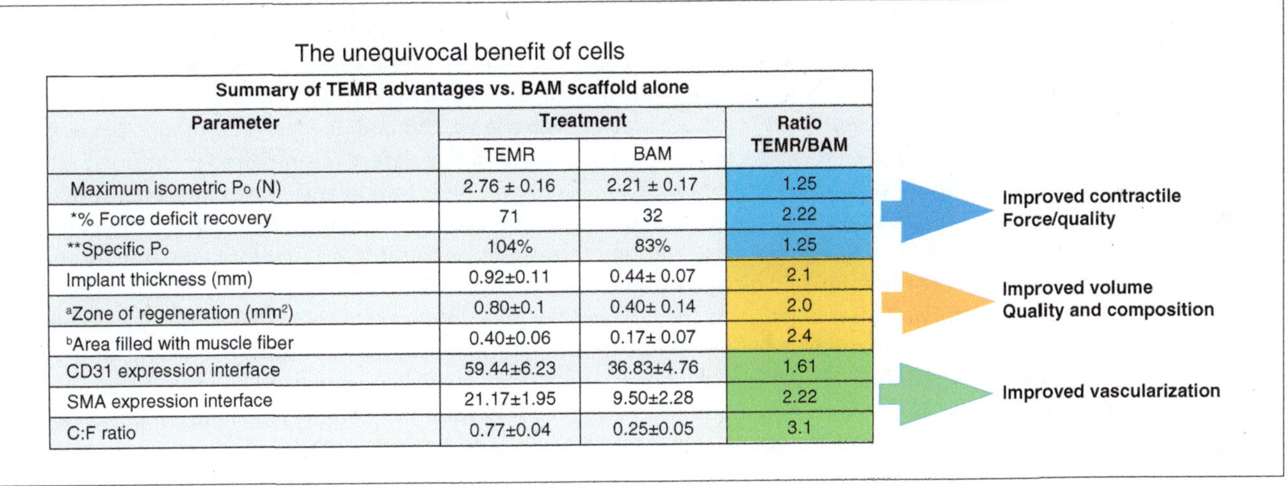

The unequivocal benefit of cells

Summary of TEMR advantages vs. BAM scaffold alone

Parameter	Treatment		Ratio TEMR/BAM
	TEMR	BAM	
Maximum isometric Po (N)	2.76 ± 0.16	2.21 ± 0.17	1.25
*% Force deficit recovery	71	32	2.22
**Specific Po	104%	83%	1.25
Implant thickness (mm)	0.92±0.11	0.44± 0.07	2.1
aZone of regeneration (mm2)	0.80±0.1	0.40± 0.14	2.0
bArea filled with muscle fiber	0.40±0.06	0.17± 0.07	2.4
CD31 expression interface	59.44±6.23	36.83±4.76	1.61
SMA expression interface	21.17±1.95	9.50±2.28	2.22
C:F ratio	0.77±0.04	0.25±0.05	3.1

FIGURE 4 Figure showing metrics for histologic assessment of tissue-engineered muscle repair (TEMR)-treated latissimus dorsi muscles retrieved 8 weeks postinjury. [a]The zone of regeneration, defined as the entire area from the native tissue interface to the most distant observable muscle fiber. [b]Area within the zone of regeneration that comprises muscle fibers. *Calculated as follows: at 2 months, no repair had a 44% force deficit relative to contralateral control (56% of control P_o [maximum force of contraction]), TEMR was 87% of control P_o for a 31% recovery of a 44% force deficit, or 71% total force deficit recovery, and BAM 70% of control P_o for a 14% recovery of the same 44% force deficit or 32% force recovery. **An assessment of the quality of contraction postinjury relative to contralateral control. Blue rows reflect improved contractile force, yellow rows reflect improved volume and quality of volume composition, and green rows reflect improved vascularization. BAM = bladder acellular matrix, C:F = capillary-to-fiber ratio, P_o = maximum force of contraction, SMA = smooth muscle actin. (Data from Passipieri JA, Hu X, Mintz E, et al: In silico and in vivo studies detect functional repair mechanisms in a volumetric muscle loss injury. *Tissue Eng Part A* 2019;25[17-18]:1272-1288.)

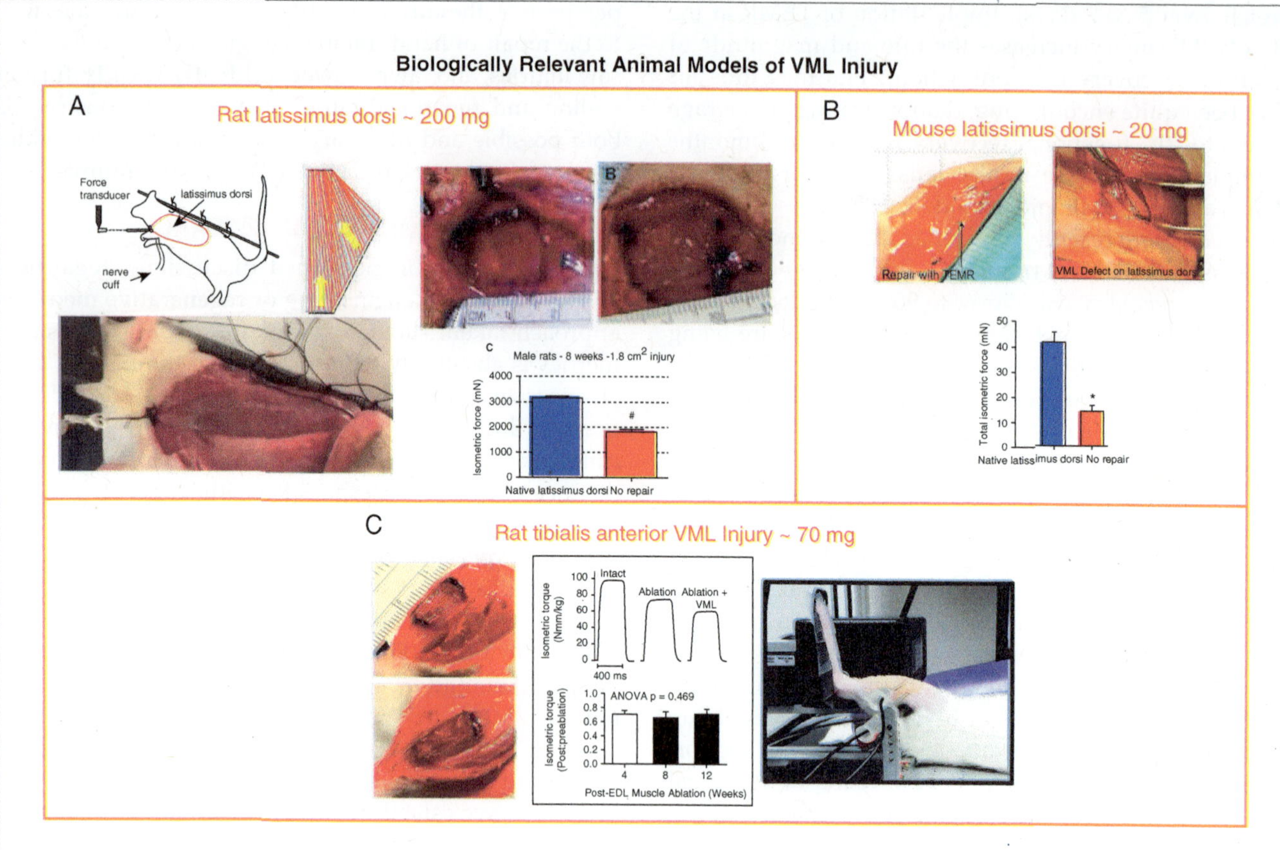

FIGURE 5 Illustration showing summary of established and biologically relevant animal models for studying volumetric muscle loss (VML) injury and repair. Injury creation and sustained contractile force deficits following VML creation are shown for various small animal injury models. **A**, Rat latissimus dorsi (LD) model. Right, Critically sized VML injury model in the rat LD muscle. (*B*) Shows a representative example of an LD VML injury in a male Lewis rat after surgical removal of 1.8 cm^2 of muscle, while (*C*) shows a folded TEMR construct sutured into the wound bed. **B**, Mouse LD model. Development and in vitro assessment of tissue-engineered muscle repair (TEMR) constructs. The defect was repaired by suturing either TEMR constructs or scaffolds without cells at the site of excised sites (arrow points to implant). VML injury was developed by excising ~50% of the native LD resulting in a volumetric muscle defect (excised area indicated by black dotted lines). **C**, Rat tibialis anterior (TA) model. *Middle*, In vivo isometric torque of the anterior crural muscles before and after TA muscle synergist ablation and VML. (*A*) Representative digitized torque tracings are presented for uninjured intact anterior crural muscles (TA, EDL, & EHL muscles), and after ablation of the EDL and EHL muscles and subsequent VML. *Note:* Following ablation (4 to 12 weeks), the TA muscle produced ≈70% of net anterior crural muscle torque. Subsequent VML of the TA muscle resulted in a further ≈20% deficit, resulting in a combined ≈50% deficit compared to preinjury (intact) torque. (*B*) TA muscle peak isometric torque (Nmm/kg body wt) normalized to preinjury values was stable from 4 to 12 weeks post-synergist ablation. EDL, extensor digitorum longus. (A, Courtesy of Amanda M. Westman. Reproduced with permission from Passipieri JA, Hu X, Mintz E, et al: In silico and in vivo studies detect functional repair mechanisms in a volumetric muscle loss injury. *Tissue Eng Part A* 2019;25[17-18]:1272-1288, Figure 1; B, Reproduced with permission from Machingal MA, Corona BT, Walters TJ, et al: A tissue-engineered muscle repair construct for functional restoration of an irrecoverable muscle injury in a murine model. *Tissue Eng Part A* 2011;17[17-18]:2291-2303, Figure 1. Passipieri JA, Baker HB, Siriwardane M, et al: Keratin hydrogel enhances in vivo skeletal muscle function in a rat model of volumetric muscle loss. *Tissue Eng Part A* 2017;23[11-12]:556-571. Mintz EL, Passipieri JA, Franklin IR, et al: Long-term evaluation of functional outcomes following rat volumetric muscle loss injury and repair. *Tissue Eng Part A* 2020;26[3-4]:140-156; Dienes J, Browne S, Farjun B, et al: Semisynthetic hyaluronic acid-based hydrogel promotes recovery of the injured tibialis anterior skeletal muscle form and function. *ACS Biomater Sci Eng* 2021;7[4]:1587-1599. C, Reproduced with permission from Corona BT, Ward CL, Baker HB, Walters TJ, Christ GJ: Implantation of in vitro tissue engineered muscle repair constructs and bladder acellular matrices partially restore in vivo skeletal muscle function in a rat model of volumetric muscle loss injury. *Tissue Eng Part A* 2014;20[3-4]:705-715.)

VML-INDUCED FUNCTIONAL DEFICITS AND REPAIR/REGENERATION

VML injuries are challenging to treat because of the variability in both volume and wound location, as well as their effects on the corresponding magnitude of the functional deficit thus produced. This fact also highlights a point of conceptual confusion in the field regarding the biomechanical mechanisms that are responsible for VML-induced functional deficits. In this setting, it is worth emphasizing that the volume of the VML injury per se is not directly linked to the corresponding magnitude of the functional deficit; as both the specific muscle(s) affected and the exact location of the injury play a key determining role. That is, the main requirement for/definition of VML is a nonrecoverable loss of muscle structure and function (**Figure 5**), and in this context, no specific volume of muscle needs be removed to define a VML injury. Further evidence for the rationale behind this critical point is provided later. Importantly, improved understanding of the mechanistic basis by which the magnitude and location of VML injuries are responsible for the resultant functional deficits is a critical knowledge gap that must be addressed to spur progress in the field. A brief summary of some of the most salient metrics is provided in the next paragraphs.

HISTOLOGIC ANALYSIS

Rigorous histologic analysis is a key tool for assessing the quality and quantity of tissue damage, wound healing, and repair. A multiscale analysis (ie, from sarcomeres to cells to tissue-level structure, orientation, and composition) is required to identify both the mechanisms responsible for VML-related functional deficits and the mechanisms that mediate functional recovery. Authors of one publication proposed some comparative histology-derived metrics that might lead to the development of a regenerative index for tissue repair using the rodent latissimus dorsi VML injury model[33] (**Figure 4**). Although this is just a first step in this direction, this list can be further expanded, and the implications to improved understanding of VML injury and therapeutic repair are discussed in the next paragraphs.

COMPUTATIONAL MODELING

Although computational models of muscle have been relatively widely used to simulate skeletal muscle function,[68-72] until recently,[33,73] they had not been applied to understanding the complex mechanisms and biomechanics of VML injury and/or wound healing. The authors of this chapter have illustrated how a novel coupled framework of in situ and in silico methods can lead to more precise understanding of the relationship between injury location and force production deficits; in this instance, in the latissimus dorsi muscle.[73] In short, to demonstrate this point, 3D finite element methods were used to model the pennate latissimus dorsi muscle in the rat and subsequently validated experimentally. Of specific relevance to this report, the predictions of the model simulation(s) accurately predicted the experimental force deficits that were measured in the latissimus dorsi muscle following surgical creation of VML injuries (**Figure 6**). For example, removal of approximately 6% of the latissimus dorsi weight near (more cranial to) the insertion of the latissimus dorsi muscle on the humerus in the rat was associated with an approximate 40% functional deficit that generated 0.8 N/g less force than a much larger VML injury. That is, although one injury was approximately 2.5-fold larger (removal of 15% of latissimus dorsi weight as opposed to 6%), the larger injury was associated with a functional deficit that was approximately one-half (20%) that of the smaller injury. The reason for the apparently disproportionate functional deficit relative to injury size is directly related to the number of end-to-end fibers that were disrupted by the creation of these two distinct injuries. In this case, although more muscle tissue was ablated in one injury than the other, the injury with the greater number of non–end-to-end fibers (eg, disrupted or damaged fibers) generated correspondingly less force. The biomechanical mechanism responsible for this finding is that disruption of end-to-end fibers makes the muscle more reliant on lateral, rather than longitudinal, force transmission, greatly compromising the shortening and force-generation ability of the muscle. This observation clearly demonstrates how important both the location and size/volume of a given VML injury are to the resultant functional deficit. Although these measurements were made on the latissimus dorsi muscle, they are applicable to any VML injury model, and thus, efforts to develop 3D finite element models for other muscles of interest can/should continue.

These findings provided clear evidence that finite element models can also be used to inform the mechanistic basis for functional recovery across VML-regenerative platforms. For example, of particular importance is the mechanistic insight that can be applied to the more recent use of biologic matrices for muscle tissue repair in patients. In these reports, the investigators have described the implantation of an acellular matrix (eg, urinary bladder matrix, porcine intestinal submucosa), a material of broad applications to various injuries, for the management of VML injuries caused by extremity trauma to the limbs.[39-41] Although these initial findings are certainly encouraging, only a relatively modest degree of functional improvement was observed,[39-41] and finite element models demonstrate that the underlying biomechanical mechanisms of the limited functional improvement observed are most likely due to volume reconstitution and passive spread of force along the length of the muscle as the surrounding muscle fibers shorten, that is, functional

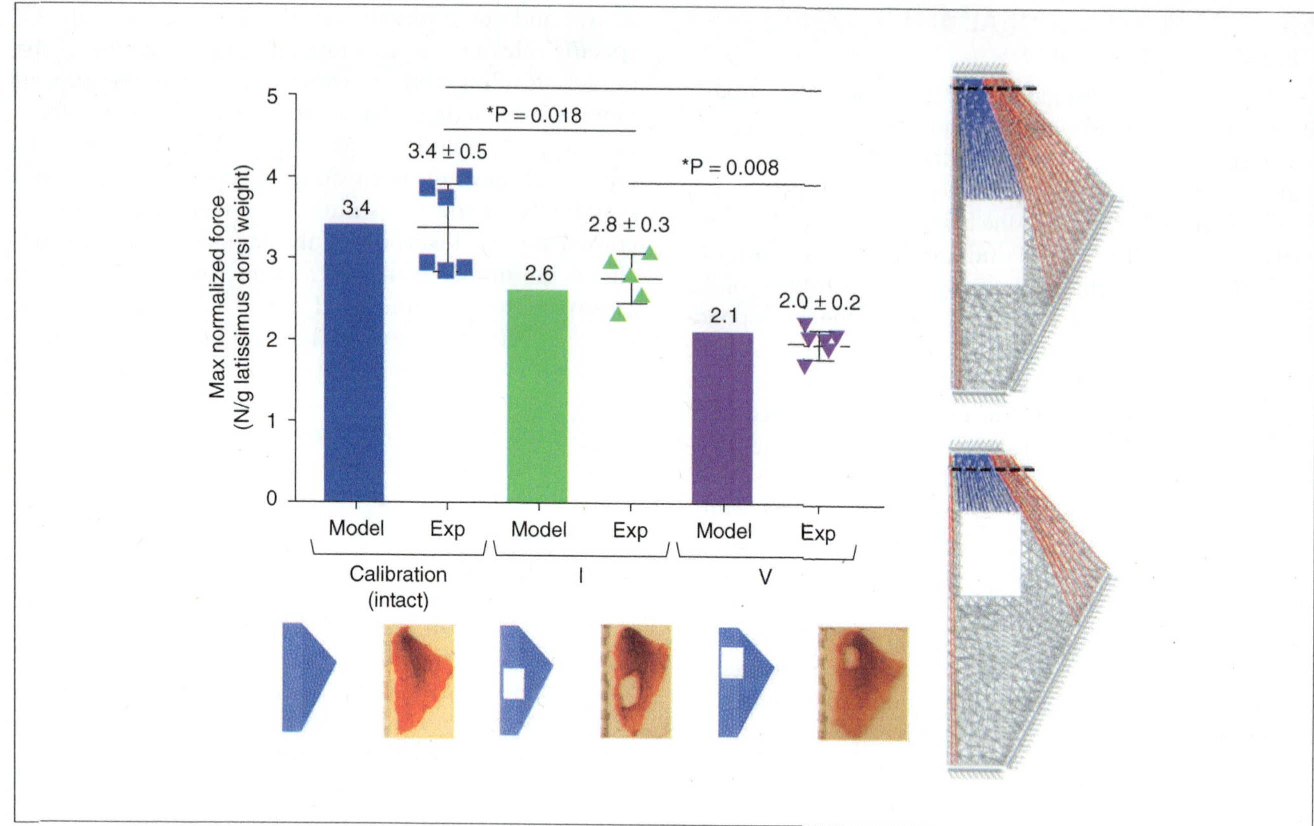

FIGURE 6 Schematic and graphic illustration shows biomechanical mechanisms of volumetric muscle loss (VML)-related functional deficits. Finite element method modeling of the rat latissimus dorsi evaluated the effect of different VML injury locations on resulting functional deficits. The model was confirmed by experimentally validating using in situ functional testing. Model I removed approximately 15% of the muscle weight and had 33% non–end-to end fibers, whereas Model V, which placed the injury closer to the insertion site, removed only approximately 6% of the latissimus dorsi weight and resulted in 45% non–end-to-end fibers. Model V subsequently resulted in greater functional deficit (40% of uninjured muscle) compared with Model I (20% deficit from uninjured muscle). (Reprinted from Westman AM, Dyer SE, Remer JD, Hu X, Christ GJ, Blemker SS: A coupled framework of in situ and in silico analysis reveals the role of lateral force transmission in force production in volumetric muscle loss injuries. *J Biomech* 2019;85:118-125. (Copyright 2016), with permission from Elsevier)

fibrosis.[37] Functional fibrosis refers to the fact that following implantation of ECM (or TEMR), volume reconstitution and tissue remodeling per se can modify the passive tissue properties of the remodeled implant area. In this setting, the finite element model indicates that, at optimal fiber length, most of the force recovery is attributable to the passive mechanical properties of the tissue in the implanted region, which, even in the presence of appreciable muscle regeneration, is still largely reflective of the larger volume of tissue reconstitution promoted by the implant. Importantly, at shorter fiber lengths and with correspondingly larger injury sizes, the presence of active tissue components, that is, regenerated skeletal muscle, will be critically required to achieve functional recovery. In short, the presence of the intervening connective tissue between the disrupted end-to-end fibers still ensures more efficient spread of contraction (compared with no repair)—permitting improved force generation, but in the absence of appreciable de novo muscle regeneration.[33] Such findings have major implications for the understanding and future development of regenerative therapeutics for VML repair and rehabilitation.

Taken together, these findings support the supposition that computational tools, such as finite element methods, can at least in part accelerate clinical translation of regenerative therapeutics via the following major avenues: (1) improvement in VML model development to customize traumatic injury profiles for desired functional deficits and lines of scientific/clinical inquiry, (2) improved insights into the biomechanical mechanisms that contribute to predicted functional deficits for muscle-specific VML injuries, and (3) development of mechanism-based, muscle-specific regenerative therapeutics. Eventually, such efforts should lead to development of personalized/precision medicine approaches that can identify and implement patient-specific, symptom-based regenerative treatment strategies for maximizing functional outcomes from distinct VML injuries.

GAIT KINEMATICS AND KINETICS

Rats are a commonly used translational model of VML extremity trauma. However, outcome analysis following injury and/or repair has traditionally been focused on histology/morphometry, and less commonly (though more frequent recently) on incorporation of force generation.[28-30,32,33] As important as force generation is to muscle function/locomotion, studies of human movement have shown that gains in strength (force-generation capacity) do not necessarily result in improvements in movement function.[74-78] In addition, as the meaning of maximum functional recovery is considered, more precisely determining the relationship between VML-related force deficits and gait biomechanics in biologically relevant preclinical animal models is yet another critical knowledge gap that must be transcended to improve the understanding, diagnosis, and treatment of VML injuries.

A method to quantify changes in gait for rats with tibialis anterior VML injuries in the absence and presence of treatment, using methods similar to those performed for human gait analysis, has recently been published.[66] More specifically, VML injuries were surgically created as previously described, with control rats running in parallel. In vivo force testing indicated, as expected, that the VML injury was associated with a significant deficit in force-generation ability. Both control rats and VML-injured rats were affixed with motion capture markers on the bony landmarks of the back and hindlimb and recorded walking on a treadmill both before injury and VML postsurgery. Data collected from the motion capture system were subsequently analyzed in OpenSim and MATLAB.

This approach allowed accurate calculation of the kinematics of the hip, knee, and ankle over complete gait cycles and compares the postinjury kinematics with baseline data from preinjury animals. In short, it was determined that the measured VML-induced functional deficits in contraction manifested as obvious differences in gait, where a vaulting gait and circumduction were noted as compensation for footdrop. Furthermore, these kinematic studies revealed gait changes both in response to injury and during recovery. Despite the limitations of a treadmill-based motion capture system, this initial study established a foundation for future work that includes protocol refinement, joint kinetics, and comparisons of efficacy of regenerative therapeutics as treatment for VML and more significant injuries. More specifically, using these same motion capture techniques on animals walking overground rather than on a treadmill would result in joint kinematics that are more reflective of natural gait patterns. Furthermore, inclusion of ground reaction forces via an instrumented walkway would permit calculation of joint moments in all three planes. In the future, the inclusion of force plates, along with the collection of contralateral limb kinematics, will provide a more comprehensive data set in the same animal. This will provide unprecedented insight into biomechanical mechanisms of VML injury and/or repair, and further, how they translate into differential strength, motion planning, and neuromuscular control strategies, both acutely and over time. In the end, it is expected that this approach will further inform evaluation of the efficacy of various regenerative therapeutics, as well as rehabilitation regimens,[27] to maximize functional outcomes for VML injury.

ROTATOR CUFF INJURY AND SKELETAL MUSCLE–FOCUSED REPAIR

Although not considered a classic VML-like injury, untreated rotator cuff tears can lead to degenerative changes within the cuff muscles. Preclinical models allow physicians to evaluate changes in the shoulder joint and rotator cuff muscles following injury,[79,80] and as a result, alterations in muscle architecture as well as increased muscle atrophy, fatty infiltration, and fibrosis have been noted. Numerous clinical studies evaluating rotator cuff repair surgeries have identified increased fatty infiltration and muscle atrophy as factors related to postoperative healing and retear.[81,82] Additionally, increased fatty infiltration of the supraspinatus muscle has been correlated with decreased contractile function.[83,84] Even after tendon repair, muscle quality has demonstrated a lack of improvement and can progressively worsen in the case of a retear.[81,82] Although much of the current research focuses on tissue engineering and scaffold-based solutions for improving tendon or enthesis quality,[85] clinical results have demonstrated a need for therapeutics that focus on addressing muscle quality in conjunction with tendon reattachment during rotator cuff repair, to reduce the risk of a retear and thereby maximize postoperative outcomes.

Several animal studies have begun to target the muscle during rotator cuff repair. Systemic administration of anti-inflammatory drugs and compounds that regulate or inhibit adipogenic and fibrotic pathways has shown promise in addressing muscle degeneration following rotator cuff injury in rodent animal models.[86,87] To target the muscle directly, and avoid any unintended effects of systemic drug administration, several studies have also explored the use of direct injections of progenitor/stem cells, or their secretome(s), into injured rotator cuff muscle to study the effect on muscle quality.[88-90] Tellier et al[91] injected microparticles loaded with stromal cell–derived factor 1 alpha into detached rat supraspinatus muscles, to attract cells to the injury site that encourage regeneration. Huynh et al[92] similarly injected ECM gel into injured rabbit supraspinatus muscle at the time of tendon reattachment and saw a reduction in muscle atrophy as well as improvements in cell signaling pathways related to reduced cuff health. Finally, Tang et al[93] applied electroconductive nanofibrous matrices directly to repaired supraspinatus muscle in a rat model and saw improvements in muscle atrophy.

In addition to imaging (MRI, CT, ultrasonography), clinical evaluations of rotator cuff muscles primarily consist of shoulder movement evaluations, such as range of motion tests and strength tests using dynamometer readings.[94] Because invasive techniques to isolate and evaluate specific muscle function in a living subject are not always feasible, especially following repair, animal models are frequently used to measure muscle function. Many preclinical models of muscle-specific treatment strategies during rotator cuff repair focus on gait changes, enthesis strength, or single fiber muscle force in conjunction with muscle histology as metrics to evaluate treatment efficacy.[87-90] Animal models have also been used to evaluate whole-muscle contractile function[95-98] in both healthy and torn animal rotator cuffs. Ditsios et al[95] conducted contractile function testing in a rat model of massive rotator cuff tear after 12 weeks and saw a decrease in muscle contractile function, as well as decreased muscle quality, with markers of injury varying by different regions of the muscle. Valencia et al[97] observed disorganized collagen and reduced contraction in a rat model of acute rotator cuff tear after 15 days, and in a separate study,[98] using a rabbit model of 12-week rotator cuff tear, they found a reduction in contractile force associated with atrophy and fatty infiltration of the muscle. Meyer et al[96] examined in situ contraction of sheep infraspinatus muscle after 16 weeks of tendon detachment and found that the injured muscles had increased atrophy and fatty infiltration, with decreased contractile function compared with the contralateral shoulder. As shown in **Figure 7**, a model of rotator cuff injury to the supraspinatus

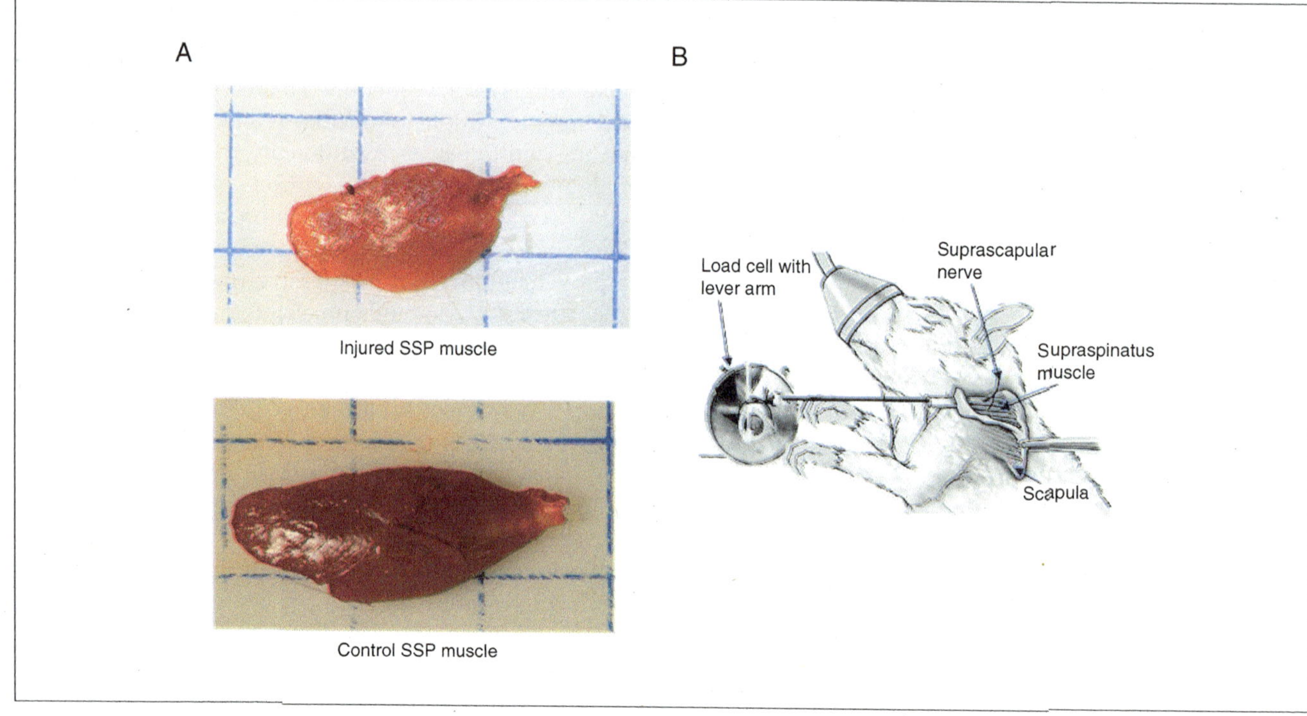

FIGURE 7 Photograph and illustration showing animal models of rotator cuff injury used to study muscle damage and inform future repair strategies and therapeutics. **A**, The supraspinatus (SSP) muscle of male Lewis rats was detached from the humeral head and the muscle was tested for contractile function and explanted 16 weeks later. Healthy, uninjured muscle from an age-matched control animal was also tested for contractile function and explanted. The injured muscle shows clear signs of atrophy at the time of explant. **B**, A setup similar to that used by other groups (Valencia et al 2017) was used to isolate the muscle and evaluate the contractile function by attaching the tendon to a force transducer, stimulating the muscle, and recording the force generated. Valencia et al (2017) saw a 20% decrease in maximal isometric force after 15 days of tendon detachment, and a 50% decrease in force was observed after 16 weeks of injury when comparing the healthy age-matched animals with the injured group. (Figure 7B reproduced from Figure 2A of Valencia AP, Iyer SR, Spangenburg EE, Gilotra MN, Lovering RM: Impaired contractile function of the supraspinatus in the acute period following a rotator cuff tear. *BMC Musculoskelet Disord* 2017;18[1]:436. This figure is licensed under a Creative Commons Attribution 4.0 International License http://creativecommons.org/licenses/by/4.0.)

muscle in rodents has been developed and validated by the chapter authors—where current work is focused on evaluating novel treatment strategies for rotator cuff muscle repair and regeneration.

SUMMARY

VML injuries represent a challenging but critical area of skeletal muscle regenerative research. Although progress with all of the regenerative technologies described herein bodes well for future treatment of VML and VML-like injuries (ie, secondary revision of cleft lip), further advancements are required before bioengineered muscle and biomaterial-based approaches can be used for more effective management of the most devastating polytraumatic VML injuries, such as those experienced by both wounded warriors and civilians. Moreover, all VML injuries are not equivalent and thus, represent a virtual continuum of magnitudes and complexities that will likely be treated by a correspondingly diverse spectrum of regenerative technologies. As with treatment of other musculoskeletal injuries, VML repair technologies will need to be scaled to address progressively larger and more challenging preclinical VML injuries (eg, porcine), to further ensure and validate clinical applicability. By comparing the efficacy of advanced regenerative therapeutic technologies/products via evaluation of comprehensive functional outcomes with robust, multiscale, computational, and biomechanical analyses, there is an opportunity to accelerate the clinical translation of regenerative therapeutics for the management of VML injuries. As with the development of all novel musculoskeletal therapeutics, these data analytics will need to be progressively scaled and conducted in biologically relevant animal models.

REFERENCES

1. Cheema U, Yang S-Y, Mudera V, Goldspink GG, Brown RA: 3-D in vitro model of early skeletal muscle development. *Cell Motil Cytoskeleton* 2003;54(3):226-236.
2. Hardy D, Besnard A, Latil M, et al: Comparative study of injury models for studying muscle regeneration in mice. *PLoS One* 2016;11(1):e0147198.
3. Järvinen TA, Järvinen M, Kalimo H: Regeneration of injured skeletal muscle after the injury. *Muscles Ligaments Tendons J* 2014;3(4):337-345.
4. Järvinen TA, Järvinen TL, Kääriäinen M, Kalimo H, Järvinen M: Muscle injuries: Biology and treatment. *Am J Sports Med* 2005;33(5):745-764.
5. McNeill Ingham SJ, de Castro Pochini A, Oliveira DA, et al: Bupivacaine injection leads to muscle force reduction and histologic changes in a murine model. *PM R* 2011;3(12):1106-1109.
6. Reali M, Serafim FG, da Cruz-Höfling MA, Fontana MD: Neurotoxic and myotoxic actions of Naja naja kaouthia venom on skeletal muscle in vitro. *Toxicon* 2003;41(6):657-665.
7. Carlson BM: Muscle regeneration in amphibians and mammals: Passing the torch. *Dev Dyn* 2003;226(2):167-181.
8. Vignaud A, Hourdé C, Butler-Browne G, Ferry A: Differential recovery of neuromuscular function after nerve/muscle injury induced by crude venom from Notechis scutatus, cardiotoxin from Naja atra and bupivacaine treatments in mice. *Neurosci Res* 2007;58(3):317-323.
9. Passipieri JA, Christ GJ: The potential of combination therapeutics for more complete repair of volumetric muscle loss injuries: The role of exogenous growth factors and/or progenitor cells in implantable skeletal muscle tissue engineering technologies. *Cells Tissues Organs* 2016;202(3-4):202-213.
10. Corona BT, Rivera JC, Owens JG, Wenke JC, Rathbone CR: Volumetric muscle loss leads to permanent disability following extremity trauma. *J Rehabil Res Dev* 2015;52(7):785-792.
11. McKinley TO, Gaski GE, Vodovotz Y, Corona BT, Billiar TR: Diagnosis and management of polytraumatized patients with severe extremity trauma. *J Orthop Trauma* 2018;32(suppl 1):S1-S6.
12. Holcomb JB, Stansbury LG, Champion HR, Wade C, Bellamy RF: Understanding combat casualty care statistics. *J Trauma* 2006;60(2):397-401.
13. Cross JD, Ficke JR, Hsu JR, Masini BD, Wenke JC: Battlefield orthopaedic injuries cause the majority of long-term disabilities. *J Am Acad Orthop Surg* 2011;19(suppl 1):S1-S7.
14. Ficke JR, Pollak AN: Extremity war injuries: Development of clinical treatment principles. *J Am Acad Orthop Surg* 2007;15(10):590-595.
15. Masini BD, Waterman SM, Wenke JC, Owens BD, Hsu JR, Ficke JR: Resource utilization and disability outcome assessment of combat casualties from Operation Iraqi Freedom and Operation Enduring Freedom. *J Orthop Trauma* 2009;23(4):261-266.
16. Owens BD, Kragh JF Jr, Wenke JC, Macaitis J, Wade CE, Holcomb JB: Combat wounds in operation Iraqi Freedom and operation Enduring Freedom. *J Trauma* 2008;64(2):295-299.
17. Hamilton PT, Jansen MS, Ganesan S, et al: Improved bone morphogenetic protein-2 retention in an injectable collagen matrix using bifunctional peptides. *PLoS One* 2013;8(8):e70715.
18. McKinley TO, Lisboa FA, Horan AD, Gaski GE, Mehta S: Precision medicine applications to manage multiply injured patients with orthopaedic trauma. *J Orthop Trauma* 2019;33(suppl 6):S25-S29.
19. Mills LA, Simpson AH: The relative incidence of fracture non-union in the Scottish population (5.17 million): A 5-year epidemiological study. *BMJ Open* 2013;3(2):e002276.
20. Papakostidis C, Kanakaris NK, Pretel J, Faour O, Morell DJ, Giannoudis PV: Prevalence of complications of open tibial shaft fractures stratified as per the Gustilo-Anderson classification. *Injury* 2011;42(12):1408-1415.
21. Hak DJ, Fitzpatrick D, Bishop JA, et al: Delayed union and nonunions: Epidemiology, clinical issues, and financial aspects. *Injury* 2014;45(suppl 2):S3-S7.
22. MacKenzie EJ, Bosse MJ, Pollak AN, et al: Long-term persistence of disability following severe lower-limb trauma. Results of a seven-year follow-up. *J Bone Joint Surg Am* 2005;87(8):1801-1809.

23. Davis KM, Griffin KS, Chu TG, et al: Muscle-bone interactions during fracture healing. *J Musculoskelet Neuronal Interact* 2015;15(1):1-9.
24. Karladani AH, Granhed H, Kärrholm J, Styf J: The influence of fracture etiology and type on fracture healing: A review of 104 consecutive tibial shaft fractures. *Arch Orthop Trauma Surg* 2001;121(6):325-328.
25. Grogan BF, Hsu JR: Volumetric muscle loss. *J Am Acad Orthop Surg* 2011;19(suppl 1):S35-S37.
26. Corona BT, Wenke JC, Ward CL: Pathophysiology of volumetric muscle loss injury. *Cells Tissues Organs* 2016;202(3-4):180-188.
27. Willett NJ, Boninger ML, Miller LJ, et al: Taking the Next steps in regenerative rehabilitation: Establishment of a new interdisciplinary field. *Arch Phys Med Rehabil* 2020;101(5):917-923.
28. Baker HB, Passipieri JA, Siriwardane M, et al: Cell and growth factor-loaded keratin hydrogels for treatment of volumetric muscle loss in a mouse model. *Tissue Eng Part A* 2017;23(11-12):572-584.
29. Corona BT, Ward CL, Baker HB, Walters TJ, Christ GJ: Implantation of in vitro tissue engineered muscle repair constructs and bladder acellular matrices partially restore in vivo skeletal muscle function in a rat model of volumetric muscle loss injury. *Tissue Eng Part A* 2014;20(3-4):705-715.
30. Machingal MA, Corona BT, Walters TJ, et al: A tissue-engineered muscle repair construct for functional restoration of an irrecoverable muscle injury in a murine model. *Tissue Eng Part A* 2011;17(17-18):2291-2303.
31. Mintz EL, Passipieri JA, Franklin IR, et al: Long-term evaluation of functional outcomes following rat volumetric muscle loss injury and repair. *Tissue Eng Part A* 2020;26(3-4):140-156.
32. Passipieri JA, Baker HB, Siriwardane M, et al: Keratin hydrogel enhances in vivo skeletal muscle function in a rat model of volumetric muscle loss. *Tissue Eng Part A* 2017;23(11-12):556-571.
33. Passipieri JA, Hu X, Mintz E, et al: In silico and in vivo studies detect functional repair mechanisms in a volumetric muscle loss injury. *Tissue Eng Part A* 2019;25(17-18):1272-1288.
34. Gilbert-Honick J, Iyer SR, Somers SM, et al: Engineering 3D skeletal muscle primed for neuromuscular regeneration following volumetric muscle loss. *Biomaterials* 2020;255:120154.
35. Shayan M, Huang NF: Pre-clinical cell therapeutic approaches for repair of volumetric muscle loss. *Bioengineering (Basel)* 2020;7(3):97.
36. Quarta M, Cromie Lear MJ, Blonigan J, Paine P, Chacon R, Rando TA: Biomechanics show stem cell necessity for effective treatment of volumetric muscle loss using bioengineered constructs. *NPJ Regen Med* 2018;3:18.
37. Corona BT, Wu X, Ward CL, McDaniel JS, Rathbone CR, Walters TJ: The promotion of a functional fibrosis in skeletal muscle with volumetric muscle loss injury following the transplantation of muscle-ECM. *Biomaterials* 2013;34(13):3324-3335.
38. Cramer MC, Badylak SF: Extracellular matrix-based biomaterials and their influence upon cell behavior. *Ann Biomed Eng* 2020;48(7):2132-2153.
39. Han N, Yabroudi MA, Stearns-Reider K, et al: Electrodiagnostic evaluation of individuals implanted with extracellular matrix for the treatment of volumetric muscle injury: Case series. *Phys Ther* 2016;96(4):540-549.
40. Mase VJ Jr, Hsu JR, Wolf SE, et al: Clinical application of an acellular biologic scaffold for surgical repair of a large, traumatic quadriceps femoris muscle defect. *Orthopedics* 2010;33(7):511.
41. Sicari BM, Rubin JP, Dearth CL, et al: An acellular biologic scaffold promotes skeletal muscle formation in mice and humans with volumetric muscle loss. *Sci Transl Med* 2014;6(234):234ra58.
42. Sicari BM, Dearth CL, Badylak SF: Tissue engineering and regenerative medicine approaches to enhance the functional response to skeletal muscle injury. *Anat Rec (Hoboken)* 2014;297(1):51-64.
43. Prestwich GD, Healy KE: Why regenerative medicine needs an extracellular matrix. *Expert Opin Biol Ther* 2015;15(1):3-7.
44. Dong R, Ma PX, Guo B: Conductive biomaterials for muscle tissue engineering. *Biomaterials* 2020;229:119584.
45. Kwee BJ, Mooney DJ: Biomaterials for skeletal muscle tissue engineering. *Curr Opin Biotechnol* 2017;47:16-22.
46. Morton AB, Jacobsen NL, Segal SS: Functionalizing biomaterials to promote neurovascular regeneration following skeletal muscle injury. *Am J Physiol Cell Physiol* 2021;320(6):C1099-C1111.
47. Smoak MM, Hogan KJ, Grande-Allen KJ, Mikos AG: Bioinspired electrospun dECM scaffolds guide cell growth and control the formation of myotubes. *Sci Adv* 2021;7(20):eabg4123.
48. Basurto IM, Mora MT, Gardner GM, Christ GJ, Caliari SR: Aligned and electrically conductive 3D collagen scaffolds for skeletal muscle tissue engineering. *Biomater Sci* 2021;9(11):4040-4053.
49. Basurto IM, Passipieri JA, Gardner GM, et al: Photoreactive hydrogel stiffness influences volumetric muscle loss repair. *Tissue Eng Part A* 2022;28(7-8):312-329.
50. Carnes ME, Pins GD: Skeletal muscle tissue engineering: Biomaterials-based strategies for the treatment of volumetric muscle loss. *Bioengineering (Basel)* 2020;7(3):85.
51. Dienes J, Browne S, Farjun B, et al: Semisynthetic hyaluronic acid-based hydrogel promotes recovery of the injured tibialis anterior skeletal muscle form and function. *ACS Biomater Sci Eng* 2021;7(4):1587-1599.
52. Dunn A, Talovic M, Patel K, Patel A, Marcinczyk M, Garg K: Biomaterial and stem cell-based strategies for skeletal muscle regeneration. *J Orthop Res* 2019;37(6):1246-1262.
53. Juhas M, Engelmayr GC, Fontanella AN, Palmer GM, Bursac N: Biomimetic engineered muscle with capacity for vascular integration and functional maturation in vivo. *Proc Natl Acad Sci USA* 2014;111(15):5508-5513.
54. Juhas M, Ye J, Bursac N: Design, evaluation, and application of engineered skeletal muscle. *Methods* 2016;99:81-90.

55. Madden L, Juhas M, Kraus WE, Truskey GA, Bursac N: Bioengineered human myobundles mimic clinical responses of skeletal muscle to drugs. *Elife* 2015;4:e04885.

56. Novakova SS, Rodriguez BL, Vega-Soto EE, et al: Repairing volumetric muscle loss in the ovine peroneus tertius following a 3-month recovery. *Tissue Eng Part A* 2020;26(15-16):837-851.

57. Nutter GP, VanDusen KW, Florida SE, Syverud BC, Larkin LM: The effects of engineered skeletal muscle on volumetric muscle loss in the tibialis anterior of rat after three months in vivo. *Regen Eng Transl Med* 2020;6(4):365-372.

58. VanDusen KW, Syverud BC, Williams ML, Lee JD, Larkin LM: Engineered skeletal muscle units for repair of volumetric muscle loss in the tibialis anterior muscle of a rat. *Tissue Eng Part A* 2014;20(21-22):2920-2930.

59. Matai I, Kaur G, Seyedsalehi A, McClinton A, Laurencin CT: Progress in 3D bioprinting technology for tissue/organ regenerative engineering. *Biomaterials* 2020;226:119536.

60. Murphy SV, De Coppi P, Atala A: Opportunities and challenges of translational 3D bioprinting. *Nat Biomed Eng* 2020 2020;4(4):370-380.

61. Thayer P, Martinez H, Gatenholm E: History and trends of 3D bioprinting. *Methods Mol Biol* 2020;2140:3-18.

62. Choi YJ, Jun YJ, Kim DY, et al: A 3D cell printed muscle construct with tissue-derived bioink for the treatment of volumetric muscle loss. *Biomaterials* 2019;206:160-169.

63. Ostrovidov S, Salehi S, Costantini M, et al: 3D bioprinting in skeletal muscle tissue engineering. *Small* 2019;15(24):1805530.

64. Russell CS, Mostafavi A, Quint JP, et al: In situ printing of adhesive hydrogel scaffolds for the treatment of skeletal muscle injuries. *ACS Appl Bio Mater* 2020;3(3):1568-1579.

65. Corona BT, Machingal MA, Criswell T, et al: Further development of a tissue engineered muscle repair construct in vitro for enhanced functional recovery following implantation in vivo in a murine model of volumetric muscle loss injury. *Tissue Eng Part A* 2012;18(11-12):1213-1228.

66. Dienes JA, Hu X, Janson KD, et al: Analysis and modeling of rat gait biomechanical deficits in response to volumetric muscle loss injury. *Front Bioeng Biotechnol* 2019;7:146.

67. Mintz EL, Passipieri JA, Lovell DY, Christ GJ: Applications of in vivo functional testing of the rat tibialis anterior for evaluating tissue engineered skeletal muscle repair. *J Vis Exp* 2016;116:54487.

68. Blemker SS, Pinsky PM, Delp SL: A 3D model of muscle reveals the causes of nonuniform strains in the biceps brachii. *J Biomech* 2005;38(4):657-665.

69. Fiorentino NM, Rehorn MR, Chumanov ES, Thelen DG, Blemker SS: Computational models predict larger muscle tissue strains at faster sprinting speeds. *Med Sci Sports Exerc* 2014;46(4):776-786.

70. Hernández-Gascón B, Grasa J, Calvo B, Rodríguez JF: A 3D electro-mechanical continuum model for simulating skeletal muscle contraction. *J Theor Biol* 2013;335:108-118.

71. Odegard GM, Donahue TL, Morrow DA, Kaufman KR: Constitutive modeling of skeletal muscle tissue with an explicit strain-energy function. *J Biomech Eng* 2008;130(6):061017.

72. Wheatley BB, Odegard GM, Kaufman KR, Haut Donahue TL: A validated model of passive skeletal muscle to predict force and intramuscular pressure. *Biomech Model Mechanobiol* 2017;16(3):1011-1022.

73. Westman AM, Dyer SE, Remer JD, Hu X, Christ GJ, Blemker SS: A coupled framework of in situ and in silico analysis reveals the role of lateral force transmission in force production in volumetric muscle loss injuries. *J Biomech* 2019;85:118-125.

74. Buchner DM, Cress ME, de Lateur BJ, et al: The effect of strength and endurance training on gait, balance, fall risk, and health services use in community-living older adults. *J Gerontol A Biol Sci Med Sci* 1997;52(4):M218-M224.

75. Damiano DL, Abel MF: Functional outcomes of strength training in spastic cerebral palsy. *Arch Phys Med Rehabil* 1998;79(2):119-125.

76. Damiano DL, Arnold AS, Steele KM, Delp SL: Can strength training predictably improve gait kinematics? A pilot study on the effects of hip and knee extensor strengthening on lower-extremity alignment in cerebral palsy. *Phys Ther* 2010;90(2):269-279.

77. Damiano DL, Prosser LA, Curatalo LA, Alter KE: Muscle plasticity and ankle control after repetitive use of a functional electrical stimulation device for foot drop in cerebral palsy. *Neurorehabil Neural Repair* 2013;27(3):200-207.

78. Topp R, Mikesky A, Wigglesworth J, Holt W Jr, Edwards JE: The effect of a 12-week dynamic resistance strength training program on gait velocity and balance of older adults. *Gerontologist* 1993;33(4):501-506.

79. Derwin KA, Baker AR, Iannotti JP, McCarron JA: Preclinical models for translating regenerative medicine therapies for rotator cuff repair. *Tissue Eng B Rev* 2010;16(1):21-30.

80. Kovacevic D, Baker AR, Staugaitis SM, Kim M-S, Ricchetti ET, Derwin KA: Development of an arthroscopic joint capsule injury model in the canine shoulder. *PLoS One* 2016;11(1):e0147949.

81. Gladstone JN, Bishop JY, Lo IK, Flatow EL: Fatty infiltration and atrophy of the rotator cuff do not improve after rotator cuff repair and correlate with poor functional outcome. *Am J Sports Med* 2007;35(5):719-728.

82. Liem D, Lichtenberg S, Magosch P, Habermeyer P: Magnetic resonance imaging of arthroscopic supraspinatus tendon repair. *J Bone Joint Surg Am* 2007;89(8):1770-1776.

83. Gerber C, Schneeberger AG, Hoppeler H, Meyer DC: Correlation of atrophy and fatty infiltration on strength and integrity of rotator cuff repairs: A study in thirteen patients. *J Shoulder Elbow Surg* 2007;16(6):691-696.

84. Yuri T, Mura N, Yuki I, Fujii H, Kiyoshige Y: Contractile property measurement of the torn supraspinatus muscle using real-time tissue elastography. *J Shoulder Elbow Surg* 2018;27(9):1700-1704.

85. Derwin KA, Badylak SF, Steinmann SP, Iannotti JP: Extracellular matrix scaffold devices for rotator cuff repair. *J Shoulder Elbow Surg* 2010;19(3):467-476.

86. Davies MR, Liu X, Lee L, et al: TGF-β small molecule inhibitor SB431542 reduces rotator cuff muscle fibrosis and fatty

infiltration by promoting fibro/adipogenic progenitor apoptosis. *PLoS One* 2016;11(5):e0155486.

87. Oak NR, Gumucio JP, Flood MD, et al: Inhibition of 5-LOX, COX-1, and COX-2 increases tendon healing and reduces muscle fibrosis and lipid accumulation after rotator cuff repair. *Am J Sports Med* 2014;42(12):2860-2868.
88. Lee C, Liu M, Agha O, Kim HT, Liu X, Feeley BT: Beige fibro-adipogenic progenitor transplantation reduces muscle degeneration and improves function in a mouse model of delayed repair of rotator cuff tears. *J Shoulder Elbow Surg* 2020;29(4):719-727.
89. Oh JH, Chung SW, Kim SH, Chung JY, Kim JY: 2013 Neer Award: Effect of the adipose-derived stem cell for the improvement of fatty degeneration and rotator cuff healing in rabbit model. *J Shoulder Elbow Surg* 2014;23(4):445-455.
90. Wang C, Hu Q, Song W, Yu W, He Y: Adipose stem cell-derived exosomes decrease fatty infiltration and enhance rotator cuff healing in a rabbit model of chronic tears. *Am J Sports Med* 2020;48(6):1456-1464.
91. Tellier LE, Krieger JR, Brimeyer AL, et al: Localized SDF-1α delivery increases pro-healing bone marrow-derived cells in the supraspinatus muscle following severe rotator cuff injury. *Regen Eng Transl Med* 2018;4(2):92-103.
92. Huynh T, Kim JT, Dunlap G, Ahmadi S, Wolchok JC: In vivo testing of an injectable matrix gel for the treatment of shoulder cuff muscle fatty degeneration. *J Shoulder Elbow Surg* 2020;29(12):e478-e490.
93. Tang X, Shemshaki NS, Vernekar VN, et al: The treatment of muscle atrophy after rotator cuff tears using electroconductive nanofibrous matrices. *Regen Eng Transl Med* 2021;7(1):1-9.
94. Jain NB, Wilcox RB III, Katz JN, Higgins LD: Clinical examination of the rotator cuff. *PM R* 2013;5(1):45-56.
95. Ditsios K, Boutsiadis A, Kapoukranidou D, et al: Chronic massive rotator cuff tear in rats: In vivo evaluation of muscle force and three-dimensional histologic analysis. *J Shoulder Elbow Surg* 2014;23(12):1822-1830.
96. Meyer DC, Gerber C, Von Rechenberg B, Wirth SH, Farshad M: Amplitude and strength of muscle contraction are reduced in experimental tears of the rotator cuff. *Am J Sports Med* 2011;39(7):1456-1461.
97. Valencia AP, Iyer SR, Spangenburg EE, Gilotra MN, Lovering RM: Impaired contractile function of the supraspinatus in the acute period following a rotator cuff tear. *BMC Musculoskelet Disord* 2017;18(1):436.
98. Valencia AP, Lai JK, Iyer SR, et al: Fatty infiltration is a prognostic marker of muscle function after rotator cuff tear. *Am J Sports Med* 2018;46(9):2161-2169.

CHAPTER 22

Measurement of Clinical Outcomes in the Upper Extremity

Vahid Entezari, MD, MSc • Jason C. Ho, MD • Joseph P. Iannotti, MD, PhD, FAAOS • Kathleen A. Derwin, PhD • Eric T. Ricchetti, MD, FAAOS

INTRODUCTION

Recently, there has been a growing interest in orthobiologics and their role in augmentation, regeneration, and healing of bone, cartilage, and soft tissues because of unmet clinical needs in bone and soft-tissue healing (eg, rotator cuff repair, fracture healing) and progression of arthritic change (eg, cartilage preservation/regeneration in early osteoarthritis). Orthobiologic products are derived from substances that naturally occur in the body, including human blood and tissue (bone marrow, adipose), extracellular matrix, placenta, and amniotic fluid. A recent survey of members of the American Orthopaedic Society for Sports Medicine revealed that 66% are using at least one orthobiologic in their practice and 72% are increasing their use,[1] although regulatory and FDA approval for the various orthobiologic agents are at various stages. Although orthobiologics are perceived as less invasive than surgery with the potential to improve healing and recovery, the lack of high-quality evidence has slowed their widespread acceptance among all practitioners. Most published studies on this topic have small sample size, lack comparative effectiveness, and have high heterogeneity in both patient characteristics and follow-up duration, as well as inconsistency in dose and preparation of orthobiologic interventions.[2] For instance, lack of standardization and high variability in the preparation, dose, frequency, and route of administration of platelet-rich plasma (PRP) have led to conflicting results and complicated the interpretation of the literature on this topic.[3] Regulatory approval may also limit the use of certain intervention and, therefore, the ability to study treatment efficacy effectively. For example, mesenchymal stem cells are not FDA approved but do have approval for use in Europe, Canada, and Australia.[4]

One of the major determinants of evaluating quality in orthobiologic studies is the selection of appropriate outcome measures. The outcome measure is defined by the World Health Organization as the change in the health of an individual, group of people, or population that is attributable to an intervention or series of interventions. The measures vary from a simple question about patient's pain level to a complex questionnaire that assigns a numeric value to patient's health status. More generalized outcome measures (eg, Short Form [SF] 36) may focus on a patient's general health status, whereas others can be specific to a disease process (eg, Western Ontario Rotator Cuff Index) or a joint in the body (eg, Constant score).[5] Also, outcome measures can be patient or physician assessed.

Wilson and Cleary combined the biomedical and social science paradigms of health outcome and proposed a conceptual model for patient outcomes that includes five main categories:[6] biologic and physiologic outcomes (eg, biomarkers), symptoms (eg, pain level), functioning (eg, return to sport), general health perception (eg, Veteran Rand 12), and overall quality of life (eg, quality-adjusted life year). One of the major attributes of good outcome measures is their relevance to patients and their experience, which explains the growing attention to patient-reported outcome measures (PROMs) in the orthopaedic literature,[7] instruments that are now widely used and encompass four of the five categories highlighted in the conceptual model of Wilson and Cleary: symptoms, functioning, general health perception, and overall quality of life. PROMs are essential to understanding the benefit of orthobiologic interventions, in addition to biologic, imaging (structural), and objective functional (strength, range of motion [ROM]) outcomes after treatment.

Dr. Entezari or an immediate family member serves as a paid consultant to or is an employee of DJ Orthopaedics and has received research or institutional support from DJ Orthopaedics and OREF. Dr. Ho or an immediate family member serves as a paid consultant to or is an employee of Biedermann Motech. Dr. Iannotti or an immediate family member has received royalties from Arthrex, Inc, DePuy, Synthes, DJ Orthopaedics, and Stryker; is a member of a speakers' bureau or has made paid presentations on behalf of DJ Orthopaedics; and serves as a paid consultant to or is an employee of DJ Orthopaedics. Dr. Derwin or an immediate family member has received royalties from Viscus Biologics; serves as a paid consultant to or is an employee of Collamedix; has stock or stock options held in Collamedix; has received research or institutional support from DJ Orthopaedics; and serves as a board member, owner, officer, or committee member of the Orthopaedic Research Society. Dr. Iannotti or an immediate family member has received royalties from DJ Orthopaedics; is a member of a speakers' bureau or has made paid presentations on behalf of DJ Orthopaedics; serves as a paid consultant to or is an employee of DJ Orthopaedics; and serves as a board member, owner, officer, or committee member of the American Academy of Orthopaedic Surgeons, the American Board of Orthopaedic Surgery, Inc., and the American Shoulder and Elbow Surgeons.

Outcomes are increasingly assessed through standardized instruments. The most important attribute of an outcome instrument is to examine whether an intervention is effective in improving symptoms or function from a patient's standpoint.[8] An outcome instrument should be reliable, valid, and responsive to change in health status relevant to the procedure or intervention it assesses.[9] Reliability refers to the extent an instrument yields the same results in repeated measurements in a cohort with stable health. This can be assessed through interrater, test-retest, and internal consistency reliability.[10] Validity is an estimate of the extent to which an instrument measures what it is designed to measure. An instrument is valid if it has face validity (relevance), content validity (covering all domains), and construct validity (correlation to other instruments). Responsiveness refers to the ability of an instrument to reflect change in a cohort of patients over time. It is critical for a responsive instrument to detect any effect that is important to the patient, even if that effect is small, and the magnitude is often referred to as the minimum clinically important difference.[11] The choice of outcome measure has important implications for all aspects of orthobiologic research, including sample size, patient compliance, feasibility, and the cost of data collection.[12] It is important to review the different outcome measures used to evaluate orthobiologic interventions in the upper extremity, including those used to assess biologic, imaging (structural), functional outcomes (strength, ROM), and PROMs.

BIOLOGIC AND PHYSIOLOGIC OUTCOMES

Orthobiologic interventions aim to improve biologic aspects of tissue healing, such as regeneration of soft tissue and articular cartilage, and they hold promise for treatment of a variety of acute and chronic orthopaedic conditions. The rationale for the clinical application of orthobiologics is that they promote or enhance a healing response in tissues that have less inherent regenerative capacity and can optimize the inflammatory response following an injury.[13] Most of the data on the biologic effects of orthobiologics are based on preclinical and in vitro laboratory studies. Clinical trials are designed with the hope that those results translate to improved outcomes for patients, but this has not always panned out because of the lack of high-quality studies and absence of true controls in many intervention studies,[14] as well as the heterogeneity of included studies in most meta-analyses.[15]

Biologic outcomes such as the evaluation of tissue biopsies and the analysis of biomarkers from serum, urine, or synovial fluid have been used in orthobiologic studies. The advantage of tissue-based outcome variables is their high sensitivity to healing or the biologic process of interest. The disadvantage of tissue biopsies is that they may fail to yield enough tissue or only small quantities that may not be representative of the tissue of interest, and the process of obtaining and analyzing tissue biopsies can be invasive and destructive, which prohibits their application in longitudinal studies. Although biomarker analysis of systemic blood or urine is not destructive and commonly can be repeated over time, there is questionable specificity and relevance to patients' local healing or inflammatory process.

Overall, the strength of the relationship between biologic outcomes and PROMs is not well understood, and the difficulty in procurement and interpretation of biologic outcome measures has limited their widespread application. Identifying prognostic biomarkers for both disease progression and response to treatment in various orthopaedic conditions would provide additional depth of assessment beyond what is captured by PROMs. For example, Carr et al[16] reported the results of a randomized clinical trial of arthroscopic acromioplasty with and without injection of autologous PRP in 60 patients with chronic rotator cuff tendinopathy. They obtained tendon biopsies at the time of surgery and at 3-month follow-up using needle biopsy under ultrasound guidance. Their study showed significant improvement in patient-reported outcomes at up to 2 years of follow-up with acromioplasty, but the PRP group showed worse tissue characteristics at 3 months, including reduced cellularity and vascularity and increased apoptosis suggesting a potential deleterious effect of PRP injection on the healing response. This example depicts a rare but effective application of a biologic outcome in orthobiologic research that adds a new dimension to the growing knowledge of these interventions.

There is a growing body of literature on the role of biomarkers in diagnosis and treatment of common upper extremity diseases such as rotator cuff disease,[17,18] glenohumeral osteoarthritis,[19] and adhesive capsulitis.[20] Although most novel biomarkers are in the early stages of preclinical validation, they are showing promising application in orthobiologic research. For example, biomarkers are able to provide information about tissue integrity by quantifying the molecular composition (such as the type and orientation of collagen fibers in tendon[21]), cellular makeup (such as the number and differentiation of regenerative cells), and healing response (such as the concentration and type of biologic mediators) in the tissue.[22] It is crucial to closely monitor the potential future application of these assays and biomarkers in orthobiologic research.

IMAGING/STRUCTURAL OUTCOMES

Imaging studies are one of the most commonly used surrogate outcome measures in orthopaedic research (**Table 1**). They provide valuable structural data that can be used in formulating the diagnosis, assessing the severity of the disease, and monitoring disease progression and the response to treatment. Examples of imaging outcome measures include the degree of joint-space

TABLE 1 Imaging Outcomes and Their Characteristics

Imaging Modality	Radiation Exposure	Resolution	Soft-Tissue Visualization	Acquisition Time	Cost	Strength	Limitations
Radiography	Yes	Low	Poor	Fast	$	Ubiquitous, low cost	Poor soft-tissue delineation
Ultrasonography	No	Average	Good	Slow	$	Low cost	Short penetration, operator dependent
CT	Yes	High	Average	Fast	$$	Three dimensional, fast, high resolution, best for bone	Radiation, poor soft-tissue delineation
MRI	No	High	Good	Slow	$$$	Three dimensional, high resolution, best for soft tissue	Slow, cost
PET/SPECT	Yes	Low	Average	Fast	$$$	Low resolution, radioactive probe	Radiation, cost

PET = positron emission tomography, SPECT = single photon emission CT

Reproduced with permission from Wallyn J, Anton N, Akram S, Vandamme TF: Biomedical imaging: Principles, technologies, clinical aspects, contrast agents, limitations and future trends in nanomedicines. *Pharm Res* 2019;36(6):78.

narrowing measured on plain radiographs, the integrity of a rotator cuff repair on ultrasonography or MRI, and the amount of fatty infiltration and atrophy of the rotator cuff muscles seen on MRI. The advantages of imaging-based outcomes include the ability to assess structural changes in a noninvasive and nondestructive manner that allows for longitudinal assessment of tissues of interest, as well as their reliability and availability as outcome measures.

There are a few universal challenges in designing studies with primary imaging outcome measures. First, exposure to radiation may pose a concern when patients undergo repeated radiographs or CT, especially at a younger age. Second, depending on the type of tissue and the intervention, an imaging-based structural effect may not be observed. For instance, several studies on the efficiency of PRP injections in rotator cuff repair have failed to show any effect on the rate of retear based on MRI evaluation.[23] This may be due to a lack of true benefit of the orthobiologic intervention, but also brings up the question of the sensitivity of imaging measures to detect change following these types of interventions, as well as the optimal timing of imaging measures to capture maximum healing response. Third, the cost of imaging studies, especially advanced imaging (eg, CT, MRI, and positron emission tomography), practically limits their use. Last, generally, there is a challenge interpreting imaging-based structural outcomes when they do not correlate with patients' symptoms and function. A classic example of this is the weak correlation between MRI-based assessment of rotator cuff integrity and PROMs in the early (1-year or at most 2-year) follow-up period after rotator cuff repair when outcomes are assessed.[24,25] Additional studies are needed to understand the relationship between poor short-term structural outcomes and longer term clinical outcomes when clinical declines are more likely to be manifest.

Plain radiography is one of the most basic and ubiquitous imaging modalities that provides useful information about bone and joint anatomy. The variables that can be assessed on radiographs include gross alignment of joints, presence and classification of fractures, fracture healing, joint space as a surrogate for cartilage height, overall bone density and cortical thickness as a crude measure of osteoporosis, and other arthritic changes, including the presence of osteophytes, joint line medialization, and bony erosion to assess the severity of osteoarthritic disease. Radiographic analysis generally has low sensitivity and long latency and provides limited data on soft tissue and its healing response while exposing patients to radiation. Although plain radiography has commonly been used as an imaging modality in cartilage restoration and osteoarthritis studies in the lower extremity, its utility in orthobiologic studies of soft tissues in the upper extremity has been limited.

Ultrasonography has dual applications both as an image guidance tool for targeted injections and a diagnostic modality for soft-tissue assessment. Ultrasound-guided injection has improved the precise and effective delivery of orthobiologics and image-guided injections have become more popular in recent years.[26] In two recent meta-analyses of the effectiveness of PRP in rotator cuff tendinopathy, almost all studies used ultrasound guidance for the injection of PRP in subacromial, intra-articular, or intratendinous applications.[27,28] As an imaging modality, ultrasonography has the advantage of not exposing patients to radiation, having reasonable cost, and being able to assess soft tissues dynamically. The limitations of ultrasonography are its user dependency, low resolution, limited depth penetration, and the effect of swelling and body habitus on its accuracy. Ultrasonography has been applied in the assessment of lateral epicondylitis[29] and rotator cuff tendinopathy and tears.[30]

CT is considered an advanced imaging study that can provide three-dimensional views of the body with high resolution, short acquisition time, and preferential visualization of bony structures. Although it is a diagnostic modality of choice in the assessment of fracture healing and has capability to quantify bone density, its application in orthobiologic studies has been limited mainly because of its decreased utility in the assessment of granular soft-tissue changes, risk of radiation exposure, and cost.

MRI is the most commonly used diagnostic imaging modality for high-resolution assessment of soft tissue, especially tendon quality, healing response, and progression of osteoarthritis. MRI has also been used frequently as an imaging outcome measure in orthobiologic studies.[28,31] It has the advantage of not exposing patients to radiation while providing detailed information about water and fat content in soft tissue, and with the help of different signal sequences, it is able to assess tendons, ligaments, muscles, cartilage, and other soft-tissue structures. In addition, it offers an enduring imaging study that can be reviewed by many and for detailed assessments. With the increased application of scaffolds to deliver orthobiologic solutions, MRI has been able to show utility in the assessment of scaffold location, integration, and integrity over time. Potential limitations of MRI-based outcome measures include long acquisition time, interference of metallic objects, and high cost. Contrast-based functional CT or MRI modalities to assess tissue quality (eg, cartilage, meniscus, tendon) or healing response around a joint are being investigated and developed,[32] but have not yet been routinely used in clinical studies to assess the benefit of orthobiologic interventions.

Positron emission tomography and single photon emission CT are advanced nuclear medicine imaging techniques that use radioactive tracers to identify areas of soft tissue and bone that are highly metabolically active.[33] They are costly, have low resolution, and require a radioactive probe and exposure to radiation, but are highly specific and can have unique applications in detection of stress fracture and intense soft-tissue healing response, and although this has not been explored, they can potentially be used in orthobiologic studies.[34]

FUNCTIONAL OUTCOMES

Assessment of function is one of the most relevant outcome measures for patients undergoing orthobiologic interventions. The functional outcome of an extremity or joint can be captured by measurement of patients' ROM and strength and can be inferred by their return to a desired level of activity at work or sports. The patient's assessment of their function is also an important part of any patient-reported outcome instrument. The advantage of functional outcomes is their objective nature and the fact that they can be quantified (eg, ROM and strength) or verified through registries or official records (eg, return to sports in professional sport leagues). The challenge in assessing functional outcomes, however, is that they are most commonly evaluated by an observer and require an in-person or virtual visit and are subjected to inaccuracies depending on the observer and the method of measurement. Although using blinded and trained observers who use standard protocols to examine and record functional outcomes can reduce the chance of error and bias, studies still show high interobserver and intraobserver variability in this setting.[8] In addition, the cause of gain of function with regard to measures such as ROM and strength can be multifactorial in nature and may be affected by a variety of mental, emotional, and physical factors.

Functional outcome measures including ROM, strength, and return to work and sports have been used in orthobiologic studies. Randelli et al[35] published a randomized controlled trial on the effect of intraoperative PRP injection after arthroscopic rotator cuff repair and showed not only better pain control in the first month and improved PROMs at 3 months, but patients' external rotation strength measured by dynamometer was also significantly higher in the treatment group at 3 months, supporting a positive effect of PRP on rotator cuff healing in this study. In contrast, Kesikburun et al[36] reported another randomized controlled trial on the effect of PRP injection on rotator cuff tendinopathy and showed at 1 year the PRP injection was no more effective than placebo in improving PROMs and pain level. In addition, no difference was found in patients' ROM at 3, 6, 12, and 24 weeks and 1 year after the PRP injection, which added more depth to the assessment of function in this study. A study by Mills et al[37] explored the ability to return to sport after PRP injection following elbow ulnar collateral ligaments injury in a cohort of 50 patients and found favorable results in type I, II, and III ulnar collateral ligament injuries, but not type IV with regard to return to sports, suggesting an effect modification by severity of the injury. As seen in these examples, functional outcomes are commonly used in orthobiologic studies and often add objectivity to the assessment of clinical outcomes.

PATIENT-REPORTED OUTCOMES

There has been a significant shift in the orthopaedic literature with increasing attention to and use of PROMs in recent years. This is mainly driven by putting patients and their experience at the center of attention, especially because many anatomic and structural outcome measures have shown low correlation with patient-reported outcomes at least in the shorter term. There has been tremendous effort in the past 2 decades to design and validate PROM instruments and establish their minimum clinically important difference for common disease processes and interventions (**Table 2**).[38-40] The advantage of these instruments is their ability to collect PROMs in a standardized fashion with known validity and reliability that allow quantification of patients' pain, function, and satisfaction.

Although utilization of PROMs has been growing steadily, their implementation in clinical research has created some challenges as well. For instance, collection of PROMs using exhaustive questionnaires over several time points may create fatigue and lack of engagement on the patient's part. Also, it is unclear as to whether PROMs are responsive enough and have enough specificity to be used in orthobiologic research. As noted previously, the association between structural and/or biologic healing and PROMs has been inconsistent in the literature, which suggests that many PROMs may lack the sensitivity to reliably detect structural and/or biologic healing and/or that poor healing does not manifest as a decline in clinical outcomes until the longer term. Similarly, the relationship between PROMs and objective measures of impairment, such as ROM and strength, can be very low. Roddey et al[41] found that in a cohort of 108 patients who participated in a randomized trial of home exercise after arthroscopic rotator cuff repair, the collected objective measures of patient impairment only explained 8% of patients' self-reported PROMs. There are also several studies that have shown a correlation between the structural healing of the rotator cuff and patient's strength in the short term, but failed to show similar relationships between strength and patient satisfaction[42] or PROMs.[43] Collectively, these studies demonstrate that sensitive assessment of outcomes requires measurement of different domains of recovery. The remainder of this section will briefly review commonly used PROMs in the upper extremity, including both general and joint-specific measures, with additional characteristics of these instruments noted in **Table 2**.

Short Form 36 and Short Form 12

The SF-36 was originally described in 1992 and has become the most commonly used tool to assess general health status.[44] It consists of 36 questions in eight domains and generates a physical component score and a mental component score. These measures are scored based on the general US population with a mean age of 50 years and SD of 10. It has been extensively validated and used in a variety of upper extremity conditions, including fracture fixation, rotator cuff repair, and shoulder arthroplasty.[45,46] Studies have shown that the physical component summary of the SF-36 improves following surgical treatment, but the mental component summary component has minimal change.[46] An abbreviated version of this instrument, the SF-12, has been introduced and demonstrated good correlation with the full physical and mental components.[47]

Disabilities of the Arm, Shoulder and Hand Score

The Disabilities of the Arm, Shoulder and Hand (DASH) score was introduced in 1996[48] as a patient-administered questionnaire consisting of 30 core questions and an optional 8 questions about return to work and sports. It is designed to assess disability of single or multiple disorders in any region of the upper extremity and has shown good test-retest reliability, minimal floor and ceiling effects,[49] and correlates well with other joint-specific PROMs.[50] In 2005, the QuickDASH, an abbreviated version of this score, was developed to reduce the responder burden with only 11 questions and has shown high correlation with the original DASH score ($r > 0.97$).[51] One of the potential shortcomings of the QuickDASH score is that if a responder misses more than one question, a total score cannot be calculated. Despite its validation and good correlation with other shoulder-specific PROMs, the DASH score is not commonly reported on in shoulder literature.[52]

Patient-Reported Outcomes Measurement Information System Upper Extremity

The Patient-Reported Outcomes Measurement Information System (PROMIS) score was developed by the National Institutes of Health in 2004 to address the need for more reliable, valid, and generalizable measures of clinical outcomes for orthopaedic patients.[53] This instrument is designed to be applicable to the general population by normalizing scores in all domains by T-score from the US general population and can be compared across different clinical scenarios without being limited to a certain diagnosis.[54] The questionnaire consists of a Physical Function domain, including social function, pain, fatigue and emotional distress, and a Global Health domain, including overall physical health, pain, fatigue, emotional distress, and social health. The PROMIS questionnaire can be applied in short form, which ranges from two to eight questions per domain or as a computer adaptive test, which uses a computer algorithm to reduce the number of questions asked and the burden on patients.[55] The PROMIS Upper Extremity score consists of 16 questions directly related to upper extremity musculoskeletal conditions and has been validated for patients undergoing shoulder instability surgery,[56] shoulder arthroplasty,[57] and rotator cuff repair.[58] The PROMIS Physical Function score is closely correlated with SF-36, whereas the PROMIS Upper Extremity score has shown good correlation with other established upper extremity PROMs, such as the American Shoulder and Elbow Surgeons (ASES) score, with generally less ceiling and floor effects.[59]

Shoulder Outcome Measures

There are several commonly used general shoulder PROMs including the ASES, Constant, Pennsylvania, Simple Assessment Numeric Evaluation, University of California Los Angeles, and Oxford shoulder scores. The commonly used ASES score has a physician-rated portion that is rarely used and a patient-rated portion that consists of a visual analog scale pain question and 10 questions related to patients' function.[60] It has been validated for a variety of shoulder problems, including rotator cuff disease, glenohumeral arthritis, shoulder instability, and following shoulder arthroplasty.[61] The minimum clinically important difference and minimally detectable change are reported as 6.7 and 9.7, respectively.[62] **Table 2** summarizes the properties of the remaining shoulder PROMs.

Disease-specific shoulder scores have been developed for the most common shoulder pathologies, including rotator cuff disease, shoulder instability, and glenohumeral arthritis. In addition to general shoulder PROMs, the rotator cuff quality of life and Western Ontario Rotator Cuff index are the two most commonly used disease-specific scores for rotator cuff disease. The Western Ontario Rotator Cuff Index has gone through more rigorous psychometric analysis and has stronger properties and hence it is more commonly used as a disease-specific outcome measure.[63] In the setting of shoulder instability, a primary limiting factor for patients following shoulder dislocation is usually not pain or lack of function but apprehension and inability to participate in certain sport activities. As a result, general shoulder PROMs focused more on pain and function have poor psychometric parameters for patients with instability.[64] This has led to the development of several instability-specific outcome measures including the Rowe score, the Western Ontario Shoulder Instability Index, and the Oxford Shoulder Instability Score. The oldest and most frequently used instrument is the Rowe score, but many of its psychometric properties have not been established. The Western Ontario Shoulder Instability Index has the strongest psychometric properties and is currently the recommended PROM for shoulder instability.[52] The Western Ontario Osteoarthritis of the Shoulder Index is the only validated PROM that is specific to shoulder arthritis and, according to its developers, also has strong psychometric properties (**Table 2**).

Elbow Outcome Measures

The joint-specific PROMs for the elbow include the ASES elbow outcome score, the Broberg and Morrey elbow scale, the Mayo elbow-performance score, the Hospital for Special Surgery assessment scale, and the Liverpool elbow score.[9,65] The Mayo Elbow Performance Score is the most commonly reported PROM in the elbow literature.[66] It consists of a physician assessment of pain, elbow ROM and stability, and patients' input on their daily function. The continuous raw score has shown good correlation to other elbow measures and has been validated for general elbow conditions.[67] The PROMs in the elbow are highly influenced by pain and all have a component of physician assessment that differentiates them from shoulder PROMs. Characteristics of the rest of the elbow PROMs are summarized in **Table 2**.

Hand Outcome Measures

Several hand-specific and wrist-specific PROMs have been developed in recent years.[68] Some of these tools are joint specific, such as the Michigan Hand Outcome Questionnaire or the Jebsen-Taylor Hand Function Test, and some are disease specific, such as the Boston Carpal Tunnel Syndrome Questionnaire.[69] The information regarding design and psychometric properties of these PROMs is summarized in **Table 2**.

SUMMARY: CHALLENGES AND OPPORTUNITIES

The choice of outcome measure(s) used to assess orthobiologic interventions has great effect on the quality of the given clinical study and should match with the goals of the study, the nature of the intervention, and the study patient characteristics. Orthobiologic treatment is a fast-growing field with the promise to improve the healing potential and regeneration of bone and soft tissues affected by injury or chronic orthopaedic conditions. There are many challenges that remain in the field, including a lack of consensus on the indication, dosage, timing, and outcomes of studies that investigate orthobiologic interventions and a lack of high-quality randomized trials with standardized treatments and robust study design.

To improve the quality of the orthobiologics literature and address the aforementioned challenges in the field, a framework should be defined to choose the appropriate outcome measures from a long list of biologic, physiologic, imaging/structural, functional, and PROMs that were reviewed. The responsiveness of many standard outcome measures, including imaging and PROMs, to orthobiologic interventions also needs to be further investigated. In addition, appropriately powered randomized controlled trials with standardization of orthobiologics by both indication and preparation and comparisons to standard-of-care interventions are needed to generate high-quality clinical evidence that establishes the true efficacy of orthobiologic treatments with regard to outcomes

TABLE 2 Patient-Reported Outcome Measures and Their Characteristics

Anatomic Region	Scale	Range of Score	Measures	Validated	Responder Burden		Target Population		MCID
					Clinician (No. of questions)	Patient (No. of questions)	Age (years)	Disorder	
None	SF-36	0-100	General health	Yes	None	36	16-74	All diagnoses	5
None	SF-12	0-100	General health	Yes	None	12	—	All diagnoses	—
Shoulder, arm, and hand	DASH	0-100	Function	Yes	None	38	18-65	All upper extremity diagnoses	10-17
Shoulder, arm, and hand	QuickDASH	0-100	Function	Yes	None	11	18-65	All upper extremity diagnoses	13-16
Shoulder, arm, and hand	PROMIS UE	Variable	Physical functional and global health	Yes	None	16 (SF), variable (CAT)	—	All upper extremity diagnoses	3-8
Shoulder	ASES	0-100	Function	Yes	Rarely used	10	20-81	All shoulder diagnoses	6.7
Shoulder	PSS	0-100	Function and satisfaction	Yes	None	24	—	All shoulder diagnoses	11.4
Shoulder	Constant	0-100	Function	Yes	6	2	14-85	RCR, shoulder arthroplasty, adhesive capsulitis, and proximal humerus fractures	6-10
Shoulder	SANE	0-100	Patient perception	No	None	1	—	All shoulder diagnoses	27
Shoulder	UCLA	0-35	Pain, function, ROM, satisfaction	No	2	3	—	All shoulder diagnoses	3
Shoulder	Oxford shoulder score	12-60	Function	No	None	12	—	All shoulder diagnoses	3
Shoulder	SST	0-12	Function	Yes	None	12	—	All shoulder diagnoses	2
Shoulder	WOOS	0-1900	Physical function, sport/recreation/work, emotional function	Yes	None	19	—	Glenohumeral osteoarthritis	—
Shoulder	WORC	0-2100	Physical function, sport/recreation/work, emotional function	Yes	None	21	20-85	Rotator cuff pathology	275

(Continued)

TABLE 2 Patient-Reported Outcome Measures and Their Characteristics (Continued)

Anatomic Region	Scale	Range of Score	Measures	Validated	Responder Burden		Target Population		MCID
					Clinician (No. of questions)	Patient (No. of questions)	Age (years)	Disorder	
Shoulder	WOSI	0-2100	Function and satisfaction	Yes	None	21	—	Shoulder instability	220
Elbow	ASES	0-100	Pain, function, satisfaction	Yes	38	19	—	All elbow diagnoses	10-17
Elbow	Broberg and Morrey	0-100	Pain, motion, strength	Yes	5	1	—	All elbow diagnoses	N/A
Elbow	Mayo elbow-performance score	0-100	Pain, motion, stability, and daily function	Yes	3	5	—	All elbow diagnoses	12-15
Elbow	HSS assessment scale	0-100	Pain, ROM, strength, duration of symptoms	Yes	6	3	—	All elbow diagnoses	12
Elbow	Liverpool elbow score	0-10	ROM, strength, ulnar nerve sensitivity, pain, ADL, and recreational activity	Yes	6	9	—	All elbow diagnoses	0.7-1.8
Hand	Boston Carpal Tunnel Questionnaire	0-100	Pain, sensitivity, weakness, function	Yes	None	19	Adult	Carpal tunnel syndrome	N/A
Hand	Jensen-Taylor	Time against standard time	Times functional task completion	Yes	Time task	7	All	General hand and wrist conditions	N/A
Hand	Michigan hand outcome	0-100	Pain, function, work	Yes	None	37	—	All hand diagnoses	11-23
Hand	PRWE	0-100	Pain, daily activities, recreation, work activities	Yes	None	15	Adult	General hand and wrist conditions	17-24

ADL = activities of daily living, ASES = American Shoulder and Elbow Surgeons, CAT = computer adaptive test, DASH = Disabilities of the Arm, Shoulder and Hand, HSS = Hospital for Special Surgery, MCID = minimum clinically important difference, PROMIS = Patient-Reported Outcomes Measurement Information System, PRWE = Patient-Rated Wrist Evaluation, PSS = Penn Shoulder Score, ROM = range of motion, SANE = Single Assessment Numeric Evaluation, SF = Short Form, SST = Simple Shoulder Test, UCLA = University of California Los Angeles, WOOS = Western Ontario Osteoarthritis of the Shoulder Index, WORC = Western Ontario Rotator Cuff Index, WOSI = Western Ontario Shoulder Instability Index

Data from Smith MV, Calfee RP, Baumgarten KM, Brophy RH, Wright RW: Upper extremity-specific measures of disability and outcomes in orthopaedic surgery. *J Bone Joint Surg Am* 2012;94(3):277-285; Wylie JD, Beckmann JT, Granger E, Tashjian RZ: Functional outcomes assessment in shoulder surgery. *World J Orthop* 2014;5(5):623-633; Xu S, Chen JY, Lie HME, Hao Y, Lie DTT: Minimal Clinically Important Difference of Oxford, Constant, and UCLA shoulder score for arthroscopic rotator cuff repair. *J Orthop* 2020;19:21-27; Jones IA, Togashi R, Heckmann N, Vangsness CT Jr. Minimal clinically important difference (MCID) for patient-reported shoulder outcomes. *J Shoulder Elbow Surg* 2020;29(7):1484-1492; and Gordon D, Pines Y, Ben-Ari E, et al: Minimal clinically important difference, substantial clinical benefit, and patient acceptable that are relevant to patients. With the continued development of sensitive and refined measures across many domains of outcomes, as well as longer follow-up, a more complete assessment of orthobiologics interventions will be possible.

REFERENCES

1. Noback PC, Donnelley CA, Yeatts NC, et al: Utilization of orthobiologics by sports medicine physicians: A survey-based study. *J Am Acad Orthop Surg Glob Res Rev* 2021;5(1):e20.00185.
2. Bowers RL, Troyer WD, Mason RA, Mautner KR: Biologics. *Tech Vasc Interv Radiol* 2020;23(4)100704.
3. Chahla J, Cinque ME, Piuzzi NS, et al: A call for standardization in platelet-rich plasma preparation protocols and composition reporting: A systematic review of the clinical orthopaedic literature. *J Bone Joint Surg Am* 2017;99(20):1769-1779.
4. Karim KE, Wu CM, Giladi AM, Murphy MS: Orthobiologics in hand surgery. *J Hand Surg Am* 2021;46(5):409-415.
5. Wright RW, Baumgarten KM: Shoulder outcomes measures. *J Am Acad Orthop Surg* 2010;18(7):436-444.
6. Wilson IB, Cleary PD: Linking clinical variables with health-related quality of life. A conceptual model of patient outcomes. *J Am Med Assoc* 1995;273(1):59-65.
7. Mosher ZA, Ewing MA, Collins CS, et al: Usage trends of patient-reported outcome measures in shoulder literature. *J Am Acad Orthop Surg* 2020;28(17):e774-e781.
8. Poolman RW, Swiontkowski MF, Fairbank JCT, Schemitsch EH, Sprague S, de Vet HCW: Outcome instruments: Rationale for their use. *J Bone Joint Surg Am* 2009;91(suppl 3):41-49.
9. Smith MV, Calfee RP, Baumgarten KM, Brophy RH, Wright RW: Upper extremity-specific measures of disability and outcomes in orthopaedic surgery. *J Bone Joint Surg Am* 2012;94(3):277-285.
10. Jackowski D, Guyatt G: A guide to health measurement. *Clin Orthop Relat Res* 2003;413:80-89.
11. Jaeschke R, Singer J, Guyatt GH: Measurement of health status. Ascertaining the minimal clinically important difference. *Control Clin Trials* 1989;10(4):407-415.
12. Bhandari M, Petrisor B, Schemitsch E: Outcome measurements in orthopedic. *Indian J Orthop* 2007;41(1):32-36.
13. Rodeo SA, Bedi A: 2019-2020 NFL and NFL physician society orthobiologics consensus statement. *Sports Health* 2020;12(1):58-60.
14. Lui M, Shih W, Yim N, Brandstater M, Ashfaq M, Tran D: Systematic review and meta-analysis of nonoperative platelet-rich plasma shoulder injections for rotator cuff pathology. *PM R* 2020;13(10):1157-1168.
15. Chen X, Jones IA, Park C, Vangsness CT Jr: The efficacy of platelet-rich plasma on tendon and ligament healing: A systematic review and meta-analysis with bias assessment. *Am J Sports Med* 2018;46(8):2020-2032.
16. Carr AJ, Murphy R, Dakin SJ, et al: Platelet-rich plasma injection with arthroscopic acromioplasty for chronic rotator cuff tendinopathy: A randomized controlled trial. *Am J Sports Med* 2015;43(12):2891-2897.
17. Ma J, Piuzzi NS, Muschler GF, Iannotti JP, Ricchetti ET, Derwin KA: Biomarkers of rotator cuff disease severity and repair healing. *JBJS Rev* 2018;6(9):e9.
18. Shih CA, Wu K-C, Shao C-J, et al: Synovial fluid biomarkers: Association with chronic rotator cuff tear severity and pain. *J Shoulder Elbow Surg* 2018;27(3):545-552.
19. Casagrande D, Stains JP, Murthi AM: Identification of shoulder osteoarthritis biomarkers: Comparison between shoulders with and without osteoarthritis. *J Shoulder Elbow Surg* 2015;24(3):382-390.
20. Page RS, McGee SL, Eng K, et al: Adhesive capsulitis of the shoulder: Protocol for the adhesive capsulitis biomarker (AdCaB) study. *BMC Musculoskelet Disord* 2019;20(1):145.
21. Docheva D, Müller SA, Majewski M, Evans CH: Biologics for tendon repair. *Adv Drug Deliv Rev* 2015;84:222-239.
22. Weber AE, Bolia IK, Trasolini NA: Biological strategies for osteoarthritis: From early diagnosis to treatment. *Int Orthop* 2021;45(2):335-344.
23. Zhao JG, Zhao L, Jiang T-X, Wang Z-L, Wang J, Zhang P: Platelet-rich plasma in arthroscopic rotator cuff repair: A meta-analysis of randomized controlled trials. *Arthroscopy* 2015;31(1):125-135.
24. Colliver J, Wang A, Brendan J, et al: Early postoperative repair status after rotator cuff repair cannot be accurately classified using questionnaires of patient function and isokinetic strength evaluation. *J Shoulder Elbow Surg* 2016;25(4):536-542.
25. Galatz LM, Ball CM, Teefey SA, Middleton WD, Yamaguchi K: The outcome and repair integrity of completely arthroscopically repaired large and massive rotator cuff tears. *J Bone Joint Surg Am* 2004;86(2):219-224.
26. An D, Black ND, Tierney S, Chan VWS, Niazi AU: Impact of an ultrasound-guided regional anesthesia workshop on participants' confidence levels and clinical practice. *Korean J Anesthesiol* 2020;73(5):465-467.
27. Lin MT, Wei KC, Wu CH: Effectiveness of platelet-rich plasma injection in rotator cuff tendinopathy: A systematic review and meta-analysis of randomized controlled trials. *Diagnostics (Basel)* 2020;10(4):189.
28. MS AH, Sazlina SG: Platelet-rich plasma for rotator cuff tendinopathy: A systematic review and meta-analysis. *PLoS One* 2021;16(5):e0251111.
29. Dones VC III, Grimmer K, Thoirs K, Suarez CG, Luker J: The diagnostic validity of musculoskeletal ultrasound in lateral epicondylalgia: A systematic review. *BMC Med Imaging* 2014;14:10.
30. Rha DW, Park G-Y, Kim Y-K, Kim MT, Lee SC: Comparison of the therapeutic effects of ultrasound-guided platelet-rich plasma injection and dry needling in rotator cuff disease: A randomized controlled trial. *Clin Rehabil* 2013;27(2):113-122.
31. Centeno C, Fausel Z, Stemper I, Azuike U, Dodson E: A randomized controlled trial of the treatment of rotator cuff tears with bone marrow concentrate and platelet products compared to exercise therapy: A midterm analysis. *Stem Cells Int* 2020;2020:5962354.

32. Bittersohl B, Miese FR, Dekkers C, et al: T2* mapping and delayed gadolinium-enhanced magnetic resonance imaging in cartilage (dGEMRIC) of glenohumeral cartilage in asymptomatic volunteers at 3 T. *Eur Radiol* 2013;23(5):1367-1374.

33. Wallyn J, Anton N, Akram S, Vandamme TF: Biomedical imaging: Principles, technologies, clinical aspects, contrast agents, limitations and future trends in nanomedicines. *Pharm Res* 2019;36(6):78.

34. Sharma AR: Nuclear medicine in sports. *Indian J Nucl Med* 2010;25(4):129-130.

35. Randelli P, Arrigoni P, Ragone V, Aliprandi A, Cabitza P: Platelet rich plasma in arthroscopic rotator cuff repair: A prospective RCT study, 2-year follow-up. *J Shoulder Elbow Surg* 2011;20(4):518-528.

36. Kesikburun S, Tan AK, Yilmaz B, Yaşar E, Yazicioğlu K: Platelet-rich plasma injections in the treatment of chronic rotator cuff tendinopathy: a randomized controlled trial with 1-year follow-up. *Am J Sports Med* 2013;41(11):2609-2616.

37. Mills FB, Misra AK, Goyeneche N, Hackel JG, Andrews MR, Joyner PW: Return to play after platelet-rich plasma injection for elbow UCL injury: Outcomes based on injury severity. *Orthop J Sports Med* 2021;9(3):2325967121991135.

38. Xu S, Chen JY, Lie HME, Hao Y, Lie DTT: Minimal clinically important difference of Oxford, Constant, and UCLA shoulder score for arthroscopic rotator cuff repair. *J Orthop* 2020;19:21-27.

39. Jones IA, Togashi R, Heckmann N, Vangsness CT Jr: Minimal clinically important difference (MCID) for patient-reported shoulder outcomes. *J Shoulder Elbow Surg* 2020;29(7):1484-1492.

40. Gordon D, Pines Y, Ben-Ari E, et al: Minimal clinically important difference, substantial clinical benefit, and patient acceptable symptom state of PROMIS upper extremity after total shoulder arthroplasty. *JSES Int* 2021;5(5):894-899.

41. Roddey TS, Cook KF, O'Malley KJ, Gartsman GM: The relationship among strength and mobility measures and self-report outcome scores in persons after rotator cuff repair surgery: Impairment measures are not enough. *J Shoulder Elbow Surg* 2005;14(suppl 1):95S-98S.

42. Shin SJ, Chung J, Lee J, Ko Y-W: Recovery of muscle strength after intact arthroscopic rotator cuff repair according to preoperative rotator cuff tear size. *Am J Sports Med* 2016;44(4):972-980.

43. Goodman J, Lau BC, Krupp RJ, et al: Clinical measurements versus patient-reported outcomes: Analysis of the American shoulder and elbow Surgeons physician assessment in patients undergoing reverse total shoulder arthroplasty. *JSES Open Access* 2018;2(2):144-149.

44. McHorney CA, Ware JE Jr, Raczek AE: The MOS 36-item short-form health survey (SF-36): II. Psychometric and clinical tests of validity in measuring physical and mental health constructs. *Med Care* 1993;31(3):247-263.

45. Castricini R, Gasparini G, Di Luggo F, De Benedetto M, De Gori M, Galasso O: Health-related quality of life and functionality after reverse shoulder arthroplasty. *J Shoulder Elbow Surg* 2013;22(12):1639-1649.

46. Yoo JH, Cho NS, Rhee YG: Effect of postoperative repair integrity on health-related quality of life after rotator cuff repair: Healed versus retear group. *Am J Sports Med* 2013;41(11):2637-2644.

47. Ware J Jr. Kosinski M, Keller SD: A 12-item short-form health survey: Construction of scales and preliminary tests of reliability and validity. *Med Care* 1996;34(3):220-233.

48. Hudak PL, Amadio PC, Bombardier C: Development of an upper extremity outcome measure: The DASH (disabilities of the arm, shoulder and hand) [corrected]. The Upper Extremity Collaborative Group (UECG). *Am J Ind Med* 1996;29(6):602-608.

49. Bot SD, Terwee C, van der Windt DAWN, Bouter L, Dekker J, de Vet HCW: Clinimetric evaluation of shoulder disability questionnaires: A systematic review of the literature. *Ann Rheum Dis* 2004;63(4):335-341.

50. Beaton DE, Katz JN, Fossel AH, Wright JG, Tarasuk V, Bombardier C: Measuring the whole or the parts? Validity, reliability, and responsiveness of the disabilities of the arm, shoulder and hand outcome measure in different regions of the upper extremity. *J Hand Ther* 2001;14(2):128-146.

51. Beaton DE, Wright JG, Katz JN: Development of the QuickDASH: Comparison of three item-reduction approaches. *J Bone Joint Surg Am* 2005;87(5):1038-1046.

52. Wylie JD, Beckmann JT, Granger E, Tashjian RZ: Functional outcomes assessment in shoulder surgery. *World J Orthop* 2014;5(5):623-633.

53. Horn ME, Reinke EK, Couce LJ, Reeve BB, Ledbetter L, George SZ: Reporting and utilization of Patient-Reported Outcomes Measurement Information System(R) (PROMIS(R)) measures in orthopedic research and practice: A systematic review. *J Orthop Surg Res* 2020;15(1):553.

54. Makhni EC, Meadows M, Hamamoto JT, Higgins JD, Romeo AA, Verma NN: Patient Reported Outcomes Measurement Information System (PROMIS) in the upper extremity: The future of outcomes reporting? *J Shoulder Elbow Surg* 2017;26(2):352-357.

55. Beckmann JT, Hung M, Bounsanga J, Wylie JD, Granger EK, Tashjian RZ: Psychometric evaluation of the PROMIS Physical Function Computerized Adaptive Test in comparison to the American Shoulder and Elbow Surgeons score and Simple Shoulder Test in patients with rotator cuff disease. *J Shoulder Elbow Surg* 2015;24(12):1961-1967.

56. Anthony CA, Glass NA, Hancock K, Bollier M, Wolf BR, Hettrich CM: Performance of PROMIS instruments in patients with shoulder instability. *Am J Sports Med* 2017;45(2):449-453.

57. Dowdle SB, Glass N, Anthony CA, Hettrich CM: Use of PROMIS for patients undergoing primary total shoulder arthroplasty. *Orthop J Sports Med* 2017;5(9):2325967117726044.

58. Patterson BM, Orvets ND, Aleem AW, et al: Correlation of Patient-Reported Outcomes Measurement Information System (PROMIS) scores with legacy patient-reported outcome scores in patients undergoing rotator cuff repair. *J Shoulder Elbow Surg* 2018;27(6 suppl):S17-S23.

59. Schwarz I, Smith JH, Houck DA, Frank RM, Bravman JT, McCarty EC: Use of the Patient-Reported Outcomes Measurement Information System (PROMIS) for operative shoulder outcomes. *Orthop J Sports Med* 2020;8(6):2325967120924345.

60. Richards RR, An KN, Bigliani LU, et al: A standardized method for the assessment of shoulder function. *J Shoulder Elbow Surg* 1994;3(6):347-352.

61. Kocher MS, Horan MP, Briggs KK, Richardson TR, O'Holleran J, Hawkins RJ: Reliability, validity, and responsiveness of the American shoulder and elbow surgeons subjective shoulder scale in patients with shoulder instability, rotator cuff disease, and glenohumeral arthritis. *J Bone Joint Surg Am* 2005;87(9):2006-2011.

62. Michener LA, McClure PW, Sennett BJ: American shoulder and elbow surgeons standardized shoulder assessment form, patient self-report section: Reliability, validity, and responsiveness. *J Shoulder Elbow Surg* 2002;11(6):587-594.

63. de Witte PB, Henseler JF, Nagels J, Vlieland TPMV, Nelissen RGHH: The Western Ontario rotator cuff index in rotator cuff disease patients: A comprehensive reliability and responsiveness validation study. *Am J Sports Med* 2012;40(7):1611-1619.

64. Dawson J, Fitzpatrick R, Carr A: The assessment of shoulder instability. The development and validation of a questionnaire. *J Bone Joint Surg Br* 1999;81(3):420-426.

65. Longo UG, Franceschi F, Loppini M, Maffulli N, Denaro V: Rating systems for evaluation of the elbow. *Br Med Bull* 2008;87:131-161.

66. Evans JP, Smith CD, Fine NF, et al: Clinical rating systems in elbow research-a systematic review exploring trends and distributions of use. *J Shoulder Elbow Surg* 2018;27(4):e98-e106.

67. Turchin DC, Beaton DE, Richards RR: Validity of observer-based aggregate scoring systems as descriptors of elbow pain, function, and disability. *J Bone Joint Surg Am* 1998;80(2):154-162.

68. Bialocerkowski AE, Grimmer KA, Bain GI: A systematic review of the content and quality of wrist outcome instruments. *Int J Qual Health Care* 2000;12(2):149-157.

69. Levine DW, Simmons BP, Koris MJ, et al: A self-administered questionnaire for the assessment of severity of symptoms and functional status in carpal tunnel syndrome. *J Bone Joint Surg Am* 1993;75(11):1585-1592.

CHAPTER 23

Summary and Perspectives

Adam Yanke, MD, PhD, FAAOS • Kevin Credille, BSE, MS • Mario Hevesi, MD, PhD • Kathleen A. Derwin, PhD

INTRODUCTION

The use of orthobiologic treatment strategies in the augmentation, regeneration, and repair of tendon, nerve, muscle, and bone injuries in the upper extremity is an area of intense research and development. A recent survey of members of the American Medical Society for Sports Medicine revealed that 66% are using at least one orthobiologic in their practice and 72% are increasing their use, although preclinical and clinical evidence for the efficacy of these treatment strategies is at various stages. Here, the current state of orthobiologic treatment strategies in the upper extremity is summarized and future research opportunities are discussed.

ROTATOR CUFF REPAIR

Despite improvements in surgical techniques for rotator cuff repair, retear following repair remains a common clinical occurrence. Orthobiologic treatment strategies have aimed to provide more consistent postoperative healing and improve outcomes. Among orthobiologics, platelet-rich plasma (PRP) has emerged as a promising augmentative therapy in rotator cuff repair in several prospective clinical trials; however, future clinical trials using standardized PRP preparations and a comparison cohort of placebo injections will be necessary to fully evaluate the efficacy of PRP. In addition to PRP, biologic and synthetic grafts are currently being used to augment repairs at the time of surgery by supplying a structural scaffold to enhance healing. The current literature suggests that at least some grafts may serve to reduce retearing after rotator cuff repair, but these reports are generally from small retrospective cohorts without controls or long-term follow-up. Without strong clinical evidence of a clear benefit of graft augmentation, which will require prospective randomized controlled trials with clinical and structural outcomes, the cost and added surgical time to apply are likely to limit the use to specific indications such as massive cuff tears. Cellular therapies such as tissue-specific activated endothelial cells, bone marrow–derived progenitor cells, and adipose-derived progenitor cells have recently emerged as potentially promising therapy modalities in preclinical models. However, because animal models do not recapitulate the complex etiology and variable presentation of rotator cuff disease, their safety and efficacy need to be further evaluated using translational studies and prospective clinical trials in humans.

TENDON MANAGEMENT, PROTECTION, AND REPAIR

Tendinopathy is a complex and multifaceted clinical disorder resulting in limb pain and disability. Highly effective treatment strategies remain elusive because the pathophysiology of tendinopathy is poorly understood, being multifactorial and clinically heterogeneous. Mechanical microtrauma or macrotrauma, hypovascularity, genomic variations, imbalance of neurogenic input, extracellular dysfunction, immune disturbances, and metabolic conditions may all contribute to varying degrees to the onset and/or progression and persistence of tendinopathy that presents itself in the clinic. Orthobiologic treatment of chronic epicondylar tendinopathy, gluteal tendinopathy, and plantar fasciitis using leukocyte-poor PRP has shown clinically meaningful improvements in pain and functional scores in level I studies. More work needs to be done to confirm the value of leukocyte-rich PRP or other formulations for other tendinopathic conditions. Other cellular and acellular biologics such as bone marrow aspirate concentrate and adipose-derived injections are currently under investigation for treating tendinopathy but presently lack enough supporting evidence to recommend wide

Dr. Yanke or an immediate family member serves as a paid consultant to or is an employee of AlloSource, CONMED Linvatec, JRF Ortho, and Olympus; serves as an unpaid consultant to Patient IQ, Smith & Nephew, and Sparta Biomedical; has stock or stock options held in Patient IQ; and has received research or institutional support from Arthrex, Inc., Organogenesis, and Vericel. Dr. Derwin or an immediate family member has received royalties from Viscus Biologics; serves as a paid consultant to or is an employee of Collamedix; has stock or stock options held in Collamedix; has received research or institutional support from DJ Orthopaedics; and serves as a board member, owner, officer, or committee member of the Orthopaedic Research Society. Neither of the following authors nor any immediate family member has received anything of value from or has stock or stock options held in a commercial company or institution related directly or indirectly to the subject of this chapter: Kevin Credille and Dr. Hevesi.

clinical use. Exercise may also be considered an effective biologic treatment and should be further investigated. Ultimately, understanding the biologic mechanisms of tendinopathy would increase the potential for more precise and effective treatment for this painful and debilitating condition. Because there are very limited animal models of naturally occurring tendinopathy, mechanistic studies are likely to require systematic and deep investigation of tendinopathic tissues biopsied from patients with these conditions.

FRESH FRACTURE, CHALLENGING BONE REPAIR, AND NONUNIONS

The biology of fracture healing is a complex, multistep, biologic process involving several gene pathways. Bone morphogenetic proteins have been the most enthusiastically investigated adjuvants for bone repair, and currently, recombinant human bone morphogenetic protein 2 is available for clinical application. However, current evidence does not support the widespread use and application of bone morphogenetic protein for improved outcomes in fracture and nonunion surgery. PRP treatment has also been investigated, yet there is currently no level I evidence to indicate that using PRP alone or in combination with other materials has a substantial effect when used for acute fractures or for nonunion augmentation. Culture-expanded autologous and even allogeneic cell–based product concepts represent a promising therapy for the augmentation of fracture and nonunion repair based on preclinical evidence, but these methodologies lack robust clinical evidence from controlled clinical trials despite widespread use of demineralized bone preparations with allogeneic cells from marrow. Bone marrow aspirate has been used as a source of bone marrow–derived mesenchymal stem cells based on its relative ease of harvest and low morbidity. However, the method of preparation, variable cell concentrations, and lack of standardized indications and outcome measures have limited the utility of cell-based therapies in bone repair to date. Although several studies have evaluated the effect of cell concentration on healing potential, an effective therapeutic range is yet to be established for nonunion treatment. Currently, there is no clear superior substantive evidence for using a specific type of bone graft substitute or bone growth adjuvants when treating complex fractures or nonunion.

PERIPHERAL NERVE REGENERATION IN THE HAND

Peripheral nerve injuries comprise potentially devastating injuries to the upper extremity that are increasingly treated with orthobiologics such as nerve conduits, stem cells, tissue engineering nerve grafts, and polyethylene glycol fusion. Vein-based and muscle-based tissues were previously well described in the basic science literature for use as nerve conduits but have been largely replaced by acellular nerve allografts (processed nerve allografts), which are processed cadaver nerves that retain the organized extracellular matrix after the immunogenic cellular components are removed. Processed nerve allografts have demonstrated a wide range of efficacy (60% to 100%) for a wide range of gap lengths (5 to 70 mm). In contrast, synthetic biologic conduits such as collagen and nonabsorbable synthetic conduits such as expanded polytetrafluoroethylene and silicone have shown lesser efficacy in smaller nerve gaps, with silicone often needing tube removal because of local tissue irritation. There have been recent developments in the creation of absorbable synthetic conduits composed of polyglycolic acid, which have shown efficacy rates of 86% for smaller nerve gaps (5 to 30 mm) and overall comparable and favorable healing compared with autogenous nerve grafting without the need for donor harvest site morbidity. Research on cellular augmentation of nerve regeneration is ongoing but at this time is mostly preclinical and translational.

SKELETAL MUSCLE REGENERATION

Skeletal muscle fatty atrophy in the upper extremity is a common consequence of unloading secondary to rotator cuff injury and has a high association with failed repairs. To date, orthobiologic treatment strategies aimed at mitigating or reversing rotator cuff muscle atrophy and fatty infiltration have been investigated only in preclinical models. Systemic administration of anti-inflammatory drugs and compounds that regulate or inhibit adipogenic and fibrotic pathways has shown promise. Local injection of progenitor/stem cells or their secretome(s) into injured rotator cuff muscle or application of electroconductive nanofibrous matrices directly to repaired muscle has been shown to improve muscle atrophy in animal studies. No biologic treatment for rotator cuff muscle regeneration has yet reached clinical trials. Although less common, volumetric muscle loss is a complex clinical issue that occurs from skeletal muscle trauma or injury that can potentially result in permanent structural and functional deficits. Such muscle injuries are difficult to treat because they often present concomitantly with neurovascular compromise as well as inflammation and fibrosis, which can create an unfavorable healing environment. In clinical trials, implantation of decellularized extracellular matrix has shown modest functional recovery but little evidence of muscle tissue regeneration at the site of injury. Although early preclinical results are promising, skeletal muscle regeneration remains in relatively early stages of translation and implementation.

MEASUREMENT OF CLINICAL OUTCOMES IN THE UPPER EXTREMITY

The role of orthobiologics in the treatment of upper extremity injuries continues to undergo rapid and expanding innovation and research. Although biologics are seen to hold substantial potential promise, currently, there is a lack of high-quality evidence regarding their benefits and best practices in most upper extremity applications. Given this, it is important to systematically document and interpret structural and clinical outcomes in upper extremity orthobiologic research. These include imaging of structural healing, objective functional assessments, and pretreatment and posttreatment (subjective) patient-reported outcome measures. Furthermore, the role of pretreatment and posttreatment biomarkers in diagnosis and assessment of orthobiologic therapies continues to evolve as the roles of these substances in initial trauma, recovery prognostication, and healing are better understood.

SUMMARY

Orthobiologic treatment strategies such as autologous or allogeneic cell therapy, tissue grafts, and PRP are commonly used in clinical practice for managing upper extremity conditions. Other biologic therapies are at earlier stages of preclinical development. The logic and advancement of successful orthobiologic therapies must be derived from the fundamental biology of the injured and healing tissues. Furthermore, demonstrating the efficacy of orthobiologic treatment strategies in clinical trials may prove elusive without patient-reported, clinical, and imaging outcomes that are sensitive to the spectrum of healing and function. These research trials should use sample sizes large enough to allow for adequate power and multivariate analyses to adjust for confounding data from the wide variability in patient and disease characteristics, which will likely require a concerted multicenter effort.

SECTION

4

Solutions for Lower Extremity Pathology

Section Editors
Robert H. Brophy, MD, FAAOS
Regis J. O'Keefe, MD, PhD, FAAOS

CHAPTER

24 Segmental Defect Repair and Nonunion

Joseph T. Patterson, MD • Jay R. Lieberman, MD, FAAOS

INTRODUCTION

Fracture nonunion and segmental bone defects represent challenging clinical problems in orthopaedic trauma surgery. Fracture nonunion at the population level occurs in 9 to 19 fracture cases per 100,000 per year.[1,2] The incidence of nonunion in long bone fractures varies with injury, treatment, and estimation methods: reported rates range from zero to 12% in femoral fractures, zero to 33% in humeral fractures, and 1% to 80% in tibial fractures.[3,4] Nonunion is associated with high-energy polytrauma; open fracture; medications including NSAIDs, opioids, anticoagulants, anticonvulsants, benzodiazepines, and diuretics; osteoarthritis; diabetes and insulin use; osteoporosis; male sex; smoking; vitamin D deficiency; and renal insufficiency.[4] Most nonunions occur in patients during their most productive years, between age 25 and 55 years.[2] Direct health care costs of nonunion treatment vary widely, with estimates ranging from $11,000 to $126,0000 USD per case.[5-9]

Segmental bone defects may be congenital, the primary result of severe trauma, or the sequelae of débridement or resection of bone for traumatic devitalization, osteomyelitis, or neoplasia.[10] The incidence of segmental bone defects is more difficult to quantify because of the variety of etiologies resulting in segmental defects. Surgical management of segmental bone defects is morbid and expensive, with amputation rates of 8% to 15% at 2 years and direct costs of treatment of $52,155 to $305,938 per case.[11]

It is important to provide context and evidence for the role of orthobiologic interventions in the treatment of fracture nonunion and segmental bone defects.

DEFINITIONS

Delayed union describes an abnormally slow or disrupted process of fracture healing. Clinical definitions vary. Specific cutoff times of 3 to 6 months after injury without bony union are described for certain injuries, whereas absence of progressive signs of healing on radiographs for 3 consecutive months is also accepted.[12] A delayed fracture union may eventually progress to union, although interventions may be required. Some areas of the body may require a longer time to achieve union, such as the tibial shaft; delayed fracture healing in the tibia is typically observed for 6 months before surgical intervention.[13] Nonunion is an arrest of fracture healing: the fracture segments have failed to unite. A nonunion is not the same as a critical-size defect: cellular and molecular signaling, with or without biomechanical instability, is altered in a nonunion. Nonunions can be classified radiographically by the apparent etiology of the failure of the fracture to unite (**Figure 1**). This radiographic classification also describes the biologic capacity of the fracture to achieve union and guides treatment (**Table 1**). An atrophic nonunion demonstrates minimal deposition of mineralized callus at the fracture site, with a "sucked candy cane" appearance of the fracture ends on plain radiographs. Atrophic nonunions result from biologic compromise, as described in the next section, and require biologic augmentation to achieve union. A hypertrophic nonunion demonstrates abundant radiographic deposition of mineralized callus but failure to achieve stability, with metaplasia of callus to fibrous tissue instead of bone at the site of the fracture. The presence of callus indicates biologic capacity to heal. The primary etiology is thought to be a cellular response to mechanical overstimulation due to inadequate fracture stabilization.

A segmental bone defect describes a section of absent bone in a limb segment. Segmental bone defects may result from trauma, neoplasia, infection, or be congenital. A critical-size defect is a defect or bone void that will be unable to spontaneously heal, even with surgical stabilization, and will require additional intervention to obtain bony union.[10,14] A precise definition of a critical-size defect is controversial because the geometry of the defect, anatomic location, etiology, integrity of the surrounding tissues, and host factors may all influence the potential of the defect to heal spontaneously.

Dr. Patterson or an immediate family member has received research or institutional support from AOTrauma North America. Dr. Lieberman or an immediate family member has received royalties from DePuy, a Johnson & Johnson Company; serves as a paid consultant to or is an employee of DePuy, a Johnson & Johnson Company; has stock or stock options held in BD Surgiphor and Hip Innovation Technology; and serves as a board member, owner, officer, or committee member of the American Academy of Orthopaedic Surgeons, the Hip Society, the Musculoskeletal Transplant Foundation, and the Western Orthopaedic Association.

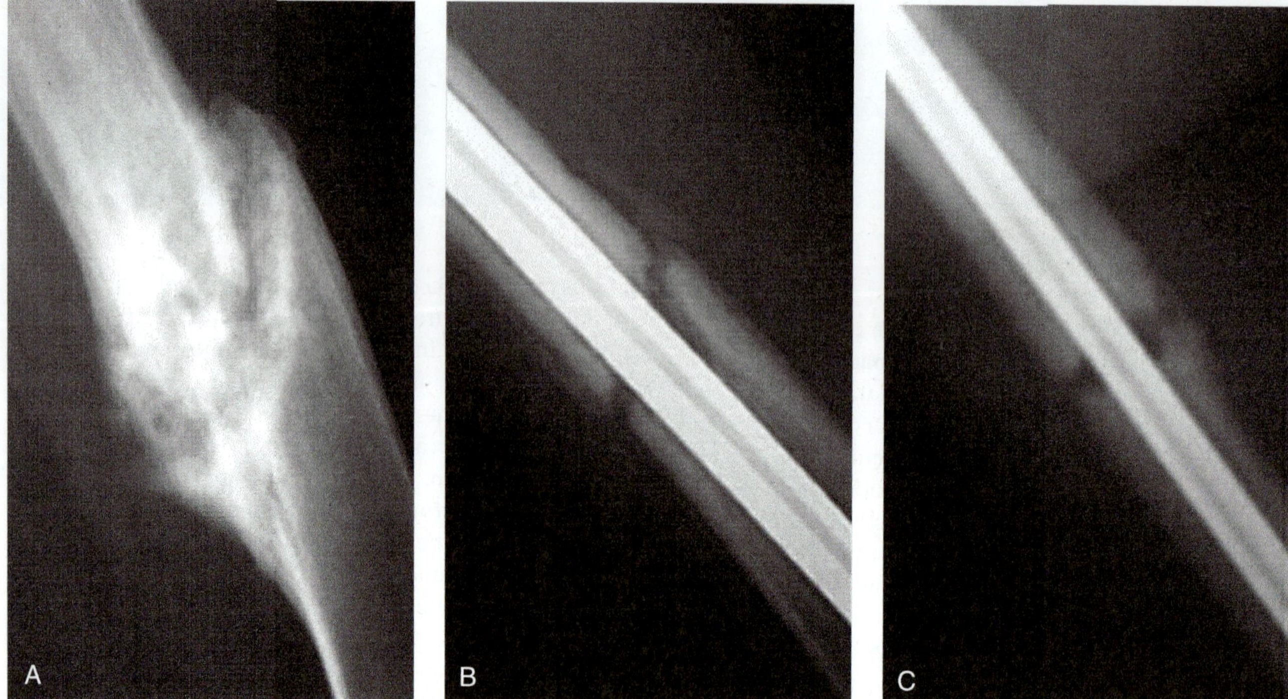

FIGURE 1 Clinical examples of diaphyseal nonunion of the femur: cropped AP radiographs of tibial hypertrophic (A), oligotrophic (B), and atrophic (C) nonunion. (Reproduced with permission from Lynch JR, Taitsman LA, Barei DP, Nork SE: Femoral nonunion: Risk factors and treatment options. *J Am Acad Orthop Surg* 2008;16[2]:88-97.)

Circumferential bone loss greater than 50% for nonsegmental defects or bone void length of greater than 1 to 2.5 cm for segmental defects has been proposed.[15-19] Conversely, spontaneous healing of femoral diaphyseal segmental defects up to 10 cm has been reported.[20] A critical-size bone defect will always require intervention to manage the defect, although fracture healing may or may not be impaired.

TABLE 1 Types and Treatment of Nonunion

Type	Biologic Characteristics	Radiographic Findings	Technetium-99 Bone Scan Findings	Treatment Options
Hypertrophic	Biologic capacity for healing	Abundant elephant foot callus Lack of bridging bone	Increased uptake	Revision internal fixation with decreased strain environment
Oligotrophic	Decreased biologic potential for healing	Little to no callus formation	Increased uptake	Rule out or treat infection Revision internal fixation with increased strain environment and biologic enhancement
Atrophic	Little to no osteogenic potential	Sclerotic, "sucked candy cane" bone ends Absence of callus	Decreased uptake	Rule out or treat infection Biologic enhancement with local bone growth factor delivery, bone marrow aspirate injection, revision internal fixation, staged management with antibiotic spacer and autografting of induced membrane, distraction osteogenesis

CLINICAL PROBLEM IN CONTEXT

Understanding the etiology of a nonunion or segmental bone defect informs the planning of interventions to address the clinical problem. It is helpful to develop a problem list of factors that contributed to the nonunion or bone defect that may also influence the choice and success of treatment options.

Similar to an acute fracture, both nonunion and segmental bone defect are the result of a soft-tissue injury with a broken bone inside. The soft tissue enveloping the problematic bone (the periosteum, adjacent musculature, innervating nerves, vascular supply, fascial covering, and cutaneous tissues) may be compromised by the congenital issue, traumatic injury, prior surgery, infection, or chemotherapy and radiation. Open fracture and extensive soft-tissue injury increase the risk of delayed fracture healing by 13% to 16% in tibial fractures, whereas associated vascular injury increases the risk to almost 50%,[21] even though the atrophic nonunion itself may not be dysvascular.[22,23] Neurologic injury may degrade the stabilizing effect of adjacent muscles, contributing to nonunion, particularly about the humeral shaft.[24] Compartment syndrome independently predicts nonunion.[25]

Modifiable patient risk factors for compromised bone healing include tobacco use, recreational drug use, and alcohol abuse.[26-29] Medications taken by the patient including corticosteroids, opioids, diuretics, benzodiazepines, anticonvulsants, and anti-inflammatories[30] and medical conditions including anemia, vitamin D deficiency, and diabetes[31,32] represent risk factors for nonunion as well as opportunities for medical optimization to improve the chance of treatment success. Previous treatment including the design of stabilization constructs,[33] prior stabilization of adjacent bones,[34,35] the presence of a fracture gap at the initial fixation,[36,37] previous radiation, chemotherapy, vascular procedures, or soft-tissue coverage procedures may also be contributing factors as well as considerations informing the management plan. Genetics may one day also play a role: single nucleotide polymorphisms in osteogenic genes have been associated with risk of delayed union following long bone fracture.[38]

Eradication of infection is critical to the treatment of nonunions and segmental bone defects. Both entities are strongly associated with fracture-related infection (FRI) as sequelae of the initial injury as well postoperative surgical site infection and osteomyelitis.[11] Similar to consensus definitions developed across societies for periprosthetic joint injection, the AO Foundation, the European Bone and Joint Infection Society, and the Orthopaedic Trauma Association have developed a consensus definition for FRI based on diagnostic criteria developed from a stepwise algorithm of history, examination, laboratory values, and surgical findings.[39] However, FRI is not always a straightforward diagnosis. Infected nonunions and segmental bone defects may be quiescent or asymptomatic and serum biomarkers associated with infection may be within normal ranges.[40,41] Clinical consensus and evidence supports the use of serum leukocyte count (white blood cell), erythrocyte sedimentation rate, and C-reactive protein to evaluate for the possibility of infection.[42-44] Clinically relevant values may be center specific, with reported cutoffs of white blood cell count (10^3 cells/µL) greater than 10.5 for men and greater than 11.0 for women; erythrocyte sedimentation rate (mm/hr) greater than 15 for men and greater than 20 for women; and C-reactive protein (mg/dL) greater than or equal to 0.9 for both men and women. However, recent data have called into question the utility of white blood cell, erythrocyte sedimentation rate, and C-reactive protein for diagnosis of FRI in nonunion and segmental bone defects as these studies demonstrated poor sensitivity and insufficient negative predictive value to rule out FRI.[41] A high index of suspicion should be maintained when the initial injury was the result of an open fracture, previous surgery has been attempted, or there is a history of previous infection.[16,40,45]

NATURAL HISTORY IF LEFT UNTREATED

The natural history of a segmental bone defect is variable, with rare reports of spontaneous healing of large long bone defects with uncompromised soft tissues.[19,20] By definition, a critical-size defect or nonunion will not heal spontaneously. Similarly, nonunion represents arrested fracture healing with no expected progress to union. Continued symptoms and failure of existing implants are to be expected.

STRUCTURE AND FUNCTIONAL CONSIDERATIONS: IS HISTOLOGICALLY PERFECT TISSUE NECESSARY FOR CLINICAL SUCCESS?

Defining clinical success after surgery for nonunion or bone defects is a process of shared decision making and goal setting between the patient and treating team. Success may relate to objective measures of physical function including needs for assistance with activities of daily living, return to prior living situation, return to same or any occupation, and return to play. However, success can be very subjective to the patient. Cosmetic considerations as well as the psychological, social, and cultural consequences of interventions such as external fixation frames or outcomes such as amputation and prosthesis wear are important to discuss with the patient.[46,47] It is important to discuss what might be the patient's desired level of function versus what might be reasonably achievable and to consider that the specific outcome desired by the patient may change with time, age, and living situation and occupational need.

Successful treatment of a nonunion or segmental bone defect usually does not require flawless reconstruction of all tissues and structures. The function of the compromised limb segment can be improved with one-bone leg[48] or one-bone forearm[49] salvage procedures, iatrogenic synostosis to bridge segmental defects,[50] or arthrodesis to address periarticular segmental bone loss.[51] In select patients with limited functional demands and/or limited life expectancy, benign neglect or deliberate nonsurgical care may lead to a useful, pain-free extremity with a functional, asymptomatic nonunion.[52]

HISTORICAL APPROACH AND ALTERNATIVES TO ORTHOBIOLOGIC SOLUTIONS

At the time of publication, no clinical practice guidelines have been published by the American Academy of Orthopaedic Surgeons, the Orthopaedic Trauma Association, or the Limb Lengthening and Reconstruction Society to guide treatment for segmental bone defects or nonunion.

In the absence of infection, nonsurgical management of nonunion or segmental bone defects may include medical optimization, immobilization, and external field bone stimulation. Medical optimization of metabolic and endocrine derangements potentially affecting bone healing is possible in 84% of patients with nonunion.[53] Functional bracing has been a historical approach to tibial union with reasonable success but may require secondary fibular osteotomy and months of orthotic use.[54] Low-intensity pulsed ultrasound (LIPUS) is an alternative to surgery for established nonunion, although the evidence is conflicting: a pooled success rate over 82% by systematic review of prospective and retrospective studies suggested LIPUS may reduce the time to radiographic fracture union,[55] but does not accelerate functional recovery.[56] Conversely, the multicenter randomized TRUST trial of LIPUS in closed and open tibial fractures found no effect on time to radiographic healing or functional recovery.[57]

Hypertrophic nonunion, characterized by little to no biologic impairment of fracture healing, may be managed by débridement, biopsy for culture, and revision internal fixation. Débridement and culture of the undesired fibrous or cartilaginous tissues interposed between the fracture fragments is performed with stabilization of the nonunion site with a stiffer construct, often with compression across the fracture or distraction osteogenesis with deformity correction.

Atrophic nonunions require additional biologic intervention to stimulate bone formation at the defect site. Overall, surgical interventions for repair of atrophic nonunion are successful in 80% of cases even after infection, although multiple interventions may be necessary.[58] Interventions can be organized along an escalating ladder of complexity and risk, beginning with dynamization of intramedullary constructs, reamed intramedullary exchange nailing, compressing plating with or without grafting, staged antibiotic spacer methods, and distraction osteogenesis techniques. Dynamization of previously statically locked intramedullary implants is 54% successful when treating femoral and tibial nonunion.[59] Exchange nailing of the tibia can achieve union in 88% to 93% of cases but may require up to five nailing attempts, and at greater cost per attempt than dynamization.[60,61] Open compression plating with or without bone grafting around existing intramedullary implants has been reported.[62] Distraction osteogenesis constructs such as external fixators or motorized intramedullary motorized devices can be used to compress a nonunion, with or without subsequent distraction to restore length.[63,64]

Aseptic segmental bone defects can be managed with bone grafting, distraction osteogenesis, acute shortening, and amputation.[10] Although indications vary, primary autologous bone grafting has been recommended for defects up to 5 cm.[10] Acute limb shortening with or without subsequent limb lengthening at the same site or via osteotomy at another level is an alternative for smaller defects. For defects greater than 5 cm, traditional alternatives include distraction osteogenesis, induced membrane staged management, and vascularized bone transfer (**Table 2**).

The induced membrane or Masquelet technique is a staged bone grafting procedure to address a segmental bone defect by first creating an environment conducive to bone formation then filling the void with graft.[65,66] A polymethyl methacrylate spacer is placed in the defect. The spacer induces the formation of a vascularized, pseudosynovial membrane, which demonstrates neovascularization, secretion of bone morphogenetic protein (BMP)-2, type I collagen, interleukin 6 and vascular endothelial growth factor, and osteoblastic precursors.[67,68] A second procedure is performed to incise the membrane, remove the spacer, and place bone graft during peak production of osteoinductive factors by the membrane around 4 to 8 weeks[68,69] (**Figure 2**).

In contrast with bone grafting, vascularized bone autografts immediately provide complete, living histologic bone architecture and mechanical integrity with a single-stage operation. Vascularized bone grafts such as the fibula, medial femoral condyle, and distal radius preserve the nutrient, metaphyseal, or other perforating vessels responsible for the primary blood supply to the osseous segment of the graft. These procedures are technically demanding and require microsurgical expertise. Complications of vascularized bone grafts include persistent defects, mechanical failure, loss of vascular supply, infection, and donor site morbidity.[70,71] Rates of union after vascularized bone grafting of segmental defects vary from 70% to 100% with a mean time to union of 6 months in case series encompassing a range of defect sizes as well as indications after trauma, infection, tumor, and prior radiation.[72-75]

Distraction osteogenesis or bone transport is the creation of new bone at a surgical osteotomy by controlled mechanical strain over time. A mechanical assembly is surgically applied such that one or more segments of

TABLE 2 Management of Segmental Bone Defects Based on Size

Management Method	Size of Defect	Advantages	Disadvantages
Autologous bone graft	<5 cm	One-stage reconstruction; no disease transmission; no immunologic rejection; low cost; standard of care with osteoinductive, osteoconductive, and osteogenic properties	Donor site morbidity, limited volume available, no structural capability
Allograft bone	Unknown	No donor site morbidity, limitless volume, structural properties with cortical allograft, volume expander	Limited graft incorporation/remodeling, potential disease transmission, no osteoinductive or osteogenic properties, cost/expense
Demineralized bone matrix	Unproven for segmental defects	Osteoinductive properties, no donor site morbidity, volume expander	No structural property, no evidence for segmental bone defect reconstruction, cost/expense
Bone morphogenetic proteins	Unproven for segmental defects	Osteoinductive, bone graft enhancer	Interferes with Masquelet technique, no structural capability, cost/expense
Induced membrane technique (Masquelet technique)	>10 cm (5-24 cm)	RIA graft harvest can provide adequate volume, internal or external fixation can be used, reconstruction time is independent of length of defect, low cost	Donor site morbidity, two-stage technique, long reconstructive period (mean, 9 month), described using external fixation, ratio of allograft to autograft cannot exceed 3:1 with theoretic defect limits
Distraction osteogenesis (Ilizarov technique)	5-10 cm (average)[a]	No donor site morbidity, no restrictions on defect length, reliable technique, can be used with a compromised soft-tissue envelope (STSG or free tissue flap), can decrease reconstructive time with multiple osteotomies and transport segments	Long reconstructive period, reconstructive period is length dependent, high rate of complications with prolonged external fixation, cost of ring or spatial external fixation frame
Acute shortening	1-3 cm	Simplest and fastest method, allows early primary closure of soft-tissue wounds, well tolerated in upper extremity, well tolerated in single bone extremity segment, no donor site morbidity, low cost	Limb dysfunction especially in lower extremities, defect length is limited may require secondary lengthening procedures to correct limb-length discrepancy
Vascularized fibular graft transfer	10-20 cm	Substantially shorter reconstruction time for large defect compared with Masquelet and Ilizarov techniques, fibular hypertrophy to support weight bearing, low cost	Donor site morbidity, requires specialized microsurgical capability, high rate of regenerate bone fracture, typically limited to tibial defects
Amputation	NA	Shorter treatment time than limb salvage/segmental defect reconstruction; good functional outcomes in young, adult trauma patient with modem prosthesis	Permanent limb loss, high rate of secondary procedures for complications, lifetime prosthetic cost

NA = not applicable, RIA = reamer-irrigator-aspirator, STSG = split-thickness skin graft

[a]Theoretically, there is no limit in terms of size.

Reproduced with permission from Mauffrey C, Barlow BT, Smith W: Management of segmental bone defects. *J Am Acad Orthop Surg* 2015;23:143-153.

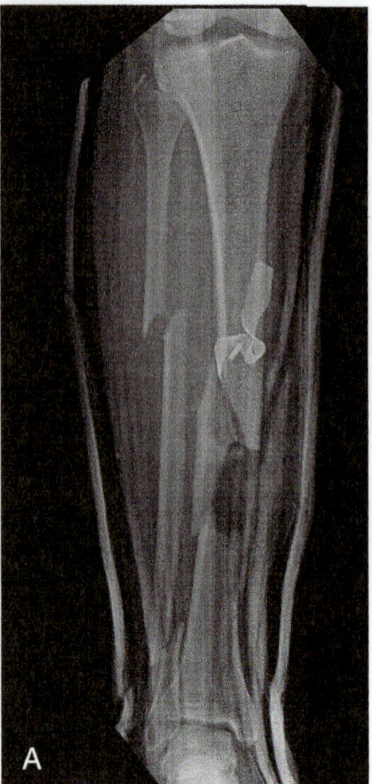

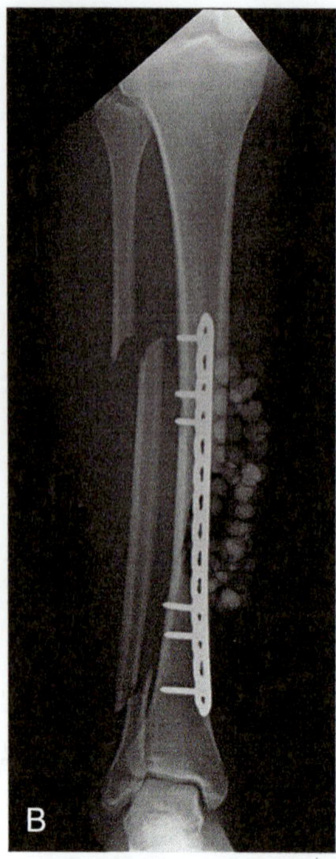

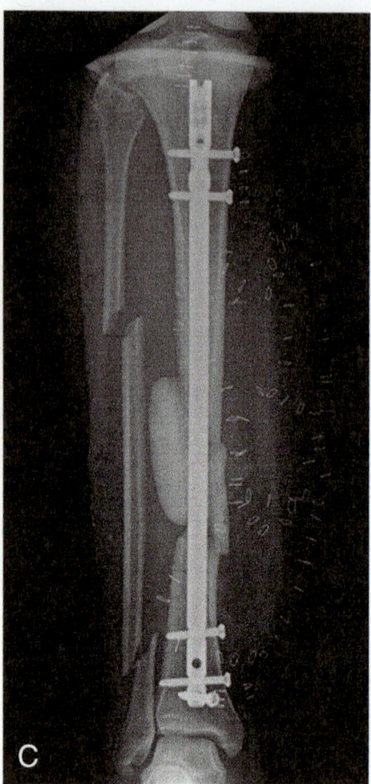

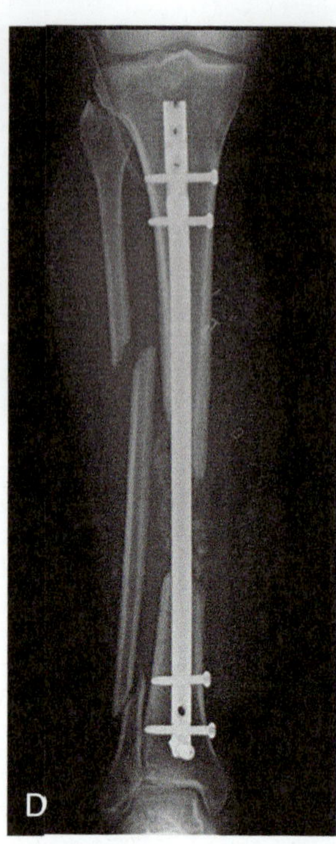

FIGURE 2 AP tibial radiographs demonstrating segmental bone defect of the tibial diaphysis following type IIIB open tibia and fibula fractures managed with induced membrane technique (**A**). Initial treatment included débridement and provisional internal fixation with antibiotic bead pouch (**B**), followed by definitive fixation with intramedullary nail and latissimus free flap coverage over a polymethyl methacrylate spacer with vancomycin and tobramycin (**C**), and subsequent autograft bone harvested from the ipsilateral femoral diaphysis with a reamer-irrigator-aspirator (**D**).

bone may be translated along the axis of the limb segment over time. Distraction osteogenesis recapitulates phases and features of both intramembranous and endochondral bone formation, including a latent phase after corticotomy, a distraction phase during bone is grown by a process demonstrating aspects of intramembranous and endochondral bone formation as well as interleukin 6, insulinlike growth factor 1, group 1 BMPs, and vascular endothelial growth factor expression,[76-78] and a consolidation phase on docking of the transported segmented into the terminal bony aspect of the limb segment. Distraction osteogenesis may be achieved with circular external fixation frames pioneered by Ilizarov[79] (**Figure 3**), monolateral external fixators,[80] cable transport frames, and motorized intramedullary transport or limb lengthening.[81] Multifocal distraction across corticotomy at multiple levels can decrease total transport time. An advantage of distraction osteogenesis is the potential for early weight bearing with a frame in place during distraction. However, distraction rates of typically 1 mm per day and the need to maintain a frame during consolidation may require fixator use for 6 to 12 months.[82] Circular frame distraction osteogenesis is associated with a refracture rate of 5% and an amputation rate of 3%, with greater risk with longer transport segments.[82]

Both the induced membrane technique and distraction osteogenesis are effective in the management of septic nonunion and bone defects. Addition of antibiotics to the initial induced membrane spacer permits high-concentration local antibiotic delivery following débridement.[66,83,84] A systematic review of case reports and series found that débridement followed by reconstruction using a staged induced membrane technique resulted in cure of infection in 91% of cases with 90% union rate.[85] A series of one-stage management of infected bone defects with radical débridement and acute bone transport via external fixation has been reported with up to 94% success rate, although these results have not been replicated.[86] When surgical cultures result in a surprise positive bacterial presence or fungal growth at an attempt at definitive nonunion surgery, the union rate is lower than when cultures are negative (73% versus 96%) and recurrent infection is more likely (12% versus 4%).[40]

EVIDENCE FOR THE CLINICAL UTILITY OF ORTHOBIOLOGICS

Commercially available orthobiologic solutions for nonunion repair and management of segmental bone defects include systemic and local medical therapy, bone graft, bone graft extenders, biologically active materials, recombinant bone growth factors, cell-based therapies, and combination products. Biomaterial solutions include inorganic materials used as bone graft extenders as well as organic scaffolds and carriers for delivery of orthobiologic

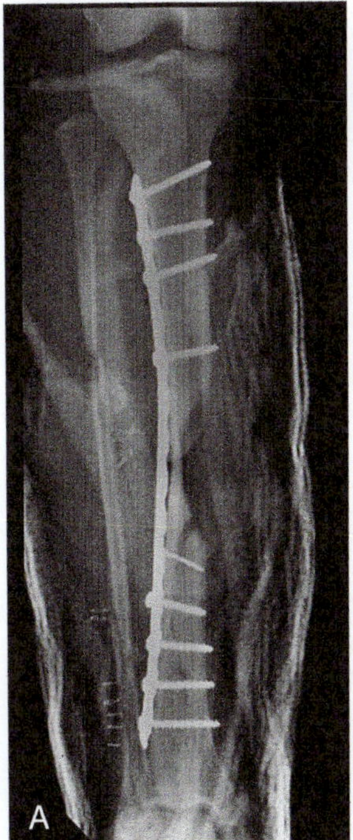

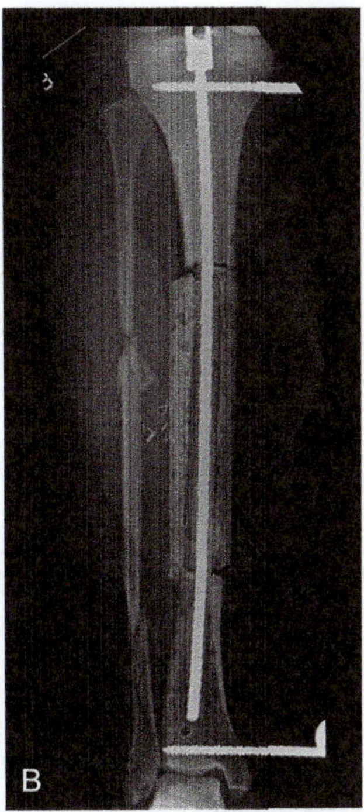

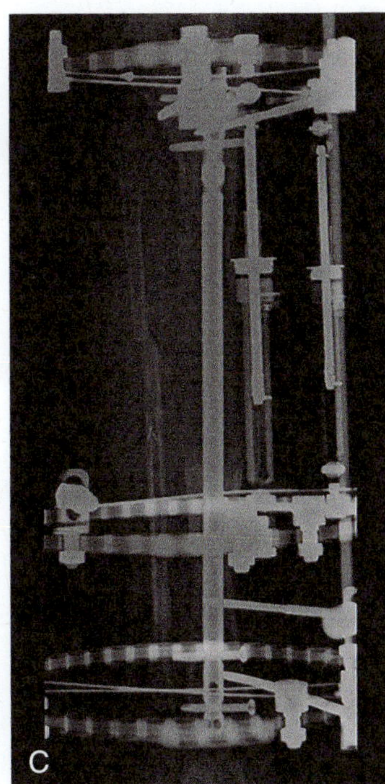

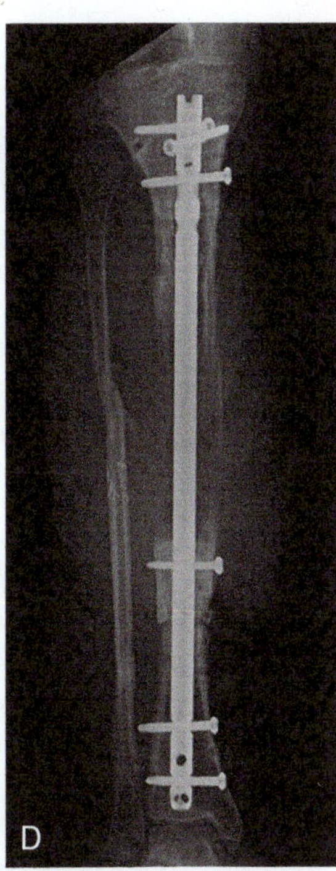

FIGURE 3 AP radiographs of the right tibia and fibula illustrating distraction osteogenesis for segmental bone defect of tibial diaphysis following management of osteomyelitis complicating type IIIB open tibia and fibula fractures (**A**). **B**, After implant removal, an antibiotic-laden cement-coated intramedullary nail was fashioned from an Ilizarov rod and surrounded by an antibiotic-laden cement spacer for management of the infection and dead space. Reconstruction of the bone defect was then staged after treatment of the infection. **C**, After removal of the antibiotic spacers, unifocal distraction osteogenesis was achieved using a circular frame to transport a proximal metadiaphyseal bone segment over a customized medullary nail with staged docking, compression, and fixation of the transport segment through an interlocking hole predrilled through the nail (**D**).

recombinant bone growth factors and cell-based therapies. Cell-based therapies and recombinant factor therapies may be used in isolation for nonunion repair, alone or in combination with delivery into the nonunion site. Conversely, bone graft substitutes, bioactive factors, and cell-based therapies are rarely used in isolation for segmental bone defects.

Medical Therapy

Presently, there are no FDA-approved systemic pharmacologic interventions for the treatment of nonunion or segmental bone defects.[87] Recombinant human parathyroid hormone (rhPTH) is a once-daily systemic injection available as teriparatide (rhPTH 1-34) and abaloparatide (rhPTH 1-34) for FDA-approved use in the prevention of fragility fracture in patients with a diagnosis of osteoporosis. Use of rhPTH systemic therapy to augment fracture healing, nonunion repair, or management of segmental bone defects is off-label. Animal data from rats, mice, and primates indicate that rhPTH accelerates fracture healing and improves union rates in delayed fracture healing models.[88] A systematic review identified 15 case reports, 4 case series, and 1 prospective study, which collectively describe 95% union rate with the use of teriparatide as medical therapy alone in the treatment of long bone delayed union and nonunion, but reporting and attribution bias are concerns and comparative evidence is not available.[89] Full-length rhPTH (1-84; NATPARA) was withdrawn from the market after the FDA issued a class I recall for a possible association with osteosarcoma in rats as well as an issue with the delivery mechanism.[90]

Bone Graft

Autologous bone graft is a reference standard orthobiologic for the management of nonunion and segmental bone defects.[91] Autologous bone grafting involves harvesting osseous matter from one site and transplanting the graft to the nonunion or bone defect. Autograft bone contains complete tissue with native histology, has full histocompatibility, and provides osteoblasts and osteogenic precursor stem cells (osteogenic), which produce new bone tissue, cytokines to encourage bone-forming activity (osteoinductive), and structural support to guide adjacent bone ingrowth (osteoconductive).[92,93] Autograft bone is authorized under 21 CFR 1271.15(b) for harvest and use in the same surgical procedure. Thus, autograft may be used for single-stage repair of nonunion as well as segmental bone defects, up to 5 cm per some authors.[10]

Autograft may be harvested from cortical bone for use as a structural graft or from cancellous bone for use as a nonstructural graft. Described cancellous autograft harvest sites include the anterior iliac crest (5 to 72 cm^3), posterior superior iliac crest (25 to 88 cm^3), femoral medullary canal (25 to 90 cm^3) or tibial medullary canal using a reamer-irrigator-aspirator (RIA) device, proximal tibia, distal radius, and olecranon.[91] Cancellous autografts can achieve similar strength to cortical bone graft in 6 to 12 months. Autograft applied to an induced membrane for segmental defects achieved union in 83% to 90% of cases at an average of 6 to 14 months after grafting.[83,94] The content, performance, and complication rate of autologous bone grafting vary with the harvest site and patient factors including age and medical comorbidities.[95] Use of autograft bone extends operating room time, may extend length of hospital stay, and is associated with complications, most frequently harvest site pain.[96]

Iliac crest harvest is associated with 2% to 9% rate of major complications, and 21% to 22% minor complications, and 40% of patients report persistent harvest site pain at 6 months postoperatively.[97,98] RIA devices involve a closed reaming system that provides continuous irrigation of the medullary canal with removal of the irrigant and reamings by suction and collection of reamed material in a mesh container. A randomized trial of medullary autograft harvest from the femur using an RIA device versus iliac crest grafting found greater graft volumes, similar union rates, similar complication rates around 6%, and lower donor-site pain with RIA.[99] RIA medullary autograft harvest has more fluidlike handling properties, a greater content of hematopoietic elements histologically and by mRNA, less organized bone structure, and greater expression of mesenchymal stem cells markers, although cell viability and osteogenic potential are similar.[100,101]

Allogeneic bone graft is derived from human tissue. Allogeneic bone grafts pose a risk of viral transmission and therefore require careful screening and preparation.[92] These grafts may be structural or nonstructural. Fresh-frozen bone allografts provide structural integrity and osteoinductive and osteoconductive properties, and can be anatomically matched to a defect including articular defects. Structural allografts obtained from the pelvis, ribs, fibula, and femur may be used as intercalary/interposition grafts. However, these grafts lack osteogenic capacity, contain immunogenic donor tissues, have limited shelf life, and provide little benefit over freeze-dried allografts for nonarticular defects.[102,103] Structural fresh-frozen allografts are associated with 54% rate of complications in the management of segmental defects.[102,103]

Allogeneic bone graft prepared from human cadaver bone by ethanol or freeze-drying followed by sterilization using gamma irradiation provides an osteoconductive scaffold composed of hydroxyapatite, type I collagen, and multiple growth factors, which guide adjacent bone ingrowth. The mechanical strength and osteoinductive properties are inferior to autograft bone. However, advantages over autograft bone include availability, low immunogenicity, and the avoidance of donor site morbidity.[104] Allograft bone is available in structural, cortical, and cancellous formulations. Cancellous bone allograft alone was inferior to autograft in the management of long bone fracture nonunion with longer time to union (416 ± 290-543 days versus 198 ± 172-225 days) and greater incidence of reoperation required to achieve union (47% versus 17%).[105,106] Cancellous bone graft reaches similar strength to cortical bone in 6 to 12 months.[107]

Bone graft substitutes, also described as bone autograft extenders, include demineralized bone matrix (DBM), calcium-based ceramics, and xenografts. Limited data support the use of bone graft substitutes alone for the management of nonunion or segmental bone defects. Direct comparative evidence between different bone graft extenders used in conjunction with autograft is not available and would be challenging to interpret in the context of heterogenous injuries and the variability of autograft between patients. Bone graft substitutes have a role in the management of osseous defects in patients unwilling to accept human tissue products and may have a role in the extension of autograft for the management of very large volume defects.

DBM is an osteogenic putty material prepared by acid extraction of the mineral component from bone allograft. DBM retains type I collagen and growth factors and is theoretically both osteoconductive and osteoinductive.[108] Methodologically poor retrospective series suggest DBM may have similar efficacy to iliac crest bone graft (ICBG) in the management of nonunion in the tibia, humerus, pelvis, and calcaneus at greater cost but without donor site morbidity.[61,109-112] An empiric investigation of the concentration of BMP-2 and BMP-7 in DBM found low overall BMP content, wide variability within lots of the same product formulation, and wide variability between DBM products.[113] The use of DBM alone for nonunion or segmental bone defects is not presently supported by level I or II evidence.

Synthetic inorganic calcium-based ceramics including calcium phosphate, tricalcium phosphate, and calcium sulfate provide a porous osteoconductive scaffold, which can be contoured to fill a defect. Calcium phosphate is mechanically 4 to 10 times stronger than cancellous allograft in compression with lower rates of subsidence in biomechanical testing[114] and clinical series of tibial plateau fracture fixation augmentation.[115] Calcium phosphate ceramics alone are not supported by clinical evidence for the treatment of nonunion or segmental bone defects.[116] Tricalcium phosphate has similar compressive strength to cancellous bone. β-Tricalcium phosphate as a bone graft extender mixed with iliac crest autograft did not perform as well as ICBG autograft alone in a retrospective series of

42 patients grafted at the second stage of induced membrane management of postinfective long bone defects, with higher rates of nonunion in the calcium phosphate group.[117] Tricalcium phosphate as a bone graft substitute in the management of nonunion was associated with 85% to 100% rate of fracture union at 1 year in uncontrolled case series.[118,119] Indications include filling of periarticular bone voids to prevent subsidence of articular reduction and internal fixation of the distal femur, proximal tibia, and distal tibial metaphysis.

Calcium sulfate is a soluble ceramic that resorbs faster than bone growth can occur.[120] Calcium sulfate is available in injectable and malleable formulations. Indications for use include filling of bone voids in the setting of débridement following infection or bone defects at high risk for infection, such as after open fracture, when bone graft or bone graft substitutes could provide a nidus for bacterial or fungal colonization. Wound drainage is reported in 4% to 51% of cases where calcium sulfate is used and correlates with the volume of calcium sulfate and proximity of the material to the skin.[121] Single-stage management of culture-positive long bone infection with tobramycin-impregnated calcium sulfate beads was successful in managing infection and achieving union in 14 of 16 patients in a prospective trial.[116] Antibiotic-impregnated calcium sulfate as a bone graft substitute without supplemental autograft or allograft bone in the management of segmental bone defects secondary to combat-related blast injuries with severe soft-tissue compromise achieved fracture union in 12 of 17 injuries, though 5 patients subsequently elected amputation for recalcitrant infection or neuropathic pain.[122]

Xenograft bone substitutes are a class of osteoconductive matrix generated by extensive processing to removal all remnants of the donor animal. Indications for use have included reconstruction of defects after resection of neoplasia as well as bone voids in patients unwilling to accept allogeneic human bone grafts. Coralline hydroxyapatite is a xenograft bone substitute produced from marine coral exoskeletons, which provide a similar three-dimensional structure and pore size to metaphyseal bone. Coralline hydroxyapatite is mechanically brittle, demonstrates slow or incomplete biodegradation, and develops mechanical properties that correlate to the degree of adjacent bony ingrowth. These features have limited its clinical application to nonunion and segmental bone defects, in which the vascularity and osteogenic potential of adjacent bone tissue may be impaired.[120] Matrices of purified bovine fibrillar collagen seeded with calcium phosphate granules, some combined with variations of hydroxyapatite and β-tricalcium phosphate, have lower compression strength than cancellous bone and are intended to extend the volume of autograft to fill a segmental defect. Level II evidence supports the use of a collagen-based matrix in conjunction with bone marrow aspirate in acute fractures, although an appropriate control group was lacking.[123] Uncontrolled case series describe the use of these products as a surface onlay graft in nonunion surgery.[124]

Cell-based therapies for the management of nonunion and bone defects include plasma-derived injections, bone marrow aspirate injection, viable bone allograft, cellular bone matrices, and combination products.

Plasma-derived mesenchymal stem cells including platelet-rich plasma (PRP) formulations are osteoinductive. The efficacy of PRP for long bone nonunion is not presently supported by randomized clinical trials, although case series suggest safety and claim efficacy.[125] PRP was inferior to rhBMP-7 injection in a randomized trial of 120 patients with long bone nonunion with regard to union rate (68% versus 87%) and median time to clinical and radiographic healing (4 versus 3.5 months, 9 versus 8 months, respectively).[126]

Bone marrow aspirate from the iliac crest is osteogenic and osteoinductive. Bone marrow aspirate by centrifugation (BMAC) does not retain the macroscopic bone architecture available with open iliac crest autograft harvest. However, BMAC is rich with osteogenic progenitor cells and mesenchymal stem cells able to undergo osteogenic differentiation in vitro without any osteogenic stimuli.[127] The concentration of osteoblast progenitor cells is improved by aspiration of multiple 1- to 2-mL aliquots from multiple sites.[128] Injection of 40 to 80 mL of marrow into and around distal tibial metadiaphyseal nonunions achieved 82% rate of union in a series of 11 patients within 6 months.[129] The number of osteogenic progenitors correlated with mineralized callus volume, clinical success, and time to union in a retrospective series of injections for nonunion repair.[130] Concentration of BMAC reduces red cell volume by one-half, increases the concentration of osteogenic cells above the densities obtained with ICBG and RIA, and concentrates platelet and leukocyte count by seven fold to ninefold.[131] A systematic review of observation studies found that percutaneous BMAC injection into long bone nonunions was associated with 89% rate of union within 2.5 to 8 months.[131] A randomized trial of BMAC in 40 patients undergoing tibial lengthening found BMAC was associated with accelerated cortical healing indices permitting earlier weight bearing, but did not permit a faster distraction rate.[132] Addition of BMAC to allograft for single-stage management of infected nonunions was associated with a higher rate of union than iliac crest bone autograft (95% versus 40%).[106] Conversely, a retrospective review of 51 patients with tibial nonunion found no difference in union rate between BMAC combined with allograft bone versus ICBG (75% versus 78%, $P = 0.8$).[133] Although BMAC combined with PRP and allograft may enhance the healing of segmental bone defects, the available evidence does not clarify whether BMAC or PRP alone or in combination mediate these eff ects.[131,132,134] Evidence supporting the efficacy of BMAC and PRP products is limited by proprietary cell processing methods and heterogeneity

Lipoaspirates are formulations of autologous mesenchymal stems derived from aspiration of adipose tissue. A level IV proof-of-concept series of three nonunion cases treated with autologous adipose-derived stem cells seeded on a DBM scaffold resulted in one union, one persistent nonunion, and one deep infection.[135]

Cultured allogeneic stem cells combined with bone graft or other materials are therapeutic biologics regulated by the FDA as class III devices or biologic products and require premarket approval. Osteocel Plus (NuVasive), Trinity Evolution (Orthofix), map3 (LifeHealthcare), and ViviGen (DePuy Synthes) are cancellous allogeneic bone graft products containing allogeneic pluripotent stem cells. A quantitative comparison of multiple Osteocel Plus lots with healthy donor iliac crest bone and bone marrow aspirate by functional assays, confocal/scanning electron microscopy, whole-genome microarray, and flow cytometry confirmed the presence of live osteocyte and osteogenic mesenchymal stem cells, an osteoinductive factor expression before culture expansion, 100-fold greater purity over ICBG, and a concentration of osteogenic mesenchymal stem cells in 1 g of cellular allograft equivalent to 45 mL of bone marrow aspirate.[136] Although in vitro studies are promising, no comparative clinical evidence supports the use of these products for nonunion or segmental bone defects. A retrospective series reported the use of map3 in fibular, navicular, and calcaneus nonunion (n = 4) without a comparison group or specific union rate for the nonunion cases.[137] A total of 10 cm^3 of ViviGen has been reported as a supplement to RIA autograft by the manufacturer for the management of posttraumatic defects of the femur, tibial metaphysis, and radial diaphysis by the manufacturer.[138,139] These allogeneic products need to be evaluated in carefully designed, appropriately powered randomized controlled trials to establish efficacy.

Bioactive factor solutions approved for clinical use include BMPs. BMPs are members of the transforming growth factor beta superfamily involved in osteogenesis and osteoblastic differentiation. rhBMP-2 is approved by the FDA for use in adults with acute open tibial shaft fractures stabilized with an intramedullary nail within 14 days of injury and no history of malignant cancer or active pregnancy; use for nonunion and segmental bone defects is off-label. rhBMP-2 combined with allograft achieved similar union rate as autograft in a randomized trial for the reconstruction of diaphyseal tibial segmental defects of 1 to 7 cm in length.[140] A retrospective series of 49 tibial nonunion cases found BMAC combined with rhBMP-2 was associated with a lower rate of union compared with BMAC injection combined with DBM.[141] rhBMP-2 used with gelatin capsules or polylactic/polyglycolic acid onlay carrier was associated with union in 11 of 12 femoral diaphyseal or metaphyseal-diaphyseal defects in an uncontrolled series.[142]

rhBMP-7 or osteogenic protein 1 requires a Humanitarian Device Exemption for use as an alternative to autograft in recalcitrant long bone nonunions where use of autograft is unfeasible and alternative treatments have failed. rhBMP-7 was associated with an 81% clinical success rate in the treatment of tibial nonunion equivalent to autograft bone without harvest site morbidity.[143] rhBMP-7 may have a synergist effect with bone autograft for nonunion repair.[144] A systematic review identified that the use of rhBMP-7 in tibial nonunion improved the rate of union, but did not find differences in union rate or time to union for application to nonunion at other anatomic sites.[145]

Overall, limited evidence is available to guide the use of BMPs in nonunion surgery. A Cochrane systematic review of randomized trials found limited data to support the use of BMPs for nonunion repair.[146] A more recent meta-analysis with considerable risk of bias included four randomized trials and four nonrandomized trials of BMP versus autologous bone grafting for the treatment of long bone nonunion, 613 cases total, and reported shorter time to healing with no differences observed in rate of healing, infection, reoperation, or limb function.[147]

PATIENT SELECTION CONSIDERATIONS

Not every patient with a nonunion or segmental bone defect may be appropriate for attempts to save or salvage the affected limb, and not every patient who pursues these procedures will reflect on their choice without regret. Persistence of nonunion or segmental bone defects and the sequelae of failed surgical procedures have major negative effects on mental health, physical function, and disability.[148] Management strategies must consider the problem in the context of the patient. Age, functional demands, goals for recovery, and self-efficacy all influence the target and final outcomes and must guide the plan for treatment. Consideration should be given to the patient's occupational requirements, social obligations, social support and resources, housing stability, transportation methods and communication capacity if frequent clinical visits or contact is required (distraction osteogenesis), tobacco and substance use, and medical comorbidities particularly diabetes and immunocompromise. The Lower Extremity Assessment Project demonstrated that outcome of severe lower trauma is influenced by the patient's socioeconomic factors more than by the technical performance of interventions.[26] Sigvard Hansen once observed, "very long treatment programs with accompanying multiple hospitalizations and operations are detrimental to many patients…the patient's life has often been drastically changed, and he or she may be demoralized, divorced, or destitute…the individual's self-image, ego, and position in the family may be forever destroyed."[149] Patient counseling about the possibility of prolonged or incomplete recuperation, treatment failure, limb amputation, and failure to achieve recovery goals is critical before making shared decision to embark on a path of surgical interventions.

Specific orthobiologic interventions may be contraindicated in specific patients. rhPTH products carry a black box warning for osteosarcoma and should not be administered in patients with a history of neoplasia. Allergies should be carefully reviewed before using bone graft extender products including coralline hydroxyapatite and collagen scaffolds or gelatin carriers derived from bovine or porcine products. Religious beliefs about human and animal tissue use should be discussed, because DBM, allogeneic bone grafts, cell-based therapies, and combination products may not be acceptable to the patient. A suggested association between BMP-2 and neoplasia remains controversial.[150]

SUMMARY—FUTURE DIRECTIONS AND CHALLENGES

Stronger clinical evidence is needed to support the use of existing orthobiologic products in the treatment of nonunion and segmental bone defects. Prospective comparative studies of conventional strategies with and without augmentation by bioactive factor solutions, cell-based therapies, and bone graft extenders with objective standardization of dosing and formulations are needed.

Future directions in the management of nonunion and segmental bone defects are thriving areas of preclinical tissue engineering research. The ideal product would provide immediate mechanical integrity sufficient for weight bearing, a volumetric match to the patient-specific defect, self-limited but accelerated osteogenic activity to promote rapid integration and union, and no immunogenic or neoplastic risks. Promising solutions include the use of patient-derived, culture-expanded osteoprogenitor lineage, hematopoietic, adipose-derived, and other mesenchymal stem/progenitor cells; gene therapy;[151] osteoconductive scaffolds seeded with osteoinductive cytokines or osteogenic lineages to accelerate defect bridging;[152] local delivery of systemic agents such as rhPTH on carriers;[153] and additive manufacturing or three-dimensional printing fabrication of defect-specific artificial bone tissue grafts, enriched with prebuilt vascular networks and seeded with osteogenic precursors.[154,155] Challenges to bringing these products into clinical use include regulatory hurdles, such as FDA policy that does not consider cell isolation and expansion as minimal manipulation, which disqualifies these products for a same surgical procedure exception and necessitates a full premarket approval pathway or biologics license application.[133]

REFERENCES

1. Mills LA, Simpson AHRW: The relative incidence of fracture non-union in the Scottish population (5.17 million): A 5-year epidemiological study. *BMJ Open* 2013;3:e002276.
2. Mills LA, Aitken SA, Simpson AHRW: The risk of nonunion per fracture: Current myths and revised figures from a population of over 4 million adults. *Acta Orthop* 2017;88:434-439.
3. Tzioupis C, Giannoudis PV: Prevalence of long-bone nonunions. *Injury* 2007;38:S3-S9.
4. Zura R, Xiong Z, Einhorn T, et al: Epidemiology of fracture nonunion in 18 human bones. *JAMA Surg* 2016;151:e162775.
5. Patil S, Montgomery R: Management of complex tibial and femoral nonunion using the Ilizarov technique, and its cost implications. *J Bone Joint Surg Br* 2006;88:928-932.
6. Dahabreh Z, Calori GM, Kanakaris NK, Nikolaou VS, Giannoudis PV: A cost analysis of treatment of tibial fracture nonunion by bone grafting or bone morphogenetic protein-7. *Int Orthop* 2009;33:1407-1414.
7. Dahabreh Z, Dimitriou R, Giannoudis PV: Health economics: A cost analysis of treatment of persistent fracture non-unions using bone morphogenetic protein-7. *Injury* 2007;38:371-377.
8. Kanakaris NK, Giannoudis PV: The health economics of the treatment of long-bone non-unions. *Injury* 2007;38:S77-S84.
9. Antonova E, Le TK, Burge R, Mershon J: Tibia shaft fractures: Costly burden of nonunions. *BMC Musculoskelet Disord* 2013;14:1-10.
10. Mauffrey C, Barlow BT, Smith W: Management of segmental bone defects. *J Am Acad Orthop Surg* 2015;23:143-153.
11. Norris BL, Vanderkarr M, Sparks C, Chitnis AS, Ray B, Holy CE: Treatments, cost and healthcare utilization of patients with segmental bone defects. *Injury* 2021;52(10):2935-2940.
12. Goulet JA, Templeman D: Delayed union and nonunion of tibial shaft fractures. *Instr Course Lect* 1997;46:281-291.
13. Bhandari M, Guyatt G, Walter SD, et al: Randomized trial of reamed and unreamed intramedullary nailing of tibial shaft fractures: By the study to prospectively evaluate reamed intramedullary nails in patients with tibial fractures (SPRINT) investigators. *J Bone Joint Surg Am* 2008;90:2567-2578.
14. Keating JF, Simpson AHRW, Robinson CM: The management of fractures with bone loss. *J Bone Joint Surg Br* 2005;87:142-150.
15. Bhandari M, Bhandari M, Tornetta P, et al: (Sample) size matters! an examination of sample size from the SPRINT trial study to prospectively evaluate reamed intramedullary nails in patients with tibial fractures. *J Orthop Trauma* 2013;27:183-188.
16. Nauth A, McKee MD, Einhorn TA, Watson JT, Li R, Schemitsch EH: Managing bone defects. *J Orthop Trauma* 2011;25:462-466.
17. Haines NM, Lack WD, Seymour RB, Bosse MJ: Defining the lower limit of a "critical bone defect" in open diaphyseal tibial fractures: *J Orthop Trauma* 2016;30:e158-e163.
18. Nauth A, Schemitsch E, Norris B, Nollin Z, Watson JT: Critical-size bone defects: Is there a consensus for diagnosis and treatment? *J Orthop Trauma* 2018;32:S7.

19. Sanders DW, Bhandari M, Guyatt G, et al: Critical-sized defect in the tibia: Is it critical? Results from the SPRINT trial. *J Orthop Trauma* 2014;28:632-635.

20. Hinsche AF, Giannoudis PV, Matthews SE, Smith RM: Spontaneous healing of large femoral cortical bone defects: Does genetic predisposition play a role? *Acta Orthop Belg* 2003;69:441-446.

21. Dickson K, Katzman S, Delgado E, Contreras D: Delayed unions and nonunions of open tibial fractures. Correlation with arteriography results. *Clin Orthop Relat Res* 1994;302:189-193.

22. Reed AAC, Joyner CJ, Brownlow HC, Simpson AHRW: Human atrophic fracture non-unions are not avascular. *J Orthop Res* 2002;20:593-599.

23. Brownlow HC, Reed A, Simpson AHRW: The vascularity of atrophic non-unions. *Injury* 2002;33:145-150.

24. Volgas DA, Stannard JP, Alonso JE: Nonunions of the humerus. *Clin Orthop Relat Res* 2004;419:46-50.

25. Reverte MM, Dimitriou R, Kanakaris NK, Giannoudis PV: What is the effect of compartment syndrome and fasciotomies on fracture healing in tibial fractures? *Injury* 2011;42:1402-1407.

26. MacKenzie EJ, Bosse MJ, Pollak AN, et al. Long-term persistence of disability following severe lower-limb trauma. Results of a seven-year follow-up. *J Bone Joint Surg Am* 2005;87:1801-1809.

27. Castillo RC, Bosse MJ, MacKenzie EJ, Patterson BM, LEAP Study Group: Impact of smoking on fracture healing and risk of complications in limb-threatening open tibia fractures. *J Orthop Trauma* 2005;19:151-157.

28. Calori GM, Albisetti W, Agus A, Iori S, Tagliabue L: Risk factors contributing to fracture non-unions. *Injury* 2007;38:S11-S18.

29. Perumal V, Roberts CS: (ii) Factors contributing to non-union of fractures. *Curr Orthop* 2007;21:258-261.

30. Pountos I, Georgouli T, Bird H, Giannoudis PV: Nonsteroidal anti-inflammatory drugs: Prostaglandins, indications, and side effects. *Int J Interferon Cytokine Mediat Res* 2011;3:19-27.

31. Heppenstall RB, Brighton CT: Fracture healing in the presence of anemia. *Clin Orthop Relat Res* 1977;123:253-258.

32. Stavrou PZ, Ciriello V, Theocharakis S, et al: Prevalence and risk factors for re-interventions following reamed intramedullary tibia nailing. *Injury* 2016;47:S49-S52.

33. Weaver MJ, Harris MB, Strom AC, et al: Fracture pattern and fixation type related to loss of reduction in bicondylar tibial plateau fractures. *Injury* 2012;43:864-869.

34. Githens M, Haller J, Agel J, Firoozabadi R: Does concurrent tibial intramedullary nailing and fibular fixation increase rates of tibial nonunion? A matched cohort study. *J Orthop Trauma* 2017;31:316-320.

35. Ko S-B, Lee S-W: Do fibula nonunions predict later tibia nonunions? *J Orthop Trauma* 2013;27:150-152.

36. Hardeman F, Bollars P, Donnelly M, Bellemans J, Nijs S: Predictive factors for functional outcome and failure in angular stable osteosynthesis of the proximal humerus. *Injury* 2012;43:153-158.

37. Claes L, Augat P, Suger G, Wilke H-J: Influence of size and stability of the osteotomy gap on the success of fracture healing. *J Orthop Res* 1997;15:577-584.

38. Sathyendra V, Donahue HJ, Vrana KE, et al: Single nucleotide polymorphisms in osteogenic genes in atrophic delayed fracture-healing: A preliminary investigation. *J Bone Joint Surg Am* 2014;96:1242-1248.

39. Govaert GAM, Kuehl R, Atkins BL, et al: Diagnosing fracture-related infection: Current concepts and recommendations. *J Orthop Trauma* 2020;34:8-17.

40. Olszewski D, Streubel PN, Stucken C, et al: Fate of patients with a "surprise" positive culture after nonunion surgery. *J Orthop Trauma* 2016;30:e19.

41. Brinker MR, Macek J, Laughlin M, Dunn WR: Utility of common biomarkers for diagnosing infection in nonunion. *J Orthop Trauma* 2021;5:121-127.

42. Glaudemans AWJM, Jutte PC, Cataldo MA, et al: Consensus document for the diagnosis of peripheral bone infection in adults: A joint paper by the EANM, EBJIS, and ESR (with ESCMID endorsement). *Eur J Nucl Med Mol Imaging* 2019;46:957-970.

43. Stucken C, Olszewski DC, Creevy WR, Murakami AM, Tornetta P: Preoperative diagnosis of infection in patients with nonunions. *J Bone Joint Surg Am* 2013;95:1409-1412.

44. Wang S, Yin P, Quan C, et al: Evaluating the use of serum inflammatory markers for preoperative diagnosis of infection in patients with nonunions. *Biomed Res Int* 2017;2017:9146317.

45. Nauth A, Lee M, Gardner MJ, et al: Principles of nonunion management: State of the art. *J Orthop Trauma* 2018;32:S52.

46. Meanley S: Different approaches and cultural considerations in third world prosthetics. *Prosthet Orthot Int* 1995;19:176-180.

47. Liu F, Williams RM, Liu H-E, Chien N-H: The lived experience of persons with lower extremity amputation. *J Clin Nurs* 2010;19:2152-2161.

48. Peterson HA: The treatment of congenital oseudarthrosis of the tibia with ipsilateral fibular transfer to make a one-bone lower leg: A review of the literature and case report with a 23-year follow-up. *J Pediatr Orthop* 2008;28:478-482.

49. Devendra A, Velmurugesan PS, Dheenadhayalan J, Venkatramani H, Sabapathy SR, Rajasekaran S: One-bone forearm reconstruction: A salvage solution for the forearm with massive bone loss. *J Bone Joint Surg Am* 2019;101:e74.

50. Konda S, Saleh H, Fisher N, Egol KA: Posterolateral bone grafting for distal tibia nonunion. *J Orthop Trauma* 2017;31:S16.

51. Bishop AT, Wood MB, Sheetz KK: Arthrodesis of the ankle with a free vascularized autogenous bone graft. Reconstruction of segmental loss of bone secondary to osteomyelitis, tumor, or trauma. *J Bone Joint Surg Am* 1995;77:1867-1875.

52. Aitken SA, Jenkins PJ, Rymaszewski L: Revisiting the 'bag of bones': Functional outcome after the conservative management of a fracture of the distal humerus. *Bone Joint J* 2015;97-B:1132-1138.

53. Brinker MR, O'Connor DP, Monla YT, Earthman TP: Metabolic and endocrine abnormalities in patients with nonunions. *J Orthop Trauma* 2007;21:14.

54. Sarmiento A, Burkhalter WE, Latta LL: Functional bracing in the treatment of delayed union and nonunion of the tibia. *Int Orthop* 2003;27:26-29.

55. Leighton R, Watson JT, Giannoudis P, Papakostidis C, Harrison A, Steen RG: Healing of fracture nonunions treated with low-intensity pulsed ultrasound (LIPUS): A systematic review and meta-analysis. *Injury* 2017;48:1339-1347.

56. Rutten S, van den Bekerom MPJ, Sierevelt IN, Nolte PA: Enhancement of bone-healing by low-intensity pulsed ultrasound: A systematic review. *JBJS Rev* 2016;4:e6.

57. TRUST Investigators writing group, Busse JW, Bhandari M, et al: Re-Evaluation of low intensity pulsed ultrasound in treatment of tibial fractures (TRUST): Randomized clinical trial. *BMJ* 2016;355:i5351.

58. Zhang JY, Tornetta P, Dale KM, et al: The fate of patients after a staged nonunion procedure for known infection. *J Orthop Trauma* 2021;35:211-216.

59. Vaughn J, Gotha H, Cohen E, et al: Nail dynamization for delayed union and nonunion in femur and tibia fractures. *Orthopedics* 2016;39:e1117-e1123.

60. Tsang STJ, Mills LA, Frantzias J, Baren JP, Keating JF, Simpson AHRW: Exchange nailing for nonunion of diaphyseal fractures of the tibia: Our results and an analysis of the risk factors for failure. *Bone Joint J* 2016;98:534-541.

61. Hierholzer C, Friederichs J, Glowalla C, Woltmann A, Bühren V, von Rüden C: Reamed intramedullary exchange nailing in the operative treatment of aseptic tibial shaft nonunion. *Int Orthop* 2017;41:1647-1653.

62. Ye J, Zheng Q: Augmentative locking compression plate Wxation for the management of long bone nonunion after intramedullary nailing. *Arch Orthop Trauma Surg* 2012;132(7):937-940.

63. Lavini F, Dall'Oca C, Bartolozzi P: Bone transport and compression-distraction in the treatment of bone loss of the lower limbs. *Injury* 2010;41:1191-1195.

64. Fragomen AT, Wellman D, Rozbruch SR: The PRECICE magnetic IM compression nail for long bone nonunions: A preliminary report. *Arch Orthop Trauma Surg* 2019;139:1551-1560.

65. Masquelet AC, Begue T: The concept of induced membrane for reconstruction of long bone defects. *Orthop Clin North Am* 2010;41:27-37.

66. Masquelet AC: Induced membrane technique: Pearls and pitfalls. *J Orthop Trauma* 2017;31:S36-S38.

67. Viateau V, Bensidhoum M, Guillemin G, et al: Use of the induced membrane technique for bone tissue engineering purposes: Animal studies. *Orthop Clin North Am* 2010;41:49-56.

68. Pelissier PH, Masquelet AC, Bareille R, Pelissier SM, Amedee J: Induced membranes secrete growth factors including vascular and osteoinductive factors and could stimulate bone regeneration. *J Orthop Res* 2004;22:73-79.

69. Aho O-M, Lehenkari P, Ristiniemi J, Lehtonen S, Risteli J, Leskelä H-V: The mechanism of action of induced membranes in bone repair. *J Bone Joint Surg Am* 2013;95:597-604.

70. Payatakes A, Sotereanos DG: Pedicled vascularized bone grafts for scaphoid and lunate reconstruction. *J Am Acad Orthop Surg* 2009;17:744-755.

71. Malizos KN, Zalavras CG, Soucacos PN, Beris AE, Urbaniak JR: Free vascularized fibular grafts for reconstruction of skeletal defects. *J Am Acad Orthop Surg* 2004;12:360-369.

72. De Boer HH, Wood MB, Hermans J: Reconstruction of large skeletal defects by vascularized fibula transfer. *Int Orthop* 1990;14:121-128.

73. Eward WC, Kontogeorgakos V, Levin LS, Brigman BE: Free vascularized fibular graft reconstruction of large skeletal defects after tumor resection. *Clin Orthop Relat Res* 2010;468:590-598.

74. Minami A, Kasashima T, Iwasaki N, Kato H, Kaneda K: Vascularised fibular grafts: An experience of 102 patients. *J Bone Joint Surg Br* 2000;82:1022-1025.

75. Nusbickel FR, Dell PC, McAndrew MP, Moore MM: Vascularized autografts for reconstruction of skeletal defects following lower extremity trauma. A review. *Clin Orthop Relat Res* 1989;243:65-70.

76. Spencer EM, Liu CC, Si EC, Howard GA: In vivo actions of insulin-like growth factor-I (IGF-I) on bone formation and resorption in rats. *Bone* 1991;12:21-26.

77. Cho T-J, Kim JA, Chung CY, et al: Expression and role of interleukin-6 in distraction osteogenesis. *Calcif Tissue Int* 2007;80:192-200.

78. Forriol F, Denaro V, Denaro L, Longo UG, Taira H: Bone lengthening osteogenesis, a combination of intramembranous and endochondral ossification: An experimental study in sheep. *Strategies Trauma Limb Reconstr* 2010;5:71-78.

79. Ilizarov GA: Basic principles of transosseous compression and distraction osteosynthesis. *Orthop Travmatol Protez* 1971;32:7-15.

80. Rohilla R, Sharma PK, Wadhwani J, et al: Prospective randomized comparison of quality of regenerate in distraction osteogenesis of ring versus monolateral fixator in patients with infected nonunion of the tibia using digital radiographs and CT. *Bone Joint J* 2019;101-B:1416-1422.

81. Rozbruch SR, Birch JG, Dahl MT, Herzenberg JE: Motorized intramedullary nail for management of limb-length discrepancy and deformity. *J Am Acad Orthop Surg* 2014;22:403-409.

82. Papakostidis C, Bhandari M, Giannoudis PV: Distraction osteogenesis in the treatment of long bone defects of the lower limbs: Effectiveness, complications and clinical results; a systematic review and meta-analysis. *Bone Joint J* 2013;95-B:1673-1680.

83. Taylor BC, Hancock J, Zitzke R, Castaneda J: Treatment of bone loss with the induced membrane technique. *J Orthop Trauma* 2015;29(12):554-557.

84. Mauffrey C, Hake ME, Chadayammuri V, Masquelet A-C: Reconstruction of long bone infections using the induced membrane technique. *J Orthop Trauma* 2016;30:e188-e193.

85. Morelli I, Drago L, George DA, Gallazzi E, Scarponi S, Romanò CL: Masquelet technique: Myth or reality? A systematic review and meta-analysis. *Injury* 2016;47:S68-S76.

86. Zhou C-H, Ren Y, Song H-J, et al: One-stage debridement and bone transport versus first-stage debridement and second-stage bone transport for the management of lower limb post-traumatic osteomyelitis. *J Orthop Translat* 2021;28:21-27.

87. Kostenuik P, Mirza FM: Fracture healing physiology and the quest for therapies for delayed healing and nonunion. *J Orthop Res* 2017;35:213-223.

88. Pietrogrande L, Raimondo E: Teriparatide in the treatment of non-unions: Scientific and clinical evidences. *Injury* 2013;44:S54-S57.

89. Canintika AF, Dilogo IH: Teriparatide for treating delayed union and nonunion: A systematic review. *J Clin Orthop Trauma* 2020;11:S107-S112.

90. United States Food and Drug Administration: *Takeda Issues US Recall of NATPARA® (parathyroid hormone) for Injection Due to the Potential for Rubber Particulate.* 5 September 2021. Available at: https://www.fda.gov/safety/recalls-market-withdrawals-safety-alerts/takeda-issues-us-recall-natparar-parathyroid-hormone-injection-due-potential-rubber-particulate.

91. Dimitriou R, Mataliotakis GI, Angoules AG, Kanakaris NK, Giannoudis PV: Complications following autologous bone graft harvesting from the iliac crest and using the RIA: A systematic review. *Injury* 2011;42:S3-S15.

92. Khan SN, Cammisa FP, Sandhu HS, Diwan AD, Girardi FP, Lane JM: The biology of bone grafting. *Am Acad Orthop Surg* 2005;13:77-86.

93. Roberts TT, Rosenbaum AJ: Bone grafts, bone substitutes and orthobiologics: The bridge between basic science and clinical advancements in fracture healing. *Organogenesis* 2012;8:114-124.

94. Karger C, Kishi T, Schneider L, Fitoussi F, Masquelet A-C: Treatment of posttraumatic bone defects by the induced membrane technique. *Orthop Traumatol Surg Res* 2012;98:97-102.

95. Zhou S, Greenberger JS, Epperly MW, et al: Age-related intrinsic changes in human bone-marrow-derived mesenchymal stem cells and their differentiation to osteoblasts. *Aging Cell* 2008;7:335-343.

96. Loeffler BJ, Kellam JF, Sims SH, Bosse MJ: Prospective observational study of donor-site morbidity following anterior iliac crest bone-grafting in orthopaedic trauma reconstruction patients. *J Bone Joint Surg Am* 2012;94:1649-1654.

97. Goulet JA, Senunas LE, DeSilva GL, Greenfield MLV: Autogenous iliac crest bone graft: Complications and functional assessment. *Clin Orthop Relat Res* 1997;339:76-81.

98. Younger EM, Chapman MW: Morbidity at bone graft donor sites. *J Orthop Trauma* 1989;3:192-195.

99. Dawson J, Kiner D, Gardner WI, Swafford R, Nowotarski PJ: The reamer–irrigator–aspirator as a device for harvesting bone graft compared with iliac crest bone graft: Union rates and complications. *J Orthop Trauma* 2014;28:584-590.

100. Sagi HC, Young ML, Gerstenfeld L, Einhorn TA, Tornetta P: Qualitative and quantitative differences between bone graft obtained from the medullary canal (with a reamer/irrigator/aspirator) and the iliac crest of the same patient. *J Bone Joint Surg Am* 2012;94:2128-2135.

101. Uppal HS, Peterson BE, Misfeldt ML, et al: The viability of cells obtained using the Reamer–Irrigator–Aspirator system and in bone graft from the iliac crest. *Bone Joint J* 2013;95-B:1269-1274.

102. De Ponte FS, Cutroneo G, Falzea R, et al: Histochemical and morphological aspects of fresh frozen bone: A preliminary study. *Eur J Histochem* 2016;60(4):2642.

103. Makley JT: The use of allografts to reconstruct intercalary defects of long bones. *Clin Orthop Relat Res* 1985;197:58-75.

104. Laurencin CT, Khan Y, Kofron M, et al: The ABJS Nicolas Andry Award: Tissue engineering of bone and ligament – A 15-year perspective. *Clin Orthop Relat Res* 2006;447:221-236.

105. Flierl MA, Smith WR, Mauffrey C, et al: Outcomes and complication rates of different bone grafting modalities in long bone fracture nonunions: A retrospective cohort study in 182 patients. *J Orthop Surg Res* 2013;8:33.

106. Hernigou P, Dubory A, Homma Y, Flouzat Lachaniette CH, Chevallier N, Rouard H: Single-stage treatment of infected tibial non-unions and osteomyelitis with bone marrow granulocytes precursors protecting bone graft. *Int Orthop* 2018;42:2443-2450.

107. Finkemeier CG: Bone-grafting and bone-graft substitutes. *J Bone Joint Surg Am* 2002;84:454-464.

108. Peterson B, Whang PG, Iglesias R, Wang JC, Lieberman JR: Osteoinductivity of commercially available demineralized bone matrix: Preparations in a spine fusion model. *J Bone Joint Surg Am* 2004;86:2243-2250.

109. Wilkins RM, Kelly CM: The effect of allomatrix injectable putty on the outcome of long bone applications. *Orthopedics* 2003;26:S567-S570.

110. Pieske O, Wittmann A, Zaspel J, et al: Autologous bone graft versus demineralized bone matrix in internal fixation of ununited long bones. *J Trauma Manag Outcomes* 2009;3:11.

111. Drosos GI, Touzopoulos P, Ververidis A, Tilkeridis K, Kazakos K: Use of demineralized bone matrix in the extremities. *World J Orthop* 2015;6:269-277.

112. Ziran BH, Smith WR, Morgan SJ: Use of calcium-based demineralized bone matrix/allograft for nonunions and posttraumatic reconstruction of the appendicular skeleton: Preliminary results and complications. *J Trauma Acute Care Surg* 2007;63:1324-1328.

113. Bae HW, Zhao L, Kanim LEA, Wong P, Delamarter RB, Dawson EG: Intervariability and intravariability of bone morphogenetic proteins in commercially available demineralized bone matrix products. *Spine* 2006;31:1299-1306.

114. Yetkinler DN, McClellan RT, Reindel ES, Carter D, Poser RD: Biomechanical comparison of conventional open reduction and internal fixation versus calcium phosphate cement fixation of a central depressed tibial plateau fracture. *J Orthop Trauma* 2001;15:197-206.

115. McDonald E, Chu T, Tufaga M, et al: tibial plateau fracture repairs augmented with calcium phosphate cement have higher in situ fatigue strength than those with autograft. *J Orthop Trauma* 2011;25:90-95.

116. McKee MD, Wild LM, Schemitsch EH, Waddell JP: The use of an antibiotic-impregnated, osteoconductive, bioabsorbable bone substitute in the treatment of infected long bone defects: Early results of a prospective trial. *J Orthop Trauma* 2002;16:622-627.

117. Gupta S, Malhotra A, Jindal R, Garg SK, Kansay R, Mittal N: Role of beta tri-calcium phosphate-based composite ceramic as bone-graft expander in Masquelet's-induced membrane technique. *Indian J Orthop* 2019;53:63-69.

118. Bucholz RW, Carlton A, Holmes RE: Hydroxyapatite and tricalcium phosphate bone graft substitutes. *Orthop Clin North Am* 1987;18:323-334.

119. McAndrew MP, Gorman PW, Lange TA: Tricalcium phosphate as a bone graft substitute in trauma: Preliminary report. *J Orthop Trauma* 1988;2:333-339.

120. Hak DJ: The use of osteoconductive bone graft substitutes in orthopaedic trauma. *J Am Acad Orthop Surg* 2007;15:525-536.

121. Beuerlein MJ, McKee MD: Calcium sulfates: What is the evidence? *J Orthop Trauma* 2010;24:S46-S51.

122. Helgeson MD, Potter BK, Tucker CJ, Frisch HM, Shawen SB: Antibiotic-impregnated calcium sulfate use in combat-related open fractures. *Orthopedics* 2009;32:323.

123. Chapman MW, Bucholz R, Cornell C: Treatment of acute fractures with a collagen-calcium phosphate graft material. A randomized clinical trial. *J Bone Joint Surg Am* 1997;79:495-502.

124. Kocialkowski A, Wallace WA, Prince HG: Clinical experience with a new artificial bone graft: Preliminary results of a prospective study. *Injury* 1990;21:142-144.

125. Andersen C, Wragg NM, Shariatzadeh M, Wilson SL: The use of platelet-rich plasma (PRP) for the management of non-union fractures. *Curr Osteoporos Rep* 2021;19:1-14.

126. Calori GM, Tagliabue L, Gala L, d'Imporzano M, Peretti G, Albisetti W: Application of rhBMP-7 and platelet-rich plasma in the treatment of long bone non-unions: A prospective randomised clinical study on 120 patients. *Injury* 2008;39:1391-1402.

127. Jäger M, Herten M, Fochtmann U, et al: Bridging the gap: Bone marrow aspiration concentrate reduces autologous bone grafting in osseous defects. *J Orthop Res* 2011;29:173-180.

128. Muschler GF, Boehm C, Easley K: Aspiration to obtain osteoblast progenitor cells from human bone marrow: The influence of aspiration volume. *J Bone Joint Surg Am* 1997;79:1699-1709.

129. Braly HL, O'Connor DP, Brinker MR: Percutaneous autologous bone marrow injection in the treatment of distal metadiaphyseal tibial nonunions and delayed unions. *J Orthop Trauma* 2013;27:527-533.

130. Hernigou P, Poignard A, Beaujean F, Rouard H: Percutaneous autologous bone-marrow grafting for nonunions: Influence of the number and concentration of progenitor cells. *J Bone Joint Surg Am* 2005;87:1430-1437.

131. Imam MA, Holton J, Ernstbrunner L, et al: A systematic review of the clinical applications and complications of bone marrow aspirate concentrate in management of bone defects and nonunions. *Int Orthop* 2017;41:2213-2220.

132. Lee DH, Ryu KJ, Kim JW, Kang KC, Choi YR: Bone marrow aspirate concentrate and platelet-rich plasma enhanced bone healing in distraction osteogenesis of the tibia. *Clin Orthop Relat Res* 2014;472:3789-3797.

133. Lin K, VandenBerg J, Putnam SM, et al: Bone marrow aspirate concentrate with cancellous allograft versus iliac crest bone graft in the treatment of long bone nonunions. *OTA Int* 2019;2:e012.

134. Kitoh H, Kitakoji T, Tsuchiya H, et al: Transplantation of marrow-derived mesenchymal stem cells and platelet-rich plasma during distraction osteogenesis—a preliminary result of three cases. *Bone* 2004;35:892-898.

135. Dufrane D, Docquier P-L, Delloye C, Poirel HA, André W, Aouassar N: Scaffold-free three-dimensional graft from autologous adipose-derived stem cells for large bone defect reconstruction: Clinical proof of concept. *Medicine (Baltimore)* 2015;94:e2220.

136. Baboolal TG, Boxall SA, El-Sherbiny YM, et al: Multipotential stromal cell abundance in cellular bone allograft: Comparison with fresh age-matched iliac crest bone and bone marrow aspirate. *Regen Med* 2014;9:593-607.

137. Dekker TJ, White P, Adams SB: Efficacy of a cellular bone allograft for foot and ankle arthrodesis and revision nonunion procedures. *Foot Ankle Int* 2017;38:277-282.

138. Apostle K: Surgical Repair of Open Femur Fracture with Bone Loss Using ViviGen® Cellular Bone Matrix. ViviGen®10. Available at: https://www.lifenethealth.org/sites/default/files/files/68-20-210.pdf

139. Kaz A: Surgical Repair of a Tibial Metaphyseal Defect Using ViviGen Formable® Cellular Bone Matrix. ViviGen®10. Available at: https://www.lifenethealth.org/sites/default/files/files/68-20-224.pdf

140. Jones AL, Bucholz RW, Bosse MJ, et al: Recombinant human BMP-2 and allograft compared with autogenous bone graft for reconstruction of diaphyseal tibial fractures with cortical defects: A randomized, controlled trial. *J Bone Joint Surg Am* 2006;88:1431-1441.

141. Desai P, Hasan SM, Zambrana L, et al: Bone mesenchymal stem cells with growth factors successfully treat nonunions and delayed unions. *HSS J* 2015;11:104-111.

142. Johnson EE, Urist MR, Finerman GA: Bone morphogenetic protein augmentation grafting of resistant femoral nonunions. A preliminary report. *Clin Orthop Relat Res* 1988;230:257-265.

143. Friedlaender GE: Osteogenic protein-1 (bone morphogenetic protein-7) in the treatment of tibial nonunions. *J Bone Joint Surg Am* 2001;83-A(suppl 1):S151-S158.

144. Giannoudis PV, Kanakaris NK, Dimitriou R, Gill I, Kolimarala V, Montgomery RJ: The synergistic effect of autograft and BMP-7 in the treatment of atrophic nonunions. *Clin Orthop Relat Res* 2009;467:3239.

145. Schenker ML, Yannascoli SM, Donegan D: Bone morphogenetic protein and fractures: A meta-analysis, in ORS 2014 Annual Meeting Poster, pp 15-18.

146. Garrison KR, Shemilt I, Donell S, et al: Bone morphogenetic protein (BMP) for fracture healing in adults. *Cochrane Database Syst Rev* 2010;2010(6):CD006950.

147. Xie C: Meta-analysis of bone morphogenetic protein versus autologous bone grafting for limb long bone nonunion. *Chin J Tissue Eng Res* 2020;53:803-810.

148. Brinker MR, Trivedi A, O'Connor DP: Debilitating effects of femoral nonunion on health-related quality of life. *J Orthop Trauma* 2017;31:e37.

149. Hansen STJ: The type-IIIC tibial fracture. Salvage or amputation. *J Bone Joint Surg Am* 1987;69:799-800.

150. James AW, LaChaud G, Shen J, et al: A review of the clinical side effects of bone morphogenetic protein-2. *Tissue Eng B Rev* 2016;22:284-297.

151. Bougioukli S, Evans CH, Alluri RK, Ghivizzani SC, Lieberman JR: Gene therapy to enhance bone and cartilage repair in orthopaedic surgery. *Curr Gene Ther* 2018;18:154-170.

152. Kir MÇ: Hyaluronic acid-based mesh add-on iliac autograft improves bone healing and functional outcomes in atrophic nonunion of clavicular midshaft: A 2-year followup. *Indian J Orthop* 2019;53:459-464.

153. Arrighi I, Mark S, Alvisi M, von Rechenberg B, Hubbell JA, Schense JC: Bone healing induced by local delivery of an engineered parathyroid hormone prodrug. *Biomaterials* 2009;30:1763-1771.

154. Tang D, Tare RS, Yang L-Y, Williams DF, Ou K-L, Oreffo ROC: Biofabrication of bone tissue: Approaches, challenges and translation for bone regeneration. *Biomaterials* 2016;83:363-382.

155. Cui H, Zhu W, Nowicki M, Zhou X, Khademhosseini A, Zhang LG: Hierarchical fabrication of engineered vascularized bone biphasic constructs via dual 3D bioprinting: Integrating regional bioactive factors into architectural design. *Adv Healthc Mater* 2016;5:2174-2181.

CHAPTER

25 Meniscal Repair and Replacement

Suhas P. Dasari, MD • Safa Gursoy, MD, PhD •
Robert F. LaPrade, MD, PhD, FAAOS • Jorge Chahla, MD, PhD

INTRODUCTION

The menisci play a critical role in preservation of the tibiofemoral joint. Their unique anisotropic structure allows them to dissipate compressive and shearing loads experienced under physiologic conditions. The menisci's hypovascularity, particularly in the more central white-white regions, gives them a relatively limited healing capacity. Because of the strong association with arthritic changes after a partial or total meniscectomy, every effort should be made to repair meniscal tears when indicated. Orthobiologic solutions have shown promising early clinical results in improving the quality of life for patients with meniscal injury. The use of scaffolds and implants has provided an alternative solution for patients with partial or total meniscectomies. Cellular solutions have also shown great promise both as an augment for meniscal repair and as an isolated therapeutic injection for patients experiencing acute traumatic tears or degenerative tears. Other orthobiologics that have received considerable interest include blood products such as platelet-rich plasma (PRP) or fibrin clots. To date, PRP has already begun to show positive preliminary results, specifically at reducing meniscal repair failure. Additionally, there is considerable potential for the translational development of growth factor augmentation in meniscal repair. Tissue engineering is the final amalgamation of these advances in the field of orthobiologics. The combination of three-dimensional (3D) printing technology, biomaterial scaffolds, progenitor cells, and biomechanical/biochemical stimulation might be the future of meniscal repair/replacement.

ANATOMY AND BIOMECHANICS OF THE MENISCI

Background

The menisci are crescent-shaped, hypocellular, hypovascular, fibrocartilaginous structures with dense collagenous extracellular matrices (ECMs) and wedge-like cross sections that function to deepen the tibial plateau, transmit load through the joint, provide shock absorption, increase joint stability, and provide lubrication of the articular cartilage between the tibial plateau and femoral condyle.[1-3] The menisci are attached to the tibial plateau via their anterior and posterior roots and are stabilized by the medial collateral ligament, the transverse ligament, the meniscotibial ligaments, and the meniscofemoral ligaments.[2,4] The roots of the meniscus are ligamentous-like structures with fibrocartilaginous entheses.[4] They are essential to function as they anchor the meniscus to prevent extrusion during joint loading.[5] The anatomy of the meniscus is outlined in detail in **Table 1**.[1,6-8]

The menisci are relatively avascular structures. This extent of the vascular zone has implications on the healing prognosis of a meniscal tear.[2] A generous estimate would approximate that 20% to 30% of the periphery of the medial meniscus and 10% to 25% of the periphery of the lateral meniscus receive direct vascular supplies.[1,3,9] The remainder of the avascular meniscus must receive nutrition via the synovial fluid and diffusion.[9,10] Based on its vascularization, the meniscus is divided into a red-red peripheral zone that is vascular, a white-white central zone that is avascular, and a red-white intermediate zone that has characteristics of the other two zones.[1] The red-red meniscal regions are thick ligamentous structures that have attachments to the joint capsule, whereas the white-white regions are thin, concave, cartilaginous structures that have unattached free edges.[1,4] Blood supply to the meniscus arises from the lateral and medial geniculate arteries, which penetrate through the joint capsule and form a perimeniscal capillary plexus with radial branches that penetrate to a depth of approximately 2 to 3 mm[11,12] (**Figure 1**). These branches supply the peripheral quarter of the meniscus, creating the red-red zone.[11-13]

Dr. LaPrade or an immediate family member has received royalties from Arthrex, Inc., Össur, and Smith & Nephew; serves as a paid consultant to or is an employee of Össur and Smith & Nephew; has received research or institutional support from Arthrex, Inc., Linvatec, Össur, and Smith & Nephew; and serves as a board member, owner, officer, or committee member of the American Orthopaedic Society for Sports Medicine and the International Society of Arthroscopy, Knee Surgery, and Orthopaedic Sports Medicine. Dr. Chahla or an immediate family member serves as a paid consultant to or is an employee of Arthrex, Inc., CONMED Linvatec, Össur, and Smith & Nephew and serves as a board member, owner, officer, or committee member of the American Orthopaedic Society for Sports Medicine, the Arthroscopy Association of North America, and the International Society of Arthroscopy, Knee Surgery, and Orthopaedic Sports Medicine. Neither of the following authors nor any immediate family member has received anything of value from or has stock or stock options held in a commercial company or institution related directly or indirectly to the subject of this chapter: Dr. Dasari and Dr. Gursoy.

TABLE 1 Anatomy of the Meniscus

Property	Medial Meniscus	Lateral Meniscus
Shape	C-shaped structure	U-shaped structure
Length × width	45.7 × 27.4 mm	35.7 × 29.3 mm
Coverage of medial tibial plateau surface area	60%	80%
Anterior root insertion	27.0 mm lateral and distal to the center of the tibial tuberosity	5.0 mm anterolateral to the center of the anterior cruciate ligament and 14.4 mm anteromedial to the lateral tibial eminence apex
Posterior root insertion	11.5 ± 0.9 mm posterior to the medial tibial eminence	5.3 ± 0.3 mm posterior to the lateral tibial eminence

Data from Kean CO, Brown RJ, Chapman J: The role of biomaterials in the treatment of meniscal tears. *PeerJ* 2017;5:e4076; Woodmass JM, LaPrade RF, Sgaglione NA, Nakamura N, Krych AJ: Meniscal repair: Reconsidering indications, techniques, and biologic augmentation. *J Bone Joint Surg Am* 2017;99(14):1222-1231; Johannsen AM, Civitarese DM, Padalecki JR, Goldsmith MT, Wijdicks CA, Laprade RF: Qualitative and quantitative anatomic analysis of the posterior root attachments of the medial and lateral menisci. *Am J Sports Med* 2012;40(10):2342-2347; and Laprade CM, Ellman MB, Rasmussen MT, et al: Anatomy of the anterior root attachments of the medial and lateral menisci. *Am J Sports Med* 2014;42(10):2386-2392.

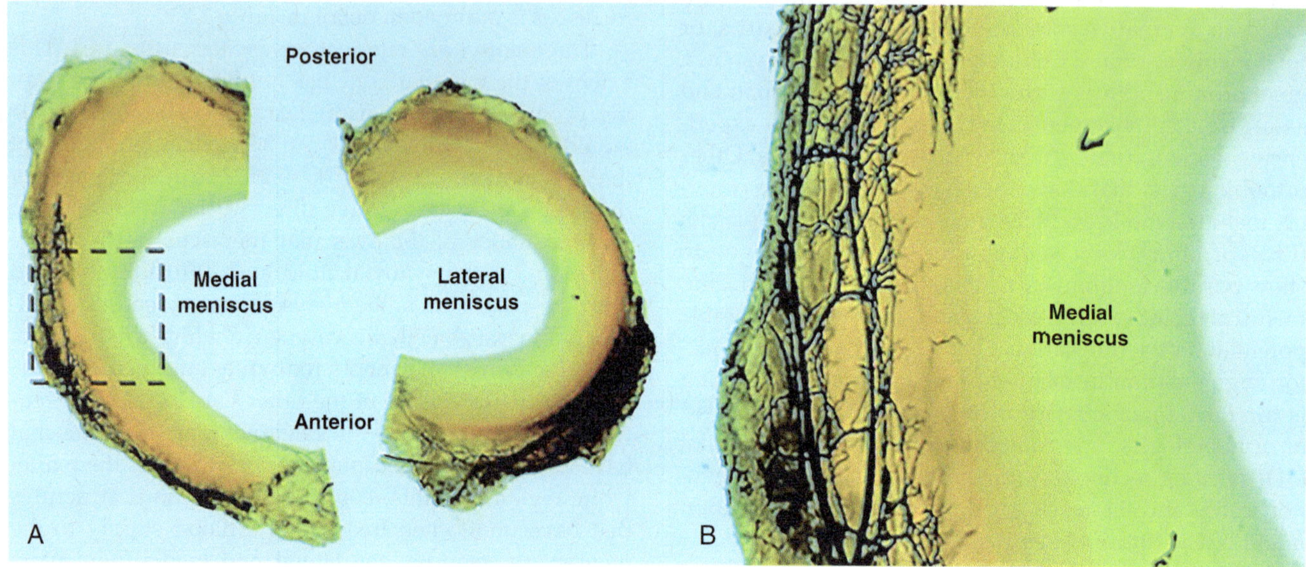

FIGURE 1 Histologic sections (**A** and **B**) of the meniscus stained with India ink showing the peripheral concentration of vasculature within the meniscus and the relative avascularity of the central regions. (Reproduced with permission from Crawford MD, Hellwinkel JE, Aman Z, Akamefula R, Singleton JT, Bahney C, LaPrade RF: Microvascular anatomy and intrinsic gene expression of menisci from young adults. *Am J Sports Med* 2020;48[13]:3147-3153.)

Biomechanics and Function

Menisci have unique anisotropic ECM arrangements, cell types, cellular distributions, and biomechanical features that provide segmental and regional variations that are specific toward their biomechanical function.[3,10] The ECM's circumferential collagen fiber arrangement is specialized to the function of the meniscus. The meniscal fibrils, fibers, and fascicles are arranged in patterns depending on the region of the tissue leading to the innermost region having a structure similar to cartilage because of its small unorganized woven radial collagen fibrils and higher proteoglycan content.[4] The outer regions consist of intertwined collagen fibers that are circumferentially oriented with radially oriented perpendicular fibers known as tie fibers that originate from the joint capsule to form a complex honeycomb network.[4] The meniscus functions by distributing compressive loads through its specialized collagen fiber arrangement.[14]

During axial loading, the forces the meniscus resists are called hoop stresses. Hoop stresses are circumferential forces that are generated when compression along the vertical axis of the meniscus is converted into a horizontal tensile force from the circumferential collagen fiber arrangement within the meniscal ECM.[4] The meniscal ECM also resists shear forces that are developed between the collagen fibers from rotational deformation of the meniscus.[4] Furthermore, the unique meniscal wedge shape is important for improving the articulation and stability between the rounded femoral condyle and the flat tibial plateau.[4] Although the lateral meniscus has been shown to be more mobile, the medial meniscus is more static and acts as a functional synergistic agonist to the anterior cruciate ligament (ACL) by assisting in the resistance of anterior tibial translation. For example, during flexion, biomechanical studies have shown increased mobility of the lateral meniscus with a posterior excursion of 11.2 mm compared with 5.1 mm for the medial meniscus.[15]

Pathology

It is widely accepted that meniscal tears do not heal spontaneously because of the tissue's inherent hypovascularity and hypocellularity. Healing is largely dictated by location of the tear because the red-red and red-white zones have some degree of vascularity and, therefore, a higher healing potential than the avascular white-white zone. The white-white zone has a poor healing capacity because diffusion of synovial fluid does not provide the proper nutrition needed for successful tissue regeneration after a meniscal repair.[16] Furthermore, degenerative tears are unlikely to heal after surgical repair because of the complex patterns of tears, the poor quality of the tissue, and the older patient profile in which they tend to occur.[16] Moreover, even tears with the ideal physical and biologic characteristics have a reported failure rate as high as 30% in young healthy patients.[16]

TEAR TYPES

The menisci can be injured through either a single traumatic event or from cumulative degenerative forces.[1] They are among the most common intra-articular knee injuries and often occur from shear loads that occur on an axially loaded knee experiencing concurrent rotational forces.[1] There is no uniformly accepted classification system for describing meniscal tears, so they are described based on their tear morphology and their anatomic location, which correlates to their vascular supply.[1,17] Cooper et al[18] described a location-based classification system for meniscal tears that attempted to divide the meniscus into circumferential zones, which would subdivide the meniscus based on its vascular supply and radial zones, which would subdivide the meniscus based on its cellularity[17] (**Figure 2, A**). Tears can also be classified based on their thickness using a gradient of 0-III with 0 indicating a normal intact meniscus and III indicating a full-thickness tear.[1]

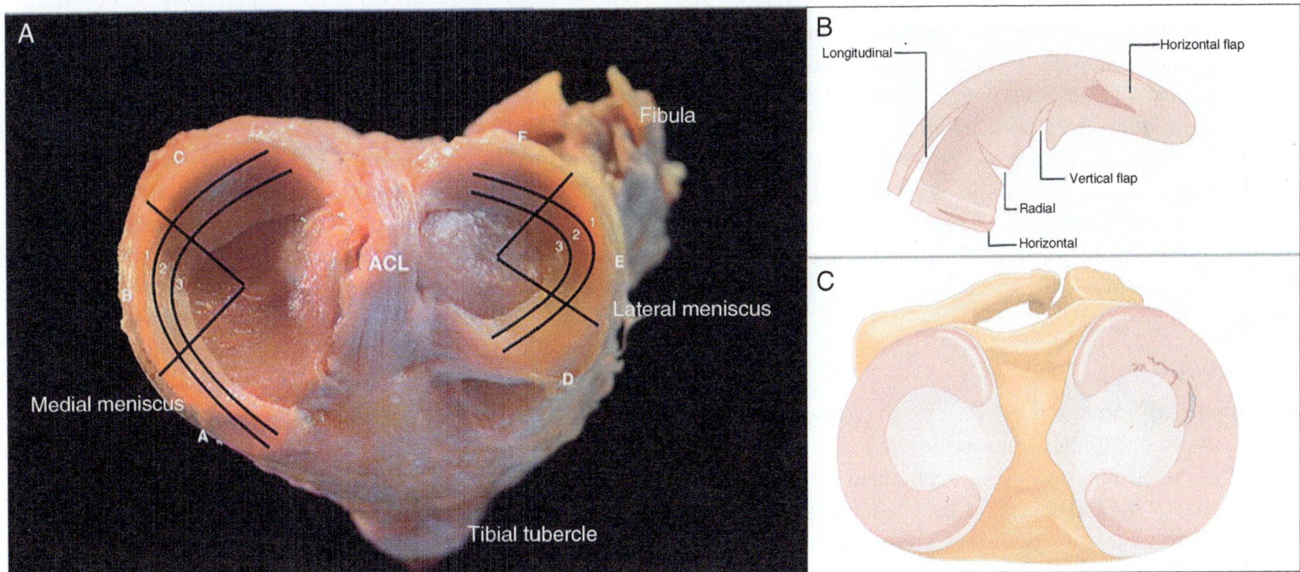

FIGURE 2 **A**, Meniscal Cooper zones. Zone 1 is the peripheral red-red zone with a higher vascular perfusion. Zone 2 is the intermediate red-white zone with a moderate level of perfusion. Zone 3 is the central white-white zone with the lowest vascular supply and healing potential. The menisci are also divided into radial zones from anterior to posterior (A, B, and C for the medial meniscus, and D, E, and F for the lateral meniscus). ACL = anterior cruciate ligament. **B**, Illustration of meniscal tear patterns including a radial tear, a longitudinal tear, a horizontal tear, a vertical flap tear, and a horizontal flap tear. **C**, Illustration of a degenerative medial meniscal tear.

Acute Tears

Acute tears typically occur from traumatic events where there is enough energy to split the meniscal tissue[3] (**Figure 2, B**). During these events, there is a combination of compressive, shear, and rotational forces from the femoral condyles across the meniscus into the tibial plateau.[4] Tear patterns caused by traumatic injuries are longitudinal tears, bucket handle tears, and radial tears.[1,3,4] These tears have the potential to progress into more complex tears and can dislodge tissue leading to locking of the knee during flexion.[4]

Degenerative Tears

Degenerative tears are due to chronic forces acting on the meniscus[4,19] (**Figure 2, C**). Examples include cavitation, fibrillation, and brittle tissue.[3] In the case of calcium pyrophosphate deposition disease, a 2015 cross-sectional study reported that patients with chondrocalcinosis had a meniscal tear rate that was 45.4% higher.[20] The authors postulated that meniscal calcium deposits, termed meniscocalcinosis, led to meniscal biomechanical functional failure, destroyed the meniscal canals, and predisposed the menisci to degenerative changes from minor trauma and simple loading. Regardless of the etiology, these chronic forces lead to horizontal tears, flap tears, and complex tear patterns, which tend to occur in the older patient population.[1,3,4] Because many of these tears remain asymptomatic, it is thought that the incidence of degenerative meniscal tears is much higher than what is currently reported.[4] Root tears can also be observed. Lateral posterior root tears tend to occur with ACL ruptures during a traumatic event, whereas medial meniscal posterior root tears usually are of a degenerative etiology.[3] These degenerative medial meniscal root tears tend to be either horizontal cleavage tears or flap tears with some element of tissue destruction.[4] Beyond just the tear morphology, the meniscal position is of clinical importance because extrusion can occur in root tears, radial tears, and the degenerative tear subtypes leading to further compromised function in regard to force transmission and hoop stresses.[4]

Root Tears

The meniscal roots are critical to the function of the meniscus. A complete tear of the root will render the meniscus nonfunctional. Biomechanical studies have shown that a medial meniscal root tear is equivalent to a total meniscectomy: there are significant increases in tibiofemoral joint contact pressures and decreased contact surface area.[5] Meniscal root tears must be repaired anatomically, because a fixation that is 5 mm off (nonanatomic) will result in the difference between a functional repair and a nonfunctional repair.[5] A nonanatomic repair has significantly decreased contact area within the joint leading to elevated contact pressures and subsequent articular cartilage damage.[5] When repaired anatomically, root repairs have been shown to restore normal contact area and contact pressure within the knee.[5] Because of the extent of altered joint biomechanics associated with meniscal root tears, surgical intervention is indicated whenever possible.[21] If a patient has severe osteoarthritis (Kellgren-Lawrence grade 3 or 4), is obese, or is a poor surgical candidate, then nonsurgical management can be pursued.[5]

Indications for Repair

The surgical treatment of meniscal tears has gradually evolved over the past 2 decades. Initially, surgical intervention aimed to resect damaged portions of the meniscus using either a partial or full meniscectomy. The loss of the meniscus can alter joint mechanics and the local biologic environment, which will promote the early development of osteoarthritis with consequent joint pain, decreased function, and impaired quality of life.[22] It has been observed that the peak contact pressure on the articular cartilage within the knee joint increases by approximately 165% after a partial meniscectomy and approximately 253% after a total meniscectomy.[1] Additionally, in these patients, there is postoperative evidence of reduced muscle strength and altered gait patterns that also contribute to worse clinical outcomes.[1] For these reasons, there has been a shift, with surgeons preferring to attempt repair when possible.[1]

A successfully repaired meniscus will lead to peak joint contact pressures that are similar to those experienced in a joint with an intact native meniscus.[1] Meniscus sutures can stabilize the tear and lead to physiologic repair via the proliferation of native cells involved in tissue regeneration, adhesion, and healing of the lesion in regions with adequate blood flow.[22] Despite this importance, physiologic healing via isolated repair has a failure rate of approximately 25% because of the low healing potential of the meniscus from its poor vascularity and the low cellularity of meniscal tissue.[22] Meniscus repair commonly provides superior clinical outcomes compared with meniscectomy, and, as a general rule, there should be an emphasis on trying to preserve meniscal tissue whenever possible.[3] There have been technical developments over the past decades that have allowed lesions previously considered irreparable (horizontal or radial tears) to have encouraging results with repair.[3] Although it is important to attempt meniscus repair whenever possible, the technique does have specific indications and its own inherent limitations. If a repair is not possible, a partial or total meniscal replacement is an adequate option.[3] The decision is made based on the type of meniscal injury, the condition and function of the joint, the cartilage condition, and the ligament status.

It has generally been considered that white-white meniscal tears could not be successfully repaired. Several studies over the past 30 years have shown that this generalized statement is not entirely true. For example, Rubman et al[23] reported that 80% of 198 white-white repairs were successful. In 2010, Gallacher et al[24] reported a 68% success rate on white-white tears repaired using the all-inside technique with a 16.8-year follow-up. In 2011, Noyes et al[25] also reported a 38% failure rate in a series of 29 white-white tear repairs. It is typically accepted that blood supply is the key factor that determines meniscus repair outcomes. Studies have also shown that the presence of viable meniscal cells plays a crucial role as well: menisci with fewer viable intrinsic cells are more prone to acute or degenerative tears.[17] Histologic examination has demonstrated reduced meniscal cellularity in patients older than 40 years.[17] Despite this, there have been studies reporting a success rate of meniscus repair as high as 86.5% to 88% in patients older than 40 years with and without concomitant anterior cruciate ligament reconstruction (ACLR).[26,27] It has been demonstrated that failure of a meniscal repair does not worsen the outcome or does not necessitate a larger volume of tissue loss should a subsequent meniscectomy be performed.[3] Thus, it is advisable to pursue meniscus repair to save the meniscus and preserve the joint whenever possible.

When this evidence is taken together, a criterion of indications and contraindications can be made. Key contraindications to meniscal repair include the presence of grade 3 to 4 osteoarthritis in the ipsilateral compartment, irreducibility of the tear because the meniscus would be under too high of a tension, and a central radial tear that is less than 25% because these small radial tears have good prognoses with resection.[17] Historically, typical patient factors to consider are the patient's age (younger than 40 years), activity level, comorbidities, body mass index (<30 kg/m^2), and willingness to comply with a postoperative rehabilitation regimen.[17] Tear characteristics to consider are that the tear should have a simple pattern and be present for less than 3 months. It had been thought that only tears in the red-white or red-red zone could be repaired and that concomitant ACLR would lead to unsuccessful repair, but the evidence suggests that meniscal repair in the white-white zone or with concomitant ACLR can be successful and should be pursued when applicable.

Historically, many surgeons would consider the inside-out technique the gold standard of meniscal repair because it allows for a more consistent suture placement that is perpendicular to the tear[17] (**Figure 3, A**). Although generally effective, this technique has been considered suboptimal for managing posterior horn tears; there have been studies suggesting meniscal repair with the inside-out technique puts the saphenous nerve and common peroneal nerve at higher risk.[28] There has been growing interest in the use of all-inside devices, which have become more popular relative to the gold standard inside-out repair[28] (**Figure 3, B**). This is largely because the use of an all-inside device is quicker, does not require a surgical assistant, and does not require an additional incision.[28] Second-generation all-inside devices are suture based with anchors and are designed to sit outside the capsule when used.[28] This allows them to act as fixation points and then the suture ends can be used to apply tension, reduce the tear, and pull the torn meniscus edges together[28] (**Figure 4**). The size and shape of the all-inside device might make it relatively difficult to handle when trying to repair the anterior or intermediate third of the meniscus, so this may be a region where the inside-out suture technique is still preferred.[28] For tears adjacent to the anterior horn, the outside-in repair may be the

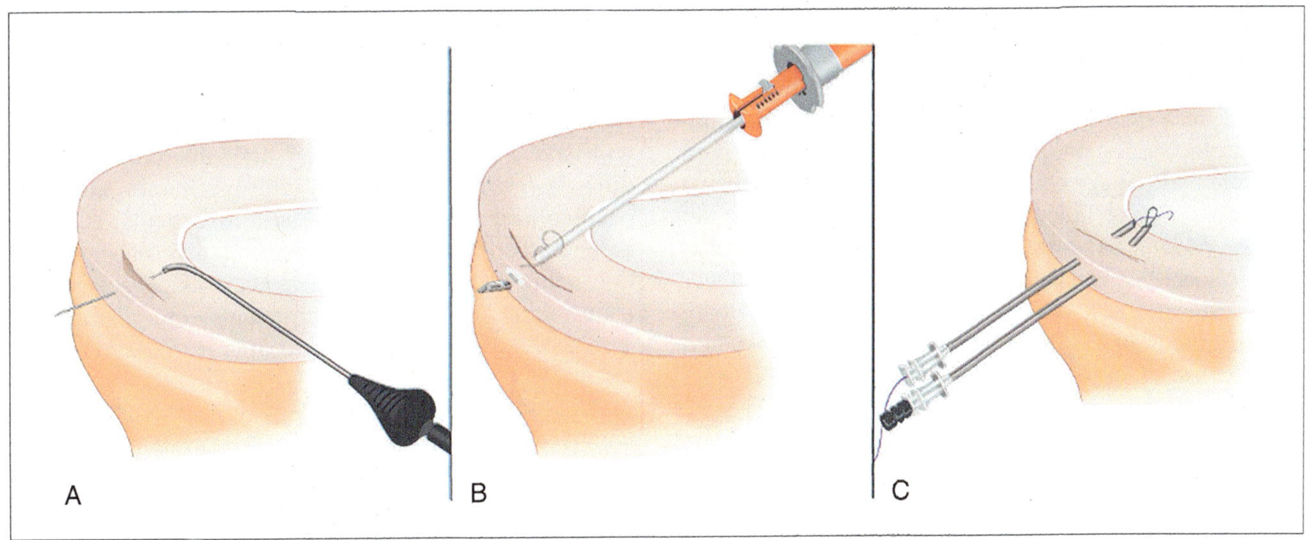

FIGURE 3 Meniscal repair techniques. Illustrations show the inside-out (**A**), all-inside (**B**), and outside-in (**C**) techniques.

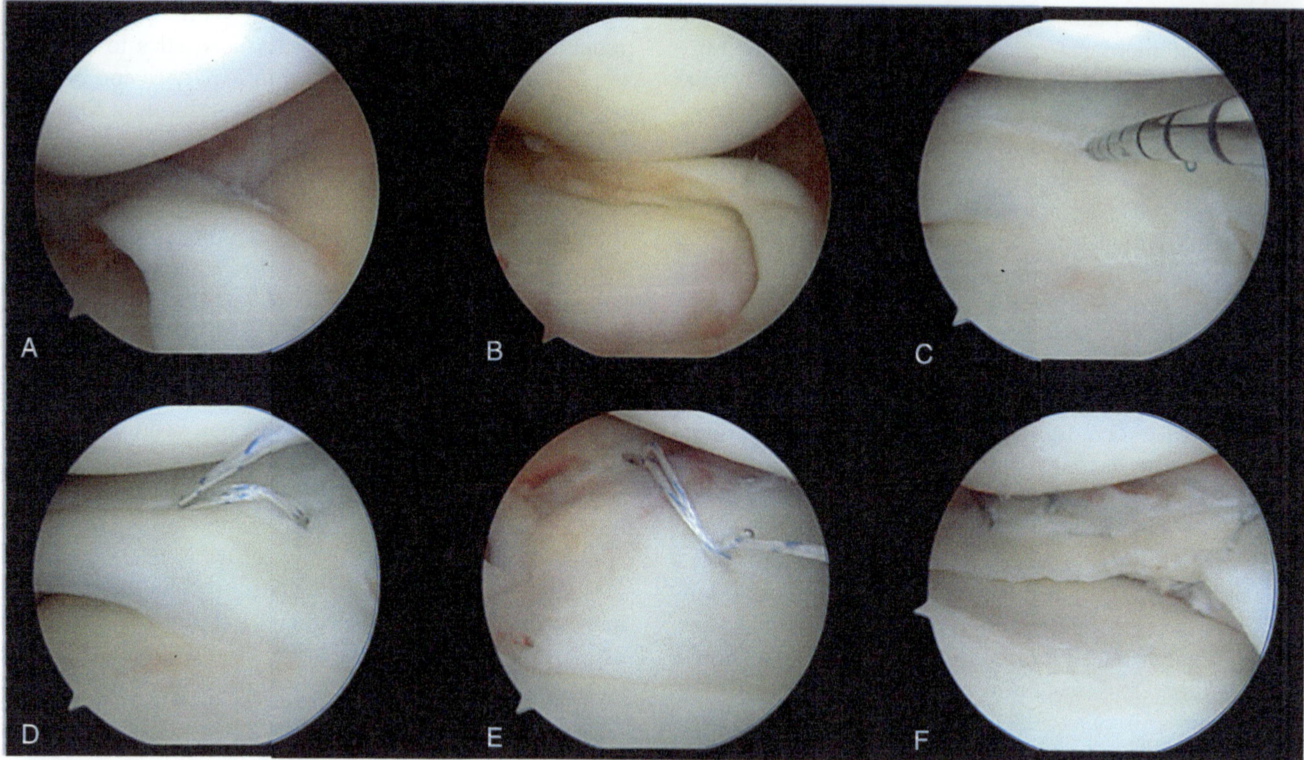

FIGURE 4 Arthroscopic images of bucket-handle tear (**A** and **B**) repaired with the all-inside technique (**C**) in horizontal mattress (**D**) and vertical mattress (**E**) configuration. Panel **F** represents the final repaired construct.

best-suited surgical technique as it will ensure the sutures are placed perpendicular to the tear to facilitate optimal healing[17,21,28] (**Figure 3, C**). This is because the technique is able to achieve adequate access to the anterior horn of the meniscus, provide a stable fixation construct, and avoid leaving prominent intra-articular material.[21] This procedure has the added benefits of small incisions, low neurovascular risk, and high success rate.[21]

An optimized rehabilitation protocol is critical for maximizing the success of a meniscal repair. Because of the lack of a clear superiority for accelerated rehabilitation protocols, the frequency of meniscal injuries with multiple tear pattern combinations, and the implications associated with a failed meniscal repair, Woodmass et al[6] proposed a standardized meniscal repair rehabilitation protocol that can be homogeneously used for all tear types. During the first 4 weeks, the patient is to remain toe-touch weight bearing, use a knee immobilizer, and have restricted range of motion (ROM) from 0° to 90°. After 4 weeks, the patient will no longer need a knee immobilizer and can now begin partial weight bearing with a loaded ROM from 0° to 90°. At 6 weeks, the patient can begin full weight bearing but must continue to maintain a restricted loaded and unloaded ROM from 0° to 90°. By 8 weeks, the patient will have no unloaded ROM restriction but should continue to maintain a loaded ROM restriction from 0° to 90°. After 16 weeks, the patient can have a full-loaded ROM with no restrictions.

CURRENT THERAPEUTIC OPTIONS FOR MENISCAL DEFICIENCY

Although meniscal repair should be considered in all patients, when possible, there are many patients with meniscal injuries who are not good candidates for repair. For patients who cannot undergo meniscal repair or who have failed a prior meniscal repair, a partial or total meniscectomy is recommended. Unfortunately, these patients will have a meniscal deficiency after this type of procedure that will lead to altered joint mechanics, increased peak contact pressures, and resulting articular cartilage damage. For this patient population, a promising solution with good clinical evidence is meniscal replacement using either an allograft for patients undergoing total meniscectomy or a scaffold for patients undergoing partial meniscectomy.

Meniscal allograft transplantation (MAT) has been widely performed after total meniscectomies (**Figure 5**). MAT is indicated for patients with ipsilateral joint line tenderness in the compartment treated with a prior meniscectomy, those in whom prior nonsurgical treatment has failed, those younger than 55 years, and those with absence of diffuse Outerbridge grade 3 or 4 cartilage

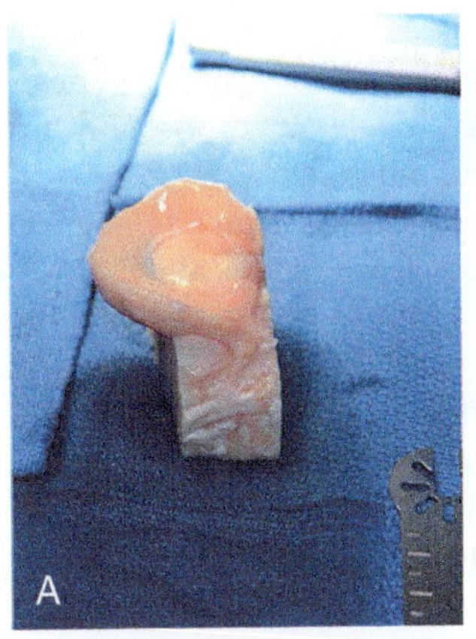

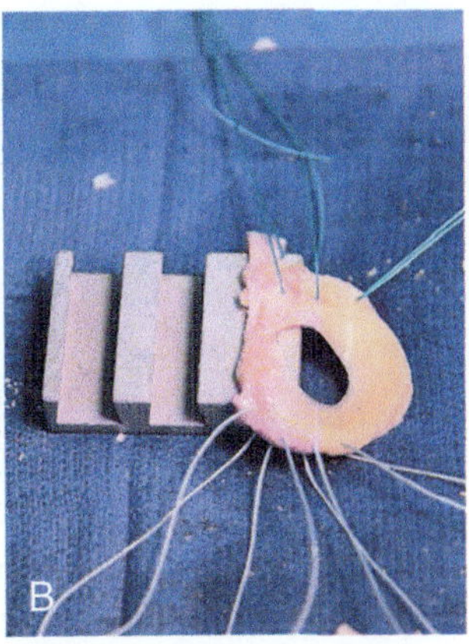

FIGURE 5 Photographs show right knee lateral meniscal allograft attached to the tibial plateau (**A**) and measurement for implantation (**B**).

damage, body mass index less than 35 kg/m^2, and a stable well-aligned knee.[2,29-31] General contraindications to MAT include older age, evidence of Outerbridge grade 3 or 4 osteoarthritis, and obesity.[2,31] Drawbacks and limitations of MAT include immunologic reaction, the risk of disease transmission, and limited donor availability.[2] There is also difficulty with the technique due to graft size matching and intricacies associated with preservation and optimal surgical technique.[2]

There is ample evidence to suggest that MAT has good clinical outcomes for patients and should be considered for patients undergoing total meniscectomy who meet the indications. Several separate systematic reviews performed from 2011 to 2019 found that MAT resulted in improved clinical outcomes for up to 14 years after surgery, that 77% to 85% of patients were able to return to their prior level of function and competition, and that concomitant procedures did not worsen MAT outcomes.[29,32-37] In an ideal candidate, an isolated MAT has greater than 70% survivorship at 10 years, leading to decreased knee pain, improved functional knee scores, and increased patient satisfaction.[31,38] A study that defined failure as transplant removal, revision, or tibiofemoral pain after daily activities evaluated 40 grafts at 5, 10, and 15 years after surgery and found survival rates of 88%, 63%, and 40%, respectively.[39]

Biomechanical studies have reported that the most important properties of MAT were proper graft sizing and secure fixation.[29,40] Appropriately sizing the allograft is essential for the long-term success of the transplant as oversized grafts unequally distribute the load, whereas undersized grafts increase the hoop stress on the meniscus, leading to a higher risk for rupture.[3,14,31] In terms of fixation, the technique used to secure the allograft depends on the author's preference and the transplantation site. Despite the plethora of grafts and fixation techniques available, with the bone fixation technique being the most commonly used, there is insufficient evidence to recommend a clinically superior fixation technique.[29-31,41] Cadaver studies have shown that bone plugs or bone blocks used for allograft attachment performed better and had increased chondroprotective effects compared with circumferential suturing.[40] Interestingly, when studied clinically, there was no significant difference in patient outcomes, failure rate, or allograft tear rates between patients who underwent MAT with soft-tissue sutures versus bone fixation.[42]

Among the bone fixation techniques, biomechanical studies have also suggested that MAT with a bone plug demonstrated superior load transmission.[14] The benefits of the bone bridge technique are to protect the collateral ligament attachments, to maintain the relationship of the anterior and posterior horns, and the ease of the insertion.[31] The bone plug is preferred for surgeons who prefer to be able to adjust the attachment site of the roots.[31] For clinical application, the bone bridge technique might be preferable for lateral MAT because of the smaller distance between the anterior and posterior horns, whereas the bone plug technique may be preferable for securing medial MAT because of the larger distance between root attachment sites, the easier fracture of the bone bridge during insertion, and the concern of disrupting the ACL tibial insertion site.[3,31]

In addition to the optimization of graft fixation constructs, there have also been substantial biologic efforts on the cellular level to maximize MAT viability and integration with the host. Unlike cryopreserved allografts, fresh allografts maintain cellular viability as the transplanted donor cells continue to have normal or near-normal function and synthesize proteoglycans as well as collagen fibers after implantation.[43] However, histologic evidence demonstrates that after transplantation, the graft undergoes rapid repopulation with host cells from the synovial membrane.[34,44,45] Despite repopulation, there remains central portions of the graft that remain largely acellular.[45,46] Subsequent studies have attempted to optimize meniscus allograft transplant viability and integration through various augmentation techniques aimed at increasing cellular repopulation of the graft. For example, Nordberg et al[47] demonstrated enhanced cellular infiltration in grafts that were needle-punched, and postulated on the potential clinical benefit their findings would have on improved postoperative remodeling. A 2022 study by Struijk et al[48] reported on the feasibility of augmenting frozen human meniscal allografts with mesenchymal stem cell injections and demonstrated robust active cell proliferation, migration, and survival within the graft. Although these preclinical studies have demonstrated a promising ability to maximize cellular infiltration and repopulation during MAT, it remains to be seen if this benefit translates to the clinical setting.

Like meniscal repair, postoperative rehabilitation is a critical component for the management of meniscal injuries with a MAT. For patients who have underwent a MAT, Saltzman et al[49] outlined a rehabilitation protocol that begins with partial weight bearing for 2 weeks while the patient's leg is kept in extension with a knee brace. The patient is allowed gentle passive and active ROM from 0° to 90°. Weight bearing is gradually increased over weeks 3 to 8 until full weight bearing and ROM are established. High-impact activities, such as running, are permitted by week 16 and a full return to activity is allowed by 6 to 9 months after surgery. The authors reported improvements in pain, function, and patient satisfaction over a minimum of 7 years follow-up using MAT supplemented with this rehabilitation protocol.

ORTHOBIOLOGICS IN MENISCAL INJURY

To further enhance the repair potential of a torn meniscus, biologic augmentation has been attempted to promote healing of these injuries. There are increasing data to support the use of scaffolds and allografts for meniscal replacement when there is a partial or total meniscus defect present, but there are limitations to these techniques.[16] This has led to the development of biologic augmentation and tissue engineering approaches to meniscus repair and replacement.[16] Biologic augmentation attempts to overcome the inherent limitations of healing from hypocellularity and poor vascularity by promoting chemotaxis, cellular proliferation, and ECM production at the repair site.[16] Much of this is based on the findings that concomitant ACLR has superior meniscal repair outcomes when compared with isolated meniscal repair.[14,16,29] This was attributed to the release of cells and growth factors from the nearby bone marrow when tunnels are drilled for ACLR.[14,29] Thus, mechanical techniques traditionally provided this by creating vascular access, stimulating cells, cytokines, and bone marrow cells in the vicinity of the repair.[2,16] Over the past 2 decades, there has been a turn to orthobiologics as a way to enhance meniscal healing and improve meniscal tear clinical outcomes. This has included the use of exogenous fibrin clots, PRP, growth factors, stem cells, scaffolds, and other tissue engineering approaches to enhance the healing on meniscal tears.

BIOMATERIALS

Biomaterials are substances that can be used to partially or completely augment or replace a tissue, organ, or function to improve the quality of life for an individual.[1] They can be synthetic or natural in origin and must be able to interact with the surrounding human tissue and/or body fluids to improve/replace an anatomical functional defect.[1] Common natural biomaterials include type I and type II collagen-based products, whereas common synthetic biomaterials include polyglycolic acid, poly-L-lactic acid, or a composite mixture.[1] Biomaterials function by providing scaffold layers for cellular attachment, growth, and differentiation.[1] They also function by facilitating the transport of proteins and genetic material to regenerate viable functional tissue.[1] Biocompatibility is a critical property of biomaterials. Biocompatibility is the ability of the substrate to exist in contact with natural tissues in vivo without causing an unacceptable degree of harm.[1] For the optimal biomaterial, a utopian state exists where the biomaterial does not adversely affect the physiologic environment nor does the inverse occur.[1] In a 2017 expert review on the role of biomaterials in the treatment of meniscal tears, Kean et al[1] proposed five criteria for the ideal biomaterial, which are outlined in **Table 2**. Currently, the primary application of biomaterials in the field of meniscal injuries is to function as an acellular scaffold that provides biomechanical support and, in certain constructs, facilitates the regeneration of meniscal tissue.

TABLE 2 The Five Criteria of an Ideal Biomaterial
1. The material must be a support structure for cells and have biomechanical functions to protect cells from damaging compressive forces when used for meniscal regeneration. It must have sufficient strength to keep the cells mechanically stable with their respective cell attachments maintained. It must maintain stability, strength, and integrity until tissue regeneration has occurred.
2. It must withstand forces during joint movement. For biomaterials used to treat meniscal injuries, compressive and tensile forces must be withstood.
3. Bioactivity should allow for cellular attachment and cellular migration to promote tissue regeneration. Chemotactic gradients can be used to provide directional guidance to allow endogenous cells to travel through the biomaterial and facilitate healing/integration with the surrounding host tissue.
4. There should be a degree of biodegradability to allow the biomaterial to remodel as novel cartilage replaces it. This requires the construct to be nontoxic and nonadhering.
5. It should be nonimmunogenic and nonstimulating to host inflammatory cells.

Adapted with permission from Kean CO, Brown RJ, Chapman J: The role of biomaterials in the treatment of meniscal tears. *PeerJ* 2017;5:e4076.

Meniscal Scaffolds

Meniscal scaffolds are a promising clinical application where orthobiologics are used to treat a challenging pathologic condition. If a patient undergoes a partial meniscectomy, there will be no natural healing response because of the meniscus' limited healing capacity. For these partial meniscal deficiencies, meniscal scaffolds can be used to overcome these remaining defects by trying to aid in the regeneration of native meniscal tissue.[9] The key challenge with scaffold-based therapy for partial meniscus injuries is finding a scaffold strong enough for suture repair yet compressible enough to avoid articular cartilage damage when weight bearing.[10]

Although there have been many scaffolds studied using in vitro and in vivo models, to date there are only two designs approved for clinical use: the collagen meniscus implant (CMI; Ivy Sports Medicine), which is FDA approved in the United States because of early promising results in Europe, and the polyurethane polymeric implant (Actifit; Orteq Ltd), which is currently only approved in Europe. These devices are available to patients with an intact peripheral rim, preserved meniscal roots, and minimally damaged cartilage after a partial meniscectomy.[2,3,14] Although these devices have shown significant improvements in pain and function with a low rate of implant failure in several studies, they have also been associated with negative outcomes such as implant resorption, hyperintensity, extrusion, and subchondral bone edema based on MRI findings.[2] Other major challenges with these implants include the technical difficulty using an arthroscopic approach, the challenge to suture them, an unproven benefit in preventing the progression of osteoarthritis, and that these implants do not regenerate meniscal tissue.[14] Despite these drawbacks, partial meniscal replacement using the CMI scaffold or the Actifit scaffold has demonstrated promising clinical results in numerous studies and is a viable treatment option for symptomatic patients who meet the adequate indications. Currently, the most recent European Society of Sports Traumatology, Knee Surgery and Arthroscopy consensus statement provided a grade A recommendation that partial meniscal replacement is only recommended for patients in whom prior meniscal surgeries have failed and for patients who have continued to report meniscal-related complaints after a partial meniscectomy.[50]

Surgical Technique

The surgical implantation of these scaffolds is done arthroscopically (**Figure 6**). The damaged meniscus is débrided until healthy tissue is reached. For the CMI device, if débridement does not extend to the red zone of the meniscus, then a microfracture awl or spinal needle is used along the peripheral rim to enhance blood supply.[51] For the Actifit scaffold, the débridement should extend to the vascular red-red zones.[51] At this point, the defect can be measured, and the scaffold is cut to match the defect. It is advised to slightly oversize the scaffold.[3] A suture is used to bring the scaffold into place, and fixation is performed.[3] For the CMI scaffold, the implant is attached to the healthy remaining meniscal tissue using standard inside-out suture technique with 2-0 nonabsorbable braided sutures.[51] For the Actifit implant, the scaffold is sutured to the peripheral rim using a hybrid suture technique with all-inside sutures and outside-in sutures.[51]

As with meniscal repair and transplantation, the ultimate success of partial meniscal replacement using a scaffold depends on the postoperative rehabilitation regimen. For the Actifit construct, nonsurgical rehabilitation protocols aim to provide an optimal environment for tissue healing and integration into the scaffold. A standardized 16- to 24-week protocol is recommended for these patients to achieve this goal.[52] Patients begin partial weight bearing at week 4. This will gradually ramp up to full weight bearing by week 9. Patients are then instructed to gradually increase their level of activity until 6 months postoperative. At this point, they can begin a gradual return to sports and higher impact activities. Similar to the Actifit implant, rehabilitation protocols with the CMI scaffold were more nonsurgical than traditional rehabilitation for meniscal repair.[53] In a protocol outlined by Zaffagnini et al,[54] patients began with a restricted ROM from 0° to 60° that can be increased to 90° of flexion by 4 weeks and a full ROM by 6 weeks. The patient is allowed to have partial weight-bearing status for the first 6 weeks before transitioning to a full weight-bearing status. The patient should plan to return to full activity by approximately 6 months. These rehabilitation protocols were developed based on the respective manufacturer recommendations. A key difference in the rehabilitation protocols between these two scaffolds is an earlier transition to partial and full weight bearing for patients treated with the CMI scaffold. This is a potential benefit that must be considered and discussed with any patient that is eligible for both constructs.

Clinically Approved Scaffolds

The CMI implant is based on a type I collagen matrix taken from bovine Achilles tendons.[3,51] It was initially designed for patients who have lost more than 50% of their meniscus but still had preserved meniscal roots and an intact peripheral rim.[55] Compared with other scaffold constructs, it theoretically has a more biocompatible profile and is designed to act as a regenerative template with which meniscal tissue can grow into.[3,51] It has a porous structure allowing for cellular infiltration to occur on implantation.[10] This mechanism requires some viable meniscal tissue from the preserved meniscal rim to be present.[51] Because there is facilitated ingrowth and regeneration of new meniscal tissue, the CMI scaffold is designed to reabsorb within 12 to 18 months of implantation.[51]

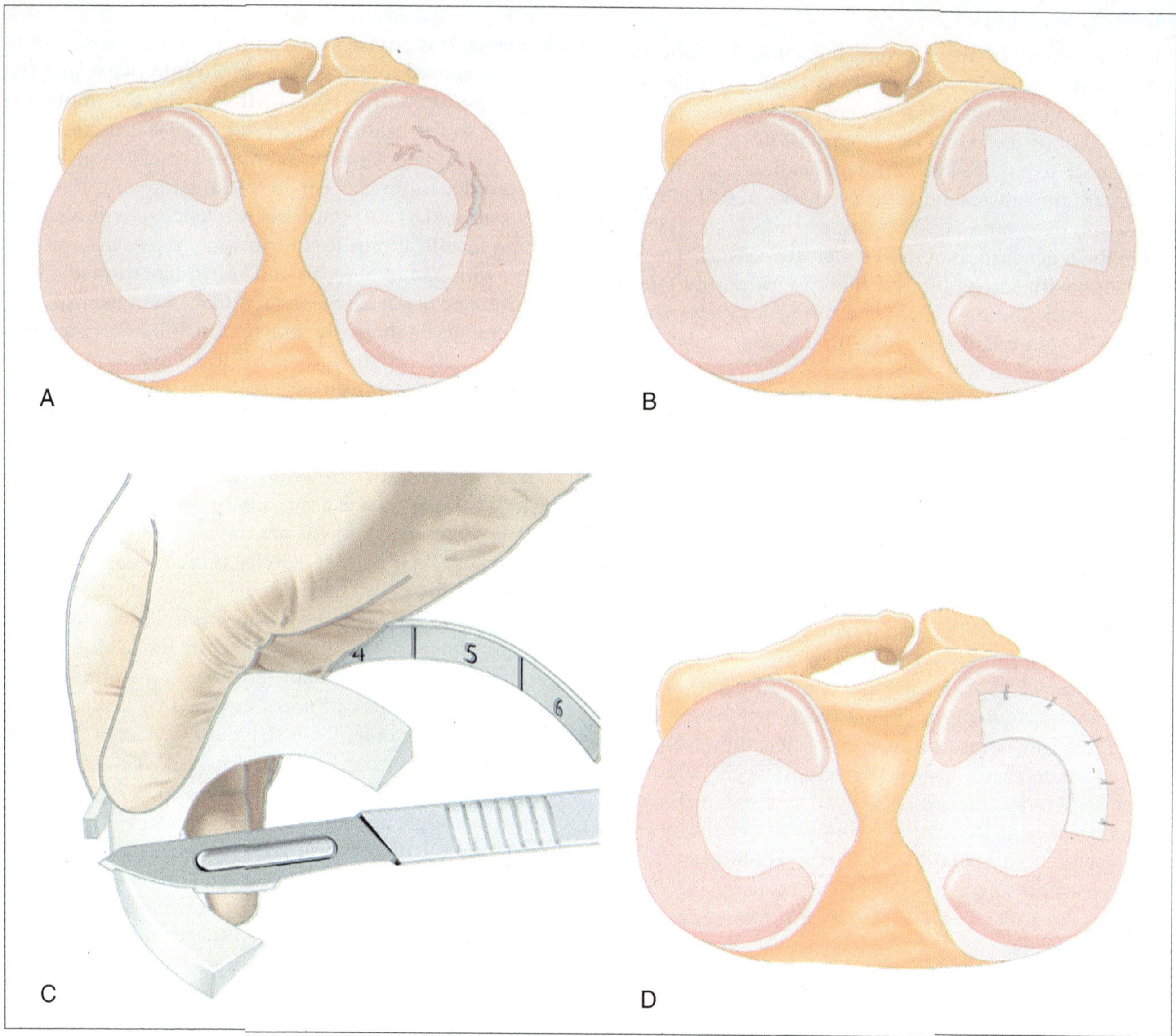

FIGURE 6 Illustrations show the step-by-step surgical technique for partial meniscus replacement using a meniscal scaffold. **A**, A degenerative, irreparable tear of the medical meniscus is shown. **B**, Débridement of the tear. **C**, A meniscal implant is then prepared according to the defect size. **D**, The implant is placed into the meniscal defect area.

The Actifit scaffold is a biodegradable construct consisting of porous synthetic poly-ε-caprolactone (80%) and urethane segments (20%). It is designed to slowly degrade over 5 years via mechanical breakdown of the urethane segments and macrophage phagocytosis.[51,55] This will provide a template for tissue ingrowth as it slowly wears away and is replaced by native tissue.[51] Unlike the CMI device, this allows it to assist with pain relief by functionally providing biomechanical support in addition to gradually restoring lost meniscal tissue as it degrades.[51] Second-look arthroscopy and histologic examination have shown that integration and immature meniscus-like tissue can be seen at approximately 1 year after implantation.[55]

A 2021 systematic review by Veronesi et al[56] sought to summarize the clinical results of the two implants. The authors identified 10 prospective studies with 593 patients who were treated with the CMI scaffold and 19 studies, of which 16 were prospective, that analyzed clinical outcomes for 777 patients treated with the Actifit scaffold. When compared with patients who underwent meniscectomy only, patients who underwent meniscectomy and were treated with the CMI scaffold consistently reported improved symptomatic relief and knee function even in cases with concomitant ACLR.[57,58] A study by Bulgheroni et al[59] evaluated the long-term efficacy of CMI implants. At a mean follow-up of 9.6 years, they found that patients who underwent partial meniscectomy and were treated with CMI implants reported substantial pain relief and functional improvement, and there was a low rate of implant failure. Efe et al[60] and Akkaya et al[61] found similarly good clinical outcome scores in patients treated with the Actifit implant. A study by Schüttler et al[62] in 2016 reported the 4-year outcomes of patients undergoing partial meniscectomy treated with Actifit implants. These authors also reported high levels of patient satisfaction with low pain scores, improved knee function, and minimal evidence of articular cartilage damage on MRI. A 2018 systematic review by Houck et al[51] attempted to compare the two implants against each other. The authors found both groups reported improvements in visual analog scale pain scores, Lysholm knee scores, Knee Injury and Osteoarthritis Outcome Score, and Tegner activity scores. They also reported a failure rate of 9.9% for the Actifit group and 6.7% for the CMI group. Additionally, when reviewed on imaging, CMI scaffolds had superior morphology and signal intensity relative to the Actifit group, whereas the Actifit group had increased coronal meniscal extrusion. On second-look arthroscopy, the CMI groups had new tissue growth that was grossly meniscal like, whereas the Actifit group revealed a yellowish scaffold that was integrated with the surrounding tissue and apparently had shrunk.[63] A separate study by Papalia et al[64] suggested that the radiologic and histologic final outcomes were similar between the two scaffold groups, leading the authors to think that both scaffolds had comparable regenerative and resorbable properties. Only one nonrandomized trial directly compared the two scaffolds and found no difference in clinical outcome scores.[65] Although there is ample clinical evidence to support the use of both techniques, there is no enough evidence to suggest one implant is superior to the other.

Other Biomaterials and Scaffolds

A variety of synthetic and natural materials have been investigated to use as scaffolds for engineering the meniscus.[14] Hydrogels are biomaterials that can be natural or synthetic and can seamlessly integrate into water matrices.[1] These constructs consist of hydrated polymer networks which absorb and retain fluids, giving them a high water-based content.[1] The key functional properties of hydrogels include their monomeric composition, their cross-linking density which makes them insoluble, and their polymerization ability.[1] The high hydration threshold and insoluble nature of hydrogels make them appealing for tissue mimetics.[1] Because they often fall short of the native meniscus properties and have limited biomechanical function, they are primarily used to deliver cells or growth factors.[16] Chitosan is another biomaterial that is used to make sutures that require exceptional integrity and physical strength.[1] Thus, they are the material of choice for sutures that improve the mechanical properties of the knee healing process.[1]

Nanofibers are electrospun scaffolds that have seen an increased role in regenerative medicine as they have the ability to mimic the anisotropy of fibrous tissues while also withstanding high load forces imposed on musculoskeletal tissues during motion.[1] A prominent example of electrospun nanofibers would be the polyethylene fibers in the NUsurface (Active Implants, LLC) implant. The fibers can also be tailored to influence cellular interactions, to control when cells will be induced to proliferate, and when/where cells will deposit ECM on the fiber network.[1] Additionally, cells prefer to align in an ordered pattern along the scaffold fibers.[1] Seeding of these nanofiber networks with cells preoperatively can then be used to develop promising tissue engineering constructs.[1]

Silk scaffolds are a natural biomaterial that were proposed for partial meniscal regeneration and can be used as acellular scaffolds or are cultivated with human bone marrow cells to form cellular scaffolds, which have been shown to possess superior biomechanical properties.[10] An example is the Fibrofix (Orthox Ltd., Abingdon, UK) meniscus scaffold, which is derived from silk. In biomechanical studies, Stein et al[66] reported improved coverage of contact areas, improved force distribution, and reduced peak pressures when comparing the Fibrofix scaffold to patients undergoing partial meniscectomy; however, the values were still inferior to the native meniscus. This construct is currently undergoing clinical trials.[10]

Biomaterials can be acellular, cell laden, biodegradable, and nonbiodegradable. Cell-free biomaterials have inherent advantages including ease of use, prolonged shelf life, availability, and cost.[10] Nonbiodegradable materials can provide extended mechanical support with gel/fluid-like components being potentially used as injectable depots for smaller defects.[10] Stiff solid constructs can support preseeded cells that facilitate cellular infiltration.[10] Cell-laden biomaterials have the advantage of living cells repairing and replenishing ECM and missing tissue to fill in the defect with components most similar to the native tissue as the scaffold gradually degrades over time.[10] It has been proven that each scaffold for meniscus regeneration has its own inherent advantages.[16] Models have shown that circumferential and axial/radial module are important determinants of the contact pressure distribution in the native meniscus and should be matched in replacement technology.[16] Ultimately, a successfully designed meniscal scaffold should primarily provide biomechanical stability in the short term and allow for cellular infiltration to facilitate generation of meniscal tissue in the long term.[16] Although there is great interest in the development of biomaterials, it is apparent that there are few studies in the literature attempting to evaluate the clinical applicability of these substances. The reduction in the number of reports available when searching for clinical studies compared with in vitro studies reflects the immense translational difficulties in turning laboratory investigation into a clinical application.[16]

CELLULAR SOLUTIONS

The complex phenotype of meniscal tissue poses a challenging problem and tissue regeneration using stem cell therapy may be the key to adequately managing meniscal tears.[4] These cellular solutions can be used directly via an injection to augment healing, or they can be used in tissue engineering constructs, where scaffolds are seeded with cells in an attempt to regenerate meniscal tissue. The cell type used to treat and develop the cartilage is crucial in the field of biomaterial development: various cell populations have been investigated for this purpose including chondrocytes, progenitor stem cells, bone marrow stromal cells, and perichondrocytes.[1] The use of meniscal and progenitor cells have been shown to be effective in regenerating meniscal tissue; however, because of its unacceptable donor morbidity and lack of intrinsic chondrogenic potential, meniscal cells have fallen out of favor as a less desirable therapeutic option.[4] Thus, most of the cellular solutions for treating meniscal injuries primarily revolve around the potential of progenitor cells.[4] Progenitor cells are promising because of their ease of availability and differentiation capabilities. Sources of progenitor cells include bone marrow aspirate, adipose tissue, and synovial tissue.

Meniscal regeneration occurs via an intrinsic and an extrinsic pathway. The intrinsic pathway is thought to have minor contributions to repair and is driven by the cellularity of the meniscus and the self-healing capability of the damaged meniscal tissue.[67] After a meniscal injury, the number of synovial progenitor cells has been shown to increase in a natural attempt to provide endogenous cells for repair.[68] Typically, for lesions with poor vascularity, this intrinsic mechanism alone is inadequate. The extrinsic pathway is dependent on the vascularity and cellularity of the damaged meniscal tissue. Growth factors and undifferentiated progenitor cells can modulate and encourage meniscal regeneration by augmenting this extrinsic pathway of meniscal repair.[4] Growth factors play a critical role in modulating meniscal vascularity but also progenitor cell's activity, differentiation, and phenotype.[4] Progenitor cells have a paracrine function where they secrete growth factors to modulate angiogenesis, cell migration, differentiation, and numerous additional localized healing processes.[69]

With regard to the intrinsic pathway of meniscus healing, recent evidence has demonstrated a clear presence of resident progenitor cells within the meniscus in both animal and human models.[70,71] This recent development has translated to clinical practice and manifested in the management of meniscal tears involving central portions of the meniscus. Historically, white-white zones were thought to have poor healing potential and were not traditionally considered amenable to successful repair.[13] A 2021 study by Chahla et al[11] demonstrated the presence of multipotent mesenchymal stromal progenitor cells in addition to vascularization in the white-white zone of the meniscus, suggesting these tears have greater healing potential than previously recognized. A 2020 study by Sun et al[70] echoed these findings using single cell RNA sequencing and demonstrated a clear, unique population of progenitor cells within the meniscus that are suitable for tissue reconstruction and tissue engineering constructs. Additionally, a prior study by Seol et al[71] demonstrated that the red-red zone of the meniscus contained a population of migratory progenitor cells that were able to mobilize to damaged white zones of the meniscus and provide strong reparative potential to the central meniscus. These recent findings would indicate that there is greater intrinsic healing potential within the meniscus than previously thought.

Extrinsic progenitor cell treatment modalities can also be implemented to augment meniscus repair. Although there is a lack of adequate clinical studies, the early data have been promising and supported the use of progenitor cells in the treatment of meniscal repair. Additionally, thus far, there have been no safety concerns or adverse effects noted with the clinical use of progenitor cell injections.[4] A double-blind randomized controlled study compared the outcomes of patients who underwent partial meniscectomy who received progenitor cell injections with a control group who received a hyaluronic acid injection.[72] The authors reported significantly higher increases in meniscal volume compared with the control group. No patient in the control group demonstrated a significant increase in meniscal volume which was defined a priori by the authors as 15%. There have also been several case reports throughout the literature of patients being successfully treated with progenitor cell injections.[4] Onoi et al[73] presented a case report of two patients who underwent partial meniscectomy for degenerative posterior horn medial meniscal tears. These patients received adipose tissue stem cell injections. At 6 months postinjection, a second-look arthroscopy showed improvement in cartilage status and partial regeneration of the resected meniscal segments for both patients. In 2019, Sekiya et al[74] performed a case series of progenitor cell injections for degenerative medial meniscal tears in five patients after arthroscopic meniscus repair. The progenitor cells were taken from synovial tissue biopsy done during the meniscus repair and were grown for 14 days before being delivered via a repeat arthroscopy.[4] The patients reported significant clinical score improvements at 2 years and 3D MRI showed no evidence of a tear at the repair site.

In contrast to the use of stem cell injections, tissue engineering attempts to regenerate tissue by combining biomaterials with cellular solutions. Tissue-engineered constructs can be designed and modified by combining various cell lines and scaffold biomaterials together. It is difficult to build a tissue-engineered construct that generates functional tissue without the appropriate stimulation.[75] Stimulation by biomechanical or biochemical sources is essential for the success of tissue-engineered constructs and can be used to enhance the maturation and remodeling of these designs.[75] Thus, the three elements of tissue engineering are the seeded cells, the scaffold used, and the biomechanical/biochemical stimulation provided. An exciting example of a tissue-engineered construct is the cell bandage described by Whitehouse et al in 2017.[76] The cell bandage is composed of autologous bone marrow–derived progenitor cells embedded in a collagen sponge that is placed between the torn edges of the native meniscus which is then sutured close.[76] At 24 months after surgery, the authors reported promising clinical results with an improvement in International Knee Documentation Committee, Tegner, and Lysholm scores. A study by Olivios-Meza et al[77] compared polyurethane meniscal scaffolds with or without autologous progenitor cell seeding. The authors found significant clinical improvements in Lysholm scores from baseline for both groups at 12 months, but there was no significant difference between the groups. When evaluating the patients' MRI findings, there was no difference noted between the groups. These early results using tissue-engineering constructs to regenerate meniscus tissue have been promising and have shown good clinical outcomes.

BLOOD-DERIVED PRODUCTS

Although the use of progenitor cells has been promising, there have also been several studies investigating the use of blood-derived products as a way to overcome the inherent poor healing capacity of the meniscus and augment the extrinsic pathway of meniscal repair. Thus far, there has been clinical evidence examining the use of PRP and fibrin clots in meniscal repair augmentation. As the understanding of the role of growth hormones in meniscal regeneration continues to evolve, there will be an increased availability of clinical studies exploring the use of growth factors such as transforming growth factor beta (TGF-ß) in this field.

Platelet-Rich Plasma

PRP is an orthobiologic that has been studied with great interest as a potential augment for meniscal repair. There is a theoretical belief that the anabolic potential of PRP can be used to enhance cellular proliferation and matrix production by increased release of growth factors and bioactive molecules.[22] It is an attractive option because it is autologous, easy to prepare, and has a high concentration of factors including platelet-derived growth factor, TGF-ß1, vascular endothelial growth factor, and insulinlike growth factor-1.[22] The clinical efficacy of PRP has been well examined with good clinical outcomes in several studies.[22]

In a 2015 prospective case-control study by Pujol et al,[78] 34 patients with horizontal meniscal tears were treated with mini-arthrotomic meniscal suture with or without PRP augmentation. The PRP group had higher clinical and MRI scores. A 2015 retrospective study by Griffin et al[79] analyzed 35 patients treated with arthroscopic meniscal repair. Fifteen of those 35 patients had suture augmented with PRP. The authors found no differences in clinical outcomes or the rate of failure between the two groups. A 2018 randomized controlled trial by Kaminski et al[80] compared 20 patients treated with meniscal suture repair augmented with PRP with 17 patients treated with meniscus repair controls augmented with placebo. The authors reported that the PRP group had a superior healing rate based on second-look arthroscopy and MRI; however, there were no differences in clinical scores between the two groups. A 2021 systematic review by Zaffagnini et al[22] included 5 studies with 111 patients treated with meniscal repair augmented with PRP and 175 patients treated with meniscal repair only. The reported failure rates were 9.9% (95% confidence interval, 4.52% to 19.1%) for PRP-augmented groups and 25.7% (95% confidence interval, 12.7% to 38.7%) in control groups. This suggested there was a significantly lower risk of failure in PRP-augmented groups (odds ratio 0.31; 95% confidence interval, 0.14 to 0.69; $P < 0.005$). A systematic review by Belk et al[81] noted a more modest difference in meniscal repair failure rates between these two groups. Belk et al found a 17.0% failure rate in patients who underwent meniscus repair treated with PRP compared with a 22.1% failure rate in patients treated with surgery only. Although a smaller improvement is seen, these results still suggested that PRP can improve meniscal healing leading to a lower failure rate. Based on the data presented thus far, it would appear that there is a potential role for PRP augmentation in meniscus repair. Patients who received PRP augmentation tended to have better outcomes, particularly with a lower rate of repair failure, and there do not seem to be any clear drawbacks with the clinical use of PRP.

Although PRP has shown clinical efficacy, it should be noted that PRP preparations are not uniform and have been shown to be variable and heterogeneous with regard to the growth factors and concentrations present. A recent systematic review by Chahla et al[82] demonstrated poor and inconsistent reporting of PRP preparations in the literature. The authors noted that only 10% of studies provided comprehensive reporting on the preparation protocol of PRP in their investigations, and only 16% of studies provided quantitative metrics regarding the composition of the PRP administered. This makes it challenging to understand the true efficacy of PRP augmentation for meniscal injuries and warrants caution when interpreting related clinical results.

Fibrin Clots

Fibrin clots are another blood-derived orthobiologic that has received considerable attention as a meniscal tear/repair augment. They have been studied because of their ability to provide chemotactic and mitogenic stimuli for reparative cells.[22] These blood-derived chemotactic factors act similar to platelet-derived growth factor and fibronectin and will stimulate local meniscal cell activity to attract synovial cells and improve the healing process.[22] Unlike PRP, the initial clinical evidence has been conflicting for the use of fibrin clot as an augmentation strategy to meniscal repair. A 2014 study by Kamimura et al[83] and a 2020 study by Nakayama et al[84] showed significant subjective clinical improvement in fibrin-augmented meniscal repairs, but there was a high failure rate of 25% to 30%. Moreover, these two studies were of low levels of evidence. There have been other examples where a fibrin clot has been used as a successful augment to meniscus repair. Jang et al[85] described a technique where they delivered an autologous fibrin clot with their inside-out sutures. They reported a success rate of 95% in 39 out of 41 patients. The same group performed a midterm follow-up study for this patient population.[86] At a mean of 30 weeks after surgery, they noted significant improvements in patient functional outcomes: there was an improvement of approximately 30 points on Lysholm score and 35 points on International Knee Documentation Committee score. Furthermore, on second-look arthroscopy, the authors noted complete healing of the meniscus in 85.71% of patients. Until higher quality comparative studies evaluating the clinical efficacy of fibrin clots become available, the potential role of fibrin clot augmentation in meniscal repair will continue to remain unclear.

Bone Marrow Aspirate Concentrate

Bone marrow aspirate concentrate (BMAC) is a potential orthobiologic adjunct to meniscal repair that may facilitate healing and regeneration of damaged meniscal tissue (**Figure 7**). In vivo models have shown improved tissue regeneration with BMAC supplementation.[87] Studies have reported the clinical efficacy of BMAC augmentation when managing chondral lesions or osteoarthritis, but there is a lack of clinical studies regarding BMAC augmentation for meniscal repair.[88] To date, there have only been reported cases and technique publications describing successful meniscal repair with concomitant BMAC augmentation.[88] Physiologically, BMAC is thought to exert a therapeutic effect through its high concentration of growth factors, which generates an anti-inflammatory and anabolic environment.[88] Although BMAC may be efficacious, the lack of comparative clinical studies makes it difficult to determine the true value of this promising therapeutic intervention.

Growth Factors

There has also been considerable interest in the use of isolated growth factors such as the TGF-ß superfamily, basic fibroblast growth factor, insulinlike growth factor 1, connective tissue growth factor, vascular endothelial growth factor, platelet-derived growth factor, and hepatocyte growth factor.[75] The desirable properties of the native meniscus are largely based on its unique ECM which is modulated by the activity of the meniscal cells.[75] Growth factors play a key role in modulating meniscal repair/regeneration via the recruitment of fibrochondrogenic cells, enhancing cell proliferation, and stimulating ECM production.[75] Therefore, the local targeted administration of growth factors can create the optimal microenvironment for promoting meniscal repair and is a promising orthobiologic adjuvant with the potential to augment meniscal tear healing. The TGF-ß superfamily, in particular, has shown great potential in the field of tissue engineering and restorative medicine. The use of TGF-ß in tissue engineering constructs has shown improved ECM protein synthesis, cell proliferation, articular cartilage regeneration, and guidance of endogenous cells.[89] Fibroblast growth factor is another peptide with promising in vitro results. In scaffold models, fibroblast growth factor–enhanced native tissue integration in tissue engineering constructs for meniscal repair.[89] Insulinlike growth factor 1 has shown similarly promising results in fibrochondrocytes.[89] Currently, there is a lack of clinical evidence examining the outcomes associated with these peptide interventions. Although the evidence regarding the potential role of growth factors in stimulating meniscal regeneration is strong, it is still limited to preclinical

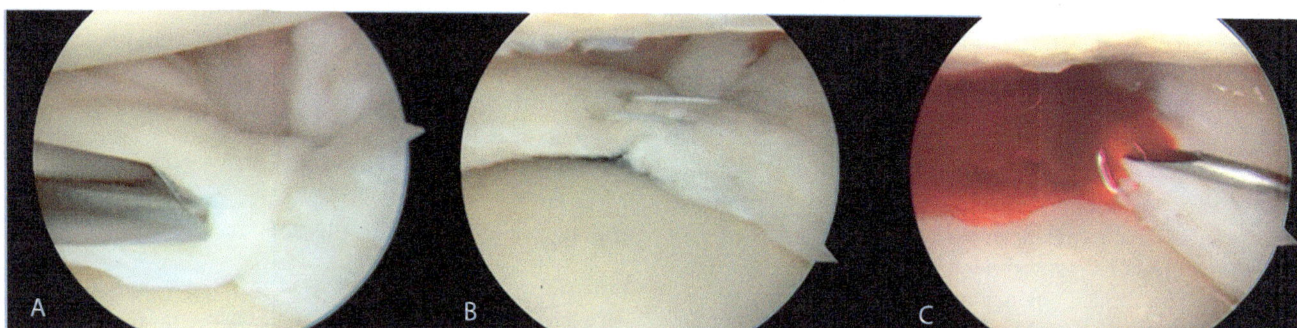

FIGURE 7 Arthroscopic images demonstrating repair of a radial meniscal tear augmented with bone marrow aspirate concentrate (BMAC). A radial tear (**A**) was repaired using an inside-out technique (**B**). BMAC was then applied to the repair site using an 18-gauge needle (**C**).

studies and adequate translation to human use will require multiple clinical trials and FDA approvals. As the field continues to advance, there is considerable potential for the translational development of growth factors augmentation strategies in meniscal repair.

FUTURE DIRECTIONS

As the field of orthobiologics continues to evolve, it is evident that an increased emphasis on translational research and well-designed clinical trials is needed to overcome the lack of high-quality published studies to provide adequate solutions to the complex pathology associated with meniscal tears. Tissue engineering constructs regenerate the meniscus by combining therapy from all three levels of orthobiologics: acellular scaffolds, progenitor cells, and biomechanical/biochemical stimulation. The recent advancements in medical imaging can allow for the construction of exact 3D objects. These can be designed to be patient specific. Moving forward, 3D printed surgical constructs will play a significant role in the visualization of pathology, surgical planning, manufacturing of patient-specific instruments and implants, and making of patient-specific scaffolds for tissue engineering approaches for meniscal repair.[2] Studies examining 3D constructs have shown that they are able to emulate the complex anisotropic circumferential meniscal fiber arrangement, which is critical to meniscal function and could theoretically improve clinical outcomes when used as a scaffold.[2] Moreover, preclinical studies have examined the combination of these anisotropic 3D constructs with spatially incorporated growth factors such as connective tissue growth factor and TGF-ß3 in ovine models.[90,91] The authors reported that endogenous cells regenerated the meniscus with zone-specific matrix phenotypes, but over long-term follow-up there was increased meniscal extrusion and articular cartilage degeneration indicating further room for improving in this promising tissue engineering technique. As 3D printing continues to gain more favor, the field of orthobiologics, scaffolds, and tissue engineering will continue to evolve and allow for more accurate patient-specific constructs and more complex designs that can be translated clinically.

SUMMARY

Orthobiologic solutions have demonstrated promising initial results in improving clinical outcomes for patients who have suffered meniscal injuries. Cellular solutions have shown promise in augmenting meniscal repair as well as isolated therapeutic interventions for both acute and degenerative meniscal tears. Blood product orthobiologic treatment modalities such PRP and fibrin clots have also been promising, with PRP demonstrating positive preliminary results. Additionally, the use of scaffolds and implants has provided an alternative solution for patients with partial or total meniscectomies. Tissue engineering is the final amalgamation of these advances in the field of orthobiologics. The combination of 3D printing technology, biomaterial scaffolds, progenitor cells, and biomechanical/biochemical stimulation might be the future of meniscal repair/replacement.

REFERENCES

1. Kean CO, Brown RJ, Chapman J: The role of biomaterials in the treatment of meniscal tears. *PeerJ*. 2017;5:e4076.
2. Shimomura K, Hamamoto S, Hart DA, Yoshikawa H, Nakamura N: Meniscal repair and regeneration: Current strategies and future perspectives. *J Clin Orthop Trauma* 2018;9(3):247-253.
3. Pereira H, Fatih Cengiz I, Gomes S, et al: Meniscal allograft transplants and new scaffolding techniques. *EFORT Open Rev* 2019;4(6):279-295.
4. Jacob G, Shimomura K, Krych AJ, Nakamura N: The meniscus tear: A review of stem cell therapies. *Cells* 2019;9(1):92.
5. LaPrade RF, Floyd ER, Carlson GB, Moatshe G, Chahla J, Monson JK: Meniscal root tears: Solving the silent epidemic. *J Arthrosc Surg Sports Med* 2020;2:47-57.
6. Woodmass JM, LaPrade RF, Sgaglione NA, Nakamura N, Krych AJ: Meniscal repair: Reconsidering indications, techniques, and biologic augmentation. *J Bone Joint Surg Am* 2017;99(14):1222-1231.
7. Laprade CM, Ellman MB, Rasmussen MT, et al: Anatomy of the anterior root attachments of the medial and lateral menisci. *Am J Sports Med* 2014;42(10):2386-2392.
8. Johannsen AM, Civitarese DM, Padalecki JR, Goldsmith MT, Wijdicks CA, Laprade RF: Qualitative and quantitative anatomic analysis of the posterior root attachments of the medial and lateral menisci. *Am J Sports Med* 2012;40(10):2342-2347.
9. Bhan K: Meniscal tears: Current understanding, diagnosis, and management. *Cureus* 2020;12(6):e8590.
10. Bilgen B, Jayasuriya CT, Owens BD: Current concepts in meniscus tissue engineering and repair. *Adv Healthc Mater* 2018;7(11):1701407.
11. Chahla J, Papalamprou A, Chan V, et al: Assessing the resident progenitor cell population and the vascularity of the adult human meniscus. *Arthroscopy* 2021;37(1):252-265.
12. Chahla J, Cinque ME, Godin JA, Geeslin AG, Moatshe G, LaPrade RF: Review of Arnoczky and Warren on the microvasculature of the human meniscus. *J ISAKOS* 2017;2(4):229-232.
13. Crawford MD, Hellwinkel JE, Aman Z, et al: Microvascular anatomy and intrinsic gene expression of menisci from young adults. *Am J Sports Med* 2020;48(13):3147-3153.
14. Kwon H, Brown WE, Lee CA, et al: Surgical and tissue engineering strategies for articular cartilage and meniscus repair. *Nat Rev Rheumatol* 2019;15(9):550-570.
15. Thompson WO, Thaete FL, Fu FH, Dye SF: Tibial meniscal dynamics using three-dimensional reconstruction of magnetic resonance images. *Am J Sports Med* 1991;19(3):210-215.

16. Moran CJ, Busilacchi A, Lee CA, Athanasiou KA, Verdonk PC: Biological augmentation and tissue engineering approaches in meniscus surgery. *Arthroscopy* 2015;31(5):944-955.

17. Karia M, Ghaly Y, Al-Hadithy N, Mordecai S, Gupte C: Current concepts in the techniques, indications and outcomes of meniscal repairs. *Eur J Orthop Surg Traumatol* 2019;29(3):509-520.

18. Cooper DE, Arnoczky SP, Warren RF: Meniscal repair. *Clin Sports Med* 1991;10(3):529-548.

19. Chahla J, Kruckeberg B, Moatshe G, LaPrade R: *Peripheral Meniscal Tears: How to Diagnose and Repair*. Springer, 2017, pp 77-91.

20. Checa A, Chun W: Rates of meniscal tearing in patients with chondrocalcinosis. *Clin Rheumatol* 2015;34(3):573-577.

21. Chahla J, Gannon J, Moatshe G, LaPrade R: *Outside-in Meniscal Repair: Technique and Outcomes*. Springer, 2017, pp 129-135.

22. Zaffagnini S, Poggi A, Reale D, Andriolo L, Flanigan DC, Filardo G: Biologic augmentation reduces the failure rate of meniscal repair: A systematic review and meta-analysis. *Orthop J Sports Med* 2021;9(2):232596712098162.

23. Rubman MH, Noyes FR, Barber-Westin SD: Arthroscopic repair of meniscal tears that extend into the avascular zone. A review of 198 single and complex tears. *Am J Sports Med* 1998;26(1):87-95.

24. Gallacher PD, Gilbert RE, Kanes G, Roberts SN, Rees D: White on white meniscal tears to fix or not to fix? *Knee* 2010;17(4):270-273.

25. Noyes FR, Chen RC, Barber-Westin SD, Potter HG: Greater than 10-year results of red-white longitudinal meniscal repairs in patients 20 years of age or younger. *Am J Sports Med* 2011;39(5):1008-1017.

26. Nishida M, Higuchi H, Kobayashi Y, Takagishi K: Histological and biochemical changes of experimental meniscus tear in the dog knee. *J Orthop Sci* 2005;10(4):406-413.

27. Noyes FR, Barber-Westin SD: Arthroscopic repair of meniscus tears extending into the avascular zone with or without anterior cruciate ligament reconstruction in patients 40 years of age and older. *Arthroscopy* 2000;16(8):822-829.

28. Vint H, Quartley M, Robinson JR: All-inside versus inside-out meniscal repair: A systematic review and meta-analysis. *Knee* 2021;28:326-337.

29. Smoak JB, Matthews JR, Vinod AV, Kluczynski MA, Bisson LJ: An up-to-date review of the meniscus literature: A systematic summary of systematic reviews and meta-analyses. *Orthop J Sports Med* 2020;8(9):232596712095030.

30. Rosso F, Bisicchia S, Bonasia DE, Amendola A: Meniscal allograft transplantation: A systematic review. *Am J Sports Med* 2015;43(4):998-1007.

31. A Cavendish P, Dibartola AC, Everhart JS, Kuzma S, Kim WJ, Flanigan DC: Meniscal allograft transplantation: A review of indications, techniques, and outcomes. *Knee Surg Sports Traumatol Arthrosc* 2020;28(11):3539-3550.

32. Myers P, Tudor F: Meniscal allograft transplantation: How should we be doing it? A systematic review. *Arthroscopy* 2015;31(5):911-925.

33. Hergan D, Thut D, Sherman O, Day MS: Meniscal allograft transplantation. *Arthroscopy* 2011;27(1):101-112.

34. Samitier G, Alentorn-Geli E, Taylor DC, et al: Meniscal allograft transplantation. Part 2: Systematic review of transplant timing, outcomes, return to competition, associated procedures, and prevention of osteoarthritis. *Knee Surg Sports Traumatol Arthrosc* 2015;23(1):323-333.

35. Lee BS, Kim HJ, Lee CR, et al: Clinical outcomes of meniscal allograft transplantation with or without other procedures: A systematic review and meta-analysis. *Am J Sports Med* 2018;46(12):3047-3056.

36. Grassi A, Bailey JR, Filardo G, Samuelsson K, Zaffagnini S, Amendola A: Return to sport activity after meniscal allograft transplantation: At what level and at what cost? A systematic review and meta-analysis. *Sports Health* 2019;11(2):123-133.

37. Smith NA, MacKay N, Costa M, Spalding T: Meniscal allograft transplantation in a symptomatic meniscal deficient knee: A systematic review. *Knee Surg Sports Traumatol Arthrosc* 2015;23(1):270-279.

38. Harris JD, Cavo M, Brophy R, Siston R, Flanigan D: Biological knee reconstruction: A systematic review of combined meniscal allograft transplantation and cartilage repair or restoration. *Arthroscopy* 2011;27(3):409-418.

39. Noyes FR, Barber-Westin SD: Meniscal transplantation in symptomatic patients under fifty years of age: Survivorship analysis. *J Bone Joint Surg Am* 2015;97(15):1209-1219.

40. Seitz AM, Dürselen L: Biomechanical considerations are crucial for the success of tendon and meniscus allograft integration-a systematic review. *Knee Surg Sports Traumatol Arthrosc* 2019;27(6):1708-1716.

41. Novaretti JV, Patel NK, Lian J, et al: Long-term survival analysis and outcomes of meniscal allograft transplantation with minimum 10-year follow-up: A systematic review. *Arthroscopy* 2019;35(2):659-667.

42. Jauregui JJ, Wu ZD, Meredith S, Griffith C, Packer JD, Henn RF III: How should we secure our transplanted meniscus? A meta-analysis. *Am J Sports Med* 2018;46(9):2285-2290.

43. Gelber PE, Verdonk P, Getgood AM, Monllau JC: Meniscal transplantation: State of the art. *J ISAKOS* 2017;2(6):339-349.

44. Jackson DW, Whelan J, Simon TM: Cell survival after transplantation of fresh meniscal allografts: DNA probe analysis in a goat model. *Am J Sports Med* 1993;21(4):540-550.

45. Rodeo SA, Seneviratne A, Suzuki K, Felker K, Wickiewicz TL, Warren RF: Histological analysis of human meniscal allografts. A preliminary report. *J Bone Joint Surg Am* 2000;82(8):1071-1082.

46. Arnoczky SP, DiCarlo EF, O'Brien SJ, Warren RF: Cellular repopulation of deep-frozen meniscal autografts: An experimental study in the dog. *Arthroscopy* 1992;8(4):428-436.

47. Nordberg RC, Charoenpanich A, Vaughn CE, et al: Enhanced cellular infiltration of human adipose-derived stem cells in allograft menisci using a needle-punch method. *J Orthop Surg Res* 2016;11(1):132.

48. Struijk C, Van Genechten W, Verdonk P, et al: Human meniscus allograft augmentation by allogeneic mesenchymal stromal/stem cell injections. *J Orthop Res* 2022;40(3):712-726.

49. Saltzman BM, Bajaj S, Salata M, et al: Prospective long-term evaluation of meniscal allograft transplantation procedure: A minimum of 7-year follow-up. *J Knee Surg* 2012;25(2):165-175.

50. Kopf S, Beaufils P, Hirschmann MT, et al: Management of traumatic meniscus tears: The 2019 ESSKA meniscus consensus. *Knee Surg Sports Traumatol Arthrosc* 2020;28(4):1177-1194.

51. Houck DA, Kraeutler MJ, Belk JW, McCarty EC, Bravman JT: Similar clinical outcomes following collagen or polyurethane meniscal scaffold implantation: A systematic review. *Knee Surg Sports Traumatol Arthrosc* 2018;26(8):2259-2269.

52. Toanen C, Dhollander A, Bulgheroni P, et al: Polyurethane meniscal scaffold for the treatment of partial meniscal deficiency: 5-year follow-up outcomes – A European multicentric study. *Am J Sports Med* 2020;48(6):1347-1355.

53. Frizziero A, Ferrari R, Giannotti E, Ferroni C, Poli P, Masiero S: The meniscus tear. State of the art of rehabilitation protocols related to surgical procedures. *Muscles Ligaments Tendons J* 2013;2(4):295-301.

54. Zaffagnini S, Giordano G, Vascellari A, et al: Arthroscopic collagen meniscus implant results at 6 to 8 years follow up. *Knee Surg Sports Traumatol Arthrosc* 2007;15(2):175-183.

55. Dangelmajer S, Familiari F, Simonetta R, Kaymakoglu M, Huri G: Meniscal transplants and scaffolds: A systematic review of the literature. *Knee Surg Relat Res* 2017;29(1):3-10.

56. Veronesi F, Di Matteo B, Vitale ND, et al: Biosynthetic scaffolds for partial meniscal loss: A systematic review from animal models to clinical practice. *Bioact Mater* 2021;6(11):3782-3800.

57. Zaffagnini S, Marcheggiani Muccioli GM, Lopomo N, et al: Prospective long-term outcomes of the medial collagen meniscus implant versus partial medial meniscectomy: A minimum 10-year follow-up study. *Am J Sports Med* 2011;39(5):977-985.

58. Rodkey WG, DeHaven KE, Montgomery WH III, et al: Comparison of the collagen meniscus implant with partial meniscectomy. A prospective randomized trial. *J Bone Joint Surg Am* 2008;90(7):1413-1426.

59. Bulgheroni E, Grassi A, Bulgheroni P, Marcheggiani Muccioli GM, Zaffagnini S, Marcacci M: Long-term outcomes of medial CMI implant versus partial medial meniscectomy in patients with concomitant ACL reconstruction. *Knee Surg Sports Traumatol Arthrosc* 2015;23(11):3221-3227.

60. Efe T, Getgood A, Schofer MD, et al: The safety and short-term efficacy of a novel polyurethane meniscal scaffold for the treatment of segmental medial meniscus deficiency. *Knee Surg Sports Traumatol Arthrosc* 2012;20(9):1822-1830.

61. Akkaya M, Şimşek ME, Gürsoy S, Çay N, Bozkurt M: Medial meniscus scaffold implantation in combination with concentrated bone marrow aspirate injection: Minimum 3-year follow-up. *J Knee Surg* 2020;33(8):838-846.

62. Schüttler KF, Haberhauer F, Gesslein M, et al: Midterm follow-up after implantation of a polyurethane meniscal scaffold for segmental medial meniscus loss: Maintenance of good clinical and MRI outcome. *Knee Surg Sports Traumatol Arthrosc* 2016;24(5):1478-1484.

63. Bulgheroni P, Bulgheroni E, Regazzola G, Mazzola C: Polyurethane scaffold for the treatment of partial meniscal tears. Clinical results with a minimum two-year follow-up. *Joints* 2013;1(4):161-166.

64. Papalia R, Franceschi F, Diaz Balzani L, D'Adamio S, Maffulli N, Denaro V: Scaffolds for partial meniscal replacement: An updated systematic review. *Br Med Bull* 2013;107:19-40.

65. Bulgheroni E, Grassi A, Campagnolo M, Bulgheroni P, Mudhigere A, Gobbi A: Comparative study of collagen versus synthetic-based meniscal scaffolds in treating meniscal deficiency in young active population. *Cartilage* 2016;7(1):29-38.

66. Stein S, Höse S, Warnecke D, et al: Meniscal replacement with a silk fibroin scaffold reduces contact stresses in the human knee. *J Orthop Res* 2019;37(12):2583-2592.

67. DeHaven KE, Lohrer WA, Lovelock JE: Long-term results of open meniscal repair. *Am J Sports Med* 1995;23(5):524-530.

68. Matsukura Y, Muneta T, Tsuji K, Koga H, Sekiya I: Mesenchymal stem cells in synovial fluid increase after meniscus injury. *Clin Orthop Relat Res* 2014;472(5):1357-1364.

69. Hofer HR, Tuan RS: Secreted trophic factors of mesenchymal stem cells support neurovascular and musculoskeletal therapies. *Stem Cell Res Ther* 2016;7(1):131.

70. Sun H, Wen X, Li H, et al: Single-cell RNA-seq analysis identifies meniscus progenitors and reveals the progression of meniscus degeneration. *Ann Rheum Dis* 2020;79(3):408-417.

71. Seol D, Zhou C, Brouillette MJ, et al: Characteristics of meniscus progenitor cells migrated from injured meniscus. *J Orthop Res* 2017;35(9):1966-1972.

72. Vangsness CTJ, Farr JI, Boyd J, Dellaero DT, Mills CR, LeRoux-Williams M: Adult human mesenchymal stem cells delivered via intra-articular injection to the knee following partial medial meniscectomy: A randomized, double-blind, controlled study. *J Bone Joint Surg Am* 2014;96(2):90-98.

73. Onoi Y, Hiranaka T, Nishida R, et al: Second-look arthroscopic findings of cartilage and meniscus repair after injection of adipose-derived regenerative cells in knee osteoarthrits: Report of two cases. *Regen Ther* 2019;11:212-216.

74. Sekiya I, Koga H, Otabe K, et al: Additional use of synovial mesenchymal stem cell transplantation following surgical repair of a complex degenerative tear of the medial meniscus of the knee: A case report. *Cell Transplant* 2019;28(11):1445-1454.

75. Chen M, Guo W, Gao S, et al: Biochemical stimulus-based strategies for meniscus tissue engineering and regeneration. *Biomed Res Int* 2018;2018:8472309.

76. Whitehouse MR, Howells NR, Parry MC, et al: Repair of torn avascular meniscal cartilage using undifferentiated autologous mesenchymal stem cells: From in vitro optimization to a first-in-human study. *Stem Cells Transl Med* 2017;6(4):1237-1248.

77. Olivos-Meza A, Pérez Jiménez FJ, Granados-Montiel J, et al: First clinical application of polyurethane meniscal scaffolds with mesenchymal stem cells and assessment of cartilage quality with T2 mapping at 12 months. *Cartilage* 2021;13(1 suppl):197S-207S.

78. Pujol N, Salle De Chou E, Boisrenoult P, Beaufils P: Platelet-rich plasma for open meniscal repair in young patients: Any benefit? *Knee Surg Sports Traumatol Arthrosc* 2015;23(1):51-58.

79. Griffin JW, Hadeed MM, Werner BC, Diduch DR, Carson EW, Miller MD: Platelet-rich plasma in meniscal repair: Does augmentation improve surgical outcomes? *Clin Orthop Relat Res* 2015;473(5):1665-1672.

80. Kaminski R, Kulinski K, Kozar-Kaminska K, et al: A prospective, randomized, double-blind, parallel-group, placebo-controlled study evaluating meniscal healing, clinical outcomes, and safety in patients undergoing meniscal repair of unstable, complete vertical meniscal tears (bucket handle) augmented with platelet-rich plasma. *Biomed Res Int* 2018;2018:9315815.

81. Belk JW, Kraeutler MJ, Thon SG, Littlefield CP, Smith JH, McCarty EC: Augmentation of meniscal repair with platelet-rich plasma: A systematic review of comparative studies. *Orthop J Sports Med* 2020;8(6):232596712092614.

82. Chahla J, Cinque ME, Piuzzi NS, et al: A call for standardization in platelet-rich plasma preparation protocols and composition reporting: A systematic review of the clinical orthopaedic literature. *J Bone Joint Surg Am* 2017;99(20):1769-1779.

83. Kamimura T, Kimura M: Meniscal repair of degenerative horizontal cleavage tears using fibrin clots: Clinical and arthroscopic outcomes in 10 cases. *Orthop J Sports Med* 2014;2(11):2325967114555678.

84. Nakayama H, Kanto R, Kambara S, Iseki T, Onishi S, Yoshiya S: Successful treatment of degenerative medial meniscal tears in well-aligned knees with fibrin clot implantation. *Knee Surg Sports Traumatol Arthrosc* 2020;28(11): 3466-3473.

85. Jang SH, Ha JK, Lee DW, Kim JG: Fibrin clot delivery system for meniscal repair. *Knee Surg Relat Res* 2011;23(3):180-183.

86. Ra HJ, Ha JK, Jang SH, Lee DW, Kim JG: Arthroscopic inside-out repair of complete radial tears of the meniscus with a fibrin clot. *Knee Surg Sports Traumatol Arthrosc* 2013;21(9):2126-2130.

87. Koch M, Hammer S, Fuellerer J, et al: Bone marrow aspirate concentrate for the treatment of avascular meniscus tears in a one-step procedure-evaluation of an in vivo model. *Int J Mol Sci* 2019;20(5):1120.

88. Muckenhirn KJ, Kruckeberg BM, Cinque ME, et al: Arthroscopic inside-out repair of a meniscus bucket-handle tear augmented with bone marrow aspirate concentrate. *Arthrosc Tech* 2017;6(4):e1221-e1227.

89. Twomey-Kozak J, Jayasuriya CT: Meniscus repair and regeneration: A systematic review from a basic and translational science perspective. *Clin Sports Med* 2020;39(1):125-163.

90. Lee CH, Rodeo SA, Fortier LA, Lu C, Erisken C, Mao JJ: Protein-releasing polymeric scaffolds induce fibrochondrocytic differentiation of endogenous cells for knee meniscus regeneration in sheep. *Sci Transl Med* 2014;6(266):266ra171.

91. Nakagawa Y, Fortier LA, Mao JJ, et al: Long-term evaluation of meniscal tissue formation in 3-dimensional–Printed scaffolds with sequential release of connective tissue growth factor and TGF-β3 in an ovine model. *Am J Sports Med* 2019;47(11):2596-2607.

CHAPTER 26

Articular Cartilage Repair—Cells and Biomaterials

Michael J. Sayegh, MD • Daniel A. Grande, PhD • Nicholas A. Sgaglione, MD, FAAOS • Kenneth R. Zaslav, MD, FAAOS

INTRODUCTION

Weight-bearing diarthrodial joints such as the knee experience constant repetitive loading and trauma throughout an individual's life. Articular cartilage is essential to provide pain-free range of motion, loading, and locomotion. As individuals age and sustain trauma/injuries, articular cartilage is prone to damage, which may or may not lead to significant clinical problems. This can be in the form of focal cartilage defects and/or osteoarthritis, often with concomitant pathologies. The subchondral bone plays an integral part in the function of this organ because it needs to be sufficiently compliant so it can absorb load, and often in the diseased or postinjury state, subchondral fractures may increase the stiffness of this important structure and cause quicker wear of the overlying cartilage. Damaged articular cartilage has limited intrinsic healing capabilities and when untreated can lead to significant pain and disability. This may ultimately lead to end-stage osteoarthritis with deformity requiring interventions such as total joint arthroplasty. For this reason, when indicated, it is important to strive to repair articular cartilage. Focal cartilage lesions have been shown to be more amenable to biologic repair with standard techniques than osteoarthritis; however, treatment strategies to repair and regenerate cartilage remain a challenge and optimal biologic treatment is yet to be defined.[1]

Although prevention of osteoarthritis has not been definitively shown to be the outcome of cartilage repair procedures, the goals of the orthopaedic surgeon should be reduction of inflammation, joint stability, and pain management in patients indicated for cartilage repair procedures. It is acknowledged, however, that successful cartilage repair, such as in the long-term follow-up studies of autologous chondrocyte implantation (ACI), has been shown to forestall the need for total joint arthroplasty.[2-5] Hence, the motivation should be the advancement of techniques that provide the optimal regenerative milieu for complete cartilage restoration.

Advancements in the field of orthobiologics have allowed surgeons to use various treatment options available to attempt to repair articular cartilage, particularly in the lower extremity. These repair strategies involve the use of cells, biomaterials, and signals to augment, regenerate, and/or replace articular cartilage defects while maintaining adequate subchondral support and load absorption. The goals of scientists are to advance the field of cartilage repair by aiming to achieve normal and healthy adult hyaline cartilage with a long-term goal of preventing posttraumatic osteoarthritis. The goals of epidemiologists are to adequately define articular cartilage injury in the population and develop treatment algorithms depending on certain patient characteristics. The patient's goals are unique and often include diminishing pain, increased stability, and personal goals. Patients generally want to resume performing activities that increase their quality of life. Although preferred, histologically perfect tissue in the form of hyaline cartilage may not always be necessary to achieve patient goals. Additionally, surgery is not always the answer as a treatment for focal articular defects. Nonsurgical interventions have historically played a large role.

Cells and biomaterials and the evolving strategies to manage articular defects of the lower extremity, which may include the hip, knee, and/or ankle, are reviewed.

ARTICULAR CARTILAGE: RESPONSE TO INJURY

Articular cartilage is avascular, aneural, and alymphatic, receiving its nutrients by diffusion from synovial fluid. Therefore, it has a limited intrinsic ability to undergo a healing response to allow repair because it does not bleed when injured.[6] Chondrocytes are also tightly bound by

Dr. Grande or an immediate family member serves as a board member, owner, officer, or committee member of ICRS. Dr. Sgaglione or an immediate family member has received royalties from Biomet and Zimmer; serves as a paid consultant to or is an employee of Biomet and Embody; has received research or institutional support from Regen Biologics and Zimmer; and serves as a board member, owner, officer, or committee member of the Arthroscopy Association of North America. Dr. Zaslav or an immediate family member serves as a paid consultant to or is an employee of Cartiheal Inc. and Lifenet; has stock or stock options held in Cartiheal Inc.; has received research or institutional support from Active Implants, Aesculap/B.Braun, Organogenesis, Regen Labs, and Zimmer; and serves as a board member, owner, officer, or committee member of Biologic Association and the International Cartilage Repair Society. Neither Dr. Sayegh nor any immediate family member has received anything of value from or has stock or stock options held in a commercial company or institution related directly or indirectly to the subject of this chapter.

extracellular matrix (ECM), which limits migration to an injured site. Injured articular cartilage does not secrete enough chemotactic factors to signal the migration of reparative cells to the area. When a defect involves penetration of the subchondral plate, there is an influx of cells and cytokines from the blood that cause a cascade of reparative inflammatory events and remodeling of ECM.[7] This is the basis of microfracture techniques, which is limited due to the formation of fibrocartilage rather than hyaline cartilage. Fibrocartilage does not exhibit properties similar to hyaline cartilage, often does not completely fill the defect, and may quickly deteriorate over time. This can be viewed as scar formation rather than pure hyaline articular cartilage regeneration.

FOCAL ARTICULAR DEFECTS

Pathologies within the joint that include articular cartilage encompass conditions such as osteoarthritis, focal chondral and osteochondral defects, chondromalacia patellae, osteochondritis dissecans, and joint malalignment. Focal chondral and osteochondral defects are areas of injury and/or degeneration that are confined to a certain area and may be the result of trauma, chronic repetitive loads, and/or disorders of bone or cartilage including subchondral osteonecrosis. Concomitant injuries such as ACL rupture or patellar instability are commonly associated with these defects.

Patients typically present with acute or chronic symptoms of pain, swelling, instability, stiffness, locking, and/or catching. Radiographs may be initially unrevealing; however, an effusion or a loose body may be present in the case of an osteochondral fracture. It is important to address the joint as a whole-organ system, and if concurrent pathology is not addressed, there is risk of failure of cartilage treatment strategies and surgery.[8] For example, a thorough ligamentous examination should be performed. Reconstruction or repair of ligaments should be performed, if indicated, before addressing chondral defects, and attempts to preserve the meniscus are also important. Lower extremity standing alignment radiographs should be analyzed, and if there is a significant mechanical axis deviation, proximal tibial or distal femoral osteotomies can be considered. In cases of patellar instability, surgery is commonly performed to address anatomic factors that place patients at risk for recurrent dislocation or failure of cartilage procedures such as patella alta, lateral patellar tilt, incompetent medial patellofemoral ligament, trochlear dysplasia, increased tibial tuberosity to trochlear groove distance, and/or coronal plane or rotational malalignment.[9] Additionally, persistent inflammation can be deleterious to any repair construct. Previous studies have demonstrated higher rates of cartilage restoration surgery failure when concurrent pathology is not addressed.[9]

MRI is the gold standard imaging modality to evaluate articular cartilage defects of the knee; however, arthroscopy provides the most precise classification of the defect with regard to depth, size, location, and quality of subchondral bone. Defects can be classified into partial-thickness chondral defects, full-thickness chondral defects extending to the subchondral bone, or osteochondral defects that also involve the subchondral bone and according to their size and geometry.[10] As per standard, a small lesion is smaller than 2 cm^2.[9] The Outerbridge classification and the International Cartilage Repair Society Classification describe these cartilage lesions based on examination during surgery including size and depth, each with a grading system of 0 to 5.[11] This has significant implications for treatment because the complex interface between cartilage and subchondral bone is essential in cartilage regeneration strategies.[12]

REPAIR STRATEGIES

Compared with 30 years ago, currently, there are many different surgical repair strategies for addressing articular defects. These techniques have goals of augmentation, regeneration, replacement, and/or substitution. Other procedures are commonly performed to address concomitant pathology, which includes distal femoral or proximal tibial osteotomies and joint distraction arthroplasty. These procedures rely on altering joint biomechanics. Patient presentation, degree, size, and location of cartilage loss, age, concomitant pathology, and functional goals all are considered when determining the optimal repair strategy.

The fixation of an unstable osteochondral fragment may be performed if the fragment has viable cartilage and at least 3 mm of bone. It has also been shown that in skeletally immature patients, large chondral fragments without attached bone may have the potential to heal with fixation.[13] Frequently, this is performed by cleaning the fibrous tissue from the osteochondral defect and the fragment, contouring the fragment and adding autologous bone graft, if necessary. Fixation can be performed with headless compression screws, countersunk headed screws, and/or bioabsorbable darts. Goals of fixation are to have a healthy and bleeding bone surface (microfracture may be performed before) and adequate compression to allow for healing.

Augmentation techniques create fibrous tissue such as fibrocartilage but do not re-create the normal hyaline cartilage structure of articular cartilage. Débridement and chondroplasty may help alleviate mechanical pain in patients with small articular cartilage defects and/or unstable cartilage flaps without concomitant pathology. This allows for faster recovery and immediate postoperative weight bearing. This procedure may also prevent propagation of the tear. The results of this procedure are controversial, with a randomized controlled study showing no benefit when performed with concomitant partial meniscectomy at 1-year follow-up.[14] Bone marrow stimulation in the form of microfracture or microdrilling of the subchondral bone stimulates an extrinsic cartilage repair response after subchondral bone penetration.[15]

The marrow clot provides a framework or provisional scaffold for cartilage repair to occur; however, this forms fibrocartilage, which is suboptimal with regard to biochemical and biomechanical properties, having a higher proportion of type I collagen than type II collagen and also with lower aggrecan content. Acellular scaffolds may be used to augment bone marrow stimulation techniques to gain a more stable clot and possibly more organized and durable repair. The use of scaffolds in articular cartilage repair is described later.

Regeneration techniques for cartilage repair aim to elicit a biologic response that may yield a more normal adult articular cartilage. With the use of cells, scaffolds, and appropriate signaling, cartilage regeneration to repair articular cartilage defects may be possible. These strategies include autologous chondrocyte transplantation, matrix-induced autologous chondrocyte implantation (MACI), and minced allogeneic cartilage products. In addition to these techniques, many next-generation strategies for cartilage regeneration are in development. However, to date, what has eluded the field is the complete regeneration of the cytoarchitecture and the Benninghoff arcade of intact native cartilage.

Osteochondral replacement in the form of allograft or autograft replacement as treatment strategies for articular cartilage defects has been used extensively. These grafts consist of full-thickness articular cartilage and a layer of attached subchondral bone and serve to replace an articular cartilage defect and restore the normal biomechanical properties. Osteochondral autograft transplant or mosaicplasty is historically best reserved to replace osteochondral defects that are smaller than 2 cm^2, typically within the knee, and is performed in a single stage with both open and arthroscopic techniques described. During this procedure, an osteochondral plug is harvested from a non–weight-bearing surface (such as the peripheral aspect of the medial or lateral trochlea or intercondylar notch). These plugs are typically smaller than 10 mm, and multiple plugs can be used in a mosaic format for large defects. Any gaps in the replacement are filled in with fibrocartilage as part of the repair. Short-term results in athletes compared with microfracture are very successful; however, at 10-year follow-up, continued participation in sports declines with 34% in patients undergoing osteochondral autograft transplantation and 17% of patients with microfracture continuing to participate in sports activities.[16] Allogeneic allograft transplantation provides great potential for chondral or osteochondral defects that are larger than 2 cm^2; however, this procedure is commonly limited by availability, waiting time, and cost. Typically, grafts are ready for implantation after a minimum of 14 days after harvesting to allow for removal of bone marrow elements by lavage and for final aerobic cultures to be negative. Once the graft is released for use, surgery is typically scheduled within 2 weeks.[17] It has been demonstrated that with prolonged storage and freezing, cartilage may fissure, delaminate, and cause chondrocyte death.[18] Replacing larger uncontained defects may be performed by the surgeon, with the placement of adjacent overlapping allografts to treat irregular or ovoid lesions or the help of instrumentation such as the BioUni System (Arthrex). Sometimes, screw fixation is used to stabilize grafts. Cartiform (Arthrex) and ProChondrix (AlloSource) are osteochondral allografts that are approved for use within the United States. Outcomes at 5 years are promising in younger patients who are not obese or have inflammatory conditions.[19] In addition, more recently available, fresh osteochondral allograft precut plugs up to 16 mm in diameter are available but limited due to shelf life; however, further research is needed to determine long-term outcomes.[20] Regardless of cartilage replacement technique by grafting, proper graft placement, chondrocyte viability, and addressing concomitant pathology are essential for success. Abnormal stresses between the graft surface, adjacent tissues, and opposing articular surface may inhibit graft healing.[21]

Substitution of the osteochondral unit with metal and/or plastic is common for articular cartilage defects of the knee in the form of total and/or partial joint arthroplasty. Focal defect resurfacing with synthetic plastic polymers has also been used. These procedures are successful in terms of pain relief and long-term outcomes in the elderly population; however, they do not have the same goals as articular cartilage repair strategies that do not include substitution. However, the emerging role of orthobiologics in the substitution of the osteochondral unit in cartilage repair includes tissue engineering of whole-joint resurfacing by bioprinting. Such technologies may eliminate the need for total joint arthroplasty with metal and/or plastic in the future but are currently in their infancy.

TISSUE ENGINEERING TRIAD

The field of tissue engineering continues to grow as potential treatment for cartilage injury as a result of greater understanding of biomaterials and cell engineering, stem cell harvesting and characterization, cell signaling and growth factors, and bioreactor technology. Scaffolds, cells, and signals in the form of biochemical or environmental cues that affect growth and phenotype of cells constitute the triad.[22] These elements may be used separately, or in combination, to treat symptomology, or affect regeneration or restoration of tissue function.[23] As understanding increases, evolving technologies involving the interaction between cells and biomaterials have led to the development of commercial products to treat cartilage injury. **Table 1** provides various marketed acellular and cellular scaffold-based therapies and cell-based therapies currently available.

Scaffolds

Scaffolds are an essential component that should provide form, fixation, and function, as well as drive tissue

TABLE 1 Cellular and Acellular Management of (Osteo) Chondral Defects of the Lower Extremities

Product	Company	Scaffold Material	Cells	Procedure Used	Market Status
Agili-C	CartiHeal	Hyaluronan and Aragonite	—	Cell-free osteochondral scaffold	Approved (USA and Europe)
BioCartilage	Arthrex	Cartilage allograft matrix	—	Microfracture augmentation	Approved (USA)
BST-CarGel	Smith & Nephew	Chitosan	—	Microfracture augmentation ± PRP	Approved (Canada and Europe)
CaReS	Arthro Kinetics	Type I collagen	Autologous chondrocytes	Autologous chondrocyte implantation (third generation)	Withdrawn
Cartiform	Arthrex	Cell-based osteochondral scaffold	Allogeneic chondrocytes	Osteochondral allograft	Approved (USA)
Cartilage allograft matrix	MTF Biologics	Cartilage allograft matrix	—	Microfracture augmentation	Approved (USA)
CartiMax	MTF Biologics	Cartilage allograft matrix	Allogeneic chondrocytes	Cell-based chondral scaffold	Approved (USA)
CARTISTEM	MEDIPOST	—	Allogeneic umbilical cord MSCs	Augmented subchondral drilling	Approved (Korea), Phase II clinical trials (USA)
Chondrofix	Zimmer Biomet	Cell-free osteochondral scaffold	—	Osteochondral allograft	Approved (USA)
Chondrosphere/ Spherox	CO.DON AG	Autologous cartilage-like extracellular matrix	Autologous chondrocytes	Autologous chondrocyte implantation (fourth generation)	Approved (Europe)
DeNovo NT	Zimmer Biomet	Minced allogeneic cartilage products	Allogeneic chondrocytes	Cell-based chondral scaffold	Approved (USA)
GelrinC	Regentis Biomaterials	Polyethylene glycol–modified fibrinogen	—	Microfracture augmentation	Approved (Europe), Phase III clinical trials (USA)
Hyalofast	Anika Therapeutics	Hyaluronan	—	Microfracture augmentation and BMAC	Approved (Europe), phase III clinical trials (USA)
Hyalograft C	Anika Therapeutics	Hyaluronic acid ester scaffold	Autologous chondrocytes	Autologous chondrocyte implantation (third generation)	Withdrawn
MACI	Vericel Corporation	Types I and III collagen	Autologous chondrocytes	Autologous chondrocyte implantation (third generation)	Approved (USA)
MaioRegen	Fin-ceramica Faenza SpA	Type I collagen and Hydroxyapatite	—	Cell-free osteochondral scaffold	Approved (Europe)
NeoCart	Histogenics	Type I collagen in honeycomb formation	Autologous chondrocytes	Autologous chondrocyte implantation (fourth generation)	Withdrawn
Novocart 3D	TETEC GmbH	Biphasic collagen scaffold, chondroitin sulfate	Autologous chondrocytes	Autologous chondrocyte implantation (third generation)	Phase III clinical trials (USA)
ProChondrix	AlloSource	Cell-based osteochondral scaffold	Allogeneic chondrocytes	Osteochondral allograft	Approved (USA)

TABLE 1 Cellular and Acellular Management of (Osteo) Chondral Defects of the Lower Extremities (Continued)

Product	Company	Scaffold Material	Cells	Procedure Used	Market Status
TissueGene-C/ Invossa	Kolon TissueGene	—	Allogeneic chondrocytes virally transduced to express TGF-β	Intra-articular injection	Phase III clinical trials (USA)
TruFit CB	Smith & Nephew	Poly(lactic-co-glycolic acid) and Calcium sulfate	—	Cell-free osteochondral scaffold	Withdrawn

BMAC = bone marrow aspirate concentrate, MSC = mesenchymal stromal cell, PRP = platelet-rich plasma

formation, whereas cells are expected to produce the desired tissue.[24] Ideally, they are cell instructive, biomimetic, resilient biomechanically, biocompatible, provoke no inflammation or immune response biodegradable, porous, and are easy to handle in a surgical environment.[25] However, as reality often limits the production of an ideal scaffold, several criteria are variably always considered in the production and analysis of scaffolds.[22] The biomechanics of a scaffold must be able to adapt and mimic the native tissue, which enables function initially, and aid in mechanical signaling. Pore size and porosity are also a particularly important consideration and can affect cell viability and mechanical function. Large pores encourage cellular migration, whereas small pores allow for better cellular attachment. Porosity is defined as the percentage of space within a scaffold, which aids in free movement of cells, nutrients, and wastes. There is a fine balance of porosity with biomechanical strength that varies depending on desired tissue. Without this balance, structural integrity may be compromised such as with increased pore size. The most optimal pore size for neovascularization is approximately 5 μm.[26] The best size for fibroblast migration is approximately 5 to 15 μm.[25] The optimal pore size for chondrocytes is 150 to 250 μm and 200 to 350 μm for osteoconduction.[27] A scaffold must also properly degrade as the desired tissue growth occurs. If this process is too slow, new tissue growth may be limited. If this process occurs too fast, function and viability may be compromised. A scaffold should also have a good biocompatibility index to avoid causing local inflammation or an immunologic response. Therefore, products including allografts or xenografts should be carefully processed as per standard protocols, and breakdown products must be nontoxic and appropriately cleared or metabolized from the body. An unsuitable local environment in and around implantation may affect healing potential in articular cartilage repair. The surface of the scaffold should mimic ECM. This is easier in natural scaffolds where small-diameter fibers with natural binding sites are typically used; however, in the case of synthetic scaffolds, natural ligands can be incorporated to facilitate cell binding.

The current state of scaffolds is one that is constantly evolving. The use of scaffolds for the management of articular cartilage defects of the knee has evolved over time from simply nonwoven polymer scaffolds to hold cells or growth factors in situ to those more sophisticated using electrospinning or three-dimensional (3D) bioprinting to more accurately represent the subtle zonal differences in articular cartilage. The ideal scaffold for chondral and osteochondral defects of the lower extremity is yet to be determined; however, many current trials in the laboratory and clinically provide a promising future.

Various types of scaffolds have included natural, synthetic, and biosynthetic composite materials with various degrees of clinical success.[1,28] Currently, natural type I collagen is widely used in scaffolds for cartilage tissue engineering products because of its ubiquitous biocompatibility and clinical approval.[29,30] An issue with type I collagen scaffolds is that they promote fibrocartilage rather than hyaline cartilage because of excess chondral calcification, lack of basal and lateral bonding, and extensive fibrillation of the articular surface.[31,32] Fibrocartilage is prone to damage over time, which questions the long-term outcomes of the commercially available collagen scaffolds.[2,20] Scaffolds that seek to more closely mimic the native cartilage microenvironment enhance chondrogenesis and hyaline cartilage production for cartilage repair.[33] Such modifications would include a specific pore size or a molecule to promote cell migration and preserve a chondrogenic phenotype.

The most common natural biodegradable polymers that are used in scaffolds include polysaccharides (hyaluronic acid derivatives, starch, alginate, or chitosan), polynucleotides (RNA or DNA), and proteins (collagen, fibrin, gels, silk, or soy).[1]

MACI is a well-studied procedure that is approved for use and often uses collagen type I and III scaffold. This multistep procedure that includes chondrocyte harvesting at index procedure has been shown to have positive clinical effects.[29] Another procedure that incorporates an ECM-derived decellularized collagen scaffold in a single procedure is autologous matrix-induced chondrogenesis, which augments procedures such as microfracture for articular cartilage defects. This acellular scaffold fills the defect void volume and allows for cellular infiltration from both the marrow and synovial cavity to assist in cartilage repair.[30]

Hydrogels have also been experimented with as potential natural scaffolds because of structural similarities to natural ECM of cartilage. These are water-swollen networks of cross-linked hydrophilic polymers and may contain polysaccharides such as hyaluronic acid derivatives of chitosan.[34] Now withdrawn from the market, Hyalograft C is composed of a hyaluronic ester (Hyaff-11, Anika Therapeutics), which was shown to have improved clinical outcomes in a single-surgeon study.[35] However, in 2013, this product was withdrawn because of a citation of an overall lack of safety and efficacy data. Another hydrogel that was studied contains water-soluble chitosan and hyaluronic acid derivatives with the goal to create a substance similar to cartilage ECM with high water content, which theoretically supports chondrocyte survival by retaining natural chondrocyte morphology.[36] In addition to supporting chondrocyte activity, chitosan-based hydrogel scaffolds are degradable in vivo by lysozyme, which is present in natural cartilage ECM.[34] An example of a chitosan-based scaffold for cartilage repair is BST-CarGel (Smith & Nephew), which is currently approved to augment microfracture in Canada and Europe. Another promising scaffold composed of a natural benzyl ester of hyaluronic acid is Hyalofast (Anika Therapeutics). This product is approved for use in Europe and currently in clinical trial phase in the United States. In a single surgery, this acellular scaffold may augment microfracture with the addition of bone marrow aspirate concentrate to attempt to regenerate hyaline cartilage rather than fibrocartilage as seen with microfracture alone. Bone marrow aspirate concentrate introduces cells that include multipotent stem cells. Strong medium-term and long-term follow-up clinical studies show promising result of this procedure compared with microfracture alone.[37,38]

The most common synthetic biodegradable polymers are poly(lactic acid), poly(glycolic acid) (PGA), poly(lactic-co-glycolic acid) (PLGA) copolymers, and polycaprolactone.[1] PLGA scaffolds seeded with mesenchymal stem cells (MSCs) have shown to be promising with regard to cartilage regeneration in vitro; however, the adhesion of chondrocytes and MSCs is limited because of hydrophobicity unlike collagen and ECM of hyaline cartilage.[39] Therefore, novel synthetic scaffolds that are modified with recognizable ligands, sodium hydroxide treatment, and collagen type II coating have been studied in vitro with short-term positive results.[40] In addition, the use of microspheres that are PLGA based and release transforming growth factor beta 3 (TGF-β3) adds to an environment that may be suitable for MSC differentiation to chondrocytes.[41] This chondroinductive factor may be a promising approach for regeneration of articular cartilage in single-stage, cell-based therapies. However, it should be noted that the degradation of these polymers can lead to local acidity and inflammation.

Composite scaffolds contain materials that include different combinations of ceramic, synthetic polymers, and natural polymers such as collagen, hydroxyapatite, gelatin, chondroitin sulfate, calcium sulfate, and hyaluronate.[22] A cell-free osteochondral scaffold that is approved for use in Europe is MaioRegen (Fin-ceramica Faenza SpA). This is a composite scaffold that uses type I collagen and hydroxyapatite and showed promising clinical results at 24-month follow-up in a 2013 comparative study.[42] Another composite synthetic scaffold used PLGA and calcium sulfate as a cell-free osteochondral scaffold, which was marketed as TruFit CB (Smith & Nephew) but withdrawn in 2012 because of high rates of revision surgery when used as treatment for patellofemoral articular cartilage defects.[43] Previously approved in Europe and recently approved by the FDA in the United States is Agili-C (CartiHeal). This is a cell-free osteochondral composite multiphasic scaffold that is made of aragonite, which is derived from coralline exoskeleton.[44] This scaffold takes advantage of MSC infiltration and healthy chondrocyte migration to regenerate healthy hyaline cartilage.[45] The plug is a biphasic plug from marine coral with pure coral or aragonite in the bottom portion and coral modified with drill holes of a specific diameter and pattern in the top portion, which has been shown to stimulate chondrogenesis and attract chondrocyte migration. Studies in a goat model have shown not only good clinical results but also biopsies with near-normal to normal hyaline cartilage according to independent pathologists.[46] A 4-year prospective single-arm multicenter study of European patients has recently been published along with a second single-arm study by Belgian authors, both of which show excellent clinical results.[47,48] In addition, a 2-year phase III randomized controlled study performed on patients in the United States, Israel, and Europe has been completed and shows exceptional clinical results both with significant Knee Injury and Osteoarthritis Outcome Score improvement of more than 30 points in the implant arm and secondary end point of significant MRI fill at 2 years.[49] Because of these successful results, the FDA has approved its use in the United States for cartilage surface lesions in the knee in all patients except severe Kellgren-Lawrence grade 4 degenerative joint disease. It is therefore the first FDA-approved technology studied in patients not only with focal chondral defects but also with Kellgren-Lawrence grade 2 and 3 arthritis, and once commercialized in the United States, it will be a major improvement in the surgeons' armamentarium.

Emerging scaffolds that are currently being studied in vitro such as nanofiber scaffolds and scaffolds that use amniotic materials may provide a treatment option for articular cartilage defects in the future. The synthetic polymers poly(glycolic acid) and poly(L-lactide-co-ε-caprolactone) are approved and have an excellent biocompatibility profile, suggesting that a novel nanofiber scaffold prepared by co-electrospinning should be examined for its chondrogenic capacity and structural integrity.[28,50,51] The structure of electrospun nanofiber membranes is remarkably similar to the ECM of cartilage and has advantages in that they have high surface area, high porosity, and adjustable pore size.[52] Dresing et al[53] demonstrated that nanofiber scaffolds have elastomeric properties that can be easily press fitted into an osteochondral defect, providing a stable matrix for tissue repair. Theoretically, this provides a high chondrogenic capacity. Recent studies have shown success with electrospun nanofiber scaffolds. Chen et al[54] demonstrated that a chondroitin sulfate nanofiber scaffold has increased potential for chondrogenic differentiation in vitro. Xu et al[55] also showed that electrospun poly(ε-caprolactone) nanofiber scaffolds increase chondrogenic gene expression of rat bone marrow MSCs compared with collagen scaffolds. Kim et al[56] demonstrated increased chondrogenic potential of adipose-derived MSCs with a poly(glycidyl methacrylate) nanofiber scaffold. Human amniotic membrane has also been recently studied as a potential scaffold for articular cartilage repair. Some clinical advantages are that it has antimicrobial, antifibrotic, antiangiogenic, and acceptable mechanical properties.[57] Studies are limited to in vitro designs but may gain more traction in the future.[58]

For stable, long-term successful cartilage reconstruction, repair, and/or regeneration, it is important to address not only the cartilage but also the underlying bone and to reestablish normal joint homeostasis. This is where bioprinted, personalized, regenerative scaffolds in the form of 3D bioprinting may provide better solutions for articular cartilage defects of the lower extremity.[59] This will allow for the fabrication of automated personalized constructs with accurately positioned cells and biologic cues to mimic the osteochondral interface and/or zone organization of cartilage. In addition, mechanical properties can be tailored by hybrid printing or reinforcement strategies to match the cartilage area that needs replacement. In orthopaedics, 3D printing technologies have the capability to provide personalized implants for cartilage defects; however, the transition from 3D printing of polymers, ceramics, and metals toward 3D bioprinting of living and biologically active constructs has not yet taken place in clinical practice.[59,60] Ongoing research in this area is promising. 3D bioprinting may also play a large role in the concept of whole-joint resurfacing by tissue engineering and may even eliminate the need for joint arthroplasty with metal and plastic in the future.

The primary objective of using scaffolds in cartilage repair lies in its ability to distribute load until such time as the cellular component, whether endogenous or extrinsic, elaborates enough ECM to transition loading to the regenerated tissue.

Cells

If cells are included in a repair strategy, they can be used as a free suspension directly added to the defect site or incorporated, for example, seeded into a solid scaffold or hydrogel. The cell type used can be a differentiated cell, such as a chondrocyte or a stem cell. Prior studies have shown that the composition of microenvironments alters cellular adhesion, differentiation, and morphology. In cartilage repair of the lower extremity, autologous or allogeneic chondrocytes are commonly used because they synthesize the requisite ECM molecules. In addition, in particulated juvenile allograft cartilage (minced), immature allogeneic chondrocytes are used. Emerging MSC sources, both from allogeneic and autogenic sources, are also being investigated for use in cartilage repair.

ACI was the first commercially marketed cell-based therapy for cartilage regeneration. This is a two-stage procedure that involves a biopsy of articular cartilage from a non–weight-bearing area, in vitro expansion, and implantation into large articular cartilage chondral or osteochondral defects (>2 cm^2). Approximately 200 to 300 mg of cartilage is harvested and sent to a Current Good Manufacturing Practice facility for chondrocyte mitotic expansion. First-generation and second-generation ACI provided a final liquid suspension of cells. Third-generation and fourth-generation ACI provided a cell-laden scaffold, approximately 2×10^6 cells/cm^2, which is extensively tested before it is sent back to the surgeon for implantation during the second stage.[61] The primary third-generation ACI technique available for use in the United States (FDA approved in 2017) is MACI (Vericel Corporation). This product uses a collagen type I/III scaffold, and at the time of implantation, fibrin glue is applied within the defect bed, and the membrane is gently pressed into the defect. A thin layer of fibrin glue is then applied over the cell-based scaffold. In a randomized prospective clinical trial of MACI compared with microfracture, there were significant better Western Ontario and McMaster Universities Osteoarthritis Index scores at 5-year follow-up.[2] CaReS (Arthro Kinetics) is a 3D type I collagen matrix purified from rat tail collagen used in single-stage surgery without cocultured cells that has been shown to have promising short-term outcomes; however, this product is available in Europe and not in the United States.[62] Hyalograft C (Anika Therapeutics) is a third-generation ACI product that has been withdrawn from clinical use from the market because of concerns of manufacturing practices and quality of comparative study submitted for approval to the European Society of Medicine.[63] Novocart 3D (TETEC GmbH) is a third-generation ACI that uses a biphasic collagen scaffold with chondroitin sulfate. Cells are distributed evenly within the 3D structure of this scaffold rather than lying only on the matrix surface. This product is currently undergoing clinical trials for use in the United States. Fourth-generation ACI techniques involve advances in bioreactor design and cell culture methods that facilitate ECM production while preserving the chondrogenic phenotype. Chondrosphere

(CO.DON AG) is a fourth-generation ACI technique approved for clinical use in Europe that cultivates chondrocytes into spheroids or chondrons containing cell aggregates and autologous cartilage-like ECM.[61] Benefits of fourth-generation techniques include the incorporation of ECM rather than isolated chondrocytes to provide structural support, more favorable cell environments, and possibly enhanced chondrogenesis.[64]

Cell-based therapies for treatment of articular cartilage defects may also use allogeneic chondrocytes seeded on scaffolds. CartiMax (MTF Biologics) uses allogeneic chondrocytes seeded on a cartilage allograft ECM. It is approved for use in the United States and has puttylike handling properties, which is useful to fill defects of different shapes and sizes. Another potential future therapy for focal articular defects and/or osteoarthritis uses allogeneic chondrocytes that are retrovirally transduced to express TGF-β to be used in the form of an intra-articular injection. TGF-β has been shown to be a vital biochemical signal contributing to cartilage regeneration.[65] TissueGene-C/Invossa (Kolon TissueGene, Inc.) is in phase III clinical trials within the United States; however, at the time of this writing, it was suspended but is now being restarted.

Particulated juvenile allograft cartilage involves implantation of minced allogeneic cartilage products, including immature chondrocytes. Juvenile cartilage has better chondrogenic activity and higher metabolic output than adult cartilage and therefore may be a good option for cartilage regeneration.[66] In a single-stage procedure, fibrin glue is applied to the bed of the articular cartilage defect, particulated juvenile allograft cartilage is applied, and a subsequent layer of fibrin glue is applied. An added benefit of this procedure is the ease of contour matching, which is useful for patellar chondral lesions; however, there has been reported graft hypertrophy.[66] The minced cartilage products act as a scaffold, providing the biochemical signals to promote cartilage repair as well as chondrocyte outmigration from the particles. DeNovo NT (Zimmer Biomet) is a particulate juvenile allograft cartilage that was approved for use in the United States, showing promising results in the knee at short-term follow-up.[66,67]

With tissue engineering, the use of various MSCs seeded on various scaffolds is gaining ground as a potential therapeutic modality for focal cartilage defects and osteoarthritis because of their strong proliferative capacity and signaling ability.[68] These cells can be differentiated into both cartilage and bone depending on the nature of biomechanical and biochemical cues.[69] They can be harvested with minimal donor-site morbidity from multiple sources (bone marrow, blood, synovium, and adipose tissue).[70] These cells may be used as a stand-alone drug or biologic in the form of an intra-articular injection, in ACI-like procedures, or as a component of future interventions along with purpose-designed scaffolds and biochemical signaling.[23] MSCs have been studied extensively as therapy for cartilage injuries; however, this is limited to animal studies and there are limited large-scale clinical data.[71] Some small sample and short-term follow-up clinical studies have shown that intra-articular injection of MSCs, as well as implantation of MSCs supported by scaffolds, results in improvement of pain and function and formation of hyaline cartilage up to 2 years following the procedure.[71] Overall, the clinical effectiveness is limited and there are also studies showing inconsistent results of MSCs for cartilage regeneration.[72] Although they may be injected alone at a particular site, it has been recognized that MSCs need a scaffold to hold them for more time, aid in differentiation without changing phenotype in the cartilage defect, and act as a mechanism for inducing cartilage regeneration and hyaline cartilage formation.[1,28,73-75] This is thought to be dependent on the type of stem cell used and the scaffold used to seed these cells. MSCs have the theoretical function of anti-inflammation and replacing local cells lost to physiologic turnover and repairing or regenerating injured tissues while showing low immunogenicity.[76] Bone marrow–derived and adipose-derived MSCs are the most extensively studied stem cell; however, studies have demonstrated that synovial fluid–derived MSCs are of greater chondrogenic potential due to the proximity to the joint.[77-79] Additionally, it was demonstrated that there are increased synovial fluid–derived MSC counts in patients with osteoarthritis compared with healthy patients, which suggests that synovial fluid may play a role in recruiting mesenchymal progenitor cells to enhance spontaneous healing, create an anti-inflammatory environment, restore homeostasis in an injured joint, and/or promote cartilage regeneration.[80,81] In addition, it has been shown that there is a significant upregulation of SOX9 in synovial fluid–derived MSCs and that there are increased amounts of regulatory proteins such as aggrecan and glycosaminoglycan content, which may be responsible for a higher chondrogenic potential than bone marrow–derived MSCs.[82] Overall, regardless of source, MSCs are emerging as a future therapeutic agent in cartilage restoration as more high-quality evidence is seen. Currently, there are no approved MSC-based therapies for cartilage restoration authorized to market within the United States. Challenges include optimizing chondrocyte differentiation and maintaining phenotypic stability.[23] The reason there are no FDA-approved MSC products lies in the fact that these approaches have used autologous tissue, usually bone marrow or adipose, and are FDA regulated as 361 use. Allogeneic MSCs have not been FDA approved as of the time of this writing.

Induced pluripotent stem cells (iPSCs) have been studied as a potential cartilage tissue engineering therapy since their discovery in 2006. iPSCs have an advantage over MSCs in that they have the capacity to derive large number of autologous cells from small starting populations.[83] As embryonic and extraembryonic tissues (placenta) divide, they become pluripotent cells, which are able to divide into cells of germ layers that distinctly form the endoderm, mesoderm, and ectoderm in embryogenesis.[84] It was originally thought that these cells were only found in the germinal ridge of the embryo; however, it was shown in 2006 that it is possible to activate a class of genes within adult cells that cause a reversion to a pluripotent state by using retroviruses to deliver and force the expression of certain transcription factors leading to what is known as iPSCs.[85] iPSCs are advantageous over embryonal stem cells because they represent an easily accessible patient-specific source and can also bypass the ethical and political issues related to the use of human embryonal stem cells because the destruction of human embryos is not needed.[83] Although some animal model in vitro and in vivo studies are promising, it is too soon to draw conclusions regarding the use of iPSCs and embryonal stem cells in cartilage regeneration, compared with other sources and methods such as MSCs.[83]

Allogeneic umbilical cord MSCs have been explored as a potential treatment of articular cartilage defects of the lower extremity. These are cultured in vitro and mixed with sodium hyaluronate before arthroscopic administration into drill holes that are created within the defect (CARTISTEM, MEDIPOST). In early phase clinical trials, there was evidence of hyaline cartilage regeneration and improved pain and function at 7 years.[86]

Signaling Molecules

Biochemical and biomechanical signaling is important for successful cartilage repair. Bioactive preparations such as platelet-rich plasma that contain fibroblast growth factor 2, insulinlike growth factor, and TGF-β are used to coat scaffolds for improved cartilage repair in vivo and induce differentiation, proliferation, and metabolic activity of cells.[22] Signaling in the form of biochemical and environmental cues affects the growth and phenotype of cells. These defined small molecular treatments have been proposed to be grouped as disease-modifying osteoarthritis drugs to enable endogenous repair mechanisms and prevent degeneration within a joint or to direct cellular behavior within an implanted construct.[23] Varying results depend on specific dosing, combinations, conditions, and mechanical cues.[87] For example, cartilage is very dense and has a charged nature. Future strategies in cartilage repair may support electrostatic interactions and dynamic loading to increase tissue penetration and residence.[88]

Proteases and cytokines may promote cartilage degradation. Blockers of these molecules have been discussed as potential combination therapy in cartilage repair. For example, the drug anakinra is an interleukin 1 receptor antagonist that has been shown to reduce pain and improve function after 2 weeks following a cartilage injury in a randomized controlled trial.[89] Brown et al[90] showed that intra-articular injection of anakinra provides benefit in knee range of motion and pain associated with persistent postsurgical effusion and inflammation. This should be considered in the clinical armamentarium for certain patients in whom oral anti-inflammatory medication and physical therapy have failed.

The use of exosomes as therapy in cartilage regeneration is also an emerging topic. Most of the mechanism of action of MSCs is due to the paracrine secretion of both trophic factors and anti-inflammatory factors, which downregulate inflammatory signals linked to cartilage destruction as well as recruitment of resident cells to a repair site.[91] One important mediator of this paracrine signaling is extracellular vesicles: vital messengers of cell-to-cell communication and a vehicle for the release of trophic factors that initiate a wide range of biologic processes and pathologic changes. A major subtype of extracellular vesicles that has received substantial attention is exosomes.[92-94] They are 30- to 150-nm-sized biphospholipid membrane–enclosed structures that contain proteins, messenger RNA, and microRNA. Exosomes are released from donor cells—such as MSCs—and carry signaling proteins and nucleic acids that induce molecular changes in nearby recipient cells.[95] The precise content of MSC-derived exosomes is a product of the tissue origin, cellular activities, and the immediate intercellular neighbors.[96] It has been shown that synovial membrane–derived exosomes have chondroprotective effects in the setting of in vivo collagenase-induced osteoarthritis.[97] Some advantages of exosomes include their small size and hypoimmunogenicity. Additionally, because exosomes are excretory vesicles secreted by cells, they do not pose the same clinical and safety concerns associated with the use of ex vivo expanded MSCs. Therefore, lower costs are involved in their maintenance and storage.

Instant MSC Product accompanying Autologous Chondron Transplantation (IMPACT) is a one-stage surgical procedure for large articular cartilage defects of the lower extremity that uses autologous recycled chondrons mixed with allogeneic bone marrow–derived MSCs in fibrin glue.[98] Chondrons may be useful for several reasons. It has been shown that débrided tissue provides chondrons that are of similar quality to those harvested from healthy tissue as seen with MACI two-stage procedures.[99,100] In addition, chondrons may have superior chondrogenic potential when compared with primary and culture-expanded chondrocytes due to retention of interactions between the ECM and chondrocytes, which provides more robust structural support.[98,99,101] This provides a more cost-effective option than MACI.[100] Chondrons are similar to exosomes in that they support the theory that MSCs are used as mediators that stimulate local tissue repair with paracrine signaling, rather than stem cells that differentiate into the desired tissue. In a 5-year randomized controlled trial comparing IMPACT with nonsurgical treatment, there were improved clinical outcomes, suggesting that one-stage cell-based cartilage repair using allogeneic MSCs and autologous chondrons is safe, clinically effective, and more cost effective than conventional cell-based therapies.[98] Additionally, there have been phase I studies investigating cocultures of chondrons and adipose tissue–derived MSCs showing increased hyaline cartilage formation in rats.[102]

TREATMENT ALGORITHM

Figure 1 illustrates the authors' treatment algorithm for the surgical treatment of chondral defects of the knee. Patients who are symptomatic are typically treated based on physical demands, age, size and location of

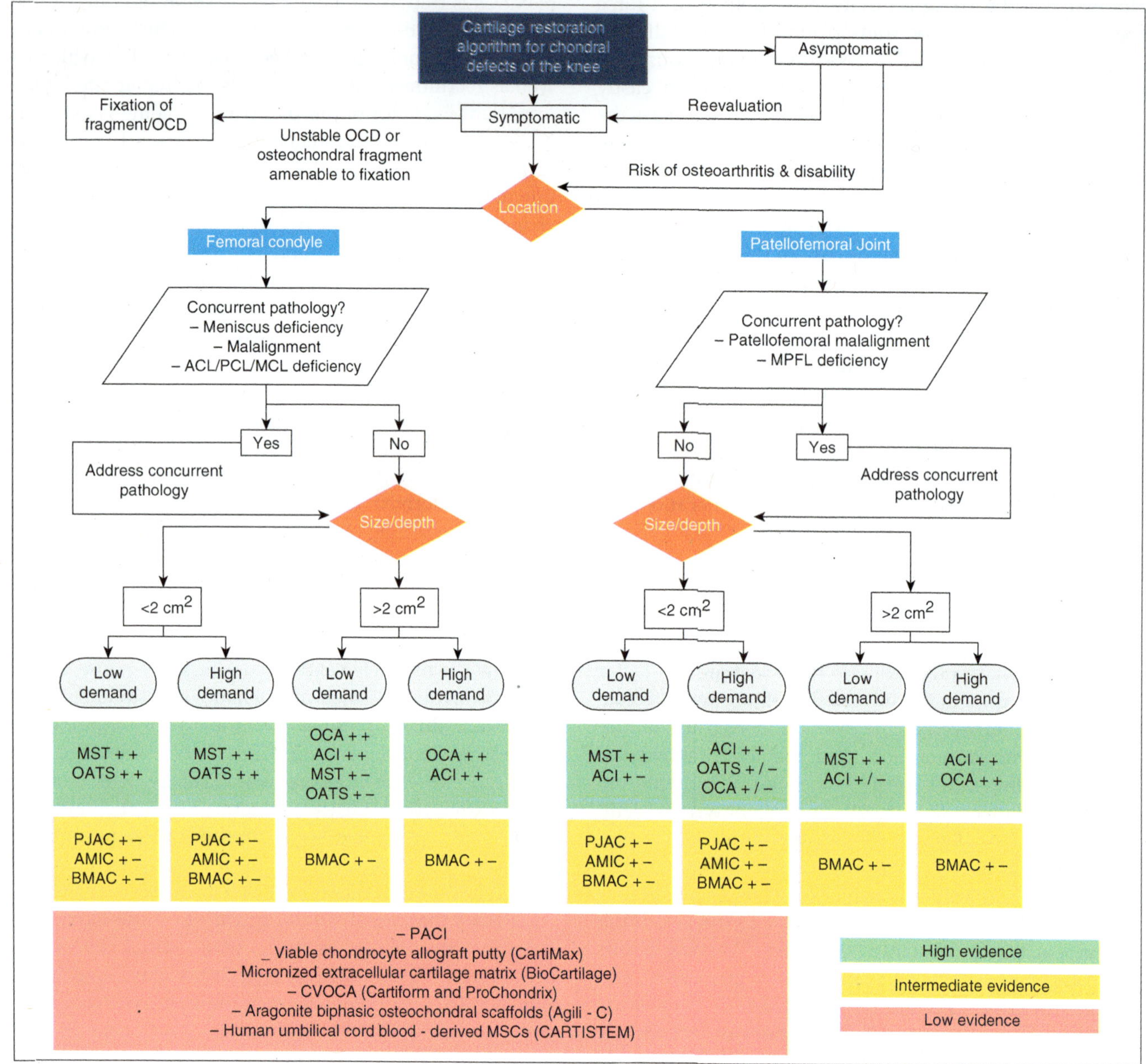

FIGURE 1 Treatment algorithm for focal chondral lesions. Before treatment, it is important to assess the presence of correctable lesions. Surgical treatment should be considered for trochlear and patellar lesions after rehabilitation programs have failed. The treatment is guided by the size and location of the defect, the patient's demands, whether it is a first-line or second-line treatment, and if there is a significant subchondral bone loss. If there is large subchondral bone loss, successful treatment strategies are typically limited to OCA, OATS, or ACI. +– = possible option depending on the patient's characteristics, ++ = best treatment option, ACI = autologous chondrocyte implantation, ACL = anterior cruciate ligament, AMIC = autologous matrix-induced chondrogenesis, BMAC = bone marrow aspirate concentrate with collagen scaffold implantation, CVOCA = cryopreserved viable osteochondral allograft, MCL = medial collateral ligament, MPFL = medial patellofemoral ligament, MSC = mesenchymal stromal cell, MST = marrow stimulation, OATS = osteochondral autograft transplant system, OCA = fresh osteochondral allograft, OCD = osteochondritis dissecans, PACI = particulated autologous cartilage implantation, PCL = posterior cruciate ligament, PJAC = particulated juvenile allograft cartilage

the defect, and whether there is a significant subchondral bone deficit. Typically, patellofemoral defects are initially treated without surgery; surgical intervention should only be considered if nonsurgical treatment fails. Concurrent pathology is very important to address for successful outcomes of cartilage restoration procedures. This is typically done in a staged manner or at the time of the cartilage restoration procedure. If there is large subchondral bone loss, successful treatment strategies are typically limited osteochondral autograft transplant implantation, ACI, and osteochondral allograft implantation. Primary and secondary surgical options must be considered and may be used concomitantly. Débridement/chondroplasty and/or removal of loose body is a possible treatment option in patients with low physical demands. If there is a fragment amendable for repair, this may be attempted, especially in patients with unstable osteochondritis dissecans.

SUMMARY

The orthopaedic surgeon now has a plethora of options available for articular cartilage repair, with decision making both complicated and important. Patient education is a significant factor specifically directed at managing patient expectations. Serious discussions must occur between the patient and surgeon concerning the expected change in lifestyle and activity from the patient's current baseline activity level to determine that these are viable potential goals. In addition, the patient needs to understand the biologic timeline for healing and regeneration and the significant rehabilitation time and potential time away from work or sports, which these procedures often necessitate to maximize long-term success.

From a preclinical perspective, the ideal scaffold-based or cell-based orthobiologic should provide a collagen cytoarchitecture reconstituting the Benninghoff arcade, have a lamina splendens at the superficial tangential surface zone, have good bonding to the subchondral plate with a reestablished tidemark, and most importantly be composed of hyaline cartilage with type II collagen and aggrecan. At the very least, a durable repair that can provide good shock absorption, healthy subchondral bone, and a low coefficient of friction with activity should be achieved. Although these are lofty goals, they should be continually strived for with future use of these technologies.

An appealing option for the near future is a readily available off-the-shelf product that would reliably recreate the bone-cartilage unit. Such a product, Agili-C (CartiHeal), was approved by the US FDA in 2022, and is a porous, biocompatible, and biodegradable bi-phasic scaffold, consisting of interconnected natural inorganic calcium carbonate (aragonite) derived from purified, inorganic, coral exoskeleton. A long-term approach would likely involve 3D bioprinting to produce patient-specific composite bone-cartilage constructs in a perioperative time frame with the initial ability to bear some load and provide a bearing surface.

REFERENCES

1. Rai V, Dilisio MF, Dietz NE, Agrawal DK: Recent strategies in cartilage repair: A systemic review of the scaffold development and tissue engineering. *J Biomed Mater Res A* 2017;105:2343-2354.
2. Brittberg M, Recker D, Ilgenfritz J, Saris DBF: Matrix-applied characterized autologous cultured chondrocytes versus microfracture: Five-year follow-up of a prospective randomized trial. *Am J Sports Med* 2018;46:1343-1351.
3. Peterson L, Vasiliadis HS, Brittberg M, Lindahl A: Autologous chondrocyte implantation: A long-term follow-up. *Am J Sports Med* 2010;38:1117-1124.
4. Gomoll AH, Gillogly SD, Cole BJ, et al: Autologous chondrocyte implantation in the patella: A multicenter experience. *Am J Sports Med* 2014;42:1074-1081.
5. Ogura T, Mosier BA, Bryant T, Minas T: A 20-year follow-up after first-generation autologous chondrocyte implantation. *Am J Sports Med* 2017;45:2751-2761.
6. Benedek TG: A history of the understanding of cartilage. *Osteoarthritis Cartilage* 2006;14:203-209.
7. Steadman JR, Rodkey WG, Briggs KK: Microfracture: Its history and experience of the developing surgeon. *Cartilage* 2010;1:78-86.
8. Krych AJ, Hevesi M, Desai VS, Camp CL, Stuart MJ, Saris DBF: Learning from failure in cartilage repair surgery: An analysis of the mode of failure of primary procedures in consecutive cases at a tertiary referral center. *Orthop J Sport Med* 2018;6:2325967118773041.
9. Krych AJ, Saris DBF, Stuart MJ, Hacken B: Cartilage injury in the knee: Assessment and treatment options. *J Am Acad Orthop Surg* 2020;28:914-922.
10. Hjelle K, Solheim E, Strand T, Muri R, Brittberg M: Articular cartilage defects in 1,000 knee arthroscopies. *Arthroscopy* 2002;18:730-734.
11. Slattery C, Kweon CY: Classifications in brief: Outerbridge classification of chondral lesions. *Clin Orthop Relat Res* 2018;476:2101-2104.
12. Deng C, Zhu H, Li J, et al: Bioactive scaffolds for regeneration of cartilage and subchondral bone interface. *Theranostics* 2018;8:1940-1955.
13. Churchill JL, Krych AJ, Lemos MJ, Redd M, Bonner KF: A case series of successful repair of articular cartilage fragments in the knee. *Am J Sports Med* 2019;47:2589-2595.
14. Bisson LJ, Kluczynski MA, Wind WM, et al: Patient outcomes after observation versus debridement of unstable chondral lesions during partial meniscectomy: The Chondral Lesions And Meniscus Procedures (ChAMP) randomized controlled trial. *J Bone Joint Surg Am* 2017;99:1078-1085.
15. Mithoefer K, McAdams T, Williams RJ, Kreuz PC, Mandelbaum BR: Clinical efficacy of the microfracture technique for articular cartilage repair in the knee: An evidence-based systematic analysis. *Am J Sports Med* 2009;37:2053-2063.

16. Gudas R, Gudaite A, Pocius A, et al: Ten-year follow-up of a prospective, randomized clinical study of mosaic osteochondral autologous transplantation versus microfracture for the treatment of osteochondral defects in the knee joint of athletes. *Am J Sports Med* 2012;40:2499-2508.
17. Hevesi M, Denbeigh JM, Paggi CA, et al: Fresh osteochondral allograft transplantation in the knee: A viability and histologic analysis for optimizing graft viability and expanding existing standard processed graft resources using a living donor cartilage program. *Cartilage* 2021;13(1 suppl):948S-956S.
18. Bugbee WD, Pallante-Kichura AL, Görtz S, Amiel D, Sah R: Osteochondral allograft transplantation in cartilage repair: Graft storage paradigm, translational models, and clinical applications. *J Orthop Res* 2016;34:31-38.
19. Chahal J, Gross AE, Gross C, et al: Outcomes of osteochondral allograft transplantation in the knee. *Arthroscopy* 2013;29:575-588.
20. Jones KJ, Mosich GM, Williams RJ: Fresh precut osteochondral allograft core transplantation for the treatment of femoral cartilage defects. *Arthrosc Tech* 2018;7:e791-e795.
21. Wu JZ, Herzog W, Hasler EM: Inadequate placement of osteochondral plugs may induce abnormal stress-strain distributions in articular cartilage – Finite element simulations. *Med Eng Phys* 2002;24:85-97.
22. Smith BD, Grande DA: The current state of scaffolds for musculoskeletal regenerative applications. *Nat Rev Rheumatol* 2015;11:213-222.
23. Aaron R: *Orthopaedic Basic Science: Foundations of Clinical Practice*, ed 5. American Academy of Orthopaedic Surgeons, 2020.
24. Voss A, McCarthy MB, Hoberman A, et al: Extracellular matrix of current biological scaffolds promotes the differentiation potential of mesenchymal stem cells. *Arthroscopy* 2016;32:2381-2392.e1.
25. Hollister SJ, Murphy WL: Scaffold translation: Barriers between concept and clinic. *Tissue Eng Part B Rev* 2011;17:459-474.
26. Brauker JH, Carr-Brendel VE, Martinson LA, Crudele J, Johnston WD, Johnson RC: Neovascularization of synthetic membranes directed by membrane microarchitecture. *J Biomed Mater Res* 1995;29:1517-1524.
27. Whang K, Healy KE, Elenz DR, et al: Engineering bone regeneration with bioabsorbable scaffolds with novel microarchitecture. *Tissue Eng* 1999;5:35-51.
28. Le H, Xu W, Zhuang X, Chang F, Wang Y, Ding J: Mesenchymal stem cells for cartilage regeneration. *J Tissue Eng* 2020;11:2041731420943839.
29. Behrens P, Bitter T, Kurz B, Russlies M: Matrix-associated autologous chondrocyte transplantation/implantation (MACT/MACI)--5-year follow-up. *Knee* 2006;13:194-202.
30. Kusano T, Jakob RP, Gautier E, Magnussen RA, Hoogewoud H, Jacobi M: Treatment of isolated chondral and osteochondral defects in the knee by autologous matrix-induced chondrogenesis (AMIC). *Knee Surg Sports Traumatol Arthrosc* 2012;20:2109-2115.
31. Lietman SA: Induced pluripotent stem cells in cartilage repair. *World J Orthop* 2016;7:149-155.
32. Wasyłeczko M, Sikorska W, Chwojnowski A: Review of synthetic and hybrid scaffolds in cartilage tissue engineering. *Membranes (Basel)* 2020;10(11):348.
33. Sawatjui N, Limpaiboon T, Schrobback K, Klein T: Biomimetic scaffolds and dynamic compression enhance the properties of chondrocyte- and MSC-based tissue-engineered cartilage. *J Tissue Eng Regen Med* 2018;12:1220-1229.
34. Jin R, Moreira Teixeira LS, Dijkstra PJ, et al: Injectable chitosan-based hydrogels for cartilage tissue engineering. *Biomaterials* 2009;30:2544-2551.
35. de Windt TS, Concaro S, Lindahl A, Saris DBF, Brittberg M: Strategies for patient profiling in articular cartilage repair of the knee: A prospective cohort of patients treated by one experienced cartilage surgeon. *Knee Surg Sports Traumatol Arthrosc* 2012;20:2225-2232.
36. Tan H, Chu CR, Payne KA, Marra KG: Injectable in situ forming biodegradable chitosan-hyaluronic acid based hydrogels for cartilage tissue engineering. *Biomaterials* 2009;30:2499-2506.
37. Gobbi A, Whyte GP: Long-term clinical outcomes of one-stage cartilage repair in the knee with hyaluronic acid-based scaffold embedded with mesenchymal stem cells sourced from bone marrow aspirate concentrate. *Am J Sports Med* 2019;47:1621-1628.
38. Gobbi A, Whyte GP: One-stage cartilage repair using a hyaluronic acid-based scaffold with activated bone marrow-derived mesenchymal stem cells compared with microfracture: Five-year follow-up. *Am J Sports Med* 2016;44:2846-2854.
39. Kay S, Thapa A, Haberstroh KM, Webster TJ: Nanostructured polymer/nanophase ceramic composites enhance osteoblast and chondrocyte adhesion. *Tissue Eng* 2002;8:753-761.
40. Park GE, Pattison MA, Park K, Webster TJ: Accelerated chondrocyte functions on NaOH-treated PLGA scaffolds. *Biomaterials* 2005;26:3075-3082.
41. Morille M, Toupet K, Montero-Menei CN, Jorgensen C, Noël D: PLGA-based microcarriers induce mesenchymal stem cell chondrogenesis and stimulate cartilage repair in osteoarthritis. *Biomaterials* 2016;88:60-69.
42. Filardo G, Kon E, Perdisa F, et al: Osteochondral scaffold reconstruction for complex knee lesions: A comparative evaluation. *Knee* 2013;20:570-576.
43. Joshi N, Reverte-Vinaixa M, Díaz-Ferreiro EW, Domínguez-Oronoz R: Synthetic resorbable scaffolds for the treatment of isolated patellofemoral cartilage defects in young patients: Magnetic resonance imaging and clinical evaluation. *Am J Sports Med* 2012;40:1289-1295.
44. Demers C, Hamdy CR, Corsi K, Chellat F, Tabrizian M, Yahia L: Natural coral exoskeleton as a bone graft substitute: A review. *Bio Med Mater Eng* 2002;12:15-35.
45. Chubinskaya S, Di Matteo B, Lovato L, Iacono F, Robinson D, Kon E: Agili-C implant promotes the regenerative capacity of articular cartilage defects in an ex vivo model. *Knee Surg Sports Traumatol Arthrosc* 2019;27:1953-1964.
46. Kon E, Filardo G, Shani J, et al: Osteochondral regeneration with a novel aragonite-hyaluronate biphasic scaffold: Up to 12-month follow-up study in a goat model. *J Orthop Surg Res* 2015;10:81.

47. Van Genechten W, Vuylsteke K, Struijk C, Swinnen L, Verdonk P: Joint surface lesions in the knee treated with an acellular aragonite-based scaffold: A 3-year follow-up case series. *Cartilage* 2021;13(1 suppl):1217S-1227S.

48. Kon E, Di Matteo B, Verdonk P, et al: Aragonite-based scaffold for the treatment of joint surface lesions in mild to moderate osteoarthritic knees: Results of a 2-year multicenter prospective study. *Am J Sports Med* 2021;49:588-598.

49. Maislin G, Kennan B: A Prospective Multicenter Open -label Randomized Controlled Trial of Agili-C(TM) vs Surgical standard of Care for the treatment of Joint Surface Lesions of the Knee: Protocol CLN0022 A Statistical Analysis Report. https://www.cartiheal.com/wp-content/uploads/2017/12/CLN0021-EU-Rev-2_Sep-18-2017-clean-2.pdf. Accessed April 2, 2022.

50. Dong Y, Yong T, Liao S, Chan CK, Stevens MM, Ramakrishna S: Distinctive degradation behaviors of electrospun polyglycolide, poly(DL-lactide-co-glycolide), and poly(L-lactide-co-epsilon-caprolactone) nanofibers cultured with/without porcine smooth muscle cells. *Tissue Eng Part A* 2010;16:283-298.

51. Place ES, George JH, Williams CK, Stevens MM: Synthetic polymer scaffolds for tissue engineering. *Chem Soc Rev* 2009;38:1139-1151.

52. Ding H, Cheng Y, Niu X, Hu Y: Application of electrospun nanofibers in bone, cartilage and osteochondral tissue engineering. *J Biomater Sci Polym Ed* 2021;32:536-561.

53. Dresing I, Zeiter S, Auer J, Alini M, Eglin D: Evaluation of a press-fit osteochondral poly(ester-urethane) scaffold in a rabbit defect model. *J Mater Sci Mater Med* 2014;25:1691-1700.

54. Chen S, Chen W, Chen Y, Mo X, Fan C: Chondroitin sulfate modified 3D porous electrospun nanofiber scaffolds promote cartilage regeneration. *Mater Sci Eng C Mater Biol Appl* 2021;118:111312.

55. Xu J, Fang Q, Liu Y, Zhou Y, Ye Z, Tan W-S: In situ ornamenting poly(ε-caprolactone) electrospun fibers with different fiber diameters using chondrocyte-derived extracellular matrix for chondrogenesis of mesenchymal stem cells. *Colloids Surf B Biointerfaces* 2021;197:111374.

56. Kim HS, Mandakhbayar N, Kim H-W, Leong KW, Yoo HS: Protein-reactive nanofibrils decorated with cartilage-derived decellularized extracellular matrix for osteochondral defects. *Biomaterials* 2021;269:120214.

57. Díaz-Prado S, Rendal-Vázquez ME, Muiños-López E, et al: Potential use of the human amniotic membrane as a scaffold in human articular cartilage repair. *Cell Tissue Bank* 2010;11:183-195.

58. Naseer N, Bashir S, Latief N, Latif F, Khan SN, Riazuddin S: Human amniotic membrane as differentiating matrix for in vitro chondrogenesis. *Regen Med* 2018;13:821-832.

59. Mouser VHM, Levato R, Bonassar LJ, et al: Three-dimensional bioprinting and its potential in the field of articular cartilage regeneration. *Cartilage* 2017;8:327-340.

60. Probst FA, Hutmacher DW, Müller DF, Machens H-G, Schantz J-T: Calvarial reconstruction by customized bioactive implant [German]. *Handchir Mikrochir Plast Chir* 2010;42:369-373.

61. Huang BJ, Hu JC, Athanasiou KA: Cell-based tissue engineering strategies used in the clinical repair of articular cartilage. *Biomaterials* 2016;98:1-22.

62. Schneider U, Rackwitz L, Andereya S, et al: A prospective multicenter study on the outcome of type I collagen hydrogel-based autologous chondrocyte implantation (CaReS) for the repair of articular cartilage defects in the knee. *Am J Sports Med* 2011;39:2558-2565.

63. Wylie JD, Hartley MK, Kapron AL, Aoki SK, Maak TG: What is the effect of matrices on cartilage repair? A systematic review. *Clin Orthop Relat Res* 2015;473:1673-1682.

64. Armoiry X, Cummins E, Connock M, et al: Autologous chondrocyte implantation with chondrosphere for treating articular cartilage defects in the knee: An evidence review group perspective of a NICE single technology appraisal. *Pharmacoeconomics* 2019;37:879-886.

65. Xu X, Zheng L, Yuan Q, et al: Transforming growth factor-β in stem cells and tissue homeostasis. *Bone Res* 2018;6:2.

66. Wang T, Belkin NS, Burge AJ, et al: Patellofemoral cartilage lesions treated with particulated juvenile allograft cartilage: A prospective study with minimum 2-year clinical and magnetic resonance imaging outcomes. *Arthroscopy* 2018;34:1498-1505.

67. Tompkins M, Hamann JC, Diduch DR, et al: Preliminary results of a novel single-stage cartilage restoration technique: Particulated juvenile articular cartilage allograft for chondral defects of the patella. *Arthroscopy* 2013;29:1661-1670.

68. Kim YS, Choi YJ, Koh YG: Mesenchymal stem cell implantation in knee osteoarthritis: An assessment of the factors influencing clinical outcomes. *Am J Sports Med* 2015;43:2293-2301.

69. Makris EA, Gomoll AH, Malizos KN, Hu JC, Athanasiou KA: Repair and tissue engineering techniques for articular cartilage. *Nat Rev Rheumatol* 2015;11:21-34.

70. Paschos NK, Sennett ML: Update on mesenchymal stem cell therapies for cartilage disorders. *World J Orthop* 2017;8:853-860.

71. Jaibaji M, Jaibaji R, Volpin A: Mesenchymal stem cells in the treatment of cartilage defects of the knee: A systematic review of the clinical outcomes. *Am J Sports Med* 2021;49(13):3716-3727.

72. Kangari P, Talaei-Khozani T, Razeghian-Jahromi I, Razmkhah M: Mesenchymal stem cells: Amazing remedies for bone and cartilage defects. *Stem Cell Res Ther* 2020;11:492.

73. Hunt NC, Grover LM: Cell encapsulation using biopolymer gels for regenerative medicine. *Biotechnol Lett* 2010;32:733-742.

74. Jorgensen C, Gordeladze J, Noel D: Tissue engineering through autologous mesenchymal stem cells. *Curr Opin Biotechnol* 2004;15:406-410.

75. ter Huurne M, Schelbergen R, Blattes R, et al: Antiinflammatory and chondroprotective effects of intraarticular injection of adipose-derived stem cells in experimental osteoarthritis. *Arthritis Rheum* 2012;64:3604-3613.

76. Chen FH, Tuan RS: Mesenchymal stem cells in arthritic diseases. *Arthritis Res Ther* 2008;10:223.

77. Fang W, Sun Z, Chen X, Han B, Vangsness CTJ: Synovial fluid mesenchymal stem cells for knee arthritis and cartilage defects: A review of the literature. *J Knee Surg* 2021;34(13):1476-1485.

78. Lee W-J, Hah Y-S, Ock S-A, et al: Cell source-dependent in vivo immunosuppressive properties of mesenchymal stem cells derived from the bone marrow and synovial fluid of minipigs. *Exp Cell Res* 2015;333:273-288.

79. Isobe Y, Koyama N, Nakao K, et al: Comparison of human mesenchymal stem cells derived from bone marrow, synovial fluid, adult dental pulp, and exfoliated deciduous tooth pulp. *Int J Oral Maxillofac Surg* 2016;45:124-131.

80. Jones EA, English A, Henshaw K, et al: Enumeration and phenotypic characterization of synovial fluid multipotential mesenchymal progenitor cells in inflammatory and degenerative arthritis. *Arthritis Rheum* 2004;50:817-827.

81. Morito T, Muneta T, Hara K, et al: Synovial fluid-derived mesenchymal stem cells increase after intra-articular ligament injury in humans. *Rheumatology* 2008;47:1137-1143.

82. Zayed M, Caniglia C, Misk N, Dhar MS: Donor-matched comparison of chondrogenic potential of equine bone marrow- and synovial fluid-derived mesenchymal stem cells: Implications for cartilage tissue regeneration. *Front Vet Sci* 2016;3:121.

83. Castro-Viñuelas R, Sanjurjo-Rodríguez C, Piñeiro-Ramil M, et al: Induced pluripotent stem cells for cartilage repair: Current status and future perspectives. *Eur Cell Mater* 2018;36:96-109.

84. Evans MJ, Kaufman MH: Establishment in culture of pluripotential cells from mouse embryos. *Nature* 1981;292:154-156.

85. Takahashi K, Yamanaka S: Induction of pluripotent stem cells from mouse embryonic and adult fibroblast cultures by defined factors. *Cell* 2006;126:663-676.

86. Park Y-B, Ha C-W, Lee C-H, Yoon YC, Park Y-G: Cartilage regeneration in osteoarthritic patients by a composite of allogeneic umbilical cord blood-derived mesenchymal stem cells and hyaluronate hydrogel: Results from a clinical trial for safety and proof-of-concept with 7 years of extended follow-Up. *Stem Cells Transl Med* 2017;6:613-621.

87. Daher RJ, Chahine NO, Greenberg AS, Sgaglione NA, Grande DA: New methods to diagnose and treat cartilage degeneration. *Nat Rev Rheumatol* 2009;5:599-607.

88. Bajpayee AG, Grodzinsky AJ: Cartilage-targeting drug delivery: Can electrostatic interactions help? *Nat Rev Rheumatol* 2017;13:183-193.

89. Kraus VB, Birmingham J, Stabler TV, et al: Effects of intraarticular IL1-Ra for acute anterior cruciate ligament knee injury: A randomized controlled pilot trial (NCT00332254). *Osteoarthritis Cartilage* 2012;20:271-278.

90. Brown C, Toth A, Magnussen R: Clinical benefits of intra-articular anakinra for persistent knee effusion. *J Knee Surg* 2011;24:61-65.

91. Mianehsaz E, Mirzaei HR, Mahjoubin-Tehran M, et al: Mesenchymal stem cell-derived exosomes: A new therapeutic approach to osteoarthritis? *Stem Cell Res Ther* 2019;10:340.

92. Schmal H, Kowal JM, Kassem M, et al: Comparison of regenerative tissue quality following matrix-associated cell implantation using amplified chondrocytes compared to synovium-derived stem cells in a rabbit model for cartilage lesions. *Stem Cells Int* 2018;2018:4142031.

93. McIntyre JA, Jones IA, Han B, Vangsness CTJ: Intra-articular mesenchymal stem cell therapy for the human joint: A systematic review. *Am J Sports Med* 2018;46:3550-3563.

94. Murphy MB, Moncivais K, Caplan AI: Mesenchymal stem cells: Environmentally responsive therapeutics for regenerative medicine. *Exp Mol Med* 2013;45:e54.

95. Chang Y-H, Wu K-C, Harn H-J, Lin S-Z, Ding D-C: Exosomes and stem cells in degenerative disease diagnosis and therapy. *Cell Transplant* 2018;27:349-363.

96. Phinney DG, Pittenger MF: Concise review: MSC-derived exosomes for cell-free therapy. *Stem Cell* 2017;35:851-858.

97. Zhu Y, Wang Y, Zhao B, et al: Comparison of exosomes secreted by induced pluripotent stem cell-derived mesenchymal stem cells and synovial membrane-derived mesenchymal stem cells for the treatment of osteoarthritis. *Stem Cell Res Ther* 2017;8:64.

98. Saris TFF, de Windt TS, Kester EC, Vonk LA, Custers RJH, Saris DBF: Five-year outcome of 1-stage cell-based cartilage repair using recycled autologous chondrons and allogenic mesenchymal stromal cells: A first-in-human clinical trial. *Am J Sports Med* 2021;49:941-947.

99. Bekkers JEJ, Tsuchida AI, van Rijen, et al: Single-stage cell-based cartilage regeneration using a combination of chondrons and mesenchymal stromal cells: Comparison with microfracture. *Am J Sports Med* 2013;41:2158-2166.

100. de Windt TS, Sorel JC, Vonk LA, Kip MMA, Ijzerman MJ, Saris DBF: Early health economic modelling of single-stage cartilage repair. Guiding implementation of technologies in regenerative medicine. *J Tissue Eng Regen Med* 2017;11:2950-2959.

101. Vonk LA, Doulabi BZ, Huang C, Helder MN, Everts V, Bank RA: Preservation of the chondrocyte's pericellular matrix improves cell-induced cartilage formation. *J Cell Biochem* 2010;110:260-271.

102. Jacer S, Shafaei H, Soleimani Rad J: An investigation on the regenerative effects of intra articular injection of co-cultured adipose derived stem cells with chondron for treatment of induced osteoarthritis. *Adv Pharm Bull* 2018;8:297-306.

CHAPTER 27

Knee and Ankle Osteoarthritis—Injectables

Hannah Bradsell, BS • Rachel M. Frank, MD, FAAOS

INTRODUCTION

Osteoarthritis is a common condition, affecting more than 10% of the US population according to the Institute for Health Metrics and Evaluation's Global Burden of Disease tool and more than 100 million people worldwide.[1,2] The prevalence of osteoarthritis increases significantly with age and it is a leading cause of disability.[1,3] Notably, these numbers are likely underestimated because models have often been based on hip and knee osteoarthritis, and the recognition of the effect and occurrence of hand/wrist and foot/ankle osteoarthritis has only recently increased.[4] In addition to the physical burden, health care spending on osteoarthritis rises annually and in 2016, it was estimated to be $80 billion, with more than half spent on patients older than 65 years.[4] There is currently no cure for osteoarthritis, but there are a multitude of treatment modalities that reduce pain and improve function. Commonly used first-line, nonbiologic injectable treatment methods include corticosteroid, hyaluronic acid, and combined hyaluronic acid–steroid solutions. Orthobiologics are a recent focus for the treatment of osteoarthritis that aim to improve longevity to the native joint and delay a total joint replacement.

OSTEOARTHRITIS

Osteoarthritis is a debilitating and chronic degenerative joint disease that is characterized by osteophyte formation and loss of cartilage. It most frequently affects older patients and appears in joints with the highest weight-bearing loads, such as the knees and ankles. Approximately 15.1 million people have symptomatic osteoarthritis at the knee and the lifetime risk of the development of osteoarthritis, or the probability of a diagnosis over the lifetime of US adults, is 13.8%.[1,5] In people older than 60 years, the prevalence of knee osteoarthritis is 37%, and this number is expected to increase with the aging population of the United States.[6] The prevalence of ankle osteoarthritis remains unclear given a historical lack of attention and research relative to other joints such as the knee, but it is estimated to affect approximately 1% of the world's adult population and a relatively younger population compared with osteoarthritis at other joints.[7,8] Compared with the knee, the ankle is rarely affected by primary osteoarthritis. Ankle osteoarthritis is more likely to develop as a result of previous trauma, with the literature showing that up to 80% of patients with ankle osteoarthritis have a history of at least one ankle joint injury. Notably, patients with posttraumatic osteoarthritis are typically younger compared with those with primary osteoarthritis.[7] Regardless of etiology and despite its lower prevalence, the severity of the disabilities associated with end-stage ankle osteoarthritis is equivalent to that of hip osteoarthritis and thus, a significant burden.[3]

End-stage osteoarthritis is indicated by a Kellgren-Lawrence (K-L) grade of 4, which is seen as bone-to-bone contact and severe joint-space narrowing in weight-bearing radiographs.[3,7] Currently, there is no definitive cure for osteoarthritis, but several treatment methods are available to modify the most common clinical symptoms of osteoarthritis, including pain and inflammation. Notably, all currently available treatment strategies for osteoarthritis that are FDA approved are considered symptom-modifying treatment strategies, as opposed to disease-modifying treatment strategies. To date, no known FDA-approved treatment has been shown to modify, halt, or reverse the progression of osteoarthritis. Typical treatment strategies for early to moderate osteoarthritis include activity modification, cryotherapy, weight loss, brace treatment, physical therapy, NSAIDs, and a variety of injections (steroid, viscosupplementation, and orthobiologics). In rare instances of osteoarthritis with associated mechanical symptoms, arthroscopy can be of some utility as well. When osteoarthritis of either the knee or ankle advances to include deformity, stiffness, and pain that no longer responds to the aforementioned treatment strategies, definitive treatment includes total joint arthroplasty

Dr. Frank or an immediate family member is a member of a speakers' bureau or has made paid presentations on behalf of Allosource, Arthrex, Inc., JRF, and Össur; serves as a paid consultant to or is an employee of Allosource, Arthrex, Inc., and JRF; has received research or institutional support from Arthrex, Inc. and Smith & Nephew; and serves as a board member, owner, officer, or committee member of the American Academy of Orthopaedic Surgeons, the American Orthopaedic Society for Sports Medicine, the American Shoulder and Elbow Surgeons, the Arthroscopy Association of North America, the International Cartilage Restoration Society, and the International Society of Arthroscopy, Knee Surgery, and Orthopaedic Sports Medicine. Neither Hannah Bradsell nor any immediate family member has received anything of value from or has stock or stock options held in a commercial company or institution related directly or indirectly to the subject of this chapter.

for either the knee or ankle or arthrodesis of the ankle.[6,8] Over the past decade, given the prevalence and disease burden associated with osteoarthritis, alternative treatment options, including orthobiologic therapies, have been introduced in an effort to delay or prevent definitive surgery such as arthroplasty or arthrodesis.

ORTHOBIOLOGIC TREATMENT OPTIONS

Biologic injectable treatment methods for osteoarthritis can be subcategorized into four types of therapies: noncellular therapies, gene therapies, point-of-care autologous cell therapies, and expanded cell therapies (**Figure 1**). Of critical importance, and as described in detail elsewhere in this text, is understanding whether a given therapy is considered approved or not approved by the FDA, as well as if the product/treatment is considered on-label or off-label. Given the ever-changing nature of the orthobiologic landscape, it is important for clinicians and researchers to understand the regulations surrounding all orthobiologic injectables, including those described in subsequent sections. As a disclaimer, the authors of this chapter are not advocating for any specific biologic treatment.

Noncellular therapies target the proinflammatory and catabolic processes that contribute to the progression of osteoarthritis and aim to correct the imbalance of catabolic and anabolic factors to promote cartilage repair. One of the major targets is interleukin 1 beta (IL-1β), which is thought to be a direct mediator in the destructive processes leading to osteoarthritis and has been shown to dedifferentiate chondrocytes.[9] The intra-articular injection of anakinra, an immunosuppressive drug and IL-1β antagonist that is used to manage rheumatoid arthritis and is also known as Kineret (Swedish Orphan Biovitrum AB), has been studied for its effectiveness in managing osteoarthritis.[10] Another major target is tumor necrosis factor (TNF), which is a proinflammatory cytokine that interacts with chondrocytes and is associated with a loss of articular cartilage. The intra-articular use of TNF inhibitors for the management of knee osteoarthritis has shown potential in early clinical investigations.[9] Growth factors are anabolic proteins that heavily influence the capacity for tissue repair and have the potential to improve cartilage and bone healing. Among their functions are chemotaxis, cell differentiation, proliferation, and cellular responses.[11] Growth factors are a target for gene therapy to enhance function or increase the expression of a particular growth factor for healing. TissueGene-C (TG-C) (Kolon TissueGene, Inc.) is an example of this, which is an injectable treatment for knee osteoarthritis containing allogeneic chondrocytes expressing transforming growth factor beta.[11,12] Recombinant human bone morphogenetic proteins are widely used growth factors and their use as an intra-articular therapy has been evaluated in clinical trials for managing knee osteoarthritis with safe and

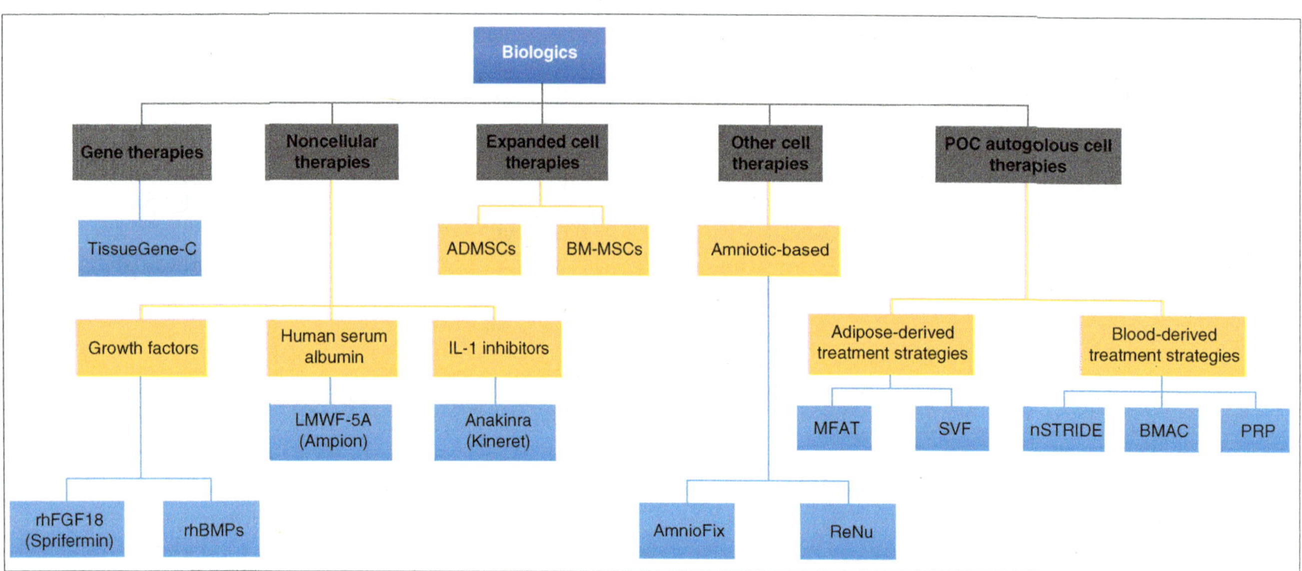

FIGURE 1 Injectable intra-articular orthobiologic solutions for the management of osteoarthritis. Schematic illustration shows current biologic treatment strategies can be subcategorized into four main types of therapies: gene, noncellular, expanded cell, and point-of-care autologous cell. Other cell-based therapies that are neither expanded nor point-of-care therapies include amniotic tissue–derived solutions. ADMSCs = adipose-derived mesenchymal stromal cells, BMAC = bone marrow aspirate concentrate, BM-MSCs = bone marrow–derived mesenchymal stromal cells, IL-1 = interleukin 1, LMWF-5A = low-molecular-weight fraction of 5% human serum albumin, MFAT = microfragmented adipose tissue, POC = point-of-care, PRP = platelet-rich plasma, rhBMPs = recombinant human bone morphogenetic proteins, rhFGF18 = recombinant human fibroblast growth factor 18, SVF = stromal vascular fraction

encouraging results.[9] Preclinical and clinical studies have also investigated recombinant human fibroblast growth factor 18, also known as Sprifermin (Merck KGaA), based on its involvement in chondrogenesis, chondrocyte proliferation, and cartilage repair.[9,12]

Point-of-care injectable autologous cell therapies include platelet-rich plasma (PRP), aspirated bone marrow concentrate, or bone marrow aspirate concentrate (BMAC), as well as adipose tissue–derived treatment strategies such as microfragmented adipose tissue (MFAT) and stromal vascular fraction (SVF). PRP is a sample of blood that is centrifuged to concentrate platelets above baseline values, which secrete several anabolic growth factors and recruit reparative cells.[13] The platelets in PRP interact with endogenous cells and intra-articular collagen within the joint, activating their healing properties and initiating the secretion of chemical mediators that act as anticatabolic and anti-inflammatory agents.[14] BMAC is obtained from bone marrow and processed similarly to PRP to concentrate its key healing components and influence cartilage restoration. It is known for its source of mesenchymal signaling or stem cells (MSCs), but it also contains chondrogenic cells, platelets, growth factors, cytokines, and numerous other bioactive factors. Together, its contents promote cartilage regeneration and induce healing responses by inhibiting inflammation, stimulating chondrogenesis, and activating cell proliferation, differentiation, and angiogenesis.[15] Autologous adipose tissue–derived injection treatment strategies are derived from lipoaspirate that undergoes either mechanical digestion to obtain MFAT or enzymatic digestion to obtain SVF.[9,16] MFAT is obtained through minimal manipulation via a manual processing device that washes and mechanically breaks down lipoaspirate without the use of enzymes or additives, resulting in a product with an intact extracellular matrix and vascular niche.[17,18] It is difficult to estimate the number of MSCs per milliliter of MFAT, but it also contains pericytes, which are MSC progenitors that are thought to differentiate into MSCs that are specific to the pathologic microenvironment after injection. In addition, MFAT is rich in angiogenic, anti-inflammatory, and immunomodulatory growth factors and cytokines and has further anti-inflammatory properties, all of which contribute to its clinical effects in combination with MSCs.[18] After the enzymatic digestion of lipoaspirate by collagenase, the product undergoes centrifugation to remove floating adipocytes and liquefied fat, resulting in a cell pellet left at the bottom of the tube, or the SVF.[19] SVF contains MSCs, macrophages, blood cells, pericytes, fibroblasts, endothelial and smooth muscle cells, and their progenitors.[19] SVF has anti-inflammatory effects through the release of growth factors and cytokines. Its mechanisms are not fully understood, but it has been suggested that SVF cells are able to detect the local environment of osteoarthritis and respond appropriately, and its regulating effects on surrounding cells can promote tissue renewal.[19] SVF and MFAT are easily accessible and efficient ways to obtain MSCs for point-of-care treatment strategies without having to undergo expansion, similar to how BMAC provides an efficient way to obtain a higher volume of MSCs from bone marrow aspirate. Each product is highly heterogeneous and, for this reason, must undergo autologous treatment strategies because of the presence of other various cell types that can cause immunologic rejection.[16]

Expanded cell therapies are derived from harvested tissue that undergoes culture expansion to allow for a more homogenous cell population in higher doses than nonexpanded, point-of-care therapies.[17] The development of these therapies requires more extensive modifications, making them subject to greater regulatory oversight, but have been shown to be safe.[9] Currently, these therapies are not permitted for use in the United States outside of an FDA-approved clinical trial. In the context of osteoarthritis, MSCs are the most frequently discussed cell types that undergo such expansion and are most commonly delivered via intra-articular injections.[17] They are multipotent and the modulation of adult MSCs can lead to chondrogenesis, osteogenesis, and adipogenesis; they are capable of differentiating into chondrocytes, osteoblasts, and adipocytes.[11,20] MSCs can be isolated and harvested via minimally invasive procedures from several different types of tissues, including bone marrow and adipose tissue, or from their respective aspirates.[11] Bone marrow–derived MSCs (BM-MSCs) are the most studied, but adipose-derived stem cells (ADSCs) have recently entered the conversation as an ideal cell source. ADSCs are multipotent cells with the capacity for self-renewal and display the same ability to differentiate toward chondrocytes and osteoblasts as BM-MSCs, despite certain fundamental differences.[20,21] They have gained recent attention as an expanded cell therapy for their regenerative potential and paracrine effects, and the MSCs contained within adipose tissue have been shown to exhibit properties that make them more efficient in regenerative medicine.[22,23] They are the most readily accessible, their capacity for proliferation and differentiation is less likely to be affected by age, they can be isolated in larger quantities and with higher cellular activity, and they have nonimmunogenic and anti-inflammatory properties.[20,22] Despite stricter regulations and a more extensive isolation process, a notable benefit to these expanded MSC and ADSC therapies is that they are useful for allogeneic treatment strategies as well as autologous treatment strategies given the isolation-based methods of processing.[16]

CLINICAL APPLICATIONS

Knee

Although PRP is routinely used in clinic for various conditions, it is not FDA approved and is considered off-label. There is a lack of standardization with respect to preparation of PRP and volume of application, leading to inconsistent results on its efficacy and indicating the need for additional high-quality studies and standardized methods. However, a significant number of studies do exist, which have evaluated the use of PRP in managing osteoarthritis. Recently, Lin et al[24] performed a randomized placebo-controlled trial including 87 osteoarthritic knees that were randomized to receive leukocyte-poor PRP (n = 31), hyaluronic acid (n = 29), or normal saline solution (n = 27). Injections were given weekly for 3 weeks and clinical outcomes (Western Ontario and McMaster Universities Osteoarthritis Index [WOMAC] and International Knee Documentation Committee [IKDC] subjective scores) were collected at baseline and at 1, 2, 6, and 12 months posttreatment with comparisons made within and between groups. At 1 month, all three groups had significant improvements in both outcome scores and baseline scores and no significant difference in scores was found between the groups. At the 12-month follow-up, only the PRP group had sustained this significant improvement in both scores. Compared with the saline group, the PRP group has consistently better WOMAC and IKDC scores at each time point throughout the study, with the exception of the 1-month follow-up. In comparison, there were no significant differences in either scores between the hyaluronic acid group and the saline group at any of the follow-up time points. On further analysis of the WOMAC scores, it was found that younger age and male sex were associated with significantly better outcomes. Body mass index and osteoarthritic severity (Ahlbäck stage) were not found to have a statistically significant influence; however, patients with less severe osteoarthritis (stage I) appeared to have smaller score improvements, and patients with stage II osteoarthritis achieved slightly better mean scores compared with patients with stage III osteoarthritis. On further analysis of IKDC scores, age was again found to be a statistically significant factor in outcomes, with younger patients exhibiting higher scores, as well as osteoarthritis severity, with patients with stage II osteoarthritis showing a significantly greater improvement compared with patients with stage III osteoarthritis. Sex and body mass index did not have a significant influence on IKDC scores. The authors concluded that leukocyte-poor PRP injections can provide clinically significant improvements for at least 1 year in patients with mild to moderate osteoarthritis.[24] In a separate randomized controlled trial comparing hyaluronic acid and leukocyte-poor PRP for the management of knee osteoarthritis, Cole et al[25] similarly found results that favored PRP over hyaluronic acid. In this study, all patients underwent 3 weekly ultrasound-guided intra-articular injections of either hyaluronic acid (n = 50) or PRP (n = 49), and measures of patient-reported outcome scores (WOMAC pain, IKDC subjective, visual analog scale [VAS] pain, and Lysholm Knee Scale assessment) and difference in intra-articular biochemical marker concentrations were recorded. Overall, no difference between groups was observed in WOMAC pain scores, but significant improvements were found in the PRP group compared with the hyaluronic acid group in IKDC and VAS scores at 24 and 52 weeks of follow-up. In addition, at 12-week follow-up, the PRP group had significantly lower concentrations of IL-1β and TNF-α, which are proinflammatory cytokines found in the knee. This decreasing trend in combination with the improved clinical outcomes that followed suggests that the anti-inflammatory properties of PRP may contribute to its clinical benefits.[25] Hyaluronic acid is an expensive, synthetically manufactured product delivered via intra-articular injection and is also known as viscosupplementation, with the goal to restore hyaluronan in the synovial fluid and its protective functions in the joint, decrease pain, and improve mobility in patients with knee osteoarthritis.[26] Although hyaluronic acid has exhibited clinical benefits, it has not been shown to reliably address the inflammatory cascade within the joint. In contrast, autologous blood products, such as PRP, are biologic alternatives that address this inflammation through growth factor stimulation and proinflammatory cytokine suppression, essentially aiming to enhance anabolic factors and inhibit catabolic factors in an affected joint.[25] As shown by Lin et al[24] and Cole et al,[25] this treatment method has been associated with significantly improved short-term results, as well as indications of significantly improved long-term results with no additional risks.[27]

Koh et al[28] studied clinical outcomes and second-look arthroscopic findings of SVF injections combined with arthroscopic lavage in 30 elderly patients (age 65 years or older) for the management of osteoarthritis. Knee Injury and Osteoarthritis Outcome Score (KOOS), VAS scores, and Lysholm scores were collected preoperatively and at 3 months, 12 months, and 2 years following treatment, and 16 patients underwent second-look arthroscopy. At final follow-up, mean VAS and Lysholm scores were significantly improved from preoperative scores, and mean KOOS scores showed statistically significant improvements at all time points compared with preoperative scores. Furthermore, mean scores of all clinical outcomes significantly improved from 1-year follow-up to 2-year follow-up. At final follow-up, K-L grade increased by one grade in only five patients. No patients underwent a second surgical procedure, such as total knee arthroplasty (TKA), during the study period and no major complications occurred. On second-look arthroscopy, 14 of 16 patients (87.5%) improved or maintained cartilage status. Overall, SVF therapy was found to improve cartilage healing, reduce pain, and improve function in elderly patients, and in addition to the safety of the procedure, the authors concluded that it appears to be an effective treatment option for osteoarthritis in this population. However, it should be noted that this was a small case series providing low-level evidence and randomized controlled trials are necessary to confirm these results. In 2019, Mautner et al[18] completed a retrospective review of prospectively collected functional outcomes following MFAT and BMAC injections in 76 patients (106 knees) with symptomatic knee osteoarthritis. KOOS, Emory Quality of Life, and VAS pain scores were completed at baseline and at a minimum follow-up of 6 months. Forty-one patients (58 knees) were treated with BMAC and had a mean follow-up time of 1.80 years, and 35 patients (48 knees) were treated with MFAT and had a mean follow-up time of 1.09 years. Overall, both groups showed significant improvements from pretreatment to posttreatment in all outcome scores measured. When comparing posttreatment scores of BMAC versus MFAT, no significant difference was observed. Based on these findings, the authors concluded that an autologous tissue source, bone marrow or adipose tissue, did not affect outcomes given that both BMAC and MFAT resulted in improved outcomes for patients with osteoarthritis. Given the lack of a control group and randomization, results should be interpreted with caution and this evidence warrants further research.

Ankle

Given the posttraumatic nature of ankle osteoarthritis, there is a significantly greater focus on the application of biologics on managing osteochondral lesions of the talus. These are defects of the cartilage surface and subchondral bone typically caused by traumatic events and are precursors to chronic symptoms and early osteoarthritis 17% to 50% of the time.[29,30] Few studies exist on injectable biologic treatment strategies for general ankle osteoarthritis. In a study by Emadedin et al[31] performed in Iran in 2015, 18 patients with knee, hip, and ankle osteoarthritis received an injection of autologous expanded BM-MSCs and were followed up for 30 months. Of the six patients with ankle osteoarthritis included in the study, all patients experienced improved outcomes over the course of the study period and no severe adverse events occurred. More specifically, mean walking distance and patient-reported outcome scores (WOMAC, Foot and Ankle Outcome Score, and VAS) all significantly improved compared with baseline measures. Furthermore, at 6-month follow-up, four patients had decreased signal intensity related to subchondral edema on MRI. Overall, the authors concluded that autologous, expanded BM-MSCs were safe and beneficial for patients with ankle osteoarthritis, but further study is warranted with larger sample sizes and longer follow-up.[31] A preliminary study performed in Thailand by Angthong et al[32] evaluated a single autologous PRP injection in 12 patients with hindfoot and ankle diseases; however, only one of these patients had a diagnosis of osteoarthritis. Improvements in clinical outcomes were reported for this patient, including improved VAS and Foot and Ankle Outcome Score at final follow-up, and posttreatment radiograph showed unchanged narrowing of the medial joint space.

Hurley et al[33] performed a systematic review of clinical studies investigating the effects of ADSCs in the form of SVF injection on managing osteoarthritis. Of the 16 studies included, only 1 study involved ankles. This study, by Kim and Koh,[34] included 49 patients with varus ankle osteoarthritis who underwent arthroscopic marrow stimulation combined with lateral sliding calcaneal osteotomy, in which 26 patients also voluntarily received an MSC injection during the marrow stimulation. The mean time to second-look arthroscopy was 12.5 months and the total mean follow-up period was 27.6 months. Second-look arthroscopy was performed to evaluate cartilage regeneration using the International Cartilage Repair Society (ICRS) grade. Clinical outcome measures were also collected, including a VAS score for pain and the American Orthopaedic Foot and Ankle Society (AOFAS) score, as well as radiologic evaluation measuring the talar tilt angle. Overall, mean VAS and AOFAS scores significantly improved for both groups at final follow-up. Both outcome scores were significantly better in the MSC group compared with the control group. Furthermore, the rate of patient satisfaction with the surgical procedure was significantly higher in the MSC group. Talar tilt angles were found to significantly improve for both groups at final follow-up; however, no significant differences between the MSC group and the control group were reported. With respect to second-look arthroscopic findings, improved ICRS grades were observed in the MSC group, but this difference was not found to be statistically significant. Interestingly, the authors found a significant correlation between VAS and AOFAS scores and ICRS grades; as ICRS repair grades worsened, the VAS pain score increased and the AOFAS score decreased. Degree of talar tilt angle correction was also found to be significantly correlated with clinical outcome scores and ICRS grades. The authors concluded that in patients who underwent lateral sliding calcaneal osteotomy and marrow stimulation, MSC injection resulted in better ICRS grades and significantly improved VAS and AOFAS scores at short-term follow-up compared with no MSC treatment.[34] There are minimal studies and a significant lack of high-level evidence regarding the use of injectable biologics for the management of general ankle osteoarthritis, indicating a need for a greater focus on this area in research to obtain a better understanding of the potential of biologic management for this impactful condition.

INJECTABLE ORTHOBIOLOGICS PIPELINE

Many of the current, more extensively studied orthobiologic treatment strategies still lack quality, high-level studies and strong evidence supporting their use, and FDA approval of these treatment strategies is scarce.

However, there remain continual efforts toward enhancing modalities and creating novel solutions to better address the symptom-inducing factors of osteoarthritis as well as the underlying degenerative mechanisms. The goal of these emerging therapies is to improve treatment by slowing or reversing the progression of osteoarthritis and potentially initiating regeneration, ultimately to achieve disease-modifying effects. TG-C, also referred to as INVOSSA, is one of the most anticipated and promising treatment strategies for osteoarthritis that is currently in development and progressing toward FDA approval. In a completed multicenter, double-blinded, phase III clinical trial, Kim et al[35] compared a TG-C injection with a placebo in 159 patients with osteoarthritis to study its clinical efficacy. Seventy-eight patients received TG-C and 81 patients received the placebo. At 26, 39, and 52 weeks, compared with baseline, patients who received the TG-C treatment had significantly greater improvement in IKDC and VAS scores compared with those who received the placebo. Improvements in total WOMAC scores and in each WOMAC category (pain, stiffness, and physical function) were greater in the TG-C group compared with the placebo group at 29, 36, and 52 weeks, with the placebo group reaching statistical significance. Similar results were found when analyzing KOOS scores, in which total KOOS score was significantly improved at all time points in the TG-C group compared with the placebo group, as well as significantly higher levels of improvement in each category at 26 and 52 weeks. At 36 weeks, however, a significant difference was observed only in the pain subscale. Structural improvements were also observed associated with TG-C, although there was no statistical significance found in these results. Overall, in this phase III clinical trial, TG-C was found to be safe and result in improved function and pain, and the authors concluded that it has significant potential for a disease-modifying osteoarthritis drug.[35]

Low-molecular-weight fraction of 5% human serum albumin (LMWF-5A), also known as Ampion (Ampio Pharmaceuticals, Inc.), is a nonsteroidal and noncellular therapy currently undergoing clinical trials to assess its efficacy in managing moderate to severe osteoarthritis. LMWF-5A is derived from human serum albumin and contains an active ingredient, aspartyl-alanyl-diketopiperazine, that has been shown to have anti-inflammatory and immune-modulating effects.[36] A randomized controlled, phase III clinical trial by Bar-Or et al[36] evaluated the safety and efficacy of two doses of an intra-articular injection of LMWF-5A. Patients were randomized to receive a single injection of 4 mL or 10 mL of either LMWF-5A or saline and followed up for 12 weeks. Pain reduction occurred as early as 4 weeks postinjection and continued to 12-week follow-up, where LMWF-5A resulted in significant decreased pain compared with saline. Comparisons of outcomes between injection volumes did not show a significant difference. The effects of LMWF-5A were most pronounced in patients with severe knee osteoarthritis (K-L grade 4), particularly resulting in a significant improvement in pain. A total of 144 patients (44%) experienced adverse events among 329 patients included in the study, which were generally mild and were similar between the LMWF-5A group (41%) and the saline control group (47%). Overall, 10% of patients in the LMWF-5A group and 13% of patients in the saline group reported treatment-related adverse events, with the most common being arthralgia and injection site pain. The authors deemed a single injection of LMWF-5A to be safe, well tolerated, and an effective treatment for knee osteoarthritis, demonstrating improved pain, function, and disease severity compared with a saline control group.[36] A long-term follow-up study of a separate, phase II clinical trial investigating three intra-articular injections of LMWF-5A[37] by Schwappach et al[38] found that at 3-year follow-up, 15 of 39 patients (38.5%) had undergone a TKA. Among these patients, those who responded well to the LMWF-5A treatment during the initial trial as indicated by a pain reduction of ≥20%, had significantly lower TKA rates (1 of 7 [14%] LMWF-5A group versus 3 of 3 [100%] saline group) and longer time to TKA compared with saline control group. Between LMWF-5A and saline, patients with severe osteoarthritis (K-L grade 4) showed a lower incidence of TKA among those who received LMWF-5A (4 of 10 [40%] LMWF-5A group versus 5 of 6 [83%] saline group) and longer delay to TKA; however, these did not reach statistical significance. Overall, there was no difference in TKA rates between patients treated with LMWF-5A (9 of 23, 39%) and patients in the saline control group (6 of 16, 38%).[38]

The nSTRIDE Autologous Protein Solution (APS) Kit (Zimmer Biomet) processes autologous blood to produce the APS output that contains high concentrations of growth factors and anti-inflammatory cytokines.[39] Compared with PRP, which contains only concentrated platelets and sometimes white blood cells, APS comprises concentrated platelets, white blood cells, and plasma proteins with anabolic growth factors and cytokines.[40] The first in-human clinical trial by Van Drumpt et al[39] included 11 patients with moderate osteoarthritis to assess safety and efficacy of the solution. By 2 weeks postinjection, mean WOMAC scores showed significant improvements compared with baseline scores. There was continual improvement until 3-month follow-up that sustained at 6 months, and at both time points, there was average WOMAC score improvement by 70%. There were no adverse events related to the device and three minor adverse events related to the injection procedure, including injection site discomfort, injection site joint pain, and procedural nausea that resolved quickly and did not require treatment.[39] A similar study performed by Hix et al,[41] including 10 patients, demonstrated a similar positive safety profile and improved WOMAC scores up to 1-year follow-up, with a mean pain score improvement of 72.5%. The authors also found a significant correlation between APS concentration of white blood cells containing anti-inflammatory cytokines and WOMAC pain improvement.[41] Following initial safety studies, a 1-year pilot randomized controlled trial was performed including 46 patients with unilateral K-L grade 2 or 3 who were randomized to receive a single ultrasound-guided injection of APS (n = 31) or saline (n = 15).[40] At 2 weeks, 1 month, 3 months, and 6 months of follow-up, there were no significant differences in WOMAC pain and VAS pain scores between the APS group and the control group. At 12-month follow-up, the APS group reported a mean 65% WOMAC score improvement compared with a mean 41% improvement reported by the saline group, which was found to be a statistically significant difference. In addition, at this time point, mean VAS pain score improved by 49% in the APS group compared with 13% in the saline group, but this was not found to be statistically significant. MRI analysis comparing findings at baseline to 12 months postinjection showed unchanged bone marrow lesions and osteophytes in the lateral zone of the femoral condyle among patients receiving APS, whereas they grew larger in control patients, and no other compartments had significant differences. No major complications were reported and no significant difference in frequency or severity of adverse events was observed between the groups.[40]

Amniotic-based biologic products are a recently evolving interest for the management of orthopaedic conditions, including osteoarthritis. Amniotic membrane–derived and amniotic fluid–derived products contain anti-inflammatory proteins. In addition, amniotic membrane tissue contains a high concentration of hyaluronic acid and amniotic fluid has the ability to differentiate into chondrocytes. Furthermore, amniotic-based products have been shown to downregulate proinflammatory cytokines.[42] A recent study by Meadows et al[42] analyzed an amniotic suspension allograft (ASA), also known as ReNu (Organogenesis), in 10 patients with symptomatic, moderate hip osteoarthritis (Tönnis grade I or II). ASA comprises micronized human amniotic membrane and cells derived from amniotic fluid from the same donor and is cryogenically preserved. Patients received a single ultrasound-guided injection of ASA and patient-reported outcomes were recorded at baseline before treatment and at 1 week and 1, 2, 3, 6, and 12 months postinjection. These outcomes included pain and function subscales of the modified Harris hip score, 12-item International Hip Outcome Tool, Medical Outcomes Study 12-Item Short Form Survey, VAS pain, and Single Assessment Numeric Evaluation. Nine patients were included in the analysis because of treatment failure in one patient who opted to undergo a total hip arthroplasty. Compared with baseline, International Hip Outcome Tool, Single Assessment Numeric Evaluation, and modified Harris hip score scores showed significant improvement at 1, 2, 3, 6, and 12 months postinjection. From baseline to 12 months, mean change in International Hip Outcome Tool (31.29) and modified Harris hip score (21.50) scores exceeded the reported minimal clinically important difference of 6.1 and 4 to 8 points, respectively. No difference in joint-space narrowing from baseline to 12 months was observed on radiographs. No patient experienced infection, effusion, or increased stiffness and no immediate postinjection complications were reported; however, two patients had elevated levels of C-reactive protein that were not correlated with clinical symptoms and normalized by 6 months postinjection.[42] A randomized controlled trial by Farr et al[43] analyzed ASA (ReNu) (n = 68) compared with hyaluronic acid (n = 64) or saline (n = 68) in 200 patients with moderate knee osteoarthritis (K-L grade 2 or 3). At 3 months postinjection, 9 patients receiving ASA (13.2%), 44 patients receiving hyaluronic acid (68.8%), and 51 patients receiving saline (75%) were considered treatment failures because of reports of unacceptable pain and were withdrawn from the study. Patient-reported outcomes were completed at baseline and at 3 and 6 months of follow-up. At 3 months compared with baseline, KOOS pain, KOOS symptoms, KOOS activities of daily living, VAS pain, and VAS pain during strenuous work were significantly improved in the ASA group compared with the hyaluronic acid group. Furthermore, compared with saline, KOOS symptoms showed significant improvement in the ASA group. At 6 months compared with baseline, all patient-reported outcomes showed significant improvement in the ASA group in comparison with the hyaluronic acid group. Compared with the saline group at 6 months, the ASA group showed significant improvements in KOOS pain, KOOS symptoms, KOOS activities of daily living, and VAS pain. Given these findings, the authors concluded that ASA is an effective and safe treatment for symptomatic knee osteoarthritis.[43] Dehydrated human amnion/chorion membrane, also known as AmnioFix (MiMedx Group Inc.), is a separate amniotic-based injectable product currently being studied for the management of osteoarthritis. Dehydrated human amnion/chorion membrane is a tissue derived from donated placentae that is microionized and suspended in saline and contains anti-inflammatory properties, promotes wound healing, and exhibits low immunogenicity, with wide-ranging clinical applications.[44,45] For its use in osteoarthritis, it was previously used in clinics to manage knee osteoarthritis as a minimally manipulated product; however, it was withdrawn after 2013 because of the FDA requiring that an Investigational New Drug Application be obtained.[9] By 2017, the phase IIb study was approved and continued, but no in-human studies investigating the osteoarthritic effects of AmnioFix have been published and only one animal study has been published, reporting promising therapeutic effects and attenuation of cartilage degeneration.[9,45] It should be noted that much of the research related to these emerging treatment strategies is limited to small pilot studies and considered preliminary evidence, and findings should therefore be interpreted carefully.

SUMMARY

Osteoarthritis is a common condition associated with high physical and financial burden and is a leading cause of disability. Biologic treatment for knee and ankle osteoarthritis, and in orthopaedics in general, has become an increasingly popular focus in research. Many injectable biologic treatment options exist, including noncellular therapies, gene therapies, point-of-care autologous cell therapies, and expanded cell therapies. Furthermore, given the lack of a definitive cure for osteoarthritis, several novel solutions are currently in development, which aim to achieve disease-modifying effects in addition to symptom-modifying effects. With continued research and additional high-level studies, obtaining more conclusive evidence can continue to expand the potential for these novel techniques and their clinical applications for the management of osteoarthritis.

REFERENCES

1. Lo J, Chan L, Flynn S: A systematic review of the incidence, prevalence, costs, and activity and work limitations of amputation, osteoarthritis, rheumatoid arthritis, back pain, multiple sclerosis, spinal cord injury, stroke, and traumatic brain injury in the United States: A 2019 update. *Arch Phys Med Rehabil* 2021;102(1):115-131.
2. Murray C, Marshall M, Rathod T, Bowen CJ, Menz HB, Roddy E: Population prevalence and distribution of ankle pain and symptomatic radiographic ankle osteoarthritis in community dwelling older adults: A systematic review and cross-sectional study. *PLoS One* 2018;13(4):e0193662.
3. Jaleel A, Golightly YM, Alvarez C, Renner JB, Nelson AE: Incidence and progression of ankle osteoarthritis: The johnston county osteoarthritis project. *Semin Arthritis Rheum* 2021;51(1):230-235.
4. Peat G, Thomas MJ: Osteoarthritis year in review 2020: Epidemiology & therapy. *Osteoarthritis Cartilage* 2021;29(2):180-189.
5. Losina E, Weinstein AM, Reichmann WM, et al: Lifetime risk and age at diagnosis of symptomatic knee osteoarthritis in the US. *Arthritis Care Res* 2013;65(5):703-711.
6. Sharma L: Osteoarthritis of the knee. *N Engl J Med* 2021;384(1):51-59.
7. Barg A, Pagenstert GI, Hügle T, et al: Ankle osteoarthritis: Etiology, diagnostics, and classification. *Foot Ankle Clin* 2013;18(3):411-426.
8. Fanelli D, Mercurio M, Castioni D, Sanzo V, Gasparini G, Galasso O: End-stage ankle osteoarthritis: Arthroplasty offers better quality of life than arthrodesis with similar complication and re-operation rates—an updated meta-analysis of comparative studies. *Int Orthop* 2021;45(9):2177-2191.
9. Jones IA, Togashi R, Wilson ML, Heckmann N, Vangsness CT: Intra-articular treatment options for knee osteoarthritis. *Nat Rev Rheumatol* 2019;15(2):77-90.
10. Chevalier X, Goupille P, Beaulieu AD, et al: Intraarticular injection of anakinra in osteoarthritis of the knee: A multicenter, randomized, double-blind, placebo-controlled study. *Arthritis Rheum* 2009;61(3):344-352.
11. Pereira H, Cengiz IF, Vilela C, et al: Emerging concepts in treating cartilage, osteochondral defects, and osteoarthritis of the knee and ankle. *Adv Exp Med Biol* 2018;1059:25-62.
12. Latourte A, Kloppenburg M, Richette P: Emerging pharmaceutical therapies for osteoarthritis. *Nat Rev Rheumatol* 2020;16(12):673-688.
13. Hall MP, Band PA, Meislin RJ, Jazrawi LM, Cardone DA: Platelet-rich plasma: Current concepts and application in sports medicine. *J Am Acad Orthop Surg* 2009;17(10):602-608.
14. Knop E, Paula LED, Fuller R: Platelet-rich plasma for osteoarthritis treatment. *Rev Bras Reumatol Engl Ed* 2016;56(2):152-164.
15. Kim GB, Seo M-S, Park WT, Lee GW: Bone marrow aspirate concentrate: Its uses in osteoarthritis. *Int J Mol Sci* 2020;21(9):3224.
16. Bora P, Majumdar AS: Adipose tissue-derived stromal vascular fraction in regenerative medicine: A brief review on biology and translation. *Stem Cell Res Ther* 2017;8(1):145.
17. Lopa S, Colombini A, Moretti M, De Girolamo L: Injective mesenchymal stem cell-based treatments for knee osteoarthritis: From mechanisms of action to current clinical evidences. *Knee Surg Sports Traumatol Arthrosc* 2019;27(6):2003-2020.
18. Mautner K, Bowers R, Easley K, Fausel Z, Robinson R: Functional outcomes following microfragmented adipose tissue versus bone marrow aspirate concentrate injections for symptomatic knee osteoarthritis. *Stem Cells Transl Med* 2019;8(11):1149-1156.
19. Zhang Y, Chen X, Tong Y, Luo J, Bi Q: Development and prospect of intra-articular injection in the treatment of osteoarthritis: A review. *J Pain Res* 2020;13:1941-1955.
20. Makris EA, Gomoll AH, Malizos KN, Hu JC, Athanasiou KA: Repair and tissue engineering techniques for articular cartilage. *Nat Rev Rheumatol* 2015;11(1):21-34.
21. Noël D, Caton D, Roche S, et al: Cell specific differences between human adipose-derived and mesenchymal–stromal cells despite similar differentiation potentials. *Exp Cell Res* 2008;314(7):1575-1584.
22. Mazini L, Rochette L, Amine M, Malka G: Regenerative capacity of Adipose Derived Stem Cells (ADSCs), comparison with Mesenchymal Stem Cells (MSCs). *Int J Mol Sci* 2019;20(10):2523.
23. Nguyen A, Guo J, Banyard DA, et al: Stromal vascular fraction: A regenerative reality? Part 1 – Current concepts and review of the literature. *J Plast Reconstr Aesthet Surg* 2016;69(2):170-179.
24. Lin KY, Yang CC, Hsu CJ, Yeh ML, Renn JH: Intra-articular injection of platelet-rich plasma is superior to hyaluronic acid or saline solution in the treatment of mild to moderate knee osteoarthritis: A randomized, double-blind, triple-parallel, placebo-controlled clinical trial. *Arthroscopy* 2019;35(1):106-117.

25. Cole BJ, Karas V, Hussey K, Pilz K, Fortier LA: Hyaluronic acid versus platelet-rich plasma: A prospective, double-blind randomized controlled trial comparing clinical outcomes and effects on intra-articular biology for the treatment of knee osteoarthritis. *Am J Sports Med* 2017;45(2):339-346.
26. Bellamy N, Campbell J, Robinson V, Gee T, Bourne R, Wells G: Viscosupplementation for the treatment of osteoarthritis of the knee. *Cochrane Database Syst Rev* 2005;2:CD005321.
27. Chen Z, Wang C, You D, Zhao S, Zhu Z, Xu M: Platelet-rich plasma versus hyaluronic acid in the treatment of knee osteoarthritis: A meta-analysis. *Medicine (Baltimore)* 2020;99(11):e19388.
28. Koh YG, Choi YJ, Kwon SK, Kim YS, Yeo JE: Clinical results and second-look arthroscopic findings after treatment with adipose-derived stem cells for knee osteoarthritis. *Knee Surg Sports Traumatol Arthrosc* 2015;23(5):1308-1316.
29. Giannini S, Buda R, Cavallo M, et al: Cartilage repair evolution in post-traumatic osteochondral lesions of the talus: From open field autologous chondrocyte to bone-marrow-derived cells transplantation. *Injury* 2010;41(11):1196-1203.
30. Giannini S, Buda R, Vannini F, Cavallo M, Grigolo B: One-step bone marrow-derived cell transplantation in talar osteochondral lesions. *Clin Orthop Relat Res* 2009;467(12):3307-3320.
31. Emadedin M, Ghorbani Liastani M, Fazeli R, et al: Long-term follow-up of intra-articular injection of autologous mesenchymal stem cells in patients with knee, ankle, or hip osteoarthritis. *Arch Iran Med* 2015;18(6):336-344.
32. Angthong C, Khadsongkram A, Angthong W: Outcomes and quality of life after platelet-rich plasma therapy in patients with recalcitrant hindfoot and ankle diseases: A preliminary report of 12 patients. *J Foot Ankle Surg* 2013;52(4):475-480.
33. Hurley ET, Yasui Y, Gianakos AL, et al: Limited evidence for adipose-derived stem cell therapy on the treatment of osteoarthritis. *Knee Surg Sports Traumatol Arthrosc* 2018;26(11):3499-3507.
34. Kim YS, Koh YG: Injection of mesenchymal stem cells as a supplementary strategy of marrow stimulation improves cartilage regeneration after lateral sliding calcaneal osteotomy for varus ankle osteoarthritis: Clinical and second-look arthroscopic results. *Arthroscopy* 2016;32(5):878-889.
35. Kim MK, Ha CW, In Y, et al: A Multicenter, double-blind, Phase III clinical trial to evaluate the efficacy and safety of a cell and gene therapy in knee osteoarthritis patients. *Hum Gene Ther Clin Dev* 2018;29(1):48-59.
36. Bar-Or D, Salottolo KM, Loose H, et al: A randomized clinical trial to evaluate two doses of an intra-articular injection of LMWF-5A in adults with pain due to osteoarthritis of the knee. *PLoS One* 2014;9(2):e87910.
37. Schwappach J, Dryden SM, Salottolo KM: Preliminary trial of intra-articular LMWF-5A for osteoarthritis of the knee. *Orthopedics* 2017;40(1):e49-e53.
38. Schwappach J, Schultz J, Salottolo K, Bar-Or D: Incidence of total knee replacement subsequent to intra-articular injection of the anti-inflammatory compound LMWF-5A versus saline: A long-term follow-up study to a randomized controlled trial. *Patient Saf Surg* 2018;12:14.
39. Van Drumpt RAM, Van Der Weegen W, King W, Toler K, Macenski MM: Safety and treatment effectiveness of a single autologous protein solution injection in patients with knee osteoarthritis. *Biores Open Access* 2016;5(1):261-268.
40. Kon E, Engebretsen L, Verdonk P, Nehrer S, Filardo G: Clinical outcomes of knee osteoarthritis treated with an autologous protein solution injection: A 1-year pilot double-blinded randomized controlled trial. *Am J Sports Med* 2018;46(1):171-180.
41. Hix J, Klaassen M, Foreman R, et al: An autologous anti-inflammatory protein solution yielded a favorable safety profile and significant pain relief in an open-label pilot study of patients with osteoarthritis. *Biores Open Access* 2017;6(1):151-158.
42. Meadows MC, Elisman K, Nho SJ, Mowry K, Safran MR: A single injection of amniotic suspension allograft is safe and effective for treatment of mild to moderate hip osteoarthritis: A prospective study. *Arthroscopy* 2021;38(2):325-331.
43. Farr J, Gomoll AH, Yanke AB, Strauss EJ, Mowry KC: A randomized controlled single-blind study demonstrating superiority of amniotic suspension allograft injection over hyaluronic acid and saline control for modification of knee osteoarthritis symptoms. *J Knee Surg* 2019;32(11):1143-1154.
44. Willett NJ, Thote T, Lin AS, et al: Intra-articular injection of micronized dehydrated human amnion/chorion membrane attenuates osteoarthritis development. *Arthritis Res Ther* 2014;16(1):R47.
45. Lei J, Priddy LB, Lim JJ, Koob TJ: Dehydrated human amnion/chorion membrane (dHACM) allografts as a therapy for orthopedic tissue repair. *Tech Orthopedics* 2017;32(3):149-157.

CHAPTER

28 Ligament Repair and Regeneration

Natalie L. Leong, MD, FAAOS • Jie Jiang, PhD

INTRODUCTION

Lower extremity ligament injuries are common and present a logical target for the application of orthobiologics. Some ligaments, such as anterior cruciate ligament (ACL) tears, are unlikely to heal without surgical intervention. Meanwhile, extra-articular ligaments, such as the medial collateral ligament (MCL), often heal without surgical intervention but require significant time lost from occupational or recreational activities. Common lower extremity ligament injuries, ligament structure and function, current evidence for the use of orthobiologics, and solutions in development for lower extremity ligament injuries are reviewed.

COMMON LOWER EXTREMITY LIGAMENT INJURIES

Natural History of Extra-articular Ligament Injuries

MCL injuries are among the most common knee injuries and, with some exceptions (interposition of pes anserinus, multiligamentous injury), are typically able to heal without surgical intervention. Likewise, isolated lateral collateral ligament sprains also have good prognosis with nonsurgical treatment.

Acute injury to an extra-articular ligament is followed by three chronologic stages of healing: inflammation, proliferation, and remodeling.[1-5] Although these stages overlap, they are characterized by distinct cytokine profiles and cellular processes. Cytokines expressed in ligament healing vary temporally and functionally, with generally proinflammatory cytokines predominating early and anti-inflammatory and restorative cytokines predominating late in the healing process.[1,6] The inflammatory stage of ligament healing begins immediately after acute injury with clot formation in damaged tissue. In this phase, a clot is formed in damaged vessels, inflammatory cells are activated, and then fibroblasts are recruited to continue the healing process.[1,2] Platelets and cells within the clot release growth factors and cytokines, causing local inflammation.[1,3,7] The clot serves as the initial scaffold for the recruited extrinsic inflammatory cells.[8] Elaboration of these growth factors recruit neutrophils, which in turn activate macrophages to phagocytose necrotic debris.[1,4,8] Approximately 2 days following injury, these cytokines released from macrophages and local cells initiate the proliferative stage by recruitment of fibroblasts.[1,3] Growth factors are responsible for roles such as regulating proteinase activity, stimulating extracellular matrix production, and later, recruiting of fibroblasts.[1,3,4,9-11] These factors work synergistically to initiate the healing process. The proliferative phase is characterized by expansion of the extracellular matrix, increased cellularity, and deposition of fibrovascular scar by fibroblasts.[1,2,8] At the site of injury, fibroblasts migrate in and proliferate.[1,2] Intrinsic local cells begin to proliferate as well.[1,2] Growth factors continue to attract fibroblasts to the site, promote angiogenesis and cell proliferation, and increase extracellular matrix production.[1,3,10-15] Collagen synthesis is a highly oxygen-dependent process, underlying the importance of synergistic angiogenic actions of growth factors in this stage of healing.[1,3,16] Approximately 2 weeks after injury, remodeling of the injured area begins with reorganization of the newly deposited collagen. This process overlaps with the proliferative phase, leading to a gradual decrease in cellularity and increase in fibrous matrix.[1,3] Both ligament fibroblasts and collagen fibers become aligned in the direction of stress, with a corresponding decrease in type III collagen, vascularity, cellularity, and water content in the forming scar.[1,8] Increased collagenase activity assists in the resorption of type III collagen and replacement with type I collagen, which has more cross-links and higher tensile strength.[1,2,17] This process continues for years following the injury; however, the newly formed tissue lacks the native biomechanical, biochemical, and ultrastructural properties of the ligament.[1,5,18] There are multiple subpopulations of cells that migrate and contribute to ligament healing. Similar to most healing processes in the body, the initial proinflammatory phase is highlighted by the presence of M1 macrophages. As the inflammation subsides, there is a transition from M1 to M2 macrophages at the injury site. During this phase, fibroblasts or connective tissue progenitors migrate in and proliferate. The origins of these fibroblasts or fibroblast progenitor cells are still a subject of debate.[1]

Dr. Leong or an immediate family member serves as a board member, owner, officer, or committee member of the Arthroscopy Association of North America. Neither Dr. Jiang nor any immediate family member has received anything of value from or has stock or stock options held in a commercial company or institution related directly or indirectly to the subject of this chapter.

Natural History of Intra-articular Ligament Injuries

ACL tears typically do not heal if managed nonsurgically. Over time, an ACL-deficient knee is more likely to have meniscus tears and posttraumatic osteoarthritis. Similar to ACL tears, complete posterior cruciate ligament tears are unlikely to heal without surgical intervention. However, isolated posterior cruciate ligament tears are often asymptomatic in nonathletes and do not require surgery as frequently. In the setting of multiligamentous knee injury, however, primary posterior cruciate ligament repair or reconstruction is commonly performed.

Although most extra-articular ligaments have at least some capacity to heal and the ability to form scar that gets remodeled over time, intra-articular ligaments generally do not have healing capacity. It has been hypothesized that access to vascular supply is the differentiating factor between those ligaments that can heal and those that cannot. This is analogous to other pathologies in sports medicine. For example, meniscal tears in the white/white zone typically do not heal, whereas tears in the red/red zone have the capacity to heal. Likewise, well-vascularized tendons such as the Achilles tendon can heal, whereas poorly vascularized tendons such as the rotator cuff are less likely to heal.

LIGAMENT STRUCTURE AND FUNCTION

Ligaments are connective tissues that have relatively low cell and vascular density compared with other tissues of the body. They are composed of an extracellular matrix that contains approximately 70% type I collagen by dry weight, 1% to 2% elastin by dry weight, and ground substance consisting of proteoglycans, glycoproteins, and water. The primary cell type found in ligaments is ligament fibroblasts. Compared with tendons, ligaments have a higher percentage of elastin and ground substance and a lower percentage of collagen, less organized collagen fibers, and round fibroblasts.[19] Of course, these are generalizations because there are variations in composition among specific ligaments and tendons that are adapted to their specific roles.[19,20]

Ligaments consist of primarily type I collagen, which is synthesized as procollagen inside the ligament fibroblasts. After being excreted into the extracellular matrix and undergoing posttranslational modification, these triple-helix collagen molecules then form collagen fibrils that bundle together to form collagen fibers.[21] These collagen fibers then are cross-linked, with the degree of cross-linking an important determinant in the stiffness of the fibers.

Ligaments function to restrict joint motion and passively stabilize joints. They also contain mechanoreceptors and free joint endings to assist with proprioception.[22-25] Ligaments can endure considerable tensile load. The ACL has been shown by Woo et al[26] to have an ultimate failure load of more than 2,000 N in younger specimens and 500 N in older specimens. The MCL and lateral collateral ligament have been shown to have ultimate tensile loads of approximately 800 and 400 N, respectively.[27]

Ligaments have mechanical properties that allow them to fulfill their functions. They demonstrate nonlinear anisotropic mechanical behavior;[21] ligaments are relatively compliant under low loading conditions (toe region on stress-strain curve) because of crimp and the properties of the individual components of ligament.[21] Then, with more load, in the linear portion of the stress-strain curve, the ligament fibers are oriented longitudinally along the direction of the load. Beyond this region, the ligament continues to absorb energy in a nonlinear manner until failure.[21] Ligaments also demonstrate stress relaxation, which is decreased stress over time in the setting of constant deformation, and creep, which is increased deformation with time under constant load.

Although the mechanical and histologic properties of ligaments have been well studied, a valid question is how closely a healing connective tissue needs to resemble normal tissue to fully restore function. For example, it has been shown that even over 2 years following Achilles tendon rupture, the healed tendon consists of less elastin, with scar that is considered biomechanically inferior.[28] And yet, it is well established that complete Achilles tendon rupture is an injury that can be successfully managed nonsurgically,[29] with most patients reporting no limitations over the long term. Similarly, MCL injuries have been shown to have persistent scar at the injury site years after the injury,[30] but return to full activity is typically on the order of weeks. Thus, a biomechanically and histologically perfect tissue may not be an absolute requirement when considering a patient's function. Rather, a scar may be functionally acceptable and may remodel to some degree over time. Although traditional dogma states that tendons and ligaments heal with scar that is mechanically inferior and can cause adhesions, perhaps this idea can be revisited to explore whether functional scar is sufficient in some applications of ligament and tendon healing. A challenge going forward will be defining when scar is sufficient, whether by patient-rated outcomes, biomechanical properties, or imaging characteristics.

HISTORICAL APPROACHES AND ALTERNATIVES TO ORTHOBIOLOGIC SOLUTIONS FOR ACL SURGERY

Historical Approaches

Currently, there are no synthetic ACL grafts available in the United States, but in the 1980s, there were several efforts to use nondegradable materials to replace the ACL. The Gore-Tex ligament, approved by the FDA in 1986, was associated with effusion, graft rupture, loosening/osteolysis, and infection. A follow-up study showed unacceptable results in 76% of patients at 4 years.[31] Similarly, the Stryker Dacron ligament, approved by the FDA in 1989, was associated with graft rupture, foreign body reactions, and poor tissue ingrowth, with a staggering failure rate of 80% after 5 years.[32]

Historically, there have also been attempts at using degradable scaffolds for ACL reconstruction. Porcine small intestine submucosa (SIS) has been considered as a biologic scaffold for tendon and ligament repair. FDA-approved as the Restore product, SIS was found to have a high failure rate when used in rotator cuff repair,[33] with marked postoperative edema. A hypothesis is that while marketed as an acellular product, there are traces of porcine DNA in the product, which could lead to an immune response. SIS has also been investigated for ACL reconstruction in small and large animal models.[34,35] In the early 1990s, DePuy conducted a small pilot study of a braided SIS construct of six patients undergoing ACL reconstruction. However, this pilot study had unacceptable results, with five out of six ACL reconstruction with SIS failing within the first 6 months postoperatively. The development team hypothesized that the postoperative rehabilitation protocol was too conservative to allow proper remodeling of the relatively short-lived graft. The experience with SIS underscores some of the challenges of biologic ACL grafts; simply having a biologic material that exceeds the initial properties of a native ACL graft at the time of implantation is not necessarily sufficient; the biologic material's remodeling and interaction with its complex in vivo environment must be considered.

The Laurencin-Cooper ligament is a braided poly-L-lactic acid–degradable synthetic ACL graft. After promising results in ovine studies,[36] a phase I clinical trial was conducted in Europe, followed by a phase II/III trial that was terminated before completion, in favor of design changes to the product.[37]

Current Approaches

Currently, autografts are considered the gold standard for ACL reconstruction. Bone–patellar tendon–bone (BPTB) grafts are harvested from the central third of the patellar tendon and include bone plugs from both the patellar and proximal tibia. Advantages include high stiffness and strength, bone-to-bone incorporation, which is often better than bone-to-soft tissue integration, and interference screw fixation. BPTB grafts are generally preferred in younger patients and high-level athletes for this reason. However, they can be associated with anterior knee pain, particularly with kneeling, patellar fracture, damage to the extensor mechanism, and patella baja. They are also obviously limited in supply, which is a consideration in multiligament injury and revision.

Another autograft option is hamstring tendon, which involves harvesting the gracilis and semitendinosus tendons, which are then doubled up to form a quadrupled hamstring graft. Biomechanically speaking, the quadrupled hamstring graft has the highest mechanical strength before implantation, although this is of questionable clinical significance as all grafts are stronger than native ACL at the time of implantation. Hamstring tendon is generally associated with less donor-site morbidity than BPTB autografts. The disadvantages are possible residual hamstring weakness and laxity if the graft stretches over time, especially in younger women. Suspensory fixation may cause a windshield wiper effect with widening of bone tunnels over time. Additionally, hamstring grafts can sometimes be of insufficient size. Quadriceps tendon autografts with and without bone from the patellar have also been gaining popularity in recent years.[38] They have the benefit of providing good graft volume, do not interfere with kneeling, but have similar disadvantages as hamstrings regarding suspensory fixation. They also have comparable success rates with other autograft options.[38,39]

As previously noted, sometimes autograft is not possible because of limited supply or a patient may be older and have lower functional demands. In that case, allograft is an option. BPTB, Achilles tendon, and quadriceps tendon are all graft options. Using allografts slightly reduces surgical time because graft harvest is not performed and avoids donor-site morbidity. However, they can also be limited in supply, may incorporate more slowly, and may become weakened during the sterilization process. In addition, while highly unlikely, there is a theoretical risk of disease transmission and immunogenicity. In addition, allografts can be limited in supply, especially internationally.

ACL Repair

Although currently much less common in the United States, primary repair of the ACL is sometimes performed rather than reconstructing the ACL. Several techniques have been developed with the goal of primary repair,[40] as detailed in the next paragraphs (**Table 1**).

In suture anchor repair, the torn ACL is anchored back to the femur, without additional construct reinforcement.

TABLE 1 Variations of Anterior Cruciate Ligament Repair

Method	Advantages	Disadvantages
Suture anchor repair	Relatively simple technique	Only for proximal tears
Internal bracing treatment	Can be used as adjunct to other techniques	Risk of joint overconstraint
Dynamic intraligamentary stabilization	Early return to sport reported	High rerupture/ reoperation rates
Bridge-enhanced ACL repair	Not inferior to hamstring autograft in randomized controlled trial	Only indicated for patients within 50 days of ACL tear

ACL = anterior cruciate ligament

The methodology is based on the observation that the proximal ACL heals similarly to the MCL, a ligament with known excellent healing capacity.[41] Thus, suture anchor repair is only indicated for Sherman type 1 proximal tears with otherwise excellent tissue quality, which accounts for only 5.7% to 9.8% of overall ACL injuries.[42,43]

Internal bracing treatment uses synthetic biomaterials to provide additional strength to the healing tissue, sharing the load of the healing ACL. These techniques include internal brace ligament augmentation, suture ligament augmentation, or suture tape augmentation. All rely on similar principles of using polyethylene tape as an internal brace within or alongside the repaired ACL. As shown in biomechanical models,[44] the suture stabilizer provides a better mechanical environment for ligament healing. Studies have reported long-term follow-up data on dozens of patients following internal brace ligament augmentation,[45,46] demonstrating a 4.8% rerupture rate. In addition to supporting primary repair, internal bracing has also been used as an adjunct to ACL reconstruction.[47]

Dynamic intraligamentary stabilization seeks to bring the two ends of the ACL stump closer together to maximize ACL healing.[48,49] Dynamic intraligamentary stabilization construct consists of a tibial preloaded spring that tensions a transosseous suture used to reduce the torn ACL to its femoral footprint.[49,50] Because of the early stability, patients return to pivoting sports as early as 3 months after surgery and competitive skiing and soccer as early as 5 months after surgery.[50] However, outcomes have been mixed, with rerupture occurring in 4% to 15% of patients and an overall reintervention rate of 40% to 50%.[51]

Overall, ACL repair has not been widely adopted, perhaps because of the limited indications and often higher rates of failure than ACL reconstruction. Current approaches to ACL repair, and more commonly, ACL reconstruction, are overall fairly successful in restoring stability to the knee and allowing patients to return to activities of daily living and sports. However, there certainly are drawbacks to current options, namely restrictive indications for ACL repair and limited graft options for ACL reconstruction. Even for ligamentous injuries that often heal without surgical intervention such as MCL tears, there is a need to expedite healing to minimize time away from work or sports participation. Thus, there has been interest in orthobiologics to develop additional options for the treatment of ligament injuries in the lower extremity.

EVIDENCE FOR THE CLINICAL UTILITY OF ORTHOBIOLOGICS

Bioactive Factor Solutions

Platelet-rich plasma (PRP) is defined as a volume of plasma containing a higher-than-average number of platelets.[52,53] Preparations of PRP traditionally have a threefold to fivefold higher platelet count than normal plasma, with some reaching 9.3 times the mean platelet concentration of whole blood.[54] To obtain PRP, venous blood is drawn from the patient and centrifuged, creating a concentrated suspension. PRP has a high concentration of platelets, which contain more than 1,100 proteins, including growth factors.[55] Platelets play a large role in the initiation of healing because they are responsible for forming the scaffolding for clot formation, which leads to chemotaxis of appropriate cytokines. Platelet alpha-granules contain growth factors and anti-inflammatory cytokines such as insulinlike growth factor (IGF)-1, IGF-2, VEGF, transforming growth factor beta (TGF-β), fibroblast growth factor (FGF), endothelial growth factor, and platelet-derived growth factor (PDGF). These are released at the healing site[56,57] and have been shown to help stimulate the growth of autologous chondrocytes and mesenchymal stem cells, as well as components of the extracellular matrix such as proteoglycans and types I and II collagen.[58-62] Following PRP injections, basic FGF, VEGF, PDGF-BB, and IGF-1 are all increased at different points over the next 96 hours, suggesting that PRP activates biologic pathways to release growth factors rather than simply delivering growth factors in the concentrate.[63] Similarly, human fibroblasts treated with leukocyte-poor PRP demonstrate a significant increase in proliferation with cytokines peaking at various time points after injection.[64] PRP has been shown to simultaneously stimulate anabolic growth factors while reducing catabolic proinflammatory cytokine concentrations.[65-67] PRP uses this dual effect to stimulate fibroblasts, mesenchymal stem cells, and autologous chondrocytes while also decreasing inflammation via inhibition of interleukin (IL)-1-mediated nuclear factor light-chain-enhancer nuclear factor kappa B activation.[68,69] There are reports of PRP use in ACL reconstruction (for allograft maturation and patellar donor-site regeneration) and for MCL injuries. However, multiple reviews and meta-analyses determined that there are insufficient data to definitively state that PRP is beneficial in these lower extremity ligament applications.[70-73] The lack of evidence supporting certain indications for PRP can present an ethical dilemma for physicians considering use outside the setting of a clinical trial, especially in the context of providing services not covered by insurance where there may be a direct financial benefit to the physician. Indeed, although PRP has evidence-based indications such as for mild knee osteoarthritis and lateral epicondylitis, there are many claims made in the community regarding indications for PRP and its regenerative properties that amount to false advertising.

Similar to PRP, autologous conditioned serum (ACS) delivers a variety of blood-derived growth factors. ACS was developed in the mid-1990s in an attempt to generate an injectable biologic enriched in endogenous anti-inflammatory cytokine IL-1Ra as a novel therapeutic for osteoarthritis. Meijer et al[74] noted that exposure of blood to glass beads elicits a vigorous, rapid increase in the synthesis of several anti-inflammatory cytokines, including IL-1Ra. In one randomized controlled trial, it was shown that ACS decreased bone tunnel widening after ACL reconstruction[75] and that Western Ontario and McMaster Universities Osteoarthritis Index and International Knee Documentation Committee 2000 score were better at 1 year postoperatively. However, the use of ACS for this application has not been widely adopted. This is likely because bone tunnel widening is only pertinent in the setting of revision ACL reconstruction, and there are many other techniques to address bone tunnel widening such as allograft bone grafting and stacking screws.

Amniotic and chorionic membrane tissue has been explored for a variety of wound healing indications and is thought to have antimicrobial and anti-inflammatory properties.[76] It is harvested after childbirth and therefore is not associated with ethical concerns. Amniotic membrane contains many biomolecules, including growth factors (hepatocyte growth factor, IGF-1, IGF-2, TGF-β1, PDGF-BB, growth-related oncogene alpha, epidermal growth factor, TGF-β2, basic FGF, TGF-α, tumor necrosis factor alpha), cytokines (IL-1RA, IL-6), chemokines (monocyte chemoattractant protein 1), and protease inhibitors (tissue inhibitors of metalloproteinase [TIMP]-2, TIMP-3, TIMP-4).[76] Amniotic membrane has been applied as a surgical adjunct to ACL reconstruction, as a wrap around the ACL graft to promote healing.[76] However, there are no high-quality studies on the efficacy of this treatment.[77]

Cellular Solutions

Bone marrow aspirate concentrate (BMAC) has been explored as a surgical adjunct used to infuse allografts used in ACL reconstruction.[78] Forsythe et al[79] demonstrated that injection of ACL BPTB allografts with BMAC demonstrated superior signal intensity ratio on patient-reported outcomes during the early postoperative period. Another mesenchymal stem cell source that is commercially available for musculoskeletal use is adipose-derived cell, such as the commercially available Lipogems, which is harvested from a patient's adipose tissue in a procedure similar to liposuction.[80] Although not a true homogenous stem cell population, there are mesenchymal stem cells in this microfragmented adipose tissue product. This product is FDA approved for same-day use for musculoskeletal applications, but currently, little evidence supports its efficacy in lower extremity ligament injuries. Other than adult stem cells such as adipose-derived stem cells and mesenchymal stem cells, no other cell types have been used in lower extremity ligament healing applications; issues such as tumorigenicity for induced pluripotent stem cells and ethical concerns for embryonic stem cells limit their use in these quality-of-life applications.

SOLUTIONS IN DEVELOPMENT

Biomaterial Scaffolds

Many efforts in the field of biomaterials have been made to develop an engineered scaffold for use in ACL reconstruction. Because type I collagen constitutes approximately 90% of the native ACL, the use of collagen-based scaffolds for engineered ACL grafts has been extensively investigated.[81] As early as the 1990s, ACL fibroblasts were seeded on collagen scaffolds in hopes of developing a graft for ACL reconstruction.[82,83] However, these constructs were limited by loss of cells over time and too-rapid scaffold degradation. Collagen-glycosaminoglycan and collagen-elastin composite scaffolds have also demonstrated the ability to support fibroblasts, but mechanical properties remained a concern.[84-86] To improve the mechanical properties of collagen scaffolds, cross-linking of collagen with ultraviolet light or chemical reagents,[87,88] braiding, twisting, or otherwise geometrically optimizing scaffold design have been attempted. Although these methods improved mechanical properties, the mechanical strength of the collagen scaffolds was still less-than ideal.[89] Additionally, the immunogenicity associated with bovine collagen[90,91] and concerns regarding leaching of chemical cross-linking agents have spurred investigation of other scaffold materials with more favorable properties, as detailed in following sections. Although collagen scaffolds are biologically favorable, they are biomechanically inadequate for most ligament replacement applications. Thus, little active work is being performed to pursue the use of collagen-based scaffolds as a graft for use in ACL reconstruction.

Similar to collagen, silk is a biologic material that has long been used as suture material and has been studied as a scaffold material for ligament tissue engineering. The most attractive feature of silk is that it is biocompatible and has tensile strength that is similar to native ACL. In addition, silk is biodegradable and loses its tensile strength in a year and undergoes complete proteolytic degradation within 2 years in vivo. Altman et al[92] developed a silk scaffold with a hierarchical structure, with silk fibers wound into strands and then twisted into cords and arranged into a three-dimensional matrix. This construct has mechanical properties similar to native ACL with an elastic modulus of 354 ± 26 N/mm, a maximum load of 2,337 ± 72 N, and a strain at failure of 38.6 ± 2.4%. The scaffolds also demonstrate the viscoelastic properties that are important for the prevention of damage because of fatigue and creep.[92,93] Silk scaffolds have been shown to support human bone marrow stromal cell attachment and proliferation in a three-dimensional environment and synthesis of fibroblastic markers with the application of dynamic mechanical loading. Chemical modification of silk has been performed to successfully increase biocompatibility, hydrophilicity, and cell proliferation.[94,95]

Although some positive results in large animal models have been reported,[96,97] silk-based scaffolds for ACL reconstruction have largely been abandoned in favor of other biomaterials. The reasons for this are not well documented in the literature, but possibilities include lack of integration into bony tunnels, immunogenicity, and mismatched biomechanical properties such as elasticity.

Other biologic materials, such as hyaluronic acid,[98] chitosan,[99-101] and alginate,[102-104] have also been used in ligament tissue engineering. To address some of the inherent weakness of these biologic materials, investigators have developed different modification methods and have formed various composites.[99,100,102-105] Although these biologic materials and their composites present interesting possibilities, they are still in an early phase of development.

Although the use of nondegradable synthetic ACL replacements in earlier decades has been largely unsuccessful, the use of synthetic biodegradable polymers has shown more promise in ACL tissue engineering. These polymers include poly(glycolic acid) (PGA), polydioxanone, poly-L-lactic acid, and polycaprolactone (PCL).[81] Many of these polymers are currently FDA approved for other surgical applications. Polymer selection and scaffold fabrication techniques can allow customization of characteristics such as mechanical properties, degradation rate, and cellular response.[90] Polymer selection is crucial to determine the mechanical properties and degradation rate of the scaffold, whereas different manufacturing methods can be used to alter the microstructure and macrostructure of the ACL graft.

Various methods of manufacturing porous scaffolds for use in tissue engineering have been proposed, including braiding, drawing, phase separation, freeze-drying, molecular self-assembly, and electrospinning.[81] Many synthetic biomaterials, composites of these biomaterials, and different fabrication techniques for these biomaterials have been investigated. These include poly(lactic-*co*-glycolic acid), poly(desaminotyrosyl-tyrosine ethyl carbonate),[106] poly(ε-caprolactone-*co*-D,L-lactide),[107] blends of hydrophobic PCL and hydrophilic PGA-PCL-PGA triblock copolymer,[108] copoly(lactic acid-*co*-ε-caprolactone) scaffold,[109] and a multitude of others.

Overall, there have been many advances in the study of biomaterials for use in ACL tissue engineering. Because of the complexity of native ligament, it is likely that composite materials will continue to be investigated because they allow the combination of advantageous traits of multiple materials and the offsetting of their weaknesses. One of the most difficult issues encountered is designing a scaffold that sufficiently mimics the complex properties of a native ACL over time in the in vivo environment while supporting the ingrowth of new ligament tissue. Further work is necessary in the development of biomaterials with in vivo mechanical properties and degradation profiles that are optimal for ligament tissue engineering.

Tissue-Engineered Grafts

Tissue-engineered grafts combine a biomaterial scaffold with cells and/or other biologic factors to encourage tissue regeneration. The chapter authors previously investigated the use of an electrospun PCL scaffold for ACL reconstruction in a rat model, with and without the addition of human foreskin fibroblasts. By 16 weeks postoperatively, the scaffold had completely degraded and biomechanically, the neoligament formed was not inferior to the gold standard autograft.[110-112] Although these results are promising, the challenge is being able to scale this technology up to the level of large animals and human studies, in which issues of vascularity and transport properties can become consequential. In one large animal study, human adipose-derived stem cells and induced pluripotent stem cells derived from human foreskin fibroblasts were implanted onto a nondegradable ACL graft, resulting in the formation of ACL-like tissue.[113]

In recent years, it has been suggested that tissue engineering has failed to live up to its promise for ligament and tendon grafts. A criticism of many techniques is that they apply an empiric approach to tissue engineering, whereby components such as biomaterials, growth factors, and cells are selected based on availability instead of scientific evidence. The understanding of ligament development and maintenance remains incomplete; ligament biology is less studied than other musculoskeletal fields such as muscle, bone, and cartilage. Increased understanding of how ligaments are formed and maintained would allow for more informed design of ACL grafts. Additionally, recent technologic developments such as three-dimensional printing of both biomaterials and cells, micromanufacturing, high-throughput screening, controlled growth factor delivery, surface modification, and nanotechnology have the potential to expedite the development of a functional tissue-engineered ACL graft.

Bridge-Enhanced ACL Repair

Instead of trying to replace a torn ACL with a graft, the bridge-enhanced ACL repair (BEAR) technique seeks to augment the poor healing response of native ACLs via a collagen scaffold[114,115] augmented with intraoperative injection of autologous blood or PRP.[116,117] In a randomized controlled study of patients with a median age of 17 years, the BEAR technique was not inferior to primarily hamstring autografts at 2-year follow-up.[118] There have been no reported complications associated with the use of bovine-derived tissue in this application. Although the BEAR implant received FDA approval in December 2020, at the time of this writing, it was not commercially available because of the COVID-19 pandemic.

PATIENT SELECTION CONSIDERATIONS

Patient selection is critical in applying orthobiologics to lower extremity ligament injuries, as it is for almost every procedure. For instance, part of the success of the BEAR implant over more traditional methods of ACL repair may be attributable to careful patient selection. Although the BEAR technique is currently approved for all skeletally mature patients at least 14 years of age, with complete ACL rupture with residual tissue attached to the tibia,[119] the clinical trials reported on the results of a relatively young patient cohort that is less likely to have comorbidities that may be seen in a more general patient population. Especially, because of the relatively young age of the patients in the BEAR cohort, long-term follow-up will be necessary. Outcomes such as patient-rated functional outcomes, rate of graft failure, development of posttraumatic osteoarthritis, and subsequent meniscal tears will be of interest in this cohort.

Similarly, clear patient guidelines are needed regarding the use of other orthobiologic therapies. For example, it is unknown whether patient characteristics such as blood count, blood type, age, sex, or comorbidities affect the efficacy of treatment strategies such as PRP or BMAC.

FUTURE DIRECTIONS/CHALLENGES

One challenge to the widespread adoption of orthobiologics for ligament injuries is financial considerations that may limit access to care and raise concerns of equity. For example, PRP injections are usually not covered by most commercial insurances, although it can be covered by the Veterans Administration and workers' compensation. With out-of-pocket charges ranging from hundreds to thousands of dollars per injection, many patients who could benefit from such therapies would not have the option. Additional commercial or venture funding for large-scale standardized studies to improve on the current body of literature supporting orthobiologics could help improve patient access to these therapies.

Looking forward, another challenge is the need for a more mechanistic-based approach to orthobiologic therapies. Currently available therapies such as PRP, BMAC, and amniotic/chorionic products are a relatively blunt instrument, with an unclear mechanism of action. Indeed, it is not even known which growth factors or cytokines are most responsible for any clinical benefit that is observed. Additionally, better understanding of the timing of therapy relative to an injury would be beneficial.

In the future, more targeted application of the exact cells and molecules that contribute to ligament healing may allow to improve the efficacy of both surgical and nonsurgical treatment strategies for ligament injures. One example of a cell type that shows promise for ligament healing is perivascular stem cells (PSCs). Several reports have identified that PSCs are at least partially responsible for tendon and ligament healing and remodeling following injury in extra-articular ligaments and tendons.[120,121] Although other stem cell–based tissue regeneration efforts manipulate stem cells with growth factors to differentiate into another cell type for nonhomologous clinical applications, applying PSCs to ligament and tendon injuries would take advantage of their natural tendency toward a fibroblast-like phenotype. In addition, PSCs can be readily isolated from lipoaspirate via fluorescence-activated cell sorting of cell surface markers, allowing the prospect of isolating enough autologous PSC via liposuction for same-day use without the need for the intervening step in vitro expansion. Ultimately, a better understanding of how extra-articular ligaments heal will hopefully facilitate the development of novel treatment strategies that harness the body's inherent ability to heal extra-articular ligaments and apply this to intra-articular ligaments such as the ACL.

SUMMARY

Orthobiologics are in a relatively early stage of clinical application but represent great promise for augmenting and expediting the ligament healing process. To develop more options for the management of ligament injuries, a better understanding of the cells and growth factors involved in the repair process is necessary.

REFERENCES

1. Leong NL, Kator JL, Clemens TL, James A, Enamoto-Iwamoto M, Jiang J: Tendon and ligament healing and current approaches to tendon and ligament regeneration. *J Orthop Res* 2020;38(1):7-12.
2. Hope M, Saxby TS: Tendon healing. *Foot Ankle Clin* 2007;12(4):553-567.
3. Molloy T, Wang Y, Murrell G: The roles of growth factors in tendon and ligament healing. *Sports Med* 2003;33(5):381-394.
4. Bedi A, Maak T, Walsh C, et al: Cytokines in rotator cuff degeneration and repair. *J Shoulder Elbow Surg* 2012;21(2):218-227.
5. Carpenter JE, Thomopoulos S, Flanagan CL, DeBano CM, Soslowsky LJ: Rotator cuff defect healing: A biomechanical and histologic analysis in an animal model. *J Shoulder Elbow Surg* 1998;7(6):599-605.
6. Thomopoulos S, Parks WC, Rifkin DB, Derwin KA: Mechanisms of tendon injury and repair. *J Orthop Res* 2015;33(6):832-839.
7. Chang J, Most D, Stelnicki E, et al: Gene expression of transforming growth factor beta-1 in rabbit zone II flexor tendon wound healing: Evidence for dual mechanisms of repair. *Plast Reconstr Surg* 1997;100(4):937-944.
8. Yang G, Rothrauff BB, Tuan RS: Tendon and ligament regeneration and repair: Clinical relevance and developmental paradigm. *Birth Defects Res C Embryo Today* 2013;99(3):203-222.
9. Marui T, Niyibizi C, Georgescu HI, et al: Effect of growth factors on matrix synthesis by ligament fibroblasts. *J Orthop Res* 1997;15(1):18-23.

10. Jones JI, Clemmons DR: Insulin-like growth factors and their binding proteins: Biological actions. *Endocr Rev* 1995;16(1):3-34.

11. Abrahamsson SO: Similar effects of recombinant human insulin-like growth factor-I and II on cellular activities in flexor tendons of young rabbits: Experimental studies in vitro. *J Orthop Res* 1997;15(2):256-262.

12. Bidder M, Towler DA, Gelberman RH, Boyer MI: Expression of mRNA for vascular endothelial growth factor at the repair site of healing canine flexor tendon. *J Orthop Res* 2000;18(2):247-252.

13. Sciore P, Boykiw R, Hart DA: Semiquantitative reverse transcription-polymerase chain reaction analysis of mRNA for growth factors and growth factor receptors from normal and healing rabbit medial collateral ligament tissue. *J Orthop Res* 1998;16(4):429-437.

14. Chang J, Most D, Thunder R, Mehrara B, Longaker MT, Lineaweaver WC: Molecular studies in flexor tendon wound healing: The role of basic fibroblast growth factor gene expression. *J Hand Surg Am* 1998;23(6):1052-1058.

15. Thomopoulos S, Harwood FL, Silva MJ, Amiel D, Gelberman RH: Effect of several growth factors on canine flexor tendon fibroblast proliferation and collagen synthesis in vitro. *J Hand Surg Am* 2005;30(3):441-447.

16. Vihersaari T, Kivisaari J, Ninikoski J: Effect of changes in inspired oxygen tension on wound metabolism. *Ann Surg* 1974;179(6):889-895.

17. Oshiro W, Lou J, Xing X, Tu Y, Manske PR: Flexor tendon healing in the rat: A histologic and gene expression study. *J Hand Surg Am* 2003;28(5):814-823.

18. Miyashita H, Ochi M, Ikuta Y: Histological and biomechanical observations of the rabbit patellar tendon after removal of its central one-third. *Arch Orthop Trauma Surg* 1997;116(8):454-462.

19. Rumian AP, Wallace AL, Birch HL: Tendons and ligaments are anatomically distinct but overlap in molecular and morphological features – A comparative study in an ovine model. *J Orthop Res* 2007;25(4):458-464.

20. Kharaz YA, Canty-Laird EG, Tew SR, Comerford EJ: Variations in internal structure, composition and protein distribution between intra- and extra-articular knee ligaments and tendons. *J Anat* 2018;232(6):943-955.

21. Frank CB: Ligament structure, physiology and function. *J Musculoskelet Neuronal Interact* 2004;4(2):199-201.

22. Morisawa Y: Morphological study of mechanoreceptors on the coracoacromial ligament. *J Orthop Sci* 1998;3(2):102-110.

23. Rebmann D, Mayr HO, Schmal H, Hernandez Latorre S, Bernstein A: Immunohistochemical analysis of sensory corpuscles in human transplants of the anterior cruciate ligament. *J Orthop Surg Res* 2020;15(1):270.

24. Leunig M, Beck M, Stauffer E, Hertel R, Ganz R: Free nerve endings in the ligamentum capitis femoris. *Acta Orthop Scand* 2000;71(5):452-454.

25. Kiter E, Karaboyun T, Tufan AC, Acar K: Immunohistochemical demonstration of nerve endings in iliolumbar ligament. *Spine (Phila Pa 1976)* 2010;35(4):E101-E104.

26. Woo SL, Hollis JM, Adams DJ, Lyon RM, Takai S: Tensile properties of the human femur-anterior cruciate ligament-tibia complex. The effects of specimen age and orientation. *Am J Sports Med* 1991;19(3):217-225.

27. Wilson WT, Deakin AH, Payne AP, Picard F, Wearing SC: Comparative analysis of the structural properties of the collateral ligaments of the human knee. *J Orthop Sports Phys Ther* 2012;42(4):345-351.

28. Frankewycz B, Penz A, Weber J, et al: Achilles tendon elastic properties remain decreased in long term after rupture. *Knee Surg Sports Traumatol Arthrosc* 2018;26(7):2080-2087.

29. Maempel JF, Clement ND, Wickramasinghe NR, Duckworth AD, Keating JF: Operative repair of acute Achilles tendon rupture does not give superior patient-reported outcomes to nonoperative management. *Bone Joint J* 2020;102-B(7):933-940.

30. Frank C, Schachar N, Dittrich D: Natural history of healing in the repaired medial collateral ligament. *J Orthop Res* 1983;1(2):179-188.

31. Paulos LE, Rosenberg TD, Grewe SR, Tearse DS, Beck CL: The GORE-TEX anterior cruciate ligament prosthesis. A long-term followup. *Am J Sports Med* 1992;20(3):246-252.

32. Wredmark T, Engström B: Five-year results of anterior cruciate ligament reconstruction with the Stryker Dacron high-strength ligament. *Knee Surg Sports Traumatol Arthrosc* 1993;1(2):71-75.

33. Chen J, Xu J, Wang A, Zheng M: Scaffolds for tendon and ligament repair: Review of the efficacy of commercial products. *Expert Rev Med Dev* 2009;6(1):61-73.

34. Badylak S, Arnoczky S, Plouhar P, et al: Naturally occurring extracellular matrix as a scaffold for musculoskeletal repair. *Clin Orthop Relat Res* 1999;367:S333-S343.

35. Lee AJ, Chung WH, Kim DH, et al: Anterior cruciate ligament reconstruction in a rabbit model using canine small intestinal submucosa and autologous platelet-rich plasma. *J Surg Res* 2012;178(1):206-215.

36. Mengsteab PY, Nair LS, Laurencin CT: The past, present and future of ligament regenerative engineering. *Regen Med* 2016;11(8):871-881.

37. L-C Ligament Versus Hamstring Autograft for Primary ACL Reconstruction. Available at: https://clinicaltrials.gov/ct2/show/NCT02183727. Updated April 26, 2017. Accessed September 15, 2021.

38. Sheean AJ, Musahl V, Slone HS, et al: Quadriceps tendon autograft for arthroscopic knee ligament reconstruction: Use it now, use it often. *Br J Sports Med* 2018;52(11): 698-701.

39. Mouarbes D, Menetrey J, Marot V, Courtot L, Berard E, Cavaignac E: Anterior cruciate ligament reconstruction: A systematic review and meta-analysis of outcomes for quadriceps tendon autograft versus bone-patellar tendon-bone and hamstring-tendon autografts. *Am J Sports Med* 2019;47(14):3531-3540.

40. Wu J, Kator JL, Zarro M, Leong NL: Rehabilitation principles to consider for anterior cruciate ligament repair. *Sports Health* 2021;14:19417381211032949.

41. Nguyen DT, Ramwadhdoebe TH, van der Hart CP, Blankevoort L, Tak PP, van Dijk CN: Intrinsic healing response of the human anterior cruciate ligament: An histological study of reattached ACL remnants. *J Orthop Res* 2014;32(2):296-301.

42. Achtnich A, Herbst E, Forkel P, et al: Acute proximal anterior cruciate ligament tears: Outcomes after arthroscopic suture anchor repair versus anatomic single-bundle reconstruction. *Arthroscopy* 2016;32(12):2562-2569.

43. DiFelice GS, Villegas C, Taylor S: Anterior cruciate ligament preservation: Early results of a novel arthroscopic technique for suture anchor primary anterior cruciate ligament repair. *Arthroscopy* 2015;31(11):2162-2171.

44. Bachmaier S, DiFelice GS, Sonnery-Cottet B, et al: Treatment of acute proximal anterior cruciate ligament tears-Part 2: The role of internal bracing on gap formation and stabilization of repair techniques. *Orthop J Sports Med* 2020;8(1):2325967119897423.

45. Heusdens CHW, Hopper GP, Dossche L, Roelant E, Mackay GM: Anterior cruciate ligament repair with Independent Suture Tape Reinforcement: A case series with 2-year follow-up. *Knee Surg Sports Traumatol Arthrosc* 2019;27(1):60-67.

46. Wilson WT, Hopper GP, Byrne PA, MacKay GM: Anterior cruciate ligament repair with internal brace ligament augmentation. *Surg Technol Int* 2016;29:273-278.

47. Smith PA, Bley JA: Allograft anterior cruciate ligament reconstruction utilizing internal brace augmentation. *Arthrosc Tech* 2016;5(5):e1143-e1147.

48. Kohl S, Evangelopoulos DS, Kohlhof H, et al: Anterior crucial ligament rupture: Self-healing through dynamic intraligamentary stabilization technique. *Knee Surg Sports Traumatol Arthrosc* 2013;21(3):599-605.

49. Kohl S, Evangelopoulos DS, Ahmad SS, et al: A novel technique, dynamic intraligamentary stabilization creates optimal conditions for primary ACL healing: A preliminary biomechanical study. *Knee* 2014;21(2):477-480.

50. Eggli S, Kohlhof H, Zumstein M, et al: Dynamic intraligamentary stabilization: Novel technique for preserving the ruptured ACL. *Knee Surg Sports Traumatol Arthrosc* 2015;23(4):1215-1221.

51. Mahapatra P, Horriat S, Anand BS: Anterior cruciate ligament repair - past, present and future. *J Exp Orthop* 2018;5(1):20.

52. Simental-Mendía MA, Vílchez-Cavazos JF, Martínez-Rodríguez HG: Platelet-rich plasma in knee osteoarthritis treatment. *Cir Cir* 2015;83(4):352-358.

53. Pourcho AM, Smith J, Wisniewski SJ, Sellon JL: Intraarticular platelet-rich plasma injection in the treatment of knee osteoarthritis: Review and recommendations. *Am J Phys Med Rehabil* 2014;93(11 suppl 3):S108-S121.

54. Southworth TM, Naveen NB, Tauro TM, Leong NL, Cole BJ: The use of platelet-rich plasma in symptomatic knee osteoarthritis. *J Knee Surg* 2019;32(1):37-45.

55. Senzel L, Gnatenko DV, Bahou WF: The platelet proteome. *Curr Opin Hematol* 2009;16(5):329-333.

56. Getgood A, Henson F, Brooks R, Fortier LA, Rushton N: Platelet-rich plasma activation in combination with biphasic osteochondral scaffolds-conditions for maximal growth factor production. *Knee Surg Sports Traumatol Arthrosc* 2011;19(11):1942-1947.

57. Bendinelli P, Matteucci E, Dogliotti G, et al: Molecular basis of anti-inflammatory action of platelet-rich plasma on human chondrocytes: Mechanisms of NF-κB inhibition via HGF. *J Cell Physiol* 2010;225(3):757-766.

58. Fortier LA, Barker JU, Strauss EJ, McCarrel TM, Cole BJ: The role of growth factors in cartilage repair. *Clin Orthop Relat Res* 2011;469(10):2706-2715.

59. Shuler FD, Georgescu HI, Niyibizi C, et al: Increased matrix synthesis following adenoviral transfer of a transforming growth factor beta1 gene into articular chondrocytes. *J Orthop Res* 2000;18(4):585-592.

60. Madry H, Zurakowski D, Trippel SB: Overexpression of human insulin-like growth factor-I promotes new tissue formation in an ex vivo model of articular chondrocyte transplantation. *Gene Ther* 2001;8(19):1443-1449.

61. Madry H, Emkey G, Zurakowski D, Trippel SB: Overexpression of human fibroblast growth factor 2 stimulates cell proliferation in an ex vivo model of articular chondrocyte transplantation. *J Gene Med* 2004;6(2):238-245.

62. Schmidt MB, Chen EH, Lynch SE: A review of the effects of insulin-like growth factor and platelet derived growth factor on in vivo cartilage healing and repair. *Osteoarthritis Cartilage* 2006;14(5):403-412.

63. Wasterlain AS, Braun HJ, Harris AH, Kim HJ, Dragoo JL: The systemic effects of platelet-rich plasma injection. *Am J Sports Med* 2013;41(1):186-193.

64. Yerlikaya M, Talay Çaliş H, Tomruk Sütbeyaz S, et al: Comparison of effects of leukocyte-rich and leukocyte-poor platelet-rich plasma on pain and functionality in patients with lateral epicondylitis. *Arch Rheumatol* 2018;33(1):73-79.

65. Cole BJ, Karas V, Hussey K, Pilz K, Fortier LA: Hyaluronic acid versus Platelet-rich plasma: A prospective, double-blind randomized controlled trial comparing clinical outcomes and effects on intra-articular biology for the treatment of knee osteoarthritis. *Am J Sports Med* 2017;45(2):339-346.

66. Kon E, Buda R, Filardo G, et al: Platelet-rich plasma: Intra-articular knee injections produced favorable results on degenerative cartilage lesions. *Knee Surg Sports Traumatol Arthrosc* 2010;18(4):472-479.

67. Patel S, Dhillon MS, Aggarwal S, Marwaha N, Jain A: Treatment with platelet-rich plasma is more effective than placebo for knee osteoarthritis: A prospective, double-blind, randomized trial. *Am J Sports Med* 2013;41(2):356-364.

68. van Buul GM, Koevoet WL, Kops N, et al: Platelet-rich plasma releasate inhibits inflammatory processes in osteoarthritic chondrocytes. *Am J Sports Med* 2011;39(11):2362-2370.

69. Pujol JP, Chadjichristos C, Legendre F, et al: Interleukin-1 and transforming growth factor-beta 1 as crucial factors in osteoarthritic cartilage metabolism. *Connect Tissue Res* 2008;49(3):293-297.

70. Bagwell MS, Wilk KE, Colberg RE, Dugas JR: The use of serial platelet rich plasma injections with early rehabilitation to expedite grade iii medial collateral ligament injury

in a professional athlete: A case report. *Int J Sports Phys Ther* 2018;13(3):520-525.

71. Moraes VY, Lenza M, Tamaoki MJ, Faloppa F, Belloti JC: Platelet-rich therapies for musculoskeletal soft tissue injuries. *Cochrane Database Syst Rev* 2014;2014(4):CD010071.
72. Braun HJ, Wasterlain AS, Dragoo JL: The use of PRP in ligament and meniscal healing. *Sports Med Arthrosc Rev* 2013;21(4):206-212.
73. Andia I, Maffulli N: Use of platelet-rich plasma for patellar tendon and medial collateral ligament injuries: Best current clinical practice. *J Knee Surg* 2015;28(1):11-18.
74. Meijer H, Reinecke J, Becker C, Tholen G, Wehling P: The production of anti-inflammatory cytokines in whole blood by physico-chemical induction. *Inflamm Res* 2003;52(10):404-407.
75. Darabos N, Haspl M, Moser C, Darabos A, Bartolek D, Groenemeyer D: Intraarticular application of autologous conditioned serum (ACS) reduces bone tunnel widening after ACL reconstructive surgery in a randomized controlled trial. *Knee Surg Sports Traumatol Arthrosc* 2011;19(suppl 1):S36-S46.
76. Woodall BM, Elena N, Gamboa JT, et al: Anterior cruciate ligament reconstruction with amnion biological augmentation. *Arthrosc Tech* 2018;7(4):e355-e360.
77. Riboh JC, Saltzman BM, Yanke AB, Cole BJ: Human amniotic membrane-derived products in sports medicine: Basic science, early results, and potential clinical applications. *Am J Sports Med* 2016;44(9):2425-2434.
78. Youn GM, Remigio Van Gogh AM, Alvarez A, et al: Stem cell-infused anterior cruciate ligament reconstruction. *Arthrosc Tech* 2019;8(11):e1313-e1317.
79. Forsythe B, Chahla J, Lavoie-Gagne O, et al: Mesenchymal Stem Cells in BTB allograft ACL reconstruction: A Prospective Randomized Controlled Trial. *Arthrosc Tech* 2021;37:E64-E65.
80. Tremolada C, Colombo V, Ventura C: Adipose tissue and mesenchymal stem cells: State of the art and Lipogems® technology development. *Curr Stem Cell Rep* 2016;2:304-312.
81. Leong NL, Petrigliano FA, McAllister DR: Current tissue engineering strategies in anterior cruciate ligament reconstruction. *J Biomed Mater Res A* 2014;102(5):1614-1624.
82. Dunn MG, Liesch JB, Tiku ML, Zawadsky JP: Development of fibroblast-seeded ligament analogs for ACL reconstruction. *J Biomed Mater Res* 1995;29(11):1363-1371.
83. Bellincampi LD, Closkey RF, Prasad R, Zawadsky JP, Dunn MG: Viability of fibroblast-seeded ligament analogs after autogenous implantation. *J Orthop Res* 1998;16(4):414-420.
84. Murray MM, Spector M: The migration of cells from the ruptured human anterior cruciate ligament into collagen-glycosaminoglycan regeneration templates in vitro. *Biomaterials* 2001;22(17):2393-2402.
85. Meaney Murray M, Rice K, Wright RJ, Spector M: The effect of selected growth factors on human anterior cruciate ligament cell interactions with a three-dimensional collagen-GAG scaffold. *J Orthop Res* 2003;21(2):238-244.
86. Mizutani N, Kawato H, Maeda Y, Takebayashi T, Miyamoto K, Horiuchi T: Multiple-type dynamic culture of highly oriented fiber scaffold for ligament regeneration. *J Artif Organs* 2013;16(1):49-58.
87. Koob TJ, Willis TA, Qiu YS, Hernandez DJ: Biocompatibility of NDGA-polymerized collagen fibers. II. Attachment, proliferation, and migration of tendon fibroblasts in vitro. *J Biomed Mater Res* 2001;56(1):40-48.
88. Caruso AB, Dunn MG: Changes in mechanical properties and cellularity during long-term culture of collagen fiber ACL reconstruction scaffolds. *J Biomed Mater Res A* 2005;73(4):388-397.
89. Walters VI, Kwansa AL, Freeman JW: Design and analysis of braid-twist collagen scaffolds. *Connect Tissue Res* 2012;53(3):255-266.
90. Petrigliano FA, McAllister DR, Wu BM: Tissue engineering for anterior cruciate ligament reconstruction: A review of current strategies. *Arthroscopy* 2006;22(4):441-451.
91. Vunjak-Novakovic G, Altman G, Horan R, Kaplan DL: Tissue engineering of ligaments. *Annu Rev Biomed Eng* 2004;6:131-156.
92. Altman GH, Horan RL, Lu HH, et al: Silk matrix for tissue engineered anterior cruciate ligaments. *Biomaterials* 2002;23(20):4131-4141.
93. Altman GH, Lu HH, Horan RL, et al: Advanced bioreactor with controlled application of multi-dimensional strain for tissue engineering. *J Biomech Eng* 2002;124(6):742-749.
94. Chen J, Altman GH, Karageorgiou V, et al: Human bone marrow stromal cell and ligament fibroblast responses on RGD-modified silk fibers. *J Biomed Mater Res A* 2003;67(2):559-570.
95. Murphy AR, St John P, Kaplan DL: Modification of silk fibroin using diazonium coupling chemistry and the effects on hMSC proliferation and differentiation. *Biomaterials* 2008;29(19):2829-2838.
96. Teuschl AH, Tangl S, Heimel P, et al: Osteointegration of a novel silk fiber-based ACL scaffold by formation of a ligament-bone interface. *Am J Sports Med* 2019;47(3):620-627.
97. Fan H, Liu H, Toh SL, Goh JC: Anterior cruciate ligament regeneration using mesenchymal stem cells and silk scaffold in large animal model. *Biomaterials* 2009;30(28):4967-4977.
98. Cristino S, Grassi F, Toneguzzi S, et al: Analysis of mesenchymal stem cells grown on a three-dimensional HYAFF 11-based prototype ligament scaffold. *J Biomed Mater Res A* 2005;73(3):275-283.
99. Hansson A, Hashom N, Falson F, Rousselle P, Jordan O, Borchard G: In vitro evaluation of an RGD-functionalized chitosan derivative for enhanced cell adhesion. *Carbohydr Polym* 2012;90(4):1494-1500.
100. Shao HJ, Lee YT, Chen CS, Wang JH, Young TH: Modulation of gene expression and collagen production of anterior cruciate ligament cells through cell shape changes on polycaprolactone/chitosan blends. *Biomaterials* 2010;31(17):4695-4705.
101. Shao HJ, Chen CS, Lee YT, Wang JH, Young TH: The phenotypic responses of human anterior cruciate ligament cells cultured on poly(epsilon-caprolactone) and chitosan. *J Biomed Mater Res A* 2010;93(4):1297-1305.

102. Masuko T, Iwasaki N, Yamane S, et al: Chitosan-RGDSGGC conjugate as a scaffold material for musculoskeletal tissue engineering. *Biomaterials* 2005;26(26):5339-5347.

103. Majima T, Funakosi T, Iwasaki N, et al: Alginate and chitosan polyion complex hybrid fibers for scaffolds in ligament and tendon tissue engineering. *J Orthop Sci* 2005;10(3):302-307.

104. Majima T, Irie T, Sawaguchi N, et al: Chitosan-based hyaluronan hybrid polymer fibre scaffold for ligament and tendon tissue engineering. *Proc Inst Mech Eng H* 2007;221(5):537-546.

105. Panas-Perez E, Gatt CJ, Dunn MG: Development of a silk and collagen fiber scaffold for anterior cruciate ligament reconstruction. *J Mater Sci Mater Med* 2013;24(1):257-265.

106. Bourke SL, Kohn J, Dunn MG: Preliminary development of a novel resorbable synthetic polymer fiber scaffold for anterior cruciate ligament reconstruction. *Tissue Eng* 2004;10(1-2):43-52.

107. Hayami JW, Surrao DC, Waldman SD, Amsden BG: Design and characterization of a biodegradable composite scaffold for ligament tissue engineering. *J Biomed Mater Res A* 2010;92(4):1407-1420.

108. Chung AS, Hwang HS, Das D, Zuk P, McAllister DR, Wu BM: Lamellar stack formation and degradative behaviors of hydrolytically degraded poly(ε-caprolactone) and poly(glycolide-ε-caprolactone) blended fibers. *J Biomed Mater Res B Appl Biomater* 2012;100(1):274-284.

109. Laurent CP, Durville D, Mainard D, Ganghoffer JF, Rahouadj R: A multilayer braided scaffold for Anterior Cruciate Ligament: Mechanical modeling at the fiber scale. *J Mech Behav Biomed Mater* 2012;12:184-196.

110. Leong NL, Kabir N, Arshi A, et al: Athymic rat model for evaluation of engineered anterior cruciate ligament grafts. *J Vis Exp* 2015;26(97):52797.

111. Leong NL, Kabir N, Arshi A, et al: Use of ultra-high molecular weight polycaprolactone scaffolds for ACL reconstruction. *J Orthop Res* 2016;34(5):828-835.

112. Leong NL, Kabir N, Arshi A, et al: Evaluation of polycaprolactone scaffold with basic fibroblast growth factor and fibroblasts in an athymic rat model for anterior cruciate ligament reconstruction. *Tissue Eng Part A* 2015;21(11-12):1859-1868.

113. Kouroupis D, Kyrkou A, Triantafyllidi E, et al: Generation of stem cell-based bioartificial anterior cruciate ligament (ACL) grafts for effective ACL rupture repair. *Stem Cell Res* 2016;17(2):448-457.

114. Fleming BC, Spindler KP, Palmer MP, Magarian EM, Murray MM: Collagen-platelet composites improve the biomechanical properties of healing anterior cruciate ligament grafts in a porcine model. *Am J Sports Med* 2009;37(8):1554-1563.

115. Joshi SM, Mastrangelo AN, Magarian EM, Fleming BC, Murray MM: Collagen-platelet composite enhances biomechanical and histologic healing of the porcine anterior cruciate ligament. *Am J Sports Med* 2009;37(12):2401-2410.

116. Perrone GS, Proffen BL, Kiapour AM, Sieker JT, Fleming BC, Murray MM: Bench-to-bedside: Bridge-enhanced anterior cruciate ligament repair. *J Orthop Res* 2017;35(12):2606-2612.

117. Murray MM, Flutie BM, Kalish LA, et al: The bridge-enhanced anterior cruciate ligament repair (BEAR) procedure: An early feasibility cohort study. *Orthop J Sports Med* 2016;4(11):2325967116672176.

118. Murray MM, Fleming BC, Badger GJ, et al: Bridge-enhanced anterior cruciate ligament repair is not inferior to autograft anterior cruciate ligament reconstruction at 2 years: Results of a prospective randomized clinical trial. *Am J Sports Med* 2020;48(6):1305-1315.

119. Bridge-Enhanced ACL Restoration (BEAR) Implant. *Miach Orthopaedics*. Available at: https://miachortho.com/medical-professionals/. Updated 7/2021. Accessed September 15, 2021.

120. Tan Q, Lui PP, Lee YW: In vivo identity of tendon stem cells and the roles of stem cells in tendon healing. *Stem Cells Dev* 2013;22(23):3128-3140.

121. Schwartz AJ, Sarver DC, Sugg KB, Dzierzawski JT, Gumucio JP, Mendias CL: p38 MAPK signaling in postnatal tendon growth and remodeling. *PLoS One* 2015;10(3):e0120044.

CHAPTER 29

Clinical Outcomes in the Hip and Knee Following Arthroplasty

Caroline Taber, AB • Robert G. Marx, MD, FAAOS • Alissa J. Burge, MD

INTRODUCTION

Measurement of clinical outcomes in orthopaedics is essential to the health of the patient, and comprehensive knowledge of outcome measures is paramount in conducting a quality orthopaedic study.[1] A baseline outcome measure is used to assess a patient's status and therefore provides data.[2] An initial outcome measure can help to guide treatment plan, and subsequent measurements can track progress.[3] Outcome measures that are used in practice can be separated into four different categories:[3]

1. Self-report measures
2. Performance-based measures
3. Observer-reported measures
4. Clinician-reported measures

Self-reported measures are usually in the form of a questionnaire. Questionnaires in which the patient is responding to give information on their health or function are known as patient-reported outcomes. Although subjective, such reports are able to objectify the patient's perspective.[4] Performance-based measurements are used to evaluate specific components of performance on certain tasks and can be quantitative or qualitative measurements.[5] Observer-reported measures come from someone who is typically caring for the patient and regularly watches them, such as a parent or in-home nurse. Finally, clinician-reported measures are those conducted by a trained health care professional and require specialized training to evaluate the patient.[6] Overall, it is a combination of these measures being used to best treat patients as well as develop new technologies for novel treatment strategies. In orthopaedics, many of these forms of measurement pertain to total hip and total knee arthroplasties, such as range of motion, Hip disability and Osteoarthritis Outcome Score (HOOS) and Knee injury and Osteoarthritis Outcome Score (KOOS) questionnaires, and Patient-Reported Outcomes Measurement Information System (PROMIS).

EVALUATING NOVEL DEVICES

In investigating novel devices for hip and knee arthroplasties, and measuring their efficacy, the FDA conducts both FDA registry studies and postmarket studies. Devices are regulated by the Center for Devices and Radiological Health at the FDA. According to the Federal Food, Drug, and Cosmetic Act, a device is an instrument, apparatus, implement, machine, contrivance, implant, or in vitro reagent that meets three conditions: (1) it is recognized in the official National Formulary or the U.S. Pharmacopeia; (2) it is intended for use in the diagnosis of disease or other conditions or the cure, mitigation, treatment, or prevention of disease; or (3) it is intended to affect the structure or function of the body of humans.[7,8] In the preclinical stages, the device undergoes preliminary bench testing and subsequent animal testing. The device is then classified into one of three groups by the FDA: class I (low risk of illness or injury), class II (moderate risk), or class III (support or sustain human life, are of substantial importance in preventing impairment of human health, or present a potential, unreasonable risk of illness or injury).[9-11] Class I and II devices typically do not need to undergo a clinical trial,[12] whereas class III devices (which include implants) pose a greater risk and require Premarket Approval (PMA).

The PMA is the strictest device marketing application and is required by the FDA for which there is no existing equivalent device or predicate. Within the PMA, the device must be shown to be safe and effective for its intended use.[13] Typically, level I or level II clinical evidence is required for class III device approval.[14] This clinical testing can range from the first time a device is used in humans to large, prospective, multicenter controlled trials and includes institutional review board approval of the clinical site.[8] The PMA application is then reviewed by the Center for Devices and Radiological Health within the FDA.

A device can also go through a fast-track process if a similar device or equivalent already exists and is

Dr. Marx or an immediate family member has stock or stock options held in MEND Nutrition Inc. and serves as a board member, owner, officer, or committee member of the American Orthopaedic Society for Sports Medicine and the International Society of Arthroscopy, Knee Surgery, and Orthopaedic Sports Medicine. Neither of the following authors nor any immediate family member has received anything of value from or has stock or stock options held in a commercial company or institution related directly or indirectly to the subject of this chapter: Caroline Taber and Dr. Burge.

approved by the FDA.[12,15] This is the case in which the creator or applicant is able to demonstrate that the device is equivalent to a predicate—a device that already exists which is similar, such as a novel hip arthroplasty implant.

POSTMARKETING STUDIES

After a device has been approved by the FDA and has begun to be produced and distributed, the FDA has postmarketing procedures in place that requires that all serious and adverse events be reported.[8] These reports are reviewed by the Office of Surveillance and Epidemiology.[16] The information in these postmarketing studies is made public and available online. Especially for devices such as implants used in total knee and total hip arthroplasties, the FDA requires that physicians, hospitals, and other users of the device report any patient incidents to both the manufacturer and the FDA, which involve patient injury, death, or any other adverse experiences.[16]

STANDARD MEASURES OF CLINICAL OUTCOMES

Radiographic Measures

There are multiple types of diagnostic imaging that serve to measure clinical outcomes. One of the oldest and most common forms of imaging is radiography, which can be particularly useful for orthopaedics. Radiographs are inexpensive; are easy to obtain; provide information about implants, bones, and joints; and can be particularly helpful for diagnosing osteoarthritis. However, one of the shortcomings of radiographs is to provide images in only two dimensions, whereas three dimensions are often needed to have a complete interpretation of the condition.

MRI is another commonly used technique to evaluate soft tissue. This is useful in investigating ligament and tendon tears. There is no radiation exposure to the patient, and it provides three-dimensional images.[17] It can be difficult to obtain clear images if the patient is unable to stay still for prolonged periods while the imaging is conducted and can be difficult for patients with metal implants because of arthroplasty and is impossible for patients with pacemakers.

Ultrasonography is the most used imaging technique for evaluating more superficial tendons, such as the Achilles tendon. Ultrasonography is safe and noninvasive and allows for dynamic assessment of joint and tendon movement and stability.[18] It is able to detect fracture, structural abnormality, infection, ligamentous injury, nerve compression, and mechanical impingement.[18,19] The real-time capability makes ultrasonography especially useful for guiding injections.

CT is analogous to radiography but generates a three-dimensional image. CT can be useful in preoperative planning, especially to see the three-dimensional structure of a bone, and gives an incredibly detailed picture of the anatomy. The shortcomings of CT include that it can be time consuming and it subjects patients to more radiation than a two-dimensional radiograph. Overall, utilization of multiple types of imaging results in the most complete depiction of the problem.

Functional Measures

The two main functional measures of outcome include physical strength and range of motion. Range of motion has classically been used to identify joint abnormalities or musculoskeletal conditions or injuries. Range of motion is also used consistently in clinical trials. However, range of motion is typically measured by the eye, rather than using a tool. For range of motion to have established reliability and validity, the evaluation should be a standardized measurement with a goniometer.[20] However, as technology advances, more complex forms of measurement can be used, such as electromagnetic tracking systems.[21]

Joint range of motion values have been established by the American Academy of Orthopaedic Surgeons.[22] However, all range of motion standards have their limitations—some studies performed of range of motion may have limited sample size or lack of standardized methodology. There are also cases of differences even between laterality because upper extremity range of motion differences between the right and left have been demonstrated.[23]

Coupled with range of motion, strength is also common as a measurement of functional outcomes. Strength is typically tested by manual muscle testing, as well as evaluation of gait and posture.[20] Manual muscle testing is most typically found in the clinical arena for evaluating muscle strength and involves testing the patient's key muscles against the examiner's resistance and rating the strength on a scale of 0 to 5.[24] The manual muscle testing scale[25] is outlined in **Table 1**.

Overall, both range of motion and strength are viewed as consistent and reliable measurements of outcome for both the hip and knee in evaluating orthopaedic patients.

TABLE 1 Manual Muscle Testing Scale

Grade	Description
5	Movement against gravity plus full resistance
4	Movement against gravity plus some resistance
3	Completes the available test range of motion against gravity, but tolerates no resistance
2	The patient completes full or partial range of motion with gravity eliminated
1	Slight contractility without any movement
0	No evidence of contractility (complete paralysis)

Modified with the permission of the Medical Research Council.

Patient-Reported Outcome Measures

Patient-reported outcome measures (PROMs) are increasingly more common in the development of treatment plans and evaluation of patients. PROMs allow for information to be collected about the patients themselves without interpretation from third parties.[26] They include patient attitudes toward functionality, symptoms, health-related quality of life, and satisfaction.[27] PROMs can range from topics being disease focused, anatomic, or generic.

The commonly used orthopaedic disease–focused PROMs are the Western Ontario and McMaster Universities Osteoarthritis Index (WOMAC) and the Knee Society Score (KSS). WOMAC is widely used in the evaluation of hip and knee osteoarthritis. It is a self-administered questionnaire that is grouped as follows:

- Pain (5 items): during walking, using stairs, in bed, sitting or lying, and standing upright
- Stiffness (2 items): after first waking and later in the day
- Physical function (17 items): using stairs, rising from sitting, standing, bending, walking, getting in/out of a car, shopping, putting on/taking off socks, rising from bed, lying in bed, getting in/out of bath, sitting, getting on/off toilet, heavy domestic duties, and light domestic duties

WOMAC questions are scored on a scale of 0 to 4: 0 = none, 1 = mild, 2 = moderate, 3 = severe, and 4 = extreme. The scores are summed, and higher total scores indicate higher levels of stiffness, pain, and functional limitation.[28]

The KSS has been shown to be a reliable and valid measurement of total knee arthroplasty outcome. The long form has four subsections: symptoms, satisfactions, expectations, and functional activities. Questions range from, "For how long can you walk (with or without aid) before stopping due to discomfort?" to "How much does your knee bother you during each of the following activities?"[29] Thorough review of the KSS provides a framework of outcomes following TKA.

Two commonly used anatomic PROMs are the HOOS and the KOOS. HOOS has 40 questions, and KOOS has 42 questions. The two questionnaires investigate five areas of lower extremity pain, joint-specific symptoms, functions in activities of daily living, sports and recreational activities, and quality of life.[30] Both HOOS and KOOS have been shown to have high validity and reliability and have high consistency for people undergoing total knee arthroplasty and total hip arthroplasty.[31,32]

One of the more generic PROMs used to review outcomes is Medical Outcomes Study 36-Item Short Form (SF-36). SF-36 is a self-administered questionnaire and takes approximately 5 minutes for the patient to finish. It has questions on eight dimensions: physical functioning, social functioning, role limitations (such as physical problems), mental health, vitality, pain, general health perceptions, and health changes.[33] SF-36 can be useful in orthopaedic settings in understanding the effect that hip and knee problems may be having on the patient's mental health and perceived effect on their life, which can be useful in determining plans of treatment.

In reviewing the usefulness of PROMs in understanding patient outcomes, as well as determining the effectiveness of procedures, there has been an increase in a set of universally adopted PROMs within the PROMIS.[34] PROMIS has been found to regularly improve coverage of the relative health domain, increase reliability, and reduce respondent burden.[35] PROMIS allows for both fixed-length questionnaires (such as SF-36) and computerized adaptive testing that tailors the length of the questionnaire depending on the responses.[36] For lower extremity issues, such as those including the hip and knee, PROMIS asks questions regarding physical function, pain interference, emotional distress (depression, anxiety, and anger), pain intensity, fatigue, satisfaction with participation in social roles, sleep disturbance, pain behavior, ability to participate in social roles and activities, global health, and physical function (mobility, upper extremity, and lower extremity). PROMIS has been shown to be useful in value-based decisions.[34,37] PROMIS also has been shown to be reliable and valid, while decreasing respondent burden because of computerized adaptive testing.

BIOLOGIC OUTCOME MEASURES

Although PROMs are incredibly useful for understanding the patient's perception of their pain and problems, biologic outcome measures are still used by the physician to have a holistic view of patient outcomes for hip and knee problems. For example, the diagnosis of periprosthetic joint infection (PJI) has been defined by the Musculoskeletal Infection Society as having three of the following five serologic markers:[38,39]

1. Increased serum C-reactive protein level (>100 mg/L in acute PJI; >10 mg/L in chronic PJI) and erythrocyte sedimentation rate (not applicable to acute PJI; >30 mm/hr in chronic PJI)
2. Increased synovial fluid white blood cell count (>10,000 cells/µL in acute PJI; >3,000 cells/µL in chronic PJI) or ++ (or greater) change on leukocyte esterase test strip of synovial fluid
3. Increased synovial fluid polymorphonuclear neutrophil percentage (PMN%) (PMN% >90% in acute PJI; PMN% >80% in chronic PJI)
4. Positive histologic analysis of periprosthetic tissue (>5 neutrophils [PMNs] per high-power field)
5. A single positive periprosthetic (tissue or fluid) culture.

Another biomarker useful in diagnosis is used to identify articular cartilage degradation and urine concentrations of cross-linked C-telopeptide fragments of type II collagen.[40,41] Urine concentrations of cross-linked C-telopeptide fragments of type II collagen are elevated in patients with knee osteoarthritis, those with focal articular cartilage lesions, and those who have undergone anterior cruciate ligament reconstruction.[42-44] Another biomarker of articular cartilage degradation is the neoepitope of type II collagen cleavage at the C-terminal three-quarter-length fragment in urine. These concentrations are elevated in patients with knee osteoarthritis[43,45] and in synovial fluid after anterior cruciate ligament injuries.[46,47]

Biopsy can also be used in orthopaedic interventions as part of the management of articular cartilage defects. Because articular cartilage has limited intrinsic healing capacity, damage or injury typically results in degradation. The field has moved in the direction of cell-based and whole-tissue transplantation.[48,49] One such example of an innovative therapy is autologous chondrocyte implantation. This technique first involves a full-thickness sample from the joint to be collected by arthroscopic biopsy to establish the chondrocyte population, which is then expanded in vitro.[50,51] The two main benefits of this technique are minimizing immune complications and viral infections by using the patient's own cells and that the small biopsy minimizes complications in general.[49]

COMBINING OBJECTIVE AND SUBJECTIVE MEASURES

Overall, both subjective and objective measures are key in creating a holistic view of the patient. PROMs, although subjective, ultimately help patients to reflect on their own health, as well as serve as prompts for open dialogues concerning issues that patients may not raise in other contexts. PROMs combined with objective measurements, such as range of motion, support patient-physician communication as well as affect the subsequent treatment process and outcomes.[52] In conjunction with PROMs and objective measures are activity rating scales, which also add to the complete picture of the patient's symptoms.

Many patients undergo hip and knee surgical procedures with the goal of returning to a particular activity such as tennis, horseback riding, or golf. Determining patient activity can be difficult, and there is no single approach that perfectly defines a patient's activity level and takes into account the duration, intensity, and frequency.[53] Some of the most commonly used activity rating scales are the Marx Activity Rating Scale, Lysholm Knee Scale, Tegner activity score, and Lower Extremity Activity Scale (LEAS).

The Marx Activity Rating Scale is for patients with knee injuries and indicates how often a patient performed an activity in their healthiest and most active state in the past year and asks about running, cutting, deceleration, and pivoting. Responses range from less than one time in a month, one time in a month, one time in a week, two or three times in a week, and four or more times in a week.[54]

The Lysholm Knee Scale score is a physician-administered questionnaire designed to measure outcomes after knee ligament surgery and serves as a measure of function. The Tegner activity scale was designed to measure activity level and be complementary to the Lysholm Knee Scale score.[55] The use of the Lysholm Knee Scale score, the Tegner activity scale, a generic measure of health-related quality of life, and a measure of patient satisfaction provides a comprehensive outcome assessment for patients with knee injuries.[56] These scales have been extremely popular for the past 25 years: the Lysholm Knee Scale score has been cited over 400 times in Pubmed for injuries, and the Tegner activity scale has been cited over 200 times.

Another scale used for assessing activity levels in patients who have undergone joint arthroplasty is the LEAS. LEAS is one of the most rigorously developed and valid activity scales in orthopaedics.[57] The LEAS scale was developed in 2005 and includes statements that cover a range of activity and include 18 statements, including "I am confined to bed all day" to "I am up and about at will in my house and outside. I also participate in vigorous physical activity such as competitive level sports daily." [58] It requires that the patient select a response that is most representative of their current activity; lower total scores correlate with lower levels of activity and higher scores with higher activity.

Overall, combining activity rating scales with subjective and objective measurements can allow for a more complete view of the problems that the patient is presenting. PROMIS can be used for these forms to make their acquisition more efficient.

As technology advances, these outcome measures have become more useful in aiding in predicting patient outcomes for hip and knee surgeries. Machine learning techniques have recently become more popular for predicting morbidity risk, revision surgery, and health-related quality of life following knee and hip arthroplasties.[59,60] Values for PROMs, activity rating scales, and functional scores can be compared with population values to predict individual outcomes.[61] Furthermore, machine learning models are highly adaptable to various clinical scenarios[62] and are expected to become even more accurate in their predictions as time goes on.

IMAGING

A variety of complementary imaging techniques are available for the assessment of outcomes following orthobiologic intervention in the hip and knee. These range from basic conventional radiographs to advanced parametric MRI sequences and may be used to generate qualitative, semiquantitative, and quantitative outcome measures.

RADIOGRAPHY

Conventional radiographs are commonly used as a first-line diagnostic imaging test for diagnosis of musculoskeletal pathology and assessment of treatment efficacy. Radiographs are relatively fast and inexpensive to obtain and provide a good overall assessment of osseous changes within a joint; however, they provide limited assessment of soft-tissue structures, without direct visualization of the ligaments, tendons, menisci, labrum, articular cartilage, and synovium. Regardless, conventional radiographs may be useful in providing an overall gross assessment of joint health, and semiquantitative grading systems, such as the Kellgren-Lawrence score, have been developed and validated for radiographic assessment of joint health.[63] Dual-energy x-ray absorptiometry is a more advanced radiographic technique using photons at two different energy levels for assessment of bone mineral density, generating density scores based on well-established age-adjusted standards.[64]

COMPUTED TOMOGRAPHY

CT, similar to radiography, is based on attenuation of x-rays, providing tissue contrast based on differing densities of various tissue types; however, per its name, CT is acquired tomographically and may be reformatted and reconstructed in various ways, allowing more detailed evaluation of osseous and soft tissues. CT is especially useful for high-resolution evaluation of mineralized bone, making it an optimal modality with which to evaluate osseous bridging following fracture or interventions such as bone grafting (**Figure 1**) with advanced CT techniques such as high-resolution peripheral quantitative CT and micro-CT providing submillimeter assessment of trabecular structure and density, allowing quantitative evaluation of bone health.[65]

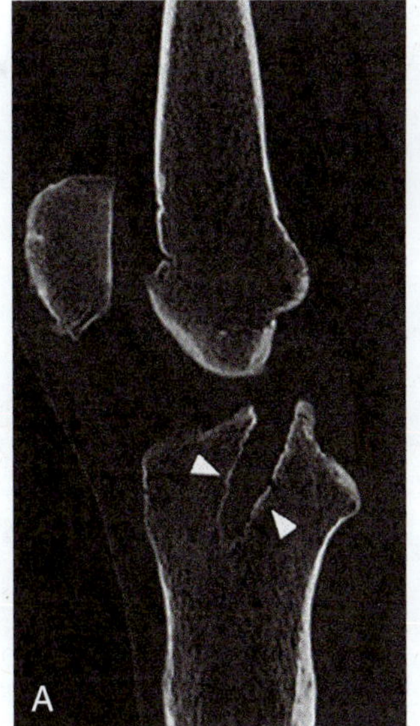

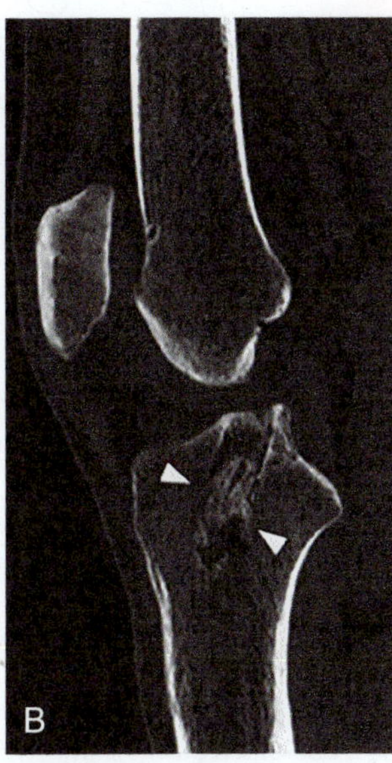

FIGURE 1 Sagittal CT image (**A**) obtained from a 19-year-old woman presenting with instability following prior anterior cruciate ligament (ACL) reconstruction demonstrates osseous tunnel (white arrowheads) within the proximal tibia related to ACL graft placement. Revision surgery with more anterior tunnel placement was planned because of instability; however, because of the risk of tunnel convergence, the patient underwent a two-stage procedure with bone marrow aspirate concentrate–augmented bone grafting of the original tibial tunnel as the first stage. Follow-up CT (**B**) performed 6 months following bone grafting demonstrates good osseous fill of the tunnel with overall good incorporation of the graft (white arrowheads).

ULTRASONOGRAPHY

Ultrasonography is based on the differential conduction of sound waves within different tissue types and provides excellent assessment of soft-tissue structures at high spatial resolution, with the added benefit of the ability to perform dynamic imaging and image-guided interventions (**Figure 2**). However, because of the limited ability of sound waves to penetrate tissues, sonographic assessment of musculoskeletal tissues is typically limited to more superficial tissues that are not obscured by osseous or gas-containing structures, and evaluation of bones is limited to the superficial cortex. Doppler ultrasonography allows assessment of tissue vascularity, but it is limited in the setting of slow blood flow. Increased sensitivity to vascular flow may be achieved through utilization of more advanced techniques such as contrast-enhanced ultrasonography and superb microvascular imaging. Another advanced sonographic technique is sonoelastography, which provides information regarding changes in tissue stiffness. Strain elastography allows qualitative and semiquantitative comparison of strain between two regions, whereas shear wave elastography allows quantitative comparison of tissue stiffness.[66]

MAGNETIC RESONANCE IMAGING

MRI is based on the interaction of protons with radiofrequency pulses and with each other within a static magnetic field, with tissue contrast arising from differences in energy transfer characteristics between protons in differing biochemical environments. Conventional MRI sequences provide superior tissue contrast when evaluating musculoskeletal soft tissues and bone marrow, although evaluation of mineralized cortical bone is limited. Advanced MRI sequences can provide more detailed assessment of tissues, which may not be optimally evaluated on conventional clinical sequences, with short echo time sequences such as ultrashort echo time allowing quantitative assessment of relaxation times within short T2 structures such as ligaments and menisci, and zero echo time (**Figure 3**) techniques allowing generation of CT-like contrast from MRI. Parametric cartilage mapping sequences such as T2 mapping, T1-rho, and delayed gadolinium-enhanced MRI

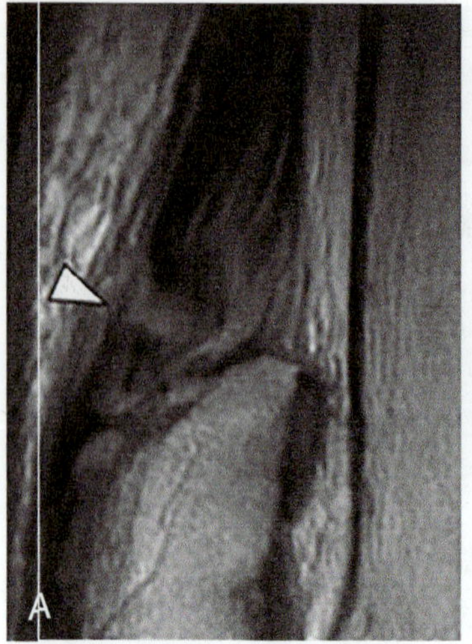

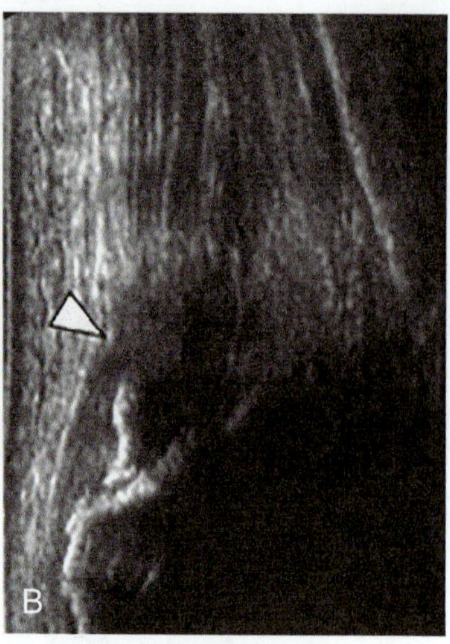

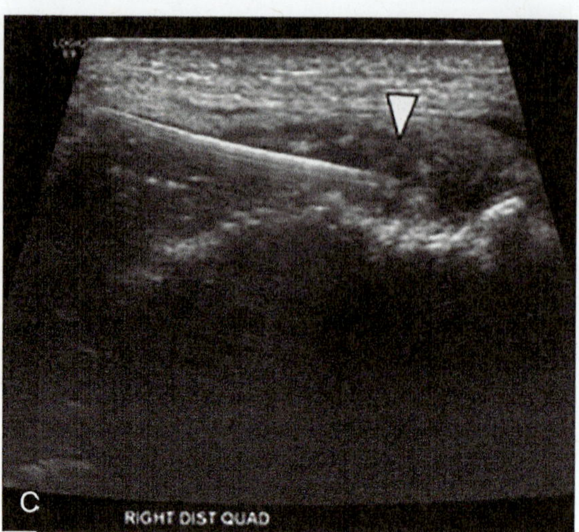

FIGURE 2 Sagittal proton density weighted magnetic resonance (**A**) and ultrasonographic (**B**) images of the knee in a 68-year-old woman demonstrate severe distal quadriceps tendinosis with enthesopathic osseous changes and a superimposed partial tear (white arrowheads). **C**, Transversely oriented ultrasound image through the distal quadriceps demonstrates needle placement in the region of pathology (white arrowhead) during ultrasound-guided platelet-rich plasma injection. (Image courtesy of Dr. Ogonna Nwawka.)

of cartilage (DGEMRIC) have been established as biomarkers for early chondral matrix depletion, with T2 mapping detecting changes in collagen orientation and mobile water content and T1-rho and DEGEMRIC detecting changes in proteoglycan content[67] (**Figure 4**); similar to the aforementioned short echo time sequences, these advanced parametric sequences provide direct quantification of relaxation times within hyaline articular cartilage.

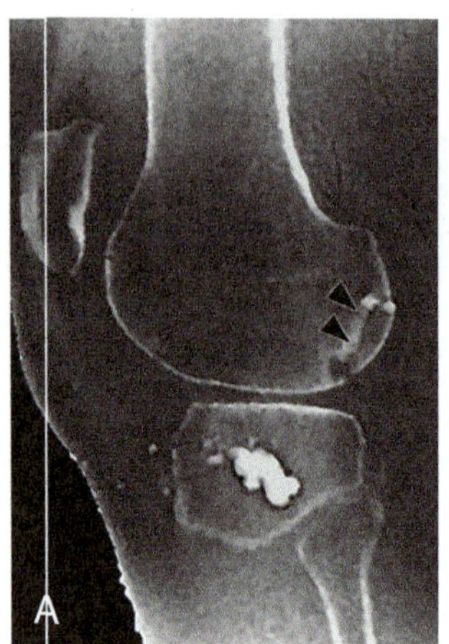

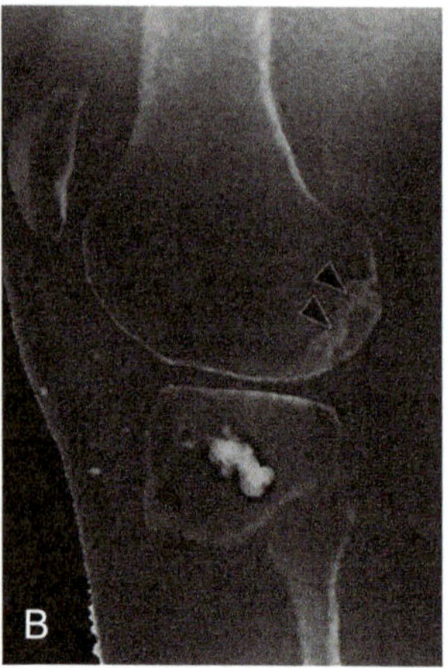

FIGURE 3 **A**, Zero echo time (ZTE) magnetic resonance image of the knee in a 51-year-old woman 6 months following lateral femoral condyle osteochondral allograft augmented with bone marrow aspirate concentrate demonstrates focal areas of osseous bridging, although there is a persistent lucent interface along the graft margin (black arrowheads). Subsequent ZTE magnetic resonance image (**B**) obtained 1 year following repair demonstrates progressive osseous incorporation of the graft (black arrowheads).

A variety of semiquantitative scoring systems have been developed and validated for assessment of joint health on conventional magnetic resonance images, incorporating grading of a variety of pertinent imaging characteristics to generate a numeric score. Examples of these include Whole-Organ Magnetic Resonance Imaging Score and MRI Osteoarthritis Knee Score, for evaluation of the native joint, as well as systems for postoperative evaluation of joint health, such as Magnetic Resonance Observation of Cartilage Repair Tissue and Osteochondral Allograft MRI Scoring System, designed for assessment following cartilage repair.[68-70]

SUMMARY

Clinical outcome measures at baseline and after surgery are important to guide treatment plans and track the progress and health of the patient. The use of a combination of these measurements provides a holistic view of the patient, allowing for the best treatment possible and innovation of new technologies. Standard measures of clinical outcomes include radiographic, functional, and PROMs. The use of a combination of radiographic measures, such as radiographs, MRI, ultrasonography, and CT, informs clinical diagnosis and evaluation of treatment efficacy. Two consistent and reliable functional outcomes used are physical strength and range of motion. PROMs are important in understanding how the patient is doing in daily life and their physical condition. A variety of PROMs questionnaires and scales are used, depending on which hip or knee problem the patient has. Another type of outcome measure is biologic outcome measures. Serologic biomarkers, biopsies, and cell-based and whole-tissue transplantation can provide information essential for treatment or be used as

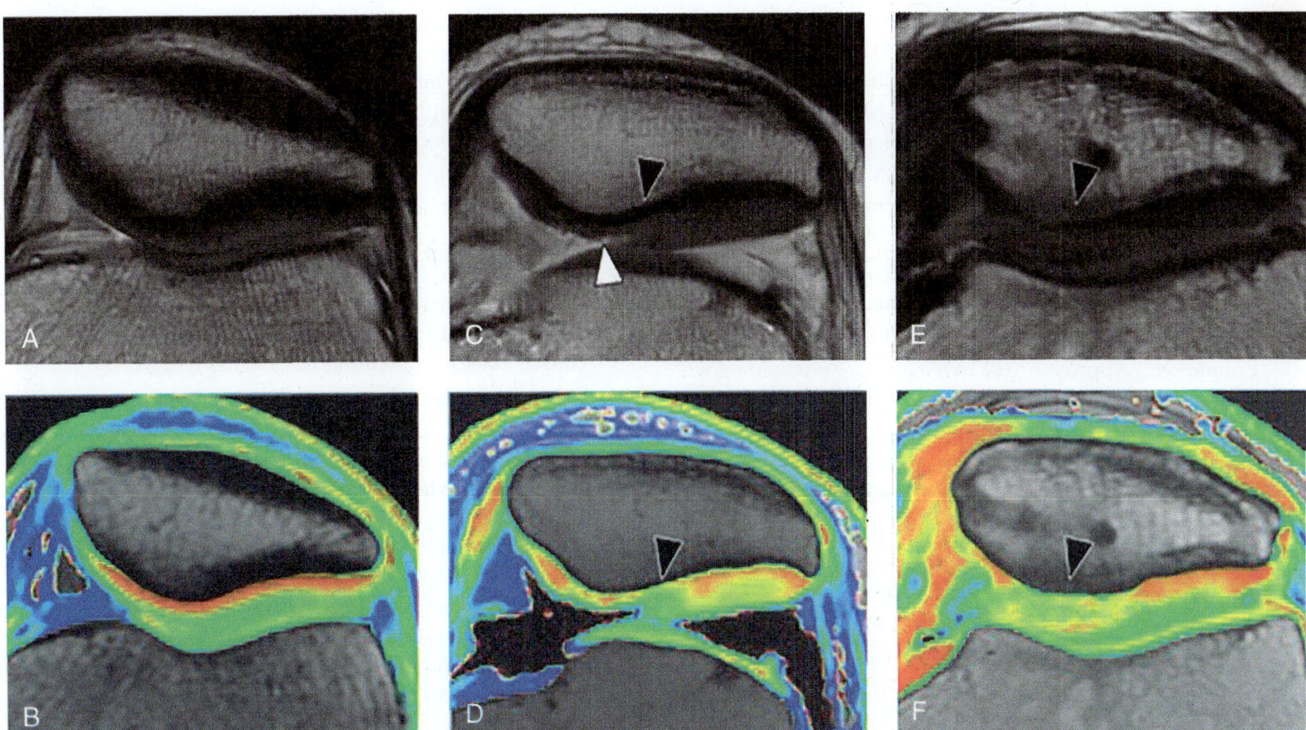

FIGURE 4 Axial proton density (**A**) and T2 mapping (**B**) images of the patella in a 30-year-old woman demonstrate normal stratified appearance of the patellar articular cartilage. Axial proton density (**C**) and T2 mapping (**D**) images of the patella in a 33-year-old woman with early patellofemoral chondral wear demonstrate focal loss of normal stratification (black arrowheads) over the patellar apex and inner aspect of the lateral facet, with focal thinning and fissuring (white arrowhead) on grayscale images. Axial proton density (**E**) and T2 mapping (**F**) images from a 26-year-old woman 1 year following repair of a full-thickness patellar apex chondral defect using particulated juvenile allograft cartilage demonstrate somewhat disorganized chondral tissue with prolongation of relaxation times over the repair site; however, there is excellent fill of the defect with restoration of the articular surface contour. This is a normal postoperative appearance in a patient with a good outcome following chondrocyte-based repair technique.

innovative therapies for orthopaedic conditions. The combination of both subjective and objective measures creates a more complete picture of patient outcomes by considering their goals and concerns, corroborated by objective measures. Different activity scales are important for determining a patient's level of activity before and after hip and knee surgery. Additionally, imaging with a variety of techniques, including radiography, MRI, ultrasonography, and CT, can increase understanding of patient outcomes after treatment with qualitative, semiquantitative, and quantitative systems used to evaluate outcome measures. Consideration of the various measurements of clinical outcomes allows the clinician to gather the whole picture of the health of the patient.

REFERENCES

1. Bhandari M, Petrisor B, Schemitsch E: Outcome measurements in orthopedic. *Indian J Orthop* 2007;41:32.
2. Fetters L, Tilson J: *Evidence Based Physical Therapy*. F.A. Davis Company, 2018.
3. Physiopedia Authors: Outcome Measures. Physiopedia.
4. Kyte DG, Calvert M, van der Wees PJ, ten Hove R, Tolan S, Hill JC: An introduction to patient-reported outcome measures (PROMs) in physiotherapy. *Physiotherapy* 2015;101:119-125.
5. Nielsen LM, Kirkegaard H, Østergaard LG, Bovbjerg K, Breinholt K, Maribo T: Comparison of self-reported and performance-based measures of functional ability in elderly patients in an emergency department: Implications for selection of clinical outcome measures. *BMC Geriatr* 2016;16:199.
6. Powers JH, Patrick DL, Walton MK, et al: Clinician-reported outcome assessments of treatment benefit: Report of the ISPOR clinical outcome assessment emerging good practices task force. *Value Health* 2017;20:2-14.
7. Federal Food Drug and Cosmetics Act 21 U.S.C. 321(h). http://uscode.house.gov/view.xhtml?path=/prelim@title21/chapter9/subchapter2&edition=prelim. Accessed May 26, 2021.
8. Van Norman GA: Drugs, Devices, and the FDA: Part 2 – An overview of approval processes – FDA approval of medical devices. *JACC Basic Transl Sci* 2016;1:277-287.
9. U.S. Food and Drug Administration: CFR-Code of Federal Regulations Title 21 vol. 8 Sec 870.3610. https://www.ecfr.gov/current/title-21/chapter-I/subchapter-H/part-870/subpart-D/section-870.3610. Accessed May 26, 2021.

10. U.S. Food and Drug Administration: CFR-Code of Federal Regulations Title 21 vol. 8. Sec 878.5020. https://www.ecfr.gov/current/title-21/chapter-I/subchapter-H/part-878/subpart-E/section-878.5020. Accessed May 26, 2021.
11. U.S. Food and Drug Administration: CFR-Code of Federal Regulations Title 21 vol. 8. Sec 880.5240. https://www.ecfr.gov/current/title-21/chapter-I/subchapter-H/part-880/subpart-F/section-880.5240. Accessed May 26, 2021.
12. Naghshineh N, Brown S, Cederna PS, et al: Demystifying the U.S. Food and Drug Administration: Understanding regulatory pathways. *Plast Reconstr Surg* 2014;134:559-569.
13. Premarket Approval (PMA): https://www.fda.gov/medical-devices/premarket-submissions/premarket-approval-pma. Accessed May 26, 2021.
14. Fargen KM, Frei D, Fiorella D, et al: The FDA approval process for medical devices: An inherently flawed system or a valuable pathway for innovation? *J Neurointerv Surg* 2013;5:269-275.
15. Kaplan AV, Baim DS, Smith JJ, et al: Medical device development: From prototype to regulatory approval. *Circulation* 2004;109:3068-3072.
16. Dabrowska A, Thaul S: How FDA Approves Drugs and Regulates Their Safety and Effectiveness. Congressional Research Service.
17. UPMC Orthopedic Care: What Are the Different Types of Orthopaedic Imaging? https://share.upmc.com/2017/03/orthopaedic-imaging/. 2017.
18. Blankstein A: Ultrasound in the diagnosis of clinical orthopedics: The orthopedic stethoscope. *World J Orthop* 2011;2:13.
19. Garcia T, Hornof WJ, Insana MF: On the ultrasonic properties of tendon. *Ultrasound Med Biol* 2003;29:1787-1797.
20. Marcano-Fernández F, Prada C, Johal H: Physical outcome measures: The role of strength and range of motion in orthopaedic research. *Injury* 2020;51:S106-S110.
21. Morphett AL, Crawford CM, Lee D: The use of electromagnetic tracking technology for measurement of passive cervical range of motion: A pilot study. *J Manipulative Physiol Ther* 2003;26:152-159.
22. Greene WB, Heckman JD: *The Clinical Measurement of Joint Motion*. American Academy of Orthopaedic Surgeons, 1994.
23. Günal I, Köse N, Erdogan O, Göktürk E, Seber S: Normal range of motion of the joints of the upper extremity in male subjects, with special reference to side. *J Bone Joint Surg Am* 1996;78:1401-1404.
24. Ciesla N, Dinglas V, Fan E, Kho M, Kuramoto J, Needham D: Manual muscle testing: A method of measuring extremity muscle strength applied to critically Ill patients. *J Vis Exp* 2011;50:2632.
25. De Jonghe B: Paresis acquired in the intensive care unit: A prospective multicenter study. *J Am Med Assoc* 2002;288:2859.
26. Knol DL, Mokkink LB, Terwee CB, De Vet HCW: *Measurement in Medicine a Practical Guide*. Cambridge University Press, 2011.
27. Gagnier JJ: Patient reported outcomes in orthopaedics: Patient reported outcome. *J Orthop Res* 2017;35:2098-2108.
28. Gandek B: Measurement properties of the Western Ontario and McMaster Universities osteoarthritis index: A systematic review. *Arthritis Care Res (Hoboken)* 2015;67:216-229.
29. Scuderi GR, Sikorskii A, Bourne RB, Lonner JH, Benjamin JB, Noble PC: The knee society short form reduces respondent burden in the assessment of patient-reported outcomes. *Clin Orthop Relat Res* 2016;474:134-142.
30. Goodman SM, Mehta BY, Mandl LA, et al: Validation of the hip disability and osteoarthritis outcome score and knee injury and osteoarthritis outcome score pain and function subscales for use in total hip replacement and total knee replacement clinical trials. *J Arthroplasty* 2020;35:1200-1207.e4.
31. Collins NJ, Misra D, Felson DT, Crossley KM, Roos EM: Measures of knee function: International Knee Documentation Committee (IKDC) Subjective Knee Evaluation Form, Knee Injury and Osteoarthritis Outcome Score (KOOS), Knee Injury and Osteoarthritis Outcome Score Physical Function Short Form (KOOS-PS), Knee Outcome Survey Activities of Daily Living Scale (KOS-ADL), Lysholm Knee Scoring Scale, Oxford Knee Score (OKS), Western Ontario and McMaster Universities Osteoarthritis Index (WOMAC), Activity Rating Scale (ARS), and Tegner Activity Score (TAS). *Arthritis Care Res (Hoboken)* 2011;63(suppl 11):S208-S228.
32. Nilsdotter A, Bremander A: Measures of hip function and symptoms: Harris Hip Score (HHS), Hip Disability and Osteoarthritis Outcome Score (HOOS), Oxford Hip Score (OHS), Lequesne Index of Severity for Osteoarthritis of the Hip (LISOH), and American Academy of Orthopedic Surgeons (AAOS) Hip and Knee Questionnaire. *Arthritis Care Res (Hoboken)* 2011;63(suppl 11):S200-S207.
33. Brazier JE, Harper R, Jones NM, et al: Validating the SF-36 health survey questionnaire: New outcome measure for primary care. *BMJ* 1992;305:160-164.
34. Horn ME, Reinke EK, Couce LJ, Reeve BB, Ledbetter L, George SZ: Reporting and utilization of Patient-Reported Outcomes Measurement Information System® (PROMIS®) measures in orthopedic research and practice: A systematic review. *J Orthop Surg Res* 2020;15:553.
35. Brodke DJ, Saltzman CL, Brodke DS: PROMIS for orthopaedic outcomes measurement: *J Am Acad Orthop Surg* 2016;24:744-749.
36. Cella D, Gershon R, Lai J-S, Choi S: The future of outcomes measurement: Item banking, tailored short-forms, and computerized adaptive assessment. *Qual Life Res* 2007;16(suppl 1):133-141.
37. Pennestrì F, Lippi G, Banfi G: Pay less and spend more—The real value in healthcare procurement. *Ann Transl Med* 2019;7:688.
38. Parvizi J, Zmistowski B, Berbari EF, et al: New definition for periprosthetic joint infection: from the Workgroup of the Musculoskeletal Infection Society. *Clin Orthop Relat Res* 2011;469:2992-2994.
39. Parvizi J, Fassihi SC, Enayatollahi MA: Diagnosis of periprosthetic joint infection following hip and knee arthroplasty. *Orthop Clin North Am* 2016;47:505-515.
40. Chmielewski TL, George SZ, Tillman SM, et al: Low- versus high-intensity plyometric exercise during rehabilitation

after anterior cruciate ligament reconstruction. *Am J Sports Med* 2016;44:609-617.

41. Ishijima M, Kaneko H, Kaneko K: The evolving role of biomarkers for osteoarthritis. *Ther Adv Musculoskelet Dis* 2014;6:144-153.
42. Chmielewski TL, Trumble TN, Joseph A-M, et al: Urinary CTX-II concentrations are elevated and associated with knee pain and function in subjects with ACL reconstruction. *Osteoarthritis Cartilage* 2012;20:1294-1301.
43. Cibere J, Zhang H, Garnero P, et al: Association of biomarkers with pre-radiographically defined and radiographically defined knee osteoarthritis in a population-based study. *Arthritis Rheum* 2009;60:1372-1380.
44. Røtterud JH, Reinholt FP, Beckstrøm KJ, Risberg MA, Årøen A: Relationship between CTX-II and patient characteristics, patient-reported outcome, muscle strength, and rehabilitation in patients with a focal cartilage lesion of the knee: A prospective exploratory cohort study of 48 patients. *BMC Musculoskelet Disord* 2014;15:99.
45. He G, Chen X, Zhang G, Lin H, Li R, Wu X: Detection of urine C2C and trace element level in patients with knee osteoarthritis. *Cell Biochem Biophys* 2014;70:475-479.
46. Yoshida H, Kojima T, Kurokouchi K, et al: Relationship between pre-radiographic cartilage damage following anterior cruciate ligament injury and biomarkers of cartilage turnover in clinical practice: A cross-sectional observational study. *Osteoarthritis Cartilage* 2013;21:831-838.
47. Kumahashi N, Swärd P, Larsson S, Lohmander LS, Frobell R, Struglics A: Type II collagen C2C epitope in human synovial fluid and serum after knee injury – Associations with molecular and structural markers of injury. *Osteoarthritis Cartilage* 2015;23:1506-1512.
48. Moran CJ, Pascual-Garrido C, Chubinskaya S, et al: Restoration of articular cartilage. *J Bone Joint Surg Am* 2014;96:336-344.
49. Makris EA, Gomoll AH, Malizos KN, Hu JC, Athanasiou KA: Repair and tissue engineering techniques for articular cartilage. *Nat Rev Rheumatol* 2015;11:21-34.
50. Saris DBF, Vanlauwe J, Victor J, et al: Characterized chondrocyte implantation results in better structural repair when treating symptomatic cartilage defects of the knee in a randomized controlled trial versus microfracture. *Am J Sports Med* 2008;36:235-246.
51. Saris DBF, Vanlauwe J, Victor J, et al: Treatment of symptomatic cartilage defects of the knee: Characterized chondrocyte implantation results in better clinical outcome at 36 months in a randomized trial compared to microfracture. *Am J Sports Med* 2009;37(suppl 1):10S-19S.
52. Greenhalgh J, Gooding K, Gibbons E, et al: How do patient reported outcome measures (PROMs) support clinician-patient communication and patient care? A realist synthesis. *J Patient Rep Outcomes* 2018;2:42.
53. Naal FD, Impellizzeri FM, Leunig M: Which is the best activity rating scale for patients undergoing total joint arthroplasty? *Clin Orthop Relat Res* 2009;467:958-965.
54. Marx RG, Stump TJ, Jones EC, Wickiewicz TL, Warren RF: Development and evaluation of an activity rating scale for disorders of the knee. *Am J Sports Med* 2001;29:213-218.
55. Tegner Y, Lysholm J: Rating systems in the evaluation of knee ligament injuries. *Clin Orthop Relat Res* 1985;198:43-49.
56. Briggs KK, Lysholm J, Tegner Y, Rodkey WG, Kocher MS, Steadman JR: The reliability, validity, and responsiveness of the Lysholm score and Tegner activity scale for anterior cruciate ligament injuries of the knee: 25 years later. *Am J Sports Med* 2009;37:890-897.
57. Terwee CB, Bouwmeester W, van Elsland SL, de Vet HCW, Dekker J: Instruments to assess physical activity in patients with osteoarthritis of the hip or knee: A systematic review of measurement properties. *Osteoarthritis Cartilage* 2011;19:620-633.
58. Saleh KJ, Mulhall KJ, Bershadsky B, et al: Development and validation of a lower-extremity activity scale. Use for patients treated with revision total knee arthroplasty. *J Bone Joint Surg Am* 2005;87:1985-1994.
59. Eneqvist T, Nemes S, Bülow E, Mohaddes M, Rolfson O: Can patient-reported outcomes predict re-operations after total hip replacement? *Int Orthop* 2018;42:273-279.
60. Wong DJN, Oliver CM, Moonesinghe SR: Predicting postoperative morbidity in adult elective surgical patients using the Surgical Outcome Risk Tool (SORT). *Br J Anaesth* 2017;119:95-105.
61. Baumhauer JF: Patient-reported outcomes – Are they living up to their potential? *N Engl J Med* 2017;377:6-9.
62. Huber M, Kurz C, Leidl R: Predicting patient-reported outcomes following hip and knee replacement surgery using supervised machine learning. *BMC Med Inform Decis Mak* 2019;19:3.
63. Kohn MD, Sassoon AA, Fernando ND: Classifications in Brief: Kellgren-Lawrence classification of osteoarthritis. *Clin Orthop Relat Res* 2016;474:1886-1893.
64. Wahner HW: Measurements of bone mass and bone density. *Endocrinol Metab Clin North Am* 1989;18:995-1012.
65. Ohs N, Collins CJ, Atkins PR: Validation of HR-pQCT against micro-CT for morphometric and biomechanical analyses: A review. *Bone Rep* 2020;13:100711.
66. Nwawka OK: Update in musculoskeletal ultrasound research. *Sports Health* 2016;8:429-437.
67. Argentieri EC, Sneag DB, Nwawka OK, Potter HG: Updates in musculoskeletal imaging. *Sports Health* 2018;10:296-302.
68. Jarraya M, Hayashi D, Roemer FW, Guermazi A: MR Imaging-based Semi-quantitative methods for knee osteoarthritis. *Magn Reson Med Sci* 2016;15:153-164.
69. Chang EY, Pallante-Kichura AL, Bae WC, et al: Development of a comprehensive Osteochondral Allograft MRI Scoring System (OCAMRISS) with histopathologic, micro-computed tomography, and biomechanical validation. *Cartilage* 2014;5:16-27.
70. Marlovits S, Singer P, Zeller P, Mandl I, Haller J, Trattnig S: Magnetic resonance observation of cartilage repair tissue (MOCART) for the evaluation of autologous chondrocyte transplantation: determination of interobserver variability and correlation to clinical outcome after 2 years. *Eur J Radiol* 2006;57:16-23.

CHAPTER 30

Biologic Considerations for Clinical Study Design: Cartilage Repair

James L. Cook, DVM, PhD • David P. Trofa, MD • Clayton W. Nuelle, MD, FAAOS • Clark T. Hung, PhD

INTRODUCTION

One of the greatest challenges faced by surgeons specializing in complex knee disorders is determining the optimal approach to manage articular cartilage lesions. This challenge is complicated by the fact that there is a paucity of high-level evidence available in the literature to help guide patient-specific and lesion-specific decision making. This is problematic given that an estimated 200,000 to 300,000 procedures are performed annually in the United States for symptomatic chondral and osteochondral defects.[1] Biologic options available to manage these lesions include arthroscopic débridement, abrasion arthroplasty, marrow stimulation procedures that may be augmented with various orthobiologic treatment strategies, osteochondral autograft transfer (OAT), osteochondral allograft (OCA) transplantation, and cell-based and matrix-based techniques. Although extensive preclinical and single-cohort outcomes studies support relative indications and potential benefits for each of these treatment strategies, robust head-to-head comparisons are unfortunately rare, usually underpowered, and statistically fragile.[2] Robust clinical trials to assess current and future options to manage articular cartilage lesions are needed to address this deficiency.

BRIEF HISTORY OF CLINICAL STUDY DESIGN IN ARTICULAR CARTILAGE REPAIR

Clinical trials are categorized into one of four basic stages:[3]

1. Feasibility—first-in-human application, primarily focused on safety
2. Clinical research—safety data are further developed and efficacy assessments are included for well-defined patient groups under close supervision of investigator/inventor
3. Validation—efficacy evaluations expanded to include multiple clinical sites
4. Acceptance—postmarket surveillance to monitor long-term outcomes and adverse events

Accordingly, clinical trial study design will reflect the intended purpose. With respect to defining the level of rigor of a clinical trial, level of evidence for clinical application is considered to graduate from case series to single-cohort studies, case-control or comparison cohort studies, and finally randomized controlled trials (RCTs), systematic reviews, and meta-analyses.[4,5] However, it is important to also consider other key aspects of the experimental design such as study population, sample size, outcome measures, and duration when determining strength and generalizability of the data. In addition, the level of evidence for systematic reviews and meta-analyses can only be considered to be as robust as the studies included in the analyses.

Despite their importance, RCTs represent 3% of orthopaedic literature.[6,7] With respect to recent level I or II clinical studies and their chosen comparator groups, 6 studies have compared OATs with autologous chondrocyte implantation (ACI),[8-13] 1 has compared OATs with matrix-induced ACI,[14] 8 have compared OAT with microfracture,[13,15-21] and 12 have compared ACI with microfracture.[22] A recently published article by Saltzman et al[23] evaluated the methodology used among level I and II studies and reported a significant heterogeneity in methodology including design, follow-up, and outcome measurements. The heterogeneity in such investigations is well demonstrated in **Table 1**.

Dr. Cook or an immediate family member has received royalties from Arthrex, Inc. and Musculoskeletal Transplant Foundation; serves as a paid consultant to or is an employee of Arthrex, Inc. and Trupanion; has received research or institutional support from Arthrex, Inc., Collagen Matrix Inc., DePuy, a Johnson & Johnson Company, Musculoskeletal Transplant Foundation, National Institutes of Health (NIAMS & NICHD), Purina, Regenosine, SITES Medical, and U.S. Department of Defense; and serves as a board member, owner, officer, or committee member of the Midwest Transplant Network and the Musculoskeletal Transplant Foundation. Dr. Nuelle or an immediate family member is a member of a speakers' bureau or has made paid presentations on behalf of Arthrex, Inc. and Vericel, Inc.; serves as a paid consultant to or is an employee of Guidepoint Consulting; has received nonincome support (such as equipment or services), commercially derived honoraria, or other non–research-related funding (such as paid travel) from AO Foundation; and serves as a board member, owner, officer, or committee member of the American Academy of Orthopaedic Surgeons, the American Orthopaedic Society for Sports Medicine, and the Arthroscopy Association of North America. Dr. Hung or an immediate family member has received royalties from Allosource and Musculoskeletal Transplant Foundation and has received research or institutional support from Musculoskeletal Transplant Foundation, National Institutes of Health, Orthopedic Science & Research Foundation and Department of Defense. Neither Dr. Trofa nor any immediate family member has received anything of value from or has stock or stock options held in a commercial company or institution related directly or indirectly to the subject of this chapter.

TABLE 1 PICO Table for Cited Studies With Functional Outcomes

Population	Intervention	Comparisons	Outcome	Studies
Patients (n = 100) with symptomatic cartilage defects in the knee (mean size, 4.7 cm^2)	Randomized to ACI or OAT-mosaicplasty (OAT-M)	Modified Cincinnati and Stanmore scores; 1-year second-look arthroscopy; 10-year treatment survivorship	Improved functional scores (88% versus 69%), postoperative arthroscopic evaluations, and failure rates (17% versus 55%) in ACI versus OAT-M	Bentley et al 2003[8], Bentley et al 2012[9]
Patients (n = 55) with isolated femoral condyle defects (2.5 to 7.5 cm^2)	Randomized to MACI (agarose-alginate scaffold) or OAT-M	IKDC score; 2 year histology (O'Driscoll score); adverse events	Significantly improved IKDC scores (81.5 versus 73.7), improved histologic characteristics, and lower adverse events in the mosaicplasty group versus MACI group	Clave et al 2016[10]
Patients (n = 23) with full-thickness chondral defects in the knee (mean, 1.9 cm^2)	Randomized to ACI or OAT-M	IKDC and Lysholm Knee Scale	No differences in average Lysholm or IKDC scales	Dozin et al 2005[11]
Patients (n = 40) with isolated femoral condyle defects (mean, 3.75 cm^2)	Randomized to ACI or OAT	2 year Lysholm, Tegner activity scale, and Meyers rating scores; histology	No difference in Tegner and Meyers scores. Improved Lysholm score after OATs versus ACI; histology demonstrated fibrocartilage repair tissue for ACI versus maintained hyaline cartilage for OAT	Horas et al 2003[12]
Patients (n = 70) with isolated cartilage defects in the knee (mean, 1.0 to 4.0 cm^2).	Microfracture, OAT, ACI cohorts	Minimum of 3-year follow-up; Lysholm, Tegner, and HSS scores; MRI using modified Outerbridge scale; 12 to 18 months second-look arthroscopy with ICRS grading system	No significant differences in functional scores, Outerbridge scale using MRI, or arthroscopy findings	Lim et al 2012[13]
Athletes (n = 60) with symptomatic articular cartilage lesions in the knee	Randomized to OAT or microfracture	3-year HSS and ICRS scores, 10-year ICRS, and Tegner scores; return to sports and failure rates; 1-year histologic biopsy; MRI	OAT demonstrated significantly better functional outcomes scores and return to sports rates and activity levels 3 and 10 years postoperatively. Histologic examination demonstrated normal hyaline cartilage in all patients undergoing OAT versus 57% of microfracture samples demonstrating fibrocartilage. There was a higher failure rate at 10 years in the microfracture (38%) versus OAT (14%) cohort. Improved chondral surface filling was found on MRI in the OAT group compared with microfracture	Gudas et al 2005[15], Gudas et al 2006[16], Gudas et al 2012[18]
Young (aged 12 to 18 months) patients (n = 50) with OCD of the femoral condyle (mean, 3.2 cm^2)	Randomized to OAT or microfracture	Follow-up of 3 to 6 years, ICRS scores, failure rates, 18-month MRI	Good to excellent outcomes in 83% OAT versus 63% microfracture; significantly higher failure rate for microfracture (41% versus zero); MRI good to excellent for 91% OAT versus 56% microfracture	Gudas et al 2009[17]
Patients (n = 102) with ACL rupture and articular cartilage damage of the medial femoral condyle	Randomized to OAT, microfracture, or débridement with ACLR and matched control (ACLR with intact cartilage)	3-year follow-up for IKDC, Tegner, and clinical assessments	IKDC: Control > OAT > microfracture or débridement; lower Tegner scores identified for the microfracture and débridement cohorts versus control and OAT group	Gudas et al 2013[19]

TABLE 1 PICO Table for Cited Studies With Functional Outcomes (Continued)

Population	Intervention	Comparisons	Outcome	Studies
Patients (n = 40) with 1 or 2 symptomatic focal full-thickness cartilage defects (2 to 6 cm^2) on the femoral condyles or trochlea	Randomized to OAT-M or microfracture	15-year follow-up for Lysholm score	Lysholm score significantly better for OAT-M at 1, 5, 10, and 15 years	Solheim et al 2018[20]
Patients (n = 25) with full-thickness chondral lesion of the distal femur (2.0 to 6.0 cm^2)	Randomized to OAT-M or microfracture	Follow-up of 5 to 11 years for Lysholm score, KOOS, and isokinetic muscle strength	No significant differences in measured outcomes	Ulstein et al 2014[21]

ACI = autologous chondrocyte implantation, ACL = anterior cruciate ligament, ACLR = anterior cruciate ligament reconstruction, HSS = Hospital for Special Surgery, ICRS = International Cartilage Repair Society, IKDC = International Knee Documentation Committee, KOOS = Knee Injury and Osteoarthritis Outcome Score, MACI = matrix-induced ACI, OAT = osteochondral autograft transfer, OCD = osteochondritis dissecans

DESIGN CONSIDERATIONS AND CHALLENGES FOR RCTs

FDA Regulatory Considerations (Device, Biologic, or HCT/P Designation)

In the United States, cartilage repair and restoration therapies can be used clinically as medical devices; biologics; drugs; or human cells, tissues, or cellular or tissue-based products (HCT/P). The specific classification in combination with the determination regarding validity greatly affects the regulatory pathway for bringing the product to market. Any product "containing or consisting of human cells or tissues that are intended for implantation, transplantation, infusion, or transfer into a human recipient"[24] that meets HCT/P criteria, including minimal manipulation and homologous use, is not subject to premarket FDA approval or clearance. Any cartilage repair or restoration device that does not meet FDA HCT/P criteria is subject to premarket FDA clearance, approval, or granting:

- Clearance: This is applicable to devices that qualify for and complete the 510(k) pathway, such that the FDA reviews and clears them for clinical use.
- Approval: Class III medical devices must be submitted for premarket approval or Humanitarian Device Exemption and then complete the rigorous review and approval process for clinical use.
- Granted: Class I and II devices may be eligible for the de novo pathway if they are considered novel such that they are not listed in the standard FDA classifications. The device must also be considered low or moderate risk to be granted for clinical use by the FDA.

Cartilage repair or restoration strategies that are considered biologics or drugs, or combination products, must go through the Center for Biologics Evaluation and Research development and approval process. This process may involve 510(k), premarket approval, Investigational New Drug, Biologics License Application, Expanded Access, or New Drug Application pathways (https://www.fda.gov/vaccines-blood-biologics/development-approval-process-cber).

Completing RCTs required by the FDA to establish safety and efficacy for novel and promising approaches to cartilage repair and restoration has been a challenge based on major barriers including costs, enrollment feasibility to meet needed sample size, and required controls.[25]

Inclusion/Exclusion Criteria

Patient-related criteria for cartilage repair interventions that often result in RCT screening failures and prolonged enrollment timelines include patient age, nature of the lesion, comorbidities, activity level, and willingness to be randomized.[26] Examples of typical criteria for patient inclusion and exclusion for cartilage repair studies gleaned from a sampling of studies on ClinicalTrials.gov are discussed in **Tables 2** and **3**.

Control Arm Selection for RCTs

The control arm is intended to include patients who are representative of the attributes of the experimental group and account for a placebo effect and to reduce selection bias where patient enrollment is skewed to individuals who are thought to respond more positively to the intervention. If clinical equipoise exists, a genuine uncertainty about the best treatment, and with preclinical data justifying human experimentation, patients can ethically be randomly assigned to an intervention to reduce the effects

TABLE 2 Sample Inclusion Criteria

Symptomatic focal or multifocal defects, often specified as contained defects
Symptomatic lesion grading International Cartilage Repair Society 3 or 4 (for osteochondral product, otherwise exclusion criteria)
Symptomatic total treatable area (eg, 1 to 7 cm^2)
Symptomatic, single or multiple, full-thickness cartilage defects of the knee with or without bone involvement
Knee pain and/or nonsurgical treatment (anti-inflammatory drugs) for a defined period (2 to 4 months)
Knee Injury and Osteoarthritis Outcome Score pain score at baseline is not less than 30 and not more than 65
Age range: Typically 18 to 55 years
Must be willing and able to undergo MRI
Must be physically and mentally willing and able to comply with postoperative rehabilitation protocol and scheduled clinical and diagnostic imaging visits
Willingness to incorporate normal standard of care or add on (nonstandard of care)
Documented informed consent

that could influence the outcome. The results observed in an RCT are more likely to be the consequence of the intervention.[7]

Ideally, the control arm will be hypothesis driven and patient and lesion oriented and will provide a valid comparison for the treatment arm such that enrollment goals are feasible and requirements of regulatory agencies are met. However, regulatory agency designation of the control arm may not align with a clinical reference standard that would inspire confidence and adoption by surgeons. For example, microfracture[27,28] serves as the current reference standard control for FDA-sanctioned cartilage repair RCTs, but is contraindicated for lesions greater than 2 cm^2 or uncontained lesions, and has been documented to burn bridges based on inferior results for subsequent cartilage restoration procedures.[29] In addition, midterm and long-term outcomes after microfracture are poor in a significant number of patients,[30] and associated failure rates and return to preinjury activities are inferior to osteochondral restoration techniques.[15,16,18,19] Therefore, comparison of experimental interventions with microfracture rather than OATs for small lesions (<2 cm^2) or OCAs for large lesions (>2 cm^2) for which good long-term outcomes have been documented[31] seems to establish a straw man comparator. Given such data, surgeons may encounter an ethical dilemma regarding the use of microfracture based on its inferior outcomes and may elect not to participate in studies that require it as the required control.

The latter is indicative of a more general problem associated with comparability, or matching, of the control and experimental groups. Case-control studies are a common method of analyzing associations between clinical outcomes and potential risk factors. Matching cases to controls based on known confounding variables (eg, age, sex, and comorbidities) can decrease bias and allow investigators to assess the association of interest with increased precision. Care should be taken in the analysis of matched data because failure to use matched statistical methods can lead to imprecise or biased results.[32,33] Nevertheless, case-control matching has been used successfully by some investigators. For example, Merkely et al[34] performed a case-control investigation evaluating primary OCA transplantation versus revision OCA transplantation following failure of ACI in a total of 26 patients. The average lesion size was 6.1 cm^2 in the revision group and 5.0 cm^2 in the primary group. Outcome measures included the pain, activities of daily living, sport/recreation, and quality of life Knee Injury and Osteoarthritis Outcome Score (KOOS) subscales, Lysholm Knee Scale and International Knee Documentation Committee scores, and reoperation and survival rates. The authors reported no significant differences in functional outcome scores, reoperation rate, or survival rates, illustrating that OCA transplantation can be an excellent salvage procedure for similar cases.[34]

Another challenge to completing RCTs for cartilage repair and restoration is feasibility for enrolling the predetermined sample size to meet thresholds for statistical power and effect size. In addition to the control arm issues and defect size considerations outlined previously, lesion-specific factors such as containment, depth, anatomic location, or the condition of surrounding, opposing, or distant

TABLE 3 Sample Exclusion Criteria

Severe osteoarthritis—Kellgren-Lawrence grade 3 or 4
Complete medial or lateral meniscus deficiency
Significant instability of the index knee according to International Knee Documentation Committee Knee Examination Form 2000, grade C (abnormal) or D (severely abnormal)
Lower extremity malalignment of certain degree—malalignment more than 5° varus OR 5° valgus according to standing radiograph
Bipolar lesions in index knee
Body mass index (eg, >35 kg/mm^2)
Previous surgery or treatment in the index knee during past 3 to 6 months
Pregnancy
Known substance abuse
Chemotherapy within 12 months
Inflammatory arthritis or degenerative joint disease
Systemic diseases (eg, insulin-dependent diabetes mellitus)
Blood disorders or coagulopathies
Bilateral joint disorders
Workers' compensation-related problem

cartilage may render a patient unsuitable for a given technique. For example, if a symptomatic lesion involves the subchondral bone, a cell-based technique may not be the ideal treatment method because it may not adequately address the pathologic bone. In contrast, cartilage lesions in the hip or shoulder may not be ideal for OAT procedures based on lack of same-joint donor tissue, and small contained defects may not be ideal for OCA transplantation based on relative cost-to-benefit ratio. Financial costs can be severely limiting because it is estimated that to-market expenses from concept to regulatory approval can potentially exceed $50 million, with RCT funding comprising a significant portion.

Single and Double Blinding

Although blinded RCTs mitigate selection bias by surgeon and patient and permit cause and effect of intervention to be determined, blinding is highly challenging in cartilage repair and restoration trials. The surgeon cannot be blinded to a subject's treatment arm, and unless a study uses a placebo or sham surgery, it is difficult to blind the patient to treatment as well. Furthermore, patients may not consent to a randomized, blinded trial because they want the best treatment possible. Blinding the rest of the evaluation team may also be difficult based on differences in single-stage versus multistage procedures, incisions, imaging findings, and postoperative rehabilitation protocols. Therefore, blinding must be carefully planned and implemented to be appropriately applied to suitable evaluators, and outcome measures should be objective and quantitative whenever possible. Karanicolas et al[35] advocate that investigators should not consider blinding as all or nothing in their study design, but instead view it as a continuum such that each component of blinding is additive to study validity. Outcomes that are typically subjective and depend on the tester (eg, range of motion) or clinical interpretation (eg, of imaging) should be prioritized for blinding. For example, simple techniques for posttreatment evaluations such as incorporating an independent assessor, concealing incisions, or masking diagnostic imaging features can blind most outcomes.[35]

Surgical Site Logistics

The Declaration of Helsinki (1964), with its subsequent amendments, defines ethical standards for performance of most clinical trials: (1) patient anonymity and safe and humane treatment with a projection of favorable risk-to-benefit ratio; (2) integrity of research process must be approved by an independent review board (eg, institutional review boards); (3) informed and uncoerced consent; and (4) only clinical researchers qualified by training and experience should conduct clinical trials.[3] These standards must be carefully considered when designing cartilage repair and restoration RCTs with respect to inclusion of sham treatment strategies and research-specific second-look arthroscopy and/or biopsy.

Protection of research subjects is paramount and the primary responsibility of the principal investigator. Sham procedures provide an ideal method for establishing efficacy of interventions and informing best practices. However, for many of the valid sham procedures related to cartilage repair and restoration techniques, the exposure of patients to risks of anesthesia and surgical interventions with no potential benefits[36] raises an ethical dilemma and is contraindicated by the principles of the Declaration of Helsinki.[3] This dilemma is heightened when considering multistage procedures and comorbidity corrections (eg, realignment osteotomies, meniscus allograft transplant, etc.) performed for a number of the current cartilage repair and restoration techniques. RCTs that include sham controls for these techniques are uncommon. Nevertheless, with truly informed consent, sham procedures can be performed with safety and can be suitably motivated when minimally invasive, low risk, and may offer research findings that significantly benefit the society.

Similarly, research-specific second-look arthroscopy and/or biopsy procedures provide data that allow for potential blinding of evaluators and critical comparisons of efficacy among treatment strategies. However, the same risk-to-benefit dilemma must be considered for inclusion of these assessments as well. Still, they can be ethically and effectively implemented for cartilage repair and restoration studies to provide pivotal data, as demonstrated by Brittberg et al,[37] Gobbi et al,[38] Jung et al,[39] and others. These assessment procedures should be considered when designing clinical studies for cartilage repair and restoration. However, modern quantitative imaging techniques such as MRI-based T2 mapping, T1rho, and volumetric analyses of cartilage repair tissue may obviate the need for these invasive assessments in some situations.[40,41]

Handling and Management of Products Under Investigation

Investigators should follow the manufacturer's recommended guidelines for storage and use of all products for cartilage repair and restoration interventions. In addition, chain of custody for all materials used must be chronologically documented with physical or electronic evidence to include collection techniques, preservation, packaging, transportation, storage, and inventory records with temperature metrics when applicable. Special considerations and documentation may be required for treatment strategies that include investigational drugs or biologics, living cells, or gene therapy interventions. Quality control assessments should also be built into the experimental design for clinical studies, whenever possible. In some studies, matched samples designated for these purposes may be included. Alternatively, unused materials that would otherwise be discarded such as portions of OCAs that are not transplanted can be analyzed. Similarly, it is possible to assay the preservation or storage media used for the product. Quality control evaluations may include cell viability, phenotype, and metabolism assays; extracellular matrix composition analyses; and/or material property assessments.[42-44]

OUTCOME MEASURES UNIQUE TO ARTICULAR CARTILAGE REPAIR

FDA Regulatory Considerations (Device, Biologic, or HCT/P Designation)

Given the challenges inherent to clinical trials for cartilage repair and restoration, primary and secondary outcome measures must be carefully selected and implemented. A 2009 USFDA Cellular, Tissue, and Gene Therapies Advisory Committee determined that both pain and function measurements should be included in the primary end point assessments for cartilage repair therapies.

Longitudinal Outcomes (Type of and Timing for Imaging or Biomarkers)

The generally accepted minimum clinical follow-up period accepted by most peer-reviewed journals is 2 years; however, long-term follow-up is generally preferred to assess treatment longevity in terms of functional survival and cost-effectiveness. For example, the outcomes associated with microfracture have been documented to significantly deteriorate after 2 to 3 years.[18] Thus, any comparative assessment to microfracture would be strengthened by planning for at least midterm (5 years) follow-up. Unfortunately, the most common time point evaluated in the literature for posttreatment analysis among cartilage procedures is 12 months, with most clinical trials having a single time point for patient evaluation.[23]

The end point pain and function outcome measures can be augmented by longitudinal assessments including diagnostic imaging; patient-reported and evaluator-assessed measures of pain, function, activity level, return to work, return to sport, physical health, mental health, and quality of life; and adverse events, complications, and morbidity. In addition, a priori definitions of success and failure should be determined and included in the protocol's documentation materials. For each of these assessments, standard-of-care methods and time points must be differentiated from research-specific methods and time points for ethical research practices and legal billing procedures (**Table 4**). Furthermore, patient privacy, security, and burden must be comprehensively addressed as foundational components of the experimental design.

Patient-reported outcome measures (PROMs) and diagnostic imaging are the mainstays of longitudinal outcome measures for cartilage repair and restoration studies. Among these, the KOOS and visual analog scale pain score have been the most commonly used in level I and II investigations.[23] Recently developed and validated PROMs including Patient-Reported Outcomes Measurement Information System computerized adaptive testing tools and abbreviated questionnaires implemented through secure electronic delivery methods have addressed patient privacy and burden considerations while also providing cost-effective quantitative and clinically relevant data.[41]

TABLE 4 Outcome Measures With Typical Standard of Care Versus Research and Adverse Events and Complications

Standard of Care	Research Only	Related Complications/ Revision Surgeries
Functional assessments	Second-look arthroscopy	Revise any cartilage procedure
Patient-reported outcome measures	Biopsy	Bone graft
Diagnostic imaging	Advanced diagnostic imaging	Conversion to unicompartmental knee arthroplasty
Return to work	Arthrocentesis + synovial fluid analysis	Conversion to total knee arthroplasty
Return to sport	Body fluid biomarkers	Arthrodesis
Patient satisfaction		Amputation
		Hardware removal/ exchange
		Irrigation and débridement
		Wound repair
		Manipulation under anesthesia
		Lysis of adhesions
		Synovectomy
		Chondroplasty
		Partial meniscectomy
		Meniscus repair

Standard-of-care diagnostic imaging can provide information that may help in determining success, failure, and functional survival, as well as for delineating adverse events, complications, and morbidity associated with cartilage repair and restoration procedures. However, these modalities often do not strongly correlate with pain, function, and clinical success or failure outcomes, such that they are not recommended to be used as a primary outcome measure or stand-alone determinant.[45] One example of a postoperative imaging investigation evaluated magnetic resonance images of patellar chondral defects managed with a particulated juvenile articular allograft cartilage (DeNovo Natural Tissue; Zimmer Biomet) transplantation.[46] As noted by the study authors, the main limitation of the investigation was the lack of clinical data to support their findings of progressive graft maturation over time. Another study performed by Jungmann et al[14] in 2018 evaluated 16 patients following surgical cartilage repair matched to 16 nonsurgical control patients and MRI was performed to assess articular degeneration. Surgical patients were found to have significantly less progression of degenerative MRI changes at 6 years of follow-up.

Such investigations provide excellent proof-of-concept evidence and support the utilization of various cartilage restoration techniques. However, both clinical and imaging outcomes represent a different domain of assessment and there should not be the expectation of concordance. Rather, each should be evaluated separately for the information each provides. More advanced quantitative and functional imaging techniques have the potential to provide compositional, metabolic, and physiologic data regarding articular cartilage and whole-joint health and should be used to augment clinical findings.[47,48] Similarly, molecular or protein biomarkers in serum, urine, and/or synovial fluid may provide mechanistic, diagnostic, and treatment monitoring data that allow for valid comparisons among treatment strategies, obviating the need for second-look arthroscopy and/or biopsies.[49] However, neither advanced imaging nor body fluid biomarkers are currently validated or accepted by regulatory bodies as unambiguous determinants of mechanisms of action (MOAs), functional outcomes, success, failure, or survivorship.

Variable Needs for Biopsy of Healing Cartilage

As mentioned previously, invasive research-specific assessments are difficult to ethically and financially justify. However, there may be opportunities for assessments such as arthrocentesis, second-look arthroscopy, and/or biopsy of tissues when subsequent treatment strategies are considered standard of care such as planned implant removal or osteotomy or those performed to address complications (eg, arthrofibrosis) or failures (eg, arthroplasty).

Unambiguous Demonstration of Proposed MOA in Patients

As physicians are recommending treatment strategies in response to pain and function deficits conveyed to them by their patients, it is appropriate that subjective pain and function measures serve as foundational patient outcomes for RCTs. This fact intrinsically increases the value and importance of any placebo (or sham surgery) effect. Randomized comparison of surgical interventions is possible, where comparison of surgical with nonsurgical interventions raises obstacles to surgeon and patient blinding and the need for sham surgery controls to truly establish intervention efficacy. Any collection of patient outcome information that introduces risk, beyond what is clinically necessary, again abuts the principles of the Declaration of Helsinki.[36] With this caveat, the MOA for cartilage repair is difficult to determine from standard imaging, such that MOA studies require quantitative or physiologic imaging, second-look arthroscopy with biopsy, synovial fluid biomarker analyses, and/or extrapolation from preclinical studies with correlations among respective mechanistic and clinical outcome measures.

In vitro and in vivo model systems can recapitulate the synovial joint and provide insights to MOA by permitting greater investigator control of experimental variables not possible in vivo. For cartilage repair, incorporation of the physical environment associated with joint loading, for example, would be critical to defining a more physiologic milieu of the synovial joint.[50] Coculture of synovium components to reestablish the native cross talk among tissues also elevates the sophistication of in vitro models.[51,52]

Animal studies not only provide a necessary proof of concept required for translation to the human but also permit opportunities to glean MOA of treatment strategies. The introduction of humanized mice models that leverage modern biology and genetic mice tools may provide significant mechanistic insights, but may not be easily scalable to the human. As such, appropriate preclinical models with size and characteristics of human patient conditions provide opportunity for sham surgery and placebo controls with narrowing of subject inhomogeneity. These models[53,54] also allow for clinically relevant comprehensive functional, imaging, and postmortem analyses, which remain an indispensable tool in the development and evaluation of cartilage repair strategies.

Specific PROMs as Historical Standard

PROMs include the KOOS and KOOS subscales (pain, symptoms, activities of daily living, sport/recreation, and quality of life), the Hospital for Special Surgery score, the International Knee Documentation Committee outcome measure, the Tegner activity scale, the Lysholm Knee Scale score, the International Cartilage Repair Society score, and the Cincinnati Knee Rating System (**Table 1**). As outlined previously, other validated PROMs that address security, privacy, and patient burden components of outcomes assessment, including PROMIS, and patient satisfaction metrics should also be considered during clinical study design.

Complications Specific to Cartilage Repair

Studies define treatment failure in a number of different ways, including fair or poor functional assessments based on the previously reviewed PROMs, graft failure based on advanced imaging, arthroscopic evidence of graft failure on a second-look arthroscopy, or revision surgery of any form including lysis of adhesions and manipulation, chondroplasty, revision cartilage transplantation, or arthroplasty. Some investigations have also included adverse events such as intra-articular effusions, hematoma, popliteus cyst, persistent patellofemoral pain, complex regional pain syndrome, and infections as treatment failures.[10]

GENERAL CONSIDERATIONS AND RECOMMENDATIONS SPECIFIC TO CARTILAGE REPAIR

After performing a sample size calculation to avoid type II error where a false difference (that might occur by chance) is detected,[6] rigorous RCTs aim for (1) true randomization of patients where individuals have an equal chance of being assigned to a particular group, (2) blinding of as many related individuals and assessments as practical (eg, patients, outcome assessors, data analysts, or surgeons), and (3) limiting patient dropout and clearly documenting losses to follow-up and study withdrawals. Following the established protocol design is critical because suboptimal adherence to the treatment regimen may compromise the study by reducing the estimates of treatment efficacy in the primary intent-to-treat analysis. Intention-to-treat analysis assumes that subjects are analyzed according to the treatment arm to which they had been randomized, regardless of the actual treatment they received. Although designed crossover studies can be useful for patient satisfaction, MOA, and cause-effect purposes, unplanned crossover from one treatment arm to another may lead to trial results that are inconclusive or even erroneous.[55]

Patient recruitment is critical to meeting the statistical power requirements of an RCT. With respect to the statistical design of an RCT, investigators must first establish the primary outcome of interest a priori and the minimal clinically important difference associated with that outcome measure. Once established, a sample size calculation can be performed before commencing a trial to ensure that investigators can correlate statistical significance to clinical significance and appropriately power their study.[4] This calculation involves the nuances of melding mathematical significance with clinically meaningful significance. In separate reviews that encompassed 105 studies, Bhandari et al[6] and Freedman et al[36] found that less than 9% and 6%, respectively, of RCTs performed calculations to ensure a properly powered study in advance of their trial. Freedman et al reported that almost half of all studies with insignificant findings were too underpowered to detect even a large treatment effect.[56]

Barriers to patient recruitment in cartilage repair studies may be imposed in part by the need to satisfy regulatory entities. In cases of premarket approval, the FDA advocates for narrower inclusion criteria, reducing eligible participants to a small fraction of patients seen by physicians, to derive a more homogeneous population. Patients in RCTs may not be representative of patients seen in orthopaedic practice.[57] This leads to longer enrollment periods and costs that often make products unmarketable on completion of the RCT.[25] Such was the case for Zimmer Biomet's DeNovo ET product whose phase III clinical trials ended after 6 years because of poor recruitment (only 14/225 patients) (ClinicalTrials.gov). The high costs associated with RCTs often reflect the need to fund both experimental and control arms of the study. Moreover, once inclusion/exclusion criteria are met, patients must be convinced to participate in the RCT without coercion. The latter may be further confounded by the sheer number of experimental treatment strategies available (and for which the surgeon may be actively recruiting subjects for multiple trials) and unwillingness of patients to be randomized because they may be seeking the best treatment and/or do not want to leave clinical care decisions up to chance. The net effect is a further reduction in the number of eligible participants from an already small subset of patients.

A related challenge is patient dropout, where a follow-up of less than 85% is looked at with concern by FDA reviewers who will consider those patients lost to follow-up as potential treatment failures.[58] Planning for a network to maintain contact with study participants is critical. Early discussions among the investigators regarding the minimum follow-up duration that would be practical and clinically meaningful would help to minimize study dropouts. Reducing the patient burden for outcome measures, such as offering study participants more convenient opportunities to complete in-person or telephone/videoconferencing visits, providing reimbursement for travel-related expenses, and modest incentive stipends for participation, may additionally serve to curtail patient attrition.[55] Establishing relevant registries for prospective longitudinal assessments provide a powerful tool for addressing these challenges.

Rates of unplanned crossover may be reduced by ensuring timely delivery of the assigned treatment (eg, surgery performed within a short period of time after enrollment in the trial and randomization), continuous monitoring of the unplanned crossover rate, and proactive discussion by the study investigators on strategies to mitigate unplanned crossover from one arm to another.[55]

SUMMARY

The take-home recommendations are as follows: (1) Determine classification, predicate, and pathway. (2) Meet with the FDA if needed. (3) Ensure valid preclinical data are in place. (4) Design the highest level of evidence ethical study possible by including surgeons, evaluators, imagers, and biostatisticians, and use Consolidated Standards of Reporting Trials (CONSORT) for RCTs.[59] If valid RCTs not feasible, consider well-designed prospective cohort studies. Register the study with clinicaltrials.gov. Also consider establishing a prospective registry. (5) Ensure patient privacy and security, and address patient burden for outcome measures. (6) Determine endpoint(s)—minimum 2 years. (7) Define standard of care versus research-specific assessments and time points a priori. (8) Determine success and failure definitions a priori. (9) Publish negative outcomes as well as positive outcomes.

REFERENCES

1. Cavendish PA, Everhart JS, Peters NJ, Sommerfeldt MF, Flanigan DC: Osteochondral allograft transplantation for knee cartilage and osteochondral defects: A review of indications, technique, rehabilitation, and outcomes. *JBJS Rev* 2019;7(6):e7.
2. Parisien RL, Constant M, Saltzman BM, et al: The fragility of statistical significance in cartilage restoration of the knee: A systematic review of randomized controlled trials. *Cartilage* 2021;13(1 suppl):147S-155S.
3. Fuson RL, Sherman M, Van Vleet J, Wendt T: The conduct of orthopaedic clinical trials. *J Bone Joint Surg Am* 1997;79(7):1089-1098.
4. Mundi R, Chaudhry H, Mundi S, Godin K, Bhandari M: Design and execution of clinical trials in orthopaedic surgery. *Bone Joint Res* 2014;3(5):161-168.
5. Wright JG, Swiontkowski MF, Heckman JD: Introducing levels of evidence to the journal. *J Bone Joint Surg Am* 2003;85(1):1-3.
6. Bhandari M, Richards RR, Sprague S, Schemitsch EH: The quality of reporting of randomized trials in the journal of bone and joint surgery from 1988 through 2000. *J Bone Joint Surg Am* 2002;84(3):388-396.
7. Campbell AJ, Bagley A, Van Heest A, James MA: Challenges of randomized controlled surgical trials. *Orthop Clin North Am* 2010;41(2):145-155.
8. Bentley G, Biant LC, Carrington RW, et al: A prospective, randomised comparison of autologous chondrocyte implantation versus mosaicplasty for osteochondral defects in the knee. *J Bone Joint Surg Br* 2003;85(2):223-230.
9. Bentley G, Biant LC, Vijayan S, Macmull S, Skinner JA, Carrington RW: Minimum ten-year results of a prospective randomised study of autologous chondrocyte implantation versus mosaicplasty for symptomatic articular cartilage lesions of the knee. *J Bone Joint Surg Br* 2012;94(4):504-509.
10. Clave A, Potel JF, Servien E, Neyret P, Dubrana F, Stindel E: Third-generation autologous chondrocyte implantation versus mosaicplasty for knee cartilage injury: 2-year randomized trial. *J Orthop Res* 2016;34(4):658-665.
11. Dozin B, Malpeli M, Cancedda R, et al: Comparative evaluation of autologous chondrocyte implantation and mosaicplasty: A multicentered randomized clinical trial. *Clin J Sport Med* 2005;15(4):220-226.
12. Horas U, Pelinkovic D, Herr G, Aigner T, Schnettler R: Autologous chondrocyte implantation and osteochondral cylinder transplantation in cartilage repair of the knee joint. A prospective, comparative trial. *J Bone Joint Surg Am* 2003;85(2):185-192.
13. Lim HC, Bae JH, Song SH, Park YE, Kim SJ: Current treatments of isolated articular cartilage lesions of the knee achieve similar outcomes. *Clin Orthop Relat Res* 2012;470(8):2261-2267.
14. Jungmann PM, Gersing AS, Baumann F, et al: Cartilage repair surgery prevents progression of knee degeneration. *Knee Surg Sports Traumatol Arthrosc* 2019;27(9):3001-3013.
15. Gudas R, Kalesinskas RJ, Kimtys V, et al: A prospective randomized clinical study of mosaic osteochondral autologous transplantation versus microfracture for the treatment of osteochondral defects in the knee joint in young athletes. *Arthroscopy* 2005;21(9):1066-1075.
16. Gudas R, Stankevicius E, Monastyreckiene E, Pranys D, Kalesinskas RJ: Osteochondral autologous transplantation versus microfracture for the treatment of articular cartilage defects in the knee joint in athletes. *Knee Surg Sports Traumatol Arthrosc* 2006;14(9):834-842.
17. Gudas R, Simonaityte R, Cekanauskas E, Tamosiūnas R: A prospective, randomized clinical study of osteochondral autologous transplantation versus microfracture for the treatment of osteochondritis dissecans in the knee joint in children. *J Pediatr Orthop* 2009;29(7):741-748.
18. Gudas R, Gudaite A, Pocius A, et al: Ten-year follow-up of a prospective, randomized clinical study of mosaic osteochondral autologous transplantation versus microfracture for the treatment of osteochondral defects in the knee joint of athletes. *Am J Sports Med* 2012;40(11):2499-2508.
19. Gudas R, Gudaitė A, Mickevičius T, et al: Comparison of osteochondral autologous transplantation, microfracture, or debridement techniques in articular cartilage lesions associated with anterior cruciate ligament injury: A prospective study with a 3-year follow-up. *Arthroscopy* 2013;29(1):89-97.
20. Solheim E, Hegna J, Strand T, Harlem T, Inderhaug E: Randomized study of long-term (15-17 Years) outcome after microfracture versus mosaicplasty in knee articular cartilage defects. *Am J Sports Med* 2018;46(4):826-831.
21. Ulstein S, Årøen A, Røtterud JH, Løken S, Engebretsen L, Heir S: Microfracture technique versus osteochondral autologous transplantation mosaicplasty in patients with articular chondral lesions of the knee: A prospective randomized trial with long-term follow-up. *Knee Surg Sports Traumatol Arthrosc* 2014;22(6):1207-1215.
22. Gou GH, Tseng FJ, Wang SH, et al: Autologous chondrocyte implantation versus microfracture in the knee: A meta-analysis and systematic review. *Arthroscopy* 2020;36(1):289-303.
23. Saltzman BM, Redondo ML, Beer A, et al: Wide variation in methodology in level I and II studies on cartilage repair: A systematic review of available clinical trials comparing patient demographics, treatment means, and outcomes reporting. *Cartilage* 2021;12(1):7-23.
24. Available at: https://www.fda.gov/regulatory-information/search-fda-guidance-documents/regulatory-considerations-human-cells-tissues-and-cellular-and-tissue-based-products-minimal.
25. Lyman S, Nakamura N, Cole BJ, Erggelet C, Gomoll AH, Farr J II: Cartilage-repair innovation at a standstill: Methodologic and regulatory pathways to breaking free. *J Bone Joint Surg Am* 2016;98(15):e63.
26. Martín AR, Patel JM, Zlotnick HM, Carey JL, Mauck RL: Emerging therapies for cartilage regeneration in currently excluded 'red knee' populations. *NPJ Regen Med* 2019;4(1):12.
27. Steadman JR, Rodkey WG, Rodrigo JJ: Microfracture: Surgical technique and rehabilitation to treat chondral defects. *Clin Orthop Relat Res* 2001;391:S362-S369.

28. Steadman JR, Rodkey WG, Briggs KK: Microfracture: Its history and experience of the developing surgeon. *Cartilage* 2010;1(2):78-86.

29. Detterline AJ, Goldberg S, Bach BRJ, Cole BJ: Treatment options for articular cartilage defects of the knee. *Orthop Nurs* 2005;24(5):1-6.

30. Knutsen G, Drogset JO, Engebretsen L, et al: A randomized trial comparing autologous chondrocyte implantation with microfracture. Findings at five years. *J Bone Joint Surg Am* 2007;89(10):2105-2112.

31. Gross AE, Shasha N, Aubin P: Long-term followup of the use of fresh osteochondral allografts for posttraumatic knee defects. *Clin Orthop Relat Res* 2005;435:79-87.

32. Jolles BM, Martin E: In brief: Statistics in brief – Study designs in orthopaedic clinical research. *Clin Orthop Relat Res* 2011;469(3):909-913.

33. LeBrun DG, Tran T, Wypij D, Kocher MS: How often do orthopaedic matched case-control studies use matched methods? A review of methodological quality. *Clin Orthop Relat Res* 2019;477(3):655-662.

34. Merkely G, Ogura T, Ackermann J, Barbieri Mestriner A, Gomoll AH: Clinical outcomes after revision of autologous chondrocyte implantation to osteochondral allograft transplantation for large chondral defects: A comparative matched-group analysis. *Cartilage* 2021;12(2):155-161.

35. Karanicolas PJ, Bhandari M, Taromi B, et al: Blinding of outcomes in trials of orthopaedic trauma: An opportunity to enhance the validity of clinical trials. *J Bone Joint Surg Am* 2008;90(5):1026-1033.

36. Mehta S, Myers TG, Lonner JH, Huffman GR, Sennett BJ: The ethics of sham surgery in clinical orthopaedic research. *J Bone Joint Surg Am* 2007;89(7):1650-1653.

37. Brittberg M, Lindahl A, Nilsson A, Ohlsson C, Isaksson O, Peterson L: Treatment of deep cartilage defects in the knee with autologous chondrocyte transplantation. *N Engl J Med* 1994;331:879-895.

38. Gobbi A, Karnatzikos G, Scotti C, Mahajan V, Mazzucco L, Grigolo B: One-step cartilage repair with bone marrow aspirate concentrated cells and collagen matrix in full-thickness knee cartilage lesions: Results at 2-year follow-up. *Cartilage* 2011;2(3):286-299.

39. Jung WH, Takeuchi R, Chun CW, et al: Second-look arthroscopic assessment of cartilage regeneration after medial opening-wedge high tibial osteotomy. *Arthroscopy* 2014;30(1):72-79.

40. Liu YW, Tran MD, Skalski MR, et al: MR imaging of cartilage repair surgery of the knee. *Clin Imaging* 2019;58:129-139.

41. Tetta C, Busacca M, Moio A, et al: Knee osteochondral autologous transplantation: Long-term MR findings and clinical correlations. *Eur J Radiol* 2010;76(1):117-123.

42. Farr J, Gracitelli GC, Shah N, Chang EY, Gomoll AH: High failure rate of a decellularized osteochondral allograft for the treatment of cartilage lesions. *Am J Sports Med* 2016;44(8):2015-2022.

43. Stoker AM, Stannard JP, Kuroki K, Bozynski CC, Pfeiffer FM, Cook JL: Validation of the Missouri osteochondral allograft preservation system for the maintenance of osteochondral allograft quality during prolonged storage. *Am J Sports Med* 2018;46(1):58-65.

44. Stoker AM, Caldwell KM, Stannard JP, Cook JL: Metabolic responses of osteochondral allografts to re-warming. *J Orthop Res* 2019;37(7):1530-1536.

45. de Windt TS, Welsch GH, Brittberg M, et al: Is magnetic resonance imaging reliable in predicting clinical outcome after articular cartilage repair of the knee? A systematic review and meta-analysis. *Am J Sports Med* 2013;41(7):1695-1702.

46. Grawe B, Burge A, Nguyen J, et al: Cartilage regeneration in full-thickness patellar chondral defects treated with particulated juvenile articular allograft cartilage: An MRI analysis. *Cartilage* 2017;8(4):374-383.

47. Kogan F, Fan AP, Monu U, Iagaru A, Hargreaves BA, Gold GE: Quantitative imaging of bone-cartilage interactions in ACL-injured patients with PET-MRI. *Osteoarthritis Cartilage* 2018;26(6):790-796.

48. Lansdown DA, Wang K, Cotter E, Davey A, Cole BJ: Relationship between quantitative MRI biomarkers and patient-reported outcome measures after cartilage repair surgery: A systematic review. *Orthop J Sports Med* 2018;6(4):2325967118765448.

49. Gabusi E, Paolella F, Manferdini C, et al: Cartilage and bone serum biomarkers as novel tools for monitoring knee osteochondritis dissecans treated with osteochondral scaffold. *Biomed Res Int* 2018;2018:9275102.

50. O'Connell GD, Lima EG, Bian L, et al: Toward engineering a biological joint replacement. *J Knee Surg* 2012;25(3):187-196.

51. Cook JL, Kuorki K, Stoker AM, Streppa H, Fox DB: Review of in vitro models and development and initial validation of a novel co-culture model for the study of osteoarthritis. *Curr Rheum Rev* 2007;3(3):172-182.

52. Stefani RM, Halder SS, Estell EG, et al: A functional tissue engineered synovium model to study osteoarthritis progression and treatment. *Tissue Eng Part A* 2019;25(7-8):538-553.

53. Cook JL, Hung CT, Kuroki K, et al: Animal models of cartilage repair. *Bone Joint Res* 2014;3(4):89-94.

54. Garner BC, Stoker AM, Kuroki K, Evans R, Cook CR, Cook JL: Using animal models in osteoarthritis biomarker research. *J Knee Surg* 2011;24(4):251-264.

55. Losina E, Wright J, Katz JN: Clinical trials in orthopaedics research. Part III. Overcoming operational challenges in the design and conduct of randomized clinical trials in orthopaedic surgery. *J Bone Joint Surg Am* 2012;94(6):e35.

56. Freedman KB, Back S, Bernstein J: Sample size and statistical power of randomised, controlled trials in orthopaedics. *J Bone Joint Surg Br* 2001;83(3):397-402.

57. Engen CN, Engebretsen L, Årøen A: Knee cartilage defect patients enrolled in randomized controlled trials are not representative of patients in orthopedic practice. *Cartilage* 2010;1(4):312-319.

58. McGowan KB, Stiegman G: Regulatory challenges for cartilage repair technologies. *Cartilage* 2013;4(1):4-11.

59. Rennie D: CONSORT revised—improving the reporting of randomized trials. *J Am Med Assoc* 2001;285(15):2006-2007.

CHAPTER

31 Summary and Perspectives

Robert H. Brophy, MD, FAAOS • Regis J. O'Keefe, MD, PhD, FAAOS

Unlike other musculoskeletal tissues that heal with scar formation, bone has high regenerative potential and repair occurs with formation of de novo bone tissue. However, in up to 10% of cases, fracture healing is impaired, and this, along with conditions of cavitary and segmental bone loss associated with severe trauma, tumors, infection, and other conditions, makes bone repair a particularly important target for orthobiologic and tissue engineering approaches. Autologous bone graft from the iliac crest has been the gold standard as an orthobiologic for bone regeneration. Autologous bone has osteoinductive properties, with cells and growth factors, as well as osteoconductive properties, with a tissue structure and matrix organization that promotes adherence, migration, and differentiation of progenitor cells. Autologous bone is effective in promoting healing in nonunion and is an effective treatment for cavitary bone defect–related tumors or trauma. In contrast, processed allograft bone has limited osteoinductive potential but retains much of the osteoconductive potential of autologous bone graft. Although not effective in the treatment of nonunion, allograft bone graft is effective for the treatment of cavitary bone defects, although the rate of incorporation of the graft is substantially delayed compared with that of autograft bone. Bone graft substitutes or extenders, which include demineralized bone matrix and calcium phosphate ceramics, have been used as an alternative to avoid the morbidity of autologous bone harvest and the potential risks associated with allograft bone. Demineralized bone matrix contains osteogenic and osteoinductive factors but does not provide structural support. In contrast, calcium phosphate ceramics provide structural support, are osteoconductive, but are only weakly osteoinductive. Cell-based therapies are another alternative that can be used alone, or more commonly in combination with other therapies, but their use is not supported by randomized controlled clinical trials. These therapies include formulations of platelet-rich plasma (PRP), bone marrow cell aspirates and concentrates, and adipose-derived progenitor cells from lipoaspirates. In addition, several companies have developed cancellous allogenic bone graft products containing allogeneic pluripotent stem cells, but efficacy has not yet been evaluated by appropriately powered randomized controlled clinical trials. Growth factor therapies harness the cells and biologic processes at the injury site and stimulate cellular proliferation, differentiation, bone formation, and healing. Bone morphogenetic protein 2 has been extensively studied and is FDA approved for the management of tibial nonunion and is delivered locally in a collagen sponge. Parathyroid hormone has been used off-label; although anecdotal, and small series evidence supports its efficacy to promote healing, randomized controlled trials have not been completed. Segmental bone loss is a particular challenge. Several surgical approaches/therapies that are based on stimulation and harnessing the reparative potential of cells in the local environment are commonly used, including bone transport procedures and the Masquelet technique. Tissue-engineered bone replacements for segmental defects that have adequate strength, durability, degradation characteristics, and osseous integration and replacement with bone with retention of mechanical strength remain a major objective of ongoing tissue engineering approaches.

Treatment of the injured meniscus may benefit from a variety of orthobiologics, primarily focused on either enhancing healing of meniscus tears or optimizing meniscal replacement. Exogenous fibrin clots, PRP, growth factors, stem cells, scaffolds, and other tissue engineering approaches have been considered to improve meniscal healing. Although various reports suggest potential benefit from augmenting meniscal repairs with PRP or fibrin clots, high-level blinded, placebo controlled clinical trials are lacking. Thus, these treatment strategies, while widely used, are not yet supported by definitive experimental evidence. Meniscal replacement requires the use of synthetic or natural biomaterials to replace part or all of an injured or deficient meniscus. Although transplantation of an entire meniscus has been performed with reasonable results for some time, synthetic options for partial meniscal replacement are coming into use, with the collagen meniscus implant (CMI; Ivy Sports Medicine GmbH) available in the United States and Europe and the polyurethane polymeric implant (Actifit 329; Orteq Ltd) available in Europe. Evidence for clinical efficacy is

Dr. Brophy or an immediate family member serves as a board member, owner, officer, or committee member of the American Academy of Orthopaedic Surgeons, the American Orthopaedic Association, and the American Orthopaedic Society for Sports Medicine. Dr. O'Keefe or an immediate family member serves as a board member, owner, officer, or committee member of the American Orthopaedic Association.

emerging. Hydrogels are another option under investigation for this application. Tissue engineering options combining scaffolds, cells, and growth factors, potentially in combination with technologies such as three-dimensional (3D) printing, could evolve and allow for more accurate patient-specific constructs and more complex designs to address meniscal injury and deficiency in the future. Regeneration and/or engineering of the meniscus is dependent on either the delivery of exogenous reparative cells or stimulation of host/resident tissue progenitor cells with the goal of differentiation into meniscal cells and tissues. Recently, preclinical studies have demonstrated a robust population of progenitor cells within meniscal tissues that have the potential to support a healing and regenerative response. Defining the appropriate signals, cells and scaffolds are the focus of ongoing tissue engineering approaches for meniscal regeneration.

An increasing number of orthobiologic options are available for restoring articular cartilage. The unique role and structure of articular cartilage makes it particularly difficult to reconstitute, and the ultimate goal of an off-the-shelf treatment option to replace or restore articular cartilage remains theoretical. However, orthobiologic options that may provide a reasonable functional substitute for articular cartilage are close to if not already under development. These can generally be thought of as scaffolds, cell-based options, signaling molecules, or some combination thereof. Scaffolds should provide form, fixation, and function while driving tissue formation. Important considerations for scaffolds include their biomechanics, biocompatibility, porosity, degradability, and ease of handling for surgery. Although a variety of natural, synthetic, and biosynthetic composite scaffolds have been considered for managing articular cartilage, the ideal approach remains elusive. A variety of cell-based approaches, autologous and allogeneic, have been tried since the introduction of autologous chondrocyte implantation, which itself has evolved to matrix-assisted chondrocyte implantation. In addition, biochemical and biomechanical signaling is important for successful cartilage repair, and modulation of this messaging is an area of great interest, although still in early stages of development. Technologies such as 3D printing could combine scaffolds, cells, and signals into an optimal package for restoring articular cartilage in the future.

Osteoarthritis of the knee and ankle is a common and debilitating problem, with few true solutions short of total joint arthroplasty, which is a well-established option for the knee and emerging option in the ankle. Thus, there is tremendous interest in the potential of injectable orthobiologics for the symptomatic and potentially disease-modifying treatment of these conditions. These are generally placed in four categories: noncellular therapies, gene therapies, point-of-care autologous cell therapies, and expanded cell therapies. Noncellular therapies such as interleukin 1 beta receptor antagonist, tumor necrosis factor inhibitors, and growth factors are intended to counteract the inflammatory and catabolic processes of osteoarthritis; currently, these are experimental approaches without wide applicability. Gene therapies have great potential, but also have special considerations in cost and safety. A key aspect of gene therapy involves the selection of an appropriate target gene that produces a protein that can maintain cartilage homeostasis. Candidate genes include the anabolic factors, such as transforming growth factor beta. TissueGene-C is an injectable treatment for osteoarthritis of the knee with allogeneic chondrocytes expressing recombinant transforming growth factor beta that has recently completed a promising phase III clinical trial as part of the process toward FDA approval. Point-of-care autologous cell therapies such as PRP, bone marrow aspirate concentrate, and adipose-derived cells are readily available and generally considered safe, with growing evidence, especially for PRP, of symptomatic clinical efficacy. Expanded cell therapies represent a more targeted approach with a more homogenous cell population but currently have additional concerns regarding safety and cost. Currently, they can only be used for approved clinical trials in the United States. More research is needed to establish and compare the efficacy of these approaches, particularly in regard to any disease-modifying potential, for the treatment of knee and ankle osteoarthritis.

Ligament injuries in the lower extremity, especially the knee, are common injuries that could benefit from orthobiologic solutions. Potential approaches to applying orthobiologics to ligament injuries include bioactive factor solutions, cellular solutions, biomaterial scaffolds, and tissue-engineered grafts. Bioactive factor solutions such as PRP, autologous conditioned serum (ACS), and amniotic and chorionic membrane tissue have been proposed as part of the treatment algorithm for lower extremity ligament injuries. The primary challenge with these approaches is that they are a relatively blunt, broad-based treatment, with little to no understanding of the precise mechanism of action. Moreover, there is no evidence of definitive benefit from PRP in the management of lower extremity ligament injuries, let alone ACS or membrane tissues. Cellular solutions such as bone marrow aspirate concentrate and adipose-derived cells have been proposed, but they lack any evidence to date for their efficacy in this application. A variety of biologic and synthetic scaffolds have been proposed and explored as treatment options for lower extremity ligament injuries. Although nondegradable synthetic scaffolds have a poor track record, degradable scaffolds are gaining attention recently for their potential utility in this application. Tissue-engineered grafts are the next step in the evolution, combining a biomaterial scaffold with cells and/or other biologic factors to facilitate ligament regeneration.

Another recent approach with a growing body of evidence is the bridge-enhanced anterior cruciate ligament repair technique that uses a collagen scaffold derived from bovine extracellular matrix proteins to augment the healing of a torn anterior cruciate ligament. Recently approved by the FDA, the optimal indications for this approach are evolving. Applying orthobiologics to the treatment of lower extremity ligament injuries is still in its early stages, facing economic and ethical, as well as scientific and clinical, challenges for the foreseeable future.

Studying the efficacy of orthobiologics presents several challenges in terms of outcome measurement and study design. Imaging may be important in addition to standard patient-reported outcomes, particularly for conditions in and around the joint. Longer follow-up and tissue biopsy are necessary for treating lower extremity conditions such as articular cartilage and meniscus pathology, despite the obvious ethical and economic challenges. Additional challenges for study design included defining the standard of care for comparison as well as randomization and blinding. Standard of care can vary widely and is often not well defined for clinical conditions treated with orthobiologics. Randomization and blinding, for the patient, provider, evaluator, or some combination thereof, can be challenging and cost prohibitive. Nevertheless, the evidence of a randomized controlled trial is the gold standard that is necessary to definitively establish the promise and pitfall of these novel treatment strategies.

Orthobiologic applications in the lower extremity face a number of common challenges. One of these challenges is the relative lack of specificity in terms of both the intended target and observed clinical effect of interventions, particularly for approaches such as PRP and bone marrow aspirate concentrate . The conceptual uncertainty is often compounded by the clinical inconsistency such as the intersubject and intrasubject variability with these techniques. Proving the efficacy of orthobiologics is not easy, even for clinical symptomatic benefit, let alone disease-modifying potential. Finally, cost is an important consideration, both in terms of development and clinical application.

Despite these challenges, great interest remains in developing these approaches for the lower extremities. The primary reason is an unmet need for reliable interventions to address important clinical problems such as nonunion, meniscal deficiency, articular cartilage defects, osteoarthritis, and ligament injuries. Advances in basic science lead to greater understanding of the problem at hand as well as novel methods to modulate the underlying biology, which make orthobiologics more feasible and potentially less expensive. Finally, the dynamics of consumer-driven healthcare demand it, encouraging scientists and clinical providers to develop solutions that appeal to the patient.

In summary, many advances in basic science and technology, such as the understanding of cell biology and the efficacy of 3D printing, are poised to move orthobiologic solutions for the lower extremity closer to clinical reality. Some of these solutions are already crossing the threshold of clinical application. Although these approaches have great potential to improve patient care, considerable effort will be needed to carefully define the indications for and assess the efficacy of these options as they come into use, with special attention to their cost-effectiveness.

SECTION

5

Solutions for Spinal Pathology

Section Editors

Wellington K. Hsu, MD, FAAOS

Kevin C. Baker, PhD

CHAPTER

32

Intervertebral Disk Repair and Regeneration—Bioactive Factors and Cell-Based Therapy

Koichi Masuda, MD • Koji Akeda, MD, PhD • Kenji Kato, MD, PhD • Jordy Schol, MSc • Daisuke Sakai, MD, PhD

INTRODUCTION

A biologic balance between the catabolic and anabolic activity of intervertebral disk (IVD) cells is the main mechanism enabling the homeostasis of the IVD. A disruption in this homeostasis, through cellular changes or cell loss, may result in disk degeneration and consequently in discogenic pain. To solve these clinical problems, new treatment strategies are specifically designed to reconstitute IVD homeostasis through transplantation of cells, growth factors, or anti-inflammatory molecules. However, the unique IVD environment, including limited nutrient availability, hypoxia, and acidic conditions, as well as reduced cellular activity and numbers, remains a potential hurdle for their therapeutic efficacy. It is important to describe the history, rationale, and current status of bioactive therapeutics aimed at alleviating discogenic pain through mitigating IVD degeneration. An overview of preclinical studies and publicly available clinical trial reports that explored the potential of growth factors, anti-inflammatory molecules, platelet-rich plasma (PRP), and (stem) cell injections toward IVD repair and regeneration is provided. The state of development, limitations, and remaining uncertainties toward the widespread application of these potential regenerative therapeutics will also be discussed.

BACKGROUND

Epidemiology of Low Back Pain

Low back pain (LBP) is one of the medical conditions that most frequently results in disability and an absence from work in many countries[1-11] (**Table 1**). The age-standardized prevalence of LBP is 7.5% of the global population, with 577 million people affected.[12] Women have a higher prevalence than men.[12] Although the prevalence of LBP decreased slightly from 1990 to 2017, the prevalence of people with LBP and years lived with disability increased, probably because of increasing population and increased age of the population.[12] The Global Burden of Diseases, Injuries, and Risk Factors Study 2017 indicated that LBP is the leading cause of years lived with disabilities.[13] The peak of years lived with disability for LBP occurred at 45 to 49 years of age and then decreased with age. Disability-adjusted life years due to LBP increased from 1990 to 2019 and were highest from 25 to 49 years of age.[14]

In the United States, 29% of the population age 18 years and older self-reported having had LBP during the past 3 months every year.[15] Importantly, LBP was reported by 33.3% of people in the active working group (45 to 64 years old) and 32.8% of people age 65 years or older.[15] Similar to the global trend, women reported at higher rates (30.5%) than men (26.4%).[15]

Health Care Visit and Economic Effects

Of 154 conditions, low back and neck pain were at the top of health care spending, with an estimated $134.5 billion in spending (57.2%; paid by private insurance, 33.7% by public insurance, and 9.2% by out-of-pocket payments); this spending is increasing 2.9% annually. Spending was concentrated on working-age adults between the ages of 20 and 64 years and increased at the highest rate compared with other disease conditions.[16] LBP health care visits are highest in those age 45 to 64 years; the 18 to 64 years age group represents 72% of the total visits. When visit numbers are adjusted by the US census population, the health care visits for LBP per 100 persons are highest for those 65 years or older[15] (**Figure 1**).

The economic effect of LBP is not limited to the direct cost of healthcare because most patients are of working age, as described previously. Work limitation or absence associated with LBP is the major cause of this economic effect. Katz[17] reported that 149 million workdays were lost because of LBP every year. In 2012, the total number of workdays lost was 234 million (11.2 days per person)

Dr. Masuda or an immediate family member serves as a paid consultant to or is an employee of Mochida Pharmaceutical Inc. and has received research or institutional support from Anges Inc. Dr. Sakai or an immediate family member serves as a paid consultant to or is an employee of DePuy, a Johnson & Johnson Company, Globus Medical, Nuvasive, Stryker, and TUNZ Pharma and has received research or institutional support from Nippon Zoki Pharmaceuticals Inc. and TUNZ Pharma. None of the following authors or any immediate family member has received anything of value from or has stock or stock options held in a commercial company or institution related directly or indirectly to the subject of this chapter: Dr. Akeda, Dr. Kato, and Jordy Schol.

TABLE 1 Clinical Characteristics of Patients With Discogenic Low Back Pain

Assessment	Clinical Presentation	Reference
Risk factor	Advanced age, but patients typically younger than those with facetogenic or sacroiliac joint pain; repetitive or acute trauma	Knezevic et al 2021
Clinical presentation	Low back pain and leg pain; pain worse with sitting	Knezevic et al 2021
Physical findings	Midline tenderness; reduced range of motion, especially bending forward; no focal neurologic findings	Knezevic et al 2021
Diagnostic imaging	Plain radiographs to evaluate disk height; MRI to detect annular tears, fissures, or high-intensity zones and Modic changes; imaging not routinely needed	Knezevic et al 2021 Vernon-Roberts et al 2007 Peng et al 2006 Teraguchi et al 2020 Mera and Hashizume 2021
Provocative diskography	An invasive diagnostic spine procedure involves the administration of contrast material into the degenerated IVDs to determine if the disk is the origin of LBP Can detect painful IVDs with relatively high specificity and sensitivity, recommended by NASS guideline although some controversies are noted in guidelines	Kreiner et al 2020 Chou et al 2009 Fujii et al 2019

IVD = intervertebral disk, NASS = North American Spine Society

for LBP alone and 104 million days (17.4 days per person) for LBP with radiating leg pain in the past 3 months. The total number of bed days was 142 million (7.7 days per patient) for LBP only and 62 million (10.8 days per person) for LBP with radiating leg pain.[18] The total cost with direct costs (one-third) and loss due to lost wages and reduced productivity (two-thirds) was estimated to be US$100 to $200 billion.[17]

Structure and Disk Environment

The IVD has three different structures with individual biochemical and biomechanical properties. The innermost

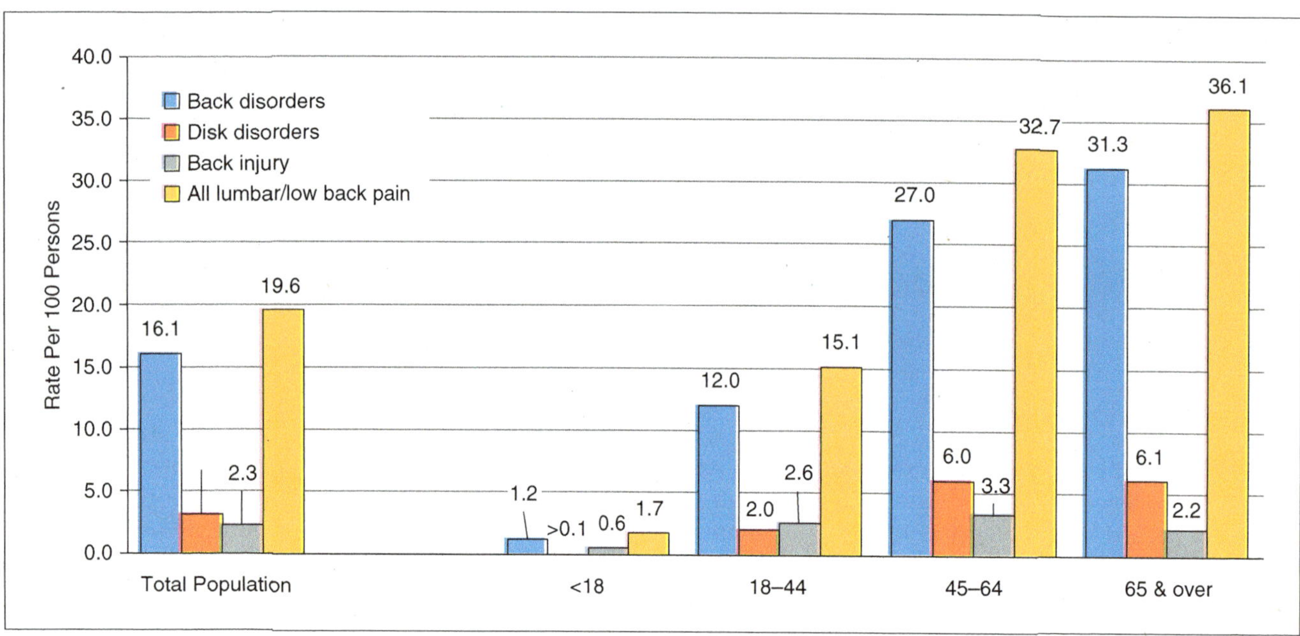

FIGURE 1 Graph showing the rate of health care visits for low back pain per 100 population, United States 2013. (Date from HCUP National Implant Sample (NIS) 2013 Agency for Healthcare Research and Quality Rockville, MD www.hcup-us.ahrg.gov/nisoverview.jsp; HCUP Nationwide Emergency Department Sample (NEDS). Healthcare Cost and Utilization Project (HCUP), 2013. Agency for Healthcare Research and Quality, Rockville MD www.hcup-us.ahrg.gov/nisoverview.jsp; National Ambulatory Medical Care Survey (NAMCS), 2013. www.cdc.gov/nchsahcd/ahcd_questionnaires.htm January 14, 2016; National Hospital Ambulatory Medical Care Survey_Outpatient Department (NHAMCS_OP), 2011. www.cdc.gov/nchsahcd/ahcd_questionnaires.htm May 23, 2016; Singh K, Andersson G, Watkins-Castillo SI: *Low Back Pain*. Available at: https://www.boneandjointburden.org/fourth-edition/iiaa0/low-back-pain. Accessed June 24, 2021.)

structure, the nucleus pulposus, is a gelatinous structure rich in proteoglycan and type II collagen. The nucleus pulposus is high in water content and resists loading by compression. Its composition and physical character change with age, going from a gellike tissue to a more fibrocartilaginous tissue with decreased proteoglycan and water content. The circumferential structure surrounding the nucleus pulposus is the anulus fibrosus that consists of concentric lamellae rich in collagen fibers and some large proteoglycans and small proteoglycans. The inner anulus fibrosus contains fibrochondrocytic cells, which produce type II collagen and proteoglycan. The outer anulus fibrosus is composed of dense collagen layers with fibroblastic cells. Cartilaginous end plates are located next to the bony end plates of two adjacent vertebral bodies and a thin layer of hyaline cartilage. These structures provide the properties of flexibility and resiliency necessary for normal spine movement and weight transfer.

LBP and Disk Degeneration

The relationship between disk degeneration and LBP is complex.[19,20] Some reviews have evaluated the correlation between LBP and degenerated IVDs.[21,22] Various pathologic conditions or injuries, including disk degeneration, facet joint arthritis, spondylolisthesis, muscle and neural pathologies, can cause LBP. Among these, it is well accepted that disk degeneration is, at least in part, one of the causes of discogenic LBP.[23,24] A recent meta-analysis showed that MRI evidence of disk bulge, degeneration, extrusion, protrusion, Modic 1 changes, and spondylolysis is more prevalent in adults age 50 years or younger with back pain, compared with asymptomatic individuals.[25]

However, disk degeneration is clinically observed in patients without LBP; thus, the relationship between IVD degeneration and pain is not fully understood. The recent review by Brinjikji et al,[26] indicated that the prevalence of disk degeneration in asymptomatic individuals increased from 37% of 20-year-old individuals to 96% of 80-year-old individuals. Other changes such as, disk protrusion, and annular fissures showed a similar trend, but to a lesser extent; these suggest the changes in MRI captured the normal aging process. Although the precise pathogenesis of discogenic pain is not totally revealed, studies have suggested that an increase in inflammatory mediators (including nerve growth factor) and nerve ingrowth into the disk are the causes of discogenic pain. As described previously, LBP is a clinical symptom and disk degeneration is not a symptom but rather the status of the disk structure mainly identified by using advanced imaging modalities. Therefore, the selection of patients for disk repair must be performed based on clinical symptoms with the aid of imaging. If multiple levels of disk degeneration are found, the precise source of pain should be carefully identified using provocative diskography. Considering the negative effect of diskography, the newly introduced magnetic resonance spectroscopy has shown high sensitivity and specificity with provocative diskography results[27] and will be suitable for patient selection when it becomes clinically available.

Mechanism of Disk Degeneration

Although the precise pathogenesis is not well known, degenerative disk disease (DDD) has been considered to be a pathologic condition that generally worsens with age.[28] DDD can possibly be initiated by mechanical factors or mediated by biologic causes with risk factors such as obesity and smoking. Adams and Roughley[29] proposed the definition "disc degeneration is an aberrant cell-mediated response to progressive structural failure." However, there are other causes of disk degeneration, such as inadequate nutrient and metabolite transfer, as well as heritability, as shown in an identical twin study.[30] Genes associated with disk degeneration and in combination with environmental factors may result in failure of disk maintenance.[31]

Clinically, disk degeneration is recognized as disk height loss or signal intensity loss on MRI. The loss of signal intensity in T2-weighted MRI reflects a loss of water content, mainly due to decreased content of the aggrecan molecule in the nucleus pulposus. The homeostasis of extracellular matrix (ECM) metabolism in the IVD is regulated by a biologic balance between the anabolic and catabolic activities of disk cells.[32] Although the ECM is constantly degraded with aging or other conditions, nucleus pulposus and anulus fibrosus cells actively synthesize and replenish tissues with the newly synthesized matrix to maintain structural integrity. On the anabolic side, polypeptide growth factors, such as insulinlike growth factor 1, transforming growth factor beta (TGF-β), and bone morphogenetic proteins (BMPs) are major players. On the catabolic side, the inflammatory cellular response plays a key role in disk degeneration.[33,34] Catabolic regulators include cytokines, such as interleukin 1 (IL-1) and tumor necrosis factor alpha (TNF-α), which induce the production of matrix-degrading enzymes.

Stage of Disk Degeneration

Thompson et al[35] introduced a 5-point grading system based on morphologic changes associated with the severity of disk degeneration using midsagittal sections of cadaver disks (**Figure 2**). Boos et al[36] developed a histologic grading system for human IVD. Clinically, the stage of disk degeneration has been assessed by using radiography and MRI. Pfirrmann et al[37] created the most widely used clinical morphologic grading system based on signal intensity in T2-weighted magnetic resonance images; this reflects the water content in tissues. This grading system uses four categories, including the appearance of the disk structure, the distinction between the nucleus and the anulus, the

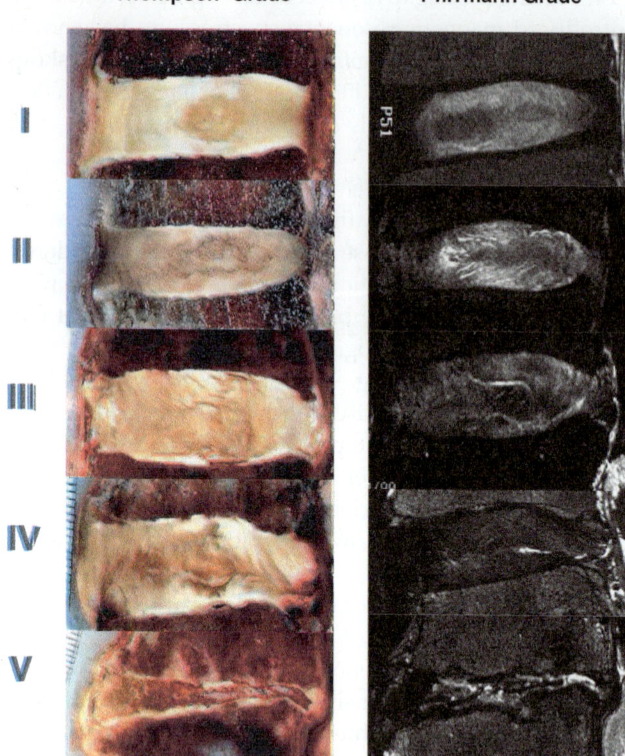

FIGURE 2 Images show Thompson (cadaver photographs) and Pfirrmann (MRIs) grading system. (Images courtesy of Dr. Howard An, Rush University.)

signal intensity, and the IVD height. Griffith et al[38] found difficulty in applying the Pfirrmann grade because most disks in patients in the older population were graded as Pfirrmann grade 3 or 4. They introduced the modified Pfirrmann grading system comprising eight grades for disk degeneration; the modified Pfirrmann grading system was commonly used in recent clinical trials for DDD.

DISK REPAIR AND DISK DEGENERATION—NONSURGICAL APPROACHES

The target patient population for disk repair is adults with chronic discogenic pain that persists for at least 3 months with nonsurgical therapies (**Table 2**). The primary aim of IVD repair is to resolve patient symptoms, mainly pain and resulting limitation of daily activity and work. Optimally, the structural repair of the disk or the prevention of further progress of disk degeneration may be achieved by treatment. Therefore, most clinical trials that evaluate the efficacy of molecules use pain as the primary outcome end point as visual analog scale (VAS) scores aim to develop symptom-modifying drugs. The structure-modifying effects, such as changes in disk height and MRI grades, are generally set as secondary outcome measures.

In 2017, the American College of Physician Guidelines established protocols for the noninvasive treatment of chronic LBP.[39] The guidelines recommend nonpharmacologic treatment with exercise, multidisciplinary rehabilitation, acupuncture, mindfulness-based stress reduction (moderate-quality evidence), tai chi, yoga, motor control exercise, progressive relaxation, electromyography biofeedback, low-level laser therapy, operant therapy, cognitive behavioral therapy, or spinal manipulation (low-quality evidence). In patients for whom nonpharmacologic treatment was unsuccessful, pharmacologic treatment with NSAIDs is recommended as a first-line therapy or tramadol or duloxetine as second-line therapy. Opioids are only an option in patients in whom the recommended treatments failed, with the patient understanding the risks and benefits. The UK National Institute for Health and Care Excellence guidelines recommend similar nonpharmacologic therapies. Radiofrequency denervation for the selected population with LBP is also recommended, although a randomized clinical trial did not show evidence.[40] The North American Spine Society recently established treatment recommendations for patients with LBP[41]: the summary of these recommendations has been published.[4] Most of these recommendations are similar to the American College of Physicians and the National Institute for Health and Care Excellence guidelines. For medical treatment, oral or intravenous steroids and antidepressants are not recommended. Topical capsicum is recommended on a short-term basis. For physical agents, ultrasound, laser acupuncture, and traction are not recommended. The addition of acupuncture to usual care and the combination of laser therapy with exercise, yoga, aerobic exercise are recommended. For invasive treatment, intradiscal electrothermal annuloplasty is suggested to improve pain and function with fair evidence. Another common procedure, intradiscal corticosteroid injection, is not recommended according to the recent guidelines from the American Pain Society.[5]

REGENERATION AND REPAIR

In regenerative medicine, repair is defined as the restoration of tissue architecture and function after an injury. Regeneration refers to a type of healing in which new growth completely restores portions of damaged tissues to their normal state.[42] In the field of disk degeneration, some researchers consider the damage irreversible, whereas a vast number of animal studies and some clinical trials showed signs of repair, such as MRI signal changes or disk height recovery. When complete regeneration is the goal, the demand for nutrition increases in a harsh environment in a degenerated disk; this may lead to cell death of the remaining functional cells. Therefore, treatment should be developed to reduce pain, preferably with some tissue repair or delaying of disease progression, without a large increase in nutrient demand and metabolic waste accumulation.

TABLE 2 Criteria of Clinical Trials for Degenerative Disk Disease

Inclusion Criteria
Has chronic low back pain for at least 6 months, where back pain is greater than leg pain
Has had inadequate response to nonsurgical medical care over a period of at least 3 months
Diagnosis of painful degenerative disk disease at one lumbar level from L1 to S1 confirmed by subject history and radiographic studies (eg, MRI, radiographs)
Radiographic studies must demonstrate the following:
A Pfirrmann score of 3 or 4 on MRI in just a single disk between L1 and S1
With or without contained disk herniations of <3 mm protrusion with no radiographic evidence of neurologic compression
Disk height loss of the symptomatic disk is less than 50% of the adjacent disks
No spondylolisthesis or instability on flexion/extension views of more than 1 to 2 mm
No evidence of sacroiliac, or extraspinal, pathology that could account for lumbar back pain
No more fluid in, or widening of, the facet joints around the symptomatic disk than is seen on the other facet joints of normal levels
Oswestry Disability Index score of at least 30 and not more than 90 on the 100-point questionnaire
Exclusion Criteria
Has a comorbid medical condition of the spine or the upper extremities that may affect neurologic and/or pain assessments as specified in the protocol, including spinal fusion, spondylolysis, and spondylolisthesis
Has evidence of hip pathology based on clinical history, physical examination, and/or radiographic imaging that could be the source of lumbar back pain
Has a history of an endocrine or metabolic disorder that affects the spine (eg, Paget disease)
Has a compressive pathology due to stenosis or frankly herniated disk or sequestered disks
Has symptomatic involvement of more than one lumbar disk, in the opinion of the investigator
Has an intact disk bulge/protrusion or focal herniation at the symptomatic level >3 mm, the presence of disk extrusion or sequestration, or a complete annular tear
Has lumbar intervertebral foraminal stenosis at the symptomatic level resulting in clinically significant spinal nerve root compression, in the opinion of the investigator
Has received any epidural steroid injection(s) within 3 months before study treatment

Data obtained from https://clinicaltrials.gov/ct2/show/NCT01124006.

Phase Ib, multicenter, double-blind, single ascending dose study designed to evaluate the safety of AMG0103 in adult male and female subjects with chronic discogenic lumbar back pain.

UNIQUE ENVIRONMENT—LIMITATIONS AND ADVANTAGES

IVD tissue has a unique avascular structure in which the nucleus pulposus is surrounded by the anulus fibrosus and cartilaginous end plate as an enclosed structure. Nutrition and cell numbers in the tissue are limited.[43] Therefore, this complex structure of the IVD has pros and cons for a repair strategy by an injection of bioactive factors or cells.

Cell Distribution and Function

In the human nucleus pulposus, there is a large population of notochordal cells in the young; these cells are replaced by, or differentiate into, a population of chondrocytelike cells with maturity. Detailed information on cell phenotype has been reviewed by Pattappa et al.[44] The density of mature nucleus pulposus cells is low and reported to be approximately 4 to 10 × 10^6 cells/cm^3.[45,46] The anulus fibrosus contains a relatively homogeneous population of cells that synthesize an ECM richer in collagen and poorer in proteoglycans than do cells from the nucleus pulposus; the resulting anulus fibrosus is a dense lamellar tissue containing fibrillar layers rich in collagen types I and II.[47] The cellularity of anulus fibrosus cells is 9 × 10^6 cells/cm^3, which is still less than that of articular cartilage (15 × 10^6 cells/cm^3).

The homeostasis of the IVD ECM is maintained by disk cells that maintain a balance between anabolic activity and catabolic activity. Although the ECM is constantly degraded by aging or other stimuli, disk cells (both nucleus pulposus and anulus fibrosus cells) actively synthesize ECM and replenish tissues with the newly synthesized matrix. However, both nucleus pulposus and anulus fibrosus cells produce many inflammatory cytokines that regulate ECM synthesis and matrix degradative enzymes in an autocrine or paracrine fashion.[48] Nucleus pulposus and anulus fibrosus cells can produce various neurotrophins, such as nerve growth factors[49] and brain-derived neurotrophic factors;[50] IL-1 and TNF-α stimulate the production of these factors, suggesting disk cells may contribute to pain regulation.

Nutrients and Diffusion

Nutrition reaching the IVD is another important factor in the pathogenesis of disk disease (see reviews and publications[31,43,51,52]). The IVD is the largest avascular tissue in the body, receiving its main supply of nutrients by diffusion from the vertebral bodies through cartilaginous end plates. In humans, cells in the center of the nucleus pulposus are 7 to 8 mm away from the closest surrounding capillaries; they encounter hypoxic and acidic conditions because of the balance between transport and metabolic demand for oxygen and glucose and the production of lactic acid even in the normal disk. An IVD that lacks proper nutrition might undergo significant degeneration by the loss of the steady-state metabolism of its cells.[53] Indeed, an increase in the cellular demand for oxygen or nutrients, or a decrease in supply, has been shown to result in cell death. Therefore, when injected molecules increase the metabolic activity of cells in a compromised nutrient transport condition, an increased demand in nutrients possibly results in further depletion of nutrients and oxygen and the increased accumulation of metabolic waste.

The MRI study by Rajasekaran et al[54] has confirmed, with the use of contrast media, the disturbance of nutrient transport, even in early disk degeneration, and a subsequent increase in transport at the advanced stage of disk degeneration, probably resulting from structural damage to the end plate. Recent MRI technology using ultrashort echo-time sequence has made it possible to evaluate the condition of end plates in detail[55-57] and the perfusion rate of solutes from the vertebral body into the IVD.[54,58] These techniques may help to identify proper target patients and to follow the consequence of therapeutic approaches.

Nerve Distribution

The posterior aspect of the IVD and the posterior longitudinal ligament are innervated through the sinuvertebral nerves. The posterolateral aspect of the IVD is innervated by branches of the ventral primary rami and the gray rami communicantes near the junction with the ventral rami. Branches to the anterior longitudinal ligament arise from the rami communicantes near the origin of the sympathetic trunk. In the healthy IVD, nerve fibers are located in the most outer layer of the anulus fibrosus at a 3-mm depth from the disk surface.[59] There are no nerve fibers in the nucleus pulposus or the inner one-third of the anulus fibrosus. In patients with severe back pain with disk height loss, proliferation of blood vessels and accompanying nerve fibers are observed in the end plate. Detailed information on nerve fibers in discs has been summarized by Ito et al.[22]

Enclosed Space and Distribution of Injected Molecules and Cells

The half-life of DNA oligonucleotide after a single intradiscal injection has recently been reported in normal rabbits. The injected oligonucleotide first disappears quickly (distribution phase, half-life: 11.9 hours), and the remaining DNA is then gradually eliminated (elimination phase, half-life: 618 hours). Because DNA may not specifically bind to the matrix and because of the unique structure of the avascular IVD enclosed by the end plate with a slow diffusion rate, these results indicate that the anulus fibrosus may have some reservoir function. Alternatively, once translocated inside the cells, the DNA oligonucleotide may remain in the cytosol or nucleus for an extended period without degradation. A similar prolonged half-life was reported for osteogenic protein 1 (OP-1), which binds to collagen.[60] This structural advantage benefits a cell-based therapy for disk degeneration. The migration of injected cells from the injection site in the IVD will be less compared with an intra-articular injection.

The elimination time of injected materials or cells depends on the binding capacity to the ECM, pathologic conditions of the disk (ie, the degree of disk degeneration and/or vascularization and annular fissures) and end plates, the injection procedure itself (ie, needle size, injection location, and volume), and characteristics of the vehicle or carrier.

SCIENTIFIC EVIDENCE FOR THE CLINICAL UTILITY OF BIOACTIVE FACTOR SOLUTIONS

In Vitro Evidence

To apply bioactive factors/drugs for the clinical treatment of human DDD, preclinical investigations to reveal the mechanism of their action are essential. The first step is to identify the efficacy of molecules using in vitro experiments with animal or human IVD cells.

In 1991, using an alginate culture system, Thompson et al[61] showed the effect of growth factors on IVD cells, opening the door for disk repair by growth factors. Subsequently, the effects of a variety of growth factors have been published, and some have been shown to have an inhibitory effect on matrix degradation or cytokine expression.[19] Detailed information from previous studies is presented in **Table 3** and can also be found in previous reviews.[19] The long list of growth factors includes TGF-β, insulinlike growth factor 1, OP-1/BMP-7, BMP-2, growth and differentiation factor (GDF-5), and more. Among these, BMP-7 and GDF-5 have been clinically tested for patients with DDD. Other molecules, including YH14618, AMG0103, and NTG-101, have recently been clinically investigated.

Table 4 includes information on recent research related to growth factors and other molecules.[62-82] The studies on growth factors focus on the combined effects of TGF-β with mesenchymal stromal cells (MSCs) and nucleus pulposus cells[62] and the effect of the BMP-2/7 heterodimer.[63] The in vitro effects of YH14618 and NTG-101 are described in the in vivo section to better understand their mode of action.

Inflammatory cytokines, such as the interleukins, are involved in IVD degeneration.[83,84] Counteracting these

TABLE 3 The In Vitro Effects of Bioactive Factors

Agent	System	Effect
TGF-β	Mature canine IVD	PG synthesis increased up to 5 times; higher in NP than AF
TGF-β	Human anulus cells, 3D culture	Cell proliferation and PG synthesis increased; reduced apoptosis with serum depletion
IGF-I	Mature canine IVD	PG synthesis marginally increased in NP
IGF-I	Young and old bovine NP cells	Cell proliferation and matrix synthesis stimulated; more IGF-I receptors
OP-1	Young rabbit NP and AF cells; alginate beads	Increased PG and collagen production and content
OP-1	Human NP and AF cells, alginate beads	Maintained cell density, increased PG synthesis and accumulation
OP-1	Rabbit IVD cells; alginate beads: IL-1α preexposure	IL-1 decreased PG and collagen; reversed and exceeded with OP-1
OP-1	Rabbit IVD cells; alginate bead: C-ABC preexposure	OP-1 upregulated PG synthesis. Greater effect on C-ABC preexposure than control
BMP-2	Rat IVD cells monolayer	Increased cell number, GAG, expression for collagen, aggrecan at higher doses
BMP-2	Human IVD cells	Increased PG synthesis, expression of aggrecan, collagen I and II; no bone formation
rhBMP-2 and 12	Human IVD cells in monolayer	PG, collagen synthesis increased in NP cells; minimal effect on AF cells
GDF-5	Bovine IVD cells; alginate bead	Increased DNA and PG content; at higher dose, PG and collagen synthesis increased
PRP	Porcine IVD cells; alginate bead	Mild increase in cell proliferation; marked increase in PG and collagen synthesis and PG accumulation
TGF-β1 and PRP	Human NP cells	NP cell proliferation and aggregation; increase in mRNA of SOX-9, collagen type II, aggrecan
Ad-TIMP-1, Ad-BMP-2	IVD cells from human degenerated IVD	2,000 pg/mL production of TIMP w/100 MOI at day 4. PG synthesis increased with both Ad-TIMP-1 and Ad-BMP-2
Dexa-methasone	Human disk herniation tissue explants	Decreased MMP-1 and MMP-3 levels
IL-1ra	Human disk herniation tissue explants	Decreased MMP-3 levels
IL-1ra	Human normal and degenerated disk tissues in situ with IL-1 treatment	IL-1ra reduced cytokine levels (MMP-3, 7, 13) and matrix degradation in all tissue types
IL-1ra/ELP	Human IVD cells (grade 2 to 3); alginate beads: IL-1ra pretreatment then IL-1β insult	Reduced ADAMTS-4, MMP-3 transcription
p38 MAPK inhibitor (SB 202190)	Rabbit NP cells pretreated with IL-1	Decreased message for collagen, aggrecan, IGF-I. Increased message for iNOS, COX-2, MMP-3, IL-6
TNF inhibitor mAb	Human IVD herniation tissue explants	Decreased MMP-3 levels
PDGF, bFGF, IGF-I	Human NP and AF cells	Increased DNA synthesis via ERK and Akt pathways
TGFb3 + Dex, notochordal conditioned media	Degenerated human NP cells	Stimulated NP cell proliferation and decreased ADAMTS-5, MMP-1 expression

(Continued)

TABLE 3 The In Vitro Effects of Bioactive Factors (Continued)

Agent	System	Effect
Lactoferricin	Bovine NP cells	Increased PG accumulation and expression of SOX-9, aggrecan, TIMP-family genes. Decreased expression of MMPs and ADAMTSs in dose-dependent manner
IGF-1, BMP-7	Bovine NP cells	Synergistically increased anabolic gene expression, PG synthesis and PG accumulation

3D = three-dimensional, ADAMTS = a disintegrin and metalloproteinase with thrombospondin motifs, Ad-BMP-2 = adenoviral vector delivering cDNA of BMP-2, Ad-TIMP-1 = adenoviral vector delivering cDNA of tissue inhibitor of matrix metalloproteinases 1, AF = anulus fibrosus, Akt = protein kinases, bFGF = basic fibroblast growth factor, BMP-2 = bone morphogenetic protein 2, C-ABC = chondroitinase-ABC, COX-2 = cyclooxygenase-2, ELP = elastinlike polypeptide, ERK = extracellular signal–regulated kinases, GAG = glycosaminoglycan, GDF-5 = growth and differentiation factor 5, IGF-I = insulinlike growth factor I, IL-1 = interleukin-1, IL-1ra = IL-1 receptor antagonist, iNOS = inducible nitric oxide synthase, IVD = intervertebral disk, mAb = monoclonal antibody, MAPK = mitogen-activated protein kinase, MMP = matrix metalloproteinase, MOI = multiplicity of infection, NP = nucleus pulposus, OP-1 = osteogenic protein 1, PDGF = platelet-derived growth factor, PG = proteoglycan, PRP = platelet-rich plasma, rh = recombinant human, SOX-9 = sex-determining region Y-box nine gene, TGF-β = transforming growth factor beta, TNF = tumor necrosis factor.

Modified by permisssion from Springer: Bae WC,Masuda K: Enhancing disc repair by growth factors and other modalities, in Shapiro IM, Risbud MV, eds: *The Intervertebral Disc*. Springer, 2014, pp 401-416.

cytokines is another approach to promote a positive disk ECM homeostasis. The inhibitory effects of IL-1 receptor antagonists (IL-1ra), including matrix metalloproteinase 3 and ADAMTS-4, have been shown.[85] Another target of inhibition is the TNF-α pathway, which is important in the process of IVD degeneration.[64,86,87]

IL-17 has been a recent focus and is reported to be elevated in nucleus pulposus cells during IVD disease. IL-17 upregulated vascular endothelial growth factor expression through the Janus kinase-signal transducer and activator of transcription pathway,[65] matrix metalloproteinase 12 expression through the NF-kB pathway,[66] and IL-6 and COX-2 expression through MAP kinase pathways.[67]

In Vivo Evidence for the Clinical Utility of Bioactive Factors

The clinical application of therapeutic agents to manage DDD is mostly considered as an intradiscal injection[32,68,72,82,88-107] (**Table 5**). Originally, a mouse caudal disk degeneration model was used to examine the effect of injection of growth factors.[88] Thereafter, many investigations have used rat or rabbit animal models to examine the efficacy of treatment materials.[60,85] This section focuses on recent developments that are at the preclinical or clinical trial stage.

Growth Factors and Related Molecules

Bone Morphogenetic Protein 7/Osteogenic Protein 1

In the rabbit annular puncture disk degeneration model, a single injection of BMP-7/OP-1 into the nucleus pulposus of a disk 4 weeks after puncture resulted in significant restoration of disk height and increased the signal intensity of the nucleus pulposus in T2-weighted MRI.[108] Biomechanical analyses of the IVDs showed that the injection of OP-1 restored dynamic viscoelastic biomechanical properties of the puncture-degenerated IVDs.[89] Clinical studies were conducted, as described in the following section.

Growth and Differentiation Factor 5

GDF-5 is also a member of the BMP family and was tested for efficacy of management of IVD disease. In the rabbit annular-puncture model, an injection of recombinant human GDF-5 resulted in the restoration of disk height and improvements in MRI and histologic grading scores with statistical significance for 12 weeks.[90] These studies led to multiple clinical studies. A recent report showed that nucleus pulposus–like cells-seeded with GDF-5-loaded polymeric gelatin microspheres could partially regenerate degenerated IVDs using a rat model.[91]

Growth and Differentiation Factor 6

GDF-6 was also tested in various species. In the rabbit annular-puncture model, an injection of GDF-6 into degenerated disks restored disk height and improved MRI findings.[92] The capacity of pain generation by the inflammatory environment of degenerated disks was tested by the two-step disk xenograft radiculopathy model. In another investigation of GDF-6 relating to the pain response, GDF-6 injection has been shown to be effective in improving mechanical and thermal-stimulated pain behavior in rats and to inhibit the expression of inflammatory factors TNF-α and IL-1β and the pain factor, calcitonin gene-related peptide in the dorsal root ganglion.[93]

NTG-101

Based on a study of notochordal cell-conditioned media,[109] NTG-101 (a combination of recombinant human connective tissue growth factor and recombinant human TGF-β1) was developed and was shown to increase cell

TABLE 4 The In Vitro Effects of Bioactive Factors

Agent	System	Effect	Reference/ Manufacturer
OP-1/BMP-7	NP	Attenuated of senescence through ROS/NF-κB pathway	Xie et al 2018
TGF-β	MSC	TGF-β3-loaded PLGA nanoparticles could induce MSCs to NP-like cells while promoting ECM-related biosynthesis	Gan et al 2016
TGF-β	Co-culture	Stimulated COL1, ACAN, and SOX9 by the interaction between MSC and NP cells	Lehmann et al 2018
GDF-6	Human ASCs	Induced NP differentiation of ASC	Hodgkinson et al 2019
BMP-2/7 heterodimer	Bovine NP cells and IVD organ culture	Upregulated the aggrecan and type II collagen gene expression, and glycosaminoglycan synthesis	Li et al 2017
TGF-β3 and IGF-1	MSC	Enhanced viability, extracellular matrix biosynthesis, and differentiation toward NP cells by the activation of the MAPK/ERK signaling pathway	Tao et al 2015
Chemokine CCL25	Micro mass pellet	Facilitated collagen type II production and induced proteoglycan and collagen type I production	Stich et al 2018
CCAAT/enhancer-binding protein β	Rat and human IVDs	TNF-α was regulated by CCAAT/enhancer-binding protein β through the MAPK pathways	Hiyama et al 2016
TAK-242	NP cell	Blocked LPS-induced hydraulic permeability and cell radius (TAK-242:Toll-like receptor-4 inhibitor)	Jacobsen et al 2021
IL-17	Rat NP cells	Upregulated VEGF expression in isolated rat NP cells through JAK/STAT pathway	Hu et al 2017
IL-17	Human NP cells	Induced upregulation of MMP-12 and extracellular matrix degradation through the NF-kB pathway	Yao et al 2016
IL-17A	Rat NP cells	Mitogen-activated protein kinase pathways were activated by stimulation and induced IL-6 and COX-2 expression	Suyama et al 2018
Gallic acid	Rat NP cells	Reduced the release of ADAMTS-4, and inhibited the TNF-α-induced apoptosis of nucleus pulposus cells through the NF-κB signaling pathways	Huang et al 2017
Resveratrol	NP cell	Inhibited IL-1β-mediated NP cell apoptosis through the PI3k/Akt pathway	Jiang et al 2021
Link N	Bovine disk culture model	Induced the increase of glycosaminoglycan and collagen content with MSC	Mwale et al 2014
Link N	Rabbit IVD cells	Binded to BMP type II receptor and upregulation of smad pathway	Wang et al 2013
siRNA of ADAMTS-5	Rabbit NP cells	Suppressed IL-1β-increased ADAMTS-5 mRNA level in NP cells and suppressed puncture-induced degradation in rabbit model	Seki et al 2009
NTG-101	Human IVD cells	Increased the variability and cell proliferation, and the expression of aggrecan, collagen 2A1, hyaluronan, and proteoglycan link protein 1 and inhibited MMP-13 and Cox-2 mRNA expression	Matta et al 2018 Notogen, Inc.
YH14618 (Peniel 2000, P2K)	Bovine IVD cells	Increased type II collagen and aggrecan by inhibition of TGF-β signaling such as downregulation of Smad1/5/8 resulted in the synthesis of ECM	Kwon et al 2013

(Continued)

TABLE 4 The In Vitro Effects of Bioactive Factors (Continued)

Agent	System	Effect	Reference/ Manufacturer
AMG0103 (NF-κB decoy oligonucleotide)	Alginate culture	Oligodeoxynucleotide containing NF-κB-binding sites, which entrap NF-κB subunits, in suppressing the PG degradation induced by IL-1 and counteract the effect IL-1 on PG accumulation	Akeda et al 2006 Anges Inc.
SM04690 (Lorecivivint)	NP and AF cell cultures	SM04690 (Wnt pathway inhibitor) inhibited senescence, decreased catabolism, and induced differentiation into chondrocyte-like cells by inhibition of Wnt pathway gene expression	Deshmukh et al 2020 Biosplice Therapeutics, Inc.

ADAMTS = a disintegrin and metalloproteinase with thrombospondin motifs, AF = anulus fibrosus, ASC = adipose stem cells, BMP = bone morphogenetic protein, IGF-1 = insulinlike growth factor 1, IL = interleukin, IVD = intervertebral disk, JAK/STAT = Janus kinase-signal transducer and activator of transcription, Link N = amino-terminal peptide of link protein (DHLSDNYTLDHDRAIH), MMP = matrix metalloproteinase, MSC = mesenchymal stromal cells, NP = nucleus pulposus, OP-1 = osteogenic protein 1, PG = proteoglycan, PLGA: poly(D,L-lactide-co-glycolide), TGF-β = transforming growth factor beta, TNF = tumor necrosis factor, VEGF = vascular endothelial growth factor

viability and proliferation of human IVD cells and induce anabolic and anticatabolic effects.[68] In vivo, NTG-101-injected IVDs maintained disk height with retention of viscoelastic properties compared with IVDs injected with phosphate-buffered saline.[68] These disks sustained the expression of healthy ECM proteins (aggrecan and collagen 2A1) and reduced the expression of inflammation-associated proteins and molecules compared with vehicle controls. These findings suggest the therapeutic potential of NTG-101 for clinical use.

YH14618

YH14618, also named Peniel 2000 (P2K), is a 7-amino-acid peptide derived from a conserved region of biglycan that binds to TGF-β1, a stimulator of IVD synthesis.[69] P2K binds to excessive TGF-β1 and partially inhibits antianabolic Smad 1/5/8, but maintains a minimal activation of Smad2. Thus, P2K induces ECM expression in IVDs.[69] In the annular-puncture model, a single injection of P2K increased disk height and improved MRI grade and histologic scores compared with control subjects.[69] This peptide has been used for clinical trials.

Other Molecules

Link N

Link N peptide is a naturally occurring 16-amino-acid peptide representing the N terminal region of link protein, a glycoprotein that stabilizes proteoglycan aggregates by binding to both hyaluronic acid and aggrecan. Link N stimulated matrix synthesis similar to that of growth factors.[110,111] The mechanism of action of Link N has been shown to be binding to BMP type II receptor and upregulation of the Smad pathway.[70] Link N inhibited IL-1 and matrix metalloproteinase 1 expression[112] and was also able to stimulate the repair of degenerated disks in organ culture.[113] In vivo, link N peptide restored disk height and the proteoglycan content and proteoglycan-to-collagen ratio of IVDs in a rabbit model.[94] Moreover, short link N also increased proteoglycan content and maintained collagen content using the rabbit annular-puncture model.[95]

AMG0103

Nuclear factor kappa B (NF-κB) is a transcription factor that regulates gene expression of inflammatory cytokines and has been shown to be involved in IVD degeneration.[64,114] AMG0103, an oligodeoxynucleotide containing NF-κB-binding sites, which entrap NF-κB subunits, is a NF-κB decoy oligodeoxynucleotide. AMG0103 has been shown to be effective in several inflammatory conditions in vivo.[115-117] In alginate culture, naked NF-κB decoy oligodeoxynucleotide was transfected successfully and the continuous transfection of decoy was effective in suppressing the proteoglycan degradation induced by IL-1 and counteracting the effect IL-1 on proteoglycan accumulation.[71,118] Injection of NF-κB decoy into degenerated IVDs using the rabbit annular-puncture model revealed that NF-κB decoy injection recovered, dose-dependently, the reduced disk height that was associated with reparative cell cloning, and morphologic changes as assessed through histology. NF-κB decoy was also found to reduce the pain response using the nude rat xenograft-radiculopathy model.[119]

SM04690

SM04690 (lorecivivint) is a small-molecule inhibitor of the Wnt pathway that has been tested in patients with

TABLE 5 The In Vivo Effects of Bioactive Factors

Agent	Species	Site	Model	Effect	Reference Author, year
IGF-I	Mice	Tail	Static compression 1wk, injected 3 wk later	Clustering of inner anulus cells after single injection	Walsh et al 2004[a]
GDF-5	Mice	Tail	Static compression 1wk, injected 3 wk later	Clustering of cells, increase in disk height (single injection)	Walsh et al 2004[a]
GDF-5	Rat	Tail	Needle puncture, injected 4 wk later	Restored disk height and increased GAG content	Yan 2014[a]
OP-1/BMP-7	Rabbit	Lumbar	None (normal)	Increased disk height and PG content in NP	An 2005[a]
OP-1/BMP-7	Rabbit	Lumbar	Needle puncture, injected 4 wk later	Increased disk height and PG content in NP and AF, improvement of MRI and histology grades	Masuda et al2006[a]
OP-1/BMP-7	Rabbit	Lumbar	Needle puncture, injected 4 wk later	Increased disk height and viscoelastic properties	Miyamoto et al, 2006[a]
GDF-5	Rabbit	Lumbar	Needle puncture, injected 4 wk later	Increased disk height, improvement of MRI and histology grades	Chujo et al 2006[a]
GDF-5	Rat	Tail	Needle puncture, injected 2 wk later	Recovered disk height and increased water content	Xia et al 2019
PRP	Rabbit	Lumbar	Nucleotomy, injected immediately	PRP + GHM group had less degeneration and increased PG	Nagae et al 2007[a]
PRP	Rabbit	Lumbar	Nucleotomy, injected immediately	PRP + GHM had greater disk height, water content, mRNA for PG core protein and type II collagen; fewer apoptotic cells in NP	Sawamura et al 2009[a]
PRP	Rabbit	Lumbar	Needle puncture, injected 4 wk later	Disk height increase, no significant MRI T2 signal	Obata et al 2012[a]
GDF-6	Sheep	Lumbar	Anular stab (3 × 6 mm), injected immediately	GDF-6 maintained disk height, MRI and histology scores, NP cell density; increased PG and collagen synthesis	Wei 2009[a]
GDF-6	Rabbit	Lumbar	Needle puncture, injected 4 wk later	Increased disk height, attenuated degenerated IVD-induced pain by the two-step disk xenograft radiculopathy model	Miyazaki et al 2018
GDF-6/ BMP13	Rat	Tail	Needle puncture, injected 1 or 2 wk later	Inhibited degeneration signal and the expression of inflammatory factors such as TNF-α and IL-1β and the pain factor calcitonin gene-related peptide	Cui et al 2021
Link N	Rabbit	Lumbar	Needle puncture, injected 2 wk later	Increased aggrecan gene expression and decreased proteinase gene expression	Mwale et al 2011[a]
Short link N	Rabbit	Lumbar	Needle puncture, injected 2 wk later	Increased proteoglycan content and maintained collagen content	Mwale et al 2018
NTG-101	Rat	Tail	Needle puncture, injected 4 wk later	Maintained disk height, viscoelastic properties, sustained expression of healthy ECM proteins and reduced expression of inflammation-associated proteins	Matta et al 2018
siRNA for ADAMTS-5	Rabbit	Lumbar	Needle puncture, injected 1 wk later	Improved degenerative parameters induced by puncture with histology score and MRI findings	Seki et al 2009[b]

(Continued)

TABLE 5 The In Vivo Effects of Bioactive Factors (Continued)

Agent	Species	Site	Model	Effect	Reference Author, year
siRNA for caspase 3	Rabbit	Lumbar	Needle puncture, injected 1 wk later	Suppressed degenerative changes fewer apoptotic nucleus pulposus cells	Sudo et al 2011
NF-κb decoy (AMG0103)	Rabbit	Lumbar	Needle puncture, injected 4 wk later	Recovered the reduced disk height with reparative cell cloning and morphologic changes, and attenuated degenerated IVD-induced pain by the two-step disk xenograft radiculopathy model	Kato et al 2021
SM04690	Rat	Tail	Needle puncture, injected 1 wk later	Increased cartilage matrix and reduced AF lamellar disorganization, fragmentation	Deshmuckh et al 2020
Lactic acid	Pig	Lumbar	None (normal)	Induced sclerozation and increased the flexural rigidity	Olmarker et al 2020
Indirect BMP Stimulation					
Lovastatin	Rat	Tail	Needle puncture injected immediately	Upregulated BMP-2, Type II collagen, and SOX9 expression. Higher GAG and cell number	Hu 2014[a]
Simvastatin	Rat	Tail	Needle puncture, injected 4 wk later	Increased aggrecan, BMP-2, Type II collagen gene expression and improved MRI and histology	Zhang 2009[a]
Simvastatin	Rat	Tail	Needle puncture, injected 6 wk later	Increased BMP-2, Aggrecan, Type II collagen gene expression, improved radiograph, MRI, and histology	Than 2014[a]

ADAMTS = a disintegrin and metalloproteinase with thrombospondin motifs, AF = anulus fibrosus, BMP = bone morphogenetic protein, ECM = extracellular matrix, GAG = glycosaminoglycan, GDF-5, GDF-6 = growth differentiation factor 5, 6, GHM = gelatin hydrogel microspheres, IGF-1 = insulinlike growth factor 1, IVD = intervertebral disk, Link N = amino-terminal peptide of link protein (DHLSDNYTLDHDRAIH), NF-κB = nuclear factor kappa-light-chain-enhancer of activated B cells, NP = nucleus pulposus, OP-1 = osteogenic protein 1, PBS = phosphate-buffered saline, PG = proteoglycan, PRP = platelet-rich plasma, SOX = SRY (sex-determining region Y)-Box Transcription Factor 9.

[a]Studies reviewed in Masuda K, Kato K: Treatment of degenerative disk disease/disk regeneration: Growth factors and platelet rich plasma, in Härtl R, Bonassar LJ, eds: *Biological Approaches* to *Spinal Disk Repair* and *Regeneration For Clinicians*. Thieme, 2017, pp 101-109.

[b]Studies reviewed in Bae WC, Masuda K: Emerging technologies for molecular therapy for intervertebral disk degeneration. *Orthop Clin North Am* 2011;42:585-601, ix.

osteoarthritis. SM04690 has been shown to inhibit Wnt pathway gene expression in both nucleus pulposus and anulus fibrosus cell cultures; in nucleus pulposus cells, SM04690 inhibited senescence, decreased catabolism, and induced differentiation into chondrocytelike cells, whereas SM04690 decreased catabolism and inhibited fibrosis in anulus fibrosus cells.[72] The efficacy of SM04690 was tested in a rat coccygeal IVD needle-puncture model. Rats in the SM04690 group qualitatively showed significantly increased cartilage matrix and reduced anulus fibrosus lamellar disorganization and fragmentation.[72]

Lactic Acid

The efficacy and toxicologic study on lactic acid–induced sclerozation were performed in pig lumbar disks by Olmarker et al.[96] The flexural rigidity of the lactic acid–injected disks was significantly less than that of the placebo-injected IVDs. The transformation of nucleus pulposus to fibroblastic tissues was noted 1 and 3 months later. Type I collagen was increased in the nucleus pulposus after the treatment.

Platelet-Rich Plasma

PRP is an autologous blood concentrate that contains a natural concentration of autologous growth factors and cytokines derived from platelets that is currently widely used in orthopaedic fields for tissue regeneration and repair.[120,121] PRP has great potential to stimulate cell proliferation and metabolic activity of IVD cells in vitro.[122] Several animal studies that evaluated the regenerative effect of the intradiscal injection of PRP have been reported.[123] A recent meta-analysis of animal studies verified that PRP treatment is potentially effective in restoring disk height in mouse, rabbit, and rat models, reducing histologic degeneration grade, and increasing MRI T2 image signals.[43]

Nagae et al[97] injected PRP-impregnated gelatin hydrogel microspheres into the IVDs of the rabbit nucleotomy disk degeneration model and showed that PRP-impregnated gelatin hydrogel microspheres was effective in slowing IVD degeneration, as assessed by histologic and biochemical analyses. Subsequently, Sawamura et al[98] reported that PRP-impregnated gelatin hydrogel microspheres had a significant effect on restoring disk height and MRI grading scores. Thereafter, several animal studies have shown that PRP or PRP-releasate[99] has the potential to restore disk height[123] or improve MRI grading scores.[124]

SCIENTIFIC EVIDENCE FOR THE CLINICAL UTILITY OF CELL-BASED THERAPIES

Cellular transplantation or cell therapy aims to confront the decline of metabolically active cells observed during IVD degeneration. It involves introducing de novo cells into the IVD to either reconstitute the IVD and the direct contribution of de novo cells to ECM repair, or indirectly through cell signaling aimed at mitigating the catabolic and inflammatory environment.[125] Nevertheless, cell therapy remains a contested strategy[51] and an optimal approach for engendering IVD repair through cell transplantation remains to be determined both from practical and regenerative perspectives[126-133] (**Table 6**). Predominant differences can be observed in the types of cells that comprise the transplantation product. Chondrogenic cell types overall demonstrate high retention following transplantation and result in strong maintenance of the disk height index and IVD architecture.[126] For example, discogenic cell products (injectable discogenic cell therapy, rebonuputemcel), based on culture-expanded human nucleus pulposus cells, have demonstrated potency in limiting induced disk degeneration, severely limiting disk height loss and supporting, at a minimum, IVD matrix

TABLE 6 Cell Types Used for the Treatment of IVD-Associated Pathologies

Cell type	NP Cells	Chondrocytes	MSC	iPSC-Derived	AF Cells	EP Cells
Advantages	High IVD survivability potential	ECM production potential	Tissue accessibility and quality	Unlimited tissue accessibility and quality	High IVD survivability potential	High IVD survivability potential
	High ECM production potential	Nonangiogenic	High expandability; scalability	High expandability; scalability	High ECM production potential	High ECM production potential
	Nonangiogenic		Strong anti-inflammatory potential	High differentiation potential		
			Differentiation potential	High ECM production potential		
Disadvantages	Low tissue accessibility and quality	Low tissue accessibility and quality	Potential undesired differentiation	Potential undesired differentiation	Low tissue accessibility and quality	Low tissue accessibility and quality
	Low expandability; scalability	Low expandability; scalability	Potential angiogenesis stimulation	Teratoma and tumorigenesis risk	Low expandability; scalability	Low expandability; scalability
		Appropriate ECM production remains undetermined	Appropriate ECM production remains undetermined	Long and costly production required	Poorly defined cell surface markers	Poorly defined cell surface markers
			Low survivability in IVD			

AF = anulus fibrosus, ECM = extracellular matrix, EP = end plate, iPSC = induced pluripotent stem cell, IVD = intervertebral disk, MSC = mesenchymal stromal cell, NP = nucleus pulposus maintenance in rabbit and canine models.[134,135] Moreover, the injectable discogenic cell therapy product showed the ability to be incorporated long term into the IVD[135] and presented an excellent safety profile.[134] Alternatively, stem and progenitor cells that are not fully differentiated, such as MSC products, are similarly being explored. These cells appear to primarily function through paracrine signaling and immune-modulation because their survival within the disk appears limited.[126,127] However, not fully differentiated stem and progenitor cells have been shown to be capable of mitigating induced disk degeneration cascades. Specifically, stromal precursor antigen-3 immuno-selected mesenchymal precursor cells are capable of limiting disk height loss and show trend for enhanced IVD matrix maintenance.[136,137] It should also be emphasized that the validity of animal models currently used for disk degeneration and treatment development remains controversial.[138] Moreover, preclinical studies examining the effect of cell therapy on discogenic pain are severely lacking.

CURRENT STATUS OF CLINICAL DEVELOPMENT

Clinical trials and clinical studies using biofactors are summarized in **Table 7**.

Clinical Trials and Clinical Studies Using Biofactors

Osteogenic Protein 1/Bone Morphogenetic Protein 7

A clinical trial of OP-1 was initiated in 2007; however, the results of the phase I trial have not been published because of the withdrawal of the trial from Clinicaltrials.gov.

Growth and Differentiation Factor 5

Since 2009, several phase Ib and phase II studies have been conducted (https://clinicaltrials.gov/ct2/show/NCT00813813, US; https://clinicaltrials.gov/ct2/show/NCT01158924, Australia; https://www.clinicaltrials.gov/ct2/show/NCT01182337, Korea), including a double-blind study (https://clinicaltrials.gov/ct2/show/NCT01124006, US). The studies were completed, and some results were posted to ClinicalTrials.gov. However, development of GDF-5 is currently halted.

AMG0103 (NF kappa B Decoy Oligo DNA)

A prospective, multicenter, double-blind, randomized controlled study with 25 patients chronic discogenic LBP (placebo and three doses) was performed (https://clinicaltrials.gov/ct2/show/NCT03263611, US); some clinical results were published as a press release.[139] As the primary outcome, the intradiscal injection of AMG0103 was well tolerated with no serious adverse effect. Administration of AMG0103 resulted in a dose-dependent and sustained reduction in back pain, measured on a 100-mm VAS. The VAS pain scores in the highest group had a median reduction of 97.5% compared with baseline, which was significantly better than that in the placebo group (15%). Other outcome measures showed similar trends. No peer-reviewed data have yet been presented.

YH14618

A phase Ib clinical trial with 48 patients was completed (https://www.clinicaltrials.gov/ct2/show/NCT01526330). The data were reported at the North American Spine Society meeting in 2015. The 50% responder rate on VAS was 41.7%, 50.0%, 30.8%, 25.0% at week 24 in the YH14618 1-, 3-, 6-mg/disk and placebo groups, respectively. A phase II clinical trial with 326 patients with placebo groups and four doses has been completed (https://clinicaltrials.gov/ct2/show/NCT02320019). The trial failed to prove a statistical significance of YH14618 treatment in Korea. The product was recently licensed to Spine Biopharma and development is continuing to start a new clinical trial in the United States.

SM04690

A clinical study was registered in ClinicalTrials.gov (https://clinicaltrials.gov/ct2/show/NCT03246399) for SM04690, but the study was stopped because of business reasons, following full enrollment of the first dose cohort in 2019.

STA363

STA363 consists of lactic acid together with a contrast agent. This agent aims to induce sclerosis of disks, resulting in spine stability. The first phase Ib study with 15 patients (three doses and placebo, 3:2) was completed, and the safety and tolerability have been shown (https://clinicaltrials.gov/ct2/show/NCT03055845). There was an indication of a lower water content of the nucleus pulposus injected with the two highest doses of STA363.[96] A phase II study with 126 patients (two doses and placebo) is currently underway (https://clinicaltrials.gov/ct2/show/NCT04673461).

Tanezumab

Tanezumab is a monoclonal antibody directed against nerve growth factor. A subcutaneous formulation of tanezumab has recently demonstrated efficacy. Clinical trials for chronic LBP have been reported with favorable effects (https://clinicaltrials.gov/ct2/show/NCT00924664). However, the long-term safety and effectiveness of tanezumab as a treatment for chronic LBP reported adverse events, such as osteonecrosis.[140]

Clinical Trials and Clinical Studies Using Cell Therapy

The number of clinical trials that are exploring the therapeutic potential of cell transplantation for IVD-related diseases is rapidly increasing.[125] Most such studies are case series or presented phase I/II trials.[141-157] Like preclinical studies, the largest number of these studies use MSC-based cell products, with a small fraction using IVD-derived cells and only one study examining articular cartilage chondrocytes (**Table 8**). It should be noted that the overall cohort size of the reported clinical trials is relatively small, lacking control groups, and involves a

TABLE 7 Clinical Trials of Bioactive Factors

Active Agent	Clinical Trial Number	Level of Target Disks	Diagnosis	Status	Study Design (Enrollment)	Title
rhGDF-5	NCT00813813	1 (L3-S1)	Standardized diskography	Completed	Phase 1/2 (n = 32)	Intradiscal rhGDF-5 phase I/II clinical trial
rhGDF-5	NCT01124006	1 (L3-S1)	Standardized diskography	Completed	Phase 2 (n = 24)	A multicenter, randomized, double-blind, placebo controlled, clinical trial to evaluate the safety, tolerability and preliminary effectiveness of 2 doses of intradiscal rhGDF-5 (single administration) for the treatment of early stage lumbar disc degeneration
rhGDF-5	NCT01182337	1 (L3-S1)	Standardized diskography	Completed	Phase 1/2 (n = 30)	A clinical trial to evaluate the safety, tolerability and preliminary effectiveness of single administration intradiscal rhGDF-5 for the treatment of early stage lumbar disc degeneration
BIOSTAT BIOLOGX	NCT01011816	1 or 2 (L1-S1)	Standard practice	Terminated	Phase 3 (n = 220), primary end point (% success): No difference between saline and BIOSTAT BIOLOGX	Treatment of symptomatic Lumbar Internal Disc Disruption with the biostat system
YH14618	NCT01526330	1 or 2 (L1-S1)	Standard practice	Completed	Phase 1/2 (n = 48): Safety and clinical efficacy confirmed	Safety, tolerability and efficacy of YH14618 in patients With degenerative disc disease YH14618: 7-Amino acid peptide derived from a conserved region of biglycan
YH14618	NCT02320019	1 or 2 (L1-S1)	Standard practice	Completed	Phase 2 (n = 326)	Clinical trial of YH14618 in patients with degenerative Disc disease YH14618: 7-Amino acid peptide derived from a conserved region of biglycan
Corticoids (Hydrocortancyl)	NCT01694134	Not described	Standard practice	Completed	Phase 3 (n = 50)	Assessment of the efficacy of an intradiscal injection of corticoids in Modic 1 Discopathies
Pamidronate	NCT01799616	Not described	Standard practice	Unknown status	Phase 2 (n = 48)	Efficiency and safety study of Pamidronate in inflammatory back pain due to degenerative disc disease

(Continued)

TABLE 7 Clinical Trials of Bioactive Factors (Continued)

Active Agent	Clinical Trial Number	Level of Target Disks	Diagnosis	Status	Study Design (Enrollment)	Title
BioDGenesis	NCT02379689	1 or 2 (L1-S1)	Standard practice	Unknown status	NA (n = 30)	Efficacy of intradiscal injection of viable placental tissue extract in subjects with one or two level, symptomatic lumbar intervertebral disc degeneration BioDGenesis: Injectable placental tissue extract
SM04690	NCT03246399	1-2 (L4-S1)	Standard practice	Terminated	Phase 1 (n = 6)	A study of the safety, tolerability, and pharmacokinetics of SM04690 injectable suspension following single intradiscal injection in subjects with degenerative disc disease SM04690: Selective inhibitor of canonical Wnt signaling
AMG0103	NCT03263611	1 (L1-S1)	Standard practice	Active, not recruiting	Phase 1 (n = 25)	AMG0103 in subjects with chronic discogenic lumbar back pain AMG0103: Nuclear factor-κB decoy oligodeoxynucleotide
Fibrin sealant	NCT04621799	Not described	Radiographically and by annulogram	Recruiting	Phase 2/3 (n = 400)	Fibrin for chronic multilevel discogenic low back pain
Platelet-rich plasma	NCT04816747	Not described	Standard practice	Not yet recruiting	Phase 3 (n = 50)	Intradiscal and intra-articular injection of autologous PRP in patients with lumbar degenerative Disc disease and facet joint Syndrome
Platelet-rich plasma	NCT04849429	Not described	Standard practice	Recruiting	Phase 1 (n = 30)	Intra-discal injection of PRP enriched with exosomes in chronic low back pain
STA363	NCT03055845	1 (L3-S1)	Standard practice	Completed	Phase 1 (n = 15)	A single ascending dose study of safety and tolerability of STA363 compared to placebo in 15 patients with chronic discogenic low back pain STA363: Lactic acid
STA363	NCT04673461	1 or 2 (L2-S1)	Standard practice	Recruiting	Phase 2 (n = 126)	Study investigating STA363 compared to placebo in patients with chronic discogenic low back pain (STA-02) STA363: Lactic acid

PRP = platelet-rich plasma, rhGDF-5 = recombinant human growth differentiation factor 5 short follow-up period of 1 to 2 years. Overall, the clinical trials suggest that cellular transplantation into a human IVD (both autologous and allogeneic) is relatively safe, with no clear evident serious adverse events (**Table 8**), although the collective sample size might remain too small to detect more rare adverse reactions.

IVD-Derived Cells and Chondrocytes

Specifically examining the IVD-derived cell products, an overall trend of improvement in pain and disability qualifiers can be detected (**Table 8**). A controlled study by Meisel et al,[150] comparing patients treated with an autologous disk-derived cell transplantation product following diskectomy with patients only treated with diskectomy, showed a trend of improved VAS and Oswestry Disability Index (ODI) scores compared with the control cohort. Notably, a significant improvement in MRI hydration values was observed. Two additional randomized placebo-controlled trials from DiscGenics aimed to examine their injectable discogenic cell therapy product to the carrier and sham injection groups are currently on-going in Japan (https://clinicaltrials.gov/ct2/show/NCT03955315) and the USA (https://clinicaltrials.gov/ct2/show/NCT03347708). Results have yet to be reported. The NuQu phase I trial examining transplantation of NuQu allogeneic juvenile chondrocytes showed a significant improvement in pain numeric rating scales and ODI scores compared with baseline and showed a trend of overall improvement through MRI.[141] Nevertheless, their follow-up phase II trial first posted in 2013 has been terminated (https://clinicaltrials.gov/ct2/show/NCT01771471) and no results have been published at this point.

Mesenchymal Stromal Cells

Examining the results obtained from MSC-based transplant products (**Table 8**) showed alleviation in pain and disability outcomes. Only the transplantation of hematopoietic stem cells did not result in any pain improvement.[142] Of particular interest are the two controlled trials, comparing bone marrow–derived MSC products with sham treatments.[143,144] First, the ITRT trial (https://clinicaltrials.gov/ct2/show/NCT01860417, Eudra-CT:2012-004444-30) examined their allogeneic MSC product and compared the respective outcomes with those of patients treated with placebo paravertebral muscle anesthetic injection. Results highlighted a significant improvement in VAS and ODI scores in their 1-year follow-up study, compared with the control cohort.[143] Also, MRI outcomes showed enhancement of Pfirrmann grades and hydration values in the cell transplant cohort, whereas the placebo control demonstrated worsened outcomes. This study followed their initial noncontrolled trial (Eudra-CT:2008-001191-68, https://clinicaltrials.gov/ct2/show/NCT02440074) examining autologous MSC transplantation, which similarly showed improvements in VAS and ODI scores, as well as significantly enhanced MRI outcomes compared with baseline.[145]

The Mesoblast phase II trial (https://clinicaltrials.gov/ct2/show/NCT01290367) compared high-dose and low-dose intradiskal injections of mesenchymal precursor cells compared with a saline and carrier injection cohort. Their results similarly highlighted the potential of mesenchymal precursor cells to significantly enhance VAS and ODI scores compared with baseline and control cohorts.[144] However, the study revealed no consistent differences in any of the groups regarding MRI observations.

A phase II randomized sham-controlled clinical trial (https://clinicaltrials.gov/ct2/show/NCT04042844) by BioRestorative Therapies with the aim to examine their hypoxia-primed bone marrow mononuclear cells combined with an autologous platelet lysate (BRTX-100) product was scheduled to start in June, 2022. Notably, a case series by Elabd et al[146] applying a similar cell product composition showed an overall trend of enhanced VAS and ODI outcomes. Centeno et al[147] followed with an extension of the study (https://clinicaltrials.gov/ct2/show/NCT03011398) and confirmed a significant improvement in numerical pain scores, with a trend of improved functional rating index outcomes. Moreover, both studies highlighted the ability of their cell products to reduce overall disk bulge sizes.

Overall, the clinical trials consistently showed cell transplantation capable of reducing LBP outcomes and disability scores. However, the ability of the transplanted cells to repair the human IVD remains to be fully elucidated, as MRI improvements were not a consistent finding in all human trials. Combining the results from animal studies with human trials, selection of the appropriate cell type and source remains a topic of debate. There is an emphasis on cell therapy products on nucleus pulposus repair, with few studies examining anulus fibrosus and end plate restoration (**Table 8**). All cell types currently examined, to some extent, were shown to be capable of forming cartilage in animal models and to alleviate pain in human trials. Nevertheless, it remains uncertain whether this formed cartilage tissue represents full nucleus pulposus tissue capable of supporting the biomechanical integrity required for full spine function. Moreover, although clinical trials showed improvement in pain and disability outcomes, it remains uncertain if these effects are long-lasting or competitive to standard care treatments. However, future cell product optimization and new techniques such as induced pluripotent stem cell technology and gene-modified cells could further enhance the potency of cellular products (**Table 8**). Ultimately, cellular products require adaptation in the clinic to be marketable; thus, their cost effectiveness requires critical examination. Other aspects could further enhance the safety and efficacy of cellular products. For example, the carrier used to transplant and retain the cells could help support the regeneration process of the IVD. Similarly, cell dosage has also been shown to be a pivotal

TABLE 8 Overview of Cell Therapy Clinical Trials

	Publication			Study Design				Outcomes			
Cell Type	**Author**	**Year**	**Registry ID**	**Cell Product**	**Cohort Size (n)**	**Maximum follow-up (Years)**	**Control Group**	**Pain**	**Disability**	**MRI**	**Safety**
IVD cells	Tschugg	2017	EudraCT 2010–023830-22, NCT01640457	NOVOCART Disc plus (ADCT) **IVD-derived cells** (autologous, PEG-HA)	20	<1	PEG-HA only	—	—	No worsening on MRI	No SAE
	Meisel	2006	—	ADCT **IVD-derived cells** (autologous, + diskectomy)	122	4	Diskectomy only	Trend improvement in VAS score compared with control	Trend of enhanced ODI scores compared with control	Significant enhancement in hydration compared with control. Disk height maintained	No SAE
	Mochida	2015	—	**NP cells** (autologous, sus)	9	3		Trend in LBP subscale improvement	Strong trend of JOA improvements	1/9 showed Pfirrmann classification. Hydration values maintained	No SAE
Chondrocytes	Coric	2013	—	NuQu allogeneic juvenile chondrocytes **Articular chondrocytes** (allogeneic, fibrin)	15	1		Significantly improved NRS	Significantly improved ODI and SF36	10/13 showed MRI improvements	No SAE

MSC[a]	Haufe	2006	—	**HSC** (autologous, sus)	10	1	—		No improvements in pain scores		—		—		No SAE
	Piccirilli	2017	—	**AD-MSC** (autologous)	8	1	—		Trend of VAS score improvement		Trend of enhanced ODI		80% of disk regained hyperintensity		No SAE
	Kumar	2017	NCT02338271	**AD-MSC** (autologous, HA)	10	1	—		Significantly improved VAS score		Significantly improved ODI and SF36		3/10 showed improved water content		No SAE
	Comella	2017	NCT02097862	Adipose stem cells **AD-MSC**[b] (autologous, sus, +PRP)	15	1	—		Trend of improvement in VAS score and pain rating		Minimal improvement in ODI, BDI, SF12 and Dallas questionnaire		—		No SAE
	Henriksson	2019	—	**BM-MSC** (autologous)	10	3	—		—		—		—		4/10 proceeded to surgery, of which 1 showed calcium deposits
	Orozco	2011	Eudra-CT:2008-001191-68, NCT02440074	**BM-MSC** (autologous, sus)	10	1	—		Significantly improved VAS score		Significantly improved ODI and SF36-physical component		DHI maintained, significant improvement in water content		No SAE

(Continued)

TABLE 8 Overview of Cell Therapy Clinical Trials (Continued)

Cell Type	Publication			Study Design				Outcomes			
	Author	Year	Registry ID	Cell Product	Cohort Size (n)	Maximum follow-up (Years)	Control Group	Pain	Disability	MRI	Safety
	Wang	2014	—	**BM-MSC** (autologous, sus)	31	<1	—	—	—	Inflammatory ankylosing spondylitis characteristics decreased	No SAE
	Yoshikawa	2010	—	**BM-MSC** (autologous, collagen sponges)	2	2	—	Trend of improved VAS score	Trend of improved JOA scores	Trend of water content increase	No SAE
	Noriega	2017	Eudra-CT:2012-004444-30, NCT01860417	**BM-MSC** (allogeneic, sus)	24	1	Paravertebral muscle anesthesia	Significantly improved VAS score, also significantly higher than control	Significantly improved ODI, also significantly higher than control	Trend of enhanced IVD hydration. Pfirrmann grading improved, got worse in control	No SAE
	Centeno	2017	NCT03011398	**BM-MSC** (autologous, sus, +PL)	33	6	—	Significant NPS improvement (long term)	Strong trend of improved FRI scores	85% of patients had reduced size of disk bulge	No SAE
	Elabd	2016	—	**BM-MSC** (autologous, sus, +PL)	5	6	—	Trend of general improvement	Trend of general improvement	4/5 showed disk bulge reduction	No SAE

	Pettine	2016	—	**BM-MSC** (autologous, sus)	26	2	—		Significantly improved VAS score		Significantly improved ODI		40% of patients reported improvement in Pfirrmann grade		No SAE, 6/26 progressed to surgery
	Amirdelfan	2021	NCT01290367	**BM-MSC** (allogeneic, HA)	100	2	Saline or HA-only		Significantly improved VAS score compared with sham, all conditions showed improvement from baseline		Significantly improved ODI compared with sham, all conditions showed improvement from baseline		No differences in Pfirrmann grades improvement between conditions. 2/60 in MSC, and 1/20 in HA improved one grade		8/60 SAE compared with 4/40 in control; SAE not specified
	Pang	2014	—	**UC-MSC** (allogeneic)	2	2	—		Trend of improved VAS score		Trend of enhanced ODI		1/2 presented higher hydration values		No SAE

ADCT = autologous disk-derived cell transplantation, AD-MSC = adipose tissue–derived mesenchymal stromal cells, BDI = Beck Depression Inventory, BM-MSC = bone marrow–derived mesenchymal stromal cell, DHI = disc height index, FRI = functional rating index, HA = hyaluronic acid, HSC = hematopoietic stem cells, IV = intravenous, IVD = intervertebral disk, JOA = Japanese Orthopaedic Association, LBP = low back pain, MSC = mesenchymal stromal cell group, NP = nucleus pulposus, NRS = numeric (pain) rating scale, ODI = Oswestry Disability Index, PEG-HA = polyethylene glycol-hyaluronic acid, PL = supplemented with platelet lysate, PRP = supplemented with platelet-rich plasma, SAE = serious adverse events, SF = Short Form (questionnaire), sus = in suspension, UC-MSC = umbilical cord–derived mesenchymal stromal cells, VAS = visual analog scale. No measurement, Worsening reported, No clear benefit reported, Trend of improvement reported, Significant improvement reported, Significant improvement reported compared to (placebo/sham/vehicle) control group.

[a]Mesenchymal stromal cells and other stem cells.

[b]Specifically stromal vascular fraction containing AD-MSC.

factor that can affect regenerative potential.[148] Moreover, patient stratification to identify optimal cell therapy patients or IVD condition candidates will likely prove critical.[125] More fully blinded, randomized, and (placebo) controlled trials are still awaited to thoroughly grasp the potential of cell therapy for discogenic pain treatment and IVD repair. Multiple randomized controlled large clinical trials are currently ongoing, and their results are highly anticipated.[158] Although IVD-targeted cell therapeutics have undergone tremendous advances in the past 2 decades, these therapeutics have not yet been developed as widespread clinical products. Challenges in manufacturing processes, product scalability, cellular batch consistency,[134] and other regulatory frameworks[159] form obstacles for development. Moreover, lack of high-quality trials, patient stratification, generally poor reporting, and lack of extensively accepted outcome parameters to determine successful treatment make comparisons and full review of cellular studies challenging. Nevertheless, initial results are promising and could hopefully engender a much-needed therapeutic alternative for patients with LBP currently without treatment options.

FUTURE DIRECTIONS/CHALLENGES

Possible Combined Therapies—Biofactors and Cells

The current target of injection therapies is generally limited to disks with early and moderate degeneration. Some studies are ongoing to use the combined application of MSCs and PRP. However, the nutrition in a degenerated disk is very limited because its end plate is often calcified and sclerotic.[160,161] The enhancement of metabolic activities with an increased number of cells may result in the further depletion of nutrients and oxygen and the accumulation of metabolic waste.

Minimize Injection Frequency—Drug Delivery System

Carragee et al[162] reported the diskography-induced disk degeneration of punctured IVDs. The contrast agents have also been reported to negatively affect cell metabolism[163-166] and induce disk degeneration in the rat model.[167] Because of the discrepancy in the guidelines by the North American Spine Society and American Pain Society, provocative diskography is a debatable procedure. Careful assessment of the necessity for diskography is required for patients requiring identification of a responsive disk that generates pain. This report by Carragee et al and the development of the disk degeneration model in animals[168,169] raised the question about the effect of needle puncture. To minimize the frequency of injection, efforts should be spent to develop a drug delivery system that prolongs the effect of the drug. When a drug with low viscosity is injected, it is possible that the injected material can be extruded from the hole created by the needle. Thus, the property of the injection substance is important to obtain proper distribution and avoidance of backflow.

SUMMARY

Various approaches aimed to reverse the IVD homeostasis dysregulations have been proven effective in a range of in vitro and in vivo studies. Preclinical animal models have emphasized the potential of growth factors, anti-inflammatory molecules, PRP, and cell product injection to limit, prevent, and even repair structural disk deterioration, as observed through histologic and imaging modalities; however, their effect on pain relief is severely lacking. However, these models have their limitations, primarily related to the differences in IVD composition and degeneration cascade (including end plate changes in animal models), which might interfere with the translation of findings to a human disk condition. Nevertheless, the subsequent advancement of growth factor and small molecule injection to the clinical trial stage has shown capable of supporting discogenic pain relief for some of the products assessed. Clinical trial reports on cell transplantation were able to report significant relief in discogenic pain, and some were able to report structural modifications. Notably, however, the current status of these bioactive factors and cells for clinical assessment remains in an early stage of development. Long-term and highly powered clinical trials are still severely lacking, and most reports did not include appropriate placebo or sham control cohorts. Nevertheless, contemporary results look promising. If these intradiscal injection therapeutics prove effective and safe, they will have an effect on patients with chronic discogenic LBP, for which currently no effective treatment options exist. Economically, the lifetime cost of treatment for these patients will be dramatically decreased by reducing the use of narcotics and preventing or delaying surgeries. Further advancements in well-designed clinical trials, new outcome measurements, such as new MRI techniques, and better patient stratification are strongly anticipated and will likely prove critical in fully assessing the therapeutic potential of these bioactive factors and cell products for patients with LBP.

REFERENCES

1. Raciborski F, Gasik R, Klak A: Disorders of the spine. A major health and social problem. *Reumatologia* 2016;54:196-200.
2. Garcia JB, Hernandez-Castro JJ, Nunez RG, et al: Prevalence of low back pain in Latin America: A systematic literature review. *Pain Physician* 2014;17:379-391.
3. Meucci RD, Fassa AG, Faria NM: Prevalence of chronic low back pain: Systematic review. *Rev Saude Publica* 2015;49:1.
4. Kreiner DS, Matz P, Bono CM, et al: Guideline summary review: An evidence-based clinical guideline for the diagnosis and treatment of low back pain. *Spine J* 2020;20:998-1024.

5. Chou R, Loeser JD, Owens DK, et al: Interventional therapies, surgery, and interdisciplinary rehabilitation for low back pain: An evidence-based clinical practice guideline from the American pain Society. *Spine (Phila Pa 1976)* 2009;34:1066-1077.
6. Knezevic NN, Candido KD, Vlaeyen JWS, Van Zundert J, Cohen SP: Low back pain. *Lancet* 2021;398(10294):78-92.
7. Vernon-Roberts B, Moore RJ, Fraser RD: The natural history of age-related disc degeneration: The pathology and sequelae of tears. *Spine (Phila Pa 1976)* 2007;32:2797-2804.
8. Peng B, Hou S, Wu W, Zhang C, Yang Y: The pathogenesis and clinical significance of a high-intensity zone (HIZ) of lumbar intervertebral disc on MR imaging in the patient with discogenic low back pain. *Eur Spine J* 2006;15:583-587.
9. Teraguchi M, Cheung JPY, Karppinen J, et al: Lumbar high-intensity zones on MRI: Imaging biomarkers for severe, prolonged low back pain and sciatica in a population-based cohort. *Spine J* 2020;20:1025-1034.
10. Mera Y, Teraguchi M, Hashizume H, et al: Association between types of modic changes in the lumbar region and low back pain in a large cohort: The Wakayama spine study. *Eur Spine J* 2021;30:1011-1017.
11. Fujii K, Yamazaki M, Kang JD, et al: Discogenic back pain: Literature review of definition, diagnosis, and treatment. *JBMR Plus* 2019;3:e10180.
12. Wu A, March L, Zheng X, et al: Global low back pain prevalence and years lived with disability from 1990 to 2017: Estimates from the global burden of disease study 2017. *Ann Transl Med* 2020;8:299.
13. GBD 2017 Disease and Injury Incidence and Prevalence Collaborators: Global, regional, and national incidence, prevalence, and years lived with disability for 354 diseases and injuries for 195 countries and territories, 1990-2017: A systematic analysis for the global burden of disease study 2017. *Lancet* 2018;392:1789-1858.
14. Vos T, Lim SS, Abbafati C, et al: Global burden of 369 diseases and injuries in 204 countries and territories, 1990-2019: A systematic analysis for the global Burden of disease study 2019. *Lancet* 2020;396:1204-1222.
15. Singh K, Andersson G, Watkins-Castillo SI: *Low Back Pain*. Available at: https://www.boneandjointburden.org/fourth-edition/iiaa0/low-back-pain. Accessed June 24, 2021.
16. Dieleman JL, Cao J, Chapin A, et al: US health care spending by payer and health condition, 1996-2016. *J Am Med Assoc* 2020;323:863-884.
17. Katz JN: Lumbar disc disorders and low-back pain: Socioeconomic factors and consequences. *J Bone Joint Surg Am* 2006;88(suppl 2):21-24.
18. Andersson G, Watkins-Castillo SI: *Bed Days/Lost Work Days*. Available at: https://www.boneandjointburden.org/2014-report/iid1/bed-dayslost-work-days. Accessed June 26, 2021.
19. Bae WC, Masuda K: Enhancing disc repair by growth factors and other modalities, in Shapiro IM, Risbud MV, eds: *The Intervertebral Disc*. Springer, 2014, pp 401-416.
20. Masuda K, Lotz JC: New challenges for intervertebral disc treatment using regenerative medicine. *Tissue Eng Part B Rev* 2010;16:147-158.
21. Samartzis D, Borthakur A, Belfer I, et al: Novel diagnostic and prognostic methods for disc degeneration and low back pain. *Spine J* 2015;15:1919-1932.
22. Ito K, Creemers L: Mechanisms of intervertebral disk degeneration/injury and pain: A review. *Global Spine J* 2013;3:145-152.
23. Andersson GB: Epidemiological features of chronic low-back pain. *Lancet* 1999;354:581-585.
24. Luoma K, Riihimäki H, Luukkonen R, Raininko R, Viikari-Juntura E, Lamminen A: Low back pain in relation to lumbar disc degeneration. *Spine (Phila Pa 1976)* 2000;25:487-492.
25. Brinjikji W, Diehn FE, Jarvik JG, et al: MRI findings of disc degeneration are more prevalent in adults with low back pain than in asymptomatic controls: A systematic review and meta-analysis. *Am J Neuroradiol* 2015;36:2394-2399.
26. Brinjikji W, Luetmer PH, Comstock B, et al: Systematic literature review of imaging features of spinal degeneration in asymptomatic populations. *Am J Neuroradiol* 2015;36:811-816.
27. Gornet MG, Peacock J, Claude J, et al: Magnetic resonance spectroscopy (MRS) can identify painful lumbar discs and may facilitate improved clinical outcomes of lumbar surgeries for discogenic pain. *Eur Spine J* 2019;28:674-687.
28. Buckwalter JA: Aging and degeneration of the human intervertebral disc. *Spine (Phila Pa 1976)* 1995;20:1307-1314.
29. Adams MA, Roughley PJ: What is intervertebral disc degeneration, and what causes it? *Spine (Phila Pa 1976)* 2006;31:2151-2161.
30. Sambrook PN, MacGregor AJ, Spector TD: Genetic influences on cervical and lumbar disc degeneration: A magnetic resonance imaging study in twins. *Arthritis Rheum* 1999;42:366-372.
31. Urban JPG, Fairbank JCT: Current perspectives on the role of biomechanical loading and genetics in development of disc degeneration and low back pain; a narrative review. *J Biomech* 2020;102:109573.
32. Masuda K, An HS: Prevention of disc degeneration with growth factors. *Eur Spine J* 2006;15(suppl 15):422-432.
33. Molinos M, Almeida CR, Caldeira J, Cunha C, Goncalves RM, Barbosa MA: Inflammation in intervertebral disc degeneration and regeneration. *J R Soc Interface* 2015;12:20150429.
34. Fontana G, See E, Pandit A: Current trends in biologics delivery to restore intervertebral disc anabolism. *Adv Drug Deliv Rev* 2015;84:146-158.
35. Thompson JP, Pearce RH, Schechter MT, Adams ME, Tsang IK, Bishop PB: Preliminary evaluation of a scheme for grading the gross morphology of the human intervertebral disc. *Spine (Phila Pa 1976)* 1990;15:411-415.
36. Boos N, Weissbach S, Rohrbach H, Weiler C, Spratt KF, Nerlich AG: Classification of age-related changes in lumbar intervertebral discs: 2002 Volvo award in basic science. *Spine (Phila Pa 1976)* 2002;27:2631-2644.
37. Pfirrmann CW, Metzdorf A, Zanetti M, Hodler J, Boos N: Magnetic resonance classification of lumbar intervertebral disc degeneration. *Spine (Phila Pa 1976)* 2001;26:1873-1878.

38. Griffith JF, Wang YX, Antonio GE, et al: Modified Pfirrmann grading system for lumbar intervertebral disc degeneration. *Spine (Phila Pa 1976)* 2007;32:E708-E712.
39. Qaseem A, Wilt TJ, McLean RM, Forciea MA: Noninvasive treatments for acute, subacute, and chronic low back pain: A clinical practice guideline from the American College of Physicians. *Ann Intern Med* 2017;166:514-530.
40. National Institute for Health and Care Excellence: *Low Back Pain and Sciatica in Over 16s: Assessment and Management*. Available at: https://www.nice.org.uk/guidance/NG59/chapter/Recommendations#non-invasive-treatments-for-low-back-pain-and-sciatica. Accessed June 30, 2021.
41. The NASS Clinical Practice Guideline Committee: *Diagnosis and Treatment of Low Back Pain (2020)*. Available at: https://www.spine.org/Research-Clinical-Care/Quality-Improvement/Clinical-Guidelines. Accessed June 30, 2021.
42. Krafts KP: Tissue repair: The hidden drama. *Organogenesis* 2010;6:225-233.
43. Bendtsen M, Bunger C, Colombier P, et al: Biological challenges for regeneration of the degenerated disc using cellular therapies. *Acta Orthop* 2016;87:39-46.
44. Pattappa G, Li Z, Peroglio M, Wismer N, Alini M, Grad S: Diversity of intervertebral disc cells: Phenotype and function. *J Anat* 2012;221:480-496.
45. Maroudas A, Stockwell RA, Nachemson A, Urban J: Factors involved in the nutrition of the human lumbar intervertebral disc: Cellularity and diffusion of glucose in vitro. *J Anat* 1975;120:113-130.
46. Chelberg MK, Banks GM, Geiger DF, Oegema TR Jr: Identification of heterogeneous cell populations in normal human intervertebral disc. *J Anat* 1995;186:43-53.
47. Schollmeier G, Lahr-Eigen R, Lewandrowski KU: Observations on fiber-forming collagens in the anulus fibrosus. *Spine (Phila Pa 1976)* 2000;25:2736-2741.
48. Masuda K: Biological repair of the degenerated intervertebral disc by the injection of growth factors. *Eur Spine J* 2008;17(suppl 4):441-451.
49. Abe Y, Pichika R, Aoki Y, et al: The prominent form of splice variants of vascular endothelial growth factor, VEGF121, was upregulated by interleukin-1β in human intervertebral disc cells. *Orthop Res Soc Trans* 2007;32:1087.
50. Purmessur D, Freemont AJ, Hoyland JA: Expression and regulation of neurotrophins in the nondegenerate and degenerate human intervertebral disc. *Arthritis Res Ther* 2008;10:R99.
51. Loibl M, Wuertz-Kozak K, Vadala G, Lang S, Fairbank J, Urban JP: Controversies in regenerative medicine: Should intervertebral disc degeneration be treated with mesenchymal stem cells? *JOR Spine* 2019;2:e1043.
52. Grunhagen T, Shirazi-Adl A, Fairbank JC, Urban JP: Intervertebral disk nutrition: A review of factors influencing concentrations of nutrients and metabolites. *Orthop Clin North Am* 2011;42:465-477, vii.
53. Urban JP, Holm S, Maroudas A, Nachemson A: Nutrition of the intervertebral disk. An in vivo study of solute transport. *Clin Orthop Relat Res* 1977;129:101-114.
54. Rajasekaran S, Babu JN, Arun R, Armstrong BR, Shetty AP, Murugan S: ISSLS prize winner: A study of diffusion in human lumbar discs – A serial magnetic resonance imaging study documenting the influence of the endplate on diffusion in normal and degenerate discs. *Spine (Phila Pa 1976)* 2004;29:2654-2667.
55. Bae WC, Statum S, Zhang Z, et al: Morphology of the cartilaginous endplates in human intervertebral disks with ultrashort echo time MR imaging. *Radiology* 2013;266:564-574.
56. Fields AJ, Han M, Krug R, Lotz JC: Cartilaginous end plates: Quantitative MR imaging with very short echo times-orientation dependence and correlation with biochemical composition. *Radiology* 2015;274:482-489.
57. Law T, Anthony M-P, Chan Q, et al: Ultrashort time-to-echo MRI of the cartilaginous endplate: Technique and association with intervertebral disc degeneration. *J Med Imaging Radiat Oncol* 2013;57:427-434.
58. Rajasekaran S, Venkatadass K, Naresh Babu J, Ganesh K, Shetty AP: Pharmacological enhancement of disc diffusion and differentiation of healthy, ageing and degenerated discs: Results from in-vivo serial post-contrast MRI studies in 365 human lumbar discs. *Eur Spine J* 2008;17:626-643.
59. Bogduk N, Tynan W, Wilson AS: The nerve supply to the human lumbar intervertebral discs. *J Anat* 1981;132:39-56.
60. Masuda K, Kato K: Treatment of degenerative disc disease/disc regeneration: Growth factors and platelet rich plasma, in Härtl R, Bonassar LJ, eds: *Biological Approaches to Spinal Disc Repair and Regeneration for Clinicians*. Thieme, 2017, pp 101-109.
61. Thompson JP, Oegema TJ, Bradford DS: Stimulation of mature canine intervertebral disc by growth factors. *Spine (Phila Pa 1976)* 1991;16:253-260.
62. Lehmann TP, Jakub G, Harasymczuk J, Jagodziński PP: Transforming growth factor β mediates communication of co-cultured human nucleus pulposus cells and mesenchymal stem cells. *J Orthop Res* 2018;36:3023-3032.
63. Li Z, Lang G, Karfeld-Sulzer LS, et al: Heterodimeric BMP-2/7 for nucleus pulposus regeneration-In vitro and ex vivo studies. *J Orthop Res* 2017;35:51-60.
64. Huang Y, Chen J, Jiang T, et al: Gallic acid inhibits the release of ADAMTS4 in nucleus pulposus cells by inhibiting p65 phosphorylation and acetylation of the NF-κB signaling pathway. *Oncotarget* 2017;8:47665-47674.
65. Hu B, Wang J, Wu X, Chen Y, Yuan W, Chen H: Interleukin-17 upregulates vascular endothelial growth factor by activating the JAK/STAT pathway in nucleus pulposus cells. *Joint Bone Spine* 2017;84:327-334.
66. Yao Z, Nie L, Zhao Y, et al: Salubrinal Suppresses IL-17-induced upregulation of MMP-13 and extracellular matrix degradation through the NF-kB pathway in human nucleus pulposus cells. *Inflammation* 2016;39:1997-2007.
67. Suyama K, Sakai D, Hirayama N, et al: Effects of interleukin-17A in nucleus pulposus cells and its small-molecule inhibitors for intervertebral disc disease. *J Cell Mol Med* 2018;22:5539-5551.
68. Matta A, Karim MZ, Gerami H, et al: NTG-101: A novel molecular therapy that halts the progression of degenerative disc disease. *Sci Rep* 2018;8:16809.

69. Kwon Y-J, Lee J-W, Moon E-J, Chung YG, Kim O-S, Kim H-J: Anabolic effects of peniel 2000, a peptide that regulates TGF-β1 signaling on intervertebral disc degeneration. *Spine (Phila Pa 1976)* 2013;38:E49-E58.

70. Wang Z, Weitzmann MN, Sangadala S, Hutton WC, Yoon ST: Link protein N-terminal peptide binds to bone morphogenetic protein (BMP) type II receptor and drives matrix protein expression in rabbit intervertebral disc cells. *J Biol Chem* 2013;288:28243-28253.

71. Akeda K, An H, Gemba T, et al: Effect of "Naked" Decoy on the IL-1-induced inhibition of matrix accumulation in alginate bead cultures of human intervertebral disc cells, in *Proceeding of International Society for the Study of the Lumber Spine*. Bergen, 2006.

72. Deshmukh V, Ibanez M, Hu H, et al: A small-molecule inhibitor of the Wnt pathway, lorecivivint (SM04690), as a potential disease-modifying agent for the treatment of degenerative disc disease. *Spine J* 2020;20:1492-1502.

73. Xie J, Li B, Zhang P, Wang L, Lu H, Song X: Osteogenic protein-1 attenuates the inflammatory cytokine-induced NP cell senescence through regulating the ROS/NF-κB pathway. *Biomed Pharmacother* 2018;99:431-437.

74. Gan Y, Li S, Li P, et al: A controlled release codelivery system of MSCs encapsulated in dextran/gelatin hydrogel with TGF-β3-loaded nanoparticles for nucleus pulposus regeneration. *Stem Cells Int* 2016;2016:9042019.

75. Hodgkinson T, Stening JZ, White LJ, Shakesheff KM, Hoyland JA, Richardson SM: Microparticles for controlled growth differentiation factor 6 delivery to direct adipose stem cell-based nucleus pulposus regeneration. *J Tissue Eng Regen Med* 2019;13:1406-1417.

76. Tao Y, Zhou X, Liang C, et al: TGF-β3 and IGF-1 synergy ameliorates nucleus pulposus mesenchymal stem cell differentiation towards the nucleus pulposus cell type through MAPK/ERK signaling. *Growth Factors* 2015;33:326-336.

77. Stich S, Möller A, Cabraja M, et al: Chemokine CCL25 induces migration and extracellular matrix production of anulus fibrosus-derived cells. *Int J Mol Sci* 2018;19:2207.

78. Hiyama A, Hiraishi S, Sakai D, Mochida J: CCAAT/enhancer binding protein β regulates the expression of tumor necrosis factor-α in the nucleus pulposus cells. *J Orthop Res* 2016;34:865-875.

79. Jacobsen TD, Hernandez PA, Chahine NO: Inhibition of toll-like receptor 4 protects against inflammation-induced mechanobiological alterations to intervertebral disc cells. *Eur Cell Mater* 2021;41:576-591.

80. Jiang Y, Xie Z, Yu J, Fu L: Resveratrol inhibits IL-1β-mediated nucleus pulposus cell apoptosis through regulating the PI3K/Akt pathway. *Biosci Rep* 2019;39.

81. Mwale F, Wang HT, Roughley P, Antoniou J, Haglund L: Link N and mesenchymal stem cells can induce regeneration of the early degenerate intervertebral disc. *Tissue Eng Part A* 2014;20:2942-2949.

82. Seki S, Asanuma-Abe Y, Masuda K, et al: Effect of small interference RNA (siRNA) for ADAMTS5 on intervertebral disc degeneration in the rabbit anular needle-puncture model. *Arthritis Res Ther* 2009;11:R166.

83. Johnson ZI, Schoepflin ZR, Choi H, Shapiro IM, Risbud MV: Disc in flames: Roles of TNF-α and IL-1β in intervertebral disc degeneration. *Eur Cell Mater* 2015;30:104-117.

84. Risbud MV, Shapiro IM: Role of cytokines in intervertebral disc degeneration: Pain and disc content. *Nat Rev Rheumatol* 2014;10:44-56.

85. Bae WC, Masuda K: Emerging technologies for molecular therapy for intervertebral disk degeneration. *Orthop Clin North Am* 2011;42:585-601, ix.

86. Kakutani K, Kanaji A, Asanuma K, et al: Effect of IL-1 receptor antagonist and soluble TNF receptor on the anabolism of human intervertebral disc cells. *Trans Orthop Res Soc* 2008;33:442.

87. Sinclair SM, Shamji MF, Chen J, et al: Attenuation of inflammatory events in human intervertebral disc cells with a tumor necrosis factor antagonist. *Spine (Phila Pa 1976)* 2011;36:1190-1196.

88. Walsh AJ, Bradford DS, Lotz JC: In vivo growth factor treatment of degenerated intervertebral discs. *Spine (Phila Pa 1976)* 2004;29:156-163.

89. Miyamoto K, Masuda K, Kim JG, et al: Intradiscal injections of osteogenic protein-1 restore the viscoelastic properties of degenerated intervertebral discs. *Spine J* 2006;6:692-703.

90. Chujo T, An HS, Akeda K, et al: Effects of growth differentiation factor-5 on the intervertebral disc--in vitro bovine study and in vivo rabbit disc degeneration model study. *Spine (Phila Pa 1976)* 2006;31:2909-2917.

91. Xia K, Zhu J, Hua J, et al: Intradiscal injection of induced pluripotent stem cell-derived nucleus pulposus-like cell-seeded polymeric microspheres promotes rat disc regeneration. *Stem Cells Int* 2019;2019:6806540.

92. Miyazaki S, Diwan AD, Kato K, et al: Issls PRIZE in basic SCIENCE 2018: Growth differentiation factor-6 attenuated pro-inflammatory molecular changes in the rabbit anular-puncture model and degenerated disc-induced pain generation in the rat xenograft radiculopathy model. *Eur Spine J* 2018;27:739-751.

93. Cui H, Zhang J, Li Z, et al: Growth differentiation factor-6 attenuates inflammatory and pain-related factors and degenerated disc-induced pain behaviors in rat model. *J Orthop Res* 2021;39:959-970.

94. Mwale F, Masuda K, Pichika R, et al: The efficacy of Link N as a mediator of repair in a rabbit model of intervertebral disc degeneration. *Arthritis Res Ther* 2011;13:R120.

95. Mwale F, Masuda K, Grant MP, et al: Short Link N promotes disc repair in a rabbit model of disc degeneration. *Arthritis Res Ther* 2018;20:201.

96. Olmarker K, Gerward A, Isberg B, Lehmann A, Berg S: Translational studies on biologic fusion of a vertebral segment as a novel treatment modality for low back pain. *Spine (Phila Pa 1976)* 2020;45:E1636-E1644.

97. Nagae M, Ikeda T, Mikami Y, et al: Intervertebral disc regeneration using platelet-rich plasma and biodegradable gelatin hydrogel microspheres. *Tissue Eng Part A* 2007;13:147-158.

98. Sawamura K, Ikeda T, Nagae M, et al: Characterization of in vivo effects of platelet-rich plasma and biodegradable

gelatin hydrogel microspheres on degenerated intervertebral discs. *Tissue Eng Part A* 2009;15:3719-3727.

99. Obata S, Akeda K, Imanishi T, et al: Effect of autologous platelet-rich plasma-releasate on intervertebral disc degeneration in the rabbit anular puncture model: A preclinical study. *Arthritis Res Ther* 2012;14:R241.
100. Sudo H, Minami A: Caspase 3 as a therapeutic target for regulation of intervertebral disc degeneration in rabbits. *Arthritis Rheum* 2011;63:1648-1657.
101. Kato K, Akeda K, Miyazaki S, et al: NF-kB decoy oligodeoxynucleotide preserves disc height in a rabbit anular-puncture model and reduces pain induction in a rat xenograft-radiculopathy model. *Eur Cell Mater* 2021;41:90-109.
102. Yan J, Yang S, Sun H, et al: Effects of releasing recombinant human growth and differentiation factor-5 from poly(lactic-co-glycolic acid) microspheres for repair of the rat degenerated intervertebral disc. *J Biomater Appl* 2014;29(1):72-80.
103. An HS, Takegami K, Kamada H, et al: Intradiscal administration of osteogenic protein-1 increases intervertebral disc height and proteoglycan content in the nucleus pulposus in normal adolescent rabbits. *Spine* 2005;30(1):25-31, discussion 31-32.
104. Wei A, Williams LA, Bhargav D, et al: BMP13 prevents the effects of annular injury in an ovine model. *Int J Biol Sci* 2009;5(5):388-396.
105. Hu MH, Yang KC, Chen YJ, Sun YH, Yang SH: Lovastatin prevents discographyassociated degeneration and maintains the functional morphology of intervertebral discs. *Spine J* 2014;14(10):2459-2466.
106. Zhang H, Wang L, Park JB, et al: Intradiscal injection of simvastatin retards progression of intervertebral disc degeneration induced by stab injury. *Arthritis Res Ther* 2009;11(6):R172.
107. Than KD, Rahman SU, Wang L, et al: Intradiscal injection of simvastatin results in radiologic, histologic, and genetic evidence of disc regeneration in a rat model of degenerative disc disease. *Spine J* 2014;14(6):1017-1028.
108. Masuda K, Imai Y, Okuma M, et al: Osteogenic protein-1 injection into a degenerated disc induces the restoration of disc height and structural changes in the rabbit anular puncture model. *Spine (Phila Pa 1976)* 2006;31:742-754.
109. Matta A, Karim MZ, Isenman DE, Erwin WM: Molecular therapy for degenerative disc disease: Clues from secretome analysis of the notochordal cell-rich nucleus pulposus. *Sci Rep* 2017;7:45623.
110. Mwale F, Demers CN, Petit A, et al: A synthetic peptide of link protein stimulates the biosynthesis of collagens II, IX and proteoglycan by cells of the intervertebral disc. *J Cell Biochem* 2003;88:1202-1213.
111. Petit A, Yao G, Rowas SA, et al: Effect of synthetic link N peptide on the expression of type I and type II collagens in human intervertebral disc cells. *Tissue Eng Part A* 2011;17:899-904.
112. Wang Z, Hutton WC, Yoon ST: ISSLS Prize winner: Effect of link protein peptide on human intervertebral disc cells. *Spine (Phila Pa 1976)* 2013;38:1501-1507.
113. AlGarni N, Grant MP, Epure LM, et al: Short link N stimulates intervertebral disc repair in a novel long-term organ culture model that includes the bony vertebrae. *Tissue Eng Part A* 2016;22:1252-1257.
114. Wang S, Liu C, Sun Z, et al: IL-1beta increases asporin expression via the NF-kappaB p65 pathway in nucleus pulposus cells during intervertebral disc degeneration. *Sci Rep* 2017;7:4112.
115. Nakamura H, Aoki M, Tamai K, et al: Prevention and regression of atopic dermatitis by ointment containing NF-kB decoy oligodeoxynucleotides in NC/Nga atopic mouse model. *Gene Ther* 2002;9:1221-1229.
116. Matsuda N, Hattori Y, Jesmin S, Gando S: Nuclear factor-kappaB decoy oligodeoxynucleotides prevent acute lung injury in mice with cecal ligation and puncture-induced sepsis. *Mol Pharmacol* 2005;67:1018-1025.
117. Morishita R, Sugimoto T, Aoki M, et al: In vivo transfection of cis element "decoy" against nuclear factor-kappaB binding site prevents myocardial infarction. *Nat Med* 1997;3:894-899.
118. Akeda K, An H, Gemba T, et al: Effect of the continuous exposure to naked NFκb decoy oligodeoxynucleotide on matrix accumulation and catabolic enzyme production by human intervertebral disc cells. *Orthop Res Soc Trans* 2007;32:321.
119. Kato K, Akeda K, Miyazaki S, et al: NF-κB decoy oligodeoxynucleotide preserves disc height in the rabbit anular-puncture model and reduces pain induction in the rat xenograft-radiculopathy model. *Eur Cell Mater* 2021;42:90-109.
120. Akeda K, Yamada J, Linn ET, Sudo A, Masuda K: Platelet-rich plasma in the management of chronic low back pain: A critical review. *J Pain Res* 2019;12:753-767.
121. Qiu S, Shi C, Anbazhagan AN, et al: Absence of VEGFR-1/Flt-1 signaling pathway in mice results in insensitivity to discogenic low back pain in an established disc injury mouse model. *J Cell Physiol* 2020;235:5305-5317.
122. Akeda K, An HS, Pichika R, et al: Platelet-rich plasma (PRP) stimulates the extracellular matrix metabolism of porcine nucleus pulposus and anulus fibrosus cells cultured in alginate beads. *Spine (Phila Pa 1976)* 2006;31:959-966.
123. Chen WH, Liu HY, Lo WC, et al: Intervertebral disc regeneration in an ex vivo culture system using mesenchymal stem cells and platelet-rich plasma. *Biomaterials* 2009;30:5523-5533.
124. Gullung GB, Woodall JW, Tucci MA, James J, Black DA, McGuire RA: Platelet-rich plasma effects on degenerative disc disease: Analysis of histology and imaging in an animal model. *Evid Based Spine Care J* 2011;2:13-18.
125. Schol J, Sakai D: Cell therapy for intervertebral disc herniation and degenerative disc disease: Clinical trials. *Int Orthop* 2019;43:1011-1025.
126. Sakai D, Andersson GB: Stem cell therapy for intervertebral disc regeneration: Obstacles and solutions. *Nat Rev Rheumatol* 2015;11:243-256.
127. Benneker LM, Andersson G, Iatridis JC, et al: Cell therapy for intervertebral disc repair: Advancing cell therapy from bench to clinics. *Eur Cell Mater* 2014;27:5-11.

128. Acosta FL Jr. Metz L, Adkisson HD, et al: Porcine intervertebral disc repair using allogeneic juvenile articular chondrocytes or mesenchymal stem cells. *Tissue Eng Part A* 2011;17:3045-3055.

129. Kusafuka K, Hiraki Y, Shukunami C, Kayano T, Takemura T: Cartilage-specific matrix protein, chondromodulin-I (ChM-I), is a strong angio-inhibitor in endochondral ossification of human neonatal vertebral tissues in vivo: Relationship with angiogenic factors in the cartilage. *Acta Histochem* 2002;104:167-175.

130. Iyer SS, Rojas M: Anti-inflammatory effects of mesenchymal stem cells: Novel concept for future therapies. *Expert Opin Biol Ther* 2008;8:569-581.

131. Planat-Benard V, Silvestre JS, Cousin B, et al: Plasticity of human adipose lineage cells toward endothelial cells: Physiological and therapeutic perspectives. *Circulation* 2004;109:656-663.

132. Takeuchi R, Katagiri W, Endo S, Kobayashi T: Exosomes from conditioned media of bone marrow-derived mesenchymal stem cells promote bone regeneration by enhancing angiogenesis. *PLoS One* 2019;14:e0225472.

133. Mwale F, Roughley P, Antoniou J: Distinction between the extracellular matrix of the nucleus pulposus and hyaline cartilage: A requisite for tissue engineering of intervertebral disc. *Eur Cell Mater* 2004;8:58-63.

134. Silverman LI, Dulatova G, Tandeski T, et al: In vitro and in vivo evaluation of discogenic cells, an investigational cell therapy for disc degeneration. *Spine J* 2020;20:138-149.

135. Hiraishi S, Schol J, Sakai D, et al: Discogenic cell transplantation directly from a cryopreserved state in an induced intervertebral disc degeneration canine model. *JOR Spine* 2018;1:e1013.

136. Ghosh P, Moore R, Vernon-Roberts B, et al: Immunoselected STRO-3+ mesenchymal precursor cells and restoration of the extracellular matrix of degenerate intervertebral discs. *J Neurosurg Spine* 2012;16:479-488.

137. Freeman BJC, Kuliwaba JS, Jones CF, et al: Allogeneic mesenchymal precursor cells promote healing in postero-lateral annular lesions and improve indices of lumbar intervertebral disc degeneration in an ovine model. *Spine (Phila Pa 1976)* 2016;41:1331-1339.

138. Alini M, Eisenstein SM, Ito K, et al: Are animal models useful for studying human disc disorders/degeneration? *Eur Spine J* 2008;17:2-19.

139. AnGes. Available at: https://www.anges.co.jp/pdf_news/public/w13OHVBcAodV5whV1pWETyvEgxH7xoE0.pdf. 2021.

140. Gimbel JS, Kivitz AJ, Bramson C, et al: Long-term safety and effectiveness of tanezumab as treatment for chronic low back pain. *Pain* 2014;155:1793-1801.

141. Coric D, Pettine K, Sumich A, Boltes MO: Prospective study of disc repair with allogeneic chondrocytes presented at the 2012 joint spine section meeting. *J Neurosurg Spine* 2013;18:85-95.

142. Haufe SM, Mork AR: Intradiscal injection of hematopoietic stem cells in an attempt to rejuvenate the intervertebral discs. *Stem Cells Dev* 2006;15:136-137.

143. Noriega DC, Ardura F, Hernandez-Ramajo R, et al: Intervertebral disc repair by allogeneic mesenchymal bone marrow cells: A randomized controlled trial. *Transplantation* 2017;101:1945-1951.

144. Amirdelfan K, Bae H, McJunkin T, et al: Allogeneic mesenchymal precursor cells treatment for chronic low back pain associated with degenerative disc disease: A prospective randomized, placebo-controlled 36-month study of safety and efficacy. *Spine J* 2021;21:212-230.

145. Orozco L, Soler R, Morera C, Alberca M, Sanchez A, Garcia-Sancho J: Intervertebral disc repair by autologous mesenchymal bone marrow cells: A pilot study. *Transplantation* 2011;92:822-828.

146. Elabd C, Centeno CJ, Schultz JR, Lutz G, Ichim T, Silva FJ: Intra-discal injection of autologous, hypoxic cultured bone marrow-derived mesenchymal stem cells in five patients with chronic lower back pain: A long-term safety and feasibility study. *J Transl Med* 2016;14:253.

147. Centeno C, Markle J, Dodson E, et al: Treatment of lumbar degenerative disc disease-associated radicular pain with culture-expanded autologous mesenchymal stem cells: A pilot study on safety and efficacy. *J Transl Med* 2017;15:197.

148. Pettine K, Suzuki R, Sand T, Murphy M: Treatment of discogenic back pain with autologous bone marrow concentrate injection with minimum two year follow-up. *Int Orthop* 2016;40:135-140.

149. Tschugg A, Diepers M, Simone S, et al: A prospective randomized multicenter phase I/II clinical trial to evaluate safety and efficacy of NOVOCART disk plus autologous disk chondrocyte transplantation in the treatment of nucleotomized and degenerative lumbar disks to avoid secondary disease: Safety results of phase I-a short report. *Neurosurg Rev* 2017;40:155-162.

150. Meisel HJ, Ganey T, Hutton WC, Libera J, Minkus Y, Alasevic O: Clinical experience in cell-based therapeutics: Intervention and outcome. *Eur Spine J* 2006;15(suppl 3):S397-S405.

151. Mochida J, Sakai D, Nakamura Y, Watanabe T, Yamamoto Y, Kato S: Intervertebral disc repair with activated nucleus pulposus cell transplantation: A three-year, prospective clinical study of its safety. *Eur Cell Mater* 2015;29:202-212.

152. Piccirilli M, Delfinis CP, Santoro A, Salvati M: Mesenchymal stem cells in lumbar spine surgery: A single institution experience about red bone marrow and fat tissue derived MSCs. *J Neurosurg Sci* 2017;61:124-133.

153. Kumar H, Ha DH, Lee EJ, et al: Safety and tolerability of intradiscal implantation of combined autologous adipose-derived mesenchymal stem cells and hyaluronic acid in patients with chronic discogenic low back pain: 1-year follow-up of a phase I study. *Stem Cell Res Ther* 2017;8:262.

154. Comella K, Silbert R, Parlo M: Effects of the intradiscal implantation of stromal vascular fraction plus platelet rich plasma in patients with degenerative disc disease. *J Transl Med* 2017;15:12.

155. Henriksson HB, Papadimitriou N, Hingert D, Baranto A, Lindahl A, Brisby H: The traceability of mesenchymal stromal cells after injection into degenerated discs in patients with low back pain. *Stem Cells Dev* 2019;28:1203-1211.

156. Yoshikawa T, Ueda Y, Miyazaki K, Koizumi M, Takakura Y: Disc regeneration therapy using marrow mesenchymal cell

transplantation: A report of two case studies. *Spine (Phila Pa 1976)* 2010;35:E475-E480.

157. Pang X, Yang H, Peng B: Human umbilical cord mesenchymal stem cell transplantation for the treatment of chronic discogenic low back pain. *Pain Physician* 2014;17:E525-E530.
158. Binch ALA, Fitzgerald JC, Growney EA, Barry F: Cell-based strategies for IVD repair: Clinical progress and translational obstacles. *Nat Rev Rheumatol* 2021;17:158-175.
159. Sakai D, Schol J: Cell therapy for intervertebral disc repair: Clinical perspective. *J Orthop Translat* 2017;9:8-18.
160. Roberts S, Menage J, Urban JP: Biochemical and structural properties of the cartilage end-plate and its relation to the intervertebral disc. *Spine (Phila Pa 1976)* 1989;14:166-174.
161. Bae WC, He J, Shieh I, Yamaguchi T, Inoue N, Masuda K: *Endplate Roughness in Human Lumbar Spines: Variations With Age, Level and Region.* The International Society for the Study of the Lumbar Spine, 2013, p GP82.
162. Carragee EJ, Don AS, Hurwitz EL, Cuellar JM, Carrino JA, Herzog R: 2009 ISSLS prize winner: Does discography cause accelerated progression of degeneration changes in the lumbar disc – A ten-year matched cohort study. *Spine (Phila Pa 1976)* 2009;34:2338-2345.
163. Gruber HE, Rhyne AL III, Hansen KJ, et al: Deleterious effects of discography radiocontrast solution on human annulus cell in vitro: Changes in cell viability, proliferation, and apoptosis in exposed cells. *Spine J* 2012;12:329-335.
164. Chee AV, Ren J, Lenart BA, Chen EY, Zhang Y, An HS: Cytotoxicity of local anesthetics and nonionic contrast agents on bovine intervertebral disc cells cultured in a three-dimensional culture system. *Spine J* 2014;14:491-498.
165. Iwasaki K, Sudo H, Yamada K, Ito M, Iwasaki N: Cytotoxic effects of the radiocontrast agent iotrolan and anesthetic agents bupivacaine and lidocaine in three-dimensional cultures of human intervertebral disc nucleus pulposus cells: Identification of the apoptotic pathways. *PLoS One* 2014;9:e92442.
166. Kim KH, Park JY, Park HS, et al: Which iodinated contrast media is the least cytotoxic to human disc cells? *Spine J* 2015;15:1021-1027.
167. Huang X, Wang W, Meng Q, et al: Effect of needle diameter, type and volume of contrast agent on intervertebral disc degeneration in rats with discography. *Eur Spine J* 2019;28:1014-1022.
168. Masuda K, Aota Y, Muehleman C, et al: A novel rabbit model of mild, reproducible disc degeneration by an anulus needle puncture: Correlation between the degree of disc injury and radiological and histological appearances of disc degeneration. *Spine (Phila Pa 1976)* 2005;30:5-14.
169. Gregory D, Bae W, Sah RL, Masuda K: Disc degeneration reduces the delamination strength of the anulus fibrosis in the rabbit anular disc puncture model. *Spine J* 2013;14(7):1265-1271.

CHAPTER 33

Spine Fusion—Bioactive Factor Based

Hyun W. Bae, MD • Michael Eng, MD • Linda E. A. Kanim, MA • Justin D. Cohen, MD • Juliane Glaeser, PhD • Julie L. Chan, MD, PhD

INTRODUCTION

An overview with current updates on bioactive materials that may be used as an adjunct in spinal fusion surgery is provided. For the purpose of this review, bioactives encompass a diverse group of compounds raging from bone grafts, synthetic materials, and even growth factors. In regard to spinal fusion, these materials can be used to increase the potential for successful fusion. Years of research have made a number of off-the-shelf preparations available, which vary widely in their material component(s), size, shape, consistency, porosity, absorbency, and strength, targeting different pathways to augment spinal fusion. Although manufacturing companies provide proprietary instructions regarding the use of bioactives during surgical procedures, the individual surgeon also introduces an added element by potentially combining more than one product to promote spinal fusion.

Historically, evidence of bony fusion has been observed and described with bone grafting material. Since then, bone grafts including autograft, allograft, and even synthetic grafts have been used in bony fusion. Although bone grafts provide excellent scaffolds for bony fusion, there may be cases where autograft alone is insufficient. To meet this need, high-quality research has developed and investigated a number of biologics such as demineralized bone matrix (DBM), cellular-based allografts, cellular bone matrix (CBM), and bone morphogenetic protein (BMP), which have been further developed into marketable products for spine fusion. In addition, there are also alternative synthetic materials including bioactive glass (BAG), growth factors, and polypeptides that may increase the efficacy of grafting in spinal fusion. Although an extensive number of bioactive factor–based products are available for use, understanding their safety and efficacy, as well as how to best optimize their use in spinal fusion, continues to be evaluated. A clearer understanding of the bioactive materials that may be used to promote bony fusion will allow spine surgeons to make an informed choice in their selection and use of bioactive materials during spinal fusion surgery. Here, a historical account of fusion-promoting materials is provided and the utility of bioactive factor–based materials that are currently being used to augment spinal fusion is discussed.

DEFINITION OF THE PATHOLOGY AND NATURAL HISTORY

The spine is subject to a wide variety of pathologies including trauma, oncologic disease, congenital anomalies, deformity, and degenerative disease. Although some spine conditions may remain asymptomatic and without clinical sequelae, many conditions affect significant pain, and if left untreated, they can lead to severe disability. These conditions often require spinal fusion to reduce pain, reduce or prevent neurologic injury, and return patients to a functional status. Following acute traumatic spinal fractures, or in the face of tumor pathology, disruption of the anatomic bony and ligamentous elements can lead to an unstable spinal column. To return spinal stability and prevent or reduce further neurologic injury, patients often undergo spinal fusion. In addition to patients who experience spine trauma, patients with insidious conditions such as spinal deformity with significant spine curvature may require correction of the abnormal angles. Curves greater than 90° have been shown to be associated with cardiopulmonary dysfunction. In addition, patients with untreated larger scoliotic curves may demonstrate signs of myelopathy, decreased mobility, and increased levels of back pain.

Although there are many patients who undergo spinal fusion for traumatic injury or deformity correction, one of the most common disease processes that may require spinal fusion is degenerative disk disease. Degenerative disk disease is a process that often develops with increasing age, and its natural history has been described in both the cervical spine and lumbar spine.[1] The stages of the degenerative

Dr. Bae or an immediate family member has received royalties from Biomet, DePuy, A Johnson & Johnson Company, Nuvasive, Prosidyan, Stryker, and Zimmer; is a member of a speakers' bureau or has made paid presentations on behalf of DePuy, A Johnson & Johnson Company, Nuvasive, Stryker, and Zimmer; serves as a paid consultant to or is an employee of Zimmer; has stock or stock options held in Medtronic and Stryker, orthovita, spinal restoration, difusion; has received research or institutional support from Empirical Spine, Medtronic, Nuvasive, OrthoRebirth, Relievant, Simplify Medical, and SpineArt; and serves as a board member, owner, officer, or committee member of KASS. Linda E. A. Kanim or an immediate family member has stock or stock options held in Abbott, Medtronic <5,000$, and Moderna. Dr. Chan or an immediate family member has received research or institutional support from Misonix and has received nonincome support (such as equipment or services), commercially derived honoraria, or other non–research-related funding (such as paid travel) from Misonix. None of the following authors or any immediate family member has received anything of value from or has stock or stock options held in a commercial company or institution related directly or indirectly to the subject of this chapter: Dr. Eng, Dr. Cohen, and Dr. Glaeser.

process are dysfunction (aged 15 to 45 years), instability (aged 35 to 70 years), and then rigid stabilization (older than 60 years).[1] Degenerative disk disease may occur anywhere throughout the spine, and it is most common in the cervical and lumbar spine. Over years, the nucleus pulposus composed mainly of water, type II collagen, and proteoglycans/aggrecan loses water and proteoglycans. This leads to a more fibrotic consistency, subsequent fissuring, and calcification of the vertebral end plates, which interrupts end plate–facilitated nutrition. In addition to the natural aging process, the intervertebral disk may undergo traumatic radial and circumferential tears, which may lead to decreases in the gellike consistency of the nucleus pulposus. In either case, disruption of the physiologic features of the intervertebral disk, which typically absorbs stress and provides motion, results in abnormal and pathologic pressure on the other components of the spine, increasing the likelihood for facet joint and end plate disruption. The body's natural response to degenerating intervertebral disk and subsequent spinal instability includes proliferation to induce bone hypertrophy in attempts to stabilize the spine.

These degenerative changes in the spine are not without clinical sequelae. As the nucleus pulposus loses its elasticity and gel-like component, it may extrude toward the spinal canal and neural foramen, causing compression of the spinal cord and/or nerve roots leading to myelopathy and radiculopathy. Furthermore, reactive hypertrophy of the ligamentum flavum, facets, and other bony anatomy may also contribute to symptomatic neural compromise or injury. Some patients may also have abnormal motion of the facet joints causing pain with motion. In addition to the physical components these pathologic degenerative processes play, there may also be concurrent ischemic and/or pro-inflammatory cascades, which increase pain related to degeneration. Degenerative changes may lead to stenosis of the central spinal canal and/or neuroforamina inducing low back pain, neurogenic claudication, and/or radiculopathy. If left untreated, these conditions can progress with increasing levels of pain, limiting function during daily activities, and ultimately reducing quality of life.

TREATMENT/MANAGEMENT

The goals for the treatment of any spinal pathology are to halt disease progression, decrease pain, increase function and mobility, and minimize the duration and/or recurrence of symptoms.[1] Initial nonsurgical management includes pharmacologic agents such as NSAIDs, steroids, and muscle relaxants; physical therapy; and occasionally temporary immobilization to reduce inflammation, pain, and disability.[1] If nonsurgical modalities fail to improve symptoms, surgical intervention often involves decompression of the involved elements and spinal fusion. Spinal arthrodesis is a surgical procedure used to stabilize the spine. It can be used to manage various spine pathologies with the overall goal to prevent further injury to the neural elements and/or reduce the risk of additional clinical sequelae by returning the spine to a more anatomic position. Although instrumentation and hardware are placed to aid in the correction of pathologic anatomy or physiology, the goal is to achieve solid bony fusion for long-term correction. To achieve spinal fusion, many graft materials and bioactive products have been developed and used to accelerate and augment this process.[2]

Bone Grafting Materials in Spinal Fusion

Although early spinal fusion dates to the early 1900s,[3] many of the same goals and principles of grafting for fracture healing and spine fusion are used in contemporary spine arthrodesis procedures.[4-6] The fundamental concepts of physiologic processes through which different grafts work include osteoinduction, osteogenesis, osteoconduction, which were described by Albee,[4] and osseointegration described and defined by Branemark et al[7] and Albrektsson et al,[8] respectively. Osteogenesis, or the formation of bone, occurs by way of osteoinduction, or the recruitment of progenitor cells, a process typically seen in healing bone. Osteoconduction, or bone growth on a surface, however, is more likely to be seen with spinal fusion with implant use. Finally, osseointegration is the process of achieving stability through contact between the bone and implant.

Successful spinal fusions are fundamentally dependent on bony fusion as evidenced by formation of bridging bone between the intended vertebral segments on radiographs. Pseudarthrosis or nonunion is considered a failure of fusion and is defined by lack of bridging bone on radiographs that correlates with persistent or recurrent symptoms. Long-term fusion rates after spine surgery vary significantly. At 1 to 2 years postoperatively, overall incidence of failure was 34.3% in lumbopelvic fixation,[9] whereas adult scoliosis demonstrates 17% nonunion in patients aged 18 to 55 years.[10] Unlike for the thoracolumbar spine, fusion rates in the cervical spine are much more robust, with some reports describing 94.7% fusion success in the cervical spine.[11]

In the interest of increasing the potential for solid spine arthrodesis following surgery, research has attempted to harness and augment the basic properties of bone growth through the development of new biologics. Osteogenic grafts including autologous bone grafts, that is, iliac crest bone graft (ICBG), local surgical site bone, bone marrow aspirate in scaffolds, and potentially cellular allografts, directly provide cells that can differentiate to form bone. Osteoinductive bone graft materials such as recombinant human bone morphogenetic protein 2 (rhBMP-2) and osteogenic protein-1 contain bioactive factors that induce differentiation of locally recruited tissue-specific progenitor cells and/or host stem cells into bone-forming cells. Specifically, these proteins can recruit and act on host cells to regulate differentiation into osteoblastic cells. Osteoconductive grafting materials such as freeze-dried crushed cancellous bone chips provide structural and/or mechanical scaffolds onto which new bone can be formed.

In practice, to achieve successful spinal fusion, surgeons may use different grafts with variable bioactive profiles to increase the likelihood of forming solid bone at the site of intended arthrodesis. **Table 1** summarizes

TABLE 1 Classifications of Bone Grafting Materials and Bone-Forming Properties

Grafting Material (Donor Site Morbidity)	Grafting Material (Typical Abbreviation)	Grafting Material Category and Description (Commercially Used Product in Spine)	Variability	Osteogenic	Osteoinductive	Osteoconductive	Immunogenicity/ Disease Transmission	Strength (Immediate)	Safety
Autograft									
Autograft (+++)	Iliac crest bone graft (ICBG)	More cancellous (mercerized and/or strut form)	Patient's self-bone quality	+++	++	+++	–	+++	+++
Autograft (+/–)	Local bone (LB, LAG)	More cortical (mostly mercerized form)		+/–	+	+	–	+/–	+++
Autograft (–)	Bone dust	Generated via high-speed burr on bone surface		+/– (less than local bone)	+/– (less than local bone)	+/– (less than local bone)	–	–	+++
Autograft (–)	[a]Platelet concentrate	Plasma preparation with increased platelet concentration	Patient's own health status`	+/–	++ (activation of growth factors)	–	–	–	+++
Autograft Bone marrow aspirate (+)	[a]Osteogenic cell with growth factors	Most common source of MSC Local surgical site (decortication) Harvested from iliac crest		+ (variable according to self-donor's condition, typically)	+ (variable according to self-donor's condition)	– (could be added to a carrier, ie, ACS)	–	–	+++
Allograft									
Allograft (–)	Fresh	1. Living donor (patient-to-patient transfer) 2. Cadaver donor (harvested within 12 hours and allotransplantation within 72 hours) → Femoral head (as osteochondral form)	Lot-to-lot variability of donor's bone condition + sterilization processing techniques Demineralization processes + particle sizes	? (no data for osteogenic graft for human)	? (no data for osteogenic graft for human)	? (no data for osteogenic graft for human)	+++ (generally causes an unacceptable host immune reaction as osteogenic graft) → Not used commercially, only animal studies		–
Allograft (–)	Fresh (osteochondral graft)	1. Living donor (patient-to-patient transfer) 2. Cadaver donor (harvested within 12 hours and allotransplantation within 24 hours) → Femoral head (as osteochondral form)		+/– (only chondrocyte viability remain)	–	++	+ (reduced/mild immune reaction by cartilaginous portion of graft) + (infection risk due to storage media)	++ (grafted at articular portion for weight supporting)	–
Allograft (–)	Fresh-frozen	From 1. Living donor 2. Cadaver donor		–	–	++ (less than autogenous bone)	+ (reported cases)	++	–

(Continued)

TABLE 1 Classifications of Bone Grafting Materials and Bone-Forming Properties (Continued)

Grafting Material (Donor Site Morbidity)	Grafting Material (Typical Abbreviation)	Grafting Material Category and Description (Commercially Used Product in Spine)	Variability	Osteogenic	Osteoinductive	Osteoconductive	Immunogenicity/ Disease Transmission	Strength (Immediate)	Safety
Allograft (–)	Freeze-dried	From 1. Living donor 2. Cadaver donor		–	–	++	+/–	+/– (significantly affected by drying process)	–
Allograft (–)	Gamma sterilization			–	–	++	+/–	+ (by radiation effect)	–
Allograft	Demineralized bone matrix (DBM, bone powder)	Mostly cadaver donors		–	+/–	++	+/–	–	+/–
Selective cell retained allografts	Osteogenic cell (eg, Cellentra, Trinity, ViviGen, Osteocel, Map3, and Bio4)		Donor characteristics	++++ (recently lots recalled due to tuberculosis contamination)	+/–	–	– (serious adverse events reported)	–	—
Allograft	Cell infused (CBMs)						—		—
Differentiation Factors (US Regulatory Approvals: HUD and HDE/Combination Products)									
Differentiation/ growth factor	rhBMP-2	Differentiation/growth factor (approved w/ ACS and/or w/ Mastergraft)	High manufacturing inconsistency	–	+++	–	–	–	+/–
	rhBMP-7	Differentiation/growth factor (no longer manufactured in the United States)		–	+++	–	–	–	+/–
Peptides	B2A	Bioactive synthetic peptide		–	–	++	–	–	+/–
	P-15	Bioactive synthetic peptide		–	–	++	–	–	+/–
[a]Synthetic Ceramics									
Tricalcium phosphate	TCP	Synthetic ceramics		–	–	++	–	–	–
Hydroxyapatite	Hydroxyapatite	Synthetic ceramics		–	–	++	–	+/–	–
Biphasic calcium phosphate	BCP	Synthetic ceramics		–	–	++	–	+/–	–
Calcium sulfate	Calcium sulfate	Synthetic ceramics		–	–	++	–	–	–
[a]Synthetic Bioactive Glasses (BAGs) (US Regulatory Approvals, FDA 510(k))									
Synthetic BAG	45S5	BAG with 45% silicate		–	+	++	–	+/–	+
	S53P4	BAG with 53% silicate			+	+ (less bioactive than 45S5)			+

Silicon nitride spinal implants	Si3N4	Inorganic, nonmetallic, nonoxide ceramic				+/–			+ (no cytotoxic effects, Fiani 2021[29])
PMMAs—new versions (antifungals)									
[a]Others Less Commonly Used									
Xenograft	Xenograft	From nonhuman species, mainly bovine-based bone graft (ie, bovine type I collagen, ACS/bACS)	Donor variability	–	+/– (sterilization process)	+	+++ (more than allograft)	++ (in spine, foot and ankle, and trauma part)	–
Type I collagen (ie, bACS)	Xenograft carrier (bovine)	Osteoconductive scaffold/hemostasis (ACS)	Anatomic source location and species	–	–	+	–	+/–	–
Combinations Mixed Grafts, Peptides, Growth Differentiating Factors, Cellularized Grafts (US Regulatory Approvals, FDA 510(k), AATB, USFDA 21 CFR, HCT/P), Combination Products									
Allograft w/growth factors or peptides (–)	Osteoconductive scaffold/putty w/ peptides	Donor variability	–	–/–	+	+++	+/–	–	–
Xenograft carrier (bovine) (–)	Osteoconductive scaffolds/hemostasis (ACS, bACS)		–	–	+	–	+/–	–	–

[a]Not discussed herein except as a composite preparation in one of the other mixed products.

+++ Characteristic is definitely observed from biologic, clinical, and preclinical studies.

++ Characteristic is somewhat observed from biologic, clinical, and preclinical studies.

+ Suggested by clinical and preclinical studies. There may be some controversy or effect is minimal.

+/– Debate status.

w/ mixed with.

– None/no effect.

21 CFR = Code of Federal Regulations Title 21, AATB = American Association of Tissue Banks, ACS = absorbable collagen sponge, and cellular and tissue-based products, CBMs = cellular bone matrices, HCT/P = human cells, HDE = Humanitarian Device Exemption, HUD = Humanitarian Use Device, IDE = Investigational Device Exemption, MSC = mesenchymal stromal cell, PMMAs = polymethylmethacrylate, rhBMP = recombinant human bone morphogenetic protein, tissues.

Adapted by permisssion from Springer: Yang JH, Glaeser JD, Kanim LEA, Battles CY, Bondre S, Bae HW: *Bone grafts and bone graft substitutes*, in *Handbook of Spine Technologies*. Springer, 2021.

the different types of grafting materials and their corresponding bone-forming characteristics.[12-28] Descriptions of classes of grafting materials for fusion and bone graft characteristics have been discussed in the literature.[30-33]

Autologous Bone Graft

The gold standard for bone grafting is autologous bone graft because it intrinsically possesses osteoinductive, osteoconductive, and osteogenic properties.[34] ICBG is one of the most commonly used autograft in orthopaedic surgery and is a viable choice for spinal fusion.[6] Autologous bone graft is cleaned of soft tissue and minced into pieces of various sizes and commonly combined with other grafting materials to increase volume.

However, autologous bone graft is not without downsides. Known iliac crest donor-site complications include pain, hematoma formation, infection, and fracture. Tuchman et al[35] reported donor-site morbidity (3.8%, 5.3%), pain (7.2%, 22%), infection (2.4%, 6.8%), and hematoma (1.6%, 4.5%) in patients who received an autograft (none in allograft) across 13 identified cervical fusion studies where there were similar number of patients fused (62% to 100% autograft versus 70% to 100% allograft). Comparison of fusion rates, pain scores, and functional outcomes between allografts and iliac crest autografts in six studies showed no difference in fusion percentages or functional results comparing local autograft or allograft with iliac crest autograft. In addition, donor-site pain and hematoma/seroma occurred more frequently in ICBG autograft group for lumbar fusion procedures.[36] Furthermore, Radcliff et al noted no significant differences in postoperative complications or reoperation rates between patients with degenerative lumbar spondylolisthesis who underwent fusion with iliac crest autograft compared with those who underwent fusion without iliac crest autograft.[37] They also detected no significant differences between scores for the groups on Medical Outcomes Study 36-Item Short Form, Oswestry Disability Index, Stenosis Bothersomeness Index, and Low Back Pain Bothersomeness Scale.

Allograft

Allografts are a popular alternative to autologous bone graft in areas where they are commercially available (the United States, parts of Europe, Korea, Australia, Latin America, India, China, and the Middle East) and frequently used by surgeons because of the ease of access. Allografts are particularly useful in cases where the need for bone-fusing materials exceeds that of reasonably obtainable autograft such as multilevel surgeries, repeat surgeries, and interbody fusion. Surgeons can take advantage of commercially available allografts to augment postoperative bony fusion while also reducing host donor-site morbidity. Allografts come in a variety of different preparations that make them useful for varying surgical applications. In general, allografts are obtained from either living or deceased donors, then processed to remove donor antigens, and sterilized. Most allografts possess osteoconductive properties with minimal osteoinductive properties because many of the osteoinductive factors are reduced during processing and sterilization. In addition, allografts typically have minimal osteogenic properties, although newer allografts may either contain, retain, or are frequently enhanced with viable cells and therefore can possess all three properties.

Fresh allograft is rarely used because of risk of immune response and disease transmission. Even with the existence of processing techniques to remove donor cells and reduce host immune responses to the graft, the risk of disease transmission is not entirely eliminated. Frozen and freeze-dried allografts have reduced immunogenicity compared with fresh allograft, yet still present risk of infection or disease transmission. The fact that classically prepared allografts contain only nonviable tissue necessitates the addition of bone-stimulating factors, such as growth factors, cells, or other materials. Allografts are frequently combined with local bone autograft in spinal surgery.

Various allografts are used during spinal fusion surgery. Cortical allografts, such as femoral ring allografts, are often used for interbody fusion because of their structural properties. Cancellous chip allografts are used as osteoconductive scaffolding in posterolateral fusions. Different forms of allograft[38-49] are presented in **Table 2**.

Demineralized Bone Matrix

DBM possesses both osteoconductive and osteoinductive properties. It is formed by processing bone in a way that removes the mineral content of bone while retaining the organic components, such as type I collagen, proteins, and various growth factors.[50] Despite having both osteoconductive and osteoinductive properties, the osteoinductive properties of DBMs are relatively decreased compared with autograft. Therefore, they are frequently used in conjunction with other graft products or augments, such as morcellized autograft, differentiation/growth factors, and bone marrow aspirate. DBM-based grafting products used in conjunction with other graft augments avoid the known morbidities associated with ICBG, while maintaining comparable outcomes. No statistical difference in fusion rates at 2 years comparing Grafton DBM matrix + local bone versus autologous ICBG in single-level posterior lumbar fusions was reported.[38] In addition, fusion rates between Grafton DBM matrix and DBX were similar at 1 and 2 years.[39]

Clinical utilization of DBM-based products is not without its challenges. Bae et al demonstrated significant variability in DBM-based products between manufacturers, product preparations, and even lot-based batches from the same manufacturer.[51,52] Variations in native BMPs, growth/differentiation factors of the donor bone, and dosages all introduce areas of variability and inconsistency that can create significant challenges for spine surgeons.

TABLE 2 Commercially Available DBM-Based Products, Allografts, and Mixed Products

Company	DBM-Based Product (Human)	Formulation	Product Composition	Peer-Reviewed Clinical Evidence/Ongoing Study ClinicalTrials.gov Identifier (NCT#)	Regulatory Clearance/ Approval FDA 510(k), K#, Month and Year Regulated Under CFR 1270, 1271 as a Human Tissue
AlloSource, Centennial, CO, USA, 1995 Allosource.org	AlloFuse Gel AlloFuse Putty (identical to StimuBlast Putty and Gel manufactured for Arthrex)	Injectable gel and putty	Demineralized bone matrix (DBM), reverse-phase medium (RPM) carrier Carrier composed of polyethylene oxide and polypropylene oxide blocks copolymer dissolved in water exhibiting reverse-phase characteristics (ie, an increase in viscosity as temperature increases)	n/a	K071849, December 2008 AATB FDA HCT/P (8 US States)
	AlloFuse Plus	Paste, putty	DBM, RPM, cancellous chips	n/a	K103036, January 2011
	AlloFlex	Strips, blocks, fillers	Cancellous bone allograft, DBM, strip form, no carriers added	n/a	Marketed as human tissue
Amend Surgical, Inc.	NanoFUSE Bioactive Matrix	Putty	DBM + 45S5 bioactive glass: bond void filler	n/a	K161996, February 2017
	NanoFUSE DBM	Putty 2 to 10 mL	45S5 bioactive glass + porcine gelatin + DBM 45S5 bioactive glass: osteoconductive Scaffold, DBM: osteoinductive potential	Kirk et al 2013[40]	K110976, May 2011 K161996 Regulated under CFR 1270, 1271 as a human tissue
Alphatec Spine, Inc., Carlsbad, CA	AlphaGRAFT DBM AlphaGRAFT ProFuse DBM	Putty or gel	An RPM spongelike DBM with superior handling characteristics and ready to use application (thickens at body temperature)	n/a	Unknown
Aziyo Biologics	OsteoGro		Cancellous bone and partially demineralized bone		
Bacterin International Holdings, Inc. → Changed to Xtant Medical Holdings, Inc.	OsetoSelect DBM	Putty	74% DBM dry weight	n/a	K091321, September 2009 K130498, May 2013
	OsteoSelect Plus DBM	Putty	74% DBM dry weight + demineralized cortical chips (1 to 4 mm)	n/a	K150621, August 2015 HCT/P (FEI 3005168462)
	OsteoSponge	The malleable sponge	DBM (100% human demineralized cancellous bone)	Shehadi and Elzein et al 2017[42]	510(k) cleared HCT/P (FEI 3005168462), November 21, 2017
	OsteoSponge SC	The malleable sponge	Demineralized cancellous bone intended to manage the pathology of damaged subchondral bone of the articulating joints	Galli et al 2015[43]	510(k) cleared HCT/P (FEI 3005168462), November 2017
	OsteoWrap	Flexible handling characteristics with a scalpel or scissors	100% human demineralized cortical bone	n/a	510(k) cleared HCT/P (FEI 3005168462), November 21, 2017
	3Demin	Various shape (fiber, boat shape, strip)	100% human demineralized cortical bone fiber Contain BMPs and other growth factor 3Demin allografts are also available as loose cortical fibers in three volume options	n/a	Compliance with FDA guidelines regarding HCT/P HCT/P 361 regulated viable allogeneic bone scaffold AATB guidelines

(Continued)

TABLE 2 Commercially Available DBM-Based Products, Allografts, and Mixed Products (Continued)

Company	DBM-Based Product (Human)	Formulation	Product Composition	Peer-Reviewed Clinical Evidence/Ongoing Study ClinicalTrials.gov Identifier (NCT#)	Regulatory Clearance/ Approval FDA 510(k), K#, Month and Year Regulated Under CFR 1270, 1271 as a Human Tissue
Berkeley Advanced Biomaterials, CA, USA	H-GENIN	Putty Matrix Sponge Powder	100% DBM putty and crush mix	n/a	510(k) cleared (as B-GENIN, R-GENIN) K092046, March 2010
Biomet Osteobiologics → Merged into Zimmer Biomet	InterGro DBM	Putty (40% DBM), paste (35% DBM)	DBM, lethicin carrier (resorbable, biocompatible, semiviscous lipid)	Prospective case series	510(k) cleared K082793, April 2009 K031399, February, 2005
Bioventus Surgical	Exponent	Putty form	DBM is composed of human DBM mixed with resorbable carrier, carboxymethyl cellulose (CMC)	n/a	AATB USFDA 21 CFR 1271 (HCT/P)
	PUREBONE	Sponge shape (available in block or strip format)	100% demineralized cancellous bone (osteoconductive matrix with osteoinductive potential that provides a natural scaffold for cellular ingrowth and revascularization) Sterilized by gamma irradiation	n/a	FDA 510(k) cleared AATB USFDA 21 CFR 1271 (HCT/P)
Bone Bank Allografts 2017/ Texas human biologics	SteriFuse DBM Putty	Flowable, formable putty	100% DBM from human bone	n/a	Regulated under 21 CFR Part 1271 (h FDA Requirements for HCT/P)
	SteriFuse Crunch	Flowable, formable crunch	SteriFuse DBM Putty with cortical cancellous bone chips (ratio composition unknown)	n/a	Regulated under 21 CFR Part 1271 (h FDA Requirements for HCT/P)
DePuy Synthes	DBX	Putty type	DBM + sodium hyaluronate	NCT02005081: RCT, no results	K103795, April 2011
	SYNTHES Dento	Powder type Granule type Putty type	Powder type: demineralized cortical powder, mineralized cancellous powder, mineralized cortical powder Granule type: demineralized cortical (80%)/cancellous granules, mineralized cortical (80%)/ cancellous granules DBM putty type: 93% DBM	n/a	Unknown
ETEX	CaP Plus	CaP Plus	Synthetic calcium phosphate, an inert carrier, CMC, and DBM	n/a	K063050, November 2007 K080329, April 2008
	EquivaBone Osteoinductive Bone Graft	Powder and hydration solution	Synthetic calcium phosphate, an inert carrier, CMC, and DBM		K090855, September 2009 K090310, March 2009
Exactech	Optecure	Injectable paste	DBM (81% by dry weight), hydrogel carrier	NCT00254852: prospective RCT	K121989, November 2012 K061668, September 2006 K050806, February 2006
	Optecure +CCC	Injectable paste	Polymer powder, DBM, cortical cancellous chips (1 to 3 mm)	NCT02127112: comparative study, allograft versus Optecure +CCC	K061668, September 2006 K121989, November 2012

TABLE 2 Commercially Available DBM-Based Products, Allografts, and Mixed Products (Continued)

Company	DBM-Based Product (Human)	Formulation	Product Composition	Peer-Reviewed Clinical Evidence/Ongoing Study ClinicalTrials.gov Identifier (NCT#)	Regulatory Clearance/ Approval FDA 510(k), K#, Month and Year Regulated Under CFR 1270, 1271 as a Human Tissue
	Optifill (OSTEOFIL DBM Paste, OSTEOFIL RT DBM Paste)	DBM paste or dry powder—hydrated to become injectable paste	DBM in gelatin carrier	n/a	K043420, February 2005
	Opteform	Putty or dry powder—hydrated to become paste	Gelatin, DBM, and cortical/ cancellous bone chips	n/a	K043421, February 2005
Integra OrthoBiologics (IsoTis OrthoBiologics), Inc., Irvine, CA/ SeaSpine 2018	Accell Connexus	Injectable putty	DBM (70% by weight), RPM	Retrospective comparative study Schizas et al, 2008 Fused 69.7% (23/33), Accell Connexus + local bone/ICBG Fused 76.9% (20/26), ICBG/local bone 1 year	K060306, March 2006 K061880, August 2007
	Accell Evo3	Injectable putty	DBM (Accell bone matrix), RPM	NCT02018445 (Accell Evo3 Demineralized Bone Matrix in Instrumented Lumbar Spine Fusion) NCT01714804 (Efficacy and Safety of Integra Accell Evo3 DBM in Instrumented Lumbar Spine Fusion) NCT01430299 Eleswarapu et al 2021[45] Fused 93.5% in posterolateral space, Accell Evo3 + local bone + allograft cancellous chips (n = 16 patients, 23 levels) Fused 100% in posterolateral space, rhBMP-2 +local bone + allograft cancellous chips (n = 21 patients, 37 levels) 2 year	K103742, March 2011
	Accell TBM	Preformed matrix (strip, square, round)	100% DBM (Accell bone matrix)	n/a	K081817, September 2008
	DynaGraft II	Injectable gel, putty	DBM (Accell bone matrix), RPM, cancellous bone chips	n/a	K040419, March 2005
	OrthoBlast II	Injectable paste, putty	DBM (Accell bone matrix), RPM, cancellous bone chips from same donor	n/a	K050642, December 2005

(Continued)

TABLE 2 Commercially Available DBM-Based Products, Allografts, and Mixed Products (Continued)

Company	DBM-Based Product (Human)	Formulation	Product Composition	Peer-Reviewed Clinical Evidence/Ongoing Study ClinicalTrials.gov Identifier (NCT#)	Regulatory Clearance/ Approval FDA 510(k), K#, Month and Year Regulated Under CFR 1270, 1271 as a Human Tissue
LifeNet Health	I/C Graft Chamber	Freeze-dried in injectable delivery chamber, can be mixed with whole blood, PRP, or BMA	DBM, cancellous chips	n/a	Regulated under CFR 1270, 1271 as a human tissue
	Optium DBM Putty	Putty	DBM, glycerol carrier	n/a	K053098, November 2005
	Optium DBM Gel	Gel	Particulate DBM, glycerol	n/a	K053098, November 2005
	Cellect DBM	Provided in a specialized cartridge	DBM fibers + cancellous chips	Case reports Lee and Goodman 2009[46]	Regulated under CFR 1270 and 1271
Medtronic Spinal and Biologics	Osteofil DBM	Injectable paste, moldable strips	DBM (24% by weight) in porcine gelatin	Prospective case series Epstein and Epstein 2007[47] Fused 98% (93/95), Osteofil + local bone (50:50 mix), one-level fusion Fused 96% (43/45), Osteofil + local bone (50:50 mix), two-level fusion 1 year	K043420, February 2005
	Progenix Plus	Putty with demineralized cortical chips	DBM in type I bovine collagen and sodium alginate	n/a	K081950, July 2008
	Progenix Putty	Injectable putty	DBM in type I bovine collagen and sodium alginate	n/a	K080462, May 2008
	Magnifuse Family Magnifuse Bone Graft substitute/ bone void filler Magnifuse II Bone Graft	—	DBM mixed with autograft in 1:1 ratio packed into polyglycolic acid resorbable mesh bag DBM + surface-demineralized chips Combination of surface-demineralized cortical chips and allograft fibers that have been processed, removing the mineral component leaving only the organic portion	NCT02684045: Retrospective case series study, results not posted	K123691, January 2013 K082615, October 2008
MTF Biologics, Edison NJ DePuy Synthes	DBX	Paste, putty mix, strip	DBM (32% by weight), sodium hyaluronate carrier (mix vary for paste, putty, mix)	Chang et al 2021[39] Fused 66.7% (18/27), DBX + local bone Fused 70.4% (19/27), Grafton matrix + local bone 2 year	K040262, March 2005 (putty, paste, matrix mix) K040501, April 2005 (putty, paste, matrix mix) K053218, December 2006 (putty, paste, matrix mix) K063676, March 2007 (putty, paste, matrix mix) K080399, October 2008 (paste) K091217, October 2009 (putty) K091218, September 2009 (putty) K103795, April 2011 (putty) K103784, April 2011 (putty) K042829, January 2006 (strip)

TABLE 2 Commercially Available DBM-Based Products, Allografts, and Mixed Products (Continued)

Company	DBM-Based Product (Human)	Formulation	Product Composition	Peer-Reviewed Clinical Evidence/Ongoing Study ClinicalTrials.gov Identifier (NCT#)	Regulatory Clearance/ Approval FDA 510(k), K#, Month and Year Regulated Under CFR 1270, 1271 as a Human Tissue
Nanotherapeutics, Inc.	Origen DBM with Biosotive Glass (NanoFUSE DBM)	A malleable, puttylike, bone void filler	Human DBM and synthetic calcium phosphosilicate particulate material particles (45S5 bioactive glass), both coated with gelatin derived from porcine skin	n/a	K120279, April 2012 K110976, May 2011
NuTech Medical, Inc.	Matrix: Osteoconductive Matrix Plus	Putty type	Allograft cancellous and demineralized cortical mixture Freeze-dried for convenient ambient temperature storage	n/a	
	Matrix: FiberOS	Putty type	Demineralized cortical fibers, mineralized cortical powder, and demineralized cortical powder Gamma sterilized for patient safety Freeze-dried for convenient ambient temperature storage		
Osteotech/ Medtronic`	Grafton A-Flex	Round flexible sheet	DBM	n/a	K051188, January 2006
	Grafton Crunch	Packable graft	DBM, demineralized cortical cubes	n/a	K051188, January 2006
	Grafton Flex	Flexible sheets, varying sizes	DBM	Retrospective comparative study	K051195, December 2005
	Grafton Gel	Injectable syringe	DBM	Cammisa et al 2004[48] PLF pedicle screw fixation, side-to-side comparison Fused 52% (42/81 sides), Grafton gel + ICBG Fused 54% (44/81 sides), ICBG 2 year An et al, 1995 ACDF: freeze-dried allograft/ tricortical graft DBM versus ICBG Fused 67% (42/63 levels), DBM Grafton Gel (pseudarthrosis developed in 33.3% levels [42.2% patients]) Fused 78% (46/59 levels), ICBG (pseudarthrosis developed in 22% levels [26.3% patients]) 1 year	K051195, December 2005
	Grafton Matrix PLF	Matrix troughs	DBM matrix troughs	Kang et al 2012[38] PLF, single level, instrumented Fused 86% (24/28) Grafton Matrix + local bone, 2 year Fused 92% (12/13), ICBG + local bone	K051195, December 2005
	Grafton Matrix Scoliosis Strips	Strips, various sizes	DBM	Retrospective case series	K051195, December 2005 (recalled 18 October, 2012; end 17 January, 2014) Multiple lots due to sterility

(Continued)

TABLE 2 Commercially Available DBM-Based Products, Allografts, and Mixed Products (Continued)

Company	DBM-Based Product (Human)	Formulation	Product Composition	Peer-Reviewed Clinical Evidence/Ongoing Study ClinicalTrials.gov Identifier (NCT#)	Regulatory Clearance/Approval FDA 510(k), K#, Month and Year Regulated Under CFR 1270, 1271 as a Human Tissue
	Grafton Orthoblend Large Defect	Packable graft	DBM, crushed cancellous chips	n/a	K051195, December 2005 (recalled 18 October, 2012; end 17 January, 2014) Multiple lots due to sterility
	Grafton Orthoblend Small Defect	Packable, moldable graft	DBM, crushed cancellous chips	n/a	K051195, December 2005 (recalled 18 October, 2012; end 17 January, 2014) Multiple lots due to sterility
	Grafton PLUS DBM Paste	Paste	Human bone allograft DBM + inert starch-based carrier has been added	n/a	K043048, November 2005 (Osteotech)—traditional K042707, November 2005 (Osteotech)
	Grafton Putty	Packable, moldable graft	DBM (17% by weight), glycerol	Park et al 2009[49] Patients undergoing ACDF, prospective case series Fused 97% (41/42 levels), Grafton Putty + local bone PEEK 1 year	K051195, December 2005
Pioneer Surgical Technology and Regeneration Technologies → All companies merged into RTI Surgical	BioSet	Injectable paste, putty, strips, and blocks with cortical cancellous chips	DBM, gelatin carrier	n/a	K060180, September 2006 Regulated under 21 CFR Part 1271 (h FDA Requirements for HCT/P)
	BioAdapt DBM	Powder form	Dried powder form (70% DBM by weight) donated from 100% donated human musculoskeletal tissue	n/a	Regulated under 21 CFR Part 1271 (h FDA Requirements for HCT/P)
	BioReady DBM Putty and Putty with Chips	Putty/putty with bone chip	Putty: 56% DBM by weight Putty with chips: 42% DBM by weight + small or large mineralized cortical cancellous chip → 100% allograft DBM	n/a	Regulated under 21 CFR Part 1271 (h FDA Requirements for HCT/P)
SeaSpine, Carlsbad, CA	OsteoBallast DBM	DBM in resorbable mesh	100% DBM	n/a	K200290, April 2020 (pouch, poly(lactic-co-glycolic acid))
	OsteoSurge 300 DBM	Moldable putty form	DBM + Accell bone matrix (it is an open-structured, dispersed form of DBM) + cancellous bone (comes OsteoSurge 100)	n/a	It is the same material as Accell Evo3 (NCT01430299) Confirm new sponsor and same material
	OsteoSurge 300c DBM	Moldable putty including cancellous chips	DBM + Accell one matrix (it is an open-structured, dispersed form of DBM) + cancellous bone + bioresorbable RPM carrier	n/a	It is the same material as Accell Evo3c SeaSpine (new sponsor, same material)
	OsteoSparx DBM	Gel or puttylike consistency	DBM + RPM carrier	n/a	It is the same material as Accell Evo3 (NCT01430299)

TABLE 2 Commercially Available DBM-Based Products, Allografts, and Mixed Products (Continued)

Company	DBM-Based Product (Human)	Formulation	Product Composition	Peer-Reviewed Clinical Evidence/Ongoing Study ClinicalTrials.gov Identifier (NCT#)	Regulatory Clearance/ Approval FDA 510(k), K#, Month and Year Regulated Under CFR 1270, 1271 as a Human Tissue
	OsteoSparx C DBM	Gel or puttylike consistency.	DBM + RPM carrier + cancellous bone	n/a	Same material as Accell Evo3c
	Accell Total Bone Matrix	Preformed shape (round or rectangular)	DBM + Accell bone matrix → 100% DBM	n/a	Same material as Accell Evo3 (NCT01430299)
	Accell Evo3c	Putty	DBM + Accell bone matrix (it is an open-structured, dispersed form of DBM) + cancellous bone + bioresorbable RPM carrier	n/a	K103742, March 2011
	Accell Evo3	Putty	DBM + Accell bone matrix (it is an open-structured, dispersed form of DBM) + bioresorbable RPM carrier.	Case study on posterolateral fusion (December 2013 ~ June 2017, NCT02018445) Prospective study on posterolateral fusion (December 2017 ~ January 2018, NCT01714804) RCT on posterolateral fusion with Accell Evo3 DBM Fused 93.5% with Accell Evo3 DBM versus fused 100% with rhBMP-2 NCT01430299	K103742, March 2011
	Capistrano	DBM + allobone	DBM + machined cortical and cancellous allograft bone	n/a	FDA 510(k) cleared
Smith & Nephew	VIAGRAF	Putty, paste, gel, crunch, and flex	DBM, glycerol	n/a	K043209, December 2005
Spinal Elements	Hero DBM	Putty, paste, and gel	DBM, RPM	n/a	Regulated under CFR 1270, 1271 as human tissue FDA registration number: FEI 3004893332 Spinal Elements, Inc. HCT/Ps: bone (store, distribute)
	Hero DBM Powder	Powder	DBM	n/a	
Wright Medical Group N.V.	ALLOMATRIX	Various volumes, consistency varies depending on proportion of cancellous chips used	DBM (86% by volume) +/− cellular bone matrix in surgical-grade calcium sulfate powder	Retrospective comparative study	K041663, September 2004
	ALLOMATRIX RCS	Formable putty	DBM, synthetic resorbable conductive scaffold (RCS), calcium sulfate, and hydroxypropyl methylcellulose	n/a	K041663, September 2004
	ALLOMATRIX C	Putty	ALLOMATRIX + small cancellous chips	n/a	K040980, July 2004

(Continued)

TABLE 2 Commercially Available DBM-Based Products, Allografts, and Mixed Products (Continued)

Company	DBM-Based Product (Human)	Formulation	Product Composition	Peer-Reviewed Clinical Evidence/Ongoing Study ClinicalTrials.gov Identifier (NCT#)	Regulatory Clearance/ Approval FDA 510(k), K#, Month and Year Regulated Under CFR 1270, 1271 as a Human Tissue
	ALLOMATRIX CUSTOM	Putty	ALLOMATRIX + large cancellous chips	n/a	K040980, July 2004
	ALLOMATRIX	Injectable	DBM (86% by volume) + OSTEOSET (surgical-grade calcium sulfate)	NCT00274378: RCT in trauma treatment	K020895, February 2004
	ALLOMATRIX DR	Putty	Calcium sulfate, DBM, and small cancellous chips	n/a	K040980, July 2004
	PRO-STIM	Injectable paste/formable putty	50% calcium sulfate, 10% calcium phosphate, and 40% DBM by weight Procedure kits: various volumes of injectable mix	n/a	K190283, March 2019
Zimmer → It merged into Zimmer Biomet	IGNITE	Percutaneous graft for fracture malunion/ nonunion	DBM in surgical-grade calcium sulfate powder to be mixed with bone marrow aspirate	n/a	K052913, November 2005
	OSTEOSET DBM Pellets	Packable pellets	3.0 mm or 4.8 mm pellets Surgical-grade calcium sulfate, DBM (53% by volume), stearic acid	n/a	K022828, April 2004 K053642, January 2006
	PRO-STIM Injectable Inductive Graft	Injectable paste/formable putty	DBM (40% by weight), calcium sulfate (50% by weight), calcium phosphate (10% by weight)	n/a	See Wright Medical Group N.V K190283, March 2019
	Puros DBM with RPM Gel and Paste	Gel, paste	DBM, RPM, ground cancellous bone (<500 μm)	n/a	Regulated under CFR 1270, 1271 as human tissue
	Puros DBM with RPM Putty and Putty with Chips	Putty	DBM, RPM, +/− cortical bone chips (850 μm to 4 mm)	n/a	Regulated under CFR 1270, 1271 as human tissue
	Puros DBM Block and Strip	Blocks, strips in varying sizes	DMB (100%)	n/a	Regulated under CFR 1270, 1271 as human tissue
	Bonus CC Matrix	Putty type	DBM + mineralized cancellous chips All-inclusive bone grafting kit	n/a	FDA registration number: FEI 1000160576 AATB and HTC/P
	StaGraft DBM Putty and Plus	—	DBM + natural lecithin carrier + resorbable coralline hydroxyapatite/ calcium carbonate granules Available as 40% DBM Putty or 35% DBM Plus	n/a	FDA registration number: FEI 1000160576, 2021 Interpore Cross International, LLC (DBA Zimmer Biomet Irvine) HCT/Ps: bone (package, process, store, label, distribute)
	StaGraft Cancellous DBM Sponge and Strips	Sponge and strips	Cancellous DBM sponge and strips are machined from a single piece of cancellous bone Osteoinductive bone, trabecular structure, spongelike handling	n/a	FDA registration number: FEI 1000160576, 2021 Interpore Cross International, LLC

TABLE 2 Commercially Available DBM-Based Products, Allografts, and Mixed Products (Continued)

Company	DBM-Based Product (Human)	Formulation	Product Composition	Peer-Reviewed Clinical Evidence/Ongoing Study ClinicalTrials.gov Identifier (NCT#)	Regulatory Clearance/ Approval FDA 510(k), K#, Month and Year Regulated Under CFR 1270, 1271 as a Human Tissue
	StaGraft Fiber	Fiber strands 2 to 10 mL sizes	100% cortical fiber DBM (demineralized to calcium content <8%)	n/a	FDA registration number: FEI 1000160576, 2021 Interpore Cross International, LLC
	FiberStack DBM	—	Manufactured entirely from cortical bone, which has been demonstrated to maintain higher osteoinductivity than cancellous bone after demineralization 100% DBM (without carrier)	—	FDA registration number: FEI 1000160576, 2021 Interpore Cross International, LLC

510(k) is a premarket submission made to the FDA to demonstrate that the device to be marketed is at least as safe and effective, that is, substantially equivalent, to a legally marketed device that is not subject to Premarket Approval. 501(k) documentation for individual products is available via FDA online database (http://www.accessdata.fda.gov).

Code of Federal Regulations (CFR) 1270 (human tissue intended for transplantation) and 1271 (human cells, tissues, and cellular and tissue-based products [HCT/Ps]) are federal regulations relating to the procurement and processing of human-derived tissues.

510(k) www.accessdata.fda.gov.

Regulated under CFR 1270, 1271 as a human tissue if indicated.

Human Tissue Banks: https://images.magnetmail.net/images/clients/AATB/attach/Bulletin_Links/18_2/AATB_Accreditation_Policies_February_08_2018.pdf (last update 2018 February).

TBI Tissue Banks International National Processing Center (an AATB-accredited tissue bank).

US Human Tissue Bank License States: California, Florida, Maryland, and New York.

AATB = American Association of Tissue Banks, ACDF = anterior cervical diskectomy and fusion, BMA = bone marrow aspirate, BMP = bone morphogenetic protein, FEI = Facility Establishment Identifier, ICBG = iliac crest bone graft, local bone (autograft obtained from the site of surgical dissection), PEEK = polyether ether ketone, PLF = posterolateral/posterior lumbar fusion, PRP = platelet-rich plasma, RCT = randomized controlled trial, rhBMP-2 = recombinant human bone morphogenetic protein-2www

Cellular-Based Allografts and CBM

CBMs are bone allografts constructed of partially demineralized cadaver bone used as matrix carriers with components of cryopreserved allogeneic cells and mesenchymal stromal cells (MSCs),[53] which avoid allogeneic rejection.[54] Manufacturers claim that the components of CBMs mimic autograft by providing the required osteoconduction, osteogenesis, and osteoinduction necessary for successful bone grafting. During surgery, CBMs are mixed with autograft from the locally prepared site and placed into the spinal fusion construct. Surgeons' use of CBMs is on the rise as the commercial availability of this class of allografts increases.

Because CBMs are commercially provided as frozen products that must be stored at −80°C, they require thawing before surgical implantation. Neither the reproducibility of cell recovery after thawing nor the cell viability following implantation has been established for commercially available products. There is currently no guideline or benchmark for threshold of number of cells, type of cells present, or even potency in CBMs.

To preserve viable cells, these products are not terminally sterilized. They rely on aseptic processing to ensure safety after thorough donor or cadaver selection via standards set by the American Association of Tissue Banks–accredited tissue banks (AATB.org). These standards have been recently updated as a result of the COVID-19 pandemic; however, historically, tissues from any donor with an active serious infection resulted in deferral of using that donor's tissues.

Table 3 presents a list of commercially available CBM products used for spinal fusion and specifics on each product. The primary studies that reported radiographic fusion rates are referenced.[55-59,61-72]

Still there are insufficient numbers of primary studies to determine clinical efficacy of viable cellular allografts in spinal fusion. Several recent reviews evaluate data from the same 12 primary studies. Non–industry-sponsored clinical studies are rare. In a retrospective study, Kerr et al[56] reported that 92.3% of consecutive patients studied had solid arthrodesis after one-level or two-level lumbar interbody fusion with Osteocel (NuVasive, San Diego, CA).

TABLE 3 Examples of Commercially Available Cellular Bone Matrices and Combination Grafting Products

Product Name (Commercial)	Commercial Company/ Manufacturer	Formulation	Product Composition	Peer-Reviewed Clinical Evidence/Ongoing study ClinicalTrials.gov (NCT#)	Regulatory Clearance/Approval: FDA 510(k), FDA 361, 21 CFR Part 1271, CFR 1270, CFR 1271, 21 CFR 3.2(e), HCT/P 361, Human Allografts (No Clinical Studies Needed), Biologic Drugs, and Devices 351 (Clinical Trials)
AlloStem Cellular Bone Autograft	AlloSource, Centennial, CO, USA, 1995 allosource.org	Strips, blocks, cubes, morcellized	Partially demineralized allograft bone combined with adipose-derived mesenchymal stromal cells (MSCs) (study adipose-derived cellular bone matrix [ACBM])	Subtalar Arthrodesis: NCT01413061, 2021 AlloSource (ACBM) versus autograft (ABG) Fused CT: ACBM 30.8% (16/52) < ABG 54.4% (31/57); nonunion: ACBM 13.5% (7/52) > ABG 8.8% (5/57) Results: Myerson et al 2019 (two studies of subtalar arthrodesis)	USFDA CFR 1270, 1271 as a human tissue
ArthroCell Viable Bone Matrices	Arthrex Naples FL/ Vivex Biologics	Moldable particulate gel	HCT/P demineralized allograft bone scaffold, cortical and cancellous components, with signaling molecules and BMPs (MIAMI cells preserved using novel DMSO-free cryoprotectant).	None	HCT/P 361, Human Allografts Registration
BIO^4 (before 2014 originally branded as OvationOS)	Stryker Corporation/ Osiris Therapeutics, Inc.	Putty type (1, 2.5, 5, 10 mL)	Allograft bone (cortical and cancellous) + periosteum A viable bone matrix containing endogenous bone-forming cells (including MSCs, osteoprogenitor cells [OPCs], and osteoblasts) as well as osteoinductive and angiogenic growth factors 70% cell viability postthaw Average 600,000 cells/mL Stored at −80°C, 2-year shelf life	NCT03077204: clinical case series study (cervical spine)	AATB USFDA 21 CFR 1271
Cellentra Advanced Allograft	Zimmer Biomet	Moldable granular putty (bone matrix)	Mixed 1:1 of cancellous bone matrix offers an interconnected trabecular structure (>750,000 cells/mL) of cancellous tissue with at least 70% cell viability (MSCs, OPCs, preosteoblasts) Cortical bone is demineralized and provides additional inherent growth factors (BMP-2, 4, 6, 7, VEGF, TGF-β, PDGF, IGF-1, and FGF1, 2)	NCT02182843, ACDF: radiographic success (grade 1 or 2) = 49.3% (35/71) at 24 mo?	AATB USFDA 21 CFR 1271
FiberCel Fiber Viable Bone Matrix	Aziyo Biologics, Inc., Richmond, CA/ Medtronic (distributor)	Moldable granular putty type	Cancellous bone particles with preserved living cells + demineralized cortical bone (DCB) fibers	n/a (none, ClinicalTrials.gov, August 2021) Postsurgical infection in 7 of 23 patients who had received FiberCel (one lot), 4 patients tested positive for tuberculosis	HCT/P per 21 CFR Part 127,1 FDA Voluntary Recall Lot number: NMDS210011 Product numbers: VBM9901, VBM9905, VBM9910

Map3 Cellular Allogeneic Bone Graft	RTI Surgical, Inc., Allendale, NJ, USA	Putty type Strip type	Cortical cancellous bone chip (or strip-shaped bone) + DBM + cryogenically preserved, viable multipotent adult progenitor cells (MAPC)	NCT02628210: lumbar interbody fusion (active status) NCT02161016: case series study in foot and ankle (results posted)	Regulations under section 361 of PHS Act (42 U.S.C. 264) and 21 CFR Part 1271.10(s)(4)(ii)(b) + FDA Act {21 U.S.C. 321(g)++) FDA ltr (November, 2017) additional requirement as a biologic, 42 U.S.C.262(a)
OsteoVive	Xtant Medical Holdings, Inc.	Putty type	A cell population that includes MIAMI cells (red and white blood cells removed) Blend of microparticulate cortical, cancellous, and demineralized cortical allograft bone (particle size range of 100 to 300 μm)	n/a (none ClinicalTrials.gov, August 2021)	FDA 510(k) cleared Compliance with FDA guidelines regarding HCT/P HCT/P 361 regulated viable allogeneic bone scaffold AATB
OsteoAMP	Advanced Biologics, Carlsbad, CA, 2009 (marketed in the United States since 2009) Bioventus Surgical, Durham, NC, USA (original developer)	Granules, sponge, putty	OsteoAMP, an allogeneic growth factor implant, exploits the angiogenic, mitogenic, and osteoinductive growth factors that are within marrow cells Growth factor–rich bone graft substitute, naturally occurring growth factors include BMP-2, BMP-7, aFGF, VEGF, ANG1, and TGF-β1: intended for homologous use, repair, replacement, or reconstruction of musculoskeletal defects	NCT02225444: lumbar spine PLF (no results posted, August 2021) Roh et al 2013 OsteoAMP + BMA (n = 132), 12 mo: 93.9%, 18 mo: 99.1% OsteoAMP (n = 94), 12 mo: 92.6%; 18 mo: 98.7%, rhBMP-2 (n = 95), 12 mo: 83.5%; 18 mo: 90.1%	FDA 510(k) cleared AATB USFDA 21 CFR 1271 Bioventus manages orders and sales of HCT/Ps (not a distributor, FDA) Regulated under CFR 1270, 1271 as a human tissue, registration held by Tissue bank Permit: Millstone Medical Outsourcing, LLC, Olive Branch, MS (bone, demineralized bone matrix, ligament, musculoskeletal tissues, tendons) Maryland New York State Tissue Bank Permit: Advanced Biologics, LLC, Carlsbad, CA (bone demineralized bone matrix)
OsteoGro ViBone	Aziyo Biologics, Inc., Richmond, CA	Cancellous bone Structural allografts Package Bone matrix	Partially DCB Preserve natural components of the matrix Viable bone matrix	NCT03425682: cervical and lumbar spine fusion (completed, no results, August 2021)	Regulated under CFR 1270, 1271 as a human tissue
OsteoVive, OsteoVive Plus	Xtant Medical Holdings, Inc., AATB	Putty type	A cell population that includes MIAMI cells (red and white blood cells removed) Blend of microparticulate cortical, cancellous, and demineralized cortical allograft bone (particle size range of 100 to 300 μm)	n/a	FDA 510(k) cleared Compliance with FDA guidelines regarding HCT/P HCT/P 361 regulated viable allogeneic bone scaffold AATB

(Continued)

TABLE 3 Examples of Commercially Available Cellular Bone Matrices and Combination Grafting Products (Continued)

Product Name (Commercial)	Commercial Company/ Manufacturer	Formulation	Product Composition	Peer-Reviewed Clinical Evidence/Ongoing study ClinicalTrials.gov (NCT#)	Regulatory Clearance/Approval: FDA 510(k), FDA 361, 21 CFR Part 1271, CFR 1270, CFR 1271, 21 CFR 3.2(e), HCT/P 361, Human Allografts (No Clinical Studies Needed), Biologic Drugs, and Devices 351 (Clinical Trials)
Osteocel, Osteocel Plus	NuVasive	Moldable bone matrix	DBM, OPC, MSC (<50,000 cells/mL, >70% viability)	Bergin et al 2021[59] Retrospective study, three centers, ACDF (326 patients) with Osteocel Pseudarthrosis: 8.4% (11/131) with structural allograft with Osteocel; 16.4% (32/195) with PEEK with Osteocel NCT00948532: Osteocel Plus in extreme lateral interbody fusion (XLIF) 12.3% versus Structural Allograft alone 5.3%; fused, Osteocel 50/57 (87.7%) versus 54/57 (94.7%); one level, Osteocel 25/29 (86.2%) versus 28/29 (96.6%); two levels, Osteocel 25/28 (89.3%) versus 25/28 (89.3%) McAnany 2016[60] NCT00942045: retrospective comparative study ACDF matched cohort analysis Fused 87.7% (50/57) Osteocel allograft Fused 94.7% (54/57) standard allograft matched controls Kerr et al 2011[56] Fused 92.3% (48/52); circumferential (67%), ALIF (17%), or TLIF (16%) Tohmeh et al, 2012 Retrospective Osteocel Plus in XLIF Fused 90.2% (55/61), 1 year. Ammerman et al 2013[63] Retrospective MITLIF 1 mL/level Osteocel Plus in PEEK Fused 92.3% (24/26) levels (n = 23 patients) at 1 year Eastlack et al 2014[64] Osteocel Plus in PEEK cage anterior plating at one or two levels in prospective case series NCT: retrospective case series, clinical trial Fused: 92% (148/161) at 2 years Hollawell et al 2019[65] Hindfoot and high-risk fractures	Regulated under CFR 1270, 1271 as a human tissue

Trinity Evolution	MTF/Orthofix	Moldable allograft fibers, varying sizes	Allogeneic DBM with OPCs, MSC (minimum of 500,000 cells/mL; 100,000 of which are MSC and/or OPC)	NCT00951938 (anterior cervical) Peppers TA 2017 doi:10.1186/s13018-017-0564-5 Fused 89.5% (34/38), two levels, ACDF PEEK + CBM (Trinity Evolution), 1 year Fused 93.4% (71/76), two levels, ACDF PEEK + CBM (Trinity Evolution), 1 year. Vanichkachorn et al 2016[66] ACDF Fused 93.5% (29/31 patients), ACDF, PEEK + CBM (Trinity Evolution), 1 year (two nonunions had obesity risk factor)	Regulated under CFR 1270, 1271 as a human tissue
	Trinity Elite	Moldable allograft fibers, varying sizes	DBM, OPCs, MSC (minimum of 500,000 cells/mL; 100,000 of which are MSC and/or OPC) Trinity Elite and/or local bone with supplemental pedicle screw fixation Allogeneic cancellous bone matrix containing viable OPCs, MSCs, and a DCB	NCT02969616 Lumbar fusion: PLF, TLIF, ALIF, XLIF, etc NCT00965380 Halalmeh and Perez-Cruet 2021[67] MITLIF Fused 98.4% (252/256), local morcellized bone autograft (LMBA) mixed with Trinity Elite or Allograft (except for three cases where LMBA was used alone)	Regulated under CRF 1270, 1271 as a human tissue
VIA Graft	Onkos Surgical/Vivex Biomedical, Inc., Marietta, GA USA	—	Microparticulate scaffold; cortical, cancellous, and demineralized cortical allograft bone; particle size range of 100 to 300 μm with MIAMI cells (cryoprotectant free of exogenous proteins and DMSO)	Tally et al 2018[68] Retrospective series MISTLIF Fused 96% (73/75) patients; 96.5% (82/85) levels at 1 year	—
ViviGen Cellular Bone Matrix, Vertigraft	DePuy Synthes/Johnson & Johnson	Cryo cortical Cortical cancellous bone matrix and demineralized bone	ViviGen Cellular Bone Matrix is composed of cryopreserved viable cortical cancellous bone matrix and demineralized bone. ViviGen Cellular Bone Matrix is an HCT/P. ViviGen Cellular Bone Matrix is processed from donated human tissue, resulting from the generous gift of an individual or their family	NCT02814825: ACDF cervical (August 2021) NCT03733626: lumbar PLF (active) NCT04007094: lumbar PLF side-by-side (active) NCT03527966: rhBMP-2 versus ViviGen (terminated early) Gibson et al 2021[69] Cohort study: Fused 92.9% (26/28) in cellular allograft ACDF Fused 84% (21/25) in decellularized allograft ACDF Elgafy et al 2021[70] Fused n = 96 patients; 91.6% (88/96) Fused: IPLF 100% (13/13) versus IPLF + TLIF 90.1% (75/83) Hall et al, 2019 V-CBA combined with local autograft in multilevel IPLF Fused: 98.7% (148/150) patients or 99.2% (608/613) levels Pseudarthrosis rate 0.8% Divi and Mikhael 2017[55] Retrospective case series, ACDF titanium plate with allograft spacer filled with CBM versus Corpectomy with CBM placed in carbon spacer, or PSF (serial radiographic data on fusion not presented) NCT04299022 (fractures)	HCT/P Divi SN 2017[55] HCT/P as defined by the USFDA in 21 CFR 1271.3(d), 21 CFR 1271

(Continued)

TABLE 3 Examples of Commercially Available Cellular Bone Matrices and Combination Grafting Products (Continued)

Product Name (Commercial)	Commercial Company/ Manufacturer	Formulation	Product Composition	Peer-Reviewed Clinical Evidence/Ongoing study ClinicalTrials.gov (NCT#)	Regulatory Clearance/Approval: FDA 510(k), FDA 361, 21 CFR Part 1271, CFR 1270, CFR 1271, 21 CFR 3.2(e), HCT/P 361, Human Allografts (No Clinical Studies Needed), Biologic Drugs, and Devices 351 (Clinical Trials)
IGNITE Power Mix	Wright Medical Group N.V	Powder	IGNITE Power Mix combines an injectable cellular CBM scaffold in DBM (IGNITE convenience kit) for mixing ALLOMATRIX powder with autologous BMA	With accessory components that are exempt from 510(k) requirements pursuant to 21 CFR 878.4800 See MAUDE for recalls	AATB USFDA 21 CFR 1271 (HCT/P) Injectable putty, K052913, November 2005 (IGNITE' Kit 510(k) SUMMARY, ALLOMATRIX, K020895, K041168) Bone Graft Syringe, K023088, 2005
NuCel Osteotech → Merged into Medtronic	Organogenesis, March 2017/NuTech Medical, Inc.	Putty type	Cryopreserved, bioactive amniotic suspension allograft Cellular, growth factor, and extracellular matrix components	ClinicalTrials.gov identifier: NCT02023372: A prospective, efficacy study (RCT) for PLF NCT02070484: NuCel versus DBM Nunley et al 2016[72] Fused 97.4 (37/38 patients), one level, 1 year Fused 100% (34/34), two levels, 1 year	NuTech Spine, Inc. HCT/P 361, Human Allografts Registration

FDA https://www.accessdata.fda.gov/scripts/cber/CFAppsPub/tiss/Index.cfm site for Human Cell And Tissue Establishment Registration—Public Query.

Status of HCT/P requires that the market product mechanism of action not be dependent on the metabolic activity of living cells, and classification does not require lot-to-lot cell composition or validation of growth factor production. Per FDA guidance documents on HCT/P, to "rely on the metabolic activity of living cells for their primary function" would render a product as a biologic drug (section 360), which would require a biologic license application and clinical trials.

US manufacturing of CBMs involves the American Association of Tissue Banks (AATB) approval processes for cadaver human bone recovery (contract with independent USFDA—registered tissue recovery groups), processing, storing, and preserving cellular components of the bone, or addition of cells, and removal of noncellular proteins. Safety is exercised by restricted donor screening. Marketed under FDA HCT wherein the regulation of product directive is safety; CBMs are not required to be terminally sterilized (unlike DBM-based allograft via 510(k)/Premarket Approval), relying on the donor screening and aseptic processing to ensure safety. The exact procedures are manufacturer specific.

510(k) is a premarket submission made to FDA to demonstrate that the device to be marketed is at least safe and effective, that is, substantially equivalent, to a legally marketed device that is not subject to Premarket Approval. 501(k) documentation for individual products is available via FDA online database (http://www.accessdata.fda.gov).

Code of Federal Regulations (CFR) 1270 (human tissue intended for transplantation) and 1271 (human cells, tissues, and tissue-based products) are federal regulations relating to the procurement and processing of human-derived tissues.

AATB = American Association of Tissue Banks, BMA = bone marrow aspirate, BMP = bone morphogenetic protein, CBM = cellular bone matrix, DBM = demineralized bone matrix, DMSO = dimethyl sulfoxide, FGF = fibroblast growth factor, HCT/P = human cells, tissues, and cellular and tissue-based products, IDE = investigational device exemption, IGF-1 = insulinlike growth factor 1, MIAMI = marrow-isolated adult multilineage inducible, MITLIF/MISTLIF = minimally invasive transforaminal lumbar interbody fusion, PDGF = platelet-derived growth factor, PEEK = polyetheretherketone, a material used for cage devices used as instrumentation in anterior interbody spinal fusion procedures, PMA = premarket approval, RCT = randomized controlled trial, rhBMP-2 = recombinant human bone morphogenetic protein-2, TGF-β = transforming growth factor beta, VEGF = vascular endothelial growth factor

There are many factors that can influence the efficacy of CBMs and therefore result in limitations to these products. Hernigou et al[73] showed that bone marrow aspirate containing fewer than 1,500 MSCs/mL was ineffective for the management of tibial nonunion, suggesting that this is the minimal MSC concentration for bony healing. Preparation of MSCs containing allograft is not standardized, and variation in donor age, donor site, and viability of remaining stem cells after thawing the allograft can all influence the effectiveness of CBMs.

Several in vivo studies demonstrated benefits of cell-seeded CBMs,[74,75] whereas others did not show any healing improvement by adding cells to CBMs.[76] Many other studies support Urist's thesis that greater demineralization of allograft bone promotes bone graft consolidation.[77]

Screening of donors, preparations, sterilization, formulation, and manufacturing processes contribute to safety, efficacy, and differences among the CBM products compared with DBM-based products. Aseptic processing may be less in CBMs (slightly less processed to preserve cells) without terminal sterilization (as in DBM-based products), resulting in less assurance of safety. Recently, a multistate outbreak of tuberculosis associated with a suspected contaminated single lot of CBM used in surgical procedures was reported by the FDA (https://www.cdc.gov/hai/outbreaks/TB-bone-allograft.html) and the American Association of Tissue Banks Bulletin 21-6 (https://www.aatb.org/bulletin-21-6). To better assess the risks for serious disease transmissions, further independent product-based testing of lot-to-lot safety even of unusual rare diseases and effectiveness should be considered and performed in the future.

Recombinant Human Bone Morphogenetic Proteins

BMPs were identified and named in 1965 by Urist, who initially identified the ability of an unknown factor in bone to induce ectopic bone formation in muscle.[50,78] BMPs constitute the largest subdivision of the transforming growth factor beta family of ligands.[79] To date, more than 20 members have been identified in humans with varying functions during processes such as embryogenesis, skeletal formation, hematopoiesis, and neurogenesis.[80] Of the BMPs identified, 12 are attributed as being involved in bone formation.[50,81-83] Osteogenic BMPs induce bone formation and healing through transmembrane serine/threonine kinase receptors such as BMP type I and type II receptors. Activated BMP type I act via the Smad complex protein pathway which involves commitment, differentiation, maturation, and proliferation of MSCs into osteogenic, osteoblast cells.[78,81-83]

For grafting in spinal fusion procedures, application of rhBMPs (eg, rhBMP-2) provides osteoinductive signals to surrounding tissue environments in the surgically prepared fusion site to promote de novo bone formation, remodeling, and healing. After over many years of bench, translation, and clinical research,[84,85] the USFDA granted in 2002 the first approval of rhBMP-2 for limited applications in single-level anterior lumbar interbody fusion (marketed as INFUSE Bone Graft, in LT-CAGE, Medtronic). Approval of rhBMP-7 was granted in 2004 (osteogenic protein-1 putty, no longer marketed in the United States).[86,87] In spinal fusion surgery, rhBMP-2 is applied to absorbable collagen sponge (rhBMP-2/absorbable collagen sponge, INFUSE, Medtronic, Inc.). A summary of growth factors used in spinal fusion is presented in **Table 3**.

Numerous studies have demonstrated the utility and benefits of rhBMP-2/absorbable collagen sponge with high rates of fused segments in various spinal fusion procedures by 12 months.[88-91] Analysis of pooled data from eight randomized controlled trials found that nonunion was two times less in the BMP versus ICBG in spinal arthrodesis at 2 years.[92] Additional FDA-approved clinical trials of other fusion procedures testing lower doses and concentrations with various carriers are still ongoing.

Over the years, because of the early success of BMP-2 in spinal fusion, off-label use became more frequent in spinal deformity.[93,94] Various groups have reported adverse complications including development of heterotopic ossification.[95] Furthermore, off-label use of rhBMP-2 in cervical fusions has resulted in severe, life-threatening swelling in the neck, leading to dyspnea and dysphagia.[96-98] Consequently, the FDA issued a warning on the use of rhBMP-2 in the cervical spine.[99] Another primary difficulty in using rhBMPs in spinal fusion is the dose-dependent efficacy of rhBMPs. BMPs have a short half-life; thus, large supraphysiologic doses of rhBMPs are needed for spinal fusion.[84] Ongoing research on combinations of BMPs, small molecules, BMP receptor–binding techniques,[100] or with various carrier materials may mitigate needed large doses for therapeutic efficacy as well as undesirable adverse effects.

INVESTIGATIONAL GROWTH FACTORS, CYTOKINES, AND PEPTIDES

Various growth factors, cytokines, and peptides are known to be crucially involved in spinal fusion. Only those with the most robust evidence, some of which are currently in preclinical phases given the novelty of their application, are presented. In 2019, Cottrill et al[101] conducted a systematic review of 14 experimental growth factors in preclinical models of spinal fusion, including AB204, angiopoietin 1, calcitonin, erythropoietin, basic fibroblast growth factor, growth differentiation factor 5, combined insulinlike growth factor 1 + transforming growth factor beta, insulin, NELL-1, noggin, P-15, peptide B2A, and secreted phosphoprotein 24. According to the reports, several growth factors had promising effects on spinal fusion rates, including calcitonin, growth differentiation factor 5, NELL-1, and P-15.

An example of peptide-enhanced bone graft is i-FACTOR Peptide Enhanced Bone Graft (CeraPedics, Inc., Westminster, Colorado; i-FACTOR Peptide Enhanced Bone Graft/anorganic bone mineral/P-15). This bone graft contains P-15, a synthetic polypeptide composed of 15 amino acids, which is meant to mimic part of the alpha-1 chain of type I collagen. It is absorbed onto calcium phosphate particles containing bovine hydroxyapatite, which are suspended in a hydrogel carrier. The polypeptide component facilitates the attachment of osteogenic cells to the calcium phosphate granule component. The calcium phosphate granules have osteoconductive properties and provide a source of calcium for new bone growth. It has been approved by the FDA for single-level anterior cervical diskectomy and fusions, C3 to C7, with an ongoing randomized clinical trial for use in the lumbar spine. Arnold et al compared autograft versus i-FACTOR in a single-level anterior cervical diskectomy and fusion for cervical radiculopathy (prospective, randomized, controlled FDA Investigational Device Exemption trial) and demonstrated safety and efficacy of both graft types.[102]

Synthetic Materials

Synthetic materials, including a variety of ceramic compounds, are a class that has been studied extensively as bone graft extenders. These have been used in combination with a wide array of other biomaterials and investigated in a variety of different spine fusion procedures.[103] Synthetic materials have a significant variability in biomechanical properties, biodegradability, microscale architecture, and surgical-handling properties.[104] The main categories include ceramics, BAG, and polymer-based compounds. **Table 4** provides a summary of commercially available bioactive synthetic bone void fillers, extenders, and substitute products.[88,102,105-112]

Bioactive Glass

BAG is used as a graft extender and mixed with local bone autograft. The consistency of nonstructural BAG-based products ranges from granules, putty, to fibrous strands. For use, these are mixed with local autograft or other grafting materials and placed into a surgically prepared site of the spine where bone growth is desired. When implanted, it reacts with bodily fluids causing it to degrade and allows specific ion exchange (Ca, P) to form a layer of hydroxyapatite, forming bonds between soft and hard tissue. This induces antimicrobial, osteoblast-stimulating, and tissue-regenerating activity for bone.

Different BAG material particle sizes and formulations are designed to alter the local site physiologic tissue environments via dissolution of surface ions that increase pH and higher osmotic pressure. This process eradicates pathogens. However, none of the new material compositions show eradication of 40 tested pathogens.[113]

BAG is available in different forms and compositions. Bioactive glass ceramic was designed as a structural cage intervertebral spacer. The bioactive glass ceramic spacer is packed with cortical local bone graft and then inserted between the two vertebral end plates with an anterior plate for cervical spine fusion.[114] Strontium ion delivery to sites of weakened bone has been able to inhibit osteoclastic mechanisms, strengthen the region within a defect, and specifically manage osteoporosis.[115] Ti-6Al-4V alloy with silica-based BAG is designed with antibacterial and bioactive surfaces by chemical doping with strontium and/or silver ions.[116] The potential to manage osteomyelitis and eradicate pathogens such as *Pseudomonas aeruginosa*, methicillin-susceptible *Staphylococcus aureus*, and methicillin-resistant *S aureus* with gentamicin-polymethylmethacrylate beads may be cost effective with better clinical outcomes given that this is a one-step treatment.[117]

There are also limitations in the use of this material. Degradation may result in strong cytotoxicity and imbalances toward osteoclasts formation that may interfere with bone induction and remodeling process, thus wear debris may have unintended consequences.[118] In addition, the pH-dependent antibacterial activity may be neutralized or lessened in vivo in patients. BAG material scaffolds tend to be brittle, and load-bearing devices for orthopaedic spine applications are not commercially available yet. BAG materials can be used as a graft extender in non–load-bearing constructs. Future development of various polymer composites and formulations that are also less brittle and flexible may increase structural functionality. There is limited literature regarding the clinical application of commercially available BAG-based products in spinal fusion. Several studies related to commercially available BAG products used for spinal fusion[41,119-125] are summarized in **Table 5**.

Discussion

Although great advances have been made in the development of biologic techniques, materials, and fusion agents, the goal is still to generate new materials with enhanced bioactivity above the gold standard of autologous bone graft. New material candidates must be well researched, approved for use, and cautiously used. They must also be evaluated for acceptable cost-benefit profiles, as well as short-term and long-term results. The ideal biologic graft should be safe and present osteoinductive, osteoconductive, and/or osteogenic properties to the site of fusion, while providing enough grafting material with minimized morbidity and surgical time.

TABLE 4 Commercially Available Bone Inductive Peptides, Proteins-Based Products, and Recombinant Versions

Company	Growth Factor Product	Formulation	Product Composition	Peer-Reviewed Clinical Evidence/ Ongoing Study	Regulatory Clearance/Approval/ PMA, FDA 510(k)
Cellumed Co., Ltd., Seoul, Korea, 2006	Rafugen BMP-2 Biosimilar rhBMP-2	Recombinant human bone morphogenetic protein (rhBMP) and ceramic	rhBMP-2 (0.036 mg/mL) + DBM + collagen gel Chinese hamster ovary cell–derived rhBMP-2	Not used in the United Studies RCT for using interbody fusion in spine (approved in 2013 by Korea FDA [KFDA])	Traumatic bone defect in upper and lower extremity (approved in Korea) GTP facility of Clean Room for tissue processing in Asia, approved by KFDA and USFDA for its safeness and effectiveness. Cellumed BMEL runs Korea's first tissue bank cellumed.en.ecplaza.net
CeraPedics, Inc.	P-15L Bone Graft	Bone graft	DBM, lethicin carrier (resorbable, biocompatible, semiviscous lipid)	Ongoing clinical trials	PMA
	i-FACTOR Bone Graft	Synthetic small peptide (P-15), peptide bone matrix used in an allograft bone ring and with supplemental anterior plate fixation C3-C4 to C6-C7 following single-level diskectomy for intractable radiculopathy (arm pain and/or a neurologic deficit), with or without neck pain, or myelopathy due to a single-level abnormality localized to the disk space	In November 2015, CeraPedics received Premarket Approval (PMA) from the FDA for the use of i-FACTOR Bone Graft in anterior cervical diskectomy and fusion (ACDF), *a composite bone substitute* consisting of a synthetic collagen fragment (P-15) bound to calcium phosphate particles As an engineered product, P-15 quantity and viability remain consistent from lot-to-lot P-15 in an anorganic bone mineral. This unique combination replicates the organic (type I human collagen) and inorganic (calcium phosphate) components of autograft bone and creates the ideal template for new bone formation	Arnold et al 2016[102] Arnold et al 2017[105]	PMA cleared, P140019 www.accessdata.fda.gov/cdrh_docs/pdf14/p140019a.pdf November 2015
CG Bio	Novosis	rhBMP and ceramic	rhBMP-2/hydroxyapatite (granule type) → Three types of composition rhBMP-2 (0.5 mg/ml)/hydroxyapatite (0.5 g/1 mL) rhBMP-2 (1.0 mg/ml)/ hydroxyapatite (1.0 g/2 mL) rhBMP-2 (3.0 mg/ml)/ hydroxyapatite (3.0 g/8 mL)	Interbody fusion in spine (rhBMP-2/β-TCP [putty type]) → ClinicalTrial.gov (NCT01764906)	Traumatic bone defect in upper and lower extremity (approved in Korea) The use of posterolateral spine fusion is permitted in June, 2017 (approved in Korea)
	Novosis-Dent	rhBMP and ceramic	rhBMP-2 (0.25 mg/ml)/ hydroxyapatite (0.25 g/0.5 mL)	For management of dental bone defect or bone formation (ClinicalTrials.gov Identifier: NCT01634308) → Results were published in PubMed → Permitted in KFDA (February, 2013)	—
Cowellmedi Co., Ltd.	COWELL BMP	rhBMP and ceramic	rhBMP-2 (0.75 mg/ml)+ BCP (mixture of hydroxyapatite and β-TCP with ratio of 3 versus 7)	RCT for using interbody fusion in spine (approved in 2012 by Cowellmedi Co., and in 2015 by OssGen company) → rhBMP-2/biphasic calcium phosphate (hydroxyapatite [60%]+ β-TCP [40%])	Traumatic bone defect in upper and lower extremity (approved in Korea)

(Continued)

TABLE 4 Commercially Available Bone Inductive Peptides, Proteins-Based Products, and Recombinant Versions (Continued)

Company	Growth Factor Product	Formulation	Product Composition	Peer-Reviewed Clinical Evidence/ Ongoing Study	Regulatory Clearance/Approval/ PMA, FDA 510(k)
Medtronic Sofamor Danek, Inc., USA	INFUSE Bone Graft/ LT-CAGE	rhBMP and a carrier/scaffold inserted into a hard LT-CAGE	rhBMP-2, absorbable collagen scaffold (ACS), filler, Ti metal prosthesis (Ti-6Al-4V)	NCT01491386 NCT01491425	Regulated under PMA P000058, July, 2002 www.accessdata.fda.gov/cdrh_docs/pdf/p000058b.pdf
	—	—	rhBMP-2/ACS/INTERFIX	NCT01491451	—
	INFUSE Bone Graft	LT-CAGE Lumbar Tapered Fusion Device and INFUSE Bone Graft	rhBMP-2, ACS, filler, Ti metal prosthesis(Ti-6Al-4V)	NCT00635843 Litrico et al 2018[106]	—
	INFUSE Bone Graft	INFUSE Bone Graft	INFUSE Bone Graft consists of two components, rhBMP-2 (known as dibotermin alfa) 1.5 mg/mL of rhBMP-2; 5.0 mg sucrose, NF; 25 mg glycine, USP; 3.7 mg L-glutamic acid, FCC; 0.1 mg sodium chloride, USP; 0.1 mg polysorbate 80, NF; and 1.0 mL of sterile water Reconstituted rhBMP-2 solution has a pH of 4.5 and is clear, colorless, and essentially free from plainly visible particulate matter. Placed on an ACS; bovine type I collagen obtained from the deep flexor (Achilles) tendon	ClinicalTrials.gov listings	Regulated under PMA P000053, March 2007 www.accessdata.fda.gov/cdrh_docs/pdf5/p050053b.pdf
	INFUSE/ MASTERGRAFT	—	Posterolateral Revision device The INFUSE/MASTERGRAFT posterolateral revision device is indicated for the repair of symptomatic, posterolateral lumbar spine pseudarthrosis. This device is intended to address a small subset of patients for whom autologous bone and/or bone marrow harvest are not feasible or are not expected to promote fusion. This includes patients with diabetes and smokers. This device is indicated to treat two or more levels of the lumbar spine. Orthopaedics Adult, October 10, 2008	NCT01491542 https://www.accessdata.fda.gov/cdrh_docs/pdf4/h040004c.pdf	INFUSE/MASTERGRAFT This device has been withdrawn at the request of the sponsor effective March 23, 2010
	INFUSE Bone Graft	Polyetheretherketone (PEEK) in oblique lateral interbody fusion (OLIF)	OLIF: 51 procedures with Divergence-L Interbody Fusion Device at a single level from L5-S1 OLIF: 25 procedures with Pivox Oblique Lateral Spine System at a single level from L2-L5 ALIF procedures with Divergence-L at a single level from L2-S1	—	2015
	INFUSE Bone Graft/ PEEK (ACDF)	—	—	NCT00485173, 2013 Zadegan et al 2017[107] IDE# G010188/NCT00642876 and IDE# G000123/NCT00437190 (www.ClinicalTrials.gov) Arnold et al 2016[105]	Not cleared

	InductOs (Medtronic Spinal and Biologics)	—	ALIF (188), PLIF (111), TLIF (4), LLIF (106), PLF (221)	NCT02280187, InductOs in Real World Spine Surgery; A Retrospective, French, Multi-centric, Study (InductOR)	—
BioAlpha, Inc.	—	—	Other Study ID Numbers: ExcelOS 14-01	NCT02714829	—
Stryker Biotech, 2004-2008	OP-1 (rhBMP-7)	Osigraft	Single-level instrumented posterolateral fusion for spondylolisthesis	Lehr et al 2021,[108] 10-year long-term follow-up rate: 73% (41/56) 78% were satisfied, no radiographs were obtained Fused 50% (10/20), OP-1, 1 year Fused 81% (17/21), ICBG, 1 year Note comparison 66% fused so 34% were classified as not fused	Utrecht, the Netherlands
Stryker Biotech, 2004	OP-1 Putty	OP-1 Putty	OP-1/BMP-7 produced Delivered on a purified type I bone collagen carrier	For revision posterior lateral intertransverse lumbar spinal fusion Vaccaro et al 2008[109] Guerado and Fuerstenberg 2011[110]	Center for Devices and Radiological Health of the FDA Humanitarian Device Exemption (2018, not sold in the United States) OP-1 implant is approved in 28 additional countries, including Australia, Canada, and the European Union
	Op-1 Putty	—	Instrumented posterolateral fusion OP-1 with local bone versus autograft OP-1/g collagen matrix versus local bone + hydroxyapatite-TCP	Delawi et al 2016[111] Fused 54% OP-1 versus fused 74% autograft ($P < 0.03$) Kanayama et al 2006[112] Surgical explorations of fusion masses Fused 57% (4/7) OP-1 versus fused 78% (7/9) LB and hydroxyapatite-TCP	Not recommended
Pfizer (Wyeth is now a wholly owned subsidiary of Pfizer)	—	rhBMP-2/CPM rhBMP-2/CPM matrix	rhBMP-2/calcium phosphate matrix (CPM)	NCT00752557 (bone mineral density) Closed fractures NCT00161629 (radius) NCT00384852 (humerus)	Not yet approved
OrthoSera GmbH, Austria	Bone Albumin	—	BoneAlbumin, a serum albumin, enhanced bone allograft that was shown to activate bone marrow stem cells leading to faster and better bone healing In R&D, growth factor–rich serum fraction (hyperacute serum or hypACT)	Not in use in United States This tissue product is already in commercial stage with two double-blinded clinical studies proving its effectiveness in sports surgery and dentistry	—

ACDF = anterior cervical diskectomy and fusion, ALIF = anterior lumbar interbody fusion, BCP = biphasic calcium phosphate, DBM = demineralized bone matrix, GTP = good tissue practice, ICBG = iliac crest bone graft, LLIF = lateral lumbar interbody fusion, OP-1 = osteogenic protein-1, PLF = posterolateral fusion, PLIF = posterior lumbar interbody fusion, RCT = randomized controlled trial, TLIF = transforaminal lumbar interbody fusion, β-TCP = beta tricalcium phosphate.

www.accessdata.fda.gov/scripts/CFappspub/tiss/Index.cfm.

www.google2.fda.gov/search?q=21CFRPart1271regulationsfor361HCT/Pslisting&client=FDAgov&proxystylesheet=FDAgov&output=xml_no_dtd&site=FDAgov&requiredfields=-archive:Yes&sort=date:D:L:d1&filter=1.

www.accessdata.fda.gov/scripts/cber/CFApps/Index.cfm.

TABLE 5 Commercially Available Bioactive Synthetic Bone Void Fillers, Extenders, and Substitute Products

Company (Synthetic)	Product	Formulation	Product Composition	Peer-Reviewed Clinical Evidence ClinicalTrials.gov/Ongoing Study Translational/Animal Studies	Regulatory Clearance/Approval FDA 510(k), #, month year CFR 1270, CFR 1271 MQV, Filler, Bone Void, Calcium Compound Common Name—Bone Grafting Material Classification Name—Bone Grafting Material, Synthetic
Bioactive glass	—	—	—	—	Regulation # CFR 888.3045 MVQ (resorbable calcium salt)
ApaTech, Ltd., Affiliated Altapore/Baxter Healthcare Corporation, Deerfield, IL	Inductigraft, Altapore	Granules in aqueous carrier	SiCaP EP, 31% to 47% enhanced strut porosity of silicate-substituted calcium phosphate–enhanced porosity, synthetic graft, 1 to 2 mm, 80% to 85% total porosity, 31% to 47% microporosity, 0.8% Si by weight	NCT01452022: posterolateral fusion (PLF) with Inductigraft Bolger et al 2019[119] Fused 86.3% (88/102 patients), 1 year Fused 90.6% (87/96), 2 years	K192363, September 2020 K191513, October 2019 K181225, August 2018 21 CFR 888.3045
Amend Surgical, Inc., FL, USA/Nanotherapeutics, Inc.®	NanoFUSE® DBM (synthetic + allograft + zenograft)	Puttylike with DBM	NanoFUSE® DBM used a patented (USPTO# 7,846,459 and 7,829,105) process to microencapsulate the DBM and bioactive glass particles in porcine gelatin NanoFUSE DBM lots produced were terminally sterilized using ionizing radiation and endotoxin free	Kirk et al 2013[41]	K142104, January 2015
	0.5 mL NanoFUSE (PLF)	Puttylike, malleable	Amend Surgical, Inc. NanoFUSE is comprised synthetic calcium phosphor-silicate particulate material particles (45S5 bioactive glass) coated with gelatin derived from porcine skin	—	K161996, February 2017 21 CFR 888.3045
	45S5 bioactive glass (1 to 10 mL)	Particulate material	45 wt% SiO_2, 24.5 wt% CaO, 24.5 wt% Na_2O, and 6.0 wt% P_2O_5, synthetic binder	—	K110368, January 2017, predicate NovaBone Products, LLC
BioMimetic Therapeutics, Inc., Franklin, TN Bioventus Surgical Bone Bank Allografts, Texas, USA Bonalive Biomaterials, Biolinja 12, 20750 Turku, Finland	OsteoMatrix	Strip type	60% hydroxyapatite + 40% beta tricalcium phosphate (β-TCP) + type I collagen Synthetic two-phase calcium phosphate embedded in a cross-linked collagen carrier	n/a	K051774, January 2006 (products name of MBCP)
	Osetoplus	Granules in delivery syringe	Biphasic calcium phosphate: 60% hydroxyapatite + 40% β-TCP Synthetic two-phase calcium phosphate granules with interconnected macropores and 3D micropores	n/a	K051774, January 2006 (products name of MBCP)

Bioventus Surgical BoneBank allografts, Texas, USA Bonalive Biomaterials, Biolinja 12, 20750 Turku, Finland BONESUPPORT HOLDING AB, Scheelevägen 19, SE-223 70 Lund, Sweden	Confirm Bioactive Confirm Gel Confirm Crunch	Gel and crunch type	*Gel type* Composition: Bioglass + hyaluronic acid + glycerol Sterile-packed in a syringe Available in three sizes: 2, 5, and 10 mL Uniform Bioglass particle sizes *Crunch type* Composition: Bioglass + hyaluronic acid + glycerol Sterile-packed in a syringe Available in three sizes: 2, 5, and 10 mL Mixture of Bioglass particle sizes	n/a, maxillofacial	K133678, August 2014
	BonAlive	Granule and putty type Various sizes	S53P4 bioactive glass (53% SiO_2, 23% Na_2O, 20% CaO, 4% P_2O)	NCT05049915 Management of tibial or femoral nonunions Malat et al 2018[120] Osteomyelitis management Aurégan and Begue 2015[121] Long bone defect management	—
Bonalive BioMaterials, Ltd./Vivoxid Ltd., Turku, Finland * US distributor, TriMed, Inc.	BonAlive	Putty Granules Plates	Bioactive glass (S53P4) as granules size 0.5 to 0.8 mm or 1.0 to 2.0 mm by weight, 53% SiO_2, 23% Na_2O, 20% CaO, and 4% P_2O_5(synthetic, osteoconductive, and bacterial growth-inhibiting material)	NCT05001893 (S53P4 bioactive glass putty, Bonalive Biomaterials, Ltd.), ongoing NCT00935870 (spine fusion and fractures) Sponsor: Turku, Finland NCT00841152 (fill contained bone defects) Bonalive Biomaterials (Vivoxid Ltd., Turku, Finland)	K191274, May 2019 (BonAlive Granules) Reclassified from K071199, February 2012 K071937, October 2007
Collagen Matrix, Inc., Oakland, NJ	Mineral Collagen Composite Bioactive Moldable	Strip Cylindrical Matrix	Calcium phosphate (anorganic bone mineral) Bioactive glass (45S5) Type I bovine collagen (Achilles tendon)	—	K182074, February 2019 21 CFR 888.3045
Globus Medical, Inc., Audubon, PA	Kinex Bioactive Kinex Plus Strip	Putty or gel Strip	Bioglass (ASTM F1538) collagen + hyaluronic acid	—	K130392, August 2013 21 CFR 888.3045
Inion, Inc., Weston FL, USA Inion Oy, Lääkärinkatu 2, 33520 Tampere, Finland	BioRestore	Cylinders, blocks, and morsels	Bioactive glass (S53P4), different sizes degradable Package sizes: syringe (5, 6, 8, and 10 mL), tube (0.25, 0.5, 1, 1.6, 2.0, 2.5, 4.6, and 5.0 mL)	NCT01304121, no results posted NCT01105026 (not spine, 2019)	K191764, July 2019 K090177, February 2009 K070998, October 2007
NovaBone, Jacksonville, FL, USA →Osteogenics Biomedical	NovaBone Putty Bioactive Synthetic Bone Graft	Soft malleable putty	Bimodal particle distribution of calcium phosphosilicate (Bioglass) + polyethylene glycol as additive + glycerin as binder Volume of active ingredient is 70%	n/a NovaBone products, LLC NovaBone Products, LLC predicate	K110368, March 2011 K082672, December 2008 CE approval

(Continued)

TABLE 5 Commercially Available Bioactive Synthetic Bone Void Fillers, Extenders, and Substitute Products (Continued)

Company (Synthetic)	Product	Formulation	Product Composition	Peer-Reviewed Clinical Evidence ClinicalTrials.gov/Ongoing Study Translational/Animal Studies	Regulatory Clearance/Approval FDA 510(k), #, month year CFR 1270, CFR 1271 MQV, Filler, Bone Void, Calcium Compound Common Name—Bone Grafting Material Classification Name—Bone Grafting Material, Synthetic
NovaBone, Jacksonville, FL, USA → Osteogenics Biomedical	NovaBone-AR	Packable graft	Synthetic calcium phosphosilicate (Bioglass) particulate, fused into a bulk porous form having a multidirectional interconnected porosity	n/a	K041613, June 2004
	NovaBone IRM	Flexible sheets, varying sizes	IRM (irrigation-resistant matrix) Bioactive calcium phosphosilicate particulate and a synthetic, absorbable binder	Retrospective comparative study	K041613, December 2005 (21 CFR 888.3045) November 19, 2016
	NovaBone Bioactive Strip	Strip type	Purified fibrillar collagen and resorbable bioactive synthetic granules (Bioglass)	n/a	K141207, May 2014
	NovaBone MacroFORM	Moldable type	Open porous structure to facilitate the absorption of bone marrow aspirate Purified collagen and resorbable bioactive synthetic granules (Bioglass)	n/a	K0140946, August 2014
	NovaBone Porous	Powder	Synthetic calcium phosphosilicate (Bioglass)	n/a	K090731, April 2009
Orthovita, Inc. → Merged into Stryker	Vitoss BA (Bioactive Bone Graft Substitute)	Various type (original, foam pack, foam strip)	Highly porous β-TCP + bioactive glass	n/a	K083033, November 2008
	Vitoss Bone Graft Substitute, Bioactive Foam Strip	Strip type	Highly porous β-TCP + bioactive glass	n/a	K072184, September 2007
	Vitoss BBTrauma	Putty type (foam pack)	Highly porous β-TCP + bioactive glass Broader range of bioactive glass particle size distribution and has a unique porosity, structure, and chemistry to help drive 3D regeneration of bone	n/a	K083033, November 2008
	Vitoss BA2X (Bioactive Bone Graft Substitute)	Putty type (foam pack)	Highly porous β-TCP + bioactive glass Increased levels of bioactive glass compared with Vitoss BA and has a unique porosity, structure, and chemistry to help drive 3D regeneration of bone	n/a	K083033, November 2008
	HydroSet HydroSet XT	Injectable type	Tetracalcium phosphate that is formulated to convert to hydroxyapatite, the principal mineral component of bone HydroSet XT is simple and easy form of HydroSet	n/a	K161447, October 2016

Prosidyan, Inc., Philadelphia, Penn, USA/ DePuy Synthes	FIBERGRAFT BG[122]	Morsels	FIBERGRAFT BG Morsels is an ultraporous synthetic bone graft substitute made entirely from crystalline 45S5 bioactive glass FIBERGRAFT BG Putty—Bone Graft Substitute Indication for use in PLF	Fortier et al 2017[122] ACDF, retrospective case series Fused 88.5% (46/52 levels, grade 1 fusion)	K132805, January 2014 K141956, August 2014 K151154, September 2015 K171284, May 2017 K143533, March 2015
	FIBERGRAFT BG Putty Bone Graft Substitute	Strip or putty	—	NCT03898232: retrospective series, CT lumbar interbody spine fusions	K170306, May 2017
	FIBERGRAFT Matrix Bone Graft Substitute	Putty (matrix)	FIBERGRAFT BG (Synthetic) mixed with extralong fibers of type I bovine collagen mixed (xenograft)	NCT03884283: prospective, posterolateral lumbar fusion, ongoing	K180080, April 2018 Regulation #CFR 888.3045 MVQ (resorbable calcium salt)
Synergy Biomedical, LLC	BioSphere Flex	—	45S5 bioactive glass sphere granules suspended in a 3D, porous scaffold carrier composed of freeze-dried collagen and sodium hyaluronate BioSphere Flex is designed to be mixed with autogenous bone marrow. The structure readily absorbs liquid and becomes flexible and moldable when fully hydrated	n/a	K173424, September 2018
Synergy Biomedical, LLC	BioSphere Putty	Putty type	80% bioactive glass spheres; 20% phospholipid carrier	Gomez and Westerlund 2021[123] Retrospective series, ACDF, PEEK filled third generation bioactive glass Fused 100% (39/39), multilevel fusion (17/17 two levels, 12/12 three level, 9/9 four level, 1/1 five level)	K122868, April 2013
Synergy Biomedical, LLC Vivoxid Ltd., Turku, Finland	BioSphere MIS Putty (BioSphere MIS)	Prefilled type	Medical-grade 45S5 bioactive glass particles + carrier (same composition of BioSphere Putty)	Westerlund and Borden 2020[124] 100% fused: 115 ACDF, 103 TLIF	K173301, January 2018
	Bioactive Glass (S53P4) as granules (BonAlive)	Granules Plates	By weight, SiO_2 53%, Na_2O 23%, CaO 20%, and P_2O_5 5 4% (synthetic, osteoconductive, and bacterial growth-inhibiting material)	*NCT00935870* Sponsor: Turku, Finland NCT00841152 Bonalive Biomaterials (Vivoxid Ltd., Turku, Finland)	K071937, October 2007
Noraker Lyon-Villeurbanne, France	Glassbone	—	45S5 BAG particle size 1 to 3 mm	Barrey and Broussolle 2019[125] Mix 50:50 BAG: local bone PF-C (n = 3 patients) Fused 81.5% (22/27), PF-L (1 year)	K000633, May 2000

Bioactive synthetics materials in this class are most always used with BMA, whole blood, serum, physiologic saline, and/or mixed with autograft (cortical or cancellous bone) or other potent grafting materials (materials that have been excluded from synthetics as not or less bioactive: porous hyper–cross-linked, polymeric carbohydrate, porous poly(lactic-co-glycolic acid)/hydroxyapatite matrix, and porous or other β-TCP).

BMA is typically added at the time of surgery to these synthetic materials for grafting into the spinal fusion surgical bed/site.

Whole blood or serum (patient's own) may be used.

ACDF = anterior cervical diskectomy and fusion, BAG = bioactive glass, BMA = bone marrow aspirate, DBM = demineralized bone matrix, PF-C = posterior fusion, cervical spine, PF-L = posterior fusion, lumbar spine

https://510k.directory/clearances/MQV/1, Accessed April-August 2021.

In the recent years, there is an increasing desire to use off-the-shelf compounds to minimize the surgical dissection and tissues destruction during the surgical procedure. The strengths and limitations of the different commercially available bioactive materials for use as adjuncts in spinal fusion surgery, including autologous bone grafts, allografts, DBM, CBM, rhBMPs, growth factors, cytokines, peptides and polypeptides, synthetic materials, and BAG, have been highlighted. A better awareness of the different options including risk-benefit assessment will help spine surgeons in making informed decisions.

As spine surgery in an aging population increases, so do the complex challenges faced by spine surgeons.[126] In spite of patient optimization, surgical innovations, including types of spinal fusion surgery, adequate surgical dissection and preparation, choice of instrumentation, spinal location of surgery, and abundant amounts of novel grafting materials, pseudarthrosis during spinal fusion remains high.

Bioactivity during spine fusion may be enhanced by critical selection of the grafting materials that are introduced into the surgical site to stimulate and support new bone growth and consolidation for fusion. Enhanced bioactive bone grafts are particularly important to consider in complex long fusion and or in nonoptimized patients with comorbidities undergoing a spinal fusion surgery. These comorbidities include risk factors, such as rheumatoid arthritis,[127] osteoporosis and osteopenia,[128,129] bone structure and quality,[88] obesity,[130] diabetes, nicotine use, nutritional status, hypovitaminosis D,[131] and decreased patient compliance with postoperative guidance.[132] Preoperative optimization of patient comorbidities and awareness of the unique properties of available bioactive agents will likely foster the development of further improved bone grafting materials, potentially improving the rate of successful fusion following spine surgery. In parallel, the safety and efficacy of new products should be monitored regularly with reporting of adverse events to an open database such as the Manufacturer and User Facility Device Experience, which is currently in use. Ongoing research and development of materials and nanomaterials that control the release of bound growth factors or similar (timed-release) to initiate improved control of inflammation and bone formation may further help to provide adequate potency to overcome critical still-existing patient comorbidities.

SUMMARY

Multiple biologic and bioactive materials exist at the disposal of the spine surgeon; many of these are now in off-the-shelf preparations. Historical literature and recent studies demonstrate that many of these substrates, used individually or in conjunction with others, may improve spinal fusion in the presence of pathologies such as acute trauma, deformity correction, and degenerative disease. Although these may improve the rate of spinal fusion under certain circumstances, there also exist conditions wherein use of these materials may induce deleterious effects. As further research into new bioactives involving combination therapies including stem cells evolves, spine surgeons should be discerning in their selection of the bioactive factor–based materials used for each patient. Spinal fusion will likely be optimized through a multifactorial approach of patient selection, specific bioactives, and surgical technique. These authors suggest prudent implementation of these factors when planning spinal fusion surgery.

REFERENCES

1. Fakhoury J, Dowling T: *Cervical Degenerative Disc Disease*. StatPearls, 2021. https://www.ncbi.nlm.nih.gov/NBK560772/.
2. Virk S, Qureshi S, Sandhu H: History of spinal fusion: Where we came from and where we are going. *HSS J* 2020;16(2):137-142.
3. Miller DJ, Vitale MG: Dr. Russell A. Hibbs: Pioneer of spinal fusion. *Spine (Phila Pa 1976)* 2015;40(16):1311-1313.
4. Albee FH: Transplantation of a portion of the tibia into the spine for Pott's disease: A preliminary report 1911. *Clin Orthop Relat Res* 2007;460:14-16.
5. Pedrero SG, Llamas-Sillero P, Serrano-Lopez J: A multidisciplinary journey towards bone tissue engineering. *Materials (Basel)* 2021;14(17):4896.
6. D'Souza M, Macdonald NA, Gendreau JL, Duddleston PJ, Feng AY, Ho AL: Graft materials and biologics for spinal interbody fusion. *Biomedicines* 2019;7(4):E75.
7. Branemark PI, Hansson BO, Adell R, et al: Osseointegrated implants in the treatment of the edentulous jaw. Experience from a 10-year period. *Scand J Plast Reconstr Surg Suppl* 1977;16:1-132.
8. Albrektsson T, Branemark PI, Hansson HA, Lindstrom J: Osseointegrated titanium implants. Requirements for ensuring a long-lasting, direct bone-to-implant anchorage in man. *Acta Orthop Scand* 1981;52(2):155-170.
9. Cho W, Mason JR, Smith JS, et al: Failure of lumbopelvic fixation after long construct fusions in patients with adult spinal deformity: Clinical and radiographic risk factors – Clinical article. *J Neurosurg Spine* 2013;19(4):445-453.
10. Kim YJ, Bridwell KH, Lenke LG, Rinella AS, Edwards C II, Edward C II: Pseudarthrosis in primary fusions for adult idiopathic scoliosis: Incidence, risk factors, and outcome analysis. *Spine (Phila Pa 1976)* 2005;30(4):468-474.
11. Oshina M, Oshima Y, Tanaka S, Riew KD: Radiological fusion criteria of postoperative anterior cervical discectomy and fusion: A systematic review. *Global Spine J* 2018;8(7):739-750.
12. Street M, Gao R, Martis W, et al: The efficacy of local autologous bone dust: A systematic review. *Spine Deform* 2017;5:231-237.
13. Gao R, Street M, Tay ML, et al: Human spinal bone dust as a potential local autograft: In vitro potent anabolic effect on human osteoblasts. *Spine (Phila Pa 1976)* 2018;43(4):E19 3-E199.

14. Elder BD, Holmes C, Goodwin CR, et al: A systematic assessment of the use of platelet-rich plasma in spinal fusion. *Ann Biomed Eng* 2015;43:1057-1070.
15. Robbins MA, Haudenschild DR, Wegner AM, Klineberg EO: Stem cells in spinal fusion. *Global Spine J* 2017;7(8):801-810.
16. Meyers MH: Resurfacing of the femoral head with fresh osteochondral allografts. Long-term results. *Clin Orthop Relat Res* 1985;197:111-114.
17. Rauck RC, Wang D, Tao M, Williams RJ: Chondral delamination of fresh osteochondral allografts after implantation in the knee: A matched cohort analysis. *Cartilage* 2019;10(4):402-407.
18. Torrie AM, Kesler WW, Elkin J, Gallo RA: Osteochondral allograft. *Curr Rev Musculoskelet Med* 2015;8(4):413-422.
19. Kawaguchi S, Hart RA: The need for structural allograft biomechanical guidelines. *Instr Course Lect* 2015;64:87-93.
20. Miyazaki M, Tsumura H, Wang JC, Alanay A: An update on bone substitutes for spinal fusion. *Eur Spine J* 2009;18(6):783-799.
21. Wheeless CR III: *Wheeless' Textbook of Orthopaedics*. Data-Trace Internet Pub., 1996. Available at: https://www.wheelessonline.com/orthopaedics-related-topics/allografts/.
22. Hamer AJ, Stockley I, Elson RA: Changes in allograft bone irradiated at different temperatures. *J Bone Joint Surg Br* 1999;81(2):342-344.
23. Morris MT, Tarpada SP, Cho W: Bone graft materials for posterolateral fusion made simple: A systematic review. *Eur Spine J* 2018;27(8):1856-1867.
24. Burke JF, Dhall SS: Bone morphogenic protein use in spinal surgery. *Neurosurg Clin N Am* 2017;28(3):331-334.
25. Glazebrook M, Young DS: B2A Polypeptide in foot and ankle fusion. *Foot Ankle Clin* 2016;21(4):803-807.
26. Hsu WK, Goldstein CL, Shamji MF, et al: Novel osteobiologics and biomaterials in the treatment of spinal disorders. *Neurosurgery* 2017;80(3 suppl):S100-S107.
27. Hench LL, Jones JR: Bioactive glasses: Frontiers and challenges. *Front Bioeng Biotechnol* 2015;3:194.
28. Shibuya N, Jupiter DC: Bone graft substitute: Allograft and xenograft. *Clin Podiatr Med Surg* 2015;32(1):21-34.
29. Fiani B, Jarrah R, Shields J, Sekhon M: Enhanced biomaterials: systematic review of alternatives to supplement spine fusion including silicon nitride, bioactive glass, amino peptide bone graft, and tantalum. *Neurosurg Focus* 2021;50(6):E10.
30. Gruskin E, Doll BA, Futrell FW, Schmitz JP, Hollinger JO: Demineralized bone matrix in bone repair: History and use. *Adv Drug Deliv Rev* 2012;64(12):1063-1077.
31. Yang JH, Glaeser JD, Kanim LE, et al: Bone grafts and bone graft substitutes, in Cheng BC, ed: *Handbook of Spine Technology*. Springer International Publishing, 2021, pp 197-273.
32. Bae H, Kanim L, Rajaee S, Yang J: Bone grafts, bone morphogenetic proteins, and bone substitutes, in Boyer MI, ed: *AAOS Comprehensive Orthopaedic Review* 2, Ch. 59. American Academy of Orthopaedic Surgeons, 2019.
33. Cohen JD, Kanim LE, Tronits AJ, Bae HW: Allografts and spinal fusion. *Int J Spine Surg* 2021;15(suppl 1):68-93.
34. Giannoudis PV, Dinopoulos H, Tsiridis E: Bone substitutes: An update. *Injury* 2005;36(suppl 3):S20-S27.
35. Tuchman A, Brodke DS, Youssef JA, et al: Autograft versus allograft for cervical spinal fusion: A systematic review. *Global Spine J* 2017;7(1):59-70.
36. Tuchman A, Brodke DS, Youssef JA, et al: Iliac crest bone graft versus local autograft or allograft for lumbar spinal fusion: A systematic review. *Global Spine J* 2016;6:592-606.
37. Radcliff K, Hwang R, Hilibrand A, et al: The effect of iliac crest autograft on the outcome of fusion in the setting of degenerative spondylolisthesis: A subgroup analysis of the Spine Patient Outcomes Research Trial (SPORT). *J Bone Joint Surg Am* 2012;94(18):1685-1692.
38. Kang J, An H, Hilibrand A, Yoon ST, Kavanagh E, Boden S: Grafton and local bone have comparable outcomes to iliac crest bone in instrumented single-level lumbar fusions. *Spine (Phila Pa 1976)* 2012;37(12):1083-1091.
39. Chang DG, Park JB, Han Y: Surgical outcomes of two kinds of demineralized bone matrix putties/local autograft composites in instrumented posterolateral lumbar fusion. *BMC Musculoskelet Disord* 2021;22(1):200.
40. An HS, Simpson JM, Glover JM, Stephany J: Comparison between allograft plus demineralized bone matrix versus autograft in anterior cervical fusion. A prospective multicenter study. *Spine (Phila Pa 1976)* 1995;20:2211-2216.
41. Kirk JF, Ritter G, Waters C, Narisawa S, Millan JL, Talton JD: Osteoconductivity and osteoinductivity of NanoFUSE(®) DBM. *Cell Tissue Bank* 2013;14(1):33-44.
42. Shehadi JA, Elzein SM: Review of commercially available demineralized bone matrix products for spinal fusions: A selection paradigm. *Surg Neurol Int* 2017;8:203.
43. Galli MM, Protzman NM, Bleazey ST, Brigido SA: Role of demineralized allograft subchondral bone in the treatment of shoulder lesions of the talus: Clinical results with two-year follow-up. *J Foot Ankle Surg* 2015;54(4):717-722.
44. Schizas C, Triantafyllopoulos D, Kosmopoulos V, Tzinieris N, Stafylas K: Posterolateral lumbar spine fusion using a novel demineralized bone matrix: A controlled case pilot study. *Arch Orthop Trauma Surg* 2008;128(6):621-625.
45. Eleswarapu A, Rowan FA, Le H, Wick JB, Roberto RF, Javidan Y, Klineberg EO: Efficacy, cost, and complications of demineralized bone matrix in instrumented lumbar fusion: Comparison With rhBMP-2. *Global Spine J* 2021;11(8):1223-1229.
46. Lee K, Goodman SB: Cell therapy for secondary osteonecrosis of the femoral condyles using the Cellect DBM system: A preliminary report. *J Arthroplasty* 2009;24(1):43-48.
47. Epstein NE, Epstein JA: SF-36 outcomes and fusion rates after multilevel laminectomies and 1 and 2-level instrumented posterolateral fusions using lamina autograft and demineralized bone matrix. *J Spinal Disord Tech* 2007;20(2):139-145.
48. Cammisa FP Jr, Lowery G, Garfin SR, et al: Two-year fusion rate equivalency between Grafton DBM gel and autograft in posterolateral spine fusion: A prospective controlled trial employing a side-by-side comparison in the same patient. *Spine (Phila Pa 1976)* 2004;29(6):660-666.

49. Park HW, Lee JK, Moon SJ, Seo SK, Lee JH, Kim SH: The efficacy of the synthetic interbody cage and Grafton for anterior cervical fusion. *Spine (Phila Pa 1976)* 2009;34(17):E591-E595.
50. Urist MR: Bone: Formation by autoinduction. *Science* 1965;150(3698):893-899.
51. Bae HW, Zhao L, Kanim LEA, Wong P, Delamarter RB, Dawson EG: Intervariability and intravariability of bone morphogenetic proteins in commercially available demineralized bone matrix products. *Spine (Phila Pa 1976)* 2006;31(12):1299-1306.
52. Bae H, Zhao L, Zhu D, Kanim LE, Wang JC, Delamarter RB: Variability across ten production lots of a single demineralized bone matrix product. *J Bone Joint Surg Am* 2010;92(2):427-435.
53. Skovrlj B, Guzman JZ, Al Maaieh M, Cho SK, Iatridis JC, Qureshi SA: Cellular bone matrices: Viable stem cell-containing bone graft substitutes. *Spine J* 2014;14(11):2763-2772.
54. Ryan JM, Barry FP, Murphy JM, Mahon BP: Mesenchymal stem cells avoid allogeneic rejection. *J Inflamm (Lond)* 2005;2:8.
55. Divi SN, Mikhael MM: Use of allogenic mesenchymal cellular bone matrix in anterior and posterior cervical spinal fusion: A case series of 21 patients. *Asian Spine J* 2017;11(3):454-462.
56. Kerr EJ III, Jawahar A, Wooten T, Kay S, Cavanaugh DA, Nunley PD: The use of osteo-conductive stem-cells allograft in lumbar interbody fusion procedures: An alternative to recombinant human bone morphogenetic protein. *J Surg Orthop Adv* 2011;20(3):193-197.
57. Myerson CL, Myerson MS, Coetzee C, McGaver RS, Giveans RS: Subtalar arthrodesis with use of adipose-derived cellular bone matrix compared with autologous bone graft. *J Bone Joint Surg Am* 2019;101(21):1904-1911. Erratum in: *J Bone Joint Surg Am* 2019;101(24):e137.
58. Roh JS, Yeung CA, Field JS, McClellan RT: Allogeneic morphogenetic protein vs. recombinant human bone morphogenetic protein-2 in lumbar interbody fusion procedures: A radiographic and economic analysis. *J Orthop Surg Res* 2013;8:49.
59. Bergin SM, Wang TY, Park C, et al: Pseudarthrosis rate following anterior cervical discectomy with fusion using an allograft cellular bone matrix: A multi-institutional analysis. *Neurosurg Focus* 2021;50(6):E6.
60. McAnany SJ, Ahn J, Elboghdady IM, et al: Mesenchymal stem cell allograft as a fusion adjunct in one- and two-level anterior cervical discectomy and fusion: a matched cohort analysis. *Spine J* 2016;16(2):163-167.
61. Pinheiro MB, Ferreira ML, Refshauge K, et al: Symptoms of depression as a prognostic factor for low back pain: A systematic review. *Spine J* 2016;16(1):105-116.
62. Tohmeh AG, Watson B, Tohmeh M, Zielinski XJ: Allograft cellular bone matrix in extreme lateral interbody fusion: Preliminary radiographic and clinical outcomes. *ScientificWorldJournal* 2012;2012:263637.
63. Ammerman JM, Libricz J, Ammerman MD: The role of Osteocel Plus as a fusion substrate in minimally invasive instrumented transforaminal lumbar interbody fusion. *Clin Neurol Neurosurg* 2013;115(7):991-994.
64. Eastlack RK, Garfin SR, Brown CR, Meyer SC: Osteocel plus cellular allograft in anterior cervical discectomy and fusion: Evaluation of clinical and radiographic outcomes from a prospective multicenter study. *Spine (Phila Pa 1976)* 2014;39(22):E1331-E1337.
65. Hollawell S, Kane B, Heisey C, Greenberg P: The role of allograft bone in foot and ankle arthrodesis and high-risk fracture management. *Foot Ankle Spec* 2019;12(5):418-425.
66. Vanichkachorn J, Peppers T, Bullard D, Stanley SK, Linovitz RJ, Ryaby JT: A prospective clinical and radiographic 12-month outcome study of patients undergoing single-level anterior cervical discectomy and fusion for symptomatic cervical degenerative disc disease utilizing a novel viable allogeneic, cancellous, bone matrix (trinity evolution™) with a comparison to historical controls. *Eur Spine J* 2016;25(7):2233-2238.
67. Halalmeh DR, Perez-Cruet MJ: Use of local morselized bone autograft in minimally invasive transforaminal lumbar interbody fusion: Cost analysis. *World Neurosurg* 2021;146:e544-e554.
68. Tally WC, Temple HT, Subhawong TY, Ganey T: Transforaminal lumbar interbody fusion with viable allograft: 75 consecutive cases at 12-month follow-up. *Int J Spine Surg* 2018;12(1):76-84.
69. Gibson AW, Feroze AH, Greil ME, et al: Cellular allograft for multilevel stand-alone anterior cervical discectomy and fusion. *Neurosurg Focus* 2021;50(6):E7.
70. Elgafy H, Wetzell B, Gillette M, et al: Lumbar spine fusion outcomes using a cellular bone allograft with lineage-committed bone-forming cells in 96 patients. *BMC Musculoskelet Disord* 2021;22(1):699.
71. Hall JF, McLean JB, Jones SM, Moore MA, Nicholson MD, Dorsch KA: Multilevel instrumented posterolateral lumbar spine fusion with an allogeneic cellular bone graft. *J Orthop Surg Res* 2019;14(1):372.
72. Nunley PD, Kerr EJ III, Utter PA, et al: Preliminary results of bioactive amniotic suspension with allograft for achieving one and two-level lumbar interbody fusion. *Int J Spine Surg* 2016;10:12.
73. Hernigou P, Mathieu G, Poignard A, Manicom O, Beaujean F, Rouard H: Percutaneous autologous bone-marrow grafting for nonunions. Surgical technique. *J Bone Joint Surg Am* 2006;88(suppl 1 pt 2):322-327.
74. Cui Q, Ming Xiao Z, Balian G, Wang G: Comparison of lumbar spine fusion using mixed and cloned marrow cells. *Spine (Phila Pa 1976)* 2001;26(21):2305-2310.
75. Gupta MC, Theerajunyaporn T, Maitra S, et al: Efficacy of mesenchymal stem cell enriched grafts in an ovine posterolateral lumbar spine model. *Spine (Phila Pa 1976)* 2007;32(7):720-726.
76. Lin C, Zhang N, Waldorff EI, et al: Comparing cellular bone matrices for posterolateral spinal fusion in a rat model. *JOR Spine* 2020;3(2):e1084.
77. Carvalho EBS, Veronesi GF, Manfredi GGP, et al: Bone demineralization improves onlay graft consolidation: A histological study in rat calvaria. *J Periodontol* 2021;92(6):1-10.
78. Kamiya N, Mishina Y: New insights on the roles of BMP signaling in bone-A review of recent mouse genetic studies. *Biofactors* 2011;37(2):75-82.

79. Lowery JW, Brookshire B, Rosen V: A survey of strategies to modulate the bone morphogenetic protein signaling pathway: Current and future perspectives. *Stem Cells Int* 2016;2016:7290686.
80. Bragdon B, Moseychuk O, Saldanha S, King D, Julian J, Nohe A: Bone morphogenetic proteins: A critical review. *Cell Signal* 2011;23(4):609-620.
81. Wozney JM, Rosen V: Bone morphogenetic protein and bone morphogenetic protein gene family in bone formation and repair. *Clin Orthop Relat Res* 1998;346:26-37.
82. Sampath TK, Reddi AH: Discovery of bone morphogenetic proteins – A historical perspective. *Bone* 2020;140:115548.
83. Lowery JW, Rosen V: Bone morphogenetic protein-based therapeutic approaches. *Cold Spring Harb Perspect Biol* 2018;10(4):a022327.
84. Presciutti S, Boden S: BMP and beyond: A 25-year historical review of translational Spine Research at Emory University. *Spine Surg Relat Res* 2018;2:1-10.
85. McKay WF, Peckham SM, Badura JM: A comprehensive clinical review of recombinant human bone morphogenetic protein-2 (INFUSE Bone Graft). *Int Orthop* 2007;31(6):729-734.
86. Vaccaro AR, Patel T, Fischgrund J, et al: A pilot safety and efficacy study of OP-1 putty (rhBMP-7) as an adjunct to iliac crest autograft in posterolateral lumbar fusions. *Eur Spine J* 2003;12(5):495-500.
87. Vaccaro AR, Patel T, Fischgrund J, et al: A pilot study evaluating the safety and efficacy of OP-1 Putty (rhBMP-7) as a replacement for iliac crest autograft in posterolateral lumbar arthrodesis for degenerative spondylolisthesis. *Spine (Phila Pa 1976)* 2004;29(17):1885-1892.
88. Liu S, Wang Y, Liang Z, Zhou M, Chen C: Comparative clinical effectiveness and safety of bone morphogenetic protein versus autologous iliac crest bone graft in lumbar fusion: A meta-analysis and systematic review. *Spine (Phila Pa 1976)* 2020;45(12):E729-E741.
89. Feng JT, Yang XG, Wang F, He X, Hu YC: Efficacy and safety of bone substitutes in lumbar spinal fusion: A systematic review and network meta-analysis of randomized controlled trials. *Eur Spine J* 2020;29(6):1261-1276.
90. Manzur M, Virk SS, Jivanelli B, et al: The rate of fusion for stand-alone anterior lumbar interbody fusion: A systematic review. *Spine J* 2019;19(7):1294-1301.
91. Manzur MK, Steinhaus ME, Virk SS, et al: Fusion rate for stand-alone lateral lumbar interbody fusion: A systematic review. *Spine J* 2020;20(11):1816-1825.
92. Noshchenko A, Hoffecker L, Lindley EM, Burger EL, Cain CMJ, Patel VV: Perioperative and long-term clinical outcomes for bone morphogenetic protein versus iliac crest bone graft for lumbar fusion in degenerative disk disease: Systematic review with meta-analysis. *J Spinal Disord Tech* 2014;27(3):117-135.
93. Bannwarth M, Smith JS, Bess S, et al: Use of rhBMP-2 for adult spinal deformity surgery: Patterns of usage and changes over the past decade. *Neurosurg Focus* 2021;50(6):E4.
94. Daniels AH, Reid DBC, Tran SN, et al: Evolution in surgical approach, complications, and outcomes in an adult spinal deformity surgery multicenter study group patient population. *Spine Deform* 2019;7(3):481-488.
95. Niu S, Anastasio AT, Faraj RR, Rhee JM: Evaluation of heterotopic ossification after using recombinant human bone morphogenetic protein-2 in transforaminal lumbar interbody fusion: A computed tomography review of 996 disc levels. *Global Spine J* 2020;10(3):280-285.
96. Shields LBE, Raque GH, Glassman SD, et al: Adverse effects associated with high-dose recombinant human bone morphogenetic protein-2 use in anterior cervical spine fusion. *Spine (Phila Pa 1976)* 2006;31(5):542-547.
97. Taylor Bellamy J, Dilbone E, Schell A, et al: Prospective comparison of dysphagia following Anterior Cervical Discectomy and Fusion (ACDF) with and without rhBMP-2. *Spine J* 2021;22(2):256-264.
98. Wen YD, Jiang WM, Yang HL, Shi JH: Exploratory meta-analysis on dose-related efficacy and complications of rhBMP-2 in anterior cervical discectomy and fusion: 1, 539, 021 cases from 2003 to 2017 studies. *J Orthop Translat* 2020;24:166-174.
99. Administration UFaD: FDA public health notification: Life-threatening complications associated with recombinant human bone morphogenetic protein in cervical spine fusion, 2008. https://www.patientsafety.va.gov/docs/alerts/AL09-13MedtronicInfuse.pdf.
100. Seeherman HJ, Wilson CG, Vanderploeg EJ, et al: A BMP/Activin a chimera induces posterolateral spine fusion in nonhuman primates at lower concentrations than BMP-2. *J Bone Joint Surg Am* 2021;103(16):e64.
101. Cottrill E, Ahmed AK, Lessing L, et al: Investigational growth factors utilized in animal models of spinal fusion: Systematic review. *World J Orthop* 2019;10:176-191.
102. Arnold PM, Sasso RC, Janssen ME, et al: Efficacy of i-factor bone graft versus autograft in anterior cervical discectomy and fusion: Results of the prospective, randomized, single-blinded food and drug administration investigational device exemption study. *Spine (Phila Pa 1976)* 2016;41(13):1075-1083.
103. Plantz MA, Gerlach EB, Hsu WK: Synthetic bone graft materials in spine fusion: Current evidence and future trends. *Int J Spine Surg* 2021;15(suppl 1):104-112.
104. Costantino PD, Friedman CD: Synthetic bone graft substitutes. *Otolaryngol Clin North Am* 1994;27(5):1037-1074.
105. Arnold PM, Anderson KK, Selim A, Dryer RF, Kenneth Burkus J: Heterotopic ossification following single-level anterior cervical discectomy and fusion: Results from the prospective, multicenter, historically controlled trial comparing allograft to an optimized dose of rhBMP-2. *J Neurosurg Spine* 2016;25(3):292-302.
106. Litrico S, Langlais T, Pennes F, Gennari A, Paquis P: Lumbar interbody fusion with utilization of recombinant human bone morphogenetic protein: A retrospective real-life study about 277 patients. *Neurosurg Rev* 2018;41(1):189-196.
107. Zadegan SA, Abedi A, Jazayeri SB, et al: Bone morphogenetic proteins in anterior cervical fusion: A systematic review and meta-analysis. *World Neurosurg* 2017;104:752-787.

108. Lehr AM, Delawi D, van Susante JLC, et al: Long-term (> 10 years) clinical outcomes of instrumented posterolateral fusion for spondylolisthesis. *Eur Spine J* 2021;30:1380-1386.

109. Vaccaro AR, Whang PG, Patel T, et al: The safety and efficacy of OP-1 (rhBMP-7) as a replacement for iliac crest autograft for posterolateral lumbar arthrodesis: Minimum 4-year follow-up of a pilot study. *Spine J* 2008;8(3):457-465.

110. Guerado E, Fuerstenberg CH: What bone graft substitutes should we use in post-traumatic spinal fusion? *Injury* 2011;42(suppl 2):S64-S71.

111. Delawi D, Jacobs W, van Susante JLC, et al: OP-1 compared with iliac crest autograft in instrumented posterolateral fusion: A randomized, multicenter non-inferiority trial. *J Bone Joint Surg Am* 2016;98(6):441-448.

112. Kanayama M, Hashimoto T, Shigenobu K, Yamane S, Bauer TW, Togawa D: A prospective randomized study of posterolateral lumbar fusion using osteogenic protein-1 (OP-1) versus local autograft with ceramic bone substitute: Emphasis of surgical exploration and histologic assessment. *Spine (Phila Pa 1976)* 2006;31(10):1067-1074.

113. Thijssen EGJ, van Gestel NAP, Bevers R, et al: Assessment of growth reduction of five clinical pathogens by injectable S53P4 bioactive glass material formulations. *Front Bioeng Biotechnol* 2020;8:634.

114. Kim HC, Oh JK, Kim DS, et al: Comparison of the effectiveness and safety of bioactive glass ceramic to allograft bone for anterior cervical discectomy and fusion with anterior plate fixation. *Neurosurg Rev* 2020;43(5):1423-1430.

115. Lee NH, Kang MS, Kim TH, et al: Dual actions of osteoclastic-inhibition and osteogenic-stimulation through strontium-releasing bioactive nanoscale cement imply biomaterial-enabled osteoporosis therapy. *Biomaterials* 2021;276:121025.

116. Cochis A, Barberi J, Ferraris S, et al: Competitive surface colonization of antibacterial and bioactive materials doped with strontium and/or silver ions. *Nanomaterials (Basel)* 2020;10(1):E120.

117. Geurts J, van Vugt T, Thijssen E, Arts JJ: Cost-effectiveness study of one-stage treatment of chronic osteomyelitis with bioactive glass S53P4. *Materials (Basel)* 2019;12(19):E3209.

118. Begum S, Johnson WE, Worthington T, Martin RA: The influence of pH and fluid dynamics on the antibacterial efficacy of 45S5 Bioglass. *Biomed Mater* 2016;11(1):015006.

119. Bolger C, Jones D, Czop S: Evaluation of an increased strut porosity silicate-substituted calcium phosphate, SiCaP EP, as a synthetic bone graft substitute in spinal fusion surgery: A prospective, open-label study. *Eur Spine J* 2019;28(7):1733-1742.

120. Malat TA, Glombitza M, Dahmen J, Hax PM, Steinhausen E: The use of bioactive glass S53P4 as bone graft substitute in the treatment of chronic osteomyelitis and infected non-unions – A retrospective study of 50 patients. *Z Orthop Unfall* 2018;156(2):152-159.

121. Auregan JC, Begue T: Bioactive glass for long bone infection: A systematic review. *Injury* 2015;46(suppl 8):S3-S7.

122. Fortier L, Bauer L, Chung E: Use Of FIBERGRAFT BG morsels mixed with bma in anterior cervical discectomy and fusion at 1, 2, 3 and 4 levels: A retrospective analysis of fusion results. *J Spine Neurosurg* 2017;6:200-205.

123. Gomez G, Westerlund LE: Clinical and radiographic outcomes using third-generation bioactive glass as a bone graft substitute for multi-level anterior cervical discectomy and fusion-a retrospective case series study. *J Spine Surg* 2021;7(2):124-131.

124. Westerlund LE, Borden M: Clinical experience with the use of a spherical bioactive glass putty for cervical and lumbar interbody fusion. *J Spine Surg* 2020;6(1):49-61.

125. Barrey C, Broussolle T: Clinical and radiographic evaluation of bioactive glass in posterior cervical and lumbar spinal fusion. *Eur J Orthop Surg Traumatol* 2019;29(8):1623-1629.

126. Martin BI, Mirza SK, Spina N, Spiker WR, Lawrence B, Brodke DS: Trends in lumbar fusion procedure rates and associated hospital costs for degenerative spinal diseases in the United States, 2004 to 2015. *Spine (Phila Pa 1976)* 2019;44(5):369-376.

127. Seki S, Hirano N, Matsushita I, et al: Lumbar spine surgery in patients with rheumatoid arthritis (RA): What affects the outcomes? *Spine J* 2018;18(1):99-106.

128. Soldozy S, Mulligan KM, Zheng DX, et al: Diagnostic, surgical, and technical considerations for lumbar interbody fusion in patients with osteopenia and osteoporosis: A systematic review. *Brain Sci* 2021;11(10):1260.

129. Varshneya K, Jokhai RT, Fatemi P, et al: Predictors of 2-year reoperation in Medicare patients undergoing primary thoracolumbar deformity surgery. *J Neurosurg Spine* 2020:1-5.

130. Puvanesarajah V, Shen FH, Cancienne JM, et al: Risk factors for revision surgery following primary adult spinal deformity surgery in patients 65 years and older. *J Neurosurg Spine* 2016;25(4):486-493.

131. Kerezoudis P, Rinaldo L, Drazin D, et al: Association between vitamin D deficiency and outcomes following spinal fusion surgery: A systematic review. *World Neurosurg* 2016;95:71-76.

132. Greenwood J, McGregor A, Jones F, Mullane J, Hurley M Rehabilitation following lumbar fusion surgery: A systematic review and meta-analysis. *Spine (Phila Pa 1976)* 2016;41(1):E28-E36.

CHAPTER 34

Measurement of Clinical Outcomes in Spine

Athan G. Zavras, BA, MD • Ishan Agarwal, BS • Bryce A. Basques, MD • Frank M. Phillips, MD, FAAOS

INTRODUCTION

There have been many advancements in biologic agents available for use in the field of spine surgery, with a corresponding increased interest in improving the reliability of patient-reported outcomes in research evaluating these agents.[1,2] Biologics in spine surgery are most commonly used to augment arthrodesis in spinal fusion procedures, and the medical device industry has continued to rapidly develop and market new agents. Biologic agents are less commonly used for other indications in spine surgery, such as to promote intervertebral disk (IVD) healing and/or reduce reherniation rates following diskectomy.[3-7] It is important for surgeons to be able to critically evaluate the evidence for the various biologic agents available because many of the commercially available agents are costly, which needs to be justified in the current health care climate.

In the context of spinal fusion procedures, the biologic agent of choice has historically been autologous bone graft from the iliac crest, which remains the gold standard graft material used to promote successful arthrodesis. However, the harvesting process poses increased risk for graft-site morbidity including infection, pain, and compromised structural integrity, in addition to increased surgical time and limited donor site material.[8-10] As an alternative, allograft bone materials such as demineralized bone matrix or exogenous growth factors including recombinant human bone morphogenetic protein 2 have been used with success.[11,12] Since its approval by the FDA in 2004 for use in titanium interbody devices in single-level anterior lumbar interbody fusion, many studies investigating the efficacy of bone morphogenetic protein 2 when compared with autograft have demonstrated similar results on patient-reported outcome measures (PROMs) and equivalent rates of successful fusion.[13,14]

Several studies have examined the efficacy of biologic agents including platelet-rich plasma, amniotic membrane, and bone marrow aspirate in improving healing of the native IVD following diskectomy.[3,7] Although potentially attractive, there are few data to support the use of biologics in playing a role in healing or regenerating human disks, and these products are yet to be approved by the FDA. There are several obstacles precluding the initiation of clinical trials, notably lack of sponsor-initiated trials and high costs that are not reimbursed by insurance companies, thus requiring the patient to pay out of pocket. Despite these obstacles, clinical trials investigating the efficacy and safety of biologics in spine surgery are necessary, especially as the public interest and resources allocated toward research and development continue to expand. To reproducibly evaluate the efficacy of various biologic agents in spine surgery, it is critical to standardize the measurement and comparison of clinical outcomes.

RADIOGRAPHIC ASSESSMENTS

Spinal imaging findings are often used as outcomes in spine surgery research, particularly in the evaluation of biologic agents. Although plain radiography is the most ubiquitous imaging modality, MRI and CT are often used to measure outcomes because of greater sensitivity and specificity for certain outcomes.

Plain Radiographs

Plain radiographs are the most frequently used measure of radiographic outcomes because of their ease of use.[15] During and following surgical intervention, radiographs are useful in the assessment of proper placement of spinal instrumentation, deformity correction, and evaluation of arthrodesis.[16-18] However, the reliability of static plain radiographs for the detection of bridging bone and solid arthrodesis is poor because of high variability in the quality of radiographs, low interobserver reliability, and a general lack of a standardized method of assessment.[17,19-21]

Dr. Phillips or an immediate family member has received royalties from NuVasive and SI Bone; serves as a paid consultant to or is an employee of Globus Medical, Medtronic, NuVasive, Orthofix, Inc., SI Bone, and Stryker; has stock or stock options held in Augmedics, Edge Surgical, Mainstay, NuVasive, Providence, SI Bone, Spinal Simplicity, Surgio, Theracell, and Vital 5; and serves as a board member, owner, officer, or committee member of the Cervical Spine Research Society, ISASS, the North American Spine Society, and Society of Minimally invasive Spine Surgery. None of the following authors or any immediate family member has received anything of value from or has stock or stock options held in a commercial company or institution related directly or indirectly to the subject of this chapter: Dr. Zavras, Ishan Agarwal, and Dr. Basques.

To improve the sensitivity for detecting motion at the fused level, which is typically assumed to be indicative of insufficient healing and the formation of a pseudarthrosis, flexion-extension dynamic radiographs are commonly used.[22,23] However, even this method of assessment is flawed because of factors such as low interobserver reliability in measurements, variability in patients' global spinal mobility, and inconsistencies throughout the literature in the set thresholds that constitute acceptable residual segmental mobility.[24-26] For example, in the cervical spine, studies have used cutoff values of greater than 2° or greater than 4° in the Cobb angle between adjacent vertebrae with flexion and extension to denote the presence of pseudarthrosis, whereas others use movement between spinous processes of greater than 1 mm or greater than 2 mm.[27-29] As might be expected, narrowing this threshold increases the specificity and positive predictive value of this mode of assessment, at the expense of decreased sensitivity. Furthermore, multiple studies have shown that, even in the presence of successful arthrodesis, persistent movement exceeding 5° may be present depending on the extent of the fusion (eg, incomplete interbody fusion), motion through the facet joints, and the inherent elasticity of bone.[19,25,30] Moreover, other confounding variables further complicate fusion assessment via plain radiographs, such as the materials of the implanted interbody device and/or graft. Modern spinal implants can encompass a wide range of biomaterials, including titanium, ceramics, and allogeneic or autologous grafts. Because of their radiopacity, these implants complicate the radiographic assessment of bony incorporation denoting arthrodesis, particularly in the early postoperative period.[31,32] Therefore, fine-cut CT is the preferred noninvasive method for detecting the presence of solid fusion.[19,33,34]

Ultrasonography

In clinical spine practice, ultrasonography is mostly used as an aid to guide injection procedures, such as epidural steroid injections, platelet-rich plasma, or bone marrow aspirate concentrate.[35] However, ultrasonography has limited applicability as an imaging modality for diagnostic or postoperative surveillance purposes.[15] Compared with plain radiographs, CT, or MRI, ultrasonography provides low-resolution imaging and is known to have greater undesired variability in image acquisition, often driven by differences in patient body habitus and user proficiency.[35] In addition, because of its uncommon use as a means to assess the outcome of an intervention, ultrasonography is subject to greater variability in image interpretation, making it less standardized than other imaging techniques.[15] Despite these disadvantages, ultrasonography has been noted to be quite effective in certain aspects of imaging.

Ultrasonography is known to be effective at imaging not only the bones of the spine and related structures but also the associated musculature, IVDs, nerve roots, and the spinal cord. Ultrasonography has even been effective at determining spinal curvature and mobility while also providing the benefit of rapid and easily obtainable dynamic images.[16] Moreover, ultrasonography more clearly delineates soft-tissue structures when compared with plain radiographs and allows for more complete visualization of the spine and surrounding structures. Compared with CT and MRI, ultrasonography may be comparable in assessing the structure of the spine and certain outcomes following spinal fusion;[36] however, lack of familiarity with this particular modality among surgeons has limited its widespread adoption. Ultrasonography may be a more convenient method of imaging in terms of affordability and accessibility compared with CT and MRI, which may make it an alternative in areas that do not have access to advanced cross-sectional imaging.[37] However, the lack of validated outcome measures for ultrasonography in the spine severely limits its potential for adoption in a clinical research setting at this time.

Computed Tomography

CT is a nearly ubiquitous imaging technique and is used very effectively to evaluate the bony structure of the spine as well as the soft tissue surrounding the spine.[34] Compared with other imaging modalities, CT provides excellent resolution to detect osseous abnormalities of the spine, such as compression or pathologic fractures, and provides visualization of adjacent soft-tissue structures.[16] In addition, when the presence of a pseudarthrosis is suspected but not confirmed via plain radiography, fine-cut CT is the preferred imaging modality to assess for bridging bone.[38] CT may also detect loosening of instrumentation that is not readily apparent on radiographs. Although materials used for older generation instrumentation, such as stainless steel, previously led to marked decrease in CT quality because of significant artifact, newer implants composed of titanium alloy, polyether ether ketone, carbon fiber, and other substances have significantly improved imaging quality and postoperative surveillance.[39] Furthermore, although the presence of metallic artifact has historically been problematic for postoperative surveillance and assessment of healing, modern protocols and design features incorporated into modern CT scanners mitigate deleterious artifact.[33,40] This includes multidetector CT, which uses multiple parallel rows of detectors rather than a single row to collect multiple slices of volumetric data at a high acquisition speed.[40,41] Artifact can be further reduced with multidetector CT via overscan and underscan techniques, as well as built-in reconstruction and artifact reduction software.[40,41] Overscan involves the addition of approximately 10% of rotation to the standard 360°, reducing motion artifact by averaging the data from repeated projections. Underscan, or partial scan modes, can similarly reduce motion artifact, although it leads to lower resolution images. Metal artifact reduction software reduces distortion caused by metallic implants through a variety of interpolation techniques, although this is imperfect because artifact at the metal-tissue interface can persist.[40]

Although CT scans provide crucial information regarding the osseous components of the spine, they provide limited detail of the neural elements.[16] CT myelography can be used to visualize compression of the neural elements; however, it has been largely replaced by MRI, except in patients for whom an MRI is contraindicated. In addition, CT exposes patients to a much higher dose of radiation when compared with plain radiographs and MRI and is contraindicated for certain patient populations, including pregnant women.[39] Despite its few drawbacks, CT remains a ubiquitous imaging modality for the spine and has become the gold standard for evaluating arthrodesis following surgery.

Magnetic Resonance Imaging

Similar to CT, MRI is one of the most popular imaging techniques used for visualization of the spine and the surrounding soft tissues.[34] Unlike CT scans or plain radiographs, MRI does not expose the patient to ionizing radiation and therefore can be generally used for all patient groups. Furthermore, MRI provides excellent detail for the soft-tissue structures around the spine, including the spinal cord, nerve roots, IVDs, and surrounding musculoligamentous structures.[16] MRI can be used for the observation of abnormalities with the bony components of the spine as well, making it a well-rounded imaging modality.[16] For acute injuries of the spine, MRI can provide full visualization of any soft-tissue or neural structural damage as well as indicate bony or soft-tissue abnormalities.[42]

When it comes to the evaluation of fusion, MRI has been demonstrated to provide clinical utility because the bridging bone between vertebrae may be visualized, particularly on coronal series, in addition to marrow changes in the vertebral body, which may signify functional instability.[39,43-46] Furthermore, MRI provides superior visualization of soft-tissue structures, thus allowing the clinician to obtain a better understanding of factors contributing to new or ongoing neurologic symptoms or underlying mechanical causes of failed back syndrome other than pseudarthrosis.[47] However, studies have demonstrated that the interrater reliability for assessing pseudarthrosis via MRI remains low.[48]

MRI evaluation in the setting of metal instrumentation has traditionally been fraught by significant artifact caused by the implanted hardware. Advances in metal subtraction sequencing have helped mitigate metal interference, including view angle tilting, off-resonance suppression, and multispectral imaging techniques such as slice encoding for metal artifact correction and multiacquisition variable-resonance image combination.[49-53] However, these advanced sequences are limited by a lower signal-to-noise ratio in addition to even higher acquisition times relative to traditional sequences, which already vastly exceed those of other radiologic assessments such as radiographs and CT.[34]

Diskography

In the presence of diskogenic pain, lumbar, thoracic, and cervical provocative diskography has been used to identify whether the underlying cause of pain stems from the disk itself or from other potential sources.[54] This technique involves disk stimulation via the injection of a contrast agent into the IVD under fluoroscopic guidance, thus providing the clinician with functional and anatomic data regarding the diseased disk. However, concerns with the invasiveness of diskography as a diagnostic procedure coupled with its low diagnostic accuracy, high rate of false-positive results, and potential associated risks, particularly in the cervical and thoracic spine, make this technique controversial with limited utility in modern clinical practice.[55-57] In the cervical spine, for example, complication rates as high as 13% have been reported, including epidural abscesses, diskitis, hematomas, and even myelopathy or quadriplegia.[58] Therefore, the major role for diskography in current clinical practice is mostly limited to the evaluation of axial lumbar back pain.[54]

In a normal disk, the contrast agent remains isolated to the nucleus pulposus, usually in a unilocular or bilocular collection, and normal disk height is observed. In degenerative disks, diskography will demonstrate loss of disk height, multiple irregular tears in the anulus fibrosus, and/or disk bulging. However, the most important indicator of diskogenic pain in diskography is the provocation of pain, although this is subject to bias because of differences in pain tolerance. Therefore, in properly indicated patients, provocative diskography may be a helpful tool in the treatment and diagnosis of patients with low back pain.

Novel software programs that work with magnetic resonance systems to leverage magnetic resonance spectroscopy have been introduced as noninvasive methods to objectively evaluate for spectral signatures of pain and degenerative biomarkers suggestive of disk degeneration.[59] A clinical trial by Gornet et al[60] investigated the efficacy of magnetic resonance spectroscopy when compared with provocative diskography, demonstrating high correlations between the two techniques and a total magnetic resonance spectroscopy accuracy of 85%, sensitivity of 82%, and specificity of 88%. As this technology continues to improve and become more widely available, it has the potential to become a viable noninvasive alternative to provocative diskography in the evaluation of chronic low back pain.

Other Radiographic Imaging Modalities

Although the most popular radiographic imaging techniques used include plain radiographs, CT, and MRI, there is documented use of other imaging methods in clinical practice to improve visualization of the spine and associated structures. Many of these additional techniques are improvements on the most common methods mentioned previously. Multidetector CT has been developed and slowly adopted for clinical use to determine subtle spinal instabilities and pick up on fusion progression that a regular CT may not detect.[16] Vertical gap open MRI scanners have been developed that allow patients to stand, providing a highly detailed look at the soft-tissue and neural elements associated with the spine when the patient is standing and load bearing.[16] There is increasing interest in artificial intelligence and machine learning for evaluating radiographs to remove the inherent subjectivity associated with radiographic assessment.[34] These advancements continue to improve the ability of the surgeon to evaluate the outcome of a spinal intervention and thus assess its effectiveness.

Although CT has demonstrated superiority over plain radiography in the detection of nonunion and formation of pseudarthrosis, plain radiographs expose the patient to less ionizing radiation while also providing useful information, particularly when taken as dynamic flexion-extension radiographs. If there is concern for poor healing, fine-cut CT is the best method to evaluate for pseudarthrosis. When evaluating soft-tissue structures such as the IVD or neural elements, MRI provides the highest resolution imaging, although ultrasonography is an alternative that lacks validated outcome measures to date. The utility of provocative diskography is confined to the assessment of diskogenic low back pain, although magnetic resonance spectroscopy offers a new and exciting noninvasive alternative that may have an increasing role going forward. **Table 1** provides a summary of advantages and disadvantages of commonly used and readily available imaging modalities.

PHYSICAL EXAMINATION

Range of Motion, Gait, and Strength

A structured physical examination provides meaningful information regarding the patient's baseline symptomatology and functional status and allows the spine surgeon to assess progress in the postoperative period. General inspection should be performed with the patient standing, if possible, while observing for signs of clear asymmetry in muscle tone, shoulder asymmetry, pelvic obliquity, and deformity in the coronal and/or sagittal plane, including potential compensatory mechanisms such as knee flexion and pelvic retroversion. If the patient presents with a report of regional pain in the neck or back, the patient should be instructed to identify the location of their pain by placing their finger on the painful region.

Assessment of range of motion should begin in the cervical spine followed by the thoracic and lumbar spine.

TABLE 1 Advantages and Disadvantages of Commonly Used and Readily Available Imaging Modalities

Modality	Advantages	Disadvantages
Plain radiography	Inexpensive Quick acquisition time Readily available Useful for diagnosing fractures, bony malformations, degenerative disease, and instability	Exposure to ionizing radiation Poor visualization of soft tissues and subtle lesions
Ultrasonography	Inexpensive Quick acquisition time Readily available Able to visualize bony and soft-tissue structures	Low resolution Image quality limited by user technique and patient body habitus Variability in user interpretation
CT	Quick acquisition time Superior visualization of bony structures Multiplanar visualization	More expensive than other readily available modalities Exposure to larger doses of ionizing radiation Limited visualization of spinal cord
MRI	No exposure to ionizing radiation Superior visualization of soft-tissue structures and spinal cord Multiplanar visualization	Expensive Long acquisition time Image limited by metal artifact (unless metal subtraction sequences are used)

Range-of-motion testing should include motion on flexion, extension, lateral bending, and rotation while noting painful movements and those that reproduce symptoms. Next, the patient's gait should be assessed for abnormal patterns (eg, spastic gait, steppage gait, and Trendelenburg sign) by asking the patient to walk 5 to 10 steps across the room and back. Balance should also be assessed via tandem gait.

Sensory, Motor, and Reflex Testing

Sensory testing involves assessment of irregularities in light touch sensation in the different dermatomes, while corroborating findings with any complaints of paresthesia or dysesthesia. Examination of strength includes manual motor testing of different muscle groups to assess for radiculopathy and for localization of affected nerve roots while noting the presence of unilateral weakness and imbalance. The reflex examination can include assessment of the biceps, triceps, extensor carpi radialis, patellar, and gastrocnemius reflexes and can be helpful for diagnosing radiculopathy (hyporeflexia) or myelopathy (hyperreflexia). Notably, reflexes can be misleadingly normal if the patient has dynamic myelopathy, which may be provoked by examining the patient with the neck in flexion or extension.

Special Testing

Additional special tests are helpful in corroborating symptoms and aiding in the diagnosis of radiculopathy or myelopathy. In the cervical spine, symptoms of radiculopathy may be reproduced via the Spurling maneuver, whereas evaluation of myelopathy can include Hoffmann sign, Lhermitte sign, Romberg test, and testing for clonus. In patients complaining of low back pain, the active straight leg raise can be used to evaluate for lumbar radiculopathy, wherein the test reproduces the symptoms or can identify other underlying etiologies for pain such as hip osteoarthritis if the patient primarily reports groin pain. Tests for spinal cord compression include the Babinski test and testing for sustained clonus.

PATIENT-REPORTED OUTCOME MEASURES

PROMs have become increasingly used in the clinical setting to subjectively assess the patient's pain and functional capacity both preoperatively and during the postoperative course, thus representing a different mode of clinical assessment than objective imaging findings.[61] Furthermore, PROMs provide a quantitative measure in multiple categories and are critical components of studies aiming to compare different interventions.

General Health Assessment Tools

PROMs that fall under the category of assessing general health are used to assess the overall well-being of a patient physically, mentally, and socially. These PROMs apply to a range of diseases/disabilities and are not solely spine focused. These allow for comparison of PROMs across various disease conditions. In general, utility scores on these general health assessment tools range from 0 to 1 (or scaled up to 0 to 100), with lower scores representing worse health states and higher scores representing better health states.[62] Commonly used general assessment PROMs include the EuroQol-5 Dimension questionnaire, Medical Outcomes Study 12-Item Short Form (SF-12), and Veterans RAND 12-Item Health Survey (VR-12).

The EuroQol-5 Dimension questionnaire is a preference-based measure that evaluates five dimensions to generate a utility score: mobility, self-care, daily activity, pain/discomfort, and depression/anxiety.[63] The EuroQol-5 Dimension questionnaire is noted for its shorter length relative to other assessments and is common in spine surgery literature.[64] The SF-12 is another widely used general health assessment tool that was created by consolidating the standard SF-36, which assessed patient health across eight different comprehensive domains and ultimately resulted in two major summary scores, a physical component summary and mental component summary.[62] The SF-12 focuses on these two summary scores and is popular because of its close similarity with the SF-36 in producing physical and mental summary scores while drastically reducing respondent burden.[62] The VR-12 is similar to SF-12, with only minor differences in the scale used to evaluate the responses to questions. The VR-12 is a generic survey adapted from the VR-36, which in turn was adapted from the SF-36 and also assesses eight different domains related to overall patient health resulting in physical and mental summary scores.[65] VR-12 is widely used when surveying patients part of the Veterans Health Administration.[66]

Lumbar-Specific Outcome Measures

Lumbar-specific outcome measures evaluate outcomes as they pertain to the lumbar spine rather than general health of the patient. A very common assessment is the visual analog scale (VAS), which is a one-dimensional continuous scale by which patients can rate their pain level.[67] Ranging from 0 to 10 with 0 being no pain and 10 being severe pain, the patient is generally asked to rate their pain level experienced over the previous 24 hours.[62] Although the VAS is a general pain scale, when localized to a specific body part such as leg pain or back pain, the VAS becomes a lumbar-specific outcome measure.[62] Another widely used lumbar-specific measure is the Oswestry Disability Index (ODI), which measures functional disability in patients with low back pain.[68] The ODI consists of 10 items regarding daily activities and is scored on a scale from 0 to 100, with lower scores indicating low levels of disability and higher scores indicating very severe disability. The ODI is extensively used in literature and is noted for its brevity as well as effectiveness at assessing disability in patients with spinal disability.[62]

There are other lumbar-specific outcome measures that are less common, such as the Roland-Morris Disability Questionnaire, which is a series of 24 yes-or-no questions with more yes answers indicating greater disability. The Roland-Morris Disability Questionnaire is advantageous over the ODI in terms of assessing patients with milder back pain as well as being a simpler survey to take for patients.[62] Other outcome measures such as the Quebec Back Pain Disability Scale and the Japanese Orthopaedic Association Back Pain Evaluation Questionnaire are much more involved for patients, and although they do provide more detail, they are burdensome for patients to complete and much less extensively used in research and clinical practice.[69]

Cervical Spine–Specific Outcome Measures

Cervical spine–specific outcome measures are used in patients with cervical spine pathology, with the most widely used being the Neck Disability Index (NDI).[62] The NDI is a brief 10-item survey with questions pertaining to pain, personal care, and other regular activities. Scores are generally represented as a percentage, with zero indicating no disability and 100% indicating complete disability.[70] Similar to its use as a lumbar-specific outcome measure, the VAS score can also be used as a cervical spine–specific outcome measure for neck and arm pain.[62] This provides detailed pain information and can be easily compared during follow-up appointments to assess the efficacy of spinal interventions. Another common neck-specific assessment is the Japanese Orthopaedic Association scale, originally developed to quantify myelopathy severity.[62] There are numerous versions, with the most extensively used in the Western world being a four-question survey assessing the domains of motor function, sensory function, and bladder function.[71] Lower Japanese Orthopaedic Association scores indicate more severe cervical myelopathy, and the survey's simplicity has translated to common use in clinical settings. The major drawback of the Japanese Orthopaedic Association scale is that unlike other measures being discussed, it has not been psychometrically validated.[62]

Less common neck-specific outcome measures include the Cervical Spine Outcomes Questionnaire, which measures disability as a result of cervical spine pathology. The Cervical Spine Outcomes Questionnaire is a comprehensive survey consisting of 35 items regarding the major domains of neck, shoulder, and arm pain; functional disability; and psychologic distress, among others.[72] Despite the detailed information obtained from the Cervical Spine Outcomes Questionnaire, it requires much more time to complete than the more widely used NDI and is also more difficult to interpret because of less published literature on the scoring algorithm.[62] The Myelopathy Disability Index is another neck-specific outcome measure that is less common in contemporary clinical practice and evaluates the degree of cervical myelopathy.[73] The Myelopathy Disability Index consists of 10 items, with a maximum score of 30 and higher scores indicating more severe myelopathy.[62]

Other Metrics

The Scoliosis Research Society 22-Item Questionnaire has become a widely used measure of health-related quality of life for patients with pediatric and adult spinal deformity.[74] The questionnaire provides outcome information regarding domains including pain, function, self-image, mental health, and satisfaction with condition management.[75]

PROMs are a continuously evolving set of surveys/questionnaires, and the ones currently used most extensively are the result of years of research and validation to determine how effective they are at assessing outcomes after spinal interventions. There are newer PROMs being developed with the goal of lowering the burden on patients while continuing to provide surgeons with detailed information regarding patient perspectives. In 2004, the National Institutes of Health formed a group called the Patient-Reported Outcomes Measurement Information System with the goal of creating new standardized PROMs for use by clinicians.[36] This group comprises multiple health domains and has both general health and pathology-specific domains. The Neuro-QoL system was developed similarly, and both these systems have led to the creation of domains that can be used based on clinician discretion. Surgeons can create their own specific or general outcome measures using these established domains to fit clinical or research goals.[36]

Most Common PROMs in Orthopaedic Surgery

Although numerous PROMs have been discussed, with some being more broadly used in clinical practice than others, it bears mentioning that PROMs are rarely used individually when assessing spinal intervention outcomes from the patient perspective. Generally, a selection of PROMs is used to achieve a holistic understanding of a patient's clinical status at each point in time and should include at least one general health assessment, pain scale, and pathology-specific metric.[76] For general health assessment, the SF-12 is the most widely used outcome measure (VR-12 for patients in the Veterans Affairs system) because it has been widely established and validated, demonstrating applicability across multiple medical disciplines. In terms of spine-specific outcome measures, the NDI, ODI, and VAS provide comprehensive data regarding the patient's pain level as well as the presence (or lack) of functional disability. These outcome measures are noted for their brevity but can still inform surgeons to a similar level as do longer item outcome measures, making them the gold standard for functional assessment based on patient perspective after spinal intervention.

Furthermore, because of their popularity and ubiquity in spinal practice, these outcome measures have been well validated with established clinically significant outcome values, such as the minimal clinically important difference. **Table 2** provides a summary of common PROMs used in current spine practice.

BIOLOGIC OUTCOME MEASURES

Although radiographic assessments, functional assessments, and PROMs are widely used in various combinations for orthobiologic interventions of the spine, collection of biologic outcome measures is less common. Collecting samples of cerebrospinal fluid (CSF) or other serologic measures is invasive and labor intensive compared with the outcome measures discussed previously and is rarely necessary for clinical research. CSF collection is more commonly performed for preclinical or translational research purposes, which has demonstrated differences in specific neurochemical markers, such as interleukins, growth factors, and tau, in CSF collected from patients with spinal cord injuries before and after surgery.[77] Assessment of biomarkers in CSF is not routinely performed in the clinical practice of spine surgery.

BIOPSY OF TARGET TISSUE AND/OR SURROUNDING TISSUES

Biopsy is an important consideration when managing neoplasia or infection of the spine; however, for degenerative or traumatic pathology, biopsy of target tissue or surrounding is less commonly performed. Tissue diagnosis is the gold standard in the management of neoplasia and is a critical part of the initial spinal tumor workup. In the setting of infection, it is important to collect intraoperative samples to identify the causative pathogen and initiate appropriate culture-directed therapy. During spine surgery for a degenerative or traumatic indication, pathologic assessment of tissue is sometimes performed to confirm retrieval of a disk herniation, for example. Although intraoperative biomarker assessment of excised tissue is not routinely performed, valuable in vivo information regarding spinal anatomy and pathology has been gleaned by the analysis of tissue collected during elective spine surgery that would otherwise have been discarded. In revision surgery, explanted devices, such as intervertebral cages, can be examined in the laboratory to determine in vivo performance, such as extent of bony ingrowth or osseointegration.

TABLE 2 Scale and Indications of Patient-Reported Outcome Measures Commonly Used in Spine Practice

Category	Outcome	Scale (Worst to Best)	Indication
General Health	SF-12/36	0-100	Any indication
	VR-12/36	0-100	Any indication
	EQ-5D	0-100	Any indication
Pain Scale	VAS back	10-0	Generalized low back pain
	VAS leg	10-0	Generalized low back pain
	VAS neck	10-0	Generalized neck pain
	VAS arm	10-0	Generalized neck pain
Pathology Specific	ODI	100-0	Generalized low back pain
	RMDQ	24-0	Generalized low back pain
	QBPDS	100-0	Generalized low back pain
	JOABPEQ	0-100	Generalized low back pain
	NDI	100-0	Generalized neck pain
	JOA	0-18	Cervical myelopathy
	CSOQ	100-0	Generalized neck pain
	MDI	30-0	Cervical myelopathy

CSOQ = Cervical Spine Outcomes Questionnaire, EQ-5D = EuroQol 5-Dimension questionnaire, JOA = Japanese Orthopaedic Association, JOABPEQ = Japanese Orthopaedic Association Back Pain Evaluation Questionnaire, MDI = Myelopathy Disability Index, NDI = Neck Disability Index, ODI = Oswestry Disability Index, QBPDS = Quebec Back Pain Disability Scale, RMDQ = Roland-Morris Disability Questionnaire, SF-12/36 = Medical Outcomes Study 12-Item/36-Item Short Form, VAS = visual analog scale, VR-12/36 = Veterans RAND 12-Item/36-Item Health Survey

RECONCILIATION OF OBJECTIVE VERSUS SUBJECTIVE OUTCOMES IN SPINE FUSION

Although subjective PROMs commonly match the objective outcomes seen radiographically, this is not always the case. Although persistent or worsening back and/or leg pain in the distribution of the surgical level may develop in patients presenting with pseudarthrosis,[78,79] patients with pseudarthrosis may also be asymptomatic, leading to a gross underestimation of true pseudarthrosis rates.[78,80] If only clinical or only radiographic outcomes were reported in this case, there could be significant variation in the interpretation of the results. Although the presence of radiographic fusion is often the primary end point for studies assessing biologic agents in spine fusion surgery,[81,82] it could be argued that the clinical outcome matters more to the patient. Given this discrepancy, it is therefore important for researchers to report both objective and subjective outcomes in these studies and highlight the need for future research to help reconcile this difference.

SUMMARY

To reproducibly evaluate the efficacy of various biologic agents in spine surgery, it is critical to standardize the measurement and comparison of clinical outcomes. When evaluating radiographically, plain radiography is the most ubiquitous imaging modality for radiographic evaluation, whereas CT and MRI are often used to measure outcomes because of greater sensitivity and specificity in detecting pseudarthrosis, sources of neurologic symptoms, or other causes of failed back syndrome. A structured physical examination provides meaningful information regarding the patient's baseline symptomatology, functional status, and clinical progression and should include motor, sensory, reflex, and disease-specific special testing. PROMs have become increasingly used in the clinical setting to subjectively assess the patient's general health status, pain, and functional capacity as a function of their disease both preoperatively and during the postoperative course. Furthermore, PROMs provide a quantitative measure in multiple categories and are critical components of studies aiming to compare different interventions.

REFERENCES

1. Rajaee SS, Bae HW, Kanim LE, Delamarter RB: Spinal fusion in the United States: Analysis of trends from 1998 to 2008. *Spine (Phila Pa 1976)* 2012;37(1):67-76.
2. Martin BI, Mirza SK, Spina N, Spiker WR, Lawrence B, Brodke DS: Trends in lumbar fusion procedure rates and associated hospital costs for degenerative spinal diseases in the United States, 2004 to 2015. *Spine (Phila Pa 1976)* 2019;44(5):369-376.
3. Anderson DG, Popov V, Raines AL, O'Connell J: Cryopreserved amniotic membrane improves clinical outcomes following microdiscectomy. *Clin Spine Surg* 2017;30(9):413-418.
4. Kubota G, Kamoda H, Orita S, et al: Platelet-rich plasma enhances bone union in posterolateral lumbar fusion: A prospective randomized controlled trial. *Spine J* 2019;19(2):e34-e40.
5. Kitchel SH: A preliminary comparative study of radiographic results using mineralized collagen and bone marrow aspirate versus autologous bone in the same patients undergoing posterior lumbar interbody fusion with instrumented posterolateral lumbar fusion. *Spine J* 2006;6(4):405-411.
6. Biehn JL, Shellock J, Guyer RD, Zigler JE: Use of amniotic membrane anti-adhesion barrier for lumbar discectomy. *Spine J* 2014;14(11):S150-S151.
7. Kamson S, Smith D: Orthobiologic Supplementation improves clinical outcomes following lumbar decompression surgery. *J Clin Med Res* 2020;12(2):64-72.
8. Arrington ED, Smith WJ, Chambers HG, Bucknell AL, Davino NA: Complications of iliac crest bone graft harvesting. *Clin Orthop Relat Res* 1996;329:300-309.
9. Dimitriou R, Mataliotakis GI, Angoules AG, Kanakaris NK, Giannoudis PV: Complications following autologous bone graft harvesting from the iliac crest and using the RIA: A systematic review. *Injury* 2011;42:S3-S15.
10. Silber JS, Anderson DG, Daffner SD, et al: Donor site morbidity after anterior iliac crest bone harvest for single-level anterior cervical discectomy and fusion. *Spine (Phila Pa 1976)* 2003;28(2):134-139.
11. Aghdasi B, Montgomery S, Daubs M, Wang J: A review of demineralized bone matrices for spinal fusion: The evidence for efficacy. *Surgeon* 2013;11(1):39-48.
12. Diaz RR, Savardekar AR, Brougham JR, Terrell D, Sin A: Investigating the efficacy of allograft cellular bone matrix for spinal fusion: A systematic review of the literature. *Neurosurg Focus* 2021;50(6):E11.
13. Chrastil J, Low JB, Whang PG, Patel AA: Complications associated with the use of the recombinant human bone morphogenetic proteins for posterior interbody fusions of the lumbar spine. *Spine (Phila Pa 1976)* 2013;38(16):E1020-E1027.
14. Parajón A, Alimi M, Navarro-Ramirez R, et al: Minimally invasive transforaminal lumbar interbody fusion: Meta-analysis of the fusion rates. What is the optimal graft material? *Neurosurgery* 2017;81(6):958-971.
15. Namjoshi S: Radiology and imaging in orthopedics. *General Principles of Orthopedics and Trauma*. Springer, 2013, pp 395-403.
16. Nouh MR: Imaging of the spine: Where do we stand? *World J Radiol* 2019;11(4):55.
17. Tuli SK, Chen P, Eichler ME, Woodard EJ: Reliability of radiologic assessment of fusion: Cervical fibular allograft model. *Spine (Phila Pa 1976)* 2004;29(8):856-860.
18. Farey I, McAfee P, Davis R, Long D: Pseudarthrosis of the cervical spine after anterior arthrodesis. Treatment by posterior nerve-root decompression, stabilization, and arthrodesis. *J Bone Joint Surg Am* 1990;72(8):1171-1177.
19. Santos ER, Goss DG, Morcom RK, Fraser RD: Radiologic assessment of interbody fusion using carbon fiber cages. *Spine (Phila Pa 1976)* 2003;28(10):997-1001.

20. Bridwell KH, Lenke LG, McEnery KW, Baldus C, Blanke K: Anterior fresh frozen structural allografts in the thoracic and lumbar spine. Do they work if combined with posterior fusion and instrumentation in adult patients with kyphosis or anterior column defects? *Spine (Phila Pa 1976)* 1995;20(12):1410-1418.
21. Blumenthal SL, Gill K: Can lumbar spine radiographs accurately determine fusion in postoperative patients? Correlation of routine radiographs with a second surgical look at lumbar fusions. *Spine (Phila Pa 1976)* 1993;18(9):1186-1189.
22. Brodsky AE, Kovalsky ES, Khalil MA: Correlation of radiologic assessment of lumbar spine fusions with surgical exploration. *Spine (Phila Pa 1976)* 1991;16(6 suppl):S261-S265.
23. Louie PK, Basques BA, Pepin NM, Shifflett GD: *Pseudarthrosis. Minimally Invasive Spine Surgery*. Springer, 2019, pp 679-686.
24. Hipp JA, Reitman CA, Wharton N: Defining pseudoarthrosis in the cervical spine with differing motion thresholds. *Spine (Phila Pa 1976)* 2005;30(2):209-210.
25. McAfee PC, Boden SD, Brantigan JW, et al: Symposium: A critical discrepancy—A criteria of successful arthrodesis following interbody spinal fusions. *Spine (Phila Pa 1976)* 2001;26(3):320-334.
26. Simmons JW, Andersson G, Russell GS, Hadjipavlou AG: A prospective study of 342 patients using transpedicular fixation instrumentation for lumbosacral spine arthrodesis. *J Spinal Disord* 1998;11(5):367-374.
27. Ploumis A, Mehbod A, Garvey T, Gilbert T, Transfeldt E, Wood K: Prospective assessment of cervical fusion status: plain radiographs versus CT-scan. *Acta Orthop Belg* 2006;72(3):342.
28. Ghiselli G, Wharton N, Hipp JA, Wong DA, Jatana S: Prospective analysis of imaging prediction of pseudarthrosis after anterior cervical discectomy and fusion: Computed tomography versus flexion-extension motion analysis with intraoperative correlation. *Spine (Phila Pa 1976)* 2011;36(6):463-468.
29. Cannada LK, Scherping SC, Yoo JU, Jones PK, Emery SE: Pseudoarthrosis of the cervical spine: A comparison of radiographic diagnostic measures. *Spine (Phila Pa 1976)* 2003;28(1):46-51.
30. Bono CM, Khandha A, Vadapalli S, Holekamp S, Goel VK, Garfin SR: Residual sagittal motion after lumbar fusion: A finite element analysis with implications on radiographic flexion-extension criteria. *Spine (Phila Pa 1976)* 2007;32(4):417-422.
31. Lerner T, Bullmann V, Schulte TL, Schneider M, Liljenqvist U: A level-1 pilot study to evaluate of ultraporous β-tricalcium phosphate as a graft extender in the posterior correction of adolescent idiopathic scoliosis. *Eur Spine J* 2009;18(2):170-179.
32. Kotwal S, Kawaguchi S, Lebl D, et al: Minimally invasive lateral lumbar interbody fusion: Clinical and radiographic outcome at a minimum 2-year follow-up. *J Spinal Disord Tech* 2015;28(4):119-125.
33. Selby MD, Clark SR, Hall DJ, Freeman BJC: Radiologic assessment of spinal fusion. *J Am Acad Orthop Surg* 2012;20(11):694-703.
34. Harada GK, Siyaji ZK, Younis S, Louie PK, Samartzis D, An HS: Imaging in spine surgery: Current concepts and future directions. *Spine Surg Relat Res* 2020;4(2):99-110.
35. Ahmed AS, Ramakrishnan R, Ramachandran V, Ramachandran SS, Phan K, Antonsen EL: Ultrasound diagnosis and therapeutic intervention in the spine. *J Spine Surg* 2018;4(2):423-432.
36. Chin KJ, Macfarlane AJ, Chan V, Brull R: The use of ultrasound to facilitate spinal anesthesia in a patient with previous lumbar laminectomy and fusion: A case report. *J Clin Ultrasound* 2009;37(8):482-485.
37. Marshburn TH, Hadfield CA, Sargsyan AE, Garcia K, Ebert D, Dulchavsky SA: New heights in ultrasound: First report of spinal ultrasound from the international space station. *J Emerg Med* 2014;46(1):61-70.
38. Kitchen D, Rao PJ, Zotti M, et al: Fusion assessment by MRI in comparison with CT in anterior lumbar interbody fusion: A prospective study. *Global Spine J* 2018;8(6):586-592.
39. Williams AL, Gornet MF, Burkus JK: CT evaluation of lumbar interbody fusion: Current concepts. *Am J Neuroradiol* 2005;26(8):2057-2066.
40. Barrett JF, Keat N: Artifacts in CT: Recognition and avoidance. *Radiographics* 2004;24(6):1679-1691.
41. Burrill J, Dabbagh Z, Gollub F, Hamady M: Multidetector computed tomographic angiography of the cardiovascular system. *Postgrad Med J* 2007;83(985):698-704.
42. Shah NG, Keraliya A, Nunez DB, et al: Injuries to the rigid spine: What the spine surgeon wants to know. *Radiographics* 2019;39(2):449-466.
43. Lang P, Chafetz N, Genant HK, Morris JM: Lumbar spinal fusion. Assessment of functional stability with magnetic resonance imaging. *Spine (Phila Pa 1976)* 1990;15(6):581-588.
44. Steinmann JC, Herkowitz HN: Pseudarthrosis of the spine. *Clin Orthop Relat Res* 1992;284:80-90.
45. Kröner AH, Eyb R, Lange A, Lomoschitz K, Mahdi T, Engel A: Magnetic resonance imaging evaluation of posterior lumbar interbody fusion. *Spine (Phila Pa 1976)* 2006;31(12):1365-1371.
46. Peters MJM, Bastiaenen CHG, Brans BT, Weijers RE, Willems PC: The diagnostic accuracy of imaging modalities to detect pseudarthrosis after spinal fusion—A systematic review and meta-analysis of the literature. *Skeletal Radiol* 2019;48(10):1499-1510.
47. Lee Y-P, Farhan SA, Musa A, Bhatia N: Pseudarthrosis in spine surgery: Diagnosis and treatment. *Contemp Spine Surg* 2019;20(8):1-7.
48. Buchowski JM, Liu G, Bunmaprasert T, Rose PS, Riew KD: Anterior cervical fusion assessment: Surgical exploration versus radiographic evaluation. *Spine (Phila Pa 1976)* 2008;33(11):1185-1191.
49. Jungmann PM, Agten CA, Pfirrmann CW, Sutter R: Advances in MRI around metal. *J Magn Reson Imaging* 2017;46(4):972-991.
50. Koch KM, Lorbiecki JE, Hinks RS, King KF: A multispectral three-dimensional acquisition technique for imaging near metal implants. *Magn Reson Med* 2009;61(2):381-390.

51. Koch K, Brau A, Chen W, et al: Imaging near metal with a MAVRIC-SEMAC hybrid. *Magn Reson Med* 2011;65(1):71-82.
52. Choi S-J, Koch KM, Hargreaves BA, Stevens KJ, Gold GE: Metal artifact reduction with MAVRIC SL at 3-T MRI in patients with hip arthroplasty. *AJR Am J Roentgenol* 2015;204(1):140.
53. Ai T, Padua A, Goerner F, et al: SEMAC-VAT and MSVAT-SPACE sequence strategies for metal artifact reduction in 1.5 T magnetic resonance imaging. *Invest Radiol* 2012;47(5):267-276.
54. Peh W: Provocative discography: Current status. *Biomed Imaging Interv J* 2005;1(1):e2.
55. Centerville O, Niagara W, Center IP, et al: An update of the systematic appraisal of the accuracy and utility of discography in chronic spinal pain. *Pain Physician* 2018;21(2):91-110.
56. Manchikanti L, Hirsch JA: An update on the management of chronic lumbar discogenic pain. *Pain Manag* 2015;5(5):373-386.
57. Bogduk N, Aprill C, Derby R: Lumbar discogenic pain: State-of-the-art review. *Pain Med* 2013;14(6):813-836.
58. Connor PM, Darden B II: Cervical discography complications and clinical efficacy. *Spine* 1993;18(14):2035-2038.
59. Keshari KR, Lotz JC, Link TM, Hu S, Majumdar S, Kurhanewicz J: Lactic acid and proteoglycans as metabolic markers for discogenic back pain. *Spine (Phila Pa 1976)* 2008;33(3):312-317.
60. Gornet MG, Peacock J, Claude J, et al: Magnetic resonance spectroscopy (MRS) can identify painful lumbar discs and may facilitate improved clinical outcomes of lumbar surgeries for discogenic pain. *Eur Spine J* 2019;28(4):674-687.
61. Stokes OM, Cole A, Breakwell L, Lloyd A, Leonard C, Grevitt M: Do we have the right PROMs for measuring outcomes in lumbar spinal surgery? *Eur Spine J* 2017;26(3):816-824.
62. Nayak NR, Coats JM, Abdullah KG, Stein SC, Malhotra NR: Tracking patient-reported outcomes in spinal disorders. *Surg Neurol Int* 2015;6(suppl 19):S490.
63. Jansson K-Å, Nemeth G, Granath F, Jönsson B, Blomqvist P: Health-related quality of life (EQ-5D) before and one year after surgery for lumbar spinal stenosis. *J Bone Joint Surg Br* 2009;91(2):210-216.
64. Mueller B, Carreon LY, Glassman SD: Comparison of the EuroQOL-5D with the oswestry disability index, back and leg pain scores in patients with degenerative lumbar spine pathology. *Spine (Phila Pa 1976)* 2013;38(9):757-761.
65. Gornet MF, Copay AG, Sorensen KM, Schranck FW: Assessment of health-related quality of life in spine treatment: Conversion from SF-36 to VR-12. *Spine J* 2018;18(7):1292-1297.
66. Selim AJ, Rogers W, Qian SX, Brazier J, Kazis LE: A preference-based measure of health: The VR-6D derived from the veterans RAND 12-item health survey. *Qual Life Res* 2011;20(8):1337-1347.
67. Parker SL, Adogwa O, Paul AR, et al: Utility of minimum clinically important difference in assessing pain, disability, and health state after transforaminal lumbar interbody fusion for degenerative lumbar spondylolisthesis. *J Neurosurg Spine* 2011;14(5):598-604.
68. Finkelstein JA, Schwartz CE: Patient-reported outcomes in spine surgery: Past, current, and future directions – JNSPG 75th anniversary invited review article. *J Neurosurg Spine* 2019;31(2):155-164.
69. Azimi P, Shahzadi S, Montazeri A: The Japanese orthopedic association back pain evaluation questionnaire (JOABPEQ) for low back disorders: A validation study from Iran. *J Orthop Sci* 2012;17(5):521-525.
70. Vernon H, Mior S: The neck disability index: A study of reliability and validity. *J Manipulative Physiol Ther* 1991;14(7):409-415.
71. Kato S, Oshima Y, Oka H, et al: Comparison of the Japanese Orthopaedic Association (JOA) score and modified JOA (mJOA) score for the assessment of cervical myelopathy: A multicenter observational study. *PLoS One* 2015;10(4):e0123022.
72. Skolasky RL, Riley LH III, Albert TJ: Psychometric properties of the cervical spine outcomes questionnaire and its relationship to standard assessment tools used in spine research. *Spine J* 2007;7(2):174-179.
73. Casey A, Bland JM, Crockard HA: Development of a functional scoring system for rheumatoid arthritis patients with cervical myelopathy. *Ann Rheum Dis* 1996;55(12):901-906.
74. Elfering A, Pellise JBF: Factor analysis of the SRS-22 outcome assessment instrument in patients with adult spinal deformity. *Eur Spine J* 2018;27(3):685-699.
75. Lee S, Kim S, Lee S: European Spine Journal: Official publication of the European Spine Society, the European Spinal Deformity Society, and the European Section of the Cervical Spine Research Society. *Eur Spine J* 2007;16(3):431-437.
76. Weldring T, Smith SMS: Patient-reported outcomes (PROs) and patient-reported outcome measures (PROMs). *Health Serv Insights* 2013;6:61-68.
77. Kwon BK, Streijger F, Fallah N, et al: Cerebrospinal fluid biomarkers to stratify injury severity and predict outcome in human traumatic spinal cord injury. *J Neurotrauma* 2017;34(3):567-580.
78. Raizman NM, O'Brien JR, Poehling-Monaghan KL, Yu WD: Pseudarthrosis of the spine. *J Am Acad Orthop Surg* 2009;17(8):494-503.
79. Chun DS, Baker KC, Hsu WK: Lumbar pseudarthrosis: A review of current diagnosis and treatment. *Neurosurg Focus* 2015;39(4):E10.
80. Crawford CH III, Carreon LY, Mummaneni P, Dryer RF, Glassman SD: Asymptomatic ACDF nonunions underestimate the true Prevalence of radiographic pseudarthrosis. *Spine (Phila Pa 1976)* 2020;45(13):E776-E780.
81. Glassman SD, Anagnost SC, Parker A, Burke D, Johnson JR, Dimar JR: The effect of cigarette smoking and smoking cessation on spinal fusion. *Spine (Phila Pa 1976)* 2000;25(20):2608-2615.
82. Bydon M, De la Garza-Ramos R, Abt NB, et al: Impact of smoking on complication and pseudarthrosis rates after single- and 2-level posterolateral fusion of the lumbar spine. *Spine (Phila Pa 1976)* 2014;39(21):1765-1770.

CHAPTER 35

Biologic Considerations for Clinical Study Design: Fusion

S. Raymond Golish, MD, PhD, MBA, FAAOS

INTRODUCTION

Two major themes emerge naturally from the topic of biologic considerations for clinical study design. The first theme is the distinction between design considerations for products that are being studied currently and those in the future versus the historical considerations from previously completed trials. Especially within regulatory affairs, the decision making that results in success is sufficiently complex that the history and rationale for why previous approaches were undertaken must be clearly understood.. Even when the approved study design for a new product departs from that of prior products, a new approach must be clearly substantiated and weighed against the potential pitfalls. To enable progress to occur, prior designs provide an essential stress test to any new approach.

With respect to past versus present, it is important to ask: Are transforaminal lumbar interbody fusion (TLIF) trials the new normal? In the past, anterior lumbar interbody fusion (ALIF) and posterolateral fusion (PLF) trials have been preferred. Currently, there are good reasons why TLIF trials are commonly performed, with multiple contemporary TLIF trials running under IDE/IND (investigational device exemption/investigational new drug). However, their design considerations are unique and must be carefully addressed because there are fewer historical guideposts compared with prior ALIF and PLF trials. The history of ALIF and PLF trials still guide decision making for a TLIF (or any other) trial.[1]

The second major theme is more complex and accentuated by the first: the three-way trade-off that exists among clinical, commercial, and regulatory considerations in product development.[2-5] It may seem obvious that all three of these are in play in a mature product development program, but they interact in nuanced ways that must be scrutinized closely to avoid circular reasoning. For example, the following, simple clinical question is considered: Is iliac crest bone graft (ICBG) donor site morbidity severe enough to warrant complex orthobiologic products as alternatives to existing local autograft, allograft, and synthetics? A clinical answer may be yes for some clinicians, whereas it might be debatable for others; that is, a qualified yes versus perhaps a strong maybe.

But the ramifications of that clinical answer should be examined. From a commercial perspective, the answer cannot be a qualified yes or a strong maybe, it must be: ICBG is absolutely unacceptable. Otherwise, there would be no rationale for a major investment in science to develop our orthobiologic product. Further, the commercial answer must also be: In addition, local autograft is either insufficient in quantity or subpar for fusion quality, and allograft and synthetic bone graft extenders are subpar for fusion quality. Otherwise, a new product will only be able to achieve commodified pricing similar to existing extenders and will not be worth the investment. Without strongly affirmative answers to these commercial questions, one cannot proceed with a risky and expensive program.

Given the regulatory implications of the aforementioned commercial reasoning, a standard experimental design would be a two-arm noninferiority trial of the experimental product compared with a fusion control. ICBG is an acknowledged gold standard for fusion, but if ICBG is rejected for donor morbidity, it cannot (or should not) be enrolled as a control arm. Therefore, if local autograft, allograft, or synthetics are chosen as the control, the commercial belief that these low-cost products are inadequate and therefore not a gold standard for a control will be contradicted. In this case, the clinician should not have a noninferiority design. If commodified products are a poorer control, perhaps the clinician should conduct a superiority study instead of a noninferiority study. But then superiority would have to be shown to an active control, a challenging task for many reasons without precedent in historical trials.

From this simple example, the complexity and interrelationship of these trade-offs become clear.[2] **Figure 1** encapsulates some of these considerations, and the others are elucidated in the sections that follow.

Dr. Golish or an immediate family member serves as a paid consultant to or is an employee of Bio2Tech, Centinel Spine, Icotec, Intrinsic Therapeutics, Kuros Biosciences, Paradigm Spine, Simplify Medical, SpineBiopharma, and Wright Medical Technology, Inc.; serves as an unpaid consultant to Cytonics; has stock or stock options held in Cytonics and Cytonics, Inc.; and serves as a board member, owner, officer, or committee member of AAOS Biomedical Engineering Committee, ASTM, and North American Spine Society.

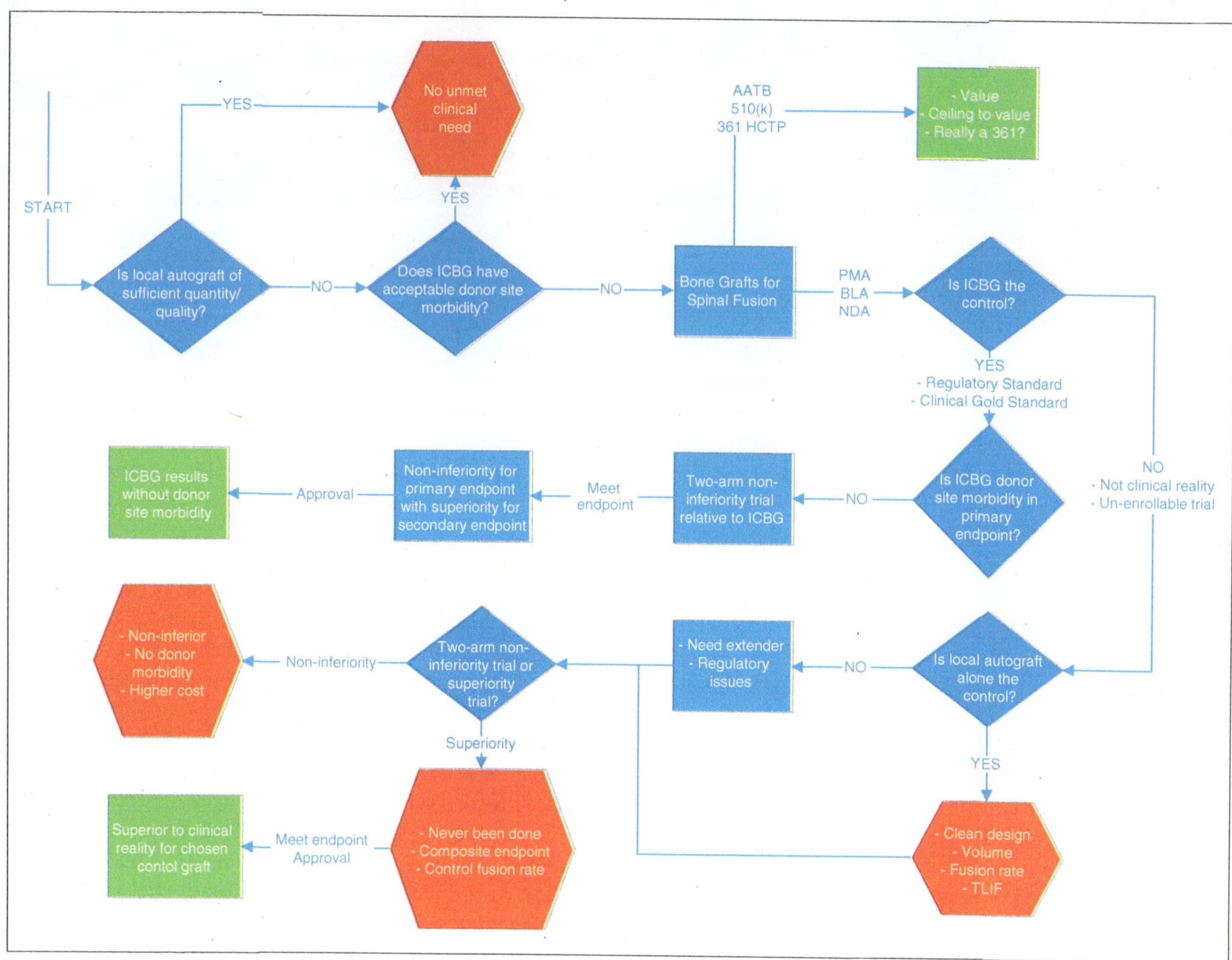

FIGURE 1 Schematic illustration shows an overview of value proposition and design considerations for fusion. AATB = American Association of Tissue Banks, BLA = biologics license application, HCTP = human cells, tissues, and cellular and tissue-based products, ICBG = iliac crest bone graft, NDA = nondisclosure agreement, PMA = premarket approval, TLIF = transforaminal lumbar interbody fusion.

ORTHOBIOLOGIC REGULATION AND COMMERCIALIZATION

To date, the most successful orthobiologics for fusion have been regulated as drug-device combinations jointly by the Center for Devices and Radiological Health (CDRH) and the Center for Drug Evaluation and Research. CDRH has acted as the lead center, with the most experience with spinal devices of all types, and the approval process was that for a class III medical device seeking premarket approval through CDRH on conducting IDE trials. Many products have been presented to CDRH's Orthopaedic and Rehabilitation Devices Panel. Sponsors who interact with the Center for Drug Evaluation and Research or Center for Biologics Evaluation and Research for spinal drugs and biologics face similar regulatory considerations, so the text applies to all biologic technologies for fusion.[6]

The regulatory, clinical, and political dimensions of orthobiologics for fusion have evolved over time.[2] **Figure 2** presents a timeline for all products that are orthobiologics for bony fusion, regardless of spinal indication; the nonspinal products are presented to paint a clear historical picture to avoid implying off-label use. In all cases, the drugs have consisted of recombinant/engineered proteins and peptides and the devices were carriers for drug delivery and release. In some cases, additional implants (which would normally be regulated as class II devices cleared through 510(k)) were included in the product, such as threaded cages in the case of Infuse. In some cases, additional implants were indicated on the label but were not formally a part of the product, such as osteosynthesis hardware for Augment.

In the early 2000s, the orthobiologic segment began inauspiciously with two humanitarian use exemptions for osteogenic protein-1 (OP-1) because the scientific evidence supported only partial regulatory success, which resulted in a commercial failure; a subsequent attempt to revitalize OP-1 for spinal indications also failed at the

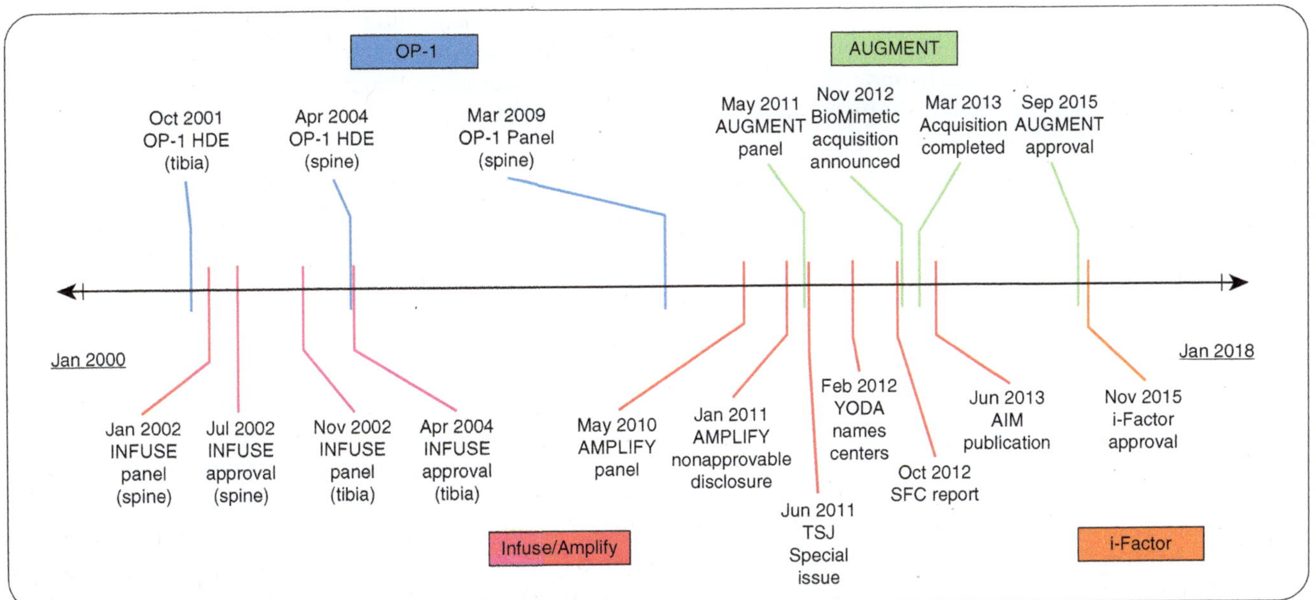

FIGURE 2 Schematic illustrations show the timeline of approvals of orthobiologics for all indications. HDE = humanitarian device exemption, OP-1 = osteogenic protein-1, TSA = The Spine Journal.

panel level in 2009. Despite the commercial failure of OP-1, this era was defined by the approval of Infuse for ALIF with a threaded cage in 2002 (and tibial osteosynthesis in 2004). A decade of unprecedented commercial success for Infuse resulted from explosive growth in clinical use, most of it off-label for numerous spinal indications.

The first signs of a backlash against Infuse came in 2010 with a contentious meeting of the orthopaedic devices panel for Amplify, the planned successor to Infuse. This resulted in a nonapprovable letter in 2011 that ultimately led to the demise of the program. Ironically, Amplify could be seen as an attempt to right much of the off-label use of Infuse, by producing a product designed for posterolateral fusion. Although some of the problems identified at the panel level were unique to Amplify, the popular response may have been partially a hangover from the exuberant adoption of Infuse and the perception of excess use associated with it. As shown in **Figure 2**, subsequent controversy and attempts to ameliorate it followed, including a special issue of *The Spine Journal*, a report from the Senate Finance Committee, the naming of the YODA centers, and their publications in the *Annals of Internal Medicine*.

At the time of this writing, Infuse might now be seen as a still successful commercial program that has been rehabilitated clinically, having withstood controversy, with its indications and its risk-benefit profile clarified over time. But the history of this product shaped the environment for contemporaneous and future products. During the height of the Infuse controversy, Biomimetic brought Augment to the FDA. After another contentious panel discussion, they received a nonapprovable letter. The company was acquired and the product ultimately received approval for hindfoot and ankle fusion. But the additional years of study and investment highlighted how risk and complexity of orthobiologics. Subsequently, iFactor was approved for a spinal indication, but for anterior cervical diskectomy and fusion, which is perceived as clinically less challenging and commercially less rewarding. Because of this, it is important to focus on lumbar fusion, the most demanding application.

Since then, approvals for orthobiologics have included label expansions for Infuse for use with more modern cages. As of the time of this writing, no major new product or indication has achieved approval in this space. It is known in the industry that many sponsors are studying new products and indications; however, making this statement precise is difficult. The presence of IDE and investigational new drug trials is not a routine matter of public record, and their disclosure requires a Freedom of Information Act filing. Although IDE and IND trials appear in clinicaltrials.gov, that database contains many trials of unclear provenance and activity. Nevertheless, the design considerations for these new products and indications, especially for TLIF, are discussed in detail in the next sections.

CONSENSUS DESIGN FOR SPINAL FUSION TRIALS

To best understand the contemporary design considerations for biologics for spinal fusion, it is essential to understand the regulatory paradigms and the history of fusion trials and products to date.[2] Of note, this includes orthobiologic products for fusion, but also motion preservation products with fusion arms as a control. The goal is to seek a consensus or guideposts for typical trial designs. Although future products may follow different regulatory and commercial paradigms, the successful regulation and commercialization of such products is sufficiently complex and risky that one must clearly understand past and present products, even if planned products differ. What emerges from the study of successful and failed products is something close to a consensus on trial design for these prior studies. Even with some variation, many trial design features have become standard.[7]

Table 1 presents new lumbar spinal devices since 2000 that were either class III devices that received premarket approval or went to the Orthopaedic Devices Panel regardless of subsequent approval; devices that were nonapprovable but did not go to panel or are still undergoing IDE trials are not publicly reportable. **Table 2** presents those trials from **Table 1** with fusion arms, including both orthobiologic products for fusion and motion preservation products with a fusion control arm.[1]

Tables 3 through **5** provide a synopsis of the major design elements of lumbar fusion trials, highlighting the similarities while accentuating the points of variation. All trials are two-arm randomized noninferiority trials to an active surgical control with 2-year final follow-up of a composite primary end point (**Table 3**). All were followed up at multiple interim timepoints prior to 2 years and subsequently out to 5 years as a condition of approval for a postapproval study. Most were asymmetrically randomized with the most common ratio being 2:1 experimental to control. All were analyzed with a noninferiority margin of 10%, although some were designed and approved with a less-stringent margin but were analyzed with 10% at the FDA's direction.[1]

With respect to the definition of the primary end point, all had four-variate or five-variate composite end points that were defined as the patient-wise logical AND of the components of the composite: each patient must succeed on all components to be considered a success (**Table 4**). All trials required no neurologic deterioration. All trials were analyzed for improvement in Oswestry Disability Index (ODI), the gold standard patient-reported outcome (PRO), of 15 points, although some were designed with other criteria and analyzed with a 15-point cutoff at the FDA's request. All required no secondary surgical interventions in some form, although their definition varied with a trend toward considering all secondary

TABLE 1 Lumbar Pivotal/IDE Trials Since 2000

Year	Approval (*Panel)	Device	Sponsor	Premarket Approval	Type[a]	Primary Endpoint	Control
2017	December 12, 2017	Barricaid Anular Closure Device *	Intrinsic Therapeutics	P160050	SU	24	Disk
2016	February 19, 2016	DIAM Spinal Stabilization System *	Medtronic Sofemor Danek	P140007	SU	12	NS
2015	June 11, 2015	ActivL Artificial Disc	Aesculap Implant Systems	P120024	NI	24	TDR
2015	May 20, 2015	Superion Interspinous Spacer	Vertiflex	P140004	NI	24	ISP
2012	October 17, 2012	Coflex Interlaminar Technology	Paradigm Spine	P110008	NI	24	PLF
2010	July 27, 2010	Amplify rhBMP Matrix *	Medtronic Sofamor Danek	P050036	NI	12/24	PLF
2009	March 31, 2009	Osteogenic protein-1 Putty *	Stryker Biotech	P060021	NI	24	PLF
2006	August 14, 2006	Prodisc L Total Disc Replacement Device	Synthes Spine	P050010	NI	24	360
2005	November 21, 2005	X-Stop Interspinous Process System	Medtronic Sofamor Danek	P040001	SU	24	NS
2004	October 26, 2004	*Charité* Artificial Disc	DePuy Spine	P040006	NI	24	ALIF
2002	July 2, 2002	Infuse Bone Graft/Lt-cage Fusion Device	Medtronic Sofamor Danek	P000058	NI	24	ALIF

ALIF = anterior lumbar interbody fusion, IDE = investigational device exemption, ISP = interspinous process spacer, NI = noninferiority, NS = nonsurgical, PLF = posterolateral fusion, RCT = randomized controlled trial, SU = superiority, TDR = total disc replacement

[a]All studies are randomized controlled trials.

TABLE 2 Lumbar Trials With Fusion Arms Since 2000

Year	Approval (*Panel)	Device	Sponsor	Premarket Approval	Primary Endpoint	Control[a]
2012	October 17,2012	Coflex Interlaminar Technology	Paradigm Spine	P110008	24	PLF
2010	July 27, 2010	Amplify rhBMP Matrix *	Medtronic Sofamor Danek	P050036	12/24	PLF
2009	March 31, 2009	Osteogenic protein-1 Putty *	Stryker Biotech	P060021	24	PLF
2006	August 14, 2006	Prodisc L Total Disc Replacement Device	Synthes Spine	P050010	24	360
2004	October 26, 2004	*Charité* Artificial Disc	DePuy Spine	P040006	24	ALIF
2002	July 2, 2002	Infuse Bone Graft/Lt-cage Fusion Device	Medtronic Sofamor Danek	P000058	24	ALIF

ALIF = anterior lumbar interbody fusion, PLF = posterolateral fusion, RCT = randomized controlled trial

[a]All trials are randomized controlled noninferiority trials.

surgical interventions as failures. Most trials considered the presence of a serious device or procedure-related serious adverse event as a failure, although the definition varied; serious adverse events are captured as safety events regardless, so whether to include them in a primary end point is a matter of debate and judgment. The radiographic criteria defining fusion varied, with a trend toward CT scans at the primary end point. Beyond the use of CT, the definition of fusion has received FDA guidance and substantial precedence (eg, number of columns, definition of bridging, definition of lucency).

Surgical technique had the greatest variation, but one common theme is stability: the use of ICBG as the gold standard for fusion in the control arm (**Table 5**). The importance of this cannot be overstated for future trial designs (as discussed in the following section on contemporary designs). Within this trend, early trials used ALIF with a threaded cage, the commonly performed procedure of that time. The Prodisc trial for lumbar arthroplasty was the most rigorous, using a front-back construct with femoral ring allograft followed by ICBG with pedicle screws. The OP-1 trial used posterolateral fusion with ICBG and without instrumentation, but that product was not approved. Amplify used posterolateral fusion with pedicle screws but without interbody grafts comparing Amplify to ICBG; use absence of interbody work was not a contentious issue in the panel debate. Perhaps the most distinct design was for Coflex, with the control arm consisting of posterolateral fusion with pedicle screws and local autograft and ICBG used as needed; however, ICBG was used in most patients.

Returning to the choice of PRO, the ODI has been the gold standard in PROs for lumbar spinal fusion (**Table 4**), with other PROs mostly subordinated to secondary end points. Currently, the psychometric properties of ODI are critiqued on the basis of stated FDA criteria: content validity,

TABLE 3 Major Design Elements of Lumbar Fusion Trials

Year	Device	Randomization[a]	Primary Endpoint	Follow-Up (months)	Noninferiority Margin	Probability
2012	Coflex Interlaminar Technology	2:1	24	6,3,6,12,18,24	10	$P = 0.975$
2010	Amplify rhBMP Matrix *	1:1	12/24	6,3,6,12,24	10	$P = 0.95$
2009	Osteogenic protein-1 Putty *	2:1	24	6,3,6,12,24	10	90% CI
2006	Prodisc L Total Disc Replacement Device	2:1	24	6,3,6,12,18,24	12.5/10	95% CI
2004	*Charité* Artificial Disc	2:1	24	6,3,6,12,24	15/10	90% CI
2002	Infuse Bone Graft/Lt-cage Fusion Device	2:1	24	6,3,6,12,24	—	95% CI

CI = confidence interval, P = posterior probability, RCT = randomized controlled trial

[a]All trials are randomized controlled noninferiority trials.

TABLE 4 The Primary End Point for Lumbar Fusion Trials

Year	Device	Composite	Components	ODI Improvement	DPR SAE	No Secondary Surgical Intervention	Radiographic Fusion	Other
2012	Coflex Interlaminar Technology	Y	4	15 points	Y	All and no LI	N	N
2010	Amplify rhBMP Matrix *	Y	5	15 points	Y	Failures/all and no LI	Y	N
2009	Osteogenic protein-1 Putty *	Y	5	20%	Y	Nonunion	Y	N
2006	Prodisc L Total Replacement Device	Y+	5	15%; 15 points	Y	Modify device/all	Y	SF-36
2004	*Charité* Artificial Disc	Y	4	25%; /15 points	Major complications	Device failure	N	N
2002	Infuse bone graft/Lt-cage Fusion Device	Y+	3	15 points	N/Y	Failure/nonunion	Y	N

ODI = Oswestry Disability Index, SAE = serious adverse event.
All trials required no neurologic deterioration.

construct validity, reliability, and sensitivity to change. As with many PROs, the patient-centered process to assure content validity is a psychological exercise in focus groups and qualitative analysis; the process for ODI looks somewhat dated for a 40-year-old instrument relative to current psychometric procedures. However, some publications have studied these properties post hoc for other instruments. Furthermore, small imperfections in this process have not resulted in major pathologies in reliability nor sensitivity over its 40-year history in multiple pivotal IDE trials and multiple publicly funded randomized controlled trials. It is important to determine whether alternative PROs such as Patient-Reported Outcomes Measurement Information System have a superior history of successful use and psychometric literature; most sponsors do not.

CONTEMPORARY DESIGN CONSIDERATIONS AND TLIF TRIALS

In the introduction, two major themes were highlighted. The thorniest design issues originate from the three-way trade-off among clinical, commercial, and regulatory considerations in product development. The contemporary trend toward TLIF designs exacerbates these commercial and clinical trade-offs and also has challenges unique to TLIF surgical technique. The following sections highlight those challenges as a series

TABLE 5 Surgical Techniques for Lumbar Fusion

Year	Device	ALIF	PLF	LLIF	TPLIF
2012	Coflex	—	PS/LA±ICBG	—	—
2010	Amplify *	—	PS/ICBG	—	—
2009	Osteogenic protein-1 Putty*	—	ICBG	—	—
2006	Prodisc L	FRA	PS/ICBG	—	—
2004	*Charité*	C/ICBG	—	—	—
2002	Infuse	C/ICBG	—	—	—

ALIF = anterior lumbar interbody fusion, C = cage, FRA = femoral ring allograft, ICBG = iliac crest bone graft, LA = local autograft, LLIF = lateral lumbar interbody fusion, PLF = posterolateral fusion, PS = pedicle screw, TPLIF = transforaminal posterior lumbar interbody fusion of dichotomies followed by the author's preferred approach to each.

ICBG Versus Other Control Grafts

The importance of the control graft has been previously discussed briefly. The question of ICBG use is central: to engage in a major development program for an orthobiologic for spinal fusion from the commercial perspective, the physician must subscribe to the notion that ICBG is unacceptable, and that alternatives are commercially commodified and clinically inferior. But the regulatory implications of that stance are substantial: a noninferiority trial relative to an inferior control graft is risky, and a superiority trial possibly more risky. This topic is highlighted further here because of its interaction with the following two topics on where to put the graft. Various sponsors have considered almost all imaginable approaches to grafting: experimental versus ICBG; experimental versus local autograft; experimental versus local autograft extended with a synthetic; experimental versus local autograft extended with a demineralized bone matrix; other permutations including cellular bone matrices. Two additional points must be considered with any design decision that includes the addition of devices beyond the experimental device: using the device on-label and the question of whether the specific device becomes part of the labeling versus just the class of devices.

The chapter author prefers a pragmatic approach to decision making. First, the ICBG should be examined closely. If the sponsor determines that ICBG is unacceptable for the reasons previously listed, a prototypical approach can be experimental graft versus local autograft in the interbody space, with remaining local autograft and a commodified extender in the gutters. Parameters can be established for graft volumes. There are several advantages to this basic design: it is as close as possible to a fusion gold standard and uses clinically accepted approaches. Further alternative combinations of grafts can be compared with the aforementioned two basic approaches.

Experimental Graft in the Cage Versus the Entire Interbody Space

Most sponsors want to see their experimental product in the cage, but depending on the formulation and dose-response considerations, this may be too little experimental graft given the limited volume of TLIF cages. Placing graft in the rest of the interbody space involves several considerations. If placed throughout, the graft needs both handling and drug-retaining properties. The handling itself is a trade-off: if too soft, the graft might extravasate ventrally or dorsally into the canal; if too hard, it might be difficult to place/inject through small TLIF annulotomies for less-invasive approaches. Some sponsors have reformulated their grafts for these considerations, a time-consuming and expensive process. Further, the preferred TLIF technique and comfort level varies widely for each surgeon. Some place the graft anteriorly and/or laterally after (or perhaps before) cage placement, relying on the anulus to retain the graft. Some avoid placing the graft dorsally after cage placement to protect the epidural space. These trade-offs are complex and are associated with scientific and patient care risk.

The chapter author's preferred approach to the decision-making process begins with experimental graft within the TLIF cage, which is uncontroversial for most sponsors. If the formulated dosing is determined to be sufficient graft, it can stand alone. More likely, additional experimental graft will be possible or desired. If handling supports it, allowing additional experimental graft in the ventral, lateral (and less likely, posterior) interbody space allows for variation in surgical technique. Reformulations are to be avoided unless strictly necessary. Parameters on graft volume are essential to control dosing.

Experimental Graft in the Interbody Space Versus Gutters

Most sponsors seeking a TLIF indication focus on the interbody space. The considerations of handling and drug retention are even more challenging in the gutters, so a graft generally cannot be applied there unless specifically designed for it; therefore, it is atypical for a sponsor to pursue experimental graft in the gutter in addition to the interbody space. The best counterexample is the failed Amplify product, which was specifically designed for and studied in the gutters for instrumented posterolateral fusion alone without interbody work.

The chapter author's preferred approach to the decision-making process is based on the observation that the absence of experimental graft in the gutters makes the choice of bone graft in the gutters even more important: typical CT-based radiographic fusion criteria examine all three columns; therefore, choosing a judicious graft for the gutters (eg, autograft, synthetic, DBM) that is balanced between arms is essential. If ICBG is being avoided, local autograft is preferred. If the autograft is to be extended with another product in the gutters, the ratio of extender to autograft ought to be balanced and recorded.

Proprietary Versus Commodified Cage and Biomaterials

For some sponsors, a proprietary cage that is labeled specifically as part of the product arises for one of two reasons: they own a cage product that is commercially or scientifically suited for their graft product or they have encountered a regulatory paradigm where the cage and biologic graft have both been adjudicated as the primary mechanism of action. In the case when the cage is commercially or scientifically suited for the graft product, some large sponsors may see value in their biologic being formally tied to their instrumentation. In the latter case where the cage and biologic graft have been adjudicated as the primary mechanism of action, the sponsor may create value around a cage product because they are required to study it, and many custom products can be designed and commissioned to fulfill this role. Multiple sponsors have encountered these scenarios. By contrast, other sponsors' commercial interests dictate that ideal label includes a commodified cage within a certain class of cages. For a sponsor defining a class of cages, the balance is to define a class that is broad enough to enroll a study and capture a commercially important class of cages but yet narrow enough to avoid too much cage heterogeneity or the impetus for subset analyses.

The chapter author's preferred approach is to avoid being boxed into proprietary cages as a regulatory stricture unless the sponsor has given a very strong scientific and commercial value to their proprietary cage. By contrast, sponsors defining a class of cages have encountered the following dichotomies: PEEK versus titanium alloy; surface coated (or treated) versus not; highly porous versus monoblock (three-dimensionally printed or otherwise); straight versus banana (transforaminal posterior lumbar interbody fusion versus TLIF). To illustrate recent decision making, porous and three-dimensionally printed titanium alloy cages are currently in vogue, but PEEK cages have commercial momentum, especially surface coated. In addition to the biomaterials and manufacturing issues, the specific vendor may be specified. The preferred approach here is to select one, two, or perhaps three vendors that capture the range of surgeon use and technologies.

Open Versus Minimally Invasive Surgery

The issue of surgical technique is most important for TLIF, but the open versus minimally invasive surgery (MIS) controversy must be handled carefully by sponsors. Although some surgeons are passionate about their MIS credentials (or dismissive of their importance), the distinction between open, mini-open, and MIS is somewhat in the eye of the beholder. Therefore, the preponderance of the literature is more ambiguous about the long-term advantages of each approach: although MIS may have shorter length of hospital stay and less blood loss (on sponges), it may have few other advantages and potentially some disadvantages (eg, lower union rate and higher neurologic injury). Some investigators may think they have conclusive answers to these questions, but that is not often the consensus opinion. Fortunately, it is not the sponsor's burden to resolve this controversy. Instead, the design should be enrollable but avoid subset analyses that make too much of the distinction.

The chapter author's preferred approach involves defining a single unified surgical approach not requiring subset analyses but allowing a range of retractors for use that includes traditional retractors (ie, open), quadrangular retractors (mini-open), and tubular retractors (MIS). One caveat about technique is critical. The side of the TLIF graft should require a partial or total facetectomy and decortication of the remaining facet joint with bone grafting for posterolateral fusion. However, the opposite side should also require at least decortication and bone grafting even for a unilateral MIS approach; it is essential to avoid unilateral posterolateral nonunions induced by surgical technique that ignores the contralateral side. This may require modification of some surgeons' preferred technique.

SUMMARY

Contemporary approaches for studying spinal fusion and orthobiologics have focused on TLIF applications, including drug-device combinations and other biologics. TLIF designs are promising commercially and clinically, but challenging scientifically and from the regulatory point of view. The history of fusion studies in ALIF and posterolateral models provides goalposts for designing successful trials and a framework for analyzing decisions unique to TLIF trials. Finally, the complex trade-offs among commercial, clinical, and regulatory decisions must be carefully analyzed to avoid circular reasoning and maximize commercial and clinical value.

REFERENCES

1. Golish SR, Reed ML: Spinal devices in the United States —— Investigational device exemption trials and premarket approval of class III devices. *Spine J* 2017;17(1):150-157.
2. Golish SR, Mihalko WM, Watson JT: *The Crisis in Orthopaedic Technology Puts Evidence-Based Medicine at Risk*. American Academy of Orthopaedic Surgeons, June 2018. Available at: https://www.aaos.org/aaosnow/issue/?issue=aaosnow/2018/jun. Accessed October 7, 2022.
3. Food and Drug Administration: Regulatory considerations for human cells, tissues, and cellular and tissue-based products: minimal manipulation and homologous use. Guidance for industry and Food and Drug Administration Staff. Available at: https://www.fda.gov/downloads/BiologicsBloodVaccines/GuidanceComplianceRegulatoryInformation/Guidances/CellularandGeneTherapy/UCM585403.pdf. Accessed June 2021.
4. U.S. Food and Drug Administration: Jurisdictional update: Human demineralized bone matrix. Available at: www.fda.gov/CombinationProducts/JurisdictionalInformation/JurisdictionalUpdates/ucm106586.htm. Accessed February 2018.
5. Golish SR, Watson JT, Mihalko WM: New FDA Guidances Tighten Regulation of Stem Cells. Available at: https://www.aaos.org/aaosnow/2018/may/research/research02/. Accessed June 2021.
6. Dubin J, Murray M: An Overview of the FDA Approval Process for Devices. Available at: https://www.aaos.org/aaosnow/2020/jul/research/research03/. Accessed June 2021.
7. Golish SR, Pezold R, Murray M, et al: *AAOS Presents the Biologics Dashboard: An Intelligent Information System*. Available at: https://www.aaos.org/aaosnow/2020/nov/research/research01/. Accessed June 2021.

CHAPTER

36 Summary and Perspectives

Kevin C. Baker, PhD • Wellington K. Hsu, MD, FAAOS

The prevalence of spinal disorders that cause dysfunction and pain to society continues to increase with each decade. Although surgical treatment options have also evolved to accommodate this growing need over time, surgeons are consistently presented with difficult decisions while weighing risks and benefits for their patients. Patients who require surgery are experiencing disorders that are more complex with associated comorbidities and structural deformity and demanding more minimally invasive options to hasten the recovery period. Regenerative technologies for a variety of tissue types have been at the forefront of innovation in spine surgery over the past 20 years. A biologic solution for degenerative disorders of the spine would be not only far-reaching but also game-changing for many patients.

As the pendulum swings toward offering invasive procedures for more challenging patients, surgeons must have at their disposal the best and most technologically evolved treatment options to achieve satisfactory outcomes. Conditions such as osteoporosis, metabolic dysfunction, and kidney disease that once precluded individuals from treatment can now be treated in a way that allows for surgical intervention. Structural deformities that previously required procedures that spanned multiple days to complete can now be corrected in a matter of hours. Further, the demand for minimally invasive approaches has steadily increased for years as both patients and surgeons look for innovative ways to decrease pain and improve function with reduced downtime. All of these factors have contributed to the demand for more-potent spinal biologics to achieve the goals of both surgical and nonsurgical treatment. Patients with associated mitigating factors require more robust actions from biologics that result in successful fusion and tissue regeneration.

The evolution and innovation of spinal biologics for fusion over recent decades has been dramatic. When allograft was the only option for surgeons to achieve bone regeneration, a high nonunion rate was the only acceptable outcome. At that time, these procedures resulted in unavoidable, high reoperation rates. The development of novel processing methods to retain biologic activity in human bone presented much better osteoinductivity and handling properties that allowed for application in more anatomic areas. Soon thereafter, the development of synthetic products that could combine the rapid scientific advancement in biomaterials and manufacturing presented additional options for surgeons to achieve the goals of surgery in patients in whom allograft is not an option for cultural and religious reasons.

This collective progress culminated in what was widely considered as the panacea of spinal biologics of the time: bone morphogenetic protein. At that moment, this revolutionary biologic regenerated bone in humans and animals that was unlike any other. However, unbridled enthusiasm quickly turned to shock when years of use revealed potential complications that left patients worse off than before surgery. The lessons learned from the introduction, adoption, and use of bone morphogenetic protein will stay with spine surgeons forever. Although being technologically savvy has certain desirable implications in the outside world, medical practitioners must exercise caution with any novel and unstudied technology where untoward effects are felt by many more than themselves; namely, their patients. These experiences have led surgeons to look critically at the proper questions and scientific data behind products that are routinely used.

More recent developments in spinal biologics have attempted to fill the clinically unmet need in bone graft substitutes but have also introduced different considerations in a more cost-conscious world. The development of a category of product called cellular bone matrices has been targeted at re-creating the potency of a growth factor such as bone morphogenetic protein without the associated adverse effects. However, the regulatory pathway, manufacturing costs, and rapid adoption in use have contributed to its existence as an expensive yet unproven biologic option. The use of these products in the setting of health care systems reducing overhead costs to remain solvent has led to additional questions

Dr. Hsu or an immediate family member has received royalties from Stryker; serves as a paid consultant to or is an employee of Asahi, Bioventus, Medtronic Sofamor Danek, and Stryker; has stock or stock options held in Amphix Bio; and serves as a board member, owner, officer, or committee member of Cervical Spine Research Society, Lumbar Spine Research Society, and North American Spine Society. Neither Dr. Baker nor any immediate family member has received anything of value from or has stock or stock options held in a commercial company or institution related directly or indirectly to the subject of this chapter.

regarding cost-effectiveness and the appropriate amount of data required for widespread use. The wide variability in its use across the country reflects the regional influence of cost, expert opinion, and availability, but more importantly, it indicates the lack of uniformity in which surgeons demand scientific data before adoption. This behavior sends inconsistent messages to industry partners who develop the portfolio of such novel products.

Similarly, there is significant preclinical research in the realm of biologics aimed at halting disk degeneration, improving symptoms, and even reversing degenerative disk disease. Autologous and allogeneic cell–based strategies have been at the forefront of this highly translational area. Because of the degradation and the inflammatory environment of a degenerative disk, there has been increasing interchange of ideas with biomaterials scientists. The development of cell encapsulation techniques and resorbable scaffolding materials aims to both sustain the viability of transplanted cells in this harsh environment and guide the structural repair of the damaged disk. Further, the delivery of bioactive factors, with or without transplantation, is a burgeoning field holding significant promise in promoting the repair and regeneration of the degenerative intervertebral disk.

As the demand for clinical data becomes more consistent, the quality of study design in the investigation of this technology becomes that much more important. Although correlating fusion with clinical outcomes will always be challenging to some degree because of the nature of the patients who suffer from spinal disorders, clinical studies must properly define the primary versus secondary outcomes of any said study. As far as fusion is concerned, weighing the relative radiation risks with the best imaging quality to assess fusion with CT will always be a challenge. For patient-reported clinical outcomes, novel developments in computerized adaptive testing will continue to push the envelope in correlating fusion and clinical outcomes. The incorporation of artificial intelligence also has the potential of identifying more specific measures that can guide the assessment and adoption of novel biologic therapies.

The future of the study of spinal biologics remains bright because of the opportunity to build on the foundation of scientific development of the recent past. Academic research groups and industry partners are incorporating expert opinion from an increasing number of associated fields such as biomaterials, biomechanical engineering, and biology that can expand the technologic options available to clinicians and their patients. However, these novel developments likely will lead to additional considerations and questions that will propel the field even further forward.

Index

Note: Page numbers followed by 'f' indicate figures and 't' indicate tables.

A

B

C

D

F

G

H

I

O

P

R

U

V

W

X